VARLEY'S
PRACTICAL CLINICAL
BIOCHEMISTRY

SIXTH EDITION

Edited by
Alan H Gowenlock
MSc, MB, ChB, PhD, CChem, FRSC, FRCPath
Formerly Consultant Chemical Pathologist, Manchester Royal Infirmary and Associated
Hospitals and Reader in Chemical Pathology, University of Manchester

With the assistance of
Janet R McMurray
MSc, MCB, MRCPath
Top Grade Biochemist, Hope Hospital, Salford

and
Donald M McLauchlan
MSc, MRCPath, FIMLS
Top Grade Biochemist, North Manchester General Hospital

CBSPD

CBS Publishers & Distributors Pvt Ltd

New Delhi • Bengaluru • Chennai • Kochi • Kolkata • Lucknow • Mumbai
Hyderabad • Jharkhand • Nagpur • Patna • Pune • Uttarakhand

VARLEY'S
PRACTICAL CLINICAL BIOCHEMISTRY

CBS Pubs   **ISBN:** 81-239-0427-4

Butterworth ISBN: 0-433-33806-7

Copyright © Alan H. Gowenlock

This edition has been published in Indian by arrangement with Butterworth-Heinemann Ltd., U.K.

First Edition: 1996

Reprint: 2002, 2011, 2012, 2014, 2016, 2019, 2020, 2022

Published by Satish Kumar Jain and produced by Varun Jain for

CBS Publishers & Distributors Pvt Ltd
4819/XI Prahlad Street, 24 Ansari Road, Daryaganj, New Delhi 110 002, India
Ph: 011-23289259, 23266861, 23266867   Website: www.cbspd.com
Fax: 011-23243014   e-mail: delhi@cbspd.com; cbspubs@airtelmail.in
Corporate Office: 204 FIE, Industrial Area, Patparganj, Delhi 110 092

Ph: 011-4934 4934   Fax: 011-4934 4935   e-mail: publishing@cbspd.com; publicity@cbspd.com

Branches

- **Bengaluru:** Seema House 2975, 17th Cross, K.R. Road, Banasankari 2nd Stage, Bengaluru 560 070, Karnataka, India
  Ph: +91-80-26771678/79   Fax: +91-80-26771680   e-mail: bangalore@cbspd.com
- **Chennai:** 7, Subbaraya Street, Shenoy Nagar, Chennai 600 030, Tamil Nadu, India
  Ph: +91-44-26680620, 26681266   Fax: +91-44-42032115   e-mail: chennai@cbspd.com
- **Kochi:** 42/1325, 1326, Power House Road, Opp. KSEB, Power House, Ernakulam 682018, Kochi, Kerala, India
  Ph: +91-484-4059061-65   Fax: +91-484-4059065   e-mail: kochi@cbspd.com
- **Kolkata:** 147, Hind Ceramics Compound, 1st Floor, Nilgunj Road, Belghoria, Kolkata-700056, West Bengal, India
  Ph: 033-25633055, 033-25633056   e-mail: kolkata@cbspd.com
- **Lucknow:** Basement, Khushnuma Complex, 7, Meerabai Marg (Behind Jawahar Bhawan), Lucknow 226001 (UP), India
  Ph: 0522-4000032   e-mail: tiwari.lucknow@cbspd.com
- **Mumbai:** PWD Shed, Gala No. 25/26, Ramchandra Bhatt Marg, Next to JJ Hospital, Gate No. 2, Opp. Union Bank of India, Noorbaug, Mumbai 400009 Maharashtra, India
  Ph: +91-22-66661880/89   e-mail: mumbai@cbspd.com

Representatives

- **Hyderabad** 0-9885175004 • **Jharkhand** 0-9811541605 • **Nagpur**   0-9421945513
- **Patna**   0-9334159340 • **Pune**   0-9623451994 • **Uttarakhand** 0-9716462459

Printed at India Binding House, Noida, UP, India

CONTENTS

PREFACE TO THE FIRST EDITION

THE rapid development of clinical biochemistry has been an outstanding feature of medicine during the past twenty to thirty years. The present book is a survey of the whole field of this subject from the standpoint of workers in hospital laboratories. It is hoped that it will appeal particularly to registrars training in clinical pathology, to hospital biochemists, and to laboratory technicians. The book should be especially useful to technicians studying for the examination in Chemical Pathological Technique of the Institute of Medical Laboratory Technology. As the tests described are also used in many laboratories not directly concerned with diagnosis and treatment, so far as possible the needs of workers in medical research laboratories have also been borne in mind.

While the purpose of the book is essentially practical, it was felt that summaries of the findings in health and disease would add considerably to its value. Although these are necessarily brief they are provided to obviate frequent reference to larger works on the interpretation of biochemical tests. No claim is made that these replace entirely such books a few examples of which are given in the short bibliography on p. 764.

My debts to other authors are many. In a rapidly developing subject such as this much is owed to the various journals which publish papers on biochemical methods. Full references to these are given. Books on practical methods which I have found valuable are also listed in the bibliography already referred to.

I wish gratefully to acknowledge permission to use material by the following: *Acta medica Scandinavica*, for material from Supplement 128 (1942) by Dr. H. O. Lagerlöf; *American Journal of Physiology* for Table XVII; Bayer Products Ltd. for Fig. 4; British Drug Houses Ltd. for the list of primary standards on p. 756; Messrs. J. and A. Churchill Ltd. for normal values for haemoglobin from "Practical Haematology", by J. V. Dacie on p. 587; Evans Electroselenium for Figs. 81 and 82; Harvard University Press for Fig. 86 adapted from "Chemical Anatomy, Physiology and Pathology of Extracellular Fluid," by J. L. Gamble; Ilford Ltd. for Figs. 9 and 10; *The Journal of Clinical Endocrinology* and Dr. S. Soskin for Fig. 36; *The Lancet* for Fig. 26a; *The Lancet* and Dr. J. D. Robertson for Table XVIII; Messrs. H. K. Lewis and Co. Ltd. for material on p. 375 from the *British Journal of Experimental Pathology*; Messrs. E. S. Livingstone for the table of Standard Weights on p. 762 from "A Textbook of Dietetics," by L. S. P. Davidson and I. A. Anderson; Dr. G. Lusk for Table XX; The Josiah Macy Jr. Foundation for material from the booklet "Copper Sulphate Method for Measuring Specific Gravities of Whole Blood and Plasma," by Phillips *et al.*; Messrs. May and Baker Ltd. for material on pp. 744–747 from their booklet "The Estimation of Sulphonamides"; Dr. M. Somogyi for Table XI; Dr. J. H. van de Kamer for Fig. 76; Drs. D. D. van Slyke and G. E. Cullen for Table XIV; Messrs. Williams and Wilkins for material on Indicators and Buffers on pp. 758–760 from "The Determination of Hydrogen Ions," by W. M. Clark (published in Great Britain by Baillière, Tindall and Cox Ltd.).

I should like especially to express my thanks to my wife who did nearly all the diagrams and formulae, and to several of my friends and colleagues from whose help I have benefited considerably. Dr. J. E. Kench has read the whole of the proofs whilst Dr. H. T. Howat, Dr. S. W. Stanbury, Mr. M. Bell and Mr. J. E. Southall have each read sections. I have received constant encouragement and advice from Dr. R. W. Fairbrother. For any errors either of omission or commission which still remain the author must accept sole responsibility.

Finally, I should like to thank my publishers for their unfailing consideration and patience during the period in which the book was being written and published.

Harold Varley, 1953

PREFACE TO THE SIXTH EDITION

The preface to the first edition, written 34 years ago, opens with a reference to the rapid development of clinical biochemistry in the previous 20 to 30 years. This development has accelerated to the present day. Such changes pose particular problems for a text book of this type and require careful reappraisal of the subject matter.

The fifth edition in 1980 involved a complete revision of that produced 13 years previously, and in consequence the book increased in size to about 1700 pages in two volumes. I was encouraged to find, however, that market research by the publishers suggested that there was still a wide-spread demand for a sixth edition.

The death of Harold Varley in 1984 deprived clinical biochemistry in Britain of one of its founder figures and meant the loss of the originator of this book and its sole author for nearly a quarter of a century. Furthermore, the retirement some time ago of Mr M. Bell effectively deprived me of my two co-authors of the fifth edition. In undertaking its revision I have been fortunate in gaining the assistance of two senior clinical biochemists in Manchester, Mrs Janet McMurray and Mr Donald McLauchlan. After joint discussions on the magnitude of the task, I have asked a number of medical and scientific colleagues in Greater Manchester, all of whom are actively working in the field of clinical biochemistry, to contribute one or more chapters. Mrs McMurray and Mr McLauchlan took on a greater individual load by revising several chapters each. By this means we have eased the burden of revision and, at the same time, kept the Mancunian tradition of this book. Two colleagues moved from Manchester while still preparing their contributions but have been regarded as honorary Mancunians nevertheless.

In preliminary discussions it was agreed to reduce the overall size of this edition to a single volume by removal of outdated matter and by combination of some chapters. With this reduction in size, it has sometimes been necessary to exclude material for which there was a moderately good case for retention. Where this has been done, there are cross references to the earlier edition. A feature of the development of instrumentation in clinical biochemistry has been the availability of a range of quite different pieces of equipment for the determination of a given analyte. When the first edition was written, the AutoAnalyzer had not yet appeared on the market but later on methods were given for this equipment as it was the basis of most automated contemporary methods. Now the availability of multi-channel analysers and of discrete analysers of different types has changed the situation greatly. Reference to external quality assurance schemes will reveal the plethora of analytical methods in use for many of the substances commonly measured in clinical biochemistry laboratories. Selection of a method for inclusion has thus been based on an assessment of current practice. Where the commonly used automated methods for a particular analyte rely on one or two instruments specifically developed for that analysis, I have felt that to give practical details would be unhelpful to the laboratory not possessing such equipment, and only of marginal assistance to those laboratories who do. On the other hand, a general purpose analyser in regular current use for the determination of several different substances has been selected for inclusion. In general, a manual technique has been included for most analytes as such methods are useful for emergency work and for the smaller or less well-equipped laboratory. A consequence of this policy has been a reduction in the number of pages devoted to practical details but this has been offset by more attention to general principles and to a more detailed appraisal of the merits of different methods in the hope that this will aid selection by the analyst.

In this revision there has been a deliberate attempt to maintain the general approach of earlier editions and I hope that the format will be familiar to previous readers of this book. In the preliminary discussion of each chapter with its author I have been responsible for suggesting the size and content of the contribution. I have been helped in this and in the preliminary editing of some of the chapters by my co-editors. I have, however, been solely responsible for the final editing of all chapters, for trying to maintain a similar style in presentation between chapters, and for a critical appraisal of their subject matter. I must therefore take personal responsibility for any defects or errors in the final version.

I hope that these results of the efforts of all the contributors and myself will prove an acceptable compromise between the many conflicting considerations which beset the person foolhardy enough to undertake the coordinating role in placing this revision before a critical audience. I also hope that it will find its traditional place as a 'bench book' in hospital biochemistry laboratories and that it will prove helpful to laboratory doctors, scientists and technologists in improving their knowledge of clinical biochemistry. It has been written by practising clinical biochemists for practising clinical biochemists. Although the title page correctly implies that I have now retired from my previous day to day involvement in the subject, this only happened a few weeks before the last manuscript was edited.

Any success the book may have will reflect the very considerable effort on the part of the contributors and I am deeply indebted to them. I must also thank many other colleagues for helpful discussions and I am sincerely grateful to my publishers for their considerable assistance and encouragement. Finally, I owe a great debt to my wife who has unselfishly facilitated my efforts to bring this new edition to fruition.

A. H. GOWENLOCK, 1987

LIST OF CONTRIBUTORS

G. M. Addison, MA, MB, BChir, PhD. Consultant Chemical Pathologist, Royal Manchester Children's Hospital, Manchester, M27 1HA.

B. Fowler, MIBiol, PhD. Principal Grade Biochemist, Royal Manchester Children's Hospital (Willinck Laboratory), Manchester M27 1HA.

A. H. Gowenlock, MSc, MB, ChB, PhD, CChem, FRSC, FRCPath. Formerly Consultant Chemical Pathologist, Manchester Royal Infirmary, Manchester M13 9WL.

E. Gowland, MB, BS, PhD, DCC, FRCPath. Consultant Chemical Pathologist, Withington Hospital, Manchester M20 8LR.

A. M. Hawks, MSc, MB, BS, PhD, MRCPath. Consultant Chemical Pathologist, Bolton Royal Infirmary, Bolton BL1 4QS.

I. B. Holbrook, BSc, PhD, MRCPath. Principal Grade Biochemist, Hope Hospital, Salford M6 8HD.

D. R. McDowell, BSc, PhD, MCB, MRCPath. Principal Grade Biochemist, Hope Hospital, Salford M6 8HD.

D. M. McLauchlan, MSc, MRCPath, FIMLS. Top Grade Biochemist, North Manchester General Hospital, Manchester M8 6RB.

Janet R. McMurray, MSc, MCB, MRCPath. Top Grade Biochemist, Hope Hospital, Salford M6 8HD.

W. McMurray, MSc, MB, ChB, MRCPath. Consultant Chemical Pathologist, Wythenshawe Hospital, Manchester M23 9LT.

J. G. Ratcliffe, MA, MSc, DM, MRCPath, FRCP. Formerly Professor of Chemical Pathology, University of Manchester; currently Professor in Clinical Chemistry, University of Birmingham and Director, Wolfson Research Laboratories, Queen Elizabeth Medical Centre, Birmingham B15 2TH.

T. Richardson, MSc, MRCPath. Senior Grade Biochemist, Manchester Royal Infirmary, Manchester M13 9WL.

E. L. Robinson, MSc, DipCB, MRCPath, FIMLS. Principal Grade Biochemist, Regional Radioimmunoassay Laboratory, Withington Hospital, Manchester M20 8LR.

C. J. Seneviratne, CChem, MRSC, MRCPath. Principal Grade Biochemist, Manchester Royal Infirmary, Manchester M13 9WL.

B. E. Senior, BSc, PhD. Top Grade Biochemist, Bolton Royal Infirmary, Bolton, BL1 4QS.

K. Wiener, BSc, PhD, CChem, MRSC, MCB. Principal Grade Biochemist, North Manchester General Hospital, M8 6RB.

C. Weinkove, BSc, MB, ChB, PhD, FCP. Senior Lecturer in Chemical Pathology, Hope Hospital, Salford M6 8HD.

F. E. Wells, BA, PhD, MCB. Formerly Principal Grade Biochemist, Booth Hall Children's Hospital, Manchester; currently Top Grade Biochemist, Pathology Laboratory, Warwick CV34 5BJ.

ABBREVIATIONS

Abbreviations for *units* appear in Chapter 2.
Where an abbreviation is used solely in one chapter, it is defined therein at its first mention, and is not included here.

A	Absorbance
AACC	American Association of Clinical Chemists
AAS	Atomic absorption spectroscopy
AC	Alternating current
ACB	Association of Clinical Biochemists
ACTH	Adrenocorticotrophic hormone
ADH	Antidiuretic hormone
ADP	Adenosine diphosphate
ALA	δ-Aminolaevulinic acid
ALT	Alanine aminotransferase, GPT
AMP	Adenosine monophosphate
AR	Analytical reagent grade
AST	Asparate aminotransferase, GOT
ATP	Adenosine triphosphate
BAIBA	β-Amino-isobutyric acid
BCG	Bromocresol green
BDH	British Drug Houses Chemicals Ltd.
BP	British Pharmacopoeia
BPB	Bromphenol blue
BSA	Bovine serum albumin
BSP	Bromsulphthalein
CCK-PZ	Cholecystokinin-pancreozymin
ChE	Choline esterase
CL	Confidence limits
CM cellulose	Carboxymethyl cellulose
CNS	Central nervous system
CPC	Cresolphthalein complexone
CoA	Coenzyme A
CSF	Cerebrospinal fluid
CV	Coefficient of variation
DC	Direct current
DEAE cellulose	Diethylaminoethyl cellulose
df	Degrees of freedom
DHA	Dehydroepiandrosterone
DHCC	1,25-Dihydroxycholecalciferol
DHSS	Department of Health and Social Security
DLE	See SLE
DNA	Deoxyribonucleic acid
Dopa	3,4-Dihydroxyphenylalanine
$\bar{\varepsilon}$	Molar absorption coefficient, molar absorptivity
ECF	Extracellular fluid
EDTA	Ethylenediamine-tetraacetic acid
EEG	Electroencephalograph
EGTA	Ethyleneglycol bis (2-aminoethyl ether) tetraacetic acid
EMF	Electromotive force
EMIT	Enzyme multiplied immunoassay technique
FAD	Flavine adenine dinucleotide
FDP	Fibrin degradation products
FFA	Free fatty acids
FMN	Flavine mononucleotide

GC	Gas chromatography
GFR	Glomerular filtration rate
GGT	Gammaglutamyl transpeptidase
GLC	Gas-liquid chromatography
GLD	Glutamate dehydrogenase
G-6-PD	Glucose-6-phosphate dehydrogenase
γ-GT	See GGT
α-HBD	α-Hydroxybutyrate dehydrogenase
HDL	High density lipoproteins
5-HIAA	5-Hydroxyindolylacetic acid
HM	Hospital Memorandum
HMMA	4-Hydroxy-3-methoxymandelic acid
HMSO	Her Majesty's Stationery Office
HPLC	High pressure (performance) liquid chromatography
HSA	Human serum albumin
5-HT	5-Hydroxytryptamine
5-HTP	5-Hydroxytryptophan
IBC	Iron binding capacity
ICF	Intracellular fluid
ICI	Imperial Chemical Industries Ltd.
ICSH	International Committee for Standardization in Hematology
i.d.	Internal diameter
IDL	Intermediate density lipoproteins
IFCC	International Federation of Clinical Chemistry
IFCC-EP	IFCC Expert Panel
Ig	Immunoglobin
IUB	International Union of Biochemistry
K_A	Dissociation constant of an acid
K_M	Michaelis constant
LCAT	Lecithin-cholesterol acyl transferase
LD	Lactate dehydrogenase
LDL	Low density lipoproteins
LPL	Lipoprotein lipase
mol wt	Molecular weight
NAD^+	Nicotinamide adenine dinucleotide
NADH	Reduced NAD^+
$NADP^+$	Nicotinamide adenine dinucleotide phosphate
NADPH	Reduced $NADP^+$
NBS	National Bureau of Standards
NEFA	Non-esterified fatty acids
NEQAS	National External Quality Assessment Scheme
NPP	4-Nitrophenyl phosphate
NTP	Normal temperature and pressure
P	Probability
P_{CO_2}	Partial pressure of carbon dioxide
P_{O_2}	Partial pressure of oxygen
PAS	p-Aminosalicylate
PBG	Porphobilinogen
PEG	Polyethylene glycol
PEP	Phosphoenol pyruvate
PGN	Proliferative glomerulonephritis
PHLA	Post-heparin lipolytic activity
pK	$-\log K_A$
PTH	Parathyroid hormone
R_f	Chromatographic mobility relative to solvent front
RBC	Red blood corpuscles
RIA	Radioimmunoassay

RNA	Ribonucleic acid
rpm	Revolutions per minute
R_t	Retention time
S	Svedberg sedimentation coefficient
$S_{20.w}$	Svedberg unit
S_f	Svedberg flotation coefficient
SD	Standard deviation
SE	Standard error of the mean
SI	Système International
SLE	Systemic lupus erythematosus
sp. gr.	Specific gravity
T3	Triiodothyronine
T4	Thyroxine
TBW	Total body water
TCA	Trichloracetic acid
TG	Triglyceride
TIBC	Total iron binding capacity
TEMED	N,N,N′,N′-Tetramethylethylenediamine
TLC	Thin layer chromatography
UIBC	Unsaturated iron binding capacity
UKEQAS	United Kingdom External Quality Assessment Scheme
ULN	Upper limit of normal
URL	Upper reference limit
UV	Ultraviolet
V_0	Void volume
VLDL	Very low density lipoproteins
w/v	Weight per unit volume

1

HAZARDS IN THE CLINICAL BIOCHEMISTRY LABORATORY

The advances in clinical practice over the last two decades have led to a steady increase in the number and range of investigations performed in the clinical biochemistry laboratory and consequently to an increase in the various hazards.

Hazards arise from three main basic causes: from dangerous chemicals, from infected specimens sent for analysis, and from faulty apparatus and instruments. The likelihood that these will lead to accidents is increased by carelessness, untidiness and faulty hygiene of the staff, and unsatisfactory buildings and working conditions. Since the increase in workload often has to be accommodated in outmoded laboratories using relatively inexperienced staff, there is considerable potential for accidents.

This chapter discusses measures which should be taken to ensure safe working practice throughout the laboratory. The Health and Safety at Work etc. Act of 1974 was passed to promote and encourage high standards of health and safety at work. A short account of this Act appears in Muir (1977). Later a working party under the chairmanship of Sir James Howie produced the 'Code of Practice for the Prevention of Infection in Clinical Laboratories and Post-mortem Rooms' (DHSS, 1978). This 'Howie Report' has been used by the Health and Safety Executive to set the standards for the prevention of infection (see also DHSS (1972), Health Services Advisory Committee (1985) and DHSS, Advisory Committee on Dangerous Pathogens (1986)).

HAZARDS FROM DANGEROUS CHEMICALS

Injury from chemicals results from:
1. Direct contact:
   (a) with the skin, e.g. when pouring reagents or from breakage of containers;
   (b) with lips or mouth when pipetting, mouth pipetting should be forbidden;
   (c) with the oesophagus and stomach if inadvertently swallowed.
2. Damage to the lungs from inhaling vapours or, less likely, fine powders.
3. Toxic effects of substances absorbed from the lungs, alimentary tract or skin on other tissues such as bone marrow, liver or kidney.

While special attention should be paid to certain groups of particularly dangerous substances there are few which may not be harmful in some circumstances. Knowledge of the effect of many organic chemicals, e.g. aromatic compounds, on the body is scanty, so care should always be taken when handling them, and spillage should be cleaned up immediately (see BDH Chemicals wall chart). All bottles containing chemicals and reagents should be clearly labelled with the name and any hazard noted. Do not lick labels.

The main groups of harmful chemicals are corrosive substances, organic solvents, explosive compounds, poisons and carcinogens. Those kept in largest quantity will be concentrated acids and flammable and toxic organic solvents. Keep only sufficient of these for current use in the laboratory itself, and store the remainder in a separate building sited near to the main laboratory. This store should conform to the building regulations for flammable solvents. Take care when transferring chemicals from this store. Trolleys, if used, should run smoothly and hold bottles in such a way that they cannot fall off it if the trolley is jolted. Never carry large bottles such as Winchesters by the neck but hold the bottle itself with two hands or, preferably, use a holder when transporting such bottles. Keep bottles in use on shelves, not higher than eye level, from which they cannot easily be dislodged or preferably in a fire-proof metal cupboard with a tray to contain spillage. When the contents have been used, empty any residue, rinse well with water and dispose of the container.

Corrosive Chemicals

Chemical burns of the skin can be caused by strong acids or alkalies, e.g. nitric, sulphuric and hydrochloric acids, sodium and potassium hydroxides and phenol (solid or strong solutions). Take great care when opening bottles containing strong acids or ammonia, particularly when previously unopened or if the stopper sticks. This is best done in a fume cupboard. When pouring from such bottles hold them firmly in both hands and, in the case of strong acids, place the receiving vessel in a sink. Always add the contents slowly to water or aqueous solutions, preferably while cooling and stirring. Avoid letting the liquid run down the outside of the bottle so that it reaches the label or gets on the hands. If a measured quantity of a corrosive liquid is needed use a safety pipette (see Fig. 1.1), a burette, or a measuring cylinder, depending on the quantity required.

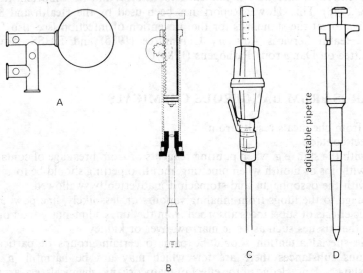

adjustable pipette

Fig. 1.1. Safety Pipettes.
A, B and C can be fitted to the top of standard pipettes. Several models of type D are available and can be adjusted to deliver volumes up to 5 or 10 ml.

Toxic Chemicals

Scheduled poisons such as cyanide and barbiturates are best kept locked in a cupboard or small store. Always measure reagents containing such poisons using a safety pipette, burette or measuring cylinder; mouth pipetting should be totally forbidden. When discarding liquids containing poisons such as cyanide down a sink, do so with a good flow of water to dilute any harmful effects. Avoid the simultaneous disposal of cyanide solutions and acids which can liberate hydrogen cyanide. A cyanide antidote kit (p. 22) should be kept in the drug cupboard of any laboratory using cyanides. Whenever possible use alternative analytical methods not using cyanide.

Organic solvents which form a commonly used group of substances may have toxic properties (see Table 1.1). Thus benzene is toxic to bone marrow, carbon tetrachloride and other halogenated hydrocarbons to the liver. Since these effects may be cumulative, keep exposure to a minimum by selecting the least toxic of alternative solvents. When using these, carry out procedures, including distillation, in a fume cupboard or under a fume hood with adequate extraction. Recovery of organic solvents is inadvisable.

When shaking to extract in separating funnels, release the pressure carefully at frequent intervals by inverting the funnel and slowly opening the tap so as to avoid solvent spraying into the air when the stopper is finally removed. Chromatographic and steroid techniques are best performed in separate rooms which can be adequately ventilated rather than in the main laboratory. So as to avoid inhaling the vapour, do not pipette toxic solvents orally. Keep only the minimum needed for daily working in the laboratory. Place bottles containing them in a cool place out of direct sunlight and in such a position that staff have free access to an exit in the event of a fire.

Mercury loses vapour into the atmosphere if exposed at ordinary temperatures. If ventilation is poor and appreciable quantities are left exposed, dangerous amounts can be inhaled. Store in properly stoppered thick-walled jars in a cool place. Spillages should be cleared up immediately. For further information see reference Mercurial Poisoning (1966).

Toxic gases most likely to be encountered are natural gas, carbon dioxide, phosgene and compressed air. The risk of carbon monoxide poisoning with natural gas is slight, unless this is burning under very abnormal conditions where the air supply is restricted. Carbon dioxide is only likely to reach hazardous concentrations where the solid form, dry ice, is stored in a poorly ventilated room. Phosgene (carbonyl chloride) may be formed in stored chloroform residues and may be liberated during distillation. The rate of formation is much reduced by the addition of a little ethanol and storage in dark bottles as is done with commercially available chloroform. Finally, compressed air supplies should be treated with respect. Never direct a jet of compressed air at the skin since severe tissue injury may occur and there is the possibility of fatal air embolism from entry into ruptured blood vessels. The same hazard can arise from a jet of gas from any high pressure source.

Carcinogens

Many chemicals have the potential to cause cancer. As the effects of carcinogens are irreversible, these substances should only be used if the work requiring them is essential and no alternative reagent is available. Those most commonly used in clinical biochemistry were aromatic amines such as benzidine and ortho-tolidine. Techniques avoiding the use of such reagents are now available. The Codes of Practice issued by the Chester Beatty Research Institute (1966, 1971) are important reading for those still handling carcinogens. It is most likely that

TABLE 1.1
Hazardous Solvents used in Clinical Biochemistry

Solvent	TLV[a] ppm	TLV[a] mg m^{-3}	Flash point[b]	Explosive limits[c]	Ignition temp.[d]	Hazards[e] Vapour	Hazards[e] Skin	Hazards[e] Explosive	Hazards[e] Fire	Hazards[e] Other
Acetic acid	10	25	43	4–16	426	I	C		F	
Acetic anhydride	5	20	54	3–10	380	I	C		F	
Acetone	1000	2400	−18	3–13	538			E	HF	
Acetonitrile	40	70	6	4–16	524	EH	HA		HF	
Amyl alcohols			19–43	1–10	300–437	I			F	P
Aniline	5	19				H	HA			
Benzene	10	32	−11	1·4–8	562	H	HA		HF	
Butanols	50–100	150–300	10–29	1·4–11	365–478	H	HA	E	F	
Carbon disulphide	20	60	−30	1–44	100	EH		E	HF	
Carbon tetrachloride	10	65				H				
Chloroform	25	120				H				
Cyclohexane	300	1050	−20	1·3–8·4	260			E	HF	
1,2-Dichloroethane	50	200	13	6·2–15·9	413	I,H	HA		HF	
Dichloromethane	100	360				H				
Diethyl ether	400	1200	−45	1·9–48	180	H		E	HF	
Dioxan	100	360	12	2–22	180	I			HF	
Ethanol	1000	1900	12	3·3–19	423	H			HF	
2-Ethoxyethanol	100	370	40	1·7–15·6	238	H		E	F	
Ethyl acetate	400	1400	−4·4	2·5–11·5	427				HF	
Heptane	400	1600	−4	1·2–6·7	223				HF	

Substance	TLV ppm	TLV mg m⁻³	Flash point	Explosive limits	Ignition temperature	Vapour hazard	Fire hazard	Other
Hexane	100	360	−23	1·2–7·5	260		HF	
Light petroleum (bp 30–160°C)	500	2 000	−17 up	1–6	290 up		HF	
Methanol	200	260	10	7·3–36·5	464	H	HF	
2-Methoxyethanol	25	80	46	2·5–14	288	H	F	P
Pentane	600	1 800	−49	1·4–8	309		HF	E
Propan-1-ol	200	500	25	2·1–13·5	433		HF	
Propan-2-ol	400	980	12	2·3–12·7	399		HF	
Pyridine	5	15	20	1·8–12·4	482		HF	
1,1,2,2-Tetrabromoethane	1	14				H		
1,1,2,2-Tetrachloroethane	5	35				EH		
Tetrachloroethylene	100	670				H		
Toluene	100	375	4·4	1·4–6·8	536	H	HF	HA
1,1,1-Trichloroethane	350	1 900				H		
Trichloroethylene	100	535				H		
Xylenes	100	435	17–25	1–7	464–529	H	F	HA

Notes. ᵃ Threshold limit value. Concentration in working environment to which most workers can be exposed repeatedly, 8 h daily, without adverse effect. ppm = ml m⁻³ of gas vapour in air at 25°C; mg m⁻³ refers to weight of solvent in air.
ᵇ Flash point (°C) determined in closed cup.
ᶜ Explosive limits: range of concentration of flammable solvent in air an explosion risk, volume of vapour per 100 volumes of mixture.
ᵈ Ignition temperature (°C) is the minimal temperature which will initiate or maintain self-sustained combustion, independent of heat source.
ᵉ Hazards: Vapour: I, irritant; H, harmful; EH, extremely harmful—if inhaled. Skin: C, corrosive on contact; HA, harmful by absorption through skin. Fire: F, flammable; HF, highly flammable; Ox, oxidising agent which may cause fire. Other: P, poison; A, asphyxiant; Explosive: E, explosion hazard. HD, harmful dust; FC, fire on contact with water.

absorption will be through the skin of the hands either from direct contact with the substances or from contaminated articles such as clothing or benches, but fine powder may be inhaled when preparing reagents as may vapour from volatile substances. Precautions include keeping them in well closed bottles, labelled 'carcinogenic' and in avoiding any contact with the skin. When handling, wear rubber or plastic gloves which are afterwards well-washed under cold running water. Should accidental skin contact occur, wash in cold running water for several minutes. After use, rinse glassware thoroughly in cold water and wash benches with cold water; impervious bench surfaces are highly desirable. After handling with full precautions, wash the hands first with cold water, then with soap. Much of this could well be the practice when handling most aromatic organic chemicals. See also George (1971) and Carcinogenic Substances Regulations (1967).

Explosive and Flammable Chemicals

Explosions may be produced when using certain chemicals, mainly oxidising agents. Especially important is *perchloric acid* used to digest organic matter. Carry out all such work with perchloric acid in a fume cupboard constructed and installed in accordance with DHSS Health Notice HN(76)95 (1976). Only use perchloric acid when there is no alternative test procedure or reagent. As *picric acid* when dry explodes on percussion, it should not be kept in ground glass stoppered bottles but stored under water in a container closed by a cork or rubber stopper . Discharge of picric acid residues down copper pipes can lead to accumulation of copper picrate, an explosion hazard—important when using it in the AutoAnalyzer. *Ammoniacal silver nitrate* should always be prepared freshly for use. Discard any surplus as on standing in light, crystals of silver azide may form which explode on shaking the bottle. *Sodium azide*, used as a bacteriostatic agent, may produce metallic azides by reacting with metal waste pipes during disposal.

Explosive hazards may arise from organic solvents. *Ether* kept in clear bottles exposed to sunlight can form peroxides. This is most likely to occur if ether residues are kept for recovery. Ether supplied commercially is usually in brown bottles and contains an antioxidant. If ether residues are redistilled the peroxides are concentrated in the unvolatilised residue and may reach sufficient concentration to produce a violent explosion. If ether is stored for recovery keep it in dark bottles and before distilling shake with freshly prepared ferrous hydroxide. Another explosive hazard from solvent residues arises from inadvertent mixing of chloroform and acetone. Under ill-defined conditions these may combine to give chloretone. The reaction is markedly exothermic and considerable pressure can build up in stoppered containers. If these solvents are to be recovered keep them separately in clearly labelled containers. An exothermic reaction also occurs when concentrated nitric acid comes into contact with alcoholic solutions. The reaction has a latent period and may then proceed with explosive violence. Extreme care should be taken if nitric acid is being used to clean glassware in which alcoholic solutions have been stored. A useful list of incompatible reagents is given in Muir (1977).

The importance of restricting the amount of flammable solvents available in the working laboratory area has already been emphasised. Fire hazards arise during the use of these limited stocks and special care should always be taken. When distilling a solvent the container must *never be heated over a naked flame* and efficient condensation of solvent vapours must be ensured at all times. The mixture of solvent vapour and air may be flammable and operations allowing escape of solvent into the air should be carefully controlled. Some solvents are of low viscosity or specific gravity and may spill easily when poured. Air–solvent vapour mixtures may be carried away by draughts to points of possible ignition, or high density vapours such as ether–air mixtures may roll for long distances along benches or floors. All operations with such flammable solvents are therefore best conducted under a fume hood.

The flash point (Table 1.1) of many solvents over a wide range of concentrations in air is below ambient working temperatures and acetone, ether, benzene and light petroleum have flash points below 0°C thus creating potentially dangerous situations in refrigerators in which such solvents are stored. Explosive ignition of solvent–air mixtures is easily achieved by naked flames and small electric sparks arising from discharge of static electricity at relay points or at switches. Refrigerators should preferably have spark-proof relay contacts.

Fire hazards may arise from exothermic oxidation reactions. Concentrated nitric acid spillages should *not* be mopped up with cotton or paper waste. Such materials may ignite after placing in a waste bin, often some time later. Preferably dilute the acid with water and neutralise with sodium carbonate before removal. Fires have arisen from the use of metallic zinc powder as a reducing agent in some procedures. The metal is often filtered off and undergoes vigorous oxidation by air when dry. This may ignite the filter paper in the waste bin some time later. The zinc may either be washed down the sink with plenty of water or destroyed by dilute acid in the fume cupboard.

Flammable gases stored in cylinders constitute a fire hazard (see Table 1.2). These gases include hydrogen, propane and acetylene. Oxygen is an additional hazard if used with any flammable chemical. Again the wide range of concentration of flammable mixtures with air or oxygen and the ease of ignition should be remembered. Keep cylinders not in use, whether full or apparently empty, outside the laboratory in a special store in racks. If possible, keep cylinders in use out of the main laboratory area and use approved leak-free tubing to convey the gas to the point of use. Where this is not feasible, transport cylinders in special trolleys and secure them firmly during use. Test the valve and blow dust etc. from the outlet *before* bringing the cylinder into the laboratory. Never use reducing valves which are damaged thereby allowing leakage of gas, and never use excessive force to open the main valve or to secure the reducing valve. Preferably this should conform to British Standard 1780 (1960). When opening the cylinder valve do so slowly; too rapid opening can cause compression heating in the regulation valve. Keep the cylinder key attached to the cylinder to allow rapid closure in an emergency. Always close the cylinder valve after use and do not rely on closing the reducing valve only. *Never* use grease or oil to lubricate the threads of reducing valves. They are likely to cause explosions when used with oxygen cylinders. Secure connections between the pressure regulator and the equipment at both ends preferably with jubilee clips. Before using any gas cylinder, *check* that it contains the gas required and that the pressure regulator is suitable. Pressure in full cylinders is now 20 MPa (3000 lb/in^2), appreciably higher than formerly. Cylinders are painted in various colour codes according to contents and gases for 'industrial' use may have a different colour code from those for 'medical' use. Many hospital laboratories use only 'medical' gas cylinders. It is good practice to have the British Standards Institution Colour Codes on display in the area where cylinders are kept but it is *always* advisable to check the written statement of contents on the label and to return unused any cylinders with illegible labels.

TABLE 1.2

Other Hazardous Chemicals used in Clinical Biochemistry

Chemical	TLV[a] ppm	TLV[a] mg m⁻³	Flash point[b]	Explosive limits[c]	Ignition temp.[d]	Hazards[e] Vapour	Skin	Explosive	Fire	Other
Acetylene				3–82	335			E	HF	A
Acrylamide		0·3					HA			HD
Aluminium lithium hydride							C		F	FC
Ammonia solution	25	18				I	C			
Butane			−60	1·9–8·5	405				HF	
Chromium trioxide		0·1					C		Ox	HD
Dimethyl sulphate	1	5				EH	HA, C	E		
Hydrochloric acid	5	7				I	C			
Hydrogen peroxide	1	1·4					C			
Lactic acid							C			
Mercury		0·1				H	HA			P
Nitric acid	2	5				I	C			
Orthophosphoric acid		1					C			
Phenol	5	19					HA, C			P
Picric acid		0·1						E (dry)		P
Potassium cyanide		5				H	HA, C			P
Potassium hydroxide							C			

Propane	1000	−104	2.2-9.5	468		E	HF
Silver nitrate	0.01				C		P
Sodium cyanide	5				H		
Sodium hydroxide	2				HA, C		
Sulphuric acid	1				C		
Trichloracetic acid					C		

Notes. *a* Threshold limit value. Concentration in working environment to which most workers can be exposed repeatedly, 8 h daily, without adverse effect. ppm = ml m⁻³ of gas vapour in air at 25°C; mg m⁻³ refers to weight of solvent in air.

b Flash point (°C) determined in closed cup.

c Explosive limits: range of concentration of flammable solvent in air an explosion risk, volume of vapour per 100 volumes of mixture.

d Ignition temperature (°C) is the minimal temperature which will initiate or maintain self-sustained combustion, independent of heat source.

e Hazards: Vapour: I, irritant; H, harmful; EH, extremely harmful—if inhaled. Skin: C, corrosive on contact; HA, harmful by absorption through skin. Explosive: E, explosion hazard. Fire: F, flammable; HF, highly flammable; HF, highly flammable; HF, highly flammable; HF, highly flammable; Ox, oxidising agent which may cause fire. Other: P, poison; A, asphyxiant; HD, harmful dust; FC, fire on contact with water.

Note. The data for Tables 1.1 and 1.2 have been obtained from Muir (1977), in which a long chapter gives a detailed description of the hazards and toxic effects possible from a wide range of gases, reagents and solvents, with information about first-aid treatment and spillage disposal in each case, thus constituting a most valuable reference book for all laboratories.

Never empty a cylinder of a flammable gas completely but discard it when a small positive pressure remains and close the valve to avoid entry of air into the cylinder. Mark the cylinder as empty.

If flammable gases are used with compressed air or oxygen, fit the gas line with a non-return valve. Taps for natural gas should be fitted towards the back of the bench to avoid turning on accidentally. Use specially modified gas burners and connect to the tap with metal-reinforced tubing preferably of non-flammable plastic which is regularly checked for wear. Do not use gas to heat ovens or water baths.

Outbreaks of Fire. If a fire breaks out, prompt, correct action will often limit the damage. The first action must be to raise the alarm. The fire alarm should be designed to alert the hospital switchboard automatically and ensure that the fire brigade is called. Only first aid fire fighting measures will be used by the laboratory staff and the area should be evacuated if the means of escape or the building structure is threatened.

The extinguishers available will usually be a fire hose, fire blankets, sand and chemical extinguishers generating a spray of halogenated hydrocarbon or dry powder intended to limit the supply of oxygen to the fire. Extinguishers should be inspected regularly and the Safety Officer should ensure that the staff is aware of their location and proper use, if necessary by regular practice. Use of the correct extinguisher is important (see Table 1.3, opposite). Avoid water near live electrical equipment, particularly if high voltages are in use. Many flammable solvents float on water and the fire may be spread by this means. Carbon tetrachloride is converted to phosgene in some circumstances and is best avoided where ventilation is poor. Carbon dioxide extinguishers are useful but high concentrations of the gas can build up in poorly ventilated areas. Small fires can often be smothered by a fire blanket or sand properly used.

If the fire is not controlled by immediate first-aid measures, reduce the air supply by closing windows and doors. The priority is then to evacuate all staff, patients and visitors. This should proceed by a pre-arranged plan without panic. A roll-call should be taken to ensure that nobody has been left in the building.

For further information see Ackroyd *et al.* (1977), and British Standard 5306, part 3 (1985).

INFECTION HAZARDS

Specimens received by pathology laboratories are all potentially infected. The main hazards in the clinical chemistry laboratory are viral hepatitis and the acquired immune deficiency syndrome (AIDS). Since a specimen of blood from a patient with these diseases may be as dangerous to handle as a specimen of faeces from a case of typhoid, precautions to prevent infection must be introduced into the clinical biochemistry laboratory. Guidelines for the prevention of infection in laboratories have been given in the Howie Code of Practice, bulletins from the DHSS, Interim Advisory Committee on Safety in Clinical Laboratories (1980, 1981), DHSS Health Circular HC (79)3 (1979), Health Service Advisory Committee (1985) and DHSS, Advisory Committee on Dangerous Pathogens (1986).

The official guidelines for the laboratory handling of material from patients with AIDS and with viral hepatitis are very similar, differing only in details. These relate particularly to the degree of containment required and to the need for agreement between laboratory staff and clinician before specimens are sent from patients with AIDS. This chapter will not attempt to present the specific details for each type of

TABLE 1.3
Selection of Appropriate Fire Extinguishers

	Type of extinguisher Water-CO_2				Halogenated
Type of fire	or soda-acid	Dry CO_2	Dry powder	Foam	hydrocarbon
Paper, wood, fabric	R		R		R
Flammable liquids	D	R	R	R	R
Flammable gases		R	R		R
Electrical	D	R	R	D	R

Note. R, recommended; D, dangerous.

infection and the reader is referred to Health Services Advisory Committee (1985) for hepatitis B and to DHSS, Advisory Committee on Dangerous Pathogens (1986) for AIDS.

The exact precautions adopted for the prevention of infection will depend on factors such as the laboratory layout, number of staff and specimens, types of patient in the hospital and the equipment used in the analysis. The general approach should concentrate attention at the most likely sources of infection and attempt to minimise spread from these by the main routes of transmission of infection (Moore, 1971).

Acquired Immune Deficiency Syndrome. AIDS is caused by human immunodeficiency virus (HIV), a retrovirus which, by damaging T cells (p. 87), reduces the ability of an affected individual to resist other infections. Exposure to the virus results in the development of HIV antibodies. The proportion of people with such antibodies which progresses to clinically-apparent AIDS is uncertain but such progression is currently invariably fatal eventually. The virus has been detected in blood and blood products, in breast milk, semen, vaginal fluid, saliva, tears, urine and brain tissue. Infection with HIV in the clinical biochemistry laboratory is most likely to occur by infection of exposed cuts, or by accidental self-inoculation with blood containing the virus. Avoidance of these hazards is essential as is prompt decontamination of areas which become accidentally infected.

High-risk specimens arise from patients with confirmed or suspected AIDS or those who are HIV antibody positive. Infected specimens are also likely from homosexual or bisexual males, intravenous drug-abusers, haemophiliacs, persons who have returned from sub-Saharan Africa during the last 5 years, and the sexual partners and babies of any of these.

Viral Hepatitis. This is an important condition causing hazards in the biochemical laboratory and precautions taken to limit hazards for this are likely to be adequate for most other infections except AIDS. Viral hepatitis occurs in three main forms and though recovery from infection by any form usually confers lasting immunity to further attacks, cross-immunity between forms does not occur. Subclinical disease may occur with development of immunity. Although workers long exposed to viral hepatitis hazards in the laboratory may have developed such immunity this cannot be relied on and is no protection to new staff.

The first form, *hepatitis A*, with an incubation period of 14 to 35 days occurs in the general population causing sporadic and epidemic cases of jaundice. The urine and faeces contain the virus and entry into a susceptible person is usually by ingestion of contaminated food or drink, or by placing contaminated fingers or other objects in the mouth. The virus also occurs in the blood which is infectious if handled, and is capable of transmitting infection if it is injected into a second person. Diagnosis of hepatitis A requires the demonstration of the virus in the faeces or the presence of hepatitis-specific IgM in the serum.

The second form of hepatitis, *hepatitis B*, has a longer incubation time of 40 to 120 days. The presence of virus particles in the blood is associated with a positive reaction for hepatitis B surface antigen (HBsAg), hepatitis B core antigen (HBcAg) and hepatitis Be antigen (HBeAg). HBeAg appears to be a component of HBcAg and is a good marker of infectivity. It is usual to confirm a diagnosis of hepatitis B by testing for the presence of HBsAg during the acute phase of the illness. Blood is highly infectious and urine and faeces are probably infected. This form of hepatitis circulates in closed communities probably by transmission via the faecal–oral route but it has been particularly associated with transfer of infected blood by direct inoculation.

The third form is *non-A non-B hepatitis*. The natural history of this condition is not clearly defined but it is also an important cause of sporadic and epidemic hepatitis. The virus occurs in the blood and non-A non-B hepatitis may be a complication of the administration of blood products. The diagnosis is made by exclusion of hepatitis A, hepatitis B, cytomegalic virus and Epstein-Barr virus infections in a patient with acute viral hepatitis.

Both hepatitis B and non-A non-B hepatitis are associated with a carrier state so blood may continue to be infectious long after the patient is well. The main source of infection in the biochemistry laboratory is blood. Possible routes of entry are by ingestion or by direct entry through breaching of the skin surface. Investigation of accidental infections in the laboratory has shown as important the hazards of sucking infected material into the mouth through a pipette, of contamination of surroundings and hence of hands and perhaps later mouth as a result of spills of infected material, of self-inoculation with needles or other sharp objects, of infection of existing cuts, and of the generation of infected aerosols. Avoidance of such hazards is obviously desirable for viral hepatitis as is prompt decontamination of areas which become accidentally infected.

High risk specimens will obviously arise from patients with frank viral hepatitis or those who are HBsAg positive. Infected specimens are also likely from drug addicts, cases in the prodromal stage of hepatitis, patients who have had multiple blood transfusions, patients receiving chronic renal dialysis treatment, cases on immunosuppressants such as post-transplant cases or patients with chronic leukaemia, and inmates with a poor standard of personal hygiene of such closed communities as mental hospitals. It is possible that all such patients are infected with Hazard Group 3 pathogens (see DHSS, 1983), and specimens from these patients should be handled separately at all stages of progress through the laboratory (pp. 14–16). This special handling of high risk specimens does not exclude the possibility that other specimens may be infected and it is wise to treat all specimens as potentially infectious.

The general precautions which should be taken are often those conducive to good laboratory work anyway. Staff locker rooms with washing facilities should be separate from the working area. Protective clothing must be provided and changed at least twice a week. The recommended pattern of coat has an overlap of several inches at the front closure, is fastened by press studs and has tight cuffs. If high risk specimens are being handled the coat should be supplemented with an impervious wrap-around apron from chest to ankles and plastic overshoes. Staff must put on laboratory coats and fasten them before entering the working laboratory and remove them before leaving the department. Such coats must not be stored in the locker used for personal clothes. An entirely separate staff room must be available where refreshments can be taken thus enabling food to be kept out of the working area. Smoking must also be forbidden except in the staff room. Hand wash basins with elbow taps and disposable paper towel dispensers must be conveniently situated in all working laboratories. Keep the hands away from the mouth and do not lick labels. Keep benches tidy so as to minimise spills. Avoid undue haste in handling liquids and clean up any spillage at once.

Tests on patients involving administration of various substances are sometimes carried out in biochemical laboratories. As a general rule it is advisable to obtain these from the Pharmacy department so as to avoid the possibility of giving the patient the wrong substance or the right substance contaminated. If, however, as for the glucose tolerance test, the glucose solution is prepared in the department, this should be done in that part of the staff room where drinks are made so that separate crockery can be kept which never enters the working laboratories.

Specimen Collection

Venepuncture. Occasionally patients are bled in the clinical biochemistry laboratory. If this is necessary, blood must be taken in separate accommodation provided for the purpose and the phlebotomist should wear protective clothing used only for taking blood. Blood must not be taken from any person known to be infected with Group 3 micro-organisms or viruses except under medical direction. Avoid spread of blood from the venepuncture site and blood escaping from the syringe or needle. Cleanse the skin with an antiseptic swab. Some workers prefer not to remove the needle from the syringe, as contamination of the fingers may occur, but to deliver the blood *slowly* through the needle with the needle touching the side of the tube to avoid aerosol formation. Alternatively, remove the needle from the syringe with needle forceps before expelling the blood through the nozzle which touches the inside of the container. In either case the empty syringe and the needle must be disposed of into a container, the walls of which cannot be penetrated by the needle.

While specimens may be collected in the laboratory it is more often done by non-laboratory staff outside the department. Whoever collects the specimen is responsible for avoiding contamination of the outside of the container and of the environment. The laboratory may have little control over this, but should be free to reject specimens which have leaked, particularly high-risk specimens.

Other Specimens. For *capillary blood* use a sterile stilette for each skin puncture and then discard this into a waste container. Avoid getting blood on the operator's fingers when collecting into glass capillaries for blood–gas determinations and take care not to scratch the skin with a roughened end of the capillary when sealing with plasticine. If blood is to be collected directly into a pipette allow it to run in by force of gravity. Place the swab used to wipe pipettes or skin in a container for autoclaving later. Use a clean pipette for each sample and place used pipettes in a hypochlorite solution containing 2500 ppm available chlorine. Pipettes can then be autoclaved and washed before re-use.

When collecting *urine, faeces or other biological specimens* use disposable containers and avoid contamination of the outside of the container.

Containers. Blood containers should be leak-proof, permit inversion if an anticoagulant is used, and be easy to close and open without contaminating the fingers. Most containers with plastic push-in stoppers are very unsatisfactory in this last respect; screw caps are much better but may not be leak-proof after use once. Re-use even after careful cleaning and sterilisation is potentially un-satisfactory, and disposable containers are preferable. Choose containers which comply with the British Standards Institution—BS 4851 (1982) and BS 6242 (1982).

Urine is best collected in screw-capped disposable plastic containers. Small volumes of urine or faeces may be sent in plastic containers with a sealed cap.

Containers from known high risk patients should be specially marked.

Transport to the Laboratory. This should not increase the risk of contamination. If collected properly the neck of the container is uncontaminated and remains so if the container remains upright. This also greatly reduces the risk of cap contamination during laboratory processing. Blood containers may be placed in racks which must be cleaned regularly either by autoclaving or by immersing in hypochlorite solution. Known high risk specimens must be placed in a two-compartment plastic bag, sealed to contain the specimen if accidental spillage occurs, and must also be kept upright. Request forms for high risk specimens are best written outside the patient treatment area and should be labelled 'High Risk' and placed in the outer pocket of the two-compartment bag.

Keep all request forms free from contamination by blood. Do not wrap them round the containers but either store them separately in an ordered fashion related to the order of the specimens in the rack, or use the two-compartment plastic bag for all specimens. The second option is preferable.

Ensure that trolleys used for delivery of specimens to the laboratory hold the racks safely and carry urine and faecal specimens upright without risk of them falling off.

Reception in the Laboratory. Specimens should be kept upright in the racks during handling. Secretarial staff can be trained to deal with specimens safely on arrival and during preliminary sorting and clerical procedures. They should report any obviously contaminated specimens or breakages to the laboratory staff. Contaminated specimens from high risk patients should be rejected and disposed of immediately and other high risk specimens passed on to a member of the laboratory staff for processing.

A specially defined and planned area should be set aside for the preliminary processing of specimens. This area must contain a bench with a smooth impervious surface which is washed daily, or after any spills, with a hypochlorite solution containing 10 000 ppm of available chlorine. Risks are reduced by using disposable gloves. Staff should not leave the specimen processing area wearing gloves and should not touch laboratory fittings unnecessarily while wearing gloves. Discard gloves in a container for incineration. A hand-wash basin must be provided in the room.

Centrifugation of specimens is particularly hazardous since infected air-borne particles may be ejected. Keep the cap on the container during centrifugation to reduce this hazard. Angle head centrifuges must not be used because they are more prone to cause aerosols. Windshields are advantageous and, if fitted, should always be used with their lids on. The centrifuge must have a lid catch, preferably interlocking, to ensure the lid is kept closed until rotation stops. Centrifuges should be sited to allow regular inspection and to allow correct positioning of trunnions to be checked.

High risk specimens must be centrifuged separately from other specimens in sealed buckets, which are then opened in an exhaust protective cabinet.

The breaking of a tube in a centrifuge is considered an incident and should be reported to the Safety Officer. The centrifuge must be kept closed for 30 minutes to allow settling of air-borne particles. The entire contents of the bowl of the centrifuge must then be autoclaved or placed in a non-corrosive disinfectant, such as glutaraldehyde (20 g/l), for 24 h. Swab the bowl with the same disinfectant immediately and again the following day. Remove the disinfectant by washing with water. If a breakage occurs in the centrifugation of a high risk specimen, loosen the cap of the bucket and autoclave the bucket and its contents.

The transfer of plasma from one container to another carries the risk of aerosol formation, splashes and spillage. This procedure should be kept to a minimum with all samples of a specimen being taken at the same time. The sample should be transferred by carefully using disposable plastic pasteur pipettes which are then autoclaved. Mouth pipetting is forbidden. The transfer of high risk material is especially hazardous. Wearing the protective clothing previously described and a visor and rubber gloves, open the sealed bucket in an exhaust protective cabinet and pipette the serum into a screw-capped container labelled 'High Risk'. The working area should be washed daily and after spills with a hypochlorite solution containing 10 000 ppm available chlorine.

The preliminary processing of urine specimens is conveniently done in the same area as specimens of blood. If this is not possible, an area of the laboratory with an easily cleaned smooth impervious surface must be provided. The volumes of 24 h specimens of urine are measured but only a small portion need be kept for the analysis. Discard the rest of the collection at once in a sluice situated close to the central processing area and disinfect the container.

Faecal specimens may be stored in a fume cupboard. If compatible with the required tests, the faecal specimen may be autoclaved. If this is not possible the preparation of the faecal suspension for fat analysis must be done in a sealed homogeniser, which must be opened in an exhaust protective cabinet. Take portions of the suspension for analysis and storage; discard the rest in the sluice. Swab the interior of the fume cupboard regularly with disinfectant. Discard faecal specimens sent for qualitative tests in the original container after removing a test portion; the collected containers can be incinerated.

Bench Organisation and Procedures

The basic requirements are tidy working methods with avoidance of unnecessary haste and careful attention to special hazards. Keep specimens from contaminating the bench by placing them in a tray or on Benchkote. Discard-buckets or similar receptacles are suitable for the disposal of used non-infected glassware and containers. Carefully empty test tubes into a sink before putting them into the buckets. Avoid skin puncture by rejecting chipped glassware and by not picking up broken glass with fingers. Avoid mouth pipetting completely, using instead automatic dilutors and dispensers for manual methods. Keep serum within its container by avoiding spillage, splashing, breakages and aerosol formation. The latter can occur when specimens are shaken, when capped containers are opened, on blowing out pipettes, and during centrifugation particularly with angle head centrifuges, centrifuge tubes with wet rims or on rapid deceleration. When mixing the contents of test tubes, stopper the tube and mix by gentle inversion or by using a vortex mixer.

Take similar care when working with urine. Aerosol formation is especially liable during extraction with organic solvents in a separating funnel. Release the pressure frequently by inverting the funnel and carefully opening the tap, preferably under a fume hood.

All automated equipment carries risks with respect to spread of infective material. Centrifugal analysers share some of the hazards of centrifugation. To achieve adequate mixing some discrete analysers expel liquids from diluters with considerable force. This causes aerosols. Such facts should be considered in deciding working practices around such instruments. Dialyser membranes in continuous flow equipment must be changed while wearing gloves, and only after the system has been thoroughly rinsed with water and then for ten minutes with a hypochlorite solution containing 2500 ppm available chlorine. The small dialysers may need individual attention during a run and are best dealt with by a careful 'no touch' technique. Analyse high risk specimens in specially marked sample cups separate from other specimens. Transfer sample cups and their contents without spillage to a plastic bag containing cellulose wadding using forceps which should then be sterilised. When tests are completed, wash the automated instrument thoroughly as instructed by the manufacturer and then with either a hypochlorite solution (2500 ppm available chlorine) or glutaraldehyde (20 g/l) if high risk specimens have been analysed. Effluent tubes from automated equipment must be inserted at least 25 cm into a sink waste pipe. Water must flow down the waste pipe while the machine is in use. Disinfect the sinks daily with about 250 ml of a hypochlorite solution (2500 ppm available chlorine). Label the traps of such sinks as 'high risk' and disinfect as above before any plumbing work is carried out on the sink or its connections.

Disposal of Specimens and Contaminated Material

Whenever possible, disposable materials are used and sent to the hospital incinerator in heavy plastic bags—specially coloured in the case of high risk materials. This is satisfactory for soiled material and plastic ware but autoclaving is preferred for blood specimens. Immerse non-disposable pasteur pipettes in hypochlorite solution (2500 ppm available chlorine) overnight before autoclaving. Disposable pasteur pipettes are preferred. Possibly infected broken glass must be autoclaved before disposal.

Disinfectants

Formalin is the name given to a 40% (w/v) solution of formaldehyde with methanol added as stabiliser. An 'x%' solution of formalin' therefore contains 0·4 x% formaldehyde. For most purposes a 5% formalin solution is effective in laboratory use for discard-containers or for swabbing contaminated surfaces. However, the vapour from formalin is more irritating to the conjunctivae and mucous membranes than hypochlorite and should only be used where there is good ventilation.

Hypochlorite solutions are active because of the free chlorine in them. Since they readily release this, their effectiveness diminishes quite quickly. Because hypochlorite is also rapidly inactivated by organic matter its effective life and useful exposure time are important in the use of hypochlorite solutions as disinfectants. The strengths and times of exposure given here are taken from the Howie Code and from Bulletins 1 and 2 of the Interim Advisory Committee on Safety in Clinical Laboratories (DHSS, 1980, 1981). The concentrations of hypochlorite solutions for disinfectant purposes are conventionally quoted in parts per million (ppm) of available chlorine.

Hypochlorite is corrosive to some metals and should not be used for disinfecting centrifuge buckets, rotors and bowls. Strong hypochlorite solutions (100 000 ppm) are a possible explosion hazard and unopened large containers must be stored in a cool place and not exposed to direct sunlight (DHSS Health Notice HN(76)189 (1976)).

Glutaraldehyde is effective against viruses and is used in a concentration of 20 g/l. The solution is non-corrosive for metals and affords a useful alternative to hypochlorite (10 000 ppm) for some purposes. It is less irritant than formaldehyde in similar concentration but is not recommended for extensive use as it is much more expensive than the alternatives. It is best used for disinfecting Auto-Analyzer modules or centrifuge parts or other metal objects where some corrosion would be detrimental to function.

Phenolic Solutions. Sudol is an example, being a lysol substitute. It contains 50% xylenols and ethyl phenols. For use add the Sudol to water to avoid gel formation; clear solutions are obtained with distilled or soft water. Phenolic disinfectants should not be used when appreciable amounts of proteins are present.

APPARATUS

Electrical Hazards

The installation and maintenance of all electrical equipment must be carried out by properly trained staff. See Hospital Technical Memorandum, No. 13 (1965) and Hospital Building Note, No. 15(revised, 1971).

The British and European colour code for electrical cables is: live, brown; neutral, blue; earth, green/yellow. Suppliers of equipment from outside Europe should be asked to ensure that the cable conforms to the local code. Cables for connecting to mains should be rubber or PVC three-core, as short as is conveniently possible and without joinings, be frequently inspected for any deterioration, and be so situated that they are not near hot pipes, or flames, or so that reagents are likely to be spilt on them. Sockets of the switchable type should be above and at the back of the bench. It is good practice as far as possible to have electrical instruments on benches supplied with adequate sockets thus avoiding the use of multiple adaptors. Wherever possible avoid gas and water supply to such a bench. Instruments should not obscure access to the switched socket and when not in use should be switched off at the socket. Do not replace blown fuses until careful inspection has been made of the instrument and circuit in use. Check that earthing arrangements are adequate and that the correct fuses have been fitted. Connections to the mains supply should only be made by a qualified electrician. Check that foreign equipment is intended for use with British mains voltages.

It is important to disconnect from the mains any equipment which is to be serviced or examined. Even then capacitors in the equipment are capable of causing unpleasant shocks. Short the terminals of such capacitors. Electrophoresis apparatus is a special hazard. Always disconnect the power supply before removing the cover to make adjustments and preferably use equipment which incorporates automatic switching off on opening the lid. Do not rely on this, however, but regard it as an additional safety device. The precautions must be especially strict where high voltage electrophoresis is being used. Earth leak circuit breakers should be used where possible.

Passage of an electric current through the body, e.g. from hand to hand or hand to foot, can be fatal. Unpleasant sensations begin at 1 mA for 50 Hz AC and 5 mA DC. Increasing the current to 15 mA 50 Hz AC or 70 mA DC causes sustained muscular contractions making it difficult for the person to release his hold. Increases beyond 20 mA 50 Hz AC or 80 mA DC produce dangerous cardiac arrhythmia and cardiac arrest occurs at about 100 mA 50 Hz AC or DC. Burning of the skin results at higher currents. For a given voltage the current varies with skin resistance which can range from 200 to 10 000 Ω depending on the dryness of the skin.

Extra care is necessary in the maintenance of equipment which operates unattended. Major fires are usually those which start when nobody is in the building.

Centrifuges

The microbiological safety of centrifugation has already been discussed (see p. 14). To prevent spread of infective material, centrifuges must also be mechanically safe and must be maintained and used correctly. Use only those centrifuges that conform to British Standard 4402 (1982).

Make sure specimen tubes are sound and of a size which allows adequate clearance when they reach the horizontal and that the pads are in position in the buckets. Before starting to centrifuge, check the load is within tolerance. Do not rely on volume if the specific gravity (sp. gr.) is greater than 1·2. Tubes should not be overfilled; the surface of the liquid should be more than 2 cm from the rim. Corrosion is a major cause of centrifuge failure. For this reason any liquid spilled in the centrifuge should be removed immediately. Very corrosive liquids should be placed in sealed containers but other solutions used in biochemistry may be sufficiently corrosive if spillage is frequent. These include mixtures of phenol or cresol with water, chloroform–isoamyl alcohol mixtures, salt solutions especially ammonium sulphate, ammoniacal solutions and solutions containing acids especially hydrochloric, perchloric or trichloracetic. Do not put water in centrifuge buckets to balance the load. Distribute the load symmetrically and evenly and increase the speed gradually on starting to spin. Centrifuge covers should preferably lock automatically during use but if this is not the case do not open until the rotor stops. Do not slow down by applying the fingers; if this does nothing more serious it can produce minor abrasions of the skin of significance in connection with hazards from infected blood. The prevention of aerosols has already been dealt with (p. 14). To keep free from such contamination disinfect the bowl and buckets regularly with a non-corrosive disinfectant such as glutaraldehyde (see p. 17). At regular intervals remove sleeves and adaptors and clean the head and accessories. Keep intact sets of accessories whose members have very similar weights. Have the centrifuge serviced every six months by an engineer and replace doubtfully sound components early and ensure that with high speed instruments, time-expired components are replaced according to instructions. See British Standard 4402 (1982).

Gas Equipment

Gas is now so much less used that it is possible to restrict the supply to certain benches in main laboratories and exclude it completely from rooms set apart for special techniques using readily flammable substances, e.g. for chromatography and steroid assays. Remember that a fully aerated bunsen burner may not be easy to see and pilot lights may not be noticed. It is safest to turn off a burner not in use.

Glass Apparatus

Cuts, sometimes severe, from broken glass still form a considerable proportion of injuries to staff. It has become all the more important to avoid these since they increase the infection hazard. A common cause was the breaking of glass tubing while threading through corks or rubber bungs. Use ground glass joints wherever possible. Never use chipped or cracked glassware, and when supporting condensers and flasks use the correct type and size of support of good quality without exerting undue pressure. Take care when disposing of broken glassware to do this in such a way that there is no danger to persons subsequently handling it. Do not pick up broken glass with bare hands. Use forceps for larger pieces; small fragments are conveniently removed with a piece of plasticine.

Dispensers

See that plastic wash bottles are properly labelled so as to distinguish clearly any containing liquids other than water, e.g. white labels for distilled water, red for all other liquids. Assume these and also aerosol dispensers contain a liquid at least as flammable as petrol and do not use near any source of ignition including electric hot plates.

Radiation Hazards

Hazards from radioactive isotopes and ionising radiations are covered by special regulations. The Ionising Radiations Regulations (1985) and the associated Approved Code of Practice (Health and Safety Commission, 1985) should be consulted if such materials are used. Staff exposed to such hazards should be specially trained and will require regular monitoring of the degree of radiation received. The discharge of radioactive waste is controlled by the Radioactive Substances Act (1960); see also Osborne (1977), Ionising Radiations Regulations (1968, 1969).

Radiation in the ultraviolet region is encountered when chromatograms are examined using the mercury discharge lamp. Direct rays from the source should be properly shielded from the eyes of the user and if chromatograms are to be examined for more than a minute or two, the eyes should be protected by glasses to reduce the risk of corneal and conjunctival irritation.

Some equipment uses a laser beam. Serious retinal damage occurs if this is allowed to enter the eye and strict precautions are needed to prevent this.

Low Pressure Systems

These are mainly met with where vacuum desiccators are in use. Injury from implosion of glass containers of this type may be minimised by using only desiccators which comply with British Standard 3423 (1962) and by enclosing them in a wire cage during evacuation. Avoid letting air enter the desiccator rapidly when re-equilibrating to atmospheric pressure. If other glassware has to be evacuated choose thick-walled round bottomed flasks and avoid the use of conical flasks unless the specially strengthened Buchner flask is used as in vacuum filtration.

NOTES ON BUILDINGS

Here are collected together a number of points to be taken into account when designing laboratories. For the sake of completeness some points already mentioned are re-included.

It should not be possible for anyone to be trapped in a room in which there is an outbreak of fire. In rooms in which this might occur there should be two exits. If the second door is kept locked the key should be in the lock, but better, an internally opening door should be fitted. Floors should have a non-slip surface.

The laboratory should be provided with first-aid and fire-fighting equipment, and fire detection and fire alarm systems in consultation with the fire protection service. Equipment should be easily reachable at all times and should not be obstructed. The major escape routes from the laboratory should be clearly marked and kept unobstructed.

There should be ample storage space with adequate shelving and plentiful room under benches for bins in which to place material for disposal, and adequate space between benches so that there is no danger of collisions leading to dropping of containers of dangerous chemicals. Likewise corridors should be kept clear. With the rapid expansion in the workload there is a great danger of putting too many articles, particularly refrigerators, large centrifuges, or cupboards in too little room. Adequate space for such articles should be planned.

A staff room should be provided and eating, drinking and smoking forbidden within the working area. The plentiful provision of wash basins with elbow taps, already mentioned, cannot be over-stressed, as frequent washing of the hands is a key measure in preventing infection. A sluice or shower should be easily accessible so that anyone who has had corrosive liquid spilt on him or herself can quickly flush the affected part with a vigorous flow of water.

Good ventilation is essential to prevent accumulation of toxic and flammable vapours. Efficient fume cupboards are also required; a useful addition is the installation of hoods with good fans. The siting of safety cabinets, the desired capacity of exhaust systems and the design and laying of trunking are discussed in PHLS Monograph No. 6 (1977).

Adequate heating should be installed so that in winter there is no need for supplementary heating and no temptation to introduce an electric fire, the use of which should not be allowed. Good lighting is also important for efficient working. The advisability of limiting the gas supply and collecting electrical instruments as far as possible on separate benches has already been mentioned as has the need to provide separate rooms for certain techniques. See Hospital Buildings Note No. 15 (revised) Pathology Department (1971).

SAFETY OFFICER

The appointment of a good safety officer is essential for the success of the safety measures adopted in a laboratory. In the clinical biochemistry laboratory it is likely that this officer will be a senior member of the staff with other duties and responsibilities also. It is thus imperative that his role as safety officer is recognised and time allowed to fulfil the necessary duties.

These duties include the maintenance of safety equipment such as fire extinguishers, first-aid outfit, hazard notices, and cyanide kit. Liaison with the fire officer, safety committee and electrician would be through the safety officer. He should be thoroughly conversant with first-aid procedures and know how to obtain medical help quickly when necessary. He should keep an accident book in which all accidents are fully and carefully described, however trivial they may appear. A record of a cut on the hand of a staff member who later developed hepatitis would give the likely mode of infection. Any change being considered within the laboratory should first be discussed with the safety officer. This is especially important if the use of a toxic chemical is envisaged but is also relevant if the structure of a room is being modified.

Whatever arrangements are made, however, satisfactory implementation will depend largely on the enthusiasm of the safety officer and the response of the staff. On appointment, all staff should be made fully aware of all safety precautions and of any legislative requirements. The induction process should also include training in the use of fire-fighting devices. These procedures give the safety officer the opportunity to impress on new staff the serious potential consequences of their failure to implement all safety precautions and to emphasise the importance of general cleanliness and tidiness and of a high standard of hygiene. Planned, controlled methods of working with avoidance of unnecessary movement around the laboratory should also be encouraged. This will only be possible if the workrate demanded of the staff is not excessive. See the Howie Report (DHSS, 1978) and Edmonds (1977) for further discussion.

FIRST-AID AND EMERGENCY TREATMENT IN THE LABORATORY

First-aid measures in the clinical biochemistry laboratory differ somewhat from those applicable to an industrial laboratory. Firstly, it is usually situated within a hospital with its own Accident and Emergency Department. Secondly, tests may be carried out on hospital patients within the laboratory. The first implies that immediate first-aid measures are all that are required in the laboratory. However, the second requires that emergency treatment of patients should be no less efficient than in other parts of the hospital. In all cases the incident should be noted by the safety officer and recorded in the accident book.

The following sections set out the treatment in general terms. For further details a first-aid manual should be consulted, and that of St John Ambulance Brigade (1975) is recommended. A wall chart giving information about first-aid procedures is available from BDH Chemicals Ltd.

Chemical Injuries

[1]. Various toxic and irritant chemicals may cause accidental injury to staff by inhalation, by contact with the eyes, skin or mouth, or by ingestion. *Speedy treatment* will often reduce the degree of injury considerably.

Inhalation injury is best treated by removal to an uncontaminated atmosphere and treating for shock. If not severe, spontaneous recovery follows. Irritation of the throat is relieved by warm, soothing drinks and bronchial irritation by inhalation over a container of hot water containing Friar's balsam if available. Accidents of the inhalation type causing serious depression or cessation of respiration are rare. Removal from the danger area and *early* institution of artificial respiration are of the utmost importance.

Chemical injuries to the eye either by vapour or by splashing require *immediate* treatment by dilution of the chemical with water. Seconds may count when particularly corrosive agents such as concentrated sulphuric acid or strong sodium hydroxide solutions are involved. The injured person will usually start treatment himself at once but may need help in opening the eye and directing the flow of water when spasm of the eyelids is severe. Wash the eye for several minutes if actual splashing has occurred using a gentle stream of water from a wash-bottle, a beaker, or eye irrigator, if available. In all cases of splashing send the injured person to the Accident and Emergency Department as soon as immediate first-aid is completed.

Splashing of the skin is similarly treated by rapid dilution with water followed by removal of any clothing involved. Further removal of immiscible chemicals is best done using soap and water. Then, where the skin shows evidence of a chemical burn, cover with a sterile dressing. Refer such cases and all others in which extensive splashing has occurred to the Accident and Emergency Department. The usual response to entry of noxious material into the mouth is prompt rejection. Swallowing is very unlikely. Immediate, repeated rinsing of the mouth with water should follow. If swallowing has occurred, dilution by drinking water followed in the case of strong acids by milk of magnesia is sensible. Do *not* give sodium bicarbonate which causes distension of the stomach by gas and can rupture the injured stomach wall. It is then better to transfer to the Accident and Emergency Department for gastric lavage rather than attempt to make the patient vomit.

[2]. Cyanide poisoning is an emergency best treated, after removal of any hydrocyanic acid gas, by intravenous therapy by a doctor. Where cyanide is used regularly, arrangements should be made to allow for oral administration of fresh ferrous hydroxide as an appropriate immediate first-aid measure before medical help arrives. The reagent is prepared by mixing two solutions:

A. 158 g $FeSO_4$, $7H_2O$ and 3 g citric acid in a litre of distilled water. Inspect regularly and reject if deteriorating.
B. 60 g anhydrous Na_2CO_3 in a litre of distilled water.

Aliquots of 50 ml of each are kept in separate stoppered bottles appropriately labelled. For use mix aliquots of A and B and swallow the mixture. This forms an insoluble iron complex with cyanide and usually causes vomiting.

Any extensive spillage of a hazardous chemical will need clearing up (see BDH Chemicals wall chart) after emergency first-aid treatment has been carried out. Other staff should avoid becoming casualties. Where a large quantity of a toxic substance has been spilled in a confined space, it may be desirable to postpone entry until breathing apparatus is available. This is the case, e.g. for halogenated hydrocarbons, benzene, ether, methanol, dimethyl sulphate or pyridine. In general wear goggles or a face mask and gloves. Extinguish all possible sources of ignition if the chemical is flammable. For water-miscible materials dilute with plenty of water and wash down a drain. Water-immiscible liquids may be removed either with water and a detergent or adsorbed on to sand, transferred to a bucket and removed. Depending on circumstances, further disposal is by evaporation, burying or chemical reaction. After removal of as much chemical as possible wash the floor with water and detergent and leave the area well-ventilated until all fumes have vanished. Strong acids can be treated with soda-ash before dilution with water. Solids should be shovelled into a bucket and brought into solution before disposal. Cyanide in solutions or as solid is best decomposed with bleaching powder or sodium hypochlorite for 24 h before disposal with plenty of water. Mercury droplets can be removed using a vacuum aspirator incorporating a trap; residual droplets are best treated by amalgam formation using zinc dust to reduce future hazardous continual evaporation.

Mechanical and Thermal Injuries

[3]. Mostly these will be minor but the possibility of serious injury exists. Wash minor cuts and abrasions, dry and cover with a sterile dressing to reduce the risk of infection. With more extensive lacerations, entry of foreign bodies and penetrating injuries, particularly from dirty objects, refer for debridement and suture and, where appropriate, anti-tetanus serum or tetanus toxoid booster dose. Foreign bodies in the eye, unless trivial and easily removed, should be dealt with in the Accident and Emergency Department after initial treatment of any coincident chemical splashing.

[4]. Severe injuries require immediate positive action by nearby staff. Summon medical help and meanwhile deal with haemorrhage, splashing by corrosive or toxic chemicals and any impairment of respiration and circulation *as a matter of urgency*. Most haemorrhages can be controlled by firm pressure over the bleeding point; if the position of pressure points is known to the rescuer the appropriate one can be used as an alternative. Avoid tourniquets except as a last resort. If the patient is unconscious ensure an adequate airway and if respirations have ceased start artificial respiration. Cardiac arrest will require institution of cardiac massage once the diagnosis is certain. Treat chemical injuries as quickly as possible as described earlier. Treat for shock but avoid giving drinks if there is a possibility of the casualty requiring an anaesthetic. Avoid moving the patient until help arrives unless his position places him in extra hazard.

[5]. Burns of the skin from chemicals have been dealt with. Thermal burns are best treated by covering with a sterile dressing. Do not puncture blisters or apply ointments, creams, etc. Extensive burns require treatment for shock and early transfer to the Accident and Emergency Department.

Electrical Injuries

[6]. Accidental electrical shocks frequently cause involuntary removal of the part of the body making contact. No further action is necessary other than to determine the cause of the accident and to correct any fault. More serious shocks involve muscular spasm preventing the electrical contact being broken and the risk of cardiac arrhythmias and severe burns. The rescuer *must* break the electrical contact before attempting further treatment. If the power supply can be switched off locally, e.g. at the socket supplying the equipment, this is all that is required. Otherwise the patient has to be detached from the electric contacts. Avoid using bare hands for this; either use rubber gloves or leverage with a non-conducting object. Once the contact is broken, the patient will need treating for shock but artificial respiration and cardiac massage may be required and should be started immediately the need is diagnosed after calling for medical assistance. Burns at the point of contact will require treatment as soon as the priorities allow.

Emergency Situations

Help from nearby staff may be all that is required immediately but in any serious case, telephone to summon professional help. For this to be mobilised efficiently it is essential that the person at the other end of the line be given the following information: the locations of the caller and the casualty, the type of injury or acute medical condition and the nature of the assistance sought. Preferably ask the recipient of the call to repeat the details to ensure there is no error. In the case of fire indicate the extent and exact location of the fire. Meanwhile it is necessary to care for the patient until medical help arrives. Ideally the safety officer should be sufficiently trained in first-aid to be able to care for an unconscious patient, carry out artificial respiration and apply external cardiac massage if necessary. If this is not necessary, keep the patient warm and lying down with feet raised. Arrest any haemorrhage. If he is conscious and there is no risk an anaesthetic will be needed to deal with the injuries, a hot sweet drink can be given. Keep the patient in this position until help arrives and if transfer to the Accident and Emergency Department is necessary arrange this by trolley or stretcher.

Care of Patients Taken Ill While Attending the Laboratory

Patients are unlikely to suffer injury in the laboratory but complications arising from the diagnostic procedure may develop or they may suffer any of the acute medical emergencies which can arise in all hospital patients. The aim of treatment is to deal rapidly with emergencies and to summon medical assistance immediately.

First-aid Boxes

The following statutory requirements for industrial laboratories form a useful guide to the contents of such boxes:

    12 small sterilised unmedicated finger dressings
    6 medium sized sterilised unmedicated dressings
    6 large sized sterilised unmedicated dressings
  24 adhesive wound dressings of assorted sizes
    4 triangular bandages
    4 sterilised eyepads.

A supply of sterilised absorbent gauze in 14 g packets, adhesive plaster, crepe bandages, safety pins.

In addition the following are suggested:

  1 500 ml irrigation bottle for washing out eyes
  1 bottle of Milk of Magnesia
  4 bottles of ferrous sulphate and sodium carbonate solutions (p. 22)
  1 bottle of dilute acetic acid (10 ml glacial acetic to 1 l with water)
  1 Porter resuscitation airway.

REFERENCES

Ackroyd G. C., Taylor H. D., Sheldon M. (1977). In *Hazards in the Chemical Laboratory*, 2nd ed (Muir, G. D., ed) p. 32. London: Royal Institute of Chemistry.

BDH Chemicals Wall Charts: *How to Deal with Spillages of Hazardous Chemicals; Laboratory First Aid; Properties of Gases.* BDH Chemicals Ltd., Poole, Dorset.

British Standard 1780. (1960). *Specification for Bourdon Tube Pressure and Vacuum Gauges.* (See also Part 2. (1971). *Metric Units.*) London: HMSO.

British Standard 3423. (1962). *Recommendations for the Design of Glass Vacuum Desiccators.* London: HMSO.

British Standard 4402. (1982). *Specification for Safety Requirements for Laboratory Centrifuges.* London: HMSO.

British Standard 4851. (1982). *Specification for Single Use Labelled Medical Specimen Containers for Haematology and Biochemistry.* London: HMSO.

British Standard 6242. (1982). *Specification for Single Use Unlabelled Medical Specimen Containers for Haematology and Biochemistry.* London: HMSO.

British Standard 5306, Part 3. (1985). *Code of Practice for Selection and Maintenance of Portable Fire Extinguishers.* London: HMSO.

Carcinogenic Substances Regulations. (1967). Statutory Instrument No. 879

Chester Beatty Research Institute. (1966). *Recommended Code of Practice for Laboratory Staff when Handling Chemicals which may cause Tumours of the Urinary Tract.* Institute of Cancer Research, Royal Cancer Hospital, London.

Chester Beatty Research Institute. (1971). *Precautions for Laboratory Workers who Handle Carcinogenic Amines.* Institute of Cancer Research, Royal Cancer Hospital, London.

Department of Health and Social Security (DHSS). (1972). *Safety in Pathology Laboratories.* London: HMSO.

DHSS. (1972). *Hepatitis and the Treatment of Chronic Renal Failure. Report of Advisory Group* (1970–72), Chairman, Lord Rosenheim. Code of Laboratory Practice Appendix III, pp. 48–54. London: HMSO.

DHSS Health Notice HN(76)95. (1976). *Use of Perchloric Acid and Treatment of Equipment affected by Perchloric Acid.* Health Services Management. London: HMSO.

DHSS Health Notice HN (76) 189. (1976). *Possible Explosion Hazard: Pressure build up in bleach disinfectant and cleansing solutions containing strong sodium hypochlorite.* London: HMSO.

DHSS. (1978). *Code of Practice for the Prevention of Infection in Clinical Laboratories and Post-mortem Rooms.* London: HMSO.

DHSS Health Circular HC (79)3. (1979). *Code of Practice for the Prevention of Infection in Clinical Laboratories and Post-mortem Rooms.* Health Services Development. London: HMSO.

DHSS. (1980). Interim Advisory Committee on Safety in Clinicial Laboratories, *Bulletin No.* 1. London: HMSO.

DHSS. (1981). Interim Advisory Committee on Safety in Clinical Laboratories, *Bulletin No.* 2. London: HMSO.

DHSS. (1983). Advisory Committee on Dangerous Pathogens, Report No. 1. *The Categorisation of Pathogens According to Risk and Categories of Containment.* London: HMSO.

DHSS. (1986). Advisory Committee on Dangerous Pathogens. *LAV/HTLVIIII—the Causative Agent of AIDS and Related Conditions—Revised Guidelines.* London: HMSO.

Edmonds, O. P. (1977). In *Safety of Biological Laboratories* (Hartree E., Booth V., eds). Biochemical Society Special Publications, No. 5. The Biochemical Society, London.

First Aid Manual, 3rd ed. (1975). St John Ambulance Association and Brigade, London.

George W. H. S. (1971). *Ann. Clin. Biochem;* **8**: 130.

Health and Safety Commission. (1985). *Approved Code of Practice. The Protection of Persons Against Ionising Radiation Arising from any Work Activity.* London: HMSO.

Health Services Advisory Committee. (1985). *Safety in Health Service Laboratories: Hepatitis B.* London: HMSO.

Hospital Building Note, No. 15 (revised 1971). *Pathology Department.* London: HMSO.

Hospital Technical Memorandum, No. 13 (1965). *Planned Preventative Maintenance. A System for Engineering Plant and Services.* London: HMSO.

Ionising Radiations Regulations. (1985). Statutory Instrument 1985/1333. London: HMSO.

Ionising Regulations. *Unsealed Radioactive Substances, Regulations* (1968). SI 780; *Sealed Sources, Regulations* (1969). SI 808. London: HMSO.

Mercurial Poisoning (1966). *Preventive Measures in Handling Liquid Mercury and Removal of Contamination.* SHW 337. London: HMSO.

Moore B. (1971). *Ann. Clin. Biochem*; **8**: 136.

Muir G. D., ed (1977). *Hazards in the Clinical Chemical Laboratory*, 2nd ed. London: Royal Institute of Chemistry.

Osborne S. B. (1977). In *Hazards in the Chemical Laboratory*, 2nd ed (Muir G. D., ed) p. 466. London: Royal Institute of Chemistry.

Public Health Laboratory Service Monograph No. 6 (1977). *The Prevention of Laboratory Acquired Infection.* London: HMSO.

Radioactive Substances Act. (1960). Ministry of Labour. *An Explanatory Memorandum for Persons Keeping Radioactive Material.* London: HMSO.

2
UNITS

A variety of units for describing the same physical quantity developed over the years in clinical biochemistry as in other branches of science and technology, but there is much to be said for a consistent system. In general the result of the measurement of any physical quantity is expressed as a numerical value and a unit. For any physical quantity the unit must be stated and never implied.

There are, of course, several systems of units including those of the metric system and different branches of science have traditionally used their own selection. The metric system has been made the basis of a coherent system of units known as SI units (Système International d'Unités). International agreement on this system was obtained in 1960 and it is the only legal system in many countries. Its use is actively encouraged in this country and it is the system now taught in educational establishments. Its adoption in biology and medicine has gradually become widespread.

The SI units are of three types—basic, supplementary and derived. The system is rational in that it defines only one unit for any physical quantity and it is coherent as units for use in a particular science or technology can be derived by combination of appropriate basic units by simple division or multiplication without the use of any numerical factor. These *basic units* apply to certain fundamental, unrelated physical quantities and are listed in Table 2.1 with their appropriate abbreviations or symbols.

These have been defined as follows:

Metre. The length equal to $1\,650\,763 \cdot 73$ wavelengths *in vacuo* of the radiation corresponding to the transition between the levels $2p_{10}$ and $5d_5$ of the krypton-86 atom. That is, the metre is no longer defined in terms of a length of precious metal but is related to a spectroscopic phenomenon.

Kilogram. The mass equal to the mass of the international prototype of the kilogram.

TABLE 2.1
Basic SI Units

Quantity	Unit	Symbol
Length	metre	m
Mass	kilogram	kg
Time	second	s
Electric current	ampere	A
Thermodynamic temperature	kelvin	K
Luminous intensity	candela	cd
Amount of substance	mole	mol

Second. The duration of 9 192 631 770 periods of the radiation corresponding to the transition between the two hyperfine levels of the ground state of the caesium-133 atom. This also is a spectroscopic definition.

Ampere. That constant current which, if maintained in two straight parallel conductors of infinite length, of negligible cross-section, and placed 1 m apart *in vacuo*, would produce between these conductors a force equal to 2×10^{-7} newton per metre of length.

Kelvin. The fraction 1/273·16 of the thermodynamic temperature of the triple point of water.

Candela. The luminous intensity, in the perpendicular direction, of a surface of 1/600 000 m^2 of black body at the temperature of freezing platinum under a pressure of 101 325 N/m^2.

Mole. The amount of substance of a system which contains as many elementary units as there are carbon atoms in 12 g of carbon-12. The elementary particle must be specified and may be atoms, molecules, ions or other particles or groups of particles. Thus the masses of 1 mol of iron, urea, Na^+, and nitrogen, are respectively 55·84, 60·06, 22·99 and 14·01 g.

The *supplementary* units are little used in clinical biochemistry; the unit for the physical quantity, plane angle, is the radian (rad) and for the physical quantity, solid angle, is the steradian (sr). Using the basic and supplementary units it is possible to define the appropriate *derived* units for other physical quantities. These units will be algebraically related to those from which they are derived and can be written in abbreviated form using the abbreviations for the basic and supplementary units. However, such forms may be rather clumsy for frequently used physical quantities and certain special names have been allocated, together with their abbreviations, for convenience, as indicated in Table 2.2. It will be noted that eponymous units in Tables 2.1 and 2.2 are spelt with a small initial letter but the symbol starts with a capital letter.

TABLE 2.2
Derived SI Units with Special Names

Physical quantity	Name of SI unit	Symbol of SI unit	Derivation of SI unit	Equivalent form
Energy	joule	J	$kg\,m^2\,s^{-2}$	N m
Force	newton	N	$kg\,m\,s^{-2}$	$J\,m^{-1}$
Pressure	pascal	Pa	$kg\,m^{-1}\,s^{-2}$	$N\,m^{-2}$
Power	watt	W	$kg\,m^2\,s^{-3}$	$J\,s^{-1}$
Electric charge	coulomb	C	A s	
Electric potential difference	volt	V	$kg\,m^2\,s^{-3}\,A^{-1}$	$J\,A^{-1}\,s^{-1}$
Electric resistance	ohm	Ω	$kg\,m^2\,s^{-3}\,A^{-2}$	$V\,A^{-1}$
Electric conductance	siemens	S	$kg^{-1}\,m^{-2}\,s^3\,A^2$	Ω^{-1}
Electric capacitance	farad	F	$A^2\,s^4\,kg^{-1}\,m^{-2}$	$A\,s\,V^{-1}$
Magnetic flux	weber	Wb	$kg\,m^2\,s^{-2}\,A^{-1}$	V s
Inductance	henry	H	$kg\,m^2\,s^{-2}\,A^{-2}$	$V\,A^{-1}\,s$
Magnetic flux density	tesla	T	$kg\,s^{-2}\,A^{-1}$	$Wb\,m^{-2}$
Luminous flux	lumen	lm	cd sr	
Illumination	lux	lx	$cd\,sr\,m^{-2}$	$lm\,m^{-2}$
Frequency	hertz	Hz	s^{-1}	
Radioactivity	becquerel	Bq	s^{-1}	

It will often happen that the units in the tables are inconveniently large or small for a particular measurement. Prefixes can then be added to the unit symbol to

TABLE 2.3
Prefixes for SI Units

Fraction	Prefix	Symbol	Multiple	Prefix	Symbol
10^{-1}	deci	d	10	deca	da
10^{-2}	centi	c	10^2	hecto	h
10^{-3}	milli	m	10^3	kilo	k
10^{-6}	micro	μ	10^6	mega	M
10^{-9}	nano	n	10^9	giga	G
10^{-12}	pico	p	10^{12}	tera	T
10^{-15}	femto	f			
10^{-18}	atto	a			

indicate decimal fractions or multiples of the same. These prefixes are listed in Table 2.3.

Thus we may have nm, μg, ms, mmol, kW, MHz, etc. Certain conventions are established. Symbols are printed in roman type, remain unaltered in the plural and are not followed by a full stop except at the end of a sentence. Thus 1 g, 5 mg are correct but not 1 g. or 5 mgs but the sentence could end as 1 g. Compound prefixes should not be used—thus nm should be used for mμm. Decimal multiples of the kg are formed by attaching the prefix to the gram, g, in spite of the fact that kg and not g is the basic SI unit. Thus mg not μkg for 10^{-6} kg. If a unit symbol carries an exponent, this raises both the factor symbol and the unit symbol to the same power. Thus cm^2 is $(10^{-2}$ m$)^2$ or 10^{-4} m^2 and not 10^{-2} m^2. When writing numbers with many digits, segregate groups of three digits either side of the decimal point by a space rather than a comma so as to improve legibility and avoid ambiguity over the decimal point. The latter in Britain will either be a full stop or a point opposite the centre of the digits but many European countries use a comma on the line. If the numerical value is less than one, the digit 0 should precede the decimal point. Thus 1 ft^2 equals 0·092 903 m^2 and 1 lb/in^2 equals 6 894·76 Pa. Where derived units incorporate quotients of basic units, ambiguity can arise. Thus the combination $a/b/c$ could mean either $(a/b)/c = ab^{-1} c^{-1}$ or $a/(b/c) = ab^{-1} c$. This can be avoided by not using more than one solidus (/) in such combinations and by using the exponent form where confusion could arise. The unit for renal clearance studies often written as ml/min/m^2 is ambiguous, but ml min^{-1} m^{-2} is not. Finally the denominator in an expression should not contain a prefix; this should appear in the numerator. Also numbers should not appear in the denominator. Thus the units mg/ml or mg/100 ml are discouraged but mg/l and g/l are acceptable.

Several derived units are not given special names or symbols, and those of particular interest to clinical biochemists are listed in Table 2.4. The rules about prefixes just outlined apply to them also. A special point arises with the choice of a suitable unit for volume. The coherent SI unit, the cubic metre (m^3), is inconveniently large for much medical work and there are considerable advantages in using the litre (l) as a convenient unit of volume. The litre was redefined in 1964 to be exactly equal to the cubic decimetre (dm^3). Previously it had been defined differently and was equal to 1·000 028 dm^3. Concentrations are best related to the litre for much medical work and these units have therefore been included in Table 2.4. Two of these units, mass fraction and volume fraction are strictly dimensionless and can be represented either with the symbol given or as a number alone. A similar situation arises with relative density (specific gravity) which is most often quoted as a number.

TABLE 2.4
Derived SI Units Used in Clinical Biochemistry

Physical quantity	SI unit	Symbol or definition
Area	square metre	m^2
Volume	cubic metre	m^3
	litre	$l = dm^3$
Density	kilogram per cubic metre	kg/m^3
Mass concentration	kilogram per litre	kg/l
Mass fraction	kilogram per kilogram	kg/kg
Molar concentration	mole per litre	mol/l
Molality	mole per kilogram	mol/kg
Mole fraction	mole per mole	mol/mol
Volume fraction	litre per litre	l/l

Atomic weight is quoted using the unit, dalton, but this usage is now not encouraged and the use of the dimensionless ratio, relative atomic mass (A_r) is preferred (see Appendix table). This is the ratio of the atomic mass (m_a) of the element in question to the atomic mass unit (unified), abbreviated as u, one twelfth the mass of the atom of ^{12}C, i.e. $m_a(^{12}C)/12$. In a similar way, molecular weight (mol. wt.) is not given in daltons but preferably as the relative molecular mass (M_r), the sum of the relative atomic masses of the constituent atoms of the molecule under consideration.

Comments on Selected Problems as Applied to Clinical Biochemistry

Time. Time units are inherently non-metric. The basic SI unit is the second (s) and for some purposes, decimal multiples of this are appropriate, e.g. ms, ks. Many biological phenomena are easily related to other familiar units of time which are given appropriate symbols. Thus we have: the minute (min) which is exactly 60 s; the hour (h), exactly 3·6 ks; the day (d), exactly 86·4 ks; the year (a) approximately 31·557 Ms. The abbreviation 'a' is unfamiliar, many people use yr but it is probably advisable not to use any abbreviation.

Radioactivity. The SI unit of radioactivity has been given the name becquerel (Bq) and corresponds to one disintegration per second. Traditionally, radioactivity has been measured in terms of the curie (Ci), originally defined as the activity of 1 g of radium and later expressed more precisely as $3·7 \times 10^{10}$ disintegrations per second. The curie is still used, often as its subdivisions, mCi and μCi. One mCi equals 37 MBq and 1 MBq equals 27 μCi.

Temperature. The customary temperature, measured in degrees Celsius (°C) which are of the same magnitude as degrees Centigrade can be defined as the excess of the thermodynamic temperature over 273·16.

Concentration. Many clinical biochemical measurements are of concentration. The appropriate units are g/l for mass concentration and mol/l for molar concentration. It is not desirable to use the abbreviation M for a molar solution (1 mol/l) as M is also in use as a prefix (mega, 10^6). The use of mol/l is clearer. Certainly M should never be used to imply a mole. For comparison of molar units, e.g. mmol/l and 'traditional' units, e.g. mg/100 ml, see the 5th edition of this book.

With simple organic molecules such as urea a choice could exist between selecting mg/l or mmol/l as the appropriate unit. There are advantages in using mmol/l in that biological systems usually react according to the number of molecules per unit volume. Furthermore, relationships between the osmotic effects of different entities are more clearly realised. Thus a serum urea of 300 mg/l and a serum glucose of 900 mg/l are both equal to 5·0 mmol/l which is insignificant compared with a serum sodium concentration of 140 mmol/l. A further advantage of molar concentration is that it may be more closely related to the actual measurement made. Thus faecal fat determinations involve a final titration of the carboxyl group in the mixture of fatty acids obtained. The answer may be reported directly as faecal fatty acid in mmol/24 h which is more logical than multiplying by an assumed and possibly erroneous mean molecular weight of mixed fatty acids in order to derive secondarily a figure in g/24 h.

For the above reasons the authors use the primary unit of concentration as mol/l or its subunits. The situation becomes less clear where macromolecules are concerned. Large molecules such as enzymes are usually measured by their biological activity (see p. 32). In the case of serum proteins, it would be possible to report in molar concentration if a single protein of known molecular weight were concerned. However this can cause difficulties where total serum protein concentration is measured routinely in that no molecular weight is applicable to the protein mixture. Accordingly we have used the units g/l and mg/l for such cases to allow easy computation of the fraction of the total applicable to different proteins. But there are positive advantages in changing to molar concentration for certain specific purposes. Thus the albumin-binding of bilirubin is more apparent in molar terms. A serum bilirubin of 232 mg/l in the presence of 34 g/l albumin gives a less clear picture than the molar equivalents of 400 μmol/l and 500 μmol/l respectively. Likewise the coexistence of serum iron concentration of 1·12 mg/l in the presence of 4·44 g/l transferrin determined immunologically does not give the same immediate picture as 20 μmol/l iron and 60 μmol/l transferrin.

Hydrogen ion concentration is often reported in terms of the pH value, a unit which is dimensionless. This is the negative exponent to the base 10 of the $[H^+]$ in mol/l. Thus pH 7·0 implies a $[H^+]$ of 10^{-7} mol/l or 0·1 μmol/l or 100 nmol/l. The range of pH in disease may vary from 6·8 to 8·0. This corresponds to a change in $[H^+]$ from 158 to 10 nmol/l. This considerable reduction is often not appreciated when thinking in logarithmic pH units and for special purposes there are some advantages in reporting in terms of molar concentration. However, the range of $[H^+]$ concentration found in buffer solutions used as reagents is very large and is more conveniently indicated on a logarithmic scale.

Energy. The coherent SI unit is the joule (J). When referring to heat energy, the traditional unit has been the calorie. In nutritional work, most people have been familiar with the kilocalorie, somewhat misleadingly transformed into the Calorie. Electrical energy has often been measured using the unit 'kilowatt hour' (kWh). All may be converted to J or multiples of the same. Thus:

$$1 \text{ calorie} = 4\cdot1868 \text{ J}$$
$$1 \text{ kilocalorie (Calorie)} = 4\cdot1868 \text{ kJ}$$
$$1 \text{ kWh} = 3\cdot6 \text{ MJ}$$

Pressure. The coherent SI unit is the pascal (Pa) or newton per square metre (N/m^2). Other units have commonly been used previously. The partial presssure of carbon dioxide in alveolar air and the blood pressure have usually been reported in conventional millimetres of mercury (mmHg). Pressure gauges on gas cylinders may be calibrated in atmospheres (atm) or pounds per square inch (lb/in^2, psi). For other work the bar and its subunit mbar have been used and the torr is often employed in high vacuum technology. The units are related as shown in Table 2.5.

TABLE 2.5
Pressure Units

Name of unit	Symbol	Equivalent
Bar	bar	10^5 Pa exactly
Atmosphere	atm	101·325 kPa (approx. 1 bar)
Torr	Torr	101·325/760 Pa (approx. 1 mmHg)
Pound/square inch	lb/in^2	6 894·76 Pa
Millimetre of mercury	mmHg	$13·595\,1 \times 980·665 \times 10^{-2}$ Pa (approx. 133 Pa) (depending on temperature)

The pascal is thus a small unit of pressure. The normal partial pressure of carbon dioxide in alveolar air is 5·32 kPa (40 mmHg) and of oxygen in atmospheric air around 20 kPa. Pressures in gas cylinders of approximately 200 atm or 3 000 lb/in^2 correspond to 20 MPa. The Royal Society of Medicine (Baron, 1977) recommended that where pressures are normally measured with a manometer, figures should be quoted in the actual units employed, with the SI equivalents in parentheses. Thus blood, intraocular and intrauterine pressures can be stated in mmHg (and Pa by multiplying by 133). Intrathecal pressures are usually recorded in cm CSF or cm water and can be so reported (and as Pa by multiplying by 98). For other pressures many instruments are now calibrated in Pa or multiples thereof. The convention used in this edition is to quote the units as read from the instrument and to give the SI unit in parentheses afterwards where necessary.

Enzyme Units. Many enzymes have been reported in arbitrary units, variously defined. In 1964, the International Union of Biochemistry defined an enzyme unit (U) as the amount of an enzyme which will catalyse the transformation of 1 μmol of the substance per minute under standard defined conditions with the proviso that in some cases it may be preferable to substitute '1 micro equivalent of the group concerned' for 1 μmol of substrate. This unit has been widely used and enzyme concentrations are then reported in U/l or subunits thereof. This enzyme unit is not a coherent unit as it uses the μmol and the min, both of which are not basic SI units. Nonetheless, the proposed coherent unit, the katal (kat), defined in terms of the mole and second, has not found much support. The authors have therefore used either the IUB unit, expressing concentrations in U/l, or arbitrary eponymous units if appropriate to give concentrations as arbitrary units/l.

FURTHER READING

Baron D. N., ed. (1977). *Units, Symbols and Abbreviations. A Guide for Biological and Medical Editors and Authors*, 3rd ed. The Royal Society of Medicine, London.

British Standards Institution. *The Use of SI Units.* P.D. 5686, British Standards Institution, London.

Broughton P. M. G. (1970). *Quantities and Units in Clinical Chemistry*. Technical Bulletin No. 20. The Association of Clinical Biochemists, London.

Broughton P. M. G., Sewell P. (1970). *Ann. Clin. Biochem*; 7: 23.

Dykbaer R., Jørgensen K. (1967). *Quantities and Units in Clinical Chemistry*, Copenhagen: Munksgaard.

McGlashan M. L. (1970) *Chemistry in Britain*; 6: 23.

International Bureau of Weights and Measures. (1970) *SI, the International System of Units*. London: HMSO.

Royal Society (1971). *Quantities, Units and Symbols*. The Royal Society, London.

3

SEPARATIVE PROCEDURES CHROMATOGRAPHY

Chromatography received its name from the work of Tswett in 1906. He adsorbed a mixture of plant pigments on to finely divided chalk and separated them into coloured bands by washing the column of chalk with solvents. Although the technique is now more often used to separate colourless substances, the original name remains and is applied to any process whereby substances are separated by a continuous redistribution between two phases, one stationary and the other mobile. Different attractive forces between the stationary phase and the substances to be separated selectively retard the latter relative to the moving phase. Under good conditions the resulting different rates of migration bring about complete separation of the substances.

Adsorption chromatography comprises systems where active adsorption occurs at the surface of the solid stationary medium. Competition for adsorptive sites occurs between molecules of the mixture to be separated and the molecules of the mobile phase, be this gas or liquid. The speed of migration of a component depends on its adsorptive affinity relative to the other species present.

Several attractive forces between the stationary phase and the substances to be separated are recognised and their mode of action provides insight into the mechanisms responsible for separation. Adsorptive forces, which are comparatively weak, include Van der Waals' forces, hydrogen bonding and those due to permanent dipoles. Van der Waals' or London dispersion forces are short-range forces of attraction between molecules, postulated by Van der Waals to explain deviations from the gas law, $PV = RT$, at high pressures and low volumes. Hydrogen bonds arise between a hydrogen atom attached to a very electronegative atom such as fluorine, oxygen or nitrogen, and an unshared electron pair on another electronegative atom. Thus hydrogen bonding occurring in water explains why it is liquid at ambient temperature whereas hydrogen sulphide with no hydrogen bonding boils at $-62\,°C$. Permanent dipoles arise, e.g. when the sharing of the electron pair between two atoms involved in a covalent bond is unequal. Thus, if in a compound $X-Y$, the electron pair is more closely related to Y than X, we get a dipole $X^+:Y^-$.

Solid adsorbents and liquids are divided into polar and non-polar types, based on the forces to which they give rise. In the case of non-polar molecules, Van der Waals' forces are the main attractive forces whereas with polar molecules, attraction is by hydrogen bonding, dipoles or ionic charges. Thus oxides such as alumina and silica are polar adsorbents showing hydrogen bonding to oxygen atoms and hydroxyl groups, while charcoal is a non-polar one. The same applies to liquids. Important polar groups include $-OH$, $-NH_2$, $-NO_2$, $-COOH$, $-CN$ and $=NH$, all of which participate in hydrogen bonding. The polarity can be roughly related to the number of hydrogen bonds which a group can form. Thus the most polar compounds are water, di- and polyhydric alcohols, hydroxyamino compounds, hydroxycarboxylic acids, followed by monohydric alcohols, mono-carboxylic acids, monoamines, then aldehydes, ketones, ethers, esters and, finally, weakly polar substances such as chloroform. Hydrocarbons are non-polar substances. The degree of polarity is influenced by the rest of the molecule to which the polar groups are attached. Thus in the homologous series of aliphatic alcohols, the increasing length of the hydrocarbon chain lessens the polarity so that methanol is the most polar.

In liquid–solid chromatography, Van der Waals' and hydrogen bonding forces occur in adsorption chromatography while in *ion-exchange chromatography*, electrostatic forces operate between charged molecules and oppositely charged groups on the particles of an ion-exchange resin, or modified cellulose or dextran. This electrostatic attraction is altered by changing the pH of the mobile phase and hence the charge on the components requiring separation.

In *partition chromatography* the separation is achieved as a consequence of the relative solubility of the substances in the stationary and mobile phases. The stationary phase is a liquid and the mobile phase a liquid or a gas. In such separations the attractive forces are largely of the hydrogen bonding and dipole types and affect the partitioning of the substance between the two phases. The liquid phase needs supporting and distributing over a large area for efficient separation to occur. The stationary phase was initially water or a polar solvent used with a relatively non-polar mobile phase. Supports are now available to hold a non-polar stationary phase. This is used with a polar mobile phase in *reverse-phase chromatography*. In gas–liquid chromatography a gaseous mobile phase passes over the stationary phase held on an inert support medium.

In *exclusion chromatography* the components are distributed between one phase contained within the solid particles (stationary phase) and the same phase flowing between the particles (mobile phase). The solid particles are porous and the pore size determines which molecules are able to enter the particle and which are excluded on the basis of a molecular size which is too large.

The physical form of the stationary phase may be columnar or laminar. In the former, the stationary phase particles are packed into a column through which the mobile phase passes. In the laminar form the stationary phase is in the form of a thin layer or sheet, through and over which the mobile phase flows. These different physical forms are used with the different physico-chemical principles of separation outlined above. Most components of a mixture will travel more slowly than the mobile phase. A characteristic property of a substance in a particular chromatographic system is the R_f value, the ratio of the distance travelled by the substance to that travelled by the mobile phase in the same time. In laminar methods, the latter is shown by the position of the solvent front.

ADSORPTION CHROMATOGRAPHY

Many solids have been used as adsorbents including charcoal, alumina, other metal oxides, silicates and silica gel. Alumina in columns was formerly much used in clinical biochemistry but more recently the use of thin layers of alumina or silica gel on plates has become commonplace. For satisfactory results the way in which the adsorbent is prepared is important. Impurities occupying active sites greatly decrease the adsorbing power of the material. Removal of water by heating (activation) improves adsorption. Another important property is the particle size which must be sufficiently small to give a large surface with rapid establishment of equilibrium without impeding the flow of solvent through the adsorbent unduly. Adsorbents are available in graded particle sizes.

For column adsorption chromatography, the adsorbent is supported by a sintered glass filter. The mixture of substances to be separated is applied in a solvent of low polarity so that the solvent does not compete with the mixture for adsorption sites. Development is carried out in several ways. In *frontal development*, which is of limited value, a large volume of the mixture to be separated is passed through the column. Pure solvent appears first, followed by the least strongly held substance, then by a mixture of this with the next least strongly held, and so on. Only the least strongly held appears in pure form. By this procedure ether may be freed from its peroxide by passage through an alumina column. In *elution development* a small volume of the mixture is applied to the column to form a narrow band at the top. An eluting solvent is chosen which competes with the forces binding the mixture to the stationary phase. In consequence the components move slowly down the column, the most weakly held in the lead and followed under optimal conditions by discrete bands of the components of the mixture, with the most tightly held coming last. Complete separation of the pure components may be possible.

In *displacement development* a liquid is used whose affinity for the stationary phase is greater than that of any component of the mixture. All components then move down the column ahead of the developing liquid and as they displace each other, the stronger driving the weaker, a series of compact bands results having the same sequence as in elution development but without developing fluid separating each band. Resolution is thus poorer. Despite this the method has certain attractions if modified so that the displacing liquid only has a higher affinity than some components which are displaced to leave the more strongly bound ones near the origin. A second development with a new displacing liquid of higher affinity will displace further components. Careful standardisation of the adsorbent and developing liquids and the use of marker substances gives useful separations. An extension of this stepwise alteration in developing fluid is a continuously changing developer giving *gradient elution* which is much used in ion-exchange chromatography.

For adsorption chromatography, solvents fall into the following approximate order of increasing eluting power and polarity: light petroleum, cyclohexane, carbon tetrachloride, toluene, benzene, ether, chloroform, acetone, ethyl acetate, pyridine, ethanol, methanol, water, acetic acid. Substances suitable for separation by the early techniques of adsorption chromatography were rather weakly polar making such methods unsuitable for the direct separation of amino acids and sugars. Their separation improved with the introduction of partition and ion-exchange methods.

Thin-layer Adsorption Chromatography

This technique, sometimes referred to as 'open column' chromatography, uses a thin layer of adsorbent on a supporting plate and is increasingly used. For reviews see Smith and Seakins (1976) and Williams (1978).

Plates. Most laboratories now use commercially prepared plates already coated with adsorbent. They are usually provided on a metal or plastic sheet, easily trimmed to the required size with scissors. If such plates are not used or are unsuitable, appropriate layers may be prepared on glass in the laboratory (see the 5th edition of this book). The adsorbents commonly used are silica gel, alumina, kieselguhr and cellulose. Gypsum may be incorporated as a binder. This calcium sulphate, however, participates actively in many separations so that adsorbents with and without binder may not be interchangeable without modification of the solvent system. Adsorbents containing gypsum are usually designated by the manufacturer by adding G to the description, e.g. Silica Gel G. Fluorescent additives may be useful if detection of separated spots by examination in ultraviolet light is intended.

Application of the Test Material. For one-dimensional runs a template is prepared from Perspex so that a straight edge bearing a 1 cm scale is supported just clear of the surface of the plate, 2 cm from its bottom edge. Apply the solution at regular intervals using a 50 µl syringe fitted with a metal needle and a 10 cm length of plastic tubing of internal diameter 0·4 mm. Volumes between 0·5 and 50 µl can easily be applied. Draw the solution into the plastic tube. It need never enter the syringe but the plastic tube can be cleaned or renewed when necessary. Large volumes are applied under a stream of warm air. For two-dimensional chromatography apply a single sample in one corner about 2 cm from each edge.

Development. Ascending development is performed with the plate held vertically in a glass tank with a flat base (Fig. 3.1). Place the solvent in the bottom of the tank using sufficient to cover the lower 0·5 cm of the plate when immersed. If necessary cover the tank and allow the solvent to equilibrate with the air space. Place the plate in the solvent and continue the run until the solvent front reaches 1–2 cm from the top of the plate, usually between 1·5 and 2 h. After removing from the tank, dry under warm air for a few minutes.

Visualisation. Details of appropriate localising reagents are given when applications to particular groups of substances are discussed. Physical or chemical methods are used. Examples of physical methods are fluorescence in ultraviolet light or the detection of radioactive components with a counter. Such methods do not change the substances on the plate so that these can be removed later for further study. In chemical methods staining is used. This is done either by dipping the plate into the developing reagent, provided the coloured product is not soluble in the reagent, or by spraying, after which the plate is dried. Such staining techniques may be sensitive enough to detect sub-microgram quantities. For quantitative work, the stained spots can be removed, eluted and measured colorimetrically Scanning instruments are available which measure the colour density in each spot. In either case, careful control of sample size, chromatographic conditions and colour reaction are needed for satisfactory precision.

Separation Enhancement. Adequate separation is often possible with a run in a single direction, but sometimes substances may have R_f values too close for satisfactory separation. A second run of the same solvent using the unsprayed plate may improve separation. Alternatively a second run of such a plate at right angles to the first using a different solvent system may be used in the technique of two-dimensional chromatography.

Various improvements in technique have been referred to as *high performance thin-layer chromatography (HPTLC)*. Improved separation of mixtures is achievable by using adsorbents with a much smaller particle diameter and narrower size distribution than conventional adsorbents. The rate of solvent flow is reduced but the increased resolution makes shorter migration distances acceptable. Thus the conventional layers may typically show 2000 theoretical plates (p. 45) over 12 cm in a 25 min run whereas the ultrafine layers can achieve 4000 theoretical plates over 3 cm distance in 10 min. A second improvement, capable of automation, is programmed multiple development in which the plate is dried after running and then re-run with the same solvent to a slightly greater distance in a repetitive fashion. As the solvent traverses a spot corresponding to a particular substance, the lower edge of the spot moves while the upper edge is still stationary. Compression of the spot to R_f times its former height occurs and the final spot

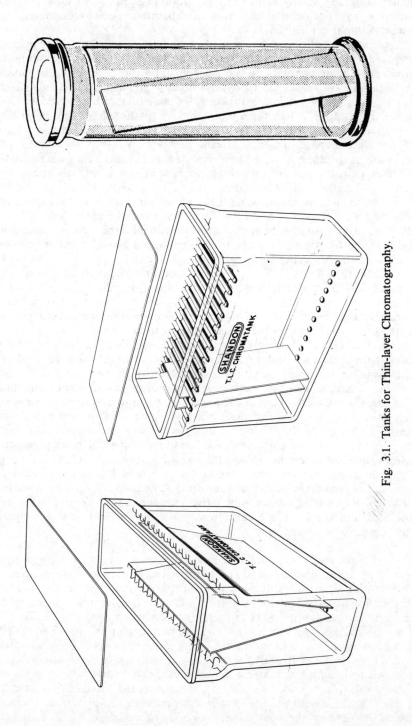

Fig. 3.1. Tanks for Thin-layer Chromatography.

width and position are independent of the size of the original spot. This is useful in compressing diffuse spots associated with the repeated application of dilute material to the starting line of the chromatogram. Such application steps can also be automated.

AFFINITY CHROMATOGRAPHY

The types of adsorption chromatography just described depend on the general physical or chemical properties of the adsorbent and the substances to be separated. In affinity chromatography use is made of bioselective adsorption which exploits the great selectivity of biological interactions between molecules in a two-component system. If one component is held on the stationary phase it can bind the required component of a complex mixture in a highly specific way, thus allowing easy separation as the unwanted materials pass by in the mobile phase. A specific displacing agent can later dislodge the required component from the column. The technique has proved particularly useful for the separation of large molecules such as enzymes, other proteins and glycoproteins, polysaccharides and nucleic acids. It can also be used to bind selected cells or cell fragments. The same principle but applied to a different physical form is made use of as a separative step in radioimmunoassay procedures (see Chapter 6). One component of an antigen–antibody system is bonded to a solid phase and the other component is adsorbed by it.

The stationary phases most often used are derived from agarose gel, either in the form of Sepharose or its cross-linked derivative Sepharose CL, produced by interacting Sepharose with 2,3-dibromopropanol. The gels are available in porous bead form with agarose concentrations of 2, 4 or 6%, designated by the suffix 2B, 4B or 6B. These beads also show some molecular sieve characteristics making them useful for gel chromatography (p. 44). Molecules above a certain size are excluded from permeation into the bead and for proteins the exclusion limits for molecular weight are: 2B, 40×10^6; 4B, 20×10^6; 6B, 4×10^6. These special agarose gels are then further modified by the insertion of reactive chemical groups which are able to form a covalent bond between the gel and the specific substance which is to be attached to it.

As shown in Table 3.1 it is possible to react such prepared gels with $-NH_2$, $-OH$, $-SH$ or $-COOH$ groups in the required molecule. Where the bound molecule is small, steric hindrance in its specific binding during affinity

TABLE 3.1

Examples of Activated Agarose Gels for Reaction with Biological Molecules

Name	Active group in gel	Group bound	Covalent linkage	Length of spacer chain
CNBr-activated Sepharose 4B	imidocarbonate	$-NH_2$	isourea	none
AH–Sepharose 4B	$-NH_2$	$-COOH$	amide	6 C atoms
CH–Sepharose 4B	$-COOH$	$-NH_2$	amide	6 C atoms
Epoxy-activated Sepharose 6B	$-CH—CH_2$ (O)	$-OH$	ether	$\equiv 12$ C atoms
		$-SH$	thioether	$\equiv 12$ C atoms
		$-NH_2$	alkylamine	$\equiv 12$ C atoms
Activated CH–Sepharose 4B	ester	$-NH_2$	amide	6 C atoms
Activated Thiol Sepharose 4B	$-S–S–$pyridyl	$-SH$	disulphide	glutathione

chromatography is minimised by inserting a spacer chain between the gel matrix and the covalent bond linking the bound molecule. Such bound molecules can then be regarded as being mounted on small stalks above the main gel surface. Once the specific substance has been bound to the gel, it can be used to prepare a chromatographic column composed of a selective adsorbent which will bind reversibly molecules showing the appropriate bioselectivity. Often only a small column is required as the specific binding is likely to be strong.

The gels just described allow the operator to prepare his own selective adsorbent with the possibility that this is highly specific for one other molecular species. Other commercially available gels already have bound to them one component of the biological system. Examples are shown in Table 3.2. Such bound substances are chosen for group specificity and will bind several components of a mixture if they share this common group property. Displacement of the separate components then relies on the use of a specific competitor for the binding sites.

Although the examples discussed above are based on the agarose gels, other matrices are available and include glass or polyacrylamide beads in graded sizes with different pore diameters, as well as cellulose. For further information on affinity chromatography see Lowe (1978).

ION-EXCHANGE CHROMATOGRAPHY

Ion-exchange resins are cross-linked polymers containing ionic groups as part of their structure. The polymer must be sufficiently cross-linked to have negligible solubility but be porous enough for the ions to diffuse freely through it. Ion-exchange resins are divisible into cation and anion exchangers and their charged groups resemble the ions of acids and bases respectively. Strong cation-exchange resins contain sulphonic acid groups $-SO_3^-$, weak ones carboxylic acid groups $-COO^-$, while strong anion-exchange resins have $-N^+(R_1R_2R_3)$ and weak ones $-N(R_1R_2)$.

The most important resins are polystyrene resins formed by condensation of styrene (vinyl benzene) and divinyl benzene, and polymethacrylic acid resins formed by condensation of methacrylic acid and divinyl benzene. Acidic or basic groups are introduced before or after polymerising. In each case the degree of cross-linking increases as the proportion of divinyl benzene increases.

Examples of resins are:

Amberlite IRC 50	weak cation	COO^-	5% cross-linked
Amberlite IRC 120	strong cation	SO_3^-	5% cross-linked
Dowex 50	strong cation	SO_3^-	8% cross-linked
Dowex 1	strong anion	$N^+(NH_3)_3$	variable
Dowex 2	strong anion	$N^+(CH_3)_2CH_2OH$	variable
Dowex 3	weak anion	polyamine	not defined
Zeocarb 225	strong cation	SO_3^-	various
Zeocarb 226	weak cation	COO^-	2·5 and 4·5%

Another family of ion-exchangers is based on cellulose and can be used in column or sheet form. Strongly alkaline cellulose treated with chloroacetic acid introduces the carboxymethyl group to give the weak cation-exchange resin carboxymethyl-cellulose (CM-cellulose) while condensation with 2-chlorotriethylamine gives the weak anion-exchanger diethylaminoethyl-cellulose (DEAE-

TABLE 3.2

Examples of Agarose Gels with Bound Ligands for Group Specific Reactions

Name	Ligand	Molecules bound
Con A–Sepharose 4B	concanavalin A	polysaccharides, glycoproteins
Poly (U)–Sepharose 4B	synthetic polyuridylate chains	polyadenylate chains of mRNA
5'-AMP–Sepharose 4B	5'-adenosine monophosphate	dehydrogenases with NAD$^+$ cofactor, kinases with ATP cofactor
2',5'-ADP–Sepharose 4B	2',5'-adenosine diphosphate	dehydrogenases with NADP$^+$ cofactor
Heparin–Sepharose CL–6B	heparin	coagulation proteins, other plasma proteins including lipoproteins and lipases, enzymes acting on nucleic acids, steroid receptors, protein synthesis factors
Blue Sepharose CL–6B	Cibachron F3G–A	serum albumin, wide variety of enzymes
Wheat germ Lectin Sepharose 6MB	wheat germ Lectin	N-acetylglucosamine residues in glycoproteins and polysaccharides
Lysine–Sepharose 4B	L-lysine	ribosomal RNA, plasminogen
Octyl–Sepharose CL–4B	n-octyloxy chain	hydrophobic parts of protein molecules
Phenyl–Sepharose CL–4B	phenoxy chain	hydrophobic parts of protein molecules

cellulose). Cellulose ion-exchange materials are particularly suitable for protein separations. A range of ion-exchangers based on polymerised dextran gels (Sephadex) or cross-linked agarose gels (Sepharose) has similar properties.

For most purposes the resins can be looked on as insoluble acids or bases which form insoluble salts. The interactions can be represented:

$$H^+\text{-resin}^- + Na^+ \rightarrow Na^+\text{-resin}^- + H^+ \qquad \text{(Cation-exchanger)}$$

and

$$Resin^+\text{-}OH^- + Cl^- \rightarrow Resin^+\text{-}Cl^- + OH^- \qquad \text{(Anion-exchanger)}.$$

The more strongly acidic the ion-exchange resin, the greater is the ionisation of the acidic group and the lower the pH at which it will exchange. A strongly acidic resin can exchange from salts, e.g. from potassium chloride as well as from potassium hydroxide, which the weakly acidic are unable to do. The strongly basic anion-exchange resins are able to take up anions at high pH, for example, Cl^- from potassium chloride, whereas the weakly basic ones can not.

Ion-exchange resins have been employed to separate amino acids and peptides. Dowex 50 in sodium or ammonium form and elution of the amino acids sequentially with buffers of increasing pH from 3·4 to 11 are used in the manual and automatic fractionation of amino acids. Resins such as Zeocarb 225 have been used to separate weak organic anions or cations from inorganic salts, the process of ion-exchange desalting to prepare urines for amino acid chromatography. Amberlite IRC 50 is used to take up amines from urine. This weak cation-exchange resin, being unable to exchange with neutral salts, allows them to pass through but takes up the amines which can be eluted later. Mixed beds of anion- and cation-exchange resins replace the cations and anions of any salts in water by equivalent amounts of H^+ and OH^- respectively in the preparation of 'deionised' water in the laboratory. Non-ionic contaminants are not removed.

For further information on ion-exchange chromatography see Stokes (1978).

PARTITION CHROMATOGRAPHY

This term is intended to cover liquid–liquid partition chromatography, gas–liquid chromatography and gel chromatography.

Liquid–Liquid Partition Chromatography

The liquid stationary phase is supported on silica gel, kieselguhr, cellulose, modified dextran or starch in column or sheet form. When the cellulose is in the form of paper sheet the term *paper chromatography* is used. The support medium may be held on a plate as in *thin-layer partition chromatography*.

If a substance is shaken with two immiscible solvents, it will distribute itself so that at equilibrium the ratio of its concentrations in the two phases is constant. This ratio, the *partition coefficient* is characteristic for a particular substance for a given pair of solvents at a stated temperature. The components of a mixture of substances with different partition coefficients will be differently distributed between two immiscible solvents. If a series of such redistributions is carried out, progressive separation of materials having dissimilar partition coefficients will result.

It is possible to construct a battery of glass extractors in which such a series of successive partitions takes place. Given sufficient extractors, substances with different partition coefficients can be separated. This complex process is an example of *countercurrent distribution*. Better resolving power occurs in liquid–liquid partition chromatography where one phase is held stationary while the other moves continuously over it. The process can be considered as a discontinuous repeated partition between successive small units or 'plates', for theoretical treatment. The number of theoretical plates represents the resolving power of the system.

Paper chromatography is now used infrequently in clinical biochemistry but details can be found, if necessary, in the 5th edition of this book. See also Smith and Seakins (1976). Thin-layer partition chromatography is carried out in a similar way to thin-layer adsorption chromatography (p. 36).

Solvent Systems. The choice has often to be made empirically. The simplest solvent is obtained by saturating an organic liquid such as butanol with water. Such solvents contain only a small proportion of water so that when they are used, polar compounds such as amino acids and sugars move slowly and may not separate. Their R_f values can be increased by adding further substances which allow more water to be included. Such tertiary mixtures, and even a few quaternary ones, are widely used in this form of chromatography. Examples of additional substances are acetic and formic acid, or bases such as ammonia or pyridine. Some tertiary mixtures are:

n-butanol–acetic acid–water	12/3/5
phenol–water–ammonia	160/40/1
butanol–pyridine–water	2/2/1
ethyl acetate–pyridine–water	12/5/4

Separation Characteristics. With these solvents the stationary phase is a polar aqueous one and under such conditions the R_f value is greater the less polar the substance. Among the neutral amino acids the R_f increases in the order: glycine, alanine, valine, leucine as the non-polar hydrocarbon chain increases in length. The inclusion of acids, bases or buffers in the mobile phase alters the ratio of ionised to non-ionised groups in ampholytes such as amino acids. As the more ionised forms have a greater affinity for the polar stationary phase, marked changes in R_f can be produced. Thus using butanol–acetic acid–water, the basic amino acids, histidine, arginine and lysine, move much more slowly than glutamic and aspartic acids with their non-ionised carboxyl groups.

Reverse-phase Operation. For separations of the more polar substances it is sometimes preferable to reverse the usual polarity of the phases. The stationary phase is made non-polar and used with a polar mobile phase which is often a mixture of water and a miscible organic solvent. Layers such as cellulose can be impregnated with long chain hydrocarbons if these are dissolved in acetone and the plate is dipped in the solution. After shaking off the excess fluid, the acetone is allowed to evaporate. It is not always easy to avoid leaching out of the non-polar material during manipulations such as the application of analytical mixtures to the plate. More recently, bonded non-polar phases have been used. Thus silica gel can be reacted with octadecylsilane in such a way that a covalent bond is formed between this non-polar material and the surface of the silica to provide a support medium which cannot lose its non-polar properties.

In clinical biochemistry, many substances of interest are relatively polar and may be analysed quantitatively using the technique of high pressure liquid chromatography (HPLC) (p. 57) with a reverse-phase column. Reverse-phase thin-layer chromatography is then useful for rapid qualitative study of the separation of mixtures by simulating various conditions which can be duplicated in HPLC work.

EXCLUSION CHROMATOGRAPHY

This form of chromatography often utilises a porous gel. It was initially introduced to separate relatively large molecules in a liquid phase but porous particles are now also used in gas chromatography. In liquid chromatography, the column is composed of the gel in the form of separate particles. The dry gel particles are first allowed to take up the chosen solvent. This is accompanied by swelling; the liquid taken up forms the stationary phase. When these swollen particles are made into a column with the same solvent, the spaces between them are filled by the solvent. This fraction of the mobile phase is the 'void volume'. The gel particles are sponge-like and the channels within them are of constant diameter (pore size) for a particular grade of gel. Molecules only enter the gel if their diameter is less than this pore size. Thus small molecules, not restricted by the pore size have the whole fluid volume (bed volume) available to them, but molecules whose size exceeds the exclusion limit of the gel are confined to the void volume and are rapidly washed through the column as the mobile phase runs through this void volume. Molecules of intermediate size have restricted access to the gel particles and thus move at an intermediate rate.

The Gels

Hydrophilic gels have been prepared from dextran, acrylamide and agarose, the first being most frequently used.

Dextran Gels. Dextran is a water-soluble polysaccharide consisting of glucose units and containing more than 90% α-1,6-glycosidic linkages. On reaction with epichlorhydrin in alkaline solution, the mixture solidifies due to the formation of crossed-linked polymers, the properties of which depend on the number of cross linkages. The Sephadex series of dextran gels are produced commercially as beads of defined particle size and pore size. The smallest particle size, superfine, is used for thin-layer chromatography while the medium and fine grades are preferred for column applications where faster flow rates are desirable. The range of separation of peptides and globular proteins is a characteristic of the pore size, designated by the symbols G-10 to G-200 (Table 3.3). The molecular weights separated vary from less than 700 for G-10 up to 800 000 for G-200, but there is appreciable overlap from one grade to the next.

In preparing gel beds, the final volume depends on the properties of the grade chosen. Adherence to the time of swelling of the gel is important in producing satisfactory columns. For proper operation the void volume should be known and although approximate values are given in Table 3.3, it is best determined using a substance with a molecular weight greater than the exclusion limit for the grade concerned. Blue Dextran, molecular weight 2 million, is convenient.

When used for thin-layer chromatography, the gel must be swollen prior to spreading on scrupulously clean glass plates which have been stored in concentrated sodium carbonate solution and rinsed with water immediately before use. Prepared plates are stored horizontally in a moist chamber over night or for periods up to three weeks, a procedure which improves the homogeneity of the layer. If Sephadex columns are kept wet, the growth of micro-organisms is inhibited by adding sodium azide (200 mg/l) to the liquid phase or by saturating this with chloroform. This may, however, induce shrinkage of the strongly swollen G-100 and G-200 gels.

TABLE 3.3

Properties of Sephadex Dextran Gels

Type	Gel bed (ml/g)	Void volume (ml/g)	Swelling time (h)	Approx. range of molecular weights ($\times 10^{-3}$) separated A	B
G-10	2	0·8	3	up to 0·7	up to 0·7
G-15	3	1·1	3	up to 1·5	up to 1·5
G-25	5	2	3	1–5	0·1–5
G-50	10	4	3	1–30	0·5–10
G-75	13	5	24	3–70	1–50
G-100	17	6	72	4–150	1–100
G-150	24	8	72	5–400	1–150
G-200	30	9	72	5–800	1–200

A—peptides and globular proteins   B—dextran fractions
The figures for gel bed and void volume refer to the weight of *dry* gel.

Other Gels. The Bio-Gel P series of cross-linked polyacrylamide gels have similar properties which are again determined by degree of swelling. The range of molecular weights covered is from 200 000 to 400 000 for globular proteins. The modified dextrans prepared by hydroxypropylation of Sephadex, namely Sephadex LH20 and LH60, or the modified agarose gels, Sepharose CL–2B, CL–4B and CL–6B, can be used for gel filtration in organic solvents and between them cover a range of molecular weights from several hundred to several million.

For further information on exclusion chromatography, see Stokes (1978).

THEORETICAL CONSIDERATION OF THE FACTORS AFFECTING CHROMATOGRAPHIC PERFORMANCE

In column chromatography the response to a single component of a mixture passing through a detector will ideally be a symmetrical Gaussian peak, the vertical component being the detector signal and the horizontal component, time. If a developed thin-layer plate is scanned in the direction of solvent flow, a similar peak should be obtained relating optical density to distance. The following discussion is based on column chromatography but the arguments are adaptable to thin-layer techniques.

Efficiency

The features of a Gaussian peak (see Chapter 10) are the mean, corresponding to the time at the top of the peak, and the standard deviation, σ, an index of peak width. The former is defined as the *retention time*, the latter is used in the calculation of the *number of theoretical plates* attributable to the system. The concept of a theoretical plate was developed in the mathematical analysis of fractional distillation and is used as the index of the efficiency of a chromatographic system.

If t_R is the time taken for a particular peak to emerge after the mixture entered the system at zero time, the number of theoretical plates, N, can be calculated from the actual chromatographic record as

$$N = (t_R/\sigma)^2$$

It is found experimentally that N is virtually independent of which peak is used in the calculation as later peaks are wider. In practice, σ is estimated from the peak width, W, which can be measured in various ways leading to the modified formula:

$$N = a^2(t_R/W)^2$$

where a is the number of standard deviations covered by the particular method of measuring W (Fig. 3.2). Four methods of measuring W are in general use: at the inflection points on the curve, 60·7% of peak height, $a^2 = 4$; at half maximum peak height, $a^2 = 5·54$; at 4·4% of peak height, $a^2 = 25$; the base line intercept defined by the intersection with the tangents to the curve, $a^2 = 16$. The last two take more cognisance of asymmetry of the peak.

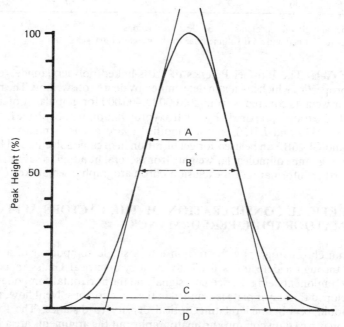

Fig. 3.2. Methods for Assessment of the Width of a Chromatographic Peak.
A—Between inflection points, approximately 2 standard deviations (SD).
B—At half peak height, approximately 2.35 SDs.
C—At 5 SDs.
D—Base line intercept, approximately 4 SDs.

From a knowledge of N and column length l (mm), it is easy to calculate either the number of theoretical plates per metre ($1000 \cdot N/l$) or the *height equivalent of a theoretical plate*, *HETP*, (l/N mm). Such figures are often quoted in relation to column efficiency which is greater, the smaller *HETP*. The retention time, t_R, is that measured from the moment of injection. In some cases it is practically more convenient to record the *net retention time*, t'_R, which is measured from the time of emergence of the solvent front. The latter also has its own retention time, t_0, when measured from the injection time so that

$$t'_R = t_R - t_0$$

Distribution Constant

Chromatographic separations depend on the distribution of a substance between two phases and this is described by a temperature-dependent distribution constant, K, where

$$K = \frac{\text{concentration in stationary phase}}{\text{concentration in mobile phase}}$$

K is also referred to as the partition, adsorption or exclusion coefficient in partition, adsorption or exclusion chromatography respectively.

Selectivity

A measure of the selectivity of the separation of two substances is the ratio, α, of their net retention times

$$\alpha = t'_{R_2}/t'_{R_1} = K_2/K_1$$

It is a characteristic of the ability of the stationary phase to discriminate between two substances. In GLC, the more selective phases are often more thermolabile thus reducing their suitability for compounds of low volatility.

Elution Volume

The elution volume V_R of a substance is related to the retention time and the volume flow rate of the mobile phase, f, as follows

$$V_R = t_R \cdot f = V_m + K \cdot V_s$$

where V_m is the volume of the mobile phase in the interstices between the discontinuous stationary phase and in other dead spaces, the *void volume*, and V_s is a feature of the stationary phase—the liquid volume in partition chromatography, the surface area in adsorption chromatography, the pore volume in exclusion chromatography or the ion exchange capacity in ion-exchange chromatography. The second component, $K \cdot V_s$, is the volume required to elute the substance.

Column Capacity Factor

The two parts of the expression for the elution volume give a measure of the column capacity, k', which is defined as

$$k' = \frac{K \cdot V_s}{V_m} = \frac{V_R - V_m}{V_m} = \frac{t_R - t_0}{t_0} = \frac{t'_R}{t_0}$$

The greater k' is, the better the separation, but the analytical time increases and the peaks become wider and lower. For HPLC columns, k' is usually between 2 and 6, and preferably above 5 for gas–liquid chromatography (GLC) columns.

Resolution

The resolution of a column for two components can now be considered. If the two peaks are regarded as two triangles with bases W_1 and W_2 and net retention times

t'_{R_1} and t'_{R_2}, the triangles will just touch when

$$(t'_{R_2} - t'_{R_1}) = (W_1 + W_2)/2$$

An index of resolution, R, can thus be defined as

$$R = 2(t'_{R_2} - t'_{R_1})/(W_1 + W_2)$$

If R exceeds one, the triangles would be separated. In the case of symmetrical Gaussian peaks, the overlap is about 2% when R is 1, and 0·3% when R equals 1·5.

The various parameters described above can be combined to give the resolution equation

$$R = \left(\frac{\sqrt{N}}{4}\right)\left(\frac{\alpha - 1}{\alpha}\right)\left(\frac{k'}{k' + 1}\right)$$

The first component in parentheses is related to column efficiency, the second to selectivity, and the third to capacity.

Column efficiency can be improved by lengthening the column or by reducing the *HETP*. The latter varies with the linear flow velocity (cm/s) of the mobile phase (liquid or gas) and is minimal at an optimal velocity which should be used if possible. *HETP* also depends on the particle size of the stationary phase and the regularity of its packing. It may be affected adversely by increasing the volume of the stationary phase. Note that when N is doubled, the resolution only increases 1.4-fold.

Column selectivity is increased by increasing the amount of stationary phase and by choosing a different, more selective stationary phase, however alteration of temperature is more likely to affect all components of a mixture similarly with only a small effect on the resolution.

Column capacity is increased by reducing the temperature and by increasing the amount of stationary phase either by increasing its liquid component in partition chromatography, the surface area in adsorption chromatography, the pore volume in exclusion chromatography or the charge density in ion-exchange chromatography.

Such considerations are important in developing good operating conditions for a particular separation. It is apparent that some changes, intended to improve resolution, may improve one factor while having an adverse effect on another. Note however that resolution may be at odds with analytical speed and capacity. Resolution is improved by sacrificing speed and by reducing sample size. The latter is important in relation to detector sensitivity. In practice the various conflicting items have to be considered and the best compromise selected for the particular problem in hand.

Quantitation in Chromatography

For many purposes, the area of the peak produced by the detector is proportional to the amount of material in that peak. Where peaks emerge at about the same time, the peak height gives a satisfactory measure, but peaks emerging later in a chromatographic separation normally become relatively wider in relation to height and a measurement of area is then essential. A simple computation is peak height multiplied by the peak width at half peak height but in many modern systems, the peaks are rather sharp and the precision of manual measurement of peak width is poor. If this is so, various devices are available to compute the peak area and an electronic integrator is very useful.

The area, or peak height if appropriate, may be compared with a standard curve of similar measurements determined from known amounts of the same substance. Alternatively, the area or height may be compared with the same measurement on the peak of an internal standard whose concentration in the original material is known.

GAS CHROMATOGRAPHY

Gas chromatography is well established as a separative technique in clinical biochemistry (Chakraborty and Lynough, 1978). In gas chromatography (Fig. 3.3) the mobile phase is an inert gas, usually nitrogen, which passes through a column containing the stationary phase. The mixture to be separated is introduced at the start of the column. Separation occurs by the distribution of the mixture in the vapour phase between the carrier gas and the stationary phase. Differing physical processes occurring on the stationary phase effect separation and include adsorption, partition and molecular sieve effects. These cause different components of the mixture to pass along the column at different rates. The analytical performance of a gas chromatograph is mainly determined by the efficiency of these separative processes in the column. The terms, gas–solid chromatography (GSC) and gas–liquid chromatography (GLC), refer to the nature of the stationary phase which is either a solid alone (GSC) or a liquid distributed on the surface of a solid (GLC).

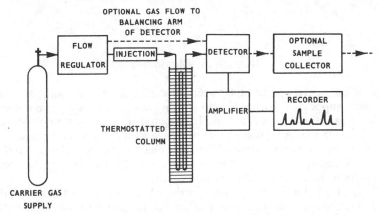

Fig. 3.3. Diagrammatic Representation of Gas Chromatography (Knox, 1962).

Gas emerging from the column contains components of the mixture in gaseous form provided the temperature is sufficiently high. The gas phase passes to a detector of high sensitivity whose output is displayed on a recorder. The characteristic behaviour of each component of a mixture is the time taken after application to the column for it to reach the detector. This *retention time* may be expressed either as an absolute time or as a relative retention time in relation to that of a reference substance.

Gas–Solid Chromatography

The stationary phase is an uncoated solid and the mode of separation depends on its properties. Some rely on adsorptive mechanisms, the more strongly adsorbed substances having the longer retention times. Activated charcoal, alumina or silica gel may be used to purify the gas phase before it enters the column by removing contaminants which are held firmly on the solid, i.e. their retention time is infinite. Where adsorption is less marked, separation of small molecules, often of gases, may be achieved. Some solid phases consist of porous particles with various total surface areas per unit weight. They may be considered as having varying pore sizes. The smaller pore sizes occur with the larger surface areas, up to $700 \, m^2/g$, and are associated with the longer retention times. Although such particles appear to behave similarly to the silica particles used in exclusion chromatography (p. 44), the physical process is largely adsorptive. Smaller molecules are usually adsorbed less strongly than larger ones and thus an increase of pore size, reducing the adsorptive area, reduces the retention of smaller molecules compared to larger ones. This is the converse of the effect of reducing the pore size in Sephadex gel chromatography which increases the rate of passage through the column of larger molecules.

Materials in use include porous silica beads (Porasil, Spherosil), cross-linked polymers such as polystyrene, polystyrene-divinylbenzene or acrylonitrile-divinylbenzene (Porapak, Chromosorb 100 series), and zeolites (aluminium silicates) in the form of their sodium and calcium salts (Molsieves). Their advantages are the lack of column 'bleed', the passage of column material into the gas phase, but columns for GSC are more readily overloaded than those for GLC. Their introduction has, however, enabled previously difficult separations to be achieved and an appropriate pore size can be selected to suit the analytical problem.

Gas–Liquid Chromatography

Separation involves partition between the carrier gas and a liquid phase held on an 'inert' support. This should ideally provide support only while presenting a large surface for the distribution of the liquid phase. The support should not interfere with the separation and when coated with its stationary phase, it should be mechanically robust allowing the solid phase to be packed easily and evenly into the column. These requirements were not met in earlier support media, and complete inertness is still difficult to achieve.

Support Media. *Diatomaceous Earths*—These commonly used media are probably the best general ones available. The natural diatomite or kieselguhr is calcined at high temperatures, sometimes with sodium carbonate, crushed and graded into particle sizes: 60–80, 80–100 or 100–120 mesh are commonly used as finer sizes increase resistance to gas flow. Examples are the Chromosorb, Anakrom, Gas-chrom and Supelcon series of supports. The crude materials show undesirable adsorption and catalytic effects which are improved if the material is washed with an acid wash (AW) to remove metallic impurities; a base wash may follow. These silicate earths possess free hydroxyl groups promoting adsorption by hydrogen bond formation and this has to be reduced. Such binding sites can be inactivated by treatment with a solution of dimethyldichlorosilane (DMCS) or hexamethyldisilazane (HMDS) which react with the hydroxyl groups. Support media so treated are usually identified by a suffix to the trade name, e.g. AW, AW/DMCS.

Other Support Media—The synthetic fluorethylene polymers, Teflon and Fluorpak-80, are the most inert support materials. A compromise is the impregnation of diatomite with a fluorohydrocarbon polymer (Gas Pack F). Such supports give relatively inefficient columns but their inertness reduces considerably the tendency of the more polar compounds to bind to the support and produce 'trailing' of peaks. Glass beads with a textured surface (Anaport, Cerabeads) provide a relatively inert support with a greater column efficiency.

Stationary Phase. Over 400 stationary phases are available commercially but the number necessary to separate most mixtures probably does not exceed ten. Attempts have been made to classify the phases into 'non-selective' and 'selective' types. On non-selective columns, separation is approximately related to molecular weight so that compounds differing by one double bond may be separated with difficulty. Selective phases have particular affinity for certain molecules, often those with groups of similar structure or polarity to those in the liquid phase. Thus the presence of phenyl groups in the stationary phase increases the affinity for compounds with one or more double bonds in their structure.

An attempt has been made to put selectivity of stationary phases on a quantitative basis by the use of McReynolds' constants (McReynolds, 1970) which are used in the form of published tables to compare separating ability for different compounds. McReynolds' constants are directly related to retention times and are listed for a series of selected test substances, namely: benzene, butan-1-ol, pentan-2-one, nitropropane, pyridine, 2-methylpentan-2-ol, 1-iodo-butane, oct-2-yne, 1,4-dioxane and *cis*-hydrindane. The constants for a particular phase are related to the least polar phase, squalene, which is given an arbitrary McReynolds' constant of zero for each of the ten substances. The average of the constants for the first five substances is usually taken as an index of polarity—the greater the figure, the greater the affinity for polar substances. For any of the ten substances, a high constant indicates a longer retention time and a big difference in constants between two test substances indicates suitability for separations of pairs of substances differing similarly in structure. Thus a large difference in constants for butan-1-ol and pentan-2-one suggests suitability for separating compounds differing only by the presence of a ketone or an alcohol group.

The choice of stationary phase depends not only on the nature of the substances to be separated, but also on the temperature at which the analytical mixture is volatile. Some phases are also volatile at higher temperatures leading to column 'bleed', while others are degraded by excessive heat. Table 3.4 lists features of some frequently used stationary phases of various chemical types. Hydrocarbons are relatively non-selective. The range of silicones whose chemical structure contains the repeating unit ($-O-SiR_2-$) changes from non-selective action where all substituents are methyl groups to increasingly selective phases as more polar substituents appear. At the same time the maximum operating temperatures fall. In the Dexasil phases, short silicone chains are linked to metacarborane units ($B_{16}H_{10}C_2$) to give greater thermal stability with the selectivity depending on the substituents in the silicone chain. Increased selectivity for polar groups is seen in the polyethylene glycol and polyester phases which are less suitable at high temperatures and are degraded by oxygen, acids or bases in the analytical mixture. The most polar phases, TCEP and BCEF are only suitable for relatively low temperature operation.

The support medium is coated by suspending it in a solution of the stationary phase in a volatile solvent. In one method, the correct amount of stationary phase for a given weight of solid medium is used and the resultant slurry is reduced to dryness in a rotary evaporator before final drying at 100°C. Alternatively, a solution of stationary phase of concentration about half that required in the final product is stirred for a while with the solid before this is removed by filtration and

TABLE 3.4

Selected Stationary Phases for Gas–Liquid Chromatography

Name	Composition	Average McReynolds constant	Approximate temperature operating range (°C)
Hydrocarbons			
Apiezon L	branched chain aliphatics	29	50–300
Silicones with different substituents			
SE–30	all methyl	43	50–350
OV–1	all methyl	44	100–350
OV–101	all methyl	46	0–325
OV–7	70% methyl, 30% phenyl	118	20–350
OV–17	50% methyl, 50% phenyl	177	0–375
OV–25	25% methyl, 75% phenyl	235	20–300
OV–210	50% CH_3, 50%–$(CH_2)_2 \cdot CF_3$	304	0–275
XE–60	50% CH_3, 50%–$(CH_2)_2 \cdot CN$	357	20–275
AN–600	75% CH_3, 25%–$(CH_2)_2 \cdot CN$	359	20–300+
OV–225	50% CH_3, 25% Ph, 25%–$(CH_2)_3 \cdot CN$	363	0–275+
OV–275	all–$(CH_2)_2 \cdot CN$	844	100–275
Silicone-metacarboranes (silicone substituents)			
Dexsil 300GC	all methyl	100	50–450 500 for short times
Dexsil 400GC	84% CH_3, 16% phenyl	117	20–400
Dexsil 410GC	84% CH_3, 16%–$(CH_2)_2 \cdot CN$	190	20–400
Polyethylene glycol			
Carbowax 20M	m.w. $15–20 \times 10^3$	462	60–225
Polyethylene glycol esters			
FFAP	PEG nitroterephthalate	509	50–250
EGA	PEG adipate	535	100–200
DEGS	poly (diethylene glycol) succinate	709	20–200 260 in stabilised form
EGS	PEG succinate	752	100–200 250 in stabilised form
Others			
TCEP	tris (cyanoethoxy) propane	829	20–175
BCEF	bis (cyanoethyl) formamide	929	10–125

dried. Many workers prefer to purchase commercially prepared materials ready for column packing.

A few 'bonded' stationary phases are available in which the organic phase is covalently bound to the support material, Porasil. Such media (Bondapak, Durapak) have varying selectivity depending on the nature of the bound molecule. They do not suffer from column bleed and column conditioning takes little time. As the coating is more even, peaks are sharper and symmetrical but some are unsuitable for high temperature operation and they are degraded by traces of water in the analytical mixture.

Columns. Two types have been used for GLC—packed columns, filled with the inert support medium holding the liquid phase, and open tubular capillary columns in which the stationary phase is on the capillary wall leaving the centre of the bore open.

Packed Columns—These are the more commonly used type with an internal diameter (ID) of 1·5 to 3 mm and length of 0·3 to 4 m, usually 1·5 to 2 m. They are made from glass or metal such as stainless steel. Interference with separation due to adsorption onto the glass column wall is reduced if the empty column is silanised before packing. Metal columns may cause catalytic destruction of trace materials, especially at high temperatures. Although glass columns are more fragile there is the added advantage of ease of inspection of the packing to see that no discontinuity has occurred which would affect column performance.

Once a column has been packed it is conditioned by heating to a temperature of 20 to 30°C above the expected operating temperature. Less firmly bound liquids are removed and thereafter a slow loss of stationary phase, referred to as column bleed, may occur. After a time the first few centimetres of column packing become disturbed by repeated sample application and impurities may collect here, requiring renewal of this part of the packing at intervals.

Capillary Columns—These have an ID of less than 1 mm, usually 0·25 or 0·5 mm, with a length of 25 to 100 m and are made of glass, silica or stainless steel. They are usually prepared commercially. A few are fully packed as in the last section but most are of the open tubular type with the stationary phase on the wall only. In the most common and most efficient form, this phase is a liquid but it is also possible to use a solid layer for GSC or a solid support coated with liquid for GLC. The open tubular construction greatly reduces the resistance to gas flow, permitting the use of much longer columns and increasing the ease of separations. In practice the most efficient columns are liquid coated. With glass columns of ID 0·25 mm there are 3000 to 5000 theoretical plates per metre falling to about half this as the ID increases to 0·5 mm, while stainless steel columns of the same sizes have somewhat lower numbers. They also have a more reactive wall surface than glass has but are mechanically stronger. Support-coated and micro-packed columns have a lower efficiency of 600 to 2000 plates per metre.

The liquid phases are those already described but such high performance reduces the need for the more selective phases used in conventional columns with the possibility of higher operating temperatures. The amount of material which can be handled by the column is considerably reduced and even for the detection of trace components the maximal sample volume is 0·5 to 2 μl, depending on the ID and nature of the column. A more elaborate injection system is required and for many purposes a sample-splitting procedure is used whereby only 1 to 5% of the injected material enters the column, the remainder being vented to the air. Careful attention to detector design is important and the analytical performance is badly affected by dead spaces near the injection and detector sites.

Carrier Gases. Nitrogen is now usually employed and is quite satisfactory. Argon is required if an argon ionisation detector is in use. The equipment includes flow rate monitors and the gas flow rate should be specified for an analytical method as it affects column efficiency.

Operating Temperatures. The distribution of a particular substance between the stationary and gaseous phases is a function of temperature, a higher proportion being volatile at higher temperatures. For a particular separation the choice of temperature is important and for compounds of high molecular weight an elevated temperature is essential. The column is therefore enclosed in a constant temperature oven. Such ovens are usually of low thermal capacity to allow rapid adjustments to be made so that the oven should not be opened during operation. The higher the temperature, the greater the column bleed when GLC is used. The degree to which this can be tolerated depends on the liquid phase, the temperature and the sensitivity of the detector to the liquid phase. This limitation is less for GSC although thermal decomposition of certain solid phases can occur at sufficiently high temperatures. Excessive bleed is undesirable as it reduces the sensitivity of detection by increasing the background signal and it causes a gradual change in column composition. For some substances GLC is only possible if they are converted into more volatile derivatives.

Sample Introduction. It is often convenient to apply the material to be separated to the column in a solvent at a concentration of 1 to 10 g/l. As the columns are relatively easily overloaded, the volume of liquid introduced must often be only 1 to 10 μl. This may be done using a micro-syringe but the precision of injection of very small volumes of volatile solvent is often rather poor. For quantitative work the material must be dissolved completely in a known, small volume of solvent preferably using a small glass conical tube to allow a reasonable depth of fluid with a small surface area to reduce evaporation. If quantitative solution or injection is difficult, an internal standard is added early in the analytical process. Application of samples to a capillary column often requires the use of a sample splitter (see p. 53).

In some cases, material in solid form has to be injected. It is sometimes possible to deposit the solid, if necessary by evaporation of liquid, on to the end of a metal wire which can then be withdrawn into a hollow needle. As with a liquid injection the needle can then be pushed through a diaphragm to reach the start of the column. Extrusion of the wire from the needle tip allows the solid sample to enter the column.

Instead of injecting straight on to the column, one may use a 'flash heater' situated above the start of the column and held at a temperature of 20 to 30°C above the column temperature. Injection into the flash heater permits rapid evaporation of the sample which is moved into the column by the carrier gas. The technique is useful for solid injections or when part of the sample is non-volatile as this remains in the flash heater and does not contaminate the column. Direct injection on to the column eventually alters the characteristics of the first few centimetres of the column packing but this can be readily renewed.

Any solvent used must be much more volatile than the components of the mixture so that the large solvent peak emerges first and returns near to the base line before other substances start to emerge. Net retention times (p. 46) are measured from the solvent peak but true retention times are measured from the time the injection was made and require a mark to be made on the base line at that moment.

Chromatographic peaks with longer retention times are wider than those emerging earlier (p. 46) but compression of later peaks with simultaneous reduction of retention time is achieved by increasing the temperature of the oven in a controlled fashion during the run. This is referred to as temperature programming. After the run is completed a rapid return to the initial temperature occurs after opening the oven.

Derivative Formation. The conversion of polar, relatively non-volatile substances into more volatile derivatives offers the possibility of determining such materials by GLC. Reactions may take place with –OH, –COOH or –NH$_2$ groups depending on the reagent used and the reaction conditions. Another use of derivatisation is to form halogenated products which are detectable in lower concentrations than the parent substance by the electron capture detector, thereby increasing the sensitivity. The reactions most often used are trimethylsilylation (introduction of a (CH$_3$)$_3$Si-or TMS group), acylation and alkylation, with the first being particularly popular.

TMS derivatives may be formed from alcohols and phenols to give TMS ethers, from carboxylic acids to form TMS esters, from both amino and carboxyl groups in amino acids, and from amides and amines. Not all groups react equally easily and selective derivatisation is possible. Reagents in more common use are: hexamethyldisilazane (Me$_3$Si–NH–SiMe$_3$), usually with trimethylchlorosilane, TMCS (Me$_3$SiCl) as a catalyst; *N,O*-bis-trimethylsilyl-acetamide (MeC(OSiMe$_3$)=NSiMe$_3$), sometimes with TMCS as catalyst; 1-trimethylsilylimidazole, particularly for hydroxyl groups selectively; trimethylsilyl diethylamine, particularly for amino acids.

Acylation of alcohols and amines is achieved using *N*-acylimidazoles to introduce acetyl, trifluoroacetyl (TFA), pentafluoropropionyl (PFP), pentafluorobenzoyl (PFB), or heptafluorobutyryl (HFB) groups. Alternatively, fluorinated acyl groups may be introduced using the appropriate acid anhydride (for TFA, PFP or HFB), acid chloride (for PFB) or *N*-methyl-bis(trifluoroacetamide) for TFA groups.

Alkylation of alcohols, phenols, carboxylic acids, amines, and amino acids by a variety of complex chemical reactions is possible using the dimethylformamide dialkyl acetals. A simpler chemical reaction is the conversion of carboxylic acids to their methyl esters by methanol and boron trifluoride. Pentafluorobenzyl bromide has been used to introduce PFB groups into phenols and carboxylic acids.

Detectors. The *katharometer*, or thermal conductivity detector, comprises two compartments each containing an electrically heated fine tungsten or platinum wire. Pure carrier gas passes through one compartment and the gas emerging from the column through the other. The thermal conductivity of the gas increases when substances emerge from the column, reducing the wire temperature and altering its resistance. The change can be detected and recorded but is a non-specific response to any substance whose thermal conductivity differs from that of the carrier gas. Early designs had a non-linear response and were relatively insensitive as most of the thermal conductivity was due to the carrier gas itself. Modern electronic developments have reduced these limitations. By using helium as the carrier gas and by controlling the filament temperature, sensitivity has increased and special amplifiers have improved linearity. Although useful for permanent gas analysis, for many purposes it has been superseded by ionisation detectors but it has the advantage of being able to detect inorganic material.

Ionisation detectors depend on the conduction of electricity by gases. Normally gases behave as perfect insulators but the introduction of charged atoms, molecules or free electrons increases the conductivity allowing a current to flow between two electrodes held at a constant electrical potential difference. Such detectors differ in the means of producing the ionisation.

In the *flame ionisation detector* (FID) the carrier gas enters a hydrogen flame burning in air. An electrical field is set up across the flame but with carrier gas only, the ionisation current is very low. When organic substances enter the flame, an increase in charged particles and hence ionisation current occurs and this current is amplified and recorded. The very low background current allows easy detection of small increases so that the sensitivity is high. This form of detector is mainly sensitive to organic compounds. Formic acid is an exception and the response is somewhat lower if oxygen or nitrogen are present in addition to carbon and hydrogen in the molecule but the response is essentially non-specific for most organic substances making it widely applicable. It is insensitive to water, permanent gases and most inorganic compounds. Its great advantages are its sensitivity, less than 1 ng/l carrier gas, and its linearity over a 10^6-fold range.

A development of the FID is the alkaline FID or *nitrogen–phosphorus detector*. Solid rubidium or caesium chloride placed in the tip of the flame reduces the ionisation of substances lacking nitrogen or phosphorus atoms but not that of compounds containing these elements. The sensitivity depends on the hydrogen flow rate and the position of the alkaline crystal in the flame which has the dual role of ionising the sample and heating the crystal to release alkali metal atoms. With use, the crystal vaporises necessitating frequent adjustment to obtain the maximal response to a standard. In more convenient developments of this detector, glass with a high rubidium content is separately heated electrically and is positioned above the flame. A collector electrode is held at a different potential from that of the flame. This electrode can be either the cathode or anode in different designs. Doubt still exists about the exact reactions which take place in the flame and at the glass surface but in practice the response is about five times greater for phosphorus-containing compounds than for nitrogenous substances. The sensitivity for compounds lacking these elements is several thousand times less and the linear range is about five decades.

Another selective detector is the *flame photometric detector* in which carrier gas plus sample is again mixed with hydrogen and burnt in air. Compared with the normal FID oxygen-rich flame, this flame is hydrogen-rich under which circumstances compounds containing sulphur and phosphorus emit characteristic radiation: sulphur, 394 nm; phosphorus, 526 nm. An interference filter is used to isolate the required emission which falls on a photomultiplier. A more sophisticated variant uses a microwave-sustained helium plasma instead of the flame. Under these conditions all elements normally found in organic molecules can be measured by their characteristic atomic emission lines. The emitted radiation is analysed using a diffraction grating and up to 12 different elements can be measured simultaneously using a separate photomultiplier and amplifier for each one.

In the *argon ionisation detector*, beta particles emitted by a ^{90}Sr or ^{3}H source collide with molecules of the carrier gas, argon, converting them into a higher energy metastable state. Such metastable atoms have sufficient energy to produce ionisation of other molecules emerging from the column and the liberated electrons are accelerated towards the detector anode held at a high voltage. These high energy electrons behave like the original beta particles, activating further argon atoms. The resultant ionisation current is amplified and recorded. The disadvantages of limitation of the carrier gas to argon, interference by water vapour and limited linearity of response has caused this detector to be mainly replaced by the FID. A modified argon detector, the *cross-section detector*, works similarly but the anode voltage is only about 100 V which reduces the sensitivity but increases the range of response. It is unselective, responding to all gases and vapours.

A selective detector also employing a radioactive source is the *electron capture detector* in which beta particles produced from a metal foil containing ^{63}Ni or ^{3}H migrate to the anode held at a fixed voltage of 2 to 30 V to produce a steady background current. When the carrier gas containing an electron-capturing substance passes through the detector, some of the electrons are removed and the current falls. Such substances include halogen compounds, nitro and carbonyl compounds, acids and esters. Carbon and hydrogen have virtually no affinity for free electrons. The selectivity increases on raising the anode potential and electron capture by appropriate groups is also facilitated by adding methane or carbon dioxide to the carrier gas to abolish the response to groups with weak electron affinity. This detector is unsuitable as a general detector but is extremely useful for halogenated compounds for which it is 1000 times more sensitive than the FID. Its simultaneous use with the FID is a very useful, informative detection system.

Two detectors offer greater possibilities for recognising the identity of substances emerging from the column. It is possible to pass the emergent gas into a heated cavity located in an *infra-red spectrophotometric detector* allowing a spectral scan to be performed and compared with reference spectra. Information about the molecular weight of emerging substances is achieved by linking the gas chromatograph to a mass spectrometer. For packed columns only part of the column output is usually sampled but the total output is satisfactory with capillary columns. The full-scale mass spectrometer is an expensive instrument, especially if solely dedicated to gas chromatographic operations, but a somewhat simpler device, the *mass selective detector*, offers reasonable performance at a lower cost. In the most elaborate systems the recorded mass spectrum can be rapidly compared in a computer with the stored spectra of over 30 000 substances and likely matches identified. (See also Hill and Whelan, 1984.)

HIGH PRESSURE LIQUID CHROMATOGRAPHY

The high resolution of gas chromatography was achieved by careful appraisal of the physical characteristics which determine the column performance (p. 45). Such considerations were later applied to liquid chromatography. It is clear that the use of small particles of absorbent as in TLC increases the resolution and thus column chromatography has been explored using smaller particles than the traditional irregular porous particles of sizes 50 μm upwards used in earlier columns. Smaller particles pack closely together leaving less space for the mobile phase to pass through and thereby increase the resistance to flow and the pressure drop along the column. This pressure drop is directly proportional to the length of the column, the velocity of flow and the viscosity of the mobile phase, but is inversely related to the *square* of the particle diameter. Thus it is no longer possible to rely on the hydrostatic pressure of the mobile phase to achieve a practically useful flow through the column and some method of applying pressure is needed. For many separations the pressure is 1000 to 5000 psi, corresponding to approximately 7 to 35 MPa, or 68 to 340 atm. This is comparable with the pressure in a full gas cylinder, about 3000 psi, hence the name *high pressure liquid chromatography (HPLC)*.

The use of much smaller particles, often 5 to 10 μm diameter, greatly increases the resolution so that alternative names are *high performance liquid chromato-*

graphy (*HPLC*) or *high resolution chromatography*. Provided that dead spaces in the system are minimised and all internal surfaces are highly polished, it is often possible to achieve efficient separations using small columns at a flow rate allowing separations to be completed within a few minutes, so that the process is also called *high speed liquid chromatography*.

The technique does not suffer from the inherent problem of gas chromatography of achieving volatility without decomposition, replacing it with the easier problem of solubility in the mobile phase and the composition of this liquid can be varied appropriately. The constituents of a mixture should emerge from the column separately and are detected and measured, usually non-destructively. They can be recovered in pure form if required so that, depending on column capacity, the technique can be preparative as well as analytical. A further advantage is the applicability to large biological molecules such as proteins for which the separation technique has been given the name, *fast protein liquid chromatography* (*FPLC*).

HPLC can be performed with different separative methods so that adsorption, partition, exclusion and ion-exchange techniques are in use. The choice depends on the size and polarity of the substances to be separated. A general guide to the type of technique which is likely to be applicable appears in Table 3.5.

TABLE 3.5

Separative Techniques Used in High Pressure Liquid Chromatography

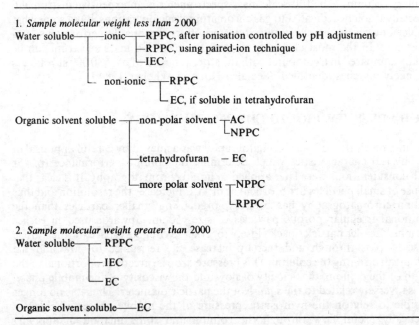

1. *Sample molecular weight less than* 2 000
Water soluble ─┬─ ionic ─┬─ RPPC, after ionisation controlled by pH adjustment
               │   ├─ RPPC, using paired-ion technique
               │   └─ IEC
               └─ non-ionic ─┬─ RPPC
                             └─ EC, if soluble in tetrahydrofuran

Organic solvent soluble ─┬─ non-polar solvent ─┬─ AC
                         │   └─ NPPC
                         ├─ tetrahydrofuran ─ EC
                         └─ more polar solvent ─┬─ NPPC
                                                └─ RPPC

2. *Sample molecular weight greater than* 2000
Water soluble ─┬─ RPPC
               ├─ IEC
               └─ EC

Organic solvent soluble ── EC

RPPC = reverse phase partition chromatography
IEC = ion-exchange chromatography
EC = exclusion chromatography
AC = adsorption chromatography
NPPC = normal phase partition chromatography

As with gas chromatography there are several different modules which comprise an HPLC system but they are arranged in a similar fashion (Fig. 3.3). Thus the gas supply and flow regulator in Fig. 3.3 are replaced by a high pressure liquid pump but the other items are arranged in the same order although their constructional details differ considerably. The optional gas flow to the reference side of the detector is replaced by an optional flow of mobile phase.

Pump

The ideal pump should deliver a pulseless, relatively low flow rate at a high pressure. The flow rate should be adjustable and then remain constant and it should be possible to change easily the solvent pumped. In some cases the solvent composition alters during an analytical run, a process referred to as gradient elution (see p. 36). Gradients can be formed in various ways but the most flexible and expensive method involves the use of two separate high pressure pumps to deliver two solvents at rates varied by an electronic controller.

High pressure pumps fall into two broad types—constant pressure and constant flow. Constant pressure pumps are simpler, cheaper and pulseless but the flow rate changes if the column resistance alters as when the packing material swells, shrinks or is contaminated with extraneous particulate matter. It can also occur if the viscosity of the mobile phase alters as a result of a change in temperature or in composition as in gradient elution. Such factors have little effect on the constant flow pump as the pump pressure alters to compensate for changes in column resistance and maintains the required flow rate so long as the pressure required does not exceed the capacity of the pump. A pulseless pump of this type is essentially a large syringe, filled with the required solvent, in which the piston is driven at a steady rate. Such pumps are wasteful of solvent if this has to be changed. The most popular pumps at present are of the reciprocating type in which the contents of a small volume chamber are expelled at a constant rate into the column feed until the chamber is emptied when, by means of valves, it is rapidly refilled and the cycle restarts. There is necessarily a pressure drop during the refilling step but this can be minimised by the use of a pulse damper. Alternatively, either a dual or multi-headed pump can be used with two or more chambers pumping asynchronously, or the pumping speed of the single chamber can be changed slightly at the beginning and end of the delivery phase by an electronic controller—electronic pulse compensation. In the reciprocating pumps it is frequently possible to use a device to alter the solvent composition simply and cheaply, and to deliver the changing mixture to the low pressure intake side of the pump if gradient elution is used.

The stainless steel inner surfaces of such pumps are easily damaged by particulate matter in the mobile phase and filters capable of removing particles above 0·2 μm diameter are required at the intake. Solvents containing strong bases or ionisable halides are best avoided as they also attack stainless steel. It is desirable to degas the mobile phase. The dissolved gas does not affect the pump action but may be released at the low pressure end of the analytical column and affect the performance of the detector.

The flow rates (ml/min) in use vary with the internal diameter (ID) of the column but typical flow rates vary from 0·5 to 2 ml/min for 2 mm ID up to 10 to 20 ml/min for 10 mm ID. Such flow rates are similar to those achieved in low pressure column chromatography and are suitable for efficient separations to be completed within 15 min. The flow rates used are often greater than those which would give the highest efficiency of the column (p. 48).

Injection of the Sample

This poses greater difficulties than with gas chromatography. It is possible to inject directly using a high pressure syringe fitted with a locking needle which is inserted through a Teflon-coated rubber septum. This becomes unsatisfactory if the pressure exceeds 1000 psi or if the sample volume exceeds 50 μl and there is a risk of dislodging small particles from the septum which then interfere with column flow. The first two difficulties may be overcome by switching devices which temporarily divert the high pressure flow of mobile phase allowing direct injection of sample volumes between 10 and 500 μl at the lowered pressure beyond the diversion.

Currently the most-favoured method employs a sampling valve, shown diagrammatically in Fig. 3.4. The sample is introduced into a sample loop at atmospheric pressure while the normal column flow continues. By rotating the valve, the mobile phase then passes through the sample loop, carrying its contents at high pressure on to the column. Depending on the design of the valve, the loop volume varies from 0·5 μl up to 5 or even 10 ml, varying with the column size and the nature of the sample, but is typically 5 to 100 μl. Such valves are usable in an automated mode.

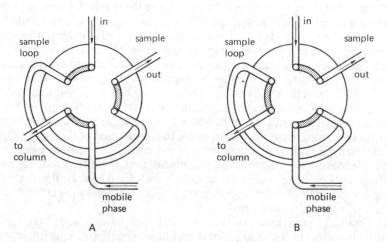

Fig. 3.4. Sampling Valve for High Pressure Liquid Chromatography.
A—Mobile phase is pumped at high pressure to column while sample loop is filled at normal pressure.
B—After rotating valve clockwise, the mobile phase carries a defined volume of sample on to the column at high pressure.

Whichever method is used, it is important that particulate matter is absent from the sample as it will degrade column performance. Samples are preferably filtered using a pore size of 0·5 μm.

Columns

These are usually made from polished stainless steel as glass columns are unsatisfactory at pressures above 600 psi. The bore depends on the intended use. For analytical work, IDs of 4 to 7 mm are common but there is increasing interest in microbore, 2 mm, or capillary, 0·5 to 1 mm, columns for economies of scale and efficient separation. For preparative work involving sample sizes between 10 and 1000 mg, the ID is 10 to 22 mm. While column lengths vary, they usually lie in the range from 10 to 100 cm, commonly 30 cm, for both analytical and preparative columns. Columns are usually straight to avoid disturbances of solvent flow and to make packing easier. If a long column is required it is best to join two or more columns together by stainless steel tubing, looped if necessary, as long columns are difficult to pack efficiently.

Column Packings

Columns may be packed with different materials enabling adsorption, partition (normal and reversed phase), exclusion or ion-exchange chromatography to be carried out.

For *adsorption chromatography*, silica gel is most frequently used and there has been a move away from using the irregular particles of size 20 μm or more, to spherical particles with a narrow range of diameter. The mean diameter varies from 3 to 10 μm and the particles are porous with an average effective pore size of 5 to 10 nm and a pore volume of 0·8 to 1·5 ml/g gel. Such particles show large surface areas (including internal surfaces) on which adsorption can take place, frequently 300 to 500 m^2/g. The most efficient columns are prepared from the smallest particles which pack closely together.

Many columns are used in the *partition chromatography* mode and for clinical biochemistry, reverse-phase partition chromatography (RPPC) is especially useful for drugs, hormones and some polypeptides and proteins. Most stationary phases are now in 'bonded' form, i.e. covalently linked to the silanol groups of silica gel of various particle sizes. This avoids the need to saturate the mobile phase with the stationary phase, excludes the latter from the column effluent, and allows gradient elution to be performed without affecting the stationary phase. Two common, non-polar media are produced by covalent bonding of an octyl or octadecyl hydrocarbon chain, usually referred to as C8 or C18 bonded phases. Not all the silica surface is covered by such chains and the residual silanol groups may show undesirable adsorption properties unless 'end-capped' by reaction with trimethyl silane. A somewhat more polar coating is produced by bonding a shorter hydrocarbon chain with a terminal phenyl group. Still more polar coatings are obtained by bonding cyanopropyl or aminopropyl chains (CN and NH2 phases), again end-capped in some cases.

The resolving power of such columns depends on the size of the initial silica particles which are similar in shape and porosity to those used for adsorption purposes. With 4 μm particles, resolution may reach 110 000 to 120 000 theoretical plates (TP)/m, falling to 30 000 to 50 000 TP/m for 10 μm particles. C8 and C18 phases are suitable for RPPC with mobile phases such as buffers, water, methanol, acetonitrile, tetrahydrofuran or mixtures thereof. It is possible to mix solvents in progressively varying proportions to alter the polarity in gradient elution. This can shorten the time for the separation of complex mixtures and in this respect is used in a similar fashion to temperature programming (p. 55) in gas chromatography. When used for protein separations, the binding forces between the macromolecules and the stationary phase will depend on the nature and extent of the non-polar side chains of the constituent amino acids. The polar CN and NH2 phases behave more like untreated silica gel but are less affected by water in the sample or mobile phase. They are used with the less polar mobile phases such as hexane, methylene dichloride, chloroform, diethyl ether or mixtures of these, using gradient elution if appropriate.

For *exclusion chromatography*, separations are performed in aqueous or organic solvents depending on the solubility of the components of the mixture. Polystyrene beads, cross-linked with divinylbenzene, are available in various particle sizes with different pore diameters to cover a range of molecular weights of analytes from 50 to 10^7. The total pore volume is commensurate with the interstitial volume between particles. For beads of less than 10 μm diameter, the resolving power is about 45 000 TP/m but this falls to 2500 TP/m with the larger 50 μm beads. Such beads are suitable for use with organic solvents.

Separations in aqueous solvents have been used for many biological molecules, particularly peptides and proteins. The column packing takes the form of rigid, porous, small (usually 10 to 20 μm) spherical particles available with different pore sizes (4 to 400 nm) to allow separation on the basis of molecular weight with exclusion limits varying from 40 000 to several million. The particle surface is hydrophilic to reduce the hydrophobic binding seen in RPPC and the particles are either based on silica with a surface-bonded organic phase containing hydroxy groups, or are cross-linked polyether or polyester resins. Care must be taken in selecting the mobile phase to avoid halides which corrode stainless steel, while slightly alkaline buffers slowly degrade silica beads. Columns using 10 μm silica beads have resolving powers up to 35 000 TP/m. However, currently available materials are not particularly satisfactory for the resolution and recovery of small peptides with molecular weights in the range of 1000 to 10 000.

Ion-exchange chromatography has been particularly useful for the rapid separation of proteins. Again, small spherical porous particles are employed with a pore size selected to give a compromise between the greater surface area and ion-exchange capacity associated with reduction in pore size and the lower exclusion limits for molecular weight imposed by smaller pore sizes. The particles, which are usually hydrophilic in nature, are available as weak (W) or strong (S), anion (AX) or cation (CX) exchangers. Some are based on polymeric resins bearing quaternary methylammonium groups (SAX) or sulphonic acid groups (SCX) while others are derived from silica either with a bonded polyethylene-imine coating (WAX) or having diethylaminoethyl (WAX) or carboxymethyl (WCX) groups attached to the silica surface. Such materials have proved invaluable for the rapid separation of peptides and proteins usually without denaturation. For the 10 μm particles the resolution may exceed 30 000 TP/m. Another advantage is that the resistance to flow through the column is such that only moderately high pressures are needed which permits the use of glass instead of stainless steel columns if the latter would be attacked by the mobile phase.

Ionic compounds present in admixture with non-ionic substances, or even on their own, may sometimes be separated by RPPC as an alternative to ion-exchange chromatography using the techniques of ion-suppression or paired-ion chromatography.

In *ion-suppression chromatography* alteration of the pH of the mobile phase, often by adding acetic acid, may sufficiently suppress ionisation and allow the non-ionised form to be separated in the usual way using RPPC.

In *paired-ion chromatography*, lipophilic counter ions are added to the mobile phase to modify the separation. Substances such as tetrabutylammonium phosphate are used to pair with anions in the mixture to be separated, while aliphatic sulphonic acids or sulphates are used to pair with cations. Three models have been suggested to explain the mode of action of, e.g., an added negatively-charged counter ion.

1. *The ion pair model.* The added ions combine with cations in the mixture to produce a neutral, lipophilic ion pair which then has an affinity for the stationary phase.
2. *The dynamic model.* The added lipophilic anion dissolves in the stationary phase causing it to act like a cation exchange system.
3. *The ion interaction model.* This more complex model (Bidlingmeyer, 1980) is preferred and explains other phenomena also. Initially some counter anions dissolve in the stationary non-polar phase with their charges protruding from it to form a negatively charged primary layer, which is covered by a secondary layer composed of an equal number of small ions such as Na^+. The mobile phase contains both cations and anions but if one of the large cations requiring separation displaces a Na^+ ion from the secondary layer it will be held by ionic attraction sufficiently long for its non-ionic part to be able to enter the stationary phase and bind this cation. This positively charged part of the surface can then attract another counter anion so that a pair of ions enter one after another, rather than as an ion pair. Depending on relative concentrations of ions in the two phases, binding to the stationary phase can either continue or desorption occurs in a stepwise way. This model exploits both ionic and non-ionic binding forces. It also allows an understanding of the fact that retention of analyte ions by the stationary phase can be modified by adding another, rather more lipophilic ion of the *same* charge. This is envisaged as entering the stationary phase preferentially and displacing the analyte ion. The technique is useful if tailing of peaks of ionic components is a problem in RPPC.

Detectors

As with GLC, these may be general, non-selective, universal detectors suitable for most substances, or specific, selective detectors, the suitability of which is restricted to substances with particular properties. The general properties required of any detector are a linear response over a wide range of concentration, adequate sensitivity, and rapid response. The detector flow cell volume is important as the volume occupied by an emergent peak may be only 50 μl. Ideally, for good resolution the detector volume should be no more than one fifth of this but the use of very small volumes is associated with loss of sensitivity and the compromise volume is usually 8 to 10 μl. The concentration of a substance producing a detector signal twice that of the baseline 'noise' is the minimal detectable concentration (MDC) but for the whole system a more important concept is the minimal detectable quantity, usually taken as MDC × peak volume, when considering sensitivity. Careful design of the detector flow cell and a low time constant of the electronic circuitry help to minimise further broadening of the peak after it leaves the column. Typically the extra broadening attributable to the detector is less than 10%. The time constant is preferably less than 10% of the time taken for a peak to emerge from the column. At a flow rate of 1 ml/min, a substance may be fully eluted in a volume of 50 μl in 3 s. This would require a time constant of 0·3 s, the lowest figure currently achievable, if peak distortion is not to occur.

General Detectors. The one in most common use is the *refractive index detector* in which the difference in refractive index, n, between the column effluent and pure mobile phase is continuously monitored. In one type, each liquid occupies a triangular cell and the path of a single light beam is so arranged that the angles of refraction produced by the cells are opposed. If both contain the mobile phase, the light beam falls at a null point, but is deflected in a positive or negative direction when n in the sample alters so that a continuous record of the light beam deflection shows positive and negative peaks. A similar record is obtained with an alternative optical arrangement which monitors the fraction of a light beam which is refracted rather than reflected at an air/liquid interface. This is also affected by n. These detectors have a linear range of 10^4 and can detect 1 μg of substance in a 10 μl volume. As n varies with temperature, thermal stability of within $\pm 0.01°C$ is essential and the system is usually unsuitable for operation with gradient elution.

The *mass spectrometer detector* (MS) has been used in conjunction with HPLC to give information both about the quantity of emergent material and about the nature of the material as judged by its mass spectrum. In the simpler, off-line mode, peaks recognised by another detector are collected separately and then prepared for analysis in a standard MS (Hill and Whelan, 1984). Difficulties have arisen in using this detector in a continuous mode when it is required to act as a general mass detector and to produce spectra of peaks of interest. It is sometimes possible to pass the column effluent on to a moving belt which is first heated to remove the solvent and then, within a confined space near the MS inlet, heated further to vaporise the analyte. An alternative, the thermospray, removes solvent from a jet of effluent by heat, and then vaporises the analytes which enter the MS. Current work suggests that the total effluent from a micro-bore analytical column can be transferred to the MS after removal of the solvent giving a system with a potential sensitivity for mass detection similar to that of the refractive index detector but with some information about the molecular structure of the substance in the peak being obtained simultaneously. There is, however, a conflict between mass detection and proper spectral identification when peaks are eluted within a few seconds and this has led to the development of the *parallel mass spectrometer* in which two ion beams are generated at the vaporiser and enter separate mass detection/resolution devices. The detector of one records total mass against time but the second beam is only subjected to a mass spectrum scan near to the centre of a definite peak.

Various cumbersome devices linked to a *flame ionisation detector* (p. 56) have been devised for substances whose boiling point is appreciably higher than that of the mobile phase. Part of the column effluent is transferred to a moving wire which first passes through a heater to remove the solvent and then enters a hot oxidising chamber to convert carbon compounds to carbon dioxide. This is then mixed with hydrogen and catalytically reduced to methane which enters the flame. The presence of salts of organic acids in the constituents of the mobile phase gives a high background. The linear range is only about 10^3 but the sensitivity is about 20 times that of the refractive index indicator.

Specific Detectors. Those in most common use are the optical detectors, the principles of which are described in greater detail in Chapter 7. In common with the refractive index indicator, such detectors allow recovery of the analyte if needed. The ability of substances to absorb light or to fluoresce is exploited.

The simplest and cheapest device is the *fixed wavelength absorption detector* which is a dual-beam colorimeter with a flow-through cuvette. A low pressure mercury arc source with a simple filter system provides essentially monochromatic light of a wavelength of 254 nm. If necessary, the lamp can be combined with a phosphor screen which increases the wavelength to 280 nm, but with a greater bandwidth. As many compounds of interest to the clinical biochemist show at least some absorption of light at one of these wavelengths, the detector is very useful and shows a wider range of applicability than might appear at first sight. For substances absorbing strongly at one of these wavelengths, the linear range is 10^4 and the sensitivity, up to 10^3 times that of the refractive index detector, allows detection of 1 ng in a 10 μl volume. The detector is also suitable for use with gradient elution.

Not all substances show absorption at these wavelengths but may be detected using the more costly *variable wavelength absorption detector* akin to a double-beam UV-visible spectrophotometer covering the range 190 to 400 nm. Substances such as carbohydrates and lipids and those containing peptide bonds absorb light in the 190 to 210 nm range and the wavelength can be adjusted to give appropriate sensitivity for the substance of interest while minimising interference from others. For work at low wavelengths, the choice of solvent is important as this may also show significant absorption below certain cut-off points, thereby reducing light intensity and increasing the detector 'noise'. Such cut-off wavelengths (nm) are: acetonitrile (190), hexane (200), methanol and propan-2-ol (205) and methylene dichloride (233).

A yet more sophisticated optical detector is the *diode array detector* (p. 139) which allows the absorption spectrum of the substance passing through the detector to be continuously monitored. *Infra-red detectors* have not found much favour for HPLC work as they have limited sensitivity while interference from solvent absorption bands is often troublesome.

For suitable substances, the *fluorescence detector*, essentially a fluorimeter with flow-through cell (see Chapter 7) offers further advantages. Not all substances fluoresce but for those which do, this yet more elaborate and costly detector offers a linear range of up to 10^6 and a further 1000-fold increase in sensitivity over that of the absorption detector, allowing measurement of 1 pg in 10 μl. While non-halogenated solvents are usually satisfactory for fluorescence work, chloroform and methylene dichloride cause quenching.

A different type of specific detector is the *electrochemical detector* which is particularly suitable for catecholamine detection. A carbon electrode in a 1 μl cell is held at a fixed electrical potential at which selected substances are oxidised or reduced at the electrode surface. The electrode current is measured as a function of time. Substances unaffected at the electrode potential used give no signal but for those which can be chemically altered, the current is proportional to the concentration present. For such substances, the sensitivity is similar to that of the optical absorption detectors while the specificity is usually higher. The system is only satisfactory with polar solvents such as water or water/methanol mixtures and is thus mainly restricted to ion-exchange chromatography and RPPC. The electrodes have often proved troublesome in practice, becoming easily contaminated with loss of sensitivity.

Other detectors of the relatively specific type have proved difficult to operate. Halogenated compounds have been detected by evaporation in a heated stainless steel capillary tube, followed by examination of the vapour using an electron capture detector (p. 57). Detection of radioactivity has usually required separate collection of peaks identified by another detector, followed by counting these fractions in a conventional counter (see Chapter 9).

Use of Derivatives

This has been much less used than in GLC but is sometimes a way of increasing the sensitivity and selectivity of the HPLC technique. As with GLC it is possible to prepare derivatives from the analytes before they are applied to the column. Ideally such derivatives should be formed rapidly and reproducibly under mild reaction conditions, while the ability to process a batch of samples simultaneously is advantageous. Any excess reagent or its further decomposition products should not interfere with the separation on the column or the operation of the detector, while the derivatives themselves should be stable during storage and analysis.

An advantage over GLC is that the derivative formation can be carried out after the analytes have been separated on the column. Reagents are added to the column effluent in a mixing device, enter a reaction chamber, heated if necessary, for derivative formation and finally pass to the detector. Derivative formation should usually reach a reproducible, advanced stage within 2 min in the reaction and detector chambers in order to minimise peak broadening and again, the reagents added should not affect the detector.

Examples of derivative formation for the detection of specific groups are:

1. *–COOH group*—formation of *p*-bromophenacyl or *p*-nitrobenzyl esters for UV detectors and formation of coumarin derivatives for fluorescence detection,
2. *–NH₂ group*—formation of *p*-nitrophenylacetamides for UV detection and reaction with dansyl chloride, fluorescamine or *o*-phthalaldehyde giving fluorescent products,
3. *–OH group*—formation of 3,5-dinitrobenzoates for UV detection.

For a general review of HPLC see Koenigsberger (1978).

RELATIVE ADVANTAGES AND DISADVANTAGES OF DIFFERENT CHROMATOGRAPHIC METHODS

The chromatographic methods used in clinical biochemistry have changed as techniques have evolved. TLC has the advantages of rapid separation of small amounts of material and can be used in adsorption and partition modes. While a visualisation step is usually required, the technique is useful for the qualitative identification of, e.g. sugars and amino acids, but it may also be used with a variety of solvents to determine quickly the best conditions for column chromatography using a similar support medium. Column chromatography has the ability to handle larger quantities of material than TLC.

A major development in chromatography has been the development of high resolution techniques, GLC, HPLC and HPTLC, which have reduced the need for two-dimensional separations on layers. Once the initial capital cost of the equipment has been met, GLC and HPLC offer complementary high resolution techniques for many substances. This is particularly so for many of the smaller molecules of interest to the clinical biochemist. The choice then depends on personal preference and the nature of the equipment currently available in that laboratory. It is sometimes possible to perform separations using HPLC without the derivatisation step needed for the same separation to be achieved by GLC and this is convenient but not essential. HPLC is much more advantageous if large molecules, or non-volatile or thermolabile compounds are to be separated. The choice of mobile phase in HPLC has a more marked effect on the separation than in GLC where the nature of the gas phase is relatively unimportant.

For some purposes when high resolution is not necessary, liquid column chromatography at atmospheric pressure has the advantages of lower cost and easy application of the analytical mixture. Selection of the column packing allows separation of a wide range of substances varying from large proteins to small molecules, or from non-polar to ionised, highly polar compounds, as exemplified by the earlier discussions in this chapter of adsorption, partition, molecular sieve, affinity and ion-exchange chromatography. Quantitation may require the collection of fractions of the column effluent using an automatic fraction collector, and later analysis of each fraction separately, although continuous monitoring is sometimes possible as with protein fractionation using an UV absorption detector.

HPLC offers, for a bigger investment in capital equipment and technical skill, the advantages of speed, resolution, sensitivity, re-use of columns and easy recovery of pure analytes for a range of substances depending on the nature of the column used. Separations are often complete within 15 to 20 min and the ability to re-use the column allows many analyses to be completed in a working day. Greater resolution may allow satisfactory separation with less initial preparation of the sample for analysis. The high sensitivity enables small samples to be analysed satisfactorily if need be while, alternatively, the use of a larger sample and column enables separation and recovery of substances of interest to be achieved.

REFERENCES

Bidlingmeyer B. A. (1980). *J. Chromatogr. Sci*; **18**: 525.

Chakraborty J., Lynough N. (1978). In *Scientific Foundations of Clinical Biochemistry, Vol. 1. Analytical Aspects.* (Williams D. L., Nunn R. F., Marks V., eds) p. 144. London: William Heinemann Medical Books.

Hill R. E., Whelan D. T. (1984). *Clin. Chim. Acta*; **139**: 231.

Knox J. H. (1962). *Gas Chromatography*. London: Methuen.

Koenigsberger R. (1978). In *Scientific Foundations of Clinical Biochemistry, Vol. 1. Analytical Aspects.* (Williams D. L., Nunn R. F., Marks V., eds) p. 165. London: William Heinemann Medical Books.

Lowe C. R. (1978). In *Scientific Foundations of Clinical Biochemistry, Vol. 1. Analytical Aspects.* (Williams D. L., Nunn R. F., Marks V., eds) p. 202. London: William Heinemann Medical Books.

McReynolds W. O. (1970). *J. Chromatogr. Sci*; **8**: 685.

Smith I., Seakins J. W. T., eds. (1976). *Chromatographic and Electrophoretic Techniques, Vol. 1. 4th ed. Paper and Thin Layer Chromatography*, p. 185. London: William Heinemann Medical Books.

Stokes A. M. (1978). In *Scientific Foundations of Clinical Biochemistry, Vol. 1. Analytical Aspects.* (Williams D. L., Nunn R. F., Marks V., eds) p. 185. London: William Heinemann Medical Books.

Williams D. L. (1978). In *Scientific Foundations of Clinical Biochemistry, Vol. 1. Analytical Aspects.* (Williams D. L., Nunn R. F., Marks V., eds) p. 123. London: William Heinemann Medical Books.

4

SEPARATIVE PROCEDURES ELECTROPHORESIS

Electrophoresis is the name given to the movement of charged particles through an electrolyte subjected to an electric field. If these are differently charged they will move in opposite directions, the positively charged to the cathode and the negatively charged to the anode. The rate of migration of particles of like charge will depend, among other things, on the number of charges each carries. Different rates of migration separate a complex mixture such as plasma proteins into a number of fractions of like mobility, the sharpness of separation depending upon the extent to which each fraction is homogeneous in its mobility.

The first technique to be introduced was that of Tiselius (1937, 1939). A buffered protein solution occupied the lower part of a quartz U-tube forming a sharp boundary with protein-free buffer solution which lay above it in both limbs of the U-tube and with which electrodes were in contact. On application of an electrical potential difference, proteins migrated to the appropriate electrode at varying speeds and the sharp boundary was disturbed. The position of the boundary for each protein could be determined by observing the change in refractive index which occurs at this point. Separation only occurs at the boundaries, the bulk of the protein remaining homogeneous. Using this technique human proteins can be resolved into albumin and three globulin zones designated α, β and γ, in order of decreasing mobility. This kind of separation in a homogeneous solution is termed *moving boundary* or *frontal electrophoresis* (Fig. 4.1(I)). The apparatus is complicated and costly and was comparatively little used. Following the introduction by Consden et al. (1946) of filter paper as supporting medium, widespread use was made of electrophoresis in clinical biochemistry. This is an example of *zone electrophoresis* (Fig. 4.1(II)). The material is applied locally as a small spot or narrow band and separation occurs into discrete spots or bands. The apparatus for zone electrophoresis is much less costly than that of Tiselius, the procedures are simpler to perform, much less material is required and many runs can be carried out at the same time. Filter paper held the field for several years, but media such as cellulose acetate, agar gel, starch block, starch gel and acrylamide gel have been used subsequently and have important advantages over paper.

In the above methods electrophoresis is carried out in a buffered medium at a fixed pH so that the charge on the particles and hence the rate of migration is stabilised. However, complex mixtures of smaller molecular weight ampholytes can be prepared in which the passage of an electric current produces a gradual increase in the pH of the system from anode to cathode as the components become arranged in order of the increasing pHs of their isoelectric points. This is the basis of the technique of *isoelectric focusing*. When a mixture of high molecular weight ampholytes such as proteins is introduced into such a system covering the pH range of their isoelectric points, the molecules migrate towards the anode or cathode until they arrive at the point at which the pH is that of their isoelectric point (Fig. 4.1(III)). Here there is no net charge so the molecule then remains stationary provided there is no disturbance from convection currents. In

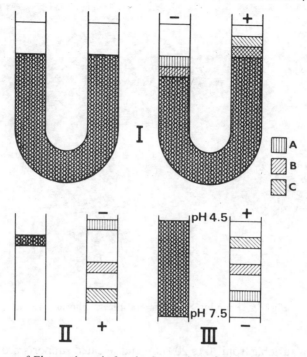

Fig. 4.1. Types of Electrophoresis for the Separation of Three Compounds—A, B, C.
I—Moving Boundary Electrophoresis; II—Zone Electrophoresis; III—Isoelectric Focusing.

association with other forms of electrophoresis this is useful for the finer resolution of mixtures such as isoenzymes and genetic variants but has not yet found a place for routine investigation of serum proteins.

ZONE ELECTROPHORESIS

Horizontal Electrophoresis Tank

The modern multi-purpose horizontal tank can be used for paper, cellulose acetate, agar, starch and acrylamide gels, as well as for immuno-electrophoresis, cross-over (p. 106) and thin-layer electrophoresis. A typical example of this kind of tank is the Shandon 600 model shown in Fig. 4.2 (Shandon Southern). This consists of a one-piece tank moulded in plastic which can be completely immersed for cleaning. It is divided into four compartments, two inner electrode compartments separated by a central partition and two outer buffer compartments separated from the electrode compartments by easily removable partitions fitting into moulded channels. Contact between the two compartments is by cambrelle wicks. The platinum electrodes run the whole length of the compartments. This arrangement prevents pH changes near the electrodes from immediately affecting the buffer in contact with the medium so that the buffer has to be changed less frequently than would otherwise be the case (see p. 74 for the effect of buffer age on cellulose acetate electrophoresis). The

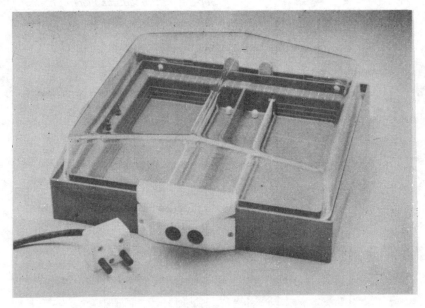

Fig. 4.2. Shandon Southern 600 Electrophoresis Tank.

bridge gap is variable from 10 to 200 mm and serrated supports provide instant and accurate positioning of the shoulder pieces parallel to each other. Quick-fit tension rods for longer strips are provided while strip support points are moulded on the central partition. A cooling platten can be added for thin-layer and gel electrophoresis. In any tank the buffer level should be the same in all compartments to prevent buffer syphoning over the strip, so the walls of the compartments are stepped for easy checking of the buffer level. In other tanks the buffer is levelled by tilting the tank so that the buffer enters all compartments before returning the tank to a horizontal position. A safety micro-switch cuts off the power when the lid is lifted. The compact Shandon 618 tank is specially designed for use with 150 mm long cellulose acetate strips. The bridge gap is constant and the integral membrane holders incorporate positioning holes for the multi-sample applicator.

Factors Influencing the Rate of Migration

Support Media. Paper, the original support medium, has been largely abandoned. Others either act only as a support (cellulose acetate and agar gel) or have properties affecting the separation in some other manner (starch and acrylamide gels).

Those in the first group and paper itself are relatively inert and have little effect on the substances being separated apart from some trailing due to adsorption. Separation depends on the net charge per molecule so that a large molecule with many charges can move the same distance as a smaller one with fewer charges. All media in this group separate plasma proteins into albumin and four or more globulin bands, the degree of resolution varying but the relative positions remaining the same.

The porous gels in the second group, however, have a pore size similar to that of the protein molecules so that a molecular sieve effect is superimposed on the electrical charge separation. Molecules with similar charge/mass ratio but of different sizes are separated, the smaller ones moving more quickly. Thus an α_2 globulin zone derived from one of the media in the first group, if inserted into a starch gel, can then be resolved into 10 to 15 bands. The pore size of acrylamide gels can be varied during polymerisation to allow separation of different ranges of molecular size, and retain molecules above a certain size at the origin. With starch gels, the standard procedure commonly used allows little variation in the pore size. Because of this and their transparency, relative chemical inertness, greater mechanical strength and shorter running times, acrylamide gels are now usually used where high resolution is required. Particular examples are the study of isoenzymes, abnormal haemoglobins, and the genetic variants of transferrin and haptoglobin. It is less satisfactory for routine use for separation of the whole range of plasma proteins.

Composition and Concentration of Buffer. Many buffers of differing composition and pH have been used. In the case of proteins the rate of migration increases as the pH of the buffer is removed from the isoelectric point. At pH 8·6 all proteins are anions and good separations are obtained. The rate of migration also increases with decrease in ionic strength of the buffer but the bands become more diffuse at low ionic strengths, probably due to impaired buffering capacity.

Note. The ionic strength (μ) of a solution is defined as

$$\mu = \tfrac{1}{2} \sum m.v^2$$

where for each ion present, m = molar concentration and v = valency. Thus for calcium chloride, 0·1 mol/l, assuming complete dissociation

$$[Ca^{2+}] = 0·1 \text{ mol/l,}$$
$$[Cl^-] = 0·2 \text{ mol/l,}$$
$$\mu = \tfrac{1}{2}(0·1 \times 2^2 + 0·2 \times 1^2) = 0·3 \text{ mol/l.}$$

Weak acids are regarded as unionised but their salts are fully dissociated. Thus for a barbiturate buffer containing 8·84 g diethylbarbituric acid and 10·3 g/l (0·05 mol/l) of the monosodium salt per litre:

$$\mu = \tfrac{1}{2}(0·05 \times 1 + 0·05 \times 1) = 0·05 \text{ mol/l.}$$

In gel electrophoresis the buffers in the electrode compartments and the medium may differ in concentration, pH or even composition giving a discontinuous buffer system. The ions from the electrode compartment move more quickly through the gel than the protein molecules and as this voltage discontinuity moves along the gel it produces narrower, sharper protein bands.

Voltage, Current, and Heating Effect. The mobility is proportional to the potential gradient along the strip. This is not the same as the voltage across the electrodes recorded on the voltmeter of the power supply. Variations in design of tanks and ionic strengths greatly modify the potential drop between electrodes and the ends of the strips. This potential drop will also vary according to the number of strips in the circuit, the more strips the greater the current passed and the greater the potential drop across the fixed resistance of the buffer compartments. The potential drop across the strip can be measured directly by a high resistance voltmeter to give the potential gradient along the strip. This value (V/cm), suitably qualified by the type of support medium and the ionic strength of the buffer, is the best way to report information concerning voltage.

It is simpler to record the current passed in terms of mA/cm width of support medium. Again the type of support and the ionic strength of the buffer must be noted. The current passed by all the strips also passes through the electrode compartments irrespective of their construction and is measured by the ammeter on the power pack. Reproducible operating conditions are obtained if the current is adjusted in proportion to the total width of the strips in use.

During the course of a run the electrical resistance (R) of the support medium decreases as buffer salts accumulate by evaporation of water due to the heating effect of the current. The current (I) and the voltage (E) cannot both remain constant as R falls as $E = IR$ (Ohm's law). If the current is kept constant the heating effect, $I^2 \times R$ watts, lessens as R falls whereas at constant voltage the heating effect, E^2/R, increases still further as R falls. A constant current device is to be preferred as the changes it introduces tend to be self limiting.

Examples of stabilised power supplies (Fig. 4.3) supplied by Shandon Southern Products include the Vokam 300/25, 400/100 and 500/150 which have continuously variable outputs up to 300, 400 or 500 V and 25, 100 or 150 mA respectively. They can be operated in either constant current or constant voltage mode. The Vokam 300/25 can supply two tanks simultaneously and the most powerful unit can supply four. The smaller units are specially designed for the Shandon Cellulose Acetate system using the electrophoresis tank described above. Upper limits for voltage or current, depending on the mode of operation, can be pre-set on the Vokam 500/150 giving further protection against overheating.

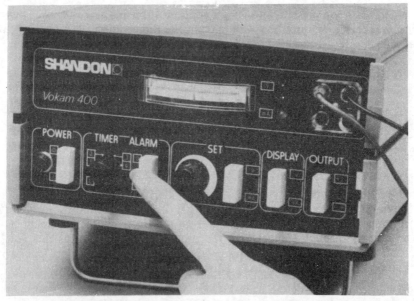

Fig. 4.3. Electrophoresis Power Supply (Shandon Southern). Vokam 400/100.

The heating effect is greater with thin cellulose strips and thick gels than with paper but the tank design minimises it as the small volume of air quickly becomes saturated and the effect of heating is reduced. There is a continuous flow of buffer along the strip towards the centre from each end. These support media normally contain carboxyl or other negatively charged groups. In an electric field these are immobile and a disproportionate flow of positively charged ions of the buffer solution occurs towards the cathode. This flow is termed *electroendosmosis* and opposes the movement of negatively charged proteins towards the anode. The effective centre of the strip is moved towards the cathode and electrophoretic migration is accelerated up to this effective centre and retarded beyond it.

Treatment Following Separation

After electrophoretic separation has ended it is necessary to prevent the separated fractions from diffusing into one another and to make them visible for further assessment. High molecular weight fractions may be prevented from diffusing by precipitation or denaturation provided enzyme activities are not being demonstrated. Such fixation is often achieved by immersion in a solution of acetic or trichloracetic acid or in alcohol or sometimes by heat denaturation by drying in an oven. Visualisation involves various chemical reactions. Many dyes bind readily to protein and may be used to stain all types of protein. Alternatively, chemical reactions may be performed leading to coloured products. These may be used to detect enzymes or may be similar to histochemical stains for selected biochemical substances, e.g. periodic acid-Schiff (PAS) staining for carbohydrate residues. Following staining, excess coloured materials are removed from the strip by washing in an appropriate solvent.

The stained zones may then either be inspected visually and compared with known substances or be cut out and eluted separately to give coloured solutions which can be measured in a colorimeter, using as blank an extract from the unstained part of the strip. The stained strip may also be subjected to scanning densitometry to obtain a permanent record of the separation and, possibly, a quantitative assessment of the different fractions. If transmitted light is used, the support medium may need to be made translucent by impregnating it with an inert liquid of similar refractive index. If reflectance scanning is used, this step is unnecessary. The areas below each section of the curve can be measured during scanning by an integrator or later by a planimeter. Each fraction can then be calculated as a percentage of the total by simple proportion. By careful attention to detail, the precision of these procedures is satisfactory. Variations of dye uptake by different proteins, different dye binding characteristics and deviations from Beer's law can affect the accuracy.

PAPER ELECTROPHORESIS

As this technique is now little used, the reader is referred to earlier editions of this book for details of low and high voltage paper electrophoretic techniques and for the important safety hazards of the latter method.

THIN LAYER ELECTROPHORESIS

The dangers of high voltage electrophoresis can be avoided and in many cases similar results obtained by employing electrophoresis using thin layers of standard adsorbents such as silica gel, alumina or cellulose on glass plates. Specially designed water-cooled thin-layer electrophoresis cells can be used but now thin-layer sheets are successfully employed for this purpose without special cooling, provided only a limited number of separations are carried out together. The Shandon tank is suitable for this.

The combination of thin-layer electrophoresis with chromatography gives a system for biological work which rivals the corresponding high voltage technique. Corrosive locating reagents can be employed when inorganic support media are used. For a review, see Ritschard (1976).

CELLULOSE ACETATE MEMBRANE ELECTROPHORESIS

The use of cellulose acetate strips was introduced by Kohn (1957, 1976), the membranes being developed from existing bacteriological membrane filters. They are white and opaque with a very smooth uniform surface. Several varieties are available. Those supplied as dry strips include Oxoid (Oxo Limited), Celagram II (Shandon), Sepraphore (Gelman, USA), Millipore (Millipore, USA) and Sartorius (Sartorius, Germany). Chemetron of Milan (UK distributors—Whatman Lab-sales Limited) developed Cellogel, a relatively tough plastic-like material in the wet state, supplied in sealed packs containing 30% methanol.

All forms have advantages over paper. The material is microporous with pore size from 1 to 5 μm for dry membranes and 0·1 to 0·5 μm for Cellogel. Such pore sizes prevent spreading of the bands or spots so that excellent separation of plasma proteins is achieved even at low voltages. The α_1 globulin band is always clearly separated from albumin and the β band splits into β_1 and β_2. Because of the higher resolution, cellulose acetate is used to separate isoenzymes, lipoproteins, haemoglobins and for immunoelectrophoresis (p. 98). Smaller samples can be examined while maintaining resolution and the greater sensitivity makes the procedure suitable for screening purposes when many samples can be applied to a single strip and run for a short time, thus facilitating visual comparison.

Minimal protein adsorption eliminates trailing and gives an almost white background after washing. The membrane can be more completely cleared than paper for subsequent assessment using Whitmore's oil or Ondine oil (Shell). Cellogel is cleared with a mixture of acetic acid/methanol/glycerol for transmittance densitometry or its whiteness can be augmented by using formaldehyde and glycerol for reflectance assessment.

Cellulose acetate is more expensive than paper and greater care is needed for satisfactory results. The strip holds little water so loss by evaporation must be minimised by using buffers of lower ionic strength to reduce the current, and thus the heating effect, at a given potential gradient. The migration rate and band width vary inversely with buffer concentration. As a result of evaporation at higher room temperatures, buffer concentration may increase leading to overheating and distorted patterns. It is advisable for buffers to be changed frequently, particularly in warm weather. For the best results, employ fresh buffer for each run by using just enough buffer to cover the bottom of the tank. Where baffles are present between compartments, use wicks which reach to the bottom of the tank.

Technique. The universal tank described earlier is used. Fill the buffer compartments equally to the appropriate mark and place the bridge frame and filter paper shoulders in position; for the best results, change these daily. Instructions on how to use the wet Cellogel strips are given with them. The technique is essentially the same as for dry strips outlined below. Buffers used are usually the lower ionic strength barbitone ones which can be varied to give the required separation. With Cellogel all separations use a 0·04 mol/l barbitone buffer (8·28 g/l). Strip size also depends on the separation required. Strips 25 × 80 mm are used for semi micro-procedures but for micro-samples using multi-applicator techniques, 60 × 150 mm strips are more economical. For any size, the strip should stretch across the bridge with 6 to 12 mm overlap.

Before impregnating with buffer, examine the strip carefully for surface irregularities. Some strips show bands which do not stain with Ponceau S but do take up nigrosin. Others which do not wet uniformly should not be used. To impregnate, float the strip on the surface of the buffer in a flat dish until the white area disappears, then submerge fully. Immersing the strip too quickly traps air bubbles producing areas which then take a long time to soak up any liquid, whether it is buffer, stain or oil. Remove the strip from the bath and blot lightly on both sides with filter paper. There should be no dry white spots; if these are present reimpregnate with buffer. A multi-applicator (Fig. 4.4) can be used to apply several samples once the strip is positioned in the tank. For larger samples apply 10 to 20 μl to each strip using a micro-pipette or capillary along a line about 1 cm on the cathodal side of the midline using a ruler to steady the applicator. The

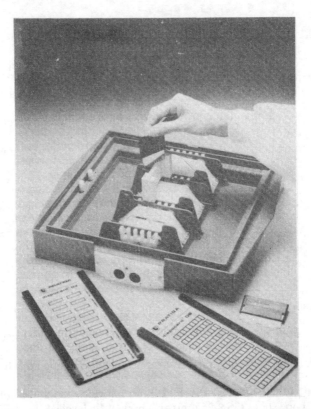

Fig. 4.4. Multi-applicator for Cellulose Acetate Electrophoresis.

streak should stop about 5 mm from the edge of the strip to limit distortion during the run. Add a trace of bromphenol blue solution which combines with the albumin to give a useful indication of the length of the run. Place the separate strips close together but without contact. Use forceps to avoid finger marks which may show up with nigrosin, ninhydrin and lipoprotein stains. Increased evaporation at the edges of the tank is best countered by using two strips carrying no samples, otherwise distorted bands may occur. Such additional strips must be included when calculating the current required in terms of mA/cm of strip.

Examples of runs given by Kohn (1976) include: a separation of 120 to 140 mm in 5 to 7 h with a barbitone buffer pH 8·6, μ 0·07, 0·4 mA/cm, and a strip 160 mm long; a serum protein separation of 50 to 60 mm in 30 to 120 min with a shoulder gap of 60 to 100 mm and a current of 0·4 mA/cm; very sharp separations using a current of 0·8 mA/cm over a 40 to 60 mm gap for 30 to 40 min. Stop the run when the bromphenol blue marker is approaching 10 mm from the bridge edge. Switch off the power and remove the strip carefully without touching the centre. Reverse the polarity for the next run.

Further treatment of the strips depends on analytical requirements. To denature proteins, transfer the strip directly into a bath of trichloracetic acid (50 g/l), then after a few minutes place in the staining solution.

Further details of techniques for individual substances are given in the appropriate sections. See also Kohn and Feinberg (1965).

AGAR GEL ELECTROPHORESIS

The use of agar gel for electrophoresis preceded by several years its use for immunoelectrophoresis (Grabar and Williams, 1953), for which it is the most common medium. Agar gel adsorbs proteins very weakly resulting in well defined bands and making it suitable for isoenzyme separation.

Agar, a dried colloid extracted from seaweed, yields D- and L- galactose and sulphate ions on hydrolysis. It consists of a mixture of molecules of which there are three extremes: neutral agar, agarose; pyruvated agar with few sulphated groups; and a sulphonated galactan (Duckworth and Yaphe, 1971; Izumi, 1971). These charged groups are responsible for the increased electroendosmotic flow with agar. Agarose, free from sulphate, is principally responsible for the gel strength of agar and is a polymer of the disaccharide agarobiose, consisting of 3,6-anhydro-L-galactose and D-galactose. Commercial agaroses contain varying amounts of pyruvate and sulphate groups (Williams, 1972). Earlier agar preparations varied appreciably in composition and it was desirable to purchase a large amount to maintain consistent results. However, the agarose now available is more consistent and is superior to other media for such purposes as the separation of lipoproteins.

Preparation of the Gel. Prepare 1 litre of a stock solution containing 5 to 10 g/l agar or agarose and 0·5 g/l sodium azide (as bacteriocide) in buffer solution. If the gel is to be used to separate isoenzymes, avoid azide. To dissolve, heat in a bacteriological steamer or on a boiling water bath for 1 h, shaking every few minutes. Place portions in 50 ml screw-capped bottles and melt in a boiling water bath as required.

Preparation of the Slides. Place 12 thoroughly cleaned and alcohol-washed glass microscope slides (76 × 26 mm) on a previously levelled sheet of plate glass. Using a warmed fast delivery pipette, layer 2 ml of molten medium onto each slide. Allow to set and store in a moist chamber at room temperature. An air-tight plastic box into which several layers of moist filter paper have been placed is satisfactory.

Wieme (1959) poured enough of the warm solution into a petri dish to cover the bottom and allowed to cool to obtain a completely flat surface. Carefully lay the microscope slides on this and add sufficient warm solution to each slide to give a layer 2 mm thick. Store in a cool place for at least a day before using.

Tanks incorporating one of the specially designed cooled thin-layer electrophoresis cells minimise heating effects.

Details of the use of agar or agarose gels are given under particular substances. For a review of methods see Feinstein (1976).

STARCH GEL ELECTROPHORESIS

Introduced by Smithies in 1955, starch gel combined the virtues of fine texture and absence of protein adsorption with a molecular sieving effect retarding proteins of larger molecular size. Its use has now been largely superseded by acrylamide gel and so details are no longer incorporated but can be found, if needed, in the 5th edition of this book.

ACRYLAMIDE GEL ELECTROPHORESIS

Acrylamide gel has the advantage over starch in that it is easier to prepare and is more inert, the pore size can be varied in a controlled manner and over a wider range, and the technique is simpler with a shorter running time.

The gel is produced by polymerisation of the acrylamide monomer with methylene bis-acrylamide (BIS) as cross-linking agent in the presence of an initiator N,N,N',N'-tetramethylethylenediamine (TEMED) or β-dimethylamino-proprionitrile (DMAP) in a buffer of selected pH and ionic strength and in the presence of a catalyst. Catalysis may be chemical, using ammonium or potassium persulphate to initiate polymerisation as soon as it is introduced into the monomer. Photochemical catalysis with riboflavin and a bright light is an alternative. The rate of polymerisation is proportional to the TEMED concentration which is adjusted so that only 10 to 30 min after mixing is needed. Variations in pore size are obtained by varying the gel concentration and the relative amounts of acrylamide and BIS. As gel concentration increases, the proportion of BIS is decreased and the pore size also decreases.

Electrophoresis has been carried out in cylindrical glass tubes (disc electrophoresis) or by using vertical or horizontal flat-bed equipment. The better resolution obtained with the tubes may be due to several factors. The firmer binding of the gel to the glass tube prevents sample creep and voltage loss down the outside of the gel, while more uniform conditions result from the sample covering the whole surface of the gel instead of being placed in a slot. The short length permits higher voltage gradients without the need for elaborate cooling devices, indeed some cooling is given by the immersion of the rod in the electrode buffer compartments. However, the migration distance for a component may vary by a few per cent in different rods run at the same time, thus introducing some uncertainty when comparing an unknown with a known of nearly the same migration.

Acrylamide Gel Disc Electrophoresis

The Shandon Polyacrylamide Gel Electrophoresis apparatus (Fig. 4.5) enables one piece of equipment to be used both for electrophoresis and destaining. A simple modification enabling it to take longer tubes allows it to be used also for isoelectric focusing (p. 81). The tubes are precision bore glass (5 × 75 mm long) so that all columns are of identical diameter, have the same resistance, pass the same current and so should give reproducible migrations. The tubes should be permanently siliconised by dipping through a solution of dimethyl dichlorosilane in chloroform (50 ml/l) to facilitate removal of the gels. Any unused holes which hold the tubes are sealed with rubber stoppers and buffer is poured in to a depth of 30 to 50 mm so as to cover the tops of the tubes. Due to the position of the lower electrode, the gas bubbles liberated during a run cannot collect in the bottom of the tubes and cut off the current.

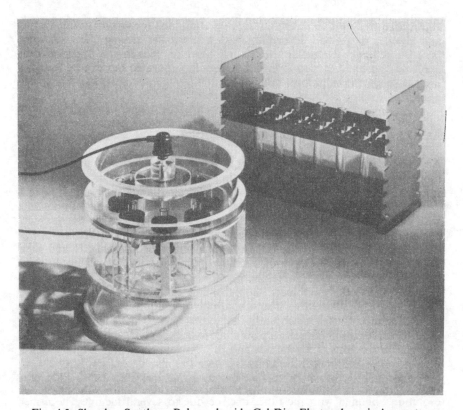

Fig. 4.5. Shandon Southern Polyacrylamide Gel Disc Electrophoresis Apparatus.

Preparation of the Gels. Concentrations of gel from 3 to 30 % have been used but mostly between 3 and 10 %. A common one, 7 %, is suitable for proteins with molecular weights from 400 000 downwards, though for those between 50 000 and 10 000, better resolution may be obtained with a gel concentration of 10 or 15 %. For peptides with molecular weights down to about 1800, 30 % gels are used, or 15 % if glycerol is added to the buffer to prevent excessive diffusion.

Three layers of gel can be used, from the top downwards: (1) a large pore gel, 3%, which contains the sample—the sample gel; (2) a large pore spacer gel, also 3%, in which concentration of the sample begun in (1) is completed; and (3) a small pore running gel, 7%, in which the electrophoresis is carried out. (1) and (2) are primarily anti-convection media, (3) is a sieving as well as anti-convection medium. These are made up as follows:

Small Pore Running Gel. Buffer: Tris-hydrochloric acid, pH 8·9. To 48 ml hydrochloric acid (1 mol/l) add 36·6 g Tris (Tris (hydroxymethyl) methylamine) and 0·23 ml TEMED and make to 100 ml with water. At 4°C in a dark bottle this is stable indefinitely.

Monomer. Dissolve 28·0 g acrylamide and 0·735 g BIS in water and make to 100 ml. Filter and store at 4°C. This has a shelf life of 2 months.

Persulphate solution. Dissolve 140 mg ammonium persulphate in 100 ml water. Store at 4°C in a dark bottle and prepare weekly.

To prepare sufficient running gel for eight tubes mix 2 ml buffer, 4 ml monomer, 2 ml water and 8 ml persulphate.

Large Pore Spacer Gel. Buffer: Tris-hydrochloric acid, pH 6·7. Dissolve 5·98 g Tris and 0·46 ml TEMED in 50 ml water and titrate to pH 6·7 with hydrochloric acid, 1·0 mol/l. Approximately 48 ml is required.

Monomer. Dissolve 10·0 g acrylamide and 2·5 g BIS in water and make to 100 ml. Filter and store at 4°C in a dark bottle.

Riboflavin. Dissolve 4·0 mg in 100 ml water.

Sucrose solution. Dissolve 40 g sucrose in water and make to 100 ml.

To prepare spacer gel mix 1·0 ml buffer, 2·0 ml monomer, 1·0 ml riboflavin and 4·0 ml sucrose.

Sample Gel. Prepare in the same way as for spacer gel and mix 150 μl portion with 2 to 5 μl of sample.

Reservoir Buffer. Tris-glycine, pH 8·3. Dissolve 6·0 g Tris and 28·8 g glycine in water and make to a litre. Dilute 1 to 10 for use and use for only one run.

Notes. Prepare all solutions with freshly distilled or boiled water since it is necessary to keep air out of the final gel. Oxygen inhibits polymerisation and bubbles of air which may form in the gelling process can become trapped in the gel and interfere with subsequent separations.

The monomers have been reported to be neurotoxic and so should be handled with care and not be allowed to come in contact with the skin.

Technique. Arrange the required number of carefully cleaned tubes vertically in a suitable stand and seal the bottom of each with a tight fitting plastic cap. Prepare running gel as described above and as polymerisation begins immediately, transfer it to the tubes within 5 min before it becomes unmanageable. It is best transferred in a syringe to which is fitted a narrow bore polythene tube. In this way the gel can be introduced right into the cap and as the polythene tubing is slowly withdrawn air is forced out of the tube ahead of the gel layer thus avoiding trapping air bubbles which would interfere with polymerisation. Carefully fill the tube to the lower scratch mark in this way. Immediately layer 20 μl of water carefully on to the top of the gel to a depth of 2 to 3 mm so that the interface, which is to be the upper boundary of the running gel, is horizontal. This is best done by using a 20 μl micro-disposable pipette which delivers the correct amount under controlled conditions. Run the water carefully down the side of the tube so that it does not penetrate the gel. Discard the tube if this happens. Leave the gel after setting for at least 30 min before use. If left overnight replace the water with the pH 8·9 buffer diluted 8-fold with water so that the gel remains covered. Then just before use, drain or flick the water or buffer from the gel surface and rinse this with spacer gel solution. Layer 100 μl of spacer gel on to the surface and photopolymerise it by placing a daylight fluorescent light close to the gel surface for 30 to 60 min. Polymerisation which begins within 10 min produces cloudiness and light scattering in the gel. Repeat this process with the sample gel containing the sample to be analysed. Carefully remove the cap which seals the bottom of the tube without detaching the gel from the tube.

As with other forms of electrophoresis it is helpful to include a marker such as bromphenol blue into the sample. In alkaline solution this gives two bands—one of albumin tagged with dye, the other of free dye which moves faster. Besides showing the best time for stopping the run, use of a marker makes it possible to see that the tubes are correctly stacked at the beginning of a run. Add 0·1 ml of bromphenol blue (10 mg/l) to the buffer in the upper reservoir, or add bromphenol blue (5 to 10 g/l) to the sucrose solution used in preparing the large pore sample gel.

Transfer the prepared tubes to the electrophoresis apparatus and place cold buffer solution in the reservoirs. The cold buffer absorbs some of the heat evolved and can eliminate the need to take elaborate cooling precautions. With the upper electrode as cathode use a current of about 1 to 2 mA per tube at the beginning of the run until the bromphenol blue is seen to enter the gel, then increase it to 5 mA. The gel should never feel more than just warm to the touch; should it do so, overheating may be occurring and a rerun at a lower current is desirable. At the end of the run the free dye should be about 10 mm from the end of the gel and about the same distance ahead of the albumin.

The gel has now to be removed from the tube for further treatment. Some practice is advisable if it is not to be damaged. The gel is removed by 'rimming'. Insert a fine needle attached to a syringe between the tube wall and the gel and detach this by gentle rotation. As the needle slowly advances inject a small quantity of water or ethylene glycol monoethyl ether to lubricate the gel tube interface as the gel is freed. The object is to free the gel from the wall without forcing it out at the other end. Care is needed to avoid damaging the gel. Slip a small tube of slightly larger diameter than the gel tube over the lower end of the latter and bring the whole vertical, the gel should then slide from the tube.

Gels are best stained in small tubes unless lengthy washing or leaching is needed. Any of the usual stains may be used. Use only a small quantity of the stain once and discard. When staining is complete it is necessary to remove the excess background dye (destaining) to make the stained bands clearly visible.

Either simple washing or electrolytic destaining is used. For the former, transfer the gels to a wash reagent such as acetic acid (70 ml/l) for proteins and allow the excess dye to diffuse out, which may take up to 24 h with four changes of acid. Electrolytic destaining is quicker, taking up to 2 h if done by passing the current down the length of the rod in the electrophoresis apparatus or as little as 15 min if the current is passed across the gel in an apparatus like the Shandon Transverse Gel Rod Destainer. The latter requires a special power supply providing 1 A DC. In both cases destain in aqueous acetic acid (70 ml/l).

The technique is useful in protein investigations where higher resolution aids separation of genetic variants or isoenzymes of, e.g. alkaline phosphatase. Cerebrospinal fluid proteins have also been usefully studied.

A continuous buffer system can be used omitting the spacer and sampler gels. The sample solution is pipetted directly on to the flat top surface of the running gel. Buffers giving good resolution are (1) barbitone, pH 8·6 (5·16 g sodium barbitone and 0·94 g barbituric acid/l) and (2) phosphate, pH 7·0 (0·883 g KH_2PO_4/l titrated to pH 7·0 with sodium hydroxide). Both gel and reservoir solutions are prepared from the same stock solution. An advantage is that current can be passed through the gels for 30 to 60 min before applying the sample so that any charged impurities pass out of the gel. The serum is diluted with an equal volume of sucrose solution (200 g/l) in distilled water containing a trace of bromphenol blue and 8 to 10 μl is applied. Then an increasing current is applied as before. The bromphenol blue moves as a diffuse streak which is allowed to flow off the gel before electrophoresis ends.

For a review of polyacrylamide gel electrophoresis in clinical biochemistry see Smith *et al.* (1976b).

ISOELECTRIC FOCUSING (ELECTRO-FOCUSING)

In isoelectric analysis a direct current passes through a series of ampholytes the pH of which increases gradually from anode to cathode. If this pH gradient remains stable, proteins and other ampholytes will be repelled from both electrodes and collect in regions where the local pH is identical with the isoelectric point (pI) of the ampholyte. There are two basic requirements: the production of a pH gradient and its stabilisation by avoiding convection currents. It has been mainly used as a research technique for investigating and separating proteins of closely similar structure such as isoenzymes, genetic variants of serum proteins, and immunoglobulins.

Production of pH Gradients

If many different low molecular weight ampholytes, e.g. a mixture of peptides, are dissolved in the electrolyte solution, when a current is passed, the ampholyte with the lowest pI, that is the most acidic, will migrate to the anode where it will be discharged and collect in its isoelectric state. Because of its buffering capacity it will give the surrounding solution a pH equal to the pI. The ampholyte with the next lowest pI, although migrating towards the anode, cannot traverse the zone occupied by the first, because at that pH its molecule would be oppositely charged. It will form an adjacent zone with pH equal to its own pI. Eventually the whole space between the cathode and anode is filled by a series of ampholytes in order of decreasing pI, creating a pH gradient each step of which is defined by one ampholyte at its isoelectric point. The pH range covered and the size and number of steps depends on the number of ampholytes, their relative amounts, pI values and buffering capacity. The technique is capable of resolving proteins with isoelectric points differing by as little as 0·02 pH units. For comprehensive reviews see Haglund (1969), Leaback and Wrigley (1976); and the shorter review by Grant and Leaback (1970).

Svensson (1961, 1962a, 1962b) decided on theoretical grounds that the two pKs of each ampholyte should differ by no more than 1·5 units, each ampholyte should have good conductivity at the pI and enough buffering power to prevent added ampholytes from distorting the pH gradient. At that time there were very few suitable substances available, but examination of the peptides in a haemoglobin hydrolysate confirmed his theoretical predictions. Peptides have disadvantages as carrier ampholytes as they are too similar to proteins and their conductivity varies too much causing heating effects at different points in the gradient. By reacting a mixture of polyethylene polyamines in aqueous solution with acrylic acid (Vesterberg and Svensson, 1966; Vesterberg, 1968) many different compounds containing amino and acid groups are produced with molecular weights between 300 and 1000. The pI range from 4 to 7 contains a large number of compounds but others extend the range to 3 and 10. These ampholytes with the general formula

$$---CH_2-\underset{\underset{NR_2}{\overset{|}{(CH_2)_x}}}{\overset{|}{N}}-(CH_2)_x-\underset{\overset{|}{R}}{N}-CH_2---$$

where x = 2 or 3 and R=H or $-(CH_2)_x-COOH$, are available as the 'Ampholine' carrier ampholytes from LKB Instruments Limited. A selection of pH ranges is available within the limits from 3 to 10, covering 0·5, 2 or 3 pH unit spans.

Stabilisation Against Convection

Of the many techniques used for this purpose (Valmet, 1968), complex density gradient methods have mainly given way to separations in gels.

Density Gradient Electrofocusing. The density gradient is prepared by mixing two solutions: a light one containing carrier ampholytes, distilled water and the sample, and the other dense containing carrier ampholytes, distilled water and a solute. This is usually sucrose, 500 g/l, but ethylene glycol or glycerol, 600 to 700 g/l, have been used, especially for enzymes which react with sucrose. Any solute selected must be non-ionic and give a minimum density difference of 0·12 g/ml between the two ends of the column. A linear gradient mixer is made by LKB Instruments Limited which gives an easily reproducible gradient much more simply than any manual method.

After the separation the liquid is run off from the column into a fraction collector and the pH and absorbance at 260 nm of each fraction is measured. On plotting the pH on the ordinate against the elution volume, the pH gradient is obtained while the absorbances similarly plotted give a series of peaks, the pI values of which are read from the pH gradient (Fig. 4.6). The technique is described in more detail for specific equipment by Haglund (1969) and Grant and Leaback (1970).

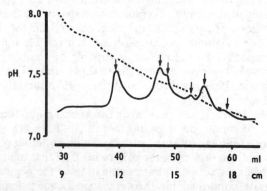

Fig. 4.6. Isoelectric Focusing of Haemoglobin (after Haglund, 1969).
Absorbance at 260 nm (——) shows peaks with pI values (↓) of 7·64, 7·46, 7·44, 7·36, 7·30 and 7·23 as determined from the pH gradient (– – – –). The abscissa shows the elution volume or distance along the column.

Gel Electrofocusing. Gel is used as the stabilising medium, usually acrylamide either in the form of a column or as a thin layer on a glass plate. Agarose has also been used. Gel electrofocusing has the advantages of simple operation, early fixation after the run ends to reduce the possibility of disturbing the bands, and greater variability in applying the sample. Several parallel runs can be made with the thin-layer technique. A disadvantage is that larger molecules such as IgM may not enter the gel.

Isoelectric focusing with acrylamide gel rods can be performed using the apparatus previously described (p. 78), preferably modified to take tubes 110 mm long. Then the upper and lower compartments are further separated by a spacer ring such as in the destainer unit normally supplied with the apparatus. Preparation of gels is as before. The sample can be included when polymerising the gel or layered between the top of the gel and a 2 to 5 mm layer of ampholyte in sucrose (50 g/l) to protect it from the electrode solution. Examples of solutions are (Dale and Latner, 1968, 1969; Leaback and Wrigley, 1976; Smith *et al.*, 1971):

1. For photopolymerisation: acrylamide solution (30 g acrylamide, 1 g BIS, in water to 100 ml) 0·6 ml; riboflavin (140 mg/l) 0·16 ml; Ampholine solution (400 g/l solution, LKB) 0·06 ml; sample 10 to 100 μl; water (containing bromphenol blue, 500 mg/l) 2·4 ml.
2. For chemical polymerisation: replace riboflavin in the above with 2 mg potassium persulphate.

If the sample is to be applied after polymerisation proceed as follows. Prepare the gel mixture as above but omitting the sample, add to the gel tube to within 5 to 10 mm of the top and allow to polymerise. Place the tube in the apparatus and add 2 ml of a freshly prepared aqueous solution containing 50 mg sucrose and 25 μl Ampholine solution (400 g/l). Layer under this 50 μl of a solution containing 1 to 5 mg of protein sample and 100 mg sucrose dissolved in 1 ml water. It is suggested that the current be passed for about 30 min before applying the sample so that the pH gradient is set up and ionic products of polymerisation are removed. Addition of bromphenol blue, best before polymerisation, is valuable since its subsequent movement shows how rapidly the pH gradient is forming as well as the minimum time for the focusing to occur. It migrates through the gel more rapidly than the proteins.

It is necessary to protect the carrier ampholytes from anodic oxidation and cathodic reduction for which purpose the electrodes are surrounded by acid (sulphuric, 2 ml/l) and base (ethanolamine, 4 ml/l) respectively. During electrolysis the acid remains in the anode vessel because of the attraction of the sulphate ions to the anode. The acid above the gel gives a positive charge to the carrier ampholytes which are repelled from the anode and so are confined to the tube; the converse occurs at the cathode. The ethanolamine is placed in the lower reservoir which is thus the cathode. Then insert the gel tubes into the upper (anode) reservoir. Arrange for electrophoresis with the spacer ring necessitated by the longer tubes. Place the sulphuric acid in the upper reservoir without disturbing any sample, if this was applied after polymerisation, and avoid trapping any air bubbles in the top of the tubes. During the run, usually carried out at room temperature, gradually increase voltage to give a maximum current of 2 mA per tube with a maximum 350 V using short tubes and 700 V with the longer ones. The time needed for a run is between 1 and 5 h. By the end of the run the current will have fallen almost to zero. The gels are then removed from the tubes by rimming as described previously (p. 80). The carrier ampholytes stain strongly with most protein stains so have to be removed before applying localising agents, which can be done as described above (p. 80) either by successive washings with trichloracetic acid (50 g/l) or electrophoretically. The carrier ampholytes may inhibit enzymes by chelating metal activators and are best removed before substrates are introduced. Dialysis against the buffer used for the enzyme system was used by Smith *et al.* (1971) for alkaline phosphatase isoenzymes. No metals were included in the buffer at this stage for the same reason.

LKB Instruments Limited now produce prepared thin-layer gels containing ampholytes as Ampholine PAG Plates.

ISOTACHOPHORESIS

Isotachophoresis is an electrophoretic technique in which charged molecules are separated on the basis of differences in net mobility. It differs from zone electrophoresis in using conditions under which the majority of the current is carried by the ions being separated. The electrical conditions in an iso-tachophoretic system produce very sharp boundaries between sample zones as well as concentrating sample components present in very small amounts. At the start of a separation a sample is introduced between two electrolytes of different mobilities. These are referred to as the leading and terminating electrolytes. During electrophoresis, anions having a mobility between those of the leading and terminating electrolytes separate into zones between these electrolytes. Variations of the technique can be used for analytical and preparative work. LKB Instruments Limited market both a capillary system for analytical separations (Tachophor) and a preparative system (Uniphor). Isotachophoresis has been used to separate complex mixtures of proteins, small ions such as ATP, ADP, pyruvate and succinate, amino acids and fatty acids. Although not generally used in clinical biochemistry as yet, it is a powerful research tool. For a review of theory and applications see Everaerts *et al.* (1976).

For general reviews on electrophoretic techniques see Morris and Morris (1976), Sargent and George (1975) and Smith (1976a).

REFERENCES

Consden R., Gordon A. H., Martin A. J. P. (1946). *Biochem. J*; **40**: 38.
Dale G., Latner A. L. (1968). *Lancet*; **1**: 847.
Dale G., Latner A. L. (1969). *Clin. Chim. Acta*; **24**: 61.
Duckworth M., Yaphe W. (1971). *Carbohydrate Research*; **16**: 189, 435.
Everaerts F. M., Beckers J. L., Verheggen T. P. (1976). *Isotachophoresis. Theory, Instrumentation and Applications.* Amsterdam: Elsevier.
Feinstein, A. (1976). In *Chromatographic and Electrophoretic Techniques*, Vol. 2, 4th ed. *Zone Electrophoresis.* (Smith I., ed). London: William Heinemann Medical Books.
Grabar P., Williams C. A. Jr. (1953). *Biochim. Biophys. Acta*; **10**: 193.
Grant G. M., Leaback D. H. (1970). Shandon Instruments Applications, No. 31. Shandon Southern Products Limited, Runcorn, Cheshire.
Haglund H. (1969). In *Methods of Biochemical Analysis*, Vol. 19 (Glick, D., ed) p. 1. London, New York: Academic Press.
Izumi K. (1971). *Carbohydrate Research*; **17**: 227.
Kohn J. (1957). *Clin. Chim. Acta*; **2**: 297.
Kohn J. (1976). In *Chromatographic and Electrophoretic Techniques*, Vol. 2, 4th ed. *Zone Electrophoresis.* (Smith, I., ed) p. 90. London: William Heinemann Medical Books.

Kohn J., Feinberg J. G. (1965). *Electrophoresis on Cellulose Acetate, Instrument Applications No.* 11. Shandon Southern Products Limited, Runcorn, Cheshire.

Leaback D. H., Wrigley C. W. (1976). In *Chromatographic and Electrophoretic Techniques,* Vol. 2, 4th ed. *Zone Electrophoresis.* (Smith I., ed) p. 272. London: William Heinemann Medical Books.

Morris C. J. O. R., Morris P. (1976). *Separation Methods in Biochemistry,* 2nd ed. London: Pitman.

Ritschard W. J. (1976). In *Chromatographic and Electrophoretic Techniques,* Vol. 2, 4th ed. *Zone Electrophoresis.* (Smith I., ed) p. 66. London: William Heinemann Medical Books.

Sargent J. R., George S. G. (1975). *Methods in Zone Electrophoresis,* 3rd ed. BDH Chemicals Limited, Poole, Dorset.

Smith I. ed. (1976a). *Chromatographic and Electrophoretic Techniques,* Vol. 2, 4th ed. *Zone Electrophoresis.* London: William Heinemann Medical Books.

Smith I., Leaback D. H., Payne J. W., Brownstone A. (1976b). In *Chromatographic and Electrophoretic Techniques,* Vol. 2, 4th ed. *Zone Electrophoresis.* (Smith I., ed) pp. 210, 250, 321, 378, 387. London: William Heinemann Medical Books.

Smith I., Lightstone P. J., Perry J. D. (1971). *Clin. Chim. Acta;* **35**: 59.

Smithies O. (1955). *Biochem. J;* **61**: 629; *Nature;* **175**, 307.

Svensson H. (1961). *Acta Chem. Scand;* **15**: 425.

Svensson H. (1962a). *Acta Chem. Scand;* **16**: 456.

Svensson H. (1962b). *Arch. Biochem. Biophys;* Suppl. **1**: 132.

Tiselius A. (1937). *Trans. Farad. Soc;* **33**: 524.

Tiselius A. (1939). *Harvey Lectures;* **35**: 57.

Valmet E. (1968). *Science Tools;* **15**: 8. LKB-Producter AB, Stockholm.

Vesterberg O. (1968). British Patent No. 1106818, July 17, 1968.

Vesterberg O., Svensson H. (1966). *Acta Chem. Scand;* **20**: 820.

Wieme R. J. (1959). *Clin. Chim. Acta;* **4**: 317.

Williams K. W. (1972). *Laboratory Practice;* **21**: 667.

5
IMMUNOCHEMICAL METHODS

Highly specific and sensitive immunological methods and reagents are now regularly used in clinical biochemistry. This chapter describes the general principles of the more common methods and gives some indication of their use. More specific examples are described elsewhere in the book in the context of the particular substance being determined by these methods.

The study of immunology arose out of the investigation of the protective mechanisms of the body to infection and was later extended to the recognition of the different blood groups. Although modern immunology has now become an autonomous laboratory discipline, use is made of the binding of antigen by antibody, directly or indirectly, in several techniques in clinical biochemistry.

GENERAL BACKGROUND

For many infectious diseases, recovery from an attack confers protection or immunity, often long-lasting, from further attacks by the same organism, or in some cases closely-related organisms, but this immunity does not extend to other infections. Such observations indicate three important aspects: there is some mechanism whereby the *memory* of the infection is retained, the protection shows *specificity* for the organism concerned, and the body recognises the introduction of foreign material into it implying a mechanism for the differentiation between 'self' and 'non-self'. Applications in clinical biochemistry have mainly exploited the specificity of the response.

The immunological responses of the body to the entry of foreign substances, *immunogens*, either in pure form, in mixtures or in the form of foreign cells fall into two main types.

Firstly there is the development of specific chemical antagonists to the immunogen, referred to as *antibodies*, which are released into the blood and other body fluids. These humoral antibodies combine with the *antigen* reducing its biological activity either directly, as in the inactivation of a bacterial toxin, or indirectly, by coating foreign organisms and making them more easily engulfed by phagocytic cells. The terms antigen and immunogen, are not synonymous. An immunogen is a preparation of a substance whose introduction into the body provokes an immune response. An antigen is a substance that will react specifically with an antibody. Thus an antigen is not necessarily immunogenic whereas all immunogens are antigens.

Secondly there is the development of *cell-mediated immunity* in which specific cells are developed which partake in more complex reactions such as the delayed hypersensitivity to the tubercle bacillus manifested in the Mantoux reaction or in the rejection of skin or organ transplants.

A central role in these immunological defence mechanisms is played by the small lymphocytes which are produced in the bone marrow and circulate in the blood and lymph. They only become immunologically competent after further processing. The thymus converts them into *T-lymphocytes* which then colonise the spleen and parts of the lymph nodes. Other lymphocytes are converted into *B-lymphocytes* at a site uncertain in man but identified in the chick as a gut-associated structure, the Bursa of Fabricius, hence the prefix B. Such B-lymphocytes form the lymphoid follicles of lymph nodes. Although the B- and T-lymphocytes cannot be differentiated by light microscopy their roles differ.

B-lymphocytes produce a humoral antibody when stimulated by an immunogen. This involves the development of rough endoplasmic reticulum, whereby the cell is transformed into a *plasma cell.* T-lymphocytes are concerned with the development of cell-mediated immunity and are transformed by immunogen exposure into larger cells, *lymphoblasts,* devoid of the rough endoplasmic reticulum characteristic of a cell synthesising and releasing protein. The cytoplasm contains many free ribosomes and the cells probably produce antibody which is retained at the cell surface. The T-lymphocytes cooperate with the B-lymphocytes, increasing their antibody production by a mechanism still obscure. It is probable that the surface antibody of the T-cells binds the immunogen and assists in its presentation to the B-lymphocyte. Although these transformed lymphocytes have important roles, some revert to small lymphocytes and become the so-called *memory cells* preserving the knowledge of the immunogenic stimulus.

For a useful account of the general background of immunology, see Roitt (1984).

Antigen–Antibody Reactions

The humoral antibodies released by the plasma cells are the immunoglobulin proteins. Parts of the molecule (Fig. 5.1) show variable amino acid sequences affording a structural explanation for antibody specificity. All the evidence indicates that formation of an antibody with a particular specificity involves the synthesis of a unique protein. According to the *clonal selection theory* a particular B-lymphocyte has the genetic information to synthesise only a unique antibody molecule. This will be of one immunoglobulin class, e.g. IgG, have one type of light chain, e.g. kappa, and have unique variable portions within the heavy and light chains. This immunoglobulin produced by the dormant cell is present in the cell surface where it acts as a receptor. If an immunogen enters the body, a particular sequence of amino acids on its molecular surface can stimulate antibody production. This part of the molecule, the antigen determinant, will be in contact with many lymphocytes but will tend to bind to the surface immunoglobulin for which it has highest affinity. This binding is thought to trigger the division of the recipient lymphocyte and its transformation into a plasma cell from which a clone of cells develops, all identical in genetic constitution and producing the same immunoglobulin as the parent cell.

Mention has been made of the *combination of antigen and antibody.* This combination does not involve the formation of a fixed chemical compound by forming covalent links, but involves rather weaker intermolecular forces. This results in an aggregation of antigen and antibody molecules in differing molecular proportions in varying circumstances, held by bonds of variable strength. There are four main types of linkages:

Coulombic forces. These arise from the electrostatic attraction between oppositely charged groups in the antigen and in the amino acid side chains of the immunoglobulin. The force varies inversely with the square of the distance between the groups.

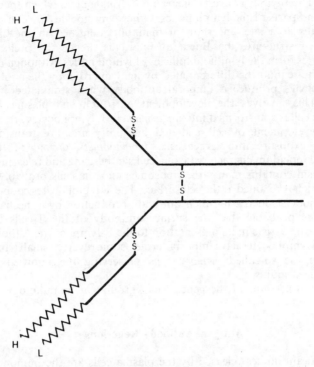

Fig. 5.1 Schematic Diagram Showing Part of the Structure of an Immunoglobulin Molecule.
L = light chain, H = heavy chain, /\/\/\ = variable region.

Hydrogen bonds. These are weak bonds produced between hydrogen-donating groups such as –OH, –NH₂, –COOH and the carbonyl groups of the peptide bonds, –CO–NH–, of a polypeptide molecule. Their formation requires the presence of the two groups at the correct spatial separation.

Hydrophobic forces. These are formed between non-polar groups which approach so closely that they exclude water molecules between them. Water molecules in contact with such groups do not form hydrogen bonds as they do with one another and their displacement from the non-polar surfaces aids such bonding thereby resulting in a lower energy state, favouring the close apposition of non-polar areas of antigen and antibody.

Van der Waals' forces. These forces depend on the interaction between electron clouds surrounding approaching molecules, probably by generating oscillating dipoles. The force of attraction varies inversely as the seventh power of the distances between the interacting parts of the molecules involved.

It will be obvious from the nature of these bonds that the binding force between the antigen and antibody will be strongest when their three-dimensional shapes are complementary thereby permitting as close an apposition as possible. The forces will be strengthened if the appropriate charged group or groups forming hydrogen bonds are also located opposite one another when this close fit is obtained. The binding sites on the immunoglobulins are located in the variable part of the light and heavy chains near their N terminal ends (Fig. 5.1). Within these sections of the chains are hypervariable regions which are thought to be brought close together by folding of the chains thereby producing a highly specific area on the immunoglobulin surface. This binding site, with dimensions about 2.5×2 nm, includes a shallow groove, 1.5×0.6 nm, similar to the substrate-combining site in an enzyme molecule.

Such a binding site will only accommodate a small determinant on the antigen. If this is a protein, the determinant will be only a few amino acids in length. As the protein polypeptide chain is folded, the determinants are amino acid sequences in those parts of the chain in the surface. One molecule will usually contain several different determinants leading to the production of antibodies combining with different parts of the antigen molecule. The determinants will differ if the antigen chain is partly unfolded by denaturation.

Antibody Affinity and Avidity. The terms *avidity* and *affinity* are often used synonymously and both relate to the energy of binding of an antigen–antibody combination. Strictly speaking, however, avidity refers specifically to the energy of reaction relating to the antibody and affinity to the energy of reaction relating to the antigen. Numerically, the avidity of the antibody for the antigen equals the affinity of the antigen for the antibody. In the simplest reaction of an antigen (Ag) with an antibody (Ab) the two combine forming a complex (Ag–Ab) which can dissociate again as the binding forces are relatively weak. Thus we can define an equilibrium constant (K_a) for the reaction

$$Ag + Ab \rightleftharpoons Ag\text{–}Ab$$

where

$$K_a = \frac{[Ag\text{–}Ab]}{[Ag][Ab]}.$$

This is similar to enzyme – substrate combination (p. 481). High avidity antibodies bind the antigen strongly and thus have a high K_a value. When half the antibody sites are occupied by antigen

$$K_a = 1/[Ag] \text{ or } [Ag] = 1/K_a.$$

Thus the antigen concentration at half saturation of the antibody will be low for high avidity antibodies and may be of the order of 100 pmol/l ($K_a = 10^{-11}$ l/mol).

This is the condition for a single antigen determinant and a particular antibody. In practice an antigen bears many determinants and the antiserum produced contains many immunoglobulins with different specificities and avidities, belonging to different classes and with both types of light chain. Not only is the antigen multivalent, but many antibody molecules have more than one binding site. Thus IgG is divalent having two binding sites (Fig. 5.1) while dimer IgA and pentameric IgM have a higher valency, at least 5 for IgM and occasionally 10 if the antigen is small enough to avoid trouble from steric hindrance. A more appropriate representation of the interaction between the antigen (Ag) and the resultant mixture of antibodies (Ab) in the antiserum would be:

$$x\, Ag + y\, Ab \rightleftharpoons Ag_x\text{–}Ab_y$$

with an equilibrium constant of

$$K = \frac{[Ag_x\text{–}Ab_y]}{[Ag]^x[Ab]^y}.$$

Again a high value for K indicates a high avidity of the antiserum for the antigen.

A further factor influencing the immunoglobulin composition of an antiserum is the dose of immunogen used. A small dose will be taken up by those B-lymphocytes whose surface immunoglobulins have a high avidity for its determinants and these will be reproduced by the resulting plasma cells. With a larger dose, some immunogen will remain to combine with lower avidity receptors, so reducing the avidity of the final mixture in the antiserum. Proteins from a particular animal species may show different responses when injected into several different species. For example, during evolution there has been gradual modification of the molecular structure of albumin and the complete albumin molecule is species-specific. However, those determinants which are immunologically identical in the albumin of different species would not be recognised as 'foreign'.

Such factors make the use of antisera as immunological reagents quite different from the use of most chemical reagents. Each antiserum raised to a particular immunogen will be a different mixture of immunoglobulins of varying individual valency and avidity. The response of an animal to repeated injection of an immunogen in an effort to produce antibodies is unpredictable and the raising of good antisera with desirable properties for analytical use is often a matter of chance. Each antiserum will vary in its avidity for a particular antigen and will show a varying tendency to react with related antigens depending on whether some of their determinants have a high affinity for particular components of the antibody mixture or not. Thus the specificity of each antiserum will vary. Such antibody heterogeneity is often a disadvantage when antisera are used as reagents. Recently, techniques for raising antibodies identical in specificity and avidity for a single antigenic determinant have become available. Such *monoclonal antibodies* (p. 113) overcome the problems of heterogeneity inherent in polyclonal antisera and provide very versatile reagents for many applications in biology and medicine.

Finally in this discussion of antigen–antibody reactions, mention should be made of *haptens*. These are small molecules (molecular weight < 500) which are not themselves immunogenic, but which are able to combine with an antibody if such is available. If the hapten is linked to a protein molecule such as bovine serum albumin (BSA) it will be present in one or more of the BSA determinants. Some of the antibodies will then react with the hapten itself as well as the hapten–BSA complex. This method has been used to raise antisera to molecules such as steroids, thyroid hormones and small peptides. The specificity of the antisera will depend on the way the hapten is covalently linked to BSA and whether its characteristic groups are thereby exposed or concealed.

Detection of the Reaction Between Antigens and Antibodies *in vitro*

In the wider field of immunology a variety of techniques are available to detect the presence of a particular antigen or antibody by demonstrating their combination. In clinical biochemistry, most of the present applications rely either on the precipitation of the antigen–antibody complex or on competition between labelled and unlabelled antigen for a limited and fixed number of antibody binding sites (saturation analysis). The latter principle is used when concentrations of reactants are too low to precipitate antigen–antibody complexes. A brief account of the principles involved in methods utilising precipitation is given below. Saturation analysis is considered in Chapter 6 (p. 110).

PRECIPITATION METHODS

General Considerations

If a multivalent antigen and a multivalent antibody are mixed, complexes of varying size are produced. Fig. 5.2 indicates diagrammatically the reaction between a trivalent antigen (Ag) and a divalent antibody (Ab), such as IgG. When there is a very large Ag excess, the complexes are mainly in the form Ag_2Ab (Fig. 5.2A) but with rather more Ab, some slightly larger complexes such as Ag_3Ab_2, Ag_4Ab_3 may exist. Such complexes are relatively small colloidal particles which remain in suspension. With better proportions of Ag and Ab, there is the possibility of forming large, lattice-like structures containing the repeating unit Ag_2Ab_3 (Fig. 5.2B). This unit corresponds to the usual ideas of valencies of atoms combining to form compounds. With a considerable excess of Ab, the complexes will again be smaller with the limiting composition $AgAb_3$ and some Ag_2Ab_5 if Ab excess is less marked (Fig. 5.2C).

When the proportion of Ag and Ab is optimal, large insoluble aggregates form as precipitates. The supernatant fluid contains virtually no Ag or Ab and the

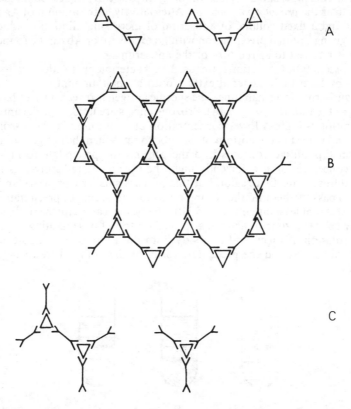

Fig. 5.2 Schematic Representation of the Combination of a Trivalent Antigen (Δ) with a Divalent Antibody (>—<).

A, Antigen excess with complexes Ag_2Ab and Ag_3Ab_2. B, Optimal proportions with the formation of a large lattice approximating to $(Ag_2Ab_3)_n$. C, Antibody excess with complexes $AgAb_3$ and Ag_2Ab_5.

amount of precipitate is maximal. As excess Ag is added, the complexes become smaller and the precipitate diminishes until eventually all the complexes are soluble and no precipitation reaction is visible. In Ag excess the supernatant fluid can combine with added Ab as unoccupied binding sites are available. With Ab excess, however, the solubility of the reaction product varies. In the simple description given (Fig. 5.2, p. 91) the Ag is considered as having three identical determinants, but in practice antigens may bear up to 50 different determinants on their surface. The Ab component is a mixture with different avidities for these determinants and some will have a higher valency than two if IgA dimer and IgM pentamer are present. The size of the complexes in Ag excess depends mainly on the Ab valency and they tend to be relatively small and soluble whereas in Ab excess, the complexes reflect the larger valency of the Ag and are frequently insoluble, particularly if rabbit antisera are used. With horse antisera, the Ab mixture is often such that the precipitate redissolves in Ab excess.

Thus if decreasing quantities of Ag are added to a series of tubes containing a fixed amount of Ab produced in the rabbit, no precipitate appears in the first tubes, then an increasing amount is apparent up to a maximum. In later tubes, where the amount of Ag diminishes, less precipitate is apparent and free Ab is present in the supernatant. This solubility in the early tubes of the series is referred to as the *prozone phenomenon*. Alternatively, if the amount of Ag is kept constant and a fixed volume of antiserum of increasing dilution is added, the dilution giving optimal precipitation with no excess Ag or Ab can be found. This dilution is referred to as the *titre* of the antiserum.

Such precipitation reactions are used in bacteriology to identify bacterial antigens by layering a bacterial extract onto a small amount of concentrated specific antiserum in a small tube. The specific antigen is revealed by a precipitate forming at the interface (Fig. 5.3A). Prozone effects are unlikely if the antiserum concentration is high. A lower concentration of antiserum may be dissolved in agar gel and placed in the bottom of the tube to set. When the antigen solution is placed on top, antigen diffuses into the gel and the precipitate forms. If the antigen concentration is sufficiently high, the precipitate redissolves as further antigen diffuses into that region but this releases smaller complexes and extra antigen to pass further into the gel and reprecipitate. A ring of precipitate moves down the tube, at least initially (Fig. 5.3B). The system can be further refined if the antibody gel has a zone of plain agar placed on top of it, separating it from the antigen solution. Antigen and antibody both diffuse into this middle zone in opposite directions and the precipitate forms at the point where their relative

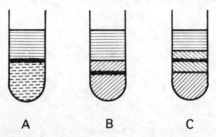

A   B   C

Fig. 5.3. Precipitin Reactions in Tubes.

A, Antigen solution layered on antibody solution. B, Antigen solution layered on antibody in agar. C, Antigen solution layered on plain agar which covers the antibody in agar gel. The precipitate forms in the plain agar.

concentrations are optimal. The lower the antigen concentration, the nearer the precipitate is to the top of the intermediate gel (Fig. 5.3C).

The methods used in clinical biochemistry can be classified in various ways. The authors have subdivided them into those in which the precipitation reaction occurs as a result of simple diffusion of antigen, antibody or both, and those in which an electric field is used to speed up the interaction. Another method uses nephelometry to measure the degree of aggregation of antigen with antibody in solution.

Methods Based on Simple Diffusion

The medium in which diffusion occurs is usually agar gel although it is possible to use cellulose acetate or Cellogel. In the simplest technique, the gel contains a constant concentration of antibody and the antigen diffuses into it. Double diffusion methods allow both antigen and antibody to pass into normal agar gel and react on contact. The antigen and antibody may be placed in separate wells in the gel as in the Ouchterlony technique. Alternatively, preliminary separation of an antigen mixture may be achieved by electrophoresis before the immunological step occurs as in immunoelectrophoresis and immunofixation.

Radial Immunodiffusion

This widely used method for antigen quantitation, introduced by Mancini *et al.* (1963, 1965), is a single diffusion type. Most reactions are carried out in agar gel but methods using cellulose acetate either unbacked (Vergani *et al.*, 1967) or backed (Nerenberg, 1972) conserve antiserum.

The agar gel incorporates a mono-specific antiserum at a dilution appropriate for the range of antigen concentration desired. A well is cut in the gel into which is placed a standard volume of antigen solution which then diffuses into the surrounding gel (Fig. 5.4). The antigen–antibody complex is revealed as a ring of precipitate. As more antigen enters the gel, its excess redissolves the precipitate (p. 92) and the soluble complexes diffuse some meeting more antibody while the size of the precipitate ring gradually increases. Eventually all the antigen has entered the gel and most has been precipitated. The ring then remains stationary. As there is less tendency for the antibody to diffuse, being present in equal

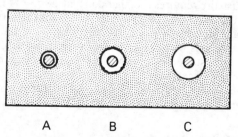

A   B   C

Fig. 5.4. Radial Immunodiffusion at Various Stages of Development with Time.

The wells (shaded) are of diameter, d. In A the precipitin ring is forming, is still increasing at B and has reached its final diameter, D, in C. To a first approximation, the clear areas within the rings have been denuded of antibody which is present at its original concentration in the stippled area. The diameter is linearly related to the logarithm of the antigen concentration in B, while D^2 is linearly related to the antigen concentration itself in C.

concentration throughout the original gel, the antibody present in the precipitate is mainly derived from the gel within the ring. If this is of diameter D, and the well is of diameter d, the amount of antibody consumed is approximately proportional to $(D^2 - d^2) \times \pi/4$, the area of gel concerned. Thus the amount of antigen (Ag) which is related to the amount of antibody consumed will be given by

$$Ag = C(D^2 - d^2) \times \pi/4 = C_1 D^2 - C_2$$

where C, C_1 and C_2 are constants if d is fixed. If the volume of antigen solution is kept constant, there is then a linear relationship between Ag concentration and the square of the diameter of the ring. If D^2 is plotted on the abscissa against concentration on the ordinate, the line should have a constant negative intercept on the latter. In practice, a series of wells is cut into a single layer of gel and standards are placed in some. The concentration of the test samples is then determined.

At high concentrations of antigen, the ring may be large and diffuse or even not apparent if gross antigen excess exists. The sample should be diluted to bring it into the concentration range suitable for the antiserum concentration in the gel. For low concentrations of antigen, the alternatives are either its preliminary concentration or the use of a lower antiserum concentration. Commercially prepared agar gel plates are available for a variety of antigens and some cover more than one concentration range. They are widely used in the determination of different classes of immunoglobulins by using antisera directed against the specific heavy chains of these molecules (p. 428). They are satisfactory for the mixture of immunoglobulins present in normal and most pathological sera, provided the standard is composed of many different immunoglobulins of the relevant class. The determination of paraproteins (p. 418) is less satisfactory as the avidity of different antisera for such a unique immunoglobulin is likely to vary (p. 431).

The time taken to reach a stable ring diameter may be 3 days so that the advantage of simplicity is offset by the delay in obtaining a result. The diffusion may be speeded up by incubation at 37°C. Alternatively, the ring diameter has been measured before equilibrium is reached. There is an empirical, linear relationship between the logarithm of the concentration and the ring diameter over a limited range. This non-equilibrium method is more difficult to control, being sensitive to temperature. Also the linearity only holds for certain stages of the diffusion process. Strict adherence to operating conditions is necessary and the reproducibility is usually less satisfactory than the method which produces a stable final ring. It usually requires a higher concentration of antiserum but has the advantage when determining immunoglobulins that the serum sample does not need preliminary dilution as is often the case with the other method. Commercially prepared gels with precut wells are again available. If all the wells are not used at once, then standards covering the required range must be included with each set of unknowns examined. In the case where the ring development is allowed to go to completion however, only one set of standards needs to be run with each plate even if the unknowns are put up in different batches.

Double Diffusion Method of Ouchterlony

In this method (Ouchterlony, 1948, 1967) wells are cut in a plate of agar gel. The antigen and antibody are placed in adjacent holes and diffuse towards one another to produce a line of precipitate where their relative concentrations are optimal. The technique is used mainly for qualitative study of antigens or antibodies. For this purpose the wells are usually arranged in a regular pattern as in Fig. 5.5 so that, e.g. up to six antigen solutions can be placed equidistant from a single antiserum located in the central well. Diffusion occurs radially from each well but the area of main interest lies between each antigen well and the central well. Fig. 5.5 shows the different reactions which can be obtained.

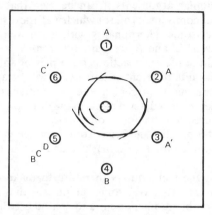

Fig. 5.5. Ouchterlony Double Diffusion Technique.
The antibody is in the centre well and the antigens in wells 1–6.

The precipitin line is a hyperbola with its concave side towards the slower diffusing substance, usually the antiserum. The arcs formed by the antigens in wells 1 and 2 are clearly completely continuous although the main part of the arc lies further from well 1 than from 2 when measured along the line joining either well to that in the centre. The difference in position indicates that the antigen concentration is higher in well 1 than in well 2 but the continuous arc, the *reaction of identity*, indicates that the antigens in the two wells are qualitatively identical in so far as the particular antiserum is concerned. The arcs join along a line defining a constant concentration of antigen derived by diffusion from both wells. Although the antigen probably has several determinants, those detected by this antiserum are identical for wells 1 and 2. Furthermore there is apparently no other antigen present which can be detected by the antiserum. This statement is made cautiously as it is possible that another antigen is present in such excess that the arc is either very weak and diffuse or fails to form at all. The arcs are only sharp when the relative amounts of antigen and antibody are near the optimum and hence it is advisable to test several dilutions of the antigen solution before concluding that other components reacting with the antiserum are indeed absent. The same argument applies to the antigens in the other wells.

In the case of the arcs derived from the antigens in wells 2 and 3 the *reaction of partial identity* is seen. The arcs are continuous as before but in addition there is a 'spur' projecting from the line towards well 2. This indicates that although the antigens share common determinants, that in well 3 has additional determinants recognised by the antiserum. The appropriate antibodies for these have not been precipitated along the main arc as it passes in front of well 2 and pass through to precipitate with antigen diffusing only from well 3. The main arc represents the reaction with the common determinants. If the antigen in wells 1 and 2 is called **A**, then that in well 3 may be designated **A'**.

The antigens in wells 3 and 4 each produce a single arc but these cross completely with no attempt at confluence. This is the *reaction of non-identity* and arises from the fact that the antigens have no common determinants and hence the specific antibodies for each diffuse past the site of reaction with the other antigen. Thus the antigen in well 4 can be called B and has nothing in common with A' or A for this antiserum. The situation may differ with a different antiserum. Using similar arguments it can be seen that the antigen in well 5 contains at least three components one of which is B, the others being called C and D. Antigen C shares some determinants with C' in well 6 but C' lacks some present in C. However, C' and A are quite different.

It is possible to find different reactions for a pair of antigens on testing with different antisera of quite different specificity. It will be apparent that this will depend on the determinants present in the two antigens and the presence or absence of antibodies to such determinants in the different antisera. Occasionally artefacts are produced in the form of duplication of precipitin lines. The duplicates are exactly parallel and arise from a change in the physico-chemical conditions during diffusion, e.g. a marked change in temperature or ionic strength.

The main role of the technique is therefore to make qualitative studies of antigens and antisera. It gives some guide to the number of separate antigen–antibody combinations present and can be used to study the purity of antigen or antibody preparations. It is less satisfactory for quantitative work although a rough assessment of concentration of antigen can be derived by comparison of the position of the arc with that from standards.

Immunoelectrophoresis

This important combination of electrophoretic separation and immunological detection was introduced by Grabar and Williams (1953, 1955). It is a delicate tool for the qualitative investigation of complex protein mixtures in biological fluids and has been especially useful in the investigation of immunoglobulins, paraproteins and complement components. For a review of the technique see Arquembourg (1975).

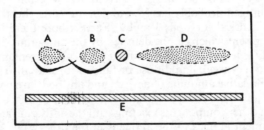

Fig. 5.6. The Principle of Immunoelectrophoresis.
The antigen mixture was originally placed in the circular well, C, cut into the agar gel while antibody was placed in the trough, E, once electrophoresis was complete. A, B and D are the areas occupied by three antigens at the end of electrophoresis and following further diffusion the arcs of precipitate are formed as shown.

Agar gel is commonly used as the medium in which electrophoretic separation is followed by reaction of the antigens with selected antisera. The electrophoretic step is performed by placing the sample to be analysed in a well (Fig. 5.6C) cut into a thin layer of buffered agar held on a glass slide, followed by application of an electric current as described earlier (p. 76). The various proteins are mainly separated in a linear direction but some diffusion also occurs as indicated by spread in a direction at right angles to that of electrophoretic migration. Once the current is discontinued the diffusion continues equally in all directions. A trough (Fig. 5.6E), cut in the gel in a direction parallel to the electrophoretic migration but separated from the electrophoretic origin, is filled with antiserum which diffuses into the gel towards the antigens. This is therefore a double diffusion technique with the difference from the Ouchterlony method that although the concentration of antigen falls off as the square of the distance from the centre of the antigen site in any direction, the concentration of antibody is the same at any particular distance from the trough, for the whole of its length and falls off linearly with the distance at right angles to the trough. Where an antibody encounters its corresponding antigen, a line of precipitate forms where the relative proportions are optimal. This results in an arc with its convex side towards the trough (Fig. 5.6).

Various features of these arcs are worthy of comment. The length of the arc reflects the variation in electrophoretic mobility of a group of proteins which are identical immunologically. Thus normal IgG gives a long arc extending from the β to the extreme slow γ region (see also Fig. 5.6D). Proteins which are electrophoretically compact occupy a slightly ovoid area when the current is switched off and give rise to a short symmetrical arc the centre of which corresponds to the average mobility (Fig. 5.6B) – a typical example is transferrin. If the mobility of the protein is mainly well defined but with a smaller fraction of somewhat different mobility, the final shape after electrophoresis is asymmetrical and the final arc is also asymmetrical or 'hooked' (Fig. 5.6A). If the protein is of high molecular weight it diffuses more slowly than the antibody and the arc is further from the trough as is seen with IgM, α_2-macroglobulin and lipoproteins. Proteins present in high concentration will form an arc early and as more antigen diffuses, antigen excess will cause the arc to move nearer to the trough and become more intense. If sufficient time is available the arc reaches the trough and produces a boat-like shape with a sharp edge remote from the trough and a less intense area connecting this to the trough. This is seen with albumin and with some paraproteins present in high concentration. If the antiserum in the trough has been raised against the whole range of proteins present in human plasma, this polyvalent antiserum will produce 30 or more arcs corresponding to the different proteins. It will be apparent that proteins with common determinants will produce the reaction of identity and a continuous precipitation line results. Many arcs will intersect one another, the reaction of non-identity, as the different proteins have no common determinants. The resulting pattern is complex especially in the α and β zones, but the situation is much clearer if the antiserum has a much narrower specificity resulting in few arcs or only a single one. Antisera available commercially may be polyvalent, or specific for a particular protein or even part of a protein as for example antisera to γ chains of IgG or κ or λ chains in different classes of immunoglobulins.

The titres of such antisera vary and the nature of the arcs will thus differ depending on the concentration of antigen in the sample. At optimal proportions the arc is sharp and intense. With increasing antigen concentration the effect described above for albumin is apparent, while with a normal antigen concentration and a weak antibody titre, a diffuse arc nearer to the trough is seen. If the antibody titre is very high the arcs are remote from the trough and less distinct. An indistinct arc is also seen with a low antigen concentration. Interpretation of the results therefore requires experience and a knowledge of the properties of the antisera used. It is helpful to use several antisera and to dilute the sample prior to electrophoresis when the arcs are heavy and near the trough. It is also convenient to utilise troughs cut on both sides of the well. If different antisera are used, the patterns can then be compared.

The technique described above uses agar gel but other media have also been employed. Kohn (1976) performed the electrophoretic separation on cellulose acetate and then cut a strip from this along the line of migration to include all the separated proteins. This strip was then laid on a slide covered with agar gel allowing the antigens to diffuse into the agar as before. Instead of cutting troughs, strips of filter paper soaked in antisera were laid on the agar gel in a similar position. Arcs form in the agar as before. It is also possible to use prepared agarose sheets supported on a plastic backing in an entirely analogous way to the standard agar gel method. Such material with pre-cut troughs and wells is available from Ciba Corning Diagnostics Limited and Beckman Instruments International.

Immunoelectrophoresis is often used to investigate an increase in γ-globulins. Such an increase may be polyclonal or monoclonal (p. 429) depending on the nature of the primary disorder. In a monoclonal paraproteinaemia there is an increase in a particular specific immunoglobulin (or paraprotein) which belongs to a single immunoglobulin class and possesses a single light chain type. Immunoelectrophoresis using antisera to different Ig classes and to kappa and lambda light chains will identify the paraprotein. Occasionally light chains only may be produced, again of one type only. In all cases the paraprotein has a sharply defined electrophoretic mobility and is usually easily seen on the electrophoretic strip. The findings are characteristically present in multiple myeloma. In contrast, in a polyclonal increase in γ-globulins, a wide variety of immunoglobulins is produced covering different classes and both types of light chain.

The antisera are chosen to include a polyvalent one, specific and separate antisera to IgG, IgA and IgM heavy chains, and anti-kappa and anti-lambda sera to investigate the light chains. In a polyclonal increase (Fig. 5.7) there are more intense arcs of one or more of the three main Ig classes. The arcs are undistorted,

---

Fig. 5.7. Polyclonal Increase in Gamma Globulins on Immunoelectrophoresis.

Serum 1 has a polyclonal increase in immunoglobulins; serum 2 shows a monoclonal band in the β-region with reduction of intensity in the usual γ-region. The positions of the samples on each immunoelectrophoresis slide correspond to the electrophoretic strips. Albumin, towards the right in each case, has been allowed to run beyond the end of the trough to extend the separation in the γ-region. In the uppermost slide the albumin arcs have joined in the reaction of identity.

In serum 1, the IgG arc, seen towards the left hand side of the slide, is particularly marked and is wider than normal towards its centre but shows no bowing. It contains both κ and λ chains throughout its length. The IgA arc can be seen projecting above the centre of the IgG arc and a shorter IgM arc lies above the right end of the IgG arc. The slight distortion towards the right ends of the κ and λ arcs probably represents reactions with κ and λ chains in the IgA.

In serum 2, only a faint IgG arc is seen. There is a faint but large arc near the trough to the right of the well. This was shown after testing against an anti-alpha serum to be an abnormal IgA. The anti-kappa serum shows a faint, short line corresponding to the reduced amount of normal IgG but the anti-lambda serum produces a markedly distorted arc. The left end corresponds to λ chains in normal IgG. This shows the reaction of identity with the bowed right end due to the presence of λ chains (but not κ chains) in the monoclonal IgA molecule which is thus of type $\alpha_2 \lambda_2$. ▶

somewhat broader than usual towards the centre and may be more diffuse on the trough side. Both κ and λ chains are present although the arcs may no longer be simple in shape as the particular light chain is present in both IgG and IgA arcs for example.

In the monoclonal type the situation differs. A very specific type of immunoglobulin is increased but there may also be suppression to a varying degree of other immunoglobulins. The final pattern depends on the amount of paraprotein and the extent of any suppression. An IgG paraprotein will produce a local increase in concentration at some part of the zone occupied by normal IgG. The resultant IgG arc is distorted by a local bulge towards the trough with an increase in intensity and width of the arc at that point—'bowing'. This is a consequence of the local increase in antigen concentration as described earlier. Other immunoglobulin arcs are undistorted but may be fainter if the total amounts of IgA and IgM are reduced. The anti-light chain sera show that the distortion is only reproduced by one type, confirming the monoclonal nature of the abnormality. The 'bow' appears in the same position as that produced by the IgG antiserum. Examples of several paraproteins appear in Figs 5.7 and 5.8.

Immunofixation

Alper and Johnson (1969) described direct immunofixation of proteins in agarose gel by precipitation with monospecific antiserum after electrophoresis. The technique was used initially to identify genetic variants of ceruloplasmin, Gc component and the conversion products of C3 but has since been applied to other fields of study. After electrophoresis in agarose gel, monospecific antiserum is applied to the surface of the gel and diffuses into the gel forming insoluble immune complexes with its respective antigen. If there is equivalence or moderate

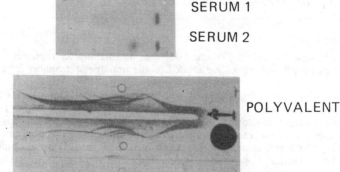

SERUM 1

SERUM 2

POLYVALENT

KAPPA

LAMBDA

antibody excess, the complexes remain in the gel on washing whereas the other unprecipitated proteins are removed. The antigen–antibody precipitate can then be stained. Other electrophoretic media used have included starch gel (Johnson *et al.*, 1969) and cellulose acetate membranes (Chang and Inglis, 1975; Kohn and Riches, 1978). Isoelectrofocusing in polyacrylamide gels has also been followed by immunofixation (Arnaud *et al.*, 1977; Constans *et al.*, 1978). Overlay techniques, particularly using cellulose acetate, can be used instead of direct application of the antiserum (Ritchie and Smith, 1976). Possibly the most widely used application of immunofixation in clinical biochemistry is the identification of paraproteins. It has several advantages over immunoelectrophoresis namely simplicity, more economical use of antisera and an immunochemically identified protein band which can be related directly to its electrophoretic position.

Immunofixation in Agarose Gel. Monospecific antisera with high titre and avidity are required. Goat or rabbit antisera such as those available from Atlantic Antibodies and Dako are recommended. The sample should be diluted to contain approximately 0·05 to 0·5 g/l of the protein under study or 0·05 to 2 g/l for heterogeneous proteins such as immunoglobulins (Johnson, 1982). Electrophoresis is performed in the usual way. Antiserum is then applied to the area of migration of the protein for 1 h using either a glass rod or a strip of cellulose acetate which has been dipped in antiserum. The concentration of antiserum used has to be assessed by trial and error. If the antiserum was applied directly, the gel surface is rinsed with sodium chloride solution, 9 g/l. The gel is then pressed by placing under moistened filter paper, overlaid with absorbent paper under a glass plate weighted with 2 kg for about 15 min. This is followed by washing in sodium chloride solution, 50 g/l, for 2 h and then the gel is pressed again and dried in air. Suitable stains include Amino Black or Coomassie Brilliant Blue. The stained antigen–antibody complex appears as a sharply defined band provided monospecific antiserum is used. Antigen excess results in wider bands or clear, unstained zones in the bands. Examples of immunofixation in the investigation of paraproteins are shown in Fig. 5.9.

Fig. 5.8. Monoclonal Increase in Gamma Globulins on Immunoelectrophoresis.

The upper electrophoretic strips are related to the immunoelectrophoretic patterns below.

A. Normal serum and serum from a patient with a monoclonal band ($\gamma_2\kappa_2$) in the slow-γ region.

The polyvalent antiserum shows a distorted IgG arc with marked 'eyebrow' bowing in its mid-zone; a second, fine arc remote from the trough is produced by a reduced amount of polyclonal $\gamma_2\lambda_2$. With anti-gamma serum, the distortion of the IgG arc is confirmed. Whereas the normal serum shows long undistorted arcs with anti-kappa and anti-lambda sera, that from the patient has relatively few λ-chains but a strong arc of κ-chains, corresponding in shape and position to the abnormal IgG arc is seen. This is continuous with a second well-defined arc with β-mobility. This is due to circulating free κ chains which can be seen as a faint but discrete band on the electrophoretic strip.

B. Normal serum and serum from a patient with a monoclonal band ($\gamma_2\kappa_2$) in the extreme slow-γ region.

In the top immunoelectrophoresis slide, the patient's serum (upper well) shows a marked distortion of the IgG arc at its left end. The fainter 'spur' projecting from this region of the arc is normal IgG with λ chains. In the anti-kappa slide, normal serum (upper well) shows an undistorted arc but the patient's serum reproduces the same shape as the IgG arc. In the anti-lambda slide, the patient's serum (upper well) gives only a faint but undistorted arc while the normal serum shows a stronger undistorted arc.

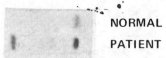

NORMAL
PATIENT

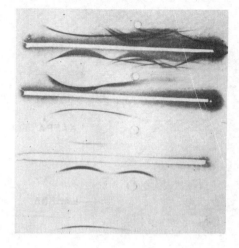

N
POLYVALENT
P

GAMMA
N

KAPPA
P

LAMBDA
N

Figure 5.8 (A)

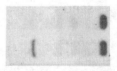

NORMAL SERUM

PATIENT'S SERUM

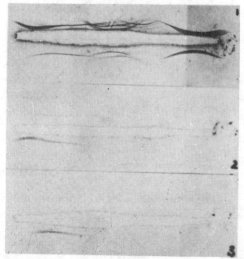

POLYVALENT

KAPPA

LAMBDA

Figure 5.8 (B)

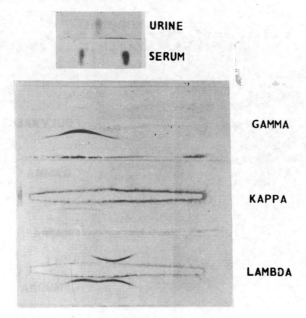

Figure 5.8 (C)

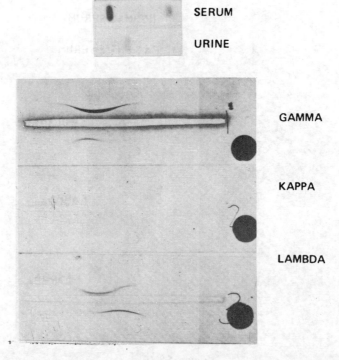

Figure 5.8 (D)

C. Urine and serum from a patient with a paraproteinaemia ($\gamma_2\lambda_2$).

The serum shows a discrete band in the mid-γ region and a fainter band in the β to fast-γ region. A single discrete band with similar mobility is present in the urine. The urine (upper well on each slide) contains only λ chains, while the serum shows a distorted IgG arc, a normal κ arc and a distorted λ arc. The left end of this corresponds to the IgG arc indicating the presence of $\gamma_2\lambda_2$. The right end continues into an arc corresponding to that in urine, indicating the presence in serum of free light chains of λ type. The patient has Bence-Jones proteinuria and the Bence-Jones protein is also detectable in the serum together with the intact paraprotein.

D. Urine and serum from a patient with a paraproteinaemia ($\gamma_2\lambda_2$).

The serum shows a discrete band in the slow-γ region with almost no other γ-globulin. The main discrete band in the urine has different mobility but there is a faint band corresponding to that in serum. On immunoelectrophoresis, the serum (upper wells) shows a distorted γ arc, no κ chains and a λ arc superimposable on the γ arc. The urine contains a small amount of the intact abnormal immunoglobulin ($\gamma_2\lambda_2$) but the main part of the λ arc is of faster electrophoretic mobility. The urine thus contains Bence-Jones protein but a small proportion of the considerable amount of the paraprotein present in the serum has passed through the glomerulus.

An alternative procedure is to produce an immunofixation print or 'immuno-print' on a cellulose acetate membrane. The method is carried out as described above but after electrophoresis, a cellulose acetate membrane soaked in antiserum is applied to the gel, glossy side up, for 15 s to 15 min. The membrane is then rinsed and stained. This method has the advantages of reduced washing time, the potential to make multiple 'prints' of different proteins from the same gel, and storage is easier. However, the sensitivity is decreased, antigen concentration is more critical and low molecular weight proteins or fragments can produce wider bands (Johnson, 1982).

Methods Based on Assisted Migration of Antigen

In these methods, diffusion is replaced by movement in an electric field. Under usual conditions antigen moves more rapidly than antibody. The medium is usually agar gel. This may be impregnated with antibody throughout as in the 'rocket' technique or the antigen and antibody may be separately introduced into plain agar gel and caused to move towards one another in the technique of counter-immunoelectrophoresis, sometimes known also as 'cross-over electrophoresis' or 'electro-immuno-endosmosis'. It is possible also to carry out preliminary electrophoretic separation before applying the rocket technique in a direction at right angles to the initial separation. For a review see Verbruggen (1975).

'Rocket' Immunoelectrophoresis

This technique, introduced by Laurell (1965, 1966) under the name 'antigen–antibody crossed electrophoresis', was later called 'electro-immunoassay' (Laurell, 1972). The term 'rocket' applies to the visual appearance once the procedure is complete.

A glass slide is covered with buffered agar gel containing an antibody specific for the antigen to be determined. Wells are cut along a line towards one end of the plate and measured amounts of standards and the samples for analysis are placed in these. Electrophoresis is then carried out in the usual way in a direction at right angles to the line of wells. The antigen is driven into the gel and reacts with

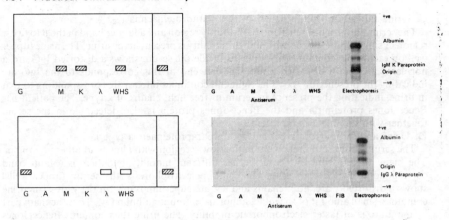

Fig. 5.9. Immunofixation in Agarose Gel.

Upper. Six samples of serum from a patient with an IgM-kappa paraproteinaemia have been electrophoresed and then each channel has been overlaid with a cellulose acetate strip containing the antiserum shown by the abbreviation. After washing, the precipitated proteins were stained. A strong band in each of the channels overlaid with anti-IgM, anti-kappa and anti-whole human serum corresponds to the paraprotein band on electrophoresis, identifying the paraprotein as IgM-kappa.

Lower. IgG-lambda paraprotein. The bands in channels overlaid with anti-IgG, anti-lambda and anti-whole human serum correspond to the paraprotein band on electrophoresis. Excess antigen has caused dissolution of the centre of the paraprotein band with anti-lambda and anti-whole human serum and of albumin with the latter also.

Abbreviations. G = anti-IgG, A = anti-IgA, M = anti-IgM, κ = anti-kappa light chains, λ = anti-lambda light chains, WHS = anti-whole human serum.

antibody to produce a precipitate. As further antigen enters, some of the precipitate redissolves and antigen moves further into the gel (see radial immunodiffusion, p. 93). Once local conditions are stable and no further antigen is available, the precipitate does not move in the field. This fixed antigen–antibody precipitate forms firstly just above the outer edges of the well and as antigen is gradually removed, the lines of precipitate gradually approach one another until the last portion of antigen to combine is precipitated where the lines converge, completing the rocket shape (Fig. 5.10).

The area within the rocket approximates to a triangle with base equal to the well diameter and height equal to the distance from the centre of the well to the rocket tip. The antibody originally within this area has been removed by the antigen to form the precipitate. As the well diameter is constant this area is directly proportional to the rocket height and hence the quantity of antigen is linearly related to the rocket height.

The method is based on a similar principle to radial immunodiffusion which has gone to completion but has the advantage that the reaction is complete within two hours compared to three days. However, it requires more complex equipment and certain antigens do not have good electrophoretic mobility. This is the case with the immunoglobulins as the conditions are chosen so that the antibody shows little migration and this must limit the movement of immunoglobulins. It is necessary to alter their electrical charge, usually by formylation by first treating the sample with formaldehyde.

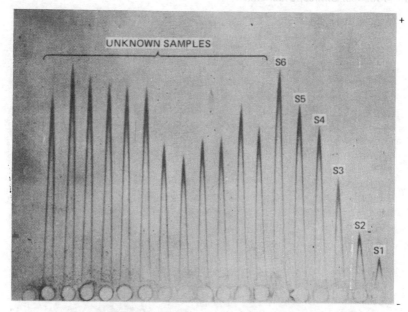

Fig. 5.10. Rocket Immunoelectrophoresis. S1–S6 = standards.

Two-dimensional Rocket Immunoelectrophoresis

The Laurell technique was modified by Clarke and Freeman (1968) by combining preliminary separation by electrophoresis with later electrophoretic migration into an agar gel containing polyvalent antiserum. They performed the first step in agarose gel and then inserted a strip of this gel containing the separated proteins into a second agarose gel containing an antiserum to all human serum proteins derived from goat, rabbit or sheep. The strip was inserted in such a way that the electric field could drive the antigens into the antiserum in a direction at right angles to the original separation.

This method produces a series of rockets of different widths and heights showing lateral displacement to one another (Fig. 5.11). The rockets correspond to the multiple arcs seen in immunoelectrophoresis (Fig. 5.7, p. 99). Their different widths reflect their original zone width in the preliminary electrophoresis and the area enclosed by the peak is a measure of the amount of the particular antigen. The method therefore has the advantage of quantitation compared with diffusion immunoelectrophoresis. The peak areas in one plate cannot be directly compared with one another as the antibody titre is different for each antigen. Comparison is made with a pooled normal serum treated similarly and hence requires careful control of the volume of sample used for the first electrophoresis and removal of an adequate width of strip from this preliminary separation. Identification of peaks may present difficulties but the position and characteristics of the peaks from known proteins can be defined using monospecific antisera in place of the polyvalent antiserum. Clarke and Freeman (1968) used the technique to study simultaneously variations in ten different proteins due to age and sex in adults. The method was also used by Abrams and Freeman (1969) to study changes in the serum proteins of infants during the first six months of life.

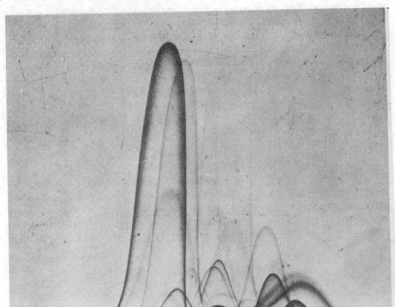

Fig. 5.11. Two Dimensional Rocket Immunoelectrophoresis.
A sample of serum was originally placed in the well just visible towards the right end of the lower margin of the figure. Electrophoresis was performed firstly from right to left. The rocket immunoelectrophoresis step was then carried out at right angles, corresponding to a vertical direction in the picture. The main peak, towards the left side, is albumin.

Although somewhat complicated, the method permits the simultaneous assessment of many proteins and allows unidentified proteins to be studied. The method is less satisfactory for the study of immunoglobulins owing to their limited mobility as discussed above (p. 104).

Counter-immunoelectrophoresis

The slow mobility of the immunoglobulins under the usual electrophoretic conditions is made use of in this procedure by placing a sample of antibody ahead of the antigen and causing this to move through the former and react to form a precipitate. Lang and Haan (1957) originally employed paper electrophoresis but agar gel is now usual, although a method using Cellogel is available commercially. The technique can detect hepatitis B surface antigen (Gocke and Howe, 1970; Prince and Burke, 1970).

In the usual method using buffered agar gel, two wells are cut (Fig. 5.12). The antibody is placed in the one nearer the anode and the antigen in the other. On applying an electric field the antigen moves towards the anode while the antibody is carried in the opposite direction by endosmotic flow. The two therefore meet in the region between the two wells and a line of precipitate forms where the proportions are optimal.

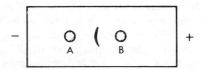

Fig. 5.12. Counter Immunoelectrophoresis.
Antigen is placed in the well A and antiserum in well B. The precipitin arc forms between the wells.

Light Scattering Techniques

The need to improve precision and to handle greater numbers of specimens for protein determination requires automation and work simplification which are not readily applicable to gel precipitation techniques. Although light scattering measurements of the antigen–antibody reaction were initially described by Libby in 1938, they were not widely used until specific antisera became available. Ritchie (1975) using a continuous flow technique demonstrated the need for high avidity antibodies and polymer enhancement of the precipitation reaction. The theoretical work of Savory *et al.* (1974) on the kinetics of the antigen–antibody reaction led to the development of discrete systems using nephelometry or turbidimetry (see Chapter 7, p. 159). Both methods of detecting light scattering have been used but nephelometry appears to be slightly more sensitive (Price *et al.*, 1983).

The shape of the immunoprecipitin curve depends on the species of origin of the antibody, its avidity for the antigen and its concentration, making evaluation of these factors important in the design of an assay. The ionic species in the reaction mixture and its ionic strength and pH also influence the kinetics of the reaction. The solubility of proteins can be reduced by exclusion of water using non-ionic polymers such as polyethylene glycol (PEG) thereby enhancing the sensitivity of the immunoprecipitin reaction (Hellsing, 1972, 1974). PEG with a molecular weight of 6000 is generally the most effective polymer although dextrans and PEG 4000 have also been used. PEG 6000 at concentrations between 20 and 40 g/l increases the sensitivity of the reaction 5- to 8-fold and reduces the time required to reach equilibrium. Polymers also enhance the effect on light scattering of substances not involved in the immunoprecipitin reaction such as lipoproteins and endogenous immune complexes thus increasing the sample blank and limiting the sensitivity of the assay in serum. Endogenous light scattering by specimens can be minimised by using a high sample dilution or by pre-treatment of the sample (Hellsing and Enstrom, 1977; Whicher and Blow, 1980). Cerebrospinal fluid and urine are not so affected by this problem.

The reaction can be followed kinetically or measured at equilibrium. The assays differ since different stages of the immunoprecipitin reaction are being used. Similarly, the observed kinetics followed by nephelometry and turbidimetry differ with the former apparently reaching equilibrium earlier than the latter (Whicher *et al.*, 1983).

Nephelometry

Several basic optical systems are employed in nephelometers as discussed in Chapter 7 (p. 160). The light source varies as does the orientation of the light beam to the cuvette and detector. Fluorimeters have been used with the primary and secondary beams at the same wavelength as in the Technicon Continuous Flow AIP System or the Multistat III F/N Microcentrifugal Analyser

(Instrumentation Laboratories Limited). Other nephelometers employ laser light sources to produce a collimated beam of high intensity light. However, the highly polarised light produces different optimal scattering angles for different sized particles making its use for kinetic measurement difficult as the complexes increase in size during the reaction. Laser light sources are employed in the Travenol-Hyland Laser Nephelometer PDQ (Travenol Laboratories, California, USA), the Behring Laser Nephelometer (Hoechst, Frankfurt, West Germany) and the Immunology Series 420 Laser Nephelometer (J. T. Baker Diagnostics, Pasadena, USA). The Beckman Immunochemistry System (Beckman Instruments International SA, Geneva, Switzerland) employs a tungsten lamp with detection of forward scattered light. The reaction is monitored kinetically and a microprocessor calculates the results.

Turbidimetry

Almost any good quality spectrophotometer can be used for turbidimetric measurements but the optical noise level is important since absorbance changes are usually small. In practice reaction rate analysers such as the LKB Instruments Limited 2086 analyser (Spencer and Price, 1979) and centrifugal analysers (Deverill, 1980; Spencer and Price, 1980) have usually been used.

　Detection of Antigen Excess. The number of light scattering immune complexes is reduced when the antigen concentration exceeds that at the equivalence point of the antigen–antibody reaction. This can cause problems particularly in immunoglobulin measurements and assay systems must be designed so that states of antigen excess are detected. This usually occurs only with paraproteins which can be present in quantities well in excess of the normal immunoglobulin concentrations. Additionally the paraprotein will only react with a few antibodies in the mixture of antibodies present in the antiserum so that antigen excess occurs at a lower concentration of antigen than for polyclonal antigens. Several approaches have been devised to detect antigen excess. Prior electrophoresis can be used to identify paraproteins. Further antigen or antibody can be added after the initial reaction resulting in a decrease or increase in light scattering respectively but this method increases the analysis time and may increase the usage of expensive antiserum. In the continuous flow method, the peak shape alters when there is antigen excess and with continuous monitoring methods a change in the rate of complex formation occurs (Deverill, 1980; Spencer and Price, 1980).

　When considering the range of immunochemical methods available, the

TABLE 5.1

Relative Sensitivities of Various Types of Specific Protein Immunoassay
(Abridged from Whicher *et al.*, 1983)

Method	ng/'cuvette'
Radial immunodiffusion	150
Rocket electrophoresis	2–10
Kinetic immunoturbidimetry, LKB 2086	75
Nephelometry—Beckman	100–200
—Hyland—diluted samples	1–2
undiluted samples	100
pretreated samples	1–5
Radioimmunoassay	0.005

sensitivity of light scattering immunoassay, which is dependent on the instrument used and the reaction conditions, can be compared with that of the other techniques (Table 5.1).

REFERENCES

Abrams B., Freeman T. (1969). *Clin. Sci*; **37**: 575.
Alper C. A., Johnson A. M. (1969). *Vox Sanguinis*; **17**: 445.
Arnaud P., Wilson G. B., Koistinen J., Fudenberg H. H. (1977). *J. Immunol. Methods*; **16**: 221.
Arquembourg P. C. (1975). *Immunoelectrophoresis. Theory, Methods, Identifications, Interpretation*, 2nd ed. Basel, London, New York: Karger.
Chang C. H., Inglis N. R. (1975). *Clin. Chim. Acta*; **65**: 91.
Clarke H. G. M., Freeman, T. (1968). *Clin. Sci*; **35**: 403.
Constans J. *et al.* (1978). *Hum. Genet*; **41**: 53.
Deverill I. (1980). In *Centrifugal Analysers in Clinical Chemistry*. (Price C. P., Spencer K. eds) p. 109. Eastbourne: Praeger.
Gocke D., Howe C. (1970). *J. Immunol*; **104**: 1031.
Grabar P., Williams C. A. (1953). *Biochim. Biophys. Acta*; **10**: 193.
Grabar P., Williams C. A. (1955). *Biochim. Biophys. Acta*; **17**: 67.
Hellsing, K. (1972). In *Automated Immunoprecipitin Reactions, Colloquium on AIP*. p. 17. Brussels: Technicon Instruments Corporation.
Hellsing K. (1974). *Protides Biol. Fluids*; **21**: 579.
Hellsing K., Enstrom H. (1977). *Scand. J. Clin. Lab. Invest*; **35**: 529.
Johnson A. M. (1982). *Clin. Chem*; **28**: 1797.
Johnson A. M., Schmid K., Alper C. A. (1969). *J. Clin. Invest*; **48**: 2293.
Kohn J. (1976). In *Chromatographic and Electrophoretic Techniques*, Vol. 2, 4th ed. *Zone Electrophoresis*. (Smith I. ed) p. 120. London: William Heinemann Medical Books.
Kohn J., Riches P. G. (1978). *J. Immunol. Methods*; **20**: 325.
Lang N., Haan J. (1957). *Allergy and Applied Immunol*; **10**: 305.
Laurell C.-B. (1965). *Analyt. Biochem*; **10**: 358.
Laurell C.-B. (1966). *Analyt. Biochem*; **15**: 45.
Laurell C.-B. (1972). *Scand. J. Clin. Lab. Invest*; **29**, Suppl. **124**: 21.
Libby R. L. (1938). *J. Immunol*; **34**: 269.
Mancini G., Carbonara A. O., Heremans J. F. (1965). *Immunochem*; **2**: 235.
Mancini G., Vaerman J. P., Carbonara A. O., Heremans J. F. (1963). *Protides Biol. Fluids*; **11**: 370.
Nerenberg S. T. (1972). *J. Lab. Clin. Med*; **79**, 673.
Ouchterlony O. (1948). *Acta Pathol. Microbiol. Scand*; **25**: 186.
Ouchterlony O. (1967). In *Handbook of Experimental Immunology*. (Weir D. ed) p. 655. Oxford: Blackwell Scientific Publications.
Price C. P., Spencer K., Whicher J. T. (1983). *Ann. Clin. Biochem*; **20**: 1.
Prince A., Burke K. (1970). *Science*; **169**: 583.
Ritchie R. F. (1975). In *The Plasma Proteins: Structure, Function and Genetic Control*. Vol. 2, 2nd ed. (Putnam F. W. ed) p. 375. London and New York: Academic Press.
Ritchie R. F. and Smith R. (1976). *Clin. Chem*; **22**: 497.
Roitt I. (1984). *Essential Immunology*, 5th ed. Oxford: Blackwell Scientific Publications.
Savory J., Buffone G. J., Reich R. (1974). *Clin. Chem*; **20**: 1071.
Spencer K., Price C. P. (1979). *Clin. Chim. Acta*; **95**: 263.
Spencer K., Price C. P. (1980). In *Centrifugal Analysers in Clinical Chemistry*. (Price C. P., Spencer K., eds) p. 457. Eastbourne: Praeger.
Verbruggen R. (1975). *Clin. Chem*; **21**: 5.
Vergani C., Stabilini R., Agostoni A. (1967). *Immunochem*; **4**: 233.
Whicher J. T., Blow C. (1980). *Ann. Clin. Biochem*; **17**: 170.
Whicher J. T., Price C. P., Spencer K. (1983). *CRC Critical Reviews in Clinical Laboratory Sciences*; **18**: 213.

6
RADIOIMMUNOASSAY AND RELATED TECHNIQUES

Several versions of the technique named *displacement analysis* by Yalow and Berson (1960) or *saturation analysis* by Ekins (1960) have been developed and diversified in recent years. These and related techniques may be applied to the measurement of antigen (Ag) or antibody (Ab) and involve the addition of a labelled reagent either as labelled Ag or labelled Ab. The final measurement is of the label following a separative step. In order to be applicable to the measurement of small quantities of Ag or Ab the properties of the label must be such that it can be detected at very low concentrations. For many purposes radioactive labels are convenient and have been widely used. More recently, alternatives to radiolabels have been used including enzymes. Other labels have been detected by the properties of fluorescence, luminescence, electron spin resonance (the label is a free radical containing an unpaired electron) or the biological properties of a bacteriophage. The label may also be a relatively large particle such as a latex particle or an erythrocyte whose properties are altered during the combination of Ag and Ab on its surface.

Specific binders other than antibodies may be used, and when these are naturally occurring plasma proteins the assay is often referred to as a *competitive protein-binding* method. An example is the use of thyroxine-binding globulin for the determination of thyroxine. Sometimes the binder is a relatively crude preparation of cell receptors for which the antigen has a biological affinity. Such methods are called *receptor assays*, e.g. the use of a rabbit uterine cytosol preparation for the assay of plasma oestrogens. In both types of assay the affinity of the binder may be less than for an antibody and the specificity variable.

Potentially greater binding affinity and specificity is obtained if the binder is an antibody raised against the desired antigen. Methods using such antibody binders are referred to collectively as *immunoassays* and are conveniently considered under sub-headings depending on the nature of the label, e.g. *radioimmunoassay* or *enzymeimmunoassay*. In all protein binding assays the material bound is called a *ligand*. However, in immunoassays the ligand may be more specifically termed an antigen.

RADIOIMMUNOASSAY

There are several reasons for the rapid growth in the use of radioimmunoassay (RIA) other than the need to replace the cumbersome and time-consuming chemical and bio-assays previously in use.

The method offers considerable *sensitivity*, perhaps best considered as the smallest amount of the substance being measured which can be distinguished from zero. With antibodies of high binding affinity and radiolabelled antigens of high specific activity, RIA has the ability to measure substances at concentrations as low as 1 pmol/l.

The method offers *specificity*, the ability to discriminate between the desired substance and related substances. This arises from the highly specific nature of the antigen–antibody interaction. Where a highly specific antiserum is available it is often possible to determine the required substance in serum without any preliminary purification procedure, thereby considerably simplifying the whole analysis.

RIA also has the advantage of a level of *precision* comparable to that of many traditional chemical methods.

Accuracy is difficult to assess since RIA can only give a measure of immunochemical activity which need not imply measurement of biological activity or complete molecular structure. In addition, high quality standard material may be difficult to obtain. Nevertheless, reasonable accuracies may be inferred from correlations with other analytical methods such as bio-assays or chemical procedures, and also from recovery experiments.

The technique is of general *applicability* to any substance against which antibodies can be produced, so that the same equipment and operating systems can be used for many different substances, and if necessary the techniques can be automated to handle larger workloads.

In RIA the essential components of the analytical system are the antigen (Ag) to be determined, a fixed amount of labelled antigen (Ag*) and a fixed limited amount of antibody (Ab). The reaction is then:

$$Ag + Ag* + Ab \rightleftharpoons AgAb + Ag*Ab$$

It will be apparent that provided the labelling procedure still allows the binding of Ag* by the antibody, then there will be competition between Ag and Ag* for the limited number of antibody binding sites. Once equilibrium has been reached, Ag and Ag* will either be present in the 'free' form (F) or combined with Ab in the 'bound' form (B). As the amounts of Ag* and Ab are constant, an increasing amount of Ag will result in less label being present in the bound form. If a satisfactory method of separating the bound and free forms is available then the radioactivity of either or both fractions can be used to produce a calibration curve. With many antigens, particularly the large peptide hormones, the sensitivity of the assay can be improved by delaying the addition of the labelled antigen. This is known as *non-equilibrium RIA or sequential saturation analysis*. The amount of label can be much greater than that which would be used for the previously described simultaneous reagent addition system. When considering the use of this assay system, the requirement for sensitivity has to be balanced against the introduction of an extra manipulation and the increased use of labelled reagent.

The following section deals specifically with RIA. However, many aspects are relevant to other assay systems which will be described later.

Technical Requirements for Radioimmunoassay

There are a number of basic requirements for establishing a satisfactory RIA, and these will be considered under separate sub-headings. Antigen is required in the preparation of all the main reagents, namely standard, label and antiserum. Antigen purification can be an exacting process especially in the case of those hormones which are labile or present in minute amounts in tissue and plasma. Such material is often expensive, or even unobtainable for all but a few specialised centres. Conversely, small antigens such as steroids and drugs are usually readily available in pure form, but difficulty may be experienced in obtaining conjugated forms of these molecules.

The Antibody

The properties of the antiserum dictate the specificity of a radioimmunoassay and therefore much attention is paid to its production.

In general, proteins having a molecular weight in excess of 5000 readily stimulate antibody production, i.e. they are immunogenic. Small molecules such as thyroid hormones, steroids, drugs and peptide hormones must be coupled to larger carrier molecules in order to become immunogenic. However, the resultant antisera will react with the free form of such molecules which are known as *haptens* (see p. 90). Examples of carrier molecules include bovine serum albumin, thyroglobulin and keyhole limpet haemocyanin. It is not entirely clear whether the choice of carrier has a significant effect upon the antibody response. It is important to consider the site of attachment of hapten to carrier and also the number of haptens per carrier, bearing in mind the need to leave important groups in the molecule accessible to antibody response. Examples of conjugation reactions include the use of carbodi-imides or the mixed anhydride reaction, both of which mediate in the formation of peptide bonds between the carboxyl residues of one molecule and the amine of the other. These reactions can also be used for haptens containing oxo or hydroxyl groups, e.g. steroids. These groups must first be converted to carboxyl residues using carboxymethyl oxime or hemisuccinate formation respectively.

A factor having a broad influence on antiserum production is the choice of animal species. There are relatively few instances where the quality of antiserum is species-dependent and the major factors to consider when selecting an animal are: the size of the animal (size being proportional to the volume of antiserum produced), the ease of handling and ease of maintenance. Most antisera for RIA have been prepared in rabbits, sheep and guinea pigs, while donkeys have been found to be very useful in fulfilling the large volume requirement for second antibody.

Immunisation generally involves the injection of antigen, held in a stable emulsion with Freund's complete adjuvant, a mixture of mineral oil, waxes and inactivated bacteria, which enhances and prolongs the antigenic response. The choice of route is usually between intramuscular, subcutaneous or intradermal immunisation, each method having its own strengths and weaknesses. Whichever route is chosen the schedule usually includes a primary injection followed by boosters at monthly intervals. Dose levels chosen range from 10 μg to 1 mg depending on such factors as the expected immunogenicity of the material being injected and the size of the animal. Peak antibody response occurs about 7 to 14 days following a booster injection, and harvesting of antisera should be timed to take advantage of this. Rabbits are bled from a lateral ear vein, guinea pigs by heart puncture and larger animals, such as sheep, by jugular vein cannulation.

Most antisera are stable at $-20°$C for at least one year or at $4°$C after treatment with a bacteriostatic agent such as azide or merthiolate. Repeated freezing and thawing should be avoided, especially if the antiserum has been diluted. Freeze drying or storage below the eutectic point of saline ($-26°$C) should be used for prolonged storage.

Once the antibody has been produced, the serum must be assessed for quantity and quality. Information must be obtained on: the titre or concentration, specificity and the avidity of the antibody. Methods for obtaining this information will be described later under assay optimisation (p. 116), since reagents other than antisera are involved.

Monoclonal Antibodies. These offer a potentially unlimited supply of identical antibodies, the ability to target specificity and the possibility of a purer antibody solution for labelling (see immunoradiometric assays, p. 124). The relatively modest avidity constants of monoclonal antibodies could limit the sensitivity of conventionally designed RIAs.

The essential stages in the production of a monoclonal antibody are:

1. A mouse or rat plasmacytoma cell line is selected for its ability to grow *in vitro* and to fuse with immunoglobulin-secreting cells, while possessing a property by means of which it can be selected against. Usually the latter involves choosing cell lines lacking the enzyme hypoxanthine phosphoribosyl transferase. When these cells are grown in a medium containing aminopterin, which blocks the main pathway of nucleic acid synthesis, they are unable to utilise an alternative pathway whereas normal cells are able to do so provided thymidine and hypoxanthine are also available. Thus, by the addition of hypoxanthine, aminopterin and thymidine to conventional media a selective (HAT) medium is produced.
2. Immunisation of mice and preliminary testing for antibody content.
3. The hybridisation or fusion step, which involves mixing spleen cells from the immunised mouse and plasmacytoma cells in the presence of a high concentration of polyethylene glycol to produce hybrid cells with the features of both parents. The cell suspension is then washed before diluting in selective growth medium and pipetting into microtitre wells.
4. At this stage any remaining non-fused cells should be incapable of growth, because mouse spleen cells do not grow *in vitro*, and plasmacytoma cells lack the necessary enzyme for growth in the selective medium, whereas the hybridoma cells possess both the ability for *in vitro* growth and the necessary enzymes as a result of the fusion of both cell types.
5. The contents of the well found to be producing antibody are recultured to separate each individual cell type. This process is known as cloning.
6. Stable clones producing antibody are then used for large-scale production of monoclonal antibody. The large-scale production can be by either *in vitro* culture or *in vivo* growth in mice or rats.

It is often desirable to obtain pure monoclonal antibody preparations especially if they are to be labelled. Unfortunately both methods for large-scale production produce a background of either serum proteins from the culture fluid or natural proteins from the mouse ascitic fluid. DEAE chromatography or affinity purification should enable a suitably pure preparation to be obtained.

Labelled Antigen

The ideal Ag* is a homogeneous preparation of the antigen which has been labelled, without any loss of affinity for the antibody being used. The choice of radioisotope in practice usually lies between ^{125}I and ^3H except in special cases. The factors influencing the final choice include the ease of introducing the radiolabel into the antigen, the chemical stability and specific activity of the product, the half-life, and the ease of counting. For further details of radioactivity and counting methods see Chapter 9. Iodine-125 has a half-life of 60 days and the labelled antigen has to be prepared every few months as a result whereas ^3H has a much longer half-life of 12.3 years. However ^{125}I can be incorporated into molecules to give a much higher specific activity than ^{3}H and its gamma radiation leads to much simpler counting procedures than those needed for the low energy beta particles emitted by ^{3}H. Tritium-labelled steroids and other small haptens are available from Amersham International, at a specific activity of 100 Ci/mmol or greater for immediate use.

Radioiodination Procedures. These are frequently used for radiolabelling polypeptides in which a tyrosine residue is present. The method of Hunter and Greenwood (1964) involves the exposure of the antigen for a defined short period of time to the oxidising agent, chloramine T, and ^{125}I in the form of carrier-free iodide. Depending on the reaction conditions, one or two ^{125}I atoms are incorporated at one or more tyrosine residues. Sometimes a histidine residue may be iodinated.

The reaction is terminated by adding sodium metabisulphite. The oxidising properties of chloramine T can also lead to oxidation of sulphydryl, thioether, imidazole and indole groups and possible denaturation of the antigen. Such products may have different affinities for the antiserum than the native antigen. Milder iodination conditions reducing the risk of denaturation include the oxidation of iodide by lactoperoxidase or electrolysis.

Immediately after iodination a purification procedure is used in order to remove excess iodide and also to separate the labelled antigen from any damaged material. Changes in the antigen can result from:

1. Exposure to reagents used in labelling, notably the oxidant.
2. The presence of the iodide group.
3. The handling and exposure to surfaces, of dilute protein solutions.
4. Radiation damage.

It is usual to assess the degree of incorporation of radioiodine into a compound by determining the specific activity (p. 213). All methods of calculating specific activity make assumptions with varying degrees of validity. For details of methods see Bolton (1985).

Some antigens contain no residue which can be iodinated or unacceptable damage may occur during the labelling process. Such molecules may be condensed at a carboxyl group with the amino group of tyrosine methyl ester, tyramine or histamine to give a product which can then be labelled with ^{125}I. Alternatively one of these three compounds can be converted to their radioiodinated forms before the condensation step. An alternative method uses 3-(4'-hydroxy-3'-iodophenyl) propionic acid N-hydroxy-succinimide ester in which the iodine atom is ^{125}I. This substance, available from Amersham International, reacts with primary amino groups in the antigen to form a covalently linked radioactive residue.

Assessment of the Quality of Radiolabels. The immunoreactivity of a labelled preparation can be assessed by determining the percentage of label capable of being bound in the presence of excess antibody. It is usual to aim for binding greater than 90%. However, labels exhibiting lower binding may prove to be acceptable. When testing a new batch of label for use in a well established assay, it is generally sufficient to demonstrate its satisfactory performance in a test assay consisting of a standard curve and quality control samples.

Storage. The stability during storage can be affected by several factors which include temperature, pH, the type and concentration of protein carrier, and the presence of protective agents, e.g. Trasylol. Commonly, iodinated preparations are stored in the presence of bovine serum albumin at $-20°C$, preferably in small aliquots each sufficient for a complete assay. Repeated freezing and thawing is to be avoided. Some antigens are better stored at $4°C$ and some may preferably be kept at temperatures below $-20°C$. Freeze-dried preparations of tracers may also be satisfactory and are the preparations of choice when they are to be distributed to other laboratories.

Safety. All radioiodination procedures must be performed in a ventilated or total enclosure and not on the open bench. It cannot be stressed too strongly that careful, organised and tidy laboratory work is required both for successful iodination and for personal safety. For current recommendations concerning the design and classification of the working area, the advice of the Radiation Protection Adviser should be sought.

Separation of Free and Bound Antigen

The separation of bound antigen (B) from free antigen (F) is an essential step in RIAs. It is time consuming, technically demanding and a major source of imprecision. There is a wide range of methods now available and the factors considered in the selection of a method for a particular RIA include efficiency and general practicability.

Efficiency. The method chosen should be capable of completely separating the B and F fractions with a reasonable margin for variation of reaction conditions, while not upsetting the distribution of Ag and Ag* between the B and F forms. The selected separation method should also have minimal sensitivity to the composition of the reaction mixture, i.e. lack of a 'matrix' effect.

Practicability. The method chosen should be quick, simple, safe, cheap, suitable for large batches and widely applicable without the need for extensive re-optimisation.

Separation Methods. These may be divided as follows:

1. *Methods based on differential migration.* Various chromatographic and electrophoretic techniques have been performed but in general such methods lack practicability.

2. *Adsorption of free antigen.* Where the properties of the free antigen permit, this may be adsorbed onto a solid support such as dextran-coated charcoal, talc or ion-exchange resins. Although reasonably practical for smaller antigens, e.g. steroids, their 'matrix' effects and interference in the primary antigen–antibody reaction militate against their continued use.

3. *Fractional precipitation of bound fraction.* This is achieved chemically if the molecular size of the B and F forms differ considerably. Ammonium sulphate, ethanol, isopropanol and polyethylene glycol have all been used. These methods, though practicable for certain analytes, still require careful optimisation.

4. *Double antibody precipitation of bound fraction.* This is a widely applicable method, whereby an antibody to the specific antibody is used to precipitate B. If the specific antiserum (first antibody) was raised in a rabbit, then an anti-rabbit antibody prepared in another animal is suitable (second antibody). This method has been shown to be both efficient and reasonably practicable. The major disadvantages are reagent cost and the prolonged incubation and centrifugation stages. These problems can be overcome to some extent by the addition of polyethylene glycol or by using second antibody attached to a solid phase.

5. *Solid phase first or second antibody.* Here the antibody is linked to a solid phase so that once equilibrium is reached, separation of B is quick and simple. Early coupling methods such as the simple adsorption of antibodies onto polystyrene tubes had some problems, including efficiency and reproducibility. Some of the practical difficulties have been overcome by materials such as finely divided celluloses and plastic beads, to which antibodies can be covalently coupled by simple and non-hazardous methods.

The choice of suitable solid phase materials facilitates the application of separation techniques such as sucrose layering or magnetic separation which lend themselves to a degree of automation not possible with centrifugation. These methods also lead to an increase in assay precision because B can easily be washed free of F.

Standards

The accuracy of a laboratory's results and the relationship to those obtained by other laboratories depend on the use of suitable common standard materials.

For small antigens such as steroids, drugs or thyroid hormones, pure preparations are readily available from commercial sources. Many polypeptide hormone standards are available from commercial companies and primary standards may be obtained from organisations such as the World Health Organisation and The National Institute of Biological Standards and Control, Holly Hill, London. These materials are particularly useful for calibrating secondary standards for routine use.

Standard preparations should be contained in a matrix as closely resembling human serum as possible. For some RIAs a suitable substitute could be peptidase-free buffered albumin solution, but for many there is no substitute for human serum. Analyte-free human serum can be obtained either by selecting a suitable human population, e.g. males where the assay is for a pregnancy-specific hormone; or by removing endogenous antigen; or by suppression of the endogenous material with, e.g. dexamethasone for the production of ad-renocorticotrophic hormone (ACTH) or cortisol-free serum. A series of standards may be diluted and stored deep frozen in small aliquots, each sufficient for a single assay. For long term storage it may be necessary to use temperatures below $-20°C$ or even lyophilisation.

Assay Optimisation

Theoretical analysis (Ekins *et al.*, 1968) would suggest that the equilibrium constant (K_a) of the antibody can be used to optimise RIA by giving an indication of the required concentration of antiserum and labelled antigen (Ag*). In practice most assayists follow a more pragmatic approach, possibly using the theoretical predictions for 'fine tuning'. The optimisation of any RIA system can be relatively complex since alteration of any reagents or conditions (time, temperature, buffer type, protein carrier, etc.) is likely to require modification of at least one other component. The following order is usual.

Assay Conditions. It is convenient initially to choose conditions which have been shown by experience to support acceptable assays for similar substances, bearing in mind that changes may be made subsequently. A moderately long incubation time could be used to reach equilibrium reasonably confidently, also a low remperature (4°C) plus inhibitors in order to lessen any damage by free radicals, oxidants, enzymes and bacteria. Also assay volumes should be kept to a minimum in order to promote an efficient immunological reaction.

Labelled Antigen Concentration (Ag*). Maximum assay sensitivity is approached when both Ag* and antibody tend towards zero. Extreme dilution, however, necessitates prolonged incubation and count-times and so a relatively arbitrary concentration of Ag* is chosen. Many workers use a concentration similar to that of the analyte at the lower end of the assay range. However, this is very much influenced by the specific activity of the label, counting time required, and any difference in affinity for the antibody between Ag* and Ag.

Separation System. A choice of separation system must first be made and then it must be optimised. In the case of a second antibody system the concentration (titre) of the first antiserum must be established before the second antibody can be titred. A convenient, preliminary approach would be to use an excess of a liquid phase second antibody bearing in mind the need to add carrier serum when the first antiserum is used at high dilution.

Antibody Concentration (Titre). Antiserum titration curves are performed by incubating increasing dilutions of antiserum with labelled antigen in the absence of unlabelled antigen. The choice of dilution range may be assisted by knowledge of previous bleeds from the same animal or from guidelines provided with commercially available antisera. In the absence of any prior indication a reasonable preliminary approach would be to use 10-fold dilutions from $1/10^2$ to $1/10^6$.

The amount of labelled antigen bound to the antibody at each dilution can be measured and expressed as a percentage of the labelled antigen added ($\% B$). The $\% B$ values can then be plotted against the antiserum dilution to produce the type of curve shown in Fig. 6.1. Conventionally the antiserum dilution giving approximately $50 \% B$ has been chosen at this stage but some of the sensitive assays have been established using antiserum dilutions far removed from this. However, when antiserum dilutions giving zero analyte binding below 50% are used, it is crucial to have a very precise separation stage in order to achieve the minimum non-specific effects.

Standard Curve. It is now necessary to investigate the response of the assay system to unlabelled antigen (standard). A series of standard solutions is

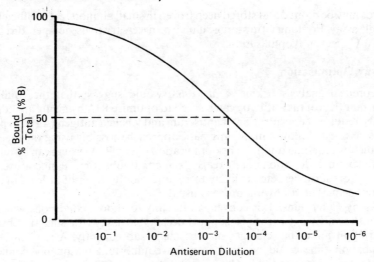

Fig. 6.1. Antiserum Dilution Curve.

constructed to span adequately the whole of the intended working range (usually a minimum of 6 points for a conventional RIA). The response ($\% B$) is plotted against the logarithm of the standard concentration.

A study of the preliminary standard curve should enable the assayist to judge the necessity to change reagent concentrations or incubation conditions. It is recommended that any changes at this stage be made one at a time and the results assessed by the use of precision profiles.

Precision Profiles

The aim of precision profiles is to assess the performance of assays throughout the whole concentration range. The experimental preparation of a precision profile requires repetitive analysis of analyte concentrations covering the whole of the assay range. Within-batch precision profiles are useful but more realistic information is gained from combining the results from several batches.

During method development a within-assay profile is sufficient, and a reasonably simple method is to analyse each standard concentration ten times and then to calculate a coefficient of variation at each concentration. The results can then be expressed graphically as shown in Fig. 6.2 (opposite).

The choice of acceptable precision when deciding the assay working range is arbitrary. The aim should be to have a coefficient of variation below 5% for the clinically critical areas of the working range, but perhaps to accept 10% for the less critical areas. If an improved precision anywhere along the standard range was required then it would be necessary to adjust reaction conditions.

The concept of precision profiles has been discussed by Ekins (1984) and the reader is referred there for a more rigorous explanation.

Validation of a Radioimmunoassay

Having optimised the assay conditions the next stage is to assess whether the assay is valid in the analytical situations for which it was designed. In the case of

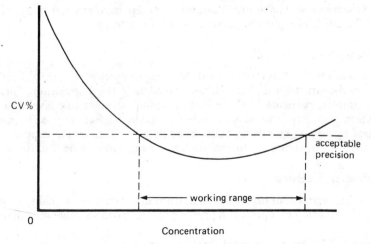

Fig. 6.2 The Precision Profile.
The horizontal broken line indicates the acceptable precision, thereby defining the working range.

'in-house' methods, validation can be considered an extension of assay optimisation, and is indeed likely to lead to minor changes in assay design. However, in the case of commercial kits, provided the protocol is being strictly observed, no assay optimisation is required.

The validation process should involve the assessment of sensitivity, specificity, precision, accuracy, linearity and stability. It is important to relate the performance of a particular assay to the specific requirements and circumstances of the individual laboratory. In the case of commercial kits, only a limited assessment is possible within the individual laboratory and this information should be augmented by the experiences of other users and if possible from more detailed evaluations performed elsewhere, possibly under the auspices of External Quality Assessment Scheme organisers.

Assessment of Sensitivity (Detection Limit)

Sensitivity is defined as the lowest concentration which can be reliably differentiated from zero concentration. A reliable but arbitrary way of assessing sensitivity involves determining the mean and standard deviation of the counts from a minimum of ten 'zero standards'. The sensitivity is taken as the concentration corresponding to the mean counts minus three standard deviations. It should be noted that routine assays do not normally employ sufficient replicates of either patients' samples or zeros for the above to be strictly valid, and that certain pathological sera can adversely affect sensitivity.

A more realistic estimate of the lowest reporting limit of an assay is gained from the precision profile (see above) or from baseline studies in External Quality Assessment schemes (see p. 122).

Assessment of Specificity

The specificity of an assay should be investigated using structurally related molecules, the choice of which is influenced both by knowledge gained from existing assays and from the probability of such substances being present in biological samples. A simple test of cross-reactivity consists of assaying a known excess of the material. The resultant assayed level expressed as a percentage of the known amount added gives a measure of cross-reactivity.

Assessment of Accuracy (Bias)

Assessment of relative bias is easily made by using samples previously assayed by another well-characterised method and calculating the correlation. Quality control samples, particularly those from national schemes can give valuable information in relation to several different methods. Recovery experiments performed by adding known amounts of analyte to either serum samples with confidently known values, or to analyte-free serum, can also be useful.

Assessment of Precision

The routine assessment of precision is described in the section on quality control (p. 307). The addition of a precision profile provides extra valuable information.

Assessment of Linearity (Parallelism)

This is normally performed by serial dilutions on sera containing high analyte concentrations to give values throughout the standard range. The assayed concentrations are then plotted against the dilutions used. The response should be linear, ideally passing through the zero position. A lack of linearity may indicate matrix interference.

Other Aspects

In addition to these technical evaluations, kits should be examined in order to check whether packaging, labelling and instructions are acceptable.

Having successfully completed the above stages, it is necessary to ensure, before routine clinical application, that:

1. A reference range is established. There is a tendency to measure the analyte on personnel drawn from the laboratory staff. These are generally young, healthy adults, and the range obtained may not be relevant for the bulk of the population under clinical investigation. Although it is considerably more difficult, it is preferable to use age- and sex-matched populations. Cooperation with other laboratories can help here.
2. There are adequate numbers of trained staff to perform the assay.
3. Adequate instrumentation exists.
4. There are adequate supplies of reagents.

Counting and Curve Fitting Procedures

The details of radioisotope counting techniques are discussed in Chapter 9 (p. 217). Many workers count each tube until a pre-set number of counts or pre-set counting time has been reached. The pre-set number of counts is often 10 000 yielding a coefficient of variation of 1 %. This strategy, although safe, can often lead to a drastic waste of counter time, possibly to the extent that a department would purchase an unnecessary extra counter. The requirement is to control error in the final analyte concentration not in the raw counts. Ekins and other workers have developed an approach, the practical impact of which can be better appreciated by considering some figures. Suppose that the experimental error in a given assay tube is 5% (not unusual in RIA!); and the counting error, assuming 10 000 counts, is 1%. However, the two errors are not simply additive, and when one uses the correct statistical formula (p. 270), the total coefficient of variation is only 5·1%. If the tube is only counted for 1000 counts, the counting error is 3·2% but the total error would be 5·9% which represents an increase of only 0·8% in imprecision at a cost of ten times as much counting time. The outcome is that one should be able to significantly reduce counting time (ideally using microprocessor controlled counters) without a significant worsening of assay performance.

Following radioactivity measurement, many curve-fitting procedures correct for non-specific binding before relating it to the concentration of analyte. Non-specific binding refers to the amount of labelled antigen which is bound in the absence of antiserum. There are many ways of relating corrected counts to the concentration of standard. Manual methods include plotting the bound counts as a fraction of the total counts on the ordinate against antigen concentration or the logarithm of concentration on the abscissa.

Automated calculation of results saves time and eliminates many potential errors. It is becoming increasingly untenable to object to automation, particularly in view of the satisfactory programs now available even for hand-held calculators. Automated curve fitting procedures may be arbitrarily divided into two categories:

1. *Empirical.* These are so named because their use is not based upon theoretical reaction mechanism, but rests entirely upon success in practice. This group includes linear interpolation, splines and logistic techniques. Many of the better packages are based on the four or five parameter logistic method.
2. *Model-based.* These procedures are based upon considerations of the law of mass action as related to ligand binding assays. The number of such models is unlimited.

Whichever technique is selected it is worth noting that good data handling does not compensate for poor raw data. Also modifying the assay design to suit the data processing technique could entail a great sacrifice in assay quality. It is a prerequisite of computerised data handling that counts be reliably entered into the computer, much of the potential advantage being lost if manual keyboard entry is used.

Quality Assessment

The quality assessment procedures required in RIA are no different in principle from those widely practised in clinical biochemistry. However, because of its extreme sensitivity and the nature of the reaction, RIA is more susceptible than most techniques to problems related to quality, particularly when comparing results between laboratories. Typical coefficient of variation figures for RIA would be 5% for within-batch and 10% for between-batch analysis.

The usual strategy for quality assessment is to have an internal system of quality control, on which are based the day-to-day assay management decisions, plus participation in external schemes for longer term independent assessment of laboratory performance, particularly assay bias.

Internal Quality Control

In common with other large batch analyses performed in clinical biochemistry, it is usual to include both within- and between-batch controls and to perform statistical analyses on these. The non-linear reaction kinetics in RIA have led most laboratories to use control samples with at least three levels of analyte concentration in order to cover more comprehensively the assay range. With some analytes the calculation of assay means can provide an extremely sensitive indicator of systematic error. However, for many substances measured by RIA, patients' means are too variable for them to be of practical use.

Aspects of quality control individual to RIA include such measures as observing the binding of label in the absence of standard (B_0), non-specific binding (NSB), and parameters relating to the curve-fit. Statistical packages are available which not only perform results calculation plus the quality control measures mentioned above, but also calculate precision profiles using data from existing assay samples. The latter is not only a sensitive means of quality control but it also enables each patient result to be accompanied by meaningful confidence limits.

Any well-designed internal quality control scheme will have a simple but effective means of recording data so that the current and past performance can be readily compared.

External Quality Assessment (EQA)

The aims of EQA schemes and their implementation are described in Chapter 12 (p. 296). The value of such schemes to the laboratory lies in providing both long term independent support for the internal procedures and in their ability to provide information which is difficult to obtain by a single laboratory. For the laboratory manager, data on assay bias is of greatest interest since precision can be more reliably assessed by the more timely and frequent internal quality control techniques. Most EQA schemes express bias relative to the mean result for all the participants, but in the absence of evidence that this is a reliable estimate of the 'true' analyte concentration, data on bias need to be interpreted with caution. For certain haptens, gas chromatography linked to mass spectrometry can be used to provide the 'true' target. Tests of base-line security and recovery experiments performed through the EQA schemes can provide invaluable information on an individual laboratory's accuracy.

EQA organisers also provide information on how certain methods perform and this can be very useful to the individual laboratory when choosing a method.

Automation

Given the success of automation in routine clinical biochemistry and the large numbers of labour intensive RIAs performed, it might be expected that the technique would become a prime candidate for automation. However, with the exception of automatic pipetting devices, this has not been the case, particularly in the UK. The reasons possibly include the type of laboratory originally involved in RIA and also the inherently difficult problems for automation, particularly the separation step.

The major advantages of automation, are: improved precision, increased sample throughput, decreased cost per sample and identical incubation times for each tube making possible the use of shorter non-equilibrium conditions. In order to remove the problem of centrifugation, separation methods such as filtration, magnetic particles, or solid phases have been used. Alternatively, a homogeneous assay system which does not require separation may be chosen, (see section on enzymeimmunoassay, p. 125).

The choice of automation as in routine clinical biochemistry is essentially between continuous flow and discrete analysers. Continuous flow has the advantages of reliability, unattended operation and limited cost with the disadvantages of limited incubation times and carry-over. Discrete systems reduce carry-over and often enable flexible incubation periods to be used, making them particularly suitable for analytes with a wide range of circulating levels, and for assays requiring high sensitivity. However, they do tend to be more expensive, particularly in maintenance costs.

Whichever instrument is chosen, the capital cost will be high and in many cases the user is tied to manufacturers' reagents and assay protocols, which can be a problem. Any prospective purchasers would be well advised to seek independent evaluation and to insist on a trial period within their own laboratories. Given the increasing use of routine immunoassay it is inevitable in the longer term that some degree of automation will occur in many laboratories. The eventual direction could be greatly influenced by developments such as labelled antibody techniques, particularly those using non-isotope labels.

Free Hormone Measurement

Certain hormones, e.g. thyroid and steroid hormones exist partially in protein-bound form. It is generally held that the concentration of free hormone in serum more closely represents the physiological activity of the hormone than the corresponding total hormone concentration. The measurement of free hormone would be expected to be particularly useful where abnormalities of binding proteins exist often leading to grossly misleading total hormone concentrations.

Several of the techniques for free hormone measurement introduce analytical principles which are conceptually different from those underlying the immunoassay of the total hormone concentrations in serum. They may usefully be divided into 'direct' and 'indirect' methods.

Indirect Methods

Indirect methods rely on the measurement of two separate and independent variables one of which is the total hormone concentration, the other being an assessment of hormone binding which can be used to sub-divide the methods which are as follows:

1. *Tracer dilution.* In this technique a known trace amount of radiolabelled hormone is added to serum. After subsequent separation of free and bound fractions by techniques such as equilibrium dialysis, the radioactivity in the free fraction in combination with measurement of the total hormone concentration gives an estimate of the free hormone concentration.
2. *Free hormone indices.* This technique is analogous to tracer dilution with the substitution of a solid adsorbent separation stage.
3. *Hormone/binding protein ratio.* This uses the relationship of the total hormone to its principal binding protein. The ratio gives a reliable and relatively simple measure of free hormone concentration. Binding proteins can be measured by several immunological techniques including RIA and immunodiffusion.

Direct Methods

These methods rely on the single direct assay of free hormone without the need for total hormone measurement. Examples of direct methods include:

1. *Equilibrium dialysis.* Serum is allowed to equilibrate in a small dialysis cell, the free hormone in the dialysate is then measured by a sensitive RIA.

2. *Direct RIA.* Such methods rely on the proposition that the introduction into serum of a 'vanishingly' small amount of antibody results in a fractional antibody occupancy which is dependent on the free hormone concentration. It is the case that even in the situation where the ratio of total hormone to antibody binding sites is in excess of 1000 there will nevertheless be free binding sites at equilibrium. The original version of this technique consists of two stages where, following the incubation of sample with a trace amount of antibody, the antibody is separated from the incubate and then back-titrated with labelled hormone in order to determine the degree of occupancy by free hormone.

   The above 'two-stage' procedure, while theoretically sound, may suffer from poor precision mainly as a result of unavoidable variation in timing, particularly in the washing and second incubation stage. More pertinently it has the practical inconvenience of a two-stage procedure with the attendant washing step.

   The introduction of a further methodological refinement which uses a *labelled hormone analogue* means that a single-step procedure can be used. The hormone derivative, while retaining the ability to bind to antibody, is unable to react with serum binding proteins thus leaving the equilibrium of free to bound hormone undisturbed. The method would be invalid if the labelled analogue were to bind to serum proteins.

3. *Other methods.* These include the use of micro-encapsulated antibody, the differential distribution of labelled antibody between free hormone and hormone analogue, and methods involving consideration of the rate of binding of free hormone by antibody. Hormone levels determined in urine and saliva have also been used to provide an indication of free hormone concentration.

TECHNIQUES RELATED TO RADIOIMMUNOASSAY

RIA is now widely used for the quantitation of many analytes in serum, however it suffers from several disadvantages. These include:

1. prolonged reaction times as a consequence of having to use reagents at high dilution;
2. problems resulting from using a gamma-emitting radioisotope, namely a relatively short shelf life and possible health hazard;
3. the need to add each reagent very precisely;
4. limited assay range;
5. lack of direct linear relationship between analyte concentration and signal response;
6. difficulty of automation;
7. lengthy counting time.

For these reasons, alternative techniques have been investigated in an attempt to retain the advantages of RIA while minimising the disadvantages.

Labelled Antibody Immunoassay

Labelled antibody assay, often referred to as *immunoradiometric assay* (IRMA), offers several advantages over RIA. In particular, the introduction of the two-site or sandwich assay procedure in which the antigen is reacted sequentially or simultaneously with solid phase antibodies and labelled antibodies, has led to improvements in specificity, sensitivity, and speed over conventional RIA.

Improvements in specificity result from the need for a substance to possess antigenic sites for both of the carefully selected antibodies in order to be measured. In RIA, the sensitivity is essentially limited by the equilibrium constant of the antibody, whereas this theoretical constraint does not apply to labelled antibody methods, the ultimate sensitivity limits of which are primarily imposed by classical considerations of signal-to-noise ratio. Rapid reactions result from the use of reagent excess, which also contributes to increased precision because only the analyte being measured needs to be added precisely. The non-competitive nature of the reaction gives a direct linear relationship between analyte concentration and response, which also leads to an extension of the useful assay range.

The main disadvantage, namely the requirement for relatively large amounts of purified antiserum, may be expected to be largely overcome by the use of monoclonal antibodies. Another constraint is the limited specific activity of ^{125}I-labelled antibodies if immunoreactivity is to be retained. This could be overcome by the use of non-isotopic labels, leading to improvements in immunoassay performance in terms of stability and sensitivity.

Enzymeimmunoassay (EIA)

Enzymes can act as labels because their catalytic properties allow the detection of extremely small quantities of labelled immune reactants. They have the advantage of a long shelf life, no radiation hazard, no requirement for specific instrumentation not already available in clinical laboratories, and no lengthy reading times.

Enzymeimmunoassay can be subdivided into *heterogeneous* and *homogeneous* assays. The former consist of assays which are analogous to RIAs or IRMAs, whereas in homogeneous assays, the reaction between enzyme-labelled antigen and antibody alters the activity of the enzyme. These assays do not require a separation step and have no analogy in RIA. Homogeneous assays are almost invariably used to quantitate smaller molecules, the key reagent being an enzyme–hapten conjugate (E–H), the activity of which is inhibited by binding to antibody.

$$E\text{–}H + Ab \rightleftharpoons E\text{–}H\text{-}Ab$$

$$\quad active \qquad\qquad inactive$$

The antibody is thought either to sterically hinder the active site or to induce conformational changes in the enzyme. Unlabelled hapten (H) competes with enzyme-labelled hapten for the limited quantity of antibody and so reduces the inhibition:

$$H + E-H + Ab \rightleftharpoons H\text{-}Ab + E-H\text{-}Ab + E-H$$

This assay has been termed the *enzyme multiplied immunoassay technique* (EMIT). Problems have occurred when trying to measure high molecular weight antigens by EMIT. It would appear that in most cases the antibody when bound to the enzyme-labelled antigen is too far removed from the enzyme's active site to cause steric hindrance.

The choice of enzyme depends on specific activity, conjugating characteristics, absence from biological fluids, availability and a satisfactory method of measurement. Alkaline phosphatase, horseradish peroxidase and β-galactosidase are the most widely used enzymes in heterogeneous EIAs. Glucose 6-phosphate dehydrogenase has been frequently used for EMIT.

Unlike radioisotopes, enzyme activity can be affected by its environment. This is likely to be a particular problem with homogeneous assays, where the enzyme activity is measured in the presence of the biological fluid under examination. In addition the critical manipulations involved in enzyme measurement can potentially lower the performance of the assay.

Homogeneous EIA (EMIT) would appear to be well suited to the measurement of haptens such as drugs, whereas heterogeneous EIAs would be useful for the semi-quantitative assay of larger molecules. Enzymeimmunoassay in the form of a two-site labelled antibody technique, immunoenzymometric assay (IEMA), may prove to be valuable in high sensitivity, quantitative measurement of high molecular weight analytes, provided that the reliability and precision prove satisfactory.

Fluoroimmunoassay (FIA)

In fluorescence or photoluminescence (Chapter 7, p. 153) light of the appropriate energy (wavelength) excites the molecule from its ground state to a higher energy state. The return to the ground state is accompanied by the release of energy in the form of light of a longer wavelength.

The use of fluorescent substances as labels offers the same advantages as enzymes without the problems inherent in biological methods of detection. Unfortunately, various factors are present in serum which can result in an apparent increase or decrease in fluorescence by phenomena such as light scattering, quenching or by the effects of endogenous fluorophores. Because of this, FIAs using conventional fluorophores and fluorimetry have failed to achieve the sensitivities accorded to RIA.

Developments have occurred in several areas which should greatly increase the impact of FIA:

1. Labelled antibody techniques have the same potential advantages as for RIA and EIA plus the ability to remove interfering factors by washing the solid phase immediately prior to reading the fluorescence.
2. Instrumental improvements have led to the use of pulsed-light, time-resolved fluorescence, by which the fluorescent signals of interest can be distinguished on the basis of their time-decay characteristics from the generally much shorter-lived background fluorescence.
3. Certain rare earth chelates, particularly those of europium, have certain advantages. They have a prolonged fluorescence decay time which helps to separate the desired signals from that of the background, and also they

possess a wide difference between the excitation and emission spectra (Stokes shift) which reduces the effects of non-specific fluorescence.
4. Fluorescence polarisation (p. 156) has been used to distinguish between fluorescent antigen bound to antibody and unbound antibody also present in the reaction mixture, thereby simplifying the immunoassay. Molecules of the large antigen–antibody complex rotate more slowly than those of the small antigen so that emitted light from the complex, but not unbound antigen, is preferentially polarised in the same plane as that of the exciting beam.

Luminescence-immunoassay (LIA)

The potential of chemiluminescence (Chapter 7, p. 158) as a label is illustrated in Table 6.1. However, before this potential is realised, certain problems have to be overcome. These include interference from serum constituents, the vigorous conditions required for labelling antigens and for producing the final luminescence, and inefficient detection of the short burst of light.

TABLE 6.1
Approximate Detection Limits for Different Immunoassay Labels

^{125}I	10^{-17} mol
Fluorescence	10^{-15} mol
Chemiluminescence	10^{-19} mol

As in the case of FIA newer developments have occurred which largely overcome the disadvantages. These include:

1. The use of solid-phase labelled antibody techniques, whereby the products of the immunological reaction can be washed free of potential interfering substances.
2. Newer chemiluminescent probes such as acridinium esters are insensitive to serum catalysts such as haem proteins, and because the mechanism involves dissociation of the excited species from the rest of the molecule the nature of the emission is largely independent of micro-environmental effects.
3. The newer labels require less vigorous conditions both for coupling and for producing the final luminescence. The latter results in a lower background and hence an improved signal-to-noise ratio.
4. As a result of using luminescence-enhancing compounds the signal is much more prolonged, with the effect of making the reagent addition and final reading steps much less critical, thus leading to more efficient luminescence measurement.

CONCLUSION

The properties of immunoassays will ensure an increase in demand for the foreseeable future. Radioisotopes will probably remain the label of choice for conventional competitive, limited-reagent immunoassay, with exceptions such as EIA for qualitative and semiquantitative assays where a visual colour change offers a very convenient end-point. However, the advantages of labelled antibody techniques, particularly when using monoclonal antibodies, will probably lead to them largely superseding competitive immunoassays. The choice of label for these assays may be dominated by non-isotopic labels such as fluorescence or luminescence, this being much influenced by the 'state of the art' in instrumentation and automation.

REFERENCES AND FURTHER READING

Bolton A. E. (1985). *Radioiodination Techniques*. Amersham International.

Butt W. R. ed (1984). *Practical Immunoassay: The State of the Art*. New York and Basel: Dekker.

Ekins R. P. (1960). *Clin. Chim. Acta*; **5**: 453.

Ekins R. P., Newman G. B., O'Riordan J. L. H. (1968). In *Radioisotopes in Medicine: In Vitro Studies* p. 59. U.S. Atomic Energy Commission, Oak Ridge, Tenn., USA.

Ekins R. P. (1984). In *Practical Immunoassay: The State of the Art*. (Butt W. R. ed) New York and Basel: Dekker.

Hunter W. M., Corrie J. E. T. eds (1983). *Immunoassays for Clinical Chemistry*, Edinburgh, London: Churchill Livingstone.

Hunter W. M., Greenwood F. C. (1964). *Biochem. J*; **91**: 43.

Jeffcoate S. L. (1981). *Efficiency and Effectiveness in the Endocrine Laboratory*. London, New York: Academic Press.

Kohler G., Milstein C. (1975). *Nature*; **256**: 495.

Midgley J. E. M., Wilkins T. A. (1981). *The Direct Estimation of Free Hormones by a Simple Equilibrium Radioimmunoassay*. p. 1. Amersham International.

O'Sullivan M. J. (1984). In *Practical Immunoassay: The State of the Art*. (Butt W. R. ed). New York and Basel: Dekker.

Selby C. (1985). *Commun. Lab. Med*; **1**: 8.

Smith D. S., Al-Hakiem M. H. H., Landon J. (1981). *Ann. Clin. Biochem*; **18**: 253.

Weeks I., *et al.* (1983). *Clin. Chem*; **29**: 1474.

Whitehead T. P. (1984). *J. Clin. Immunol*; **7**: 82.

Woodhead J. S., Addison G. M., Hales C. N. (1974) *Br. Med. Bull*; **30**: 44.

Yalow R. S., Berson S. A. (1960). *J. Clin. Invest*; **39**: 1157.

7

INSTRUMENTS USING MEASUREMENT OF LIGHT INTENSITY

The development 50 years ago of photoelectric instruments for measuring light intensity marked an important advance in the history of clinical biochemistry and made possible the subsequent production of the wide range of instruments now used—colorimeters, spectrophotometers, fluorimeters, flame photometers, electrophoretic and chromatographic scanners, in both manual and automated form. The low concentration of many substances in body fluids and the difficulty of isolating them from such complex mixtures make colorimetric methods based on specific chemical reactions particularly suitable and they have been extensively used.

Considerations of space preclude a full account of the theory of the subject and of all the instruments but full descriptions of most instruments are available from the manufacturers. (See also Lee and Schmidt, 1983.)

THE LAWS OF LIGHT ABSORPTION

When light passes through a solution some may be absorbed. Two fundamental laws describing such absorption give rise to the equation

$$I_E/I_O = e^{-kct}$$

in which I_E = intensity of the emergent light, I_O = intensity of the incident light, k = a constant, c = concentration of absorbing substance, t = path length of light passing through the solution, e = 2·718, the base of natural logarithms. The equation indicates that when monochromatic light passes through a solution, the intensity of light transmitted decreases exponentially with increasing path length (Lambert's law) and with increasing concentration of the absorbing substance (Beer's law). The combination is often termed the Beer–Lambert law.

From Lambert's law, the proportion of light absorbed, $(I_O - I_E)/I_O$, or transmitted, I_E/I_O, is independent of the intensity of light entering the solution, I_O. A constant proportion of the light entering each successive layer of the solution is absorbed, although the absolute amount in each layer diminishes progressively. For a very small layer, dt, then

$$dI/dt = -k_1 \cdot I$$

where I = light intensity and k_1 = a constant related to the rate at which the absorption diminishes. Integration of the equation gives

$$\ln I_E - \ln I_O = -k_1 t \quad \text{or} \quad I_E/I_O = e^{-k_1 t}$$

Similarly, Beer's law relating to concentration, c, gives

$$I_E/I_O = e^{-k_2 c}$$

Combined, these two give the expression for the Beer–Lambert law.

The ratio I_E/I_O is known as the *transmission* (T), *transmittance* or *transmittancy*. Transmission $\times 100$ is the *percentage transmission* ($\%T$). Hence

$$T = e^{-kct}$$

or

$$\ln T = -kct$$

or

$$-\log T = Kct \quad \text{where K is another constant.}$$

This quantity, $-\log T$, $\log(1/T)$ or $\log(100/\%T)$ is termed the *extinction*, *optical density* or *absorbance* (A). Thus

$$A = \log(I_O/I_E) = Kct = 2 - \log \%T$$

Several terms for the absorbance measured under defined conditions are recognised. The *absorption coefficient* is the absorbance with a path length of 1 cm and the *specific extinction coefficient*, $E_1^{1\%}$ cm, or *absorptivity index* is that at a path length of 1 cm and a concentration of 1 % (10 g/l). Its dimensions are $1\,cm^{-1}g^{-1} \times 10^{-1}$ or $m^2 \cdot g^{-1} \times 10^{-2}$. The *molar absorption coefficient* (ε) or *molar absorptivity* refers to a path length of 1 cm and a concentration of 1 mol/l and has the dimensions $1\,cm^{-1}\,mol^{-1}$, $10^3 \times cm^2/mol$ or $10^{-1} \times m^2/mol$. The nearest derived SI unit is m^2/mol.

Confusion can arise if the units used for ε are not clearly stated. Thus, ε for NADH is $6.30 \times 10^6\,cm^2/mol$ which is $6.30 \times 10^2\,m^2/mol$. Thus, as A equals εct, if c is in molar units, then for a concentration of 1 mol/l ($10^3\,mol/m^3$ or $10^{-3}\,mol/cm^3$) and path length of 1 cm (10^{-2} m) the value of A can be calculated as either

$$A = 6.30 \times 10^6 \times 10^{-3} \times 1 \quad \frac{cm^2}{mol} \cdot \frac{mol}{cm^3} \cdot cm$$

$$= 6.30 \times 10^3$$

or

$$A = 6.30 \times 10^2 \times 10^3 \times 10^{-2} \quad \frac{m^2}{mol} \cdot \frac{mol}{m^3} \cdot m$$

$$= 6.30 \times 10^3$$

If the concentration is altered to 1 mmol/l or 1 μmol in 1 ml, then A is 6.30. This factor is useful in methods for the study of enzyme reaction rates (Chapter 22).

Some photoelectric instruments are provided with two scales (Fig. 7.1), one from 0 to 100 showing $\%T$, the other from ∞ to 0 showing the absorbance. In practice the instrument is set to zero absorbance with the appropriate blank in position. The test solution is then introduced and the absorbance is read again. In most cases the path length is constant so that provided Beer's law is obeyed, absorbance is linearly related to concentration. On the other hand, if $\%T$ is read from the scale and is plotted against concentration, a curve results. The percentage transmission must be plotted on the vertical, logarithmic scale of semi-

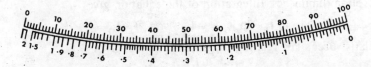

Fig. 7.1. Scales Used on Photoelectric Colorimeters.
The upper is for $\%T$, the lower for absorbance.

logarithmic paper against concentration on the horizontal, linear scale in order to achieve a straight line.

If a suitable standard is prepared and the absorbances of this and the unknown solution are read, then provided Beer's law is obeyed

$$\frac{\text{Concentration of unknown}}{\text{Concentration of standard}} = \frac{\text{Absorbance of unknown}}{\text{Absorbance of standard}}$$

and therefore

Concentration of unknown =
$$\frac{\text{Absorbance of unknown}}{\text{Absorbance of standard}} \times \text{Concentration of standard.}$$

Throughout the book this has been expressed as:

Concentration of unknown =
$$\frac{\text{Reading of unknown}}{\text{Reading of standard}} \times \text{Concentration of standard}$$

Reflectance Spectroscopy

This technique is becoming increasingly used in clinical biochemistry in relation to 'dry chemistries' or 'stick' tests (pp. 182–4). The intensity of light reflected from a coloured layer is measured and related to the concentration of the substance participating in the colour reaction developed in an initially white layer. If I_o is the intensity of the incident light and I_R that of the reflected light then the *reflecting power, $R = I_R/I_o$*.

Two limiting cases for reflection of an incident beam are *specular reflection* at a shiny (mirror) surface, with the angle of reflection equal to the angle of incidence, and *diffuse reflection* (*reflectance*) arising from scattering of the beam in all directions, either at a matt, particulate surface or by particles within the irradiated layer. The optical geometry can be arranged to prevent any specular reflection reaching the detector while the remainder of the light, scattered over a 2π solid angle is collected and focused onto the detector.

Theoretical considerations applied to the ideal case where the layer particles are very small in relation to the layer thickness and are uniform in size and distribution, the irradiating light is diffuse, the layer is opaque and sufficiently thick to prevent any transmitted background radiation, indicate that the absorption coefficient, K, of the coloured substance absorbing light is given by

$$K = S \cdot (1 - R_\infty)^2 / 2R_\infty$$

where S is the scattering coefficient and R_∞ is the diffuse reflectance of the opaque layer and is related in concept to R above. If there are excess scattering particles, S is constant and the concentration, c, is proportional to K so that

$$K = \varepsilon_R \cdot c$$

where ε_R is an absorption coefficient similar to the absorption coefficient in transmission spectroscopy (p. 130). These expressions combine to give the Kubelka–Munk function

$$c = -\frac{S}{\varepsilon_R} + \left(\frac{S}{2\varepsilon_R}\right) R_\infty + \left(\frac{S}{2\varepsilon_R}\right) R_\infty^{-1} = -A + \frac{A}{2} \cdot R + \frac{A}{2} \cdot R^{-1}$$

In practice, the relationship between c and R can often be better expressed by a more general, non-linear function with similar features such as

$$c = A_0 + A_1 \cdot R + A_2 \cdot R^{-1}$$

although with some instruments (e.g. Boehringer Reflotron) a further refinement gives

$$c = A_0 + A_1 \cdot R + A_2 \cdot R^{-1} + A_3 \cdot e^{nR}$$

If n is positive, a sigmoid relationship is produced; if n is zero or negative, a hyperbolic curve results. In practice, therefore, calibration is achieved by using as many pairs of (c, R) values as there are coefficients in the expression. This is a bare minimum and more paired observations are preferable in order to derive the arbitrary expression which most closely describes the rather complex relationship between c and R. Once this is established, any R measurement can then be transformed into a measurement of concentration.

In transmission photometry (p. 130) the relationship between transmittance and concentration is also non-linear but is further dependent on the thickness of the absorbing layer. Reflectance photometry is independent of sample thickness and this allows the use of undiluted samples with less stringent requirements for the sample volume. As with transmission photometry the technique is applicable either to the measurement of rates of development of colour, of colour intensity at a fixed time after the reaction commences, or final colour intensity after the reaction has gone to completion.

SPECTROPHOTOMETRY

The essential parts of photoelectric instruments are a light source, a means of selecting near monochromatic light of suitable wavelength, a series of lenses, mirrors and slits to improve the resolution and sensitivity of the instrument, sample-holders, a means of detecting the light leaving the sample and a display of the output of the detector. (See also Parlett (1978).)

1. Light Sources

For most purposes in clinical biochemistry only the ultraviolet, visible and near infrared parts of the spectrum, 200 to 1200 nm, need to be covered. Different sources are necessary depending on the wavelength and intensity of radiation required. For the visible region a tungsten filament lamp is often used. It emits most of its energy in the near infrared with a peak at about 1000 nm and has only 15% emission in the visible region. Increasing the operating temperature lowers the wavelength maximum and increases the energy output, but the lamp life is shortened. In practice the minimum operating wavelength is about 340 nm. Quartz halogen lamps have greater emission at the near ultraviolet and blue end of the spectrum compared with the filament lamp. For ultraviolet work, high pressure hydrogen or deuterium discharge lamps are used. Hydrogen lamps emit a continuous spectrum down to 200 nm with a quartz envelope or to 185 nm if fused silica is used. The upper limit of usefulness is about 400 nm. The deuterium lamp has similar spectral characteristics but over twice the radiant energy output. The radiation intensity from filament and deuterium sources is similar around 370 nm. Infrared spectrophotometers use a silicon carbon rod heated to 1200°C.

High·stability of these sources is needed, particularly in single beam instruments. The lamp voltage should not change more than a few millivolts for the detector response to vary less than 0·2%. Optimal and reproducible conditions require accurate positioning of the lamp in the optical axis, particularly with diffraction grating instruments. This is achieved by using pre-focused lamps and locating the brightest part of the image in an optimal position by mechanical adjustments.

2. Wavelength Selection

This may be made by absorption or interference filters, prisms or diffraction gratings incorporated in a monochromator. Filters are characterised by (1) the wavelength at peak transmission; (2) the bandwidth—the range of wavelength between two points at which transmission is half the peak transmission and hence the narrower the greater the resolution; (3) the peak transmission.

Absorption filters consist either of tinted glass or of gelatin impregnated with organic dyes, held between two plates of glass, and function by selective absorption of unwanted wavelengths. Their peak transmission varies from 5 to over 50% and they have bandwidths of 30 to 50 nm. Tables giving the transmission characteristics of such filters are available from the manufacturers.

With detectors of limited sensitivity it may be necessary, in order to get full scale deflection of the galvanometer, to use filters with wider bandwidths as they transmit more light. The choice of a filter is usually a compromise between bandwidth and peak transmission of which the former should be as narrow and the latter as high as possible.

Tinted glass filters have the advantage of high %T at peak wavelength but the bandwidth is much greater than for gelatin film filters, ranging from 90 nm in the ultraviolet to about 300 nm in the visible range. Glass filters are now rarely used as primary filters but are still usefully employed as cut-off filters to eliminate light above or below a given wavelength or where the coloured solution obeys Beer's Law at the bandwidth achievable. They are also used under circumstances where high intensity light sources are required; in bright light the gelatin slowly deteriorates and the colours are bleached.

Interference filters consist of two semi-transparent metallic-coated mirrors whose metallic surfaces are opposed and separated by a transparent, thin, intermediate film. The coating on most semi-transparent mirrors is silver and the spacer (or dielectric) is commonly magnesium fluoride. Light incident at 90° to the plane of the filter partly passes directly through the filter and is partly reflected at the half-silvered surfaces. Any such light emerging in the same direction as the original beam will have traversed a path two thicknesses of the spacer longer than the direct path (Fig. 7.2). Where this thickness equals the wavelength of the light transmitted the two beams, direct and extended path, reinforce one another. Light of wavelengths which are further from this particularly favoured wave length will cause progressive interference between the two beams with low intensity of the resultant light beam. However, reinforcement will again occur at a wavelength equal to twice the thickness of the spacer, the path lengths then differing by exactly one wavelength. This second wavelength can often be excluded using a cut-off filter with strong absorption for the longer wavelength and high transmission for the shorter one. While the thickness of the spacer determines the central wavelength of the transmission band, the optical characteristics of the mirrors largely determine %T and the evenness of the

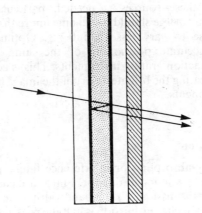

Fig. 7.2. The Principle of the Interference Filter.
The thick vertical lines are the half-silvered surfaces, the stippled area is the spacer and the hatched zone is the cut-off filter (see text). In order to show the beams clearly, the incident angle is not the right angle normally used. At 90° the difference in the path length is twice the spacer thickness.

spacer is related to the bandwidth. In contrast to absorption filters almost any wavelength can be manufactured.

A variety of interference filters is available. The peak transmission wavelength is within 1·0% of the stated value under 340 nm and over 1200 nm, within 0·5% at 800 to 1200 nm, and falls to 0·3% over the commonly used range of 340 to 800 nm. The better filters have peak %T of 20 to 40 with bandwidths of 2 to 10 nm. The greater transmission and resolution of such filters compared with gelatin filters are apparent.

Interference filters should always be used with the mirrored surface facing the light source and at right angles to the light beam which must be parallel. A change in angle of incidence of 10 degrees decreases the peak wavelength by about 0·5% so that a non-parallel incident beam will increase the bandwidth. Above 40°C, keep the exposure time as short as possible to protect the silver surfaces, and never exceed 70°C. As unwanted wavelengths are removed by internal reflection rather than absorption, these filters do not deteriorate when used with high energy sources. The advantages of endurance, selectivity and high transmission are offset by increased cost, particularly if a variety of wavelengths is needed. The total cost may then be comparable with a monochromator.

A compromise between cost and availability for many wavelengths is afforded by the wedge interference filter in which the spacer between the two semi-transparent mirrors is wedge shaped. By altering the position of the filter in relation to a narrow light beam, the spacer thickness and hence wavelength are varied. Interference wedges are available for wavelengths from 260 to 700 nm. Those with greater %T show bandwidths up to 40 nm but these can be reduced to 10 or 20 nm if the %T is less. Thus the resolution falls between that of gelatin and conventional interference filters. They are convenient but as the transmitted light is far from monochromatic, high resolution for spectrum measurements is not possible.

3. Associated Optical Systems and Slits

Instruments using filters as wavelength selectors require lenses to focus correctly the light from the source through the filter and cuvette to the detector. For work in the ultraviolet such optics are made from quartz. In order to regulate the amount of light reaching the detector and hence to set the instrument to zero absorbance with the blank solution, a variable slit or iris diaphragm is inserted into the optical pathway.

For instruments which use a prism or diffraction grating, the optical requirements are more stringent. The dispersion device and associated optical system constitute the monochromator whose function is to produce 'monochromatic' light, i.e. with a minimum bandwidth. The dispersion device is a prism or diffraction grating and a narrow beam of light, derived by focusing an image of the radiation source on to the entrance slit of the monochromator, is allowed to fall on it. The beam is split into a spectrum and the optical system is such that the spectrum is focused and can be made to move in relation to the exit slit of the monochromator which lies at the focal point. By increasing the width of this slit an increased amount of radiation will be produced. The requirements are therefore adequate radiant energy for the detector with as narrow a bandwidth as possible to increase the resolution of the instrument. The two requirements are in opposition. For a given focal length, the brightness of the image formed by a lens depends on its diameter. The ratio focal length/aperture is the f-number and the lower the f-number, the brighter the image. Light is also lost at reflecting surfaces along the light path so that image brightness can be improved by an optical design that reduces the number of surfaces and by delaying the tarnishing of these metallic surfaces by coating with a thin layer of silica. The f-number is decreased by increasing the size of the mirrors, lenses, prisms or gratings and hence the cost of the instrument. Alternatively, by careful design of the optical path its focal length can be reduced with consequent reduction in f-number. With a lower f-number the slit width and hence the bandwidth of the radiation can be reduced thereby improving the resolution. This is the ability to discriminate between two wavelengths of radiation. The spectrum emitted by an element in a discharge lamp or flame (see pages 160, 167) contains very sharply defined 'lines' of characteristic wavelengths. As the spectrum is moved across the exit slit, the finite slit width broadens the line into a peak, the centre of which is at the characteristic wavelength. If two lines occur close together their peaks will tend to overlap but if the height of the point of overlap is less than half the height of the smaller peak, the peaks are said to be 'resolved'. Resolution will depend on peak width and can be expressed as the distance between the centres of two peaks which are just resolved. It is often quoted in nanometres; the smaller the value the better will the monochromator differentiate between two closely similar wavelengths. High resolution usually implies a low f-number, a sensitive detector and hence a more costly instrument. As the light energy of a source varies with wavelength and as the detector sensitivity is similarly variable, the resolution depends on wavelength.

Resolution is important when measuring the shape and maximal absorbance of a sharp absorption peak as the detector averages the signal across the whole bandwidth. For good results the ratio, peak width/bandwidth, should be greater than 5. For most substances in solution, any absorption peaks have widths of 5 to 50 nm, requiring the spectrometer bandwidth to be 1 nm for the most critical case. Further reduction of bandwidth reduces the light energy reaching the detector and increases the effect of noise in the recorded signal until this reaches an unacceptable level.

The dispersive device in the monochromator is a prism or a diffraction grating.

Prisms refract light thereby separating it into component wavelengths, the shortest being refracted most. The prism material, glass, quartz, fused silica or salt crystal, depends on the wavelength range needed. Glass absorbs strongly below

310 nm but quartz can be used down to about 200 nm and fused silica to 185 nm. For the visible region glass is preferable, having three times the dispersive power of quartz. Salt crystal prisms are used for the infrared region. Sodium chloride covers the range 2·5 to 15·4 μm and this is extended to 25 μm using potassium bromide and to 38 μm using caesium iodide. For all prisms the angular dispersion varies with wavelength so that at the focal point the linear dispersion also varies causing crowding of longer wavelengths which becomes serious beyond 600 nm for quartz. The actual separation depends on the refractive index of the prism material and the length of the prism base. The mounting is of the Littrow type in which the light, which passes through a 30° prism, is reflected back through it by a mirror thus doubling the dispersion with a more compact optical system and cancelling the double refraction produced with a quartz prism. Only one spectrum is obtained from a prism unlike a diffraction grating thereby conserving radiant energy. However, the prism material itself may absorb some light and is also relatively costly. Because of the varying dispersion, the width of the monochromator's exit slit requires continuous adjustment to keep a constant bandwidth and even then the resolution is often inferior to that of a good diffraction grating, especially at higher wavelengths. These features of the use of prisms have resulted in their almost complete replacement by diffraction gratings for instruments used in the ultraviolet and visible regions.

Diffraction gratings were originally produced by cutting parallel grooves on a highly polished metal surface. For work in the visible/ultraviolet region 600 to 2000 lines/mm are needed and the machines required to produce such conventional gratings are heavy, costly and slow. They are used to produce master gratings from which replica gratings are made by allowing a thin layer of plastic to evaporate on its surface. The plastic film, mounted on an optical flat, is coated with aluminium to give a working diffraction grating of the reflector type. Despite every care there are small variations in the shape, straightness and position of the individual grooves produced mechanically. *Holographic gratings* which greatly reduce these variations are produced by optical methods. A glass blank covered with a thin photoresistive surface is exposed to the parallel interference fringes produced by the interaction of two collimated beams from a laser source. The resistance of the exposed surface to an etching solution depends on the intensity of light reaching it. It is thus possible to develop a surface pattern of etched surface grooves corresponding to the interference fringes which is inherently more uniform than that produced by mechanical cutting. Simpler, quicker production allows master gratings to be used for the highest performance. Holographic gratings produce much less stray light (p. 151) than those produced by mechanical means.

The wave theory of light requires that a beam of light falling on the grating will leave in several different directions. The angles of the reflected light bear a simple relation to its wavelength and the distance between the grating lines. Thus radiation containing different wavelengths produces several spectra referred to as first order, second order, etc. with the higher orders overlapping markedly. The dispersion of radiant energy over several spectra can be modified greatly by making the original cuts in the conventional master grating in a saw-tooth fashion. The final grating then has its reflecting surfaces set at an angle to the optical flat—the 'blaze angle'. By selecting the angle, about 90 % of the reflected light can be concentrated in the first order spectrum. The percentage varies with wavelength and gratings are therefore blazed for a particular optimal wavelength. It is also possible to produce blazed holographic gratings. In use, the spectrum is made to move across the exit slit of the monochromator by rotating the grating mounting. Diffraction gratings give constant angular dispersion over the whole wavelength range and give better discrimination at longer wavelengths than prisms. This constant dispersion eliminates the need for constant readjustment of slit width necessary for prism instruments. The resolution depends on the *total* number of lines on the grating and the constancy of the distance between adjacent lines. Good gratings are capable of high resolution (less than 0·1 nm) and this is relatively constant over the whole visible and ultraviolet spectrum.

Gratings can be used in infrared instruments in which, in order to cover the whole spectrum, they are usually employed in pairs. They are ruled from 50 to 250 lines/mm and may be used alone or in place of the mirror in Littrow type mountings incorporating sodium chloride prisms.

In all diffraction gratings there is overlap of the shorter wavelengths of the second order spectrum and longer wavelengths of the first order spectrum. Blazing reduces the intensity of the second order and residual interfering wavelengths can be easily removed by cut-off filters as they are only half the wavelength of the band selected from the first order spectrum.

4. Sample Holders, Cells or Cuvettes

For visible wavelengths, glass or plastic cells are convenient but below 340 nm silica or quartz must be used. The shape of the sample holder may vary. Cylindrical cells are simple to construct and are relatively cheap. They have the disadvantage that they may not be perfectly round, thus altering the path length as the cell is rotated. Where the light beam width is significant in relation to the cell diameter the path length varies across the light beam. Cylindrical cells also focus the light beam and the focal point will depend on the refractive index of the solution in the cell. Rectangular cells, incorporating two parallel, optically flat, flawless faces provide a constant path length and refraction is not a problem. Such cells are usually more expensive than the cylindrical type. For an account of available cuvettes and their properties, see Brown and Gowenlock (1971).

Manual filling of cells or cuvettes is associated with the risk of scratching or contaminating the outer optical surfaces. Unless the cell is well drained between samples one sample will contaminate the next—the phenomenon of carry-over. Replacement of cylindrical cells may not be exactly the same each time leading to difficulties if the cell is not exactly round. All such errors can be avoided by the use of a carefully designed 'flow-through' cuvette which is not removed from the instrument but is emptied by mechanical means. Such cells may have better 'carry-over' characteristics and allow rapid sampling of a series of coloured solutions. They are an inherent part of instruments used in continuous flow systems.

5. Single Beam and Double Beam Optical Paths

The simpler instruments use a single beam of light to pass through the cuvette and reach the detector. In the double beam system, the light emerging from the monochromator is split into two identical beams, each of which passes through its own cuvette. Usually a modulating or 'chopping' device allows the two beams to fall alternately onto a single detector which must be a photomultiplier (p.139) as high sensitivity, short response time and linear response over a wide range are required. Its alternating signal can then be processed electronically.

The double beam method has several advantages which result from the ability to compare the ratio of the detector responses. Alterations in the intensity of the light source affect both responses similarly and do not alter the ratio. If the cuvette in one beam (the reference beam) contains the blank solution and the cuvette in the other (sample) beam contains the sample under investigation, the intensity of light reaching the reference beam detector will be I_O, and that reaching the sample beam detector will be I_E, using the symbols on (p. 129). Thus the transmittance (I_E/I_O) is obtained directly from the ratio of the detector responses. Furthermore, it is possible by electronic means to convert this to log (I_O/I_E) and to obtain a reading of absorbance directly. In the manually-operated single beam instrument, alteration in wavelength necessitates readjustment of the output device to zero absorbance for the blank solution before an absorbance measurement on the sample is possible. This requirement is no longer present for the double beam instrument as the ratio method is independent of the absolute value of the intensity in the reference beam. This permits automatic change of wavelength and continuous display of absorbance, a facility used in recording spectrophotometers.

Although the photometric accuracy and precision of the earlier double beam instruments were inferior to that of the single beam models, this is no longer the case. The increased versatility of double beam operation allows a greater flexibility in the use of output devices (p. 140).

6. Photosensitive Detectors

(a) **Barrier Layer Cells**. In these photovoltaic cells a thin layer of selenium is deposited on a copper or iron plate (the positive electrode), and is itself covered with a thin, transparent layer of gold (the negative electrode). This thin layer is protected by a clear lacquer except for the periphery where the gold is in contact with a thicker metal edge from which a connection is made to a galvanometer. The other terminal of the galvanometer is connected to the positive plate. Light passes through the lacquer and thin metal coat to the layer of selenium beneath. Here it liberates electrons which pass across the 'barrier' between the selenium and the thin metal layer, which thus becomes negatively charged in relation to the base plate. The potential difference is several volts and provided the resistance of the external circuit including the galvanometer coil is small, a current will flow of strength proportional to the intensity of light falling on the detector. The sensitivity of the cells to different wavelengths is adjustable during manufacture. As the output cannot be readily amplified, the barrier cell has been mainly used in filter photometers where the light energy falling on the detector is sufficient to produce an adequate current. Barrier cells show fatigue on continuous exposure and thus tend to drift. They are temperature sensitive and the cell response is slow, but they have the advantage of cheapness and do not need an expensive amplifier or power supply. The output is proportional to the light intensity reaching the detector but this linearity is disturbed at high intensities or high circuit resistance.

(b) **Photoconductive Cells**. The resistance of these cells changes with the intensity of light falling on them. Various semiconductor materials are used, some sulphides being particularly useful. Wavelengths for maximal sensitivity vary: cadmium sulphide (520 nm), plumbous sulphide (800 nm), cadmium selenide (720 nm) and cadmium telluride (840 nm). These cells differ from barrier layer cells in that a small external potential difference applied across the cell allows changes in resistance to produce larger current changes for operating the measuring device. The output is more stable than that from the barrier layer cell but the earlier cells showed some temperature sensitivity and somewhat sluggish response times.

Silicon diodes are available with similar photoresistive properties. Their small size enables an array of several hundred photodiodes to be constructed which is only 1 cm long. The exit slit in a grating spectrophotometer may be replaced by such a diode array with a spacing between elements similar to the usual exit slit width. The spectrum then falls across it enabling simultaneous readings to be made at several hundred different wavelengths so allowing a full range spectrum to be measured in one second or less. Such *photodiode array spectrophotometers* show promise in rapid spectral scanning, e.g. in monitoring the outflow from chromatography columns.

(c) **Photoemissive Tubes**. These glass phototubes, either evacuated or containing an inert gas at low pressure, have a cathode formed from a half-cylinder metal plate coated on its inner surface with a light sensitive substance—lithium, potassium, caesium, rubidium or their alloys. A thin wire along the axis of the cylinder forms the anode. Photons striking the cathode surface release electrons from it and these move towards the anode, held at about 90 V above the cathode potential. In an argon-filled tube the increased energy of the electrons ionises the gas, further increasing the current. Gas-filled tubes are more sensitive but less stable than vacuum tubes. The current from either is amplified before reading. These detectors have the advantage of increased sensitivity, quicker response and less liability to fatigue. Varying the cathode material changes the wavelength for maximum sensitivity. Although tubes are available for wavelengths well beyond both ends of the visible spectrum, two tubes are often needed to cover the range 200 to 800 nm. With relatively high anode voltages, electrons can pass to the anode even when light is excluded producing a detectable current—the 'dark current'. This must be offset when making measurements of light intensity by using a variable resistance thereby preventing this small current from affecting the output device. Alternatively, a 'chopper' inserted in the light beam varies the light reaching the detector in a cyclical fashion to give an alternating current output. This can be amplified using an AC amplifier while excluding the DC signal due to the dark current.

(d) **Photomultiplier Tubes**. These vacuum tube photoemissive devices have a cathode coated with photosensitive material and a series of similar but positively charged electrodes (dynodes), 9 to 16 in number. The voltage jump between adjacent dynodes is fixed at about 100 V. Each electron emitted from the cathode when light falls on it is accelerated to the first dynode and strikes this, releasing 4 or 5 electrons from its surface. These are then attracted to the next dynode in the series and the process is repeated at each stage. This set of multiplication steps produces a great increase in the number of electrons leaving the last dynode, often 10^6 or more times the original number of photoemissive electrons. The output current can then be further amplified.

Photomultipliers are particularly useful at low light intensities. The response is linear with intensity under normal conditions, the response time is short and fatigue is minimal but an inherent dark current has to be allowed for. A very stable, high voltage and low current supply is required which adds to the cost. As with other detectors the response differs with wavelength but a single tube can often be used over the whole visible and ultraviolet range. Photomultipliers are used in most instruments but the cheapest, and have been responsible for advances in photometric measurements.

As the photomultiplier detects light intensities 200 times weaker than those affecting the simple phototube, it must be shielded from stray light. In fluorimeters, the light intensity emitted from highly fluorescent solutions can produce damage if too great an amplification is inadvertently used. The short response time enables the photomultiplier to be used as a photon counter in scintillation counters; light pulses separated by 1 μs duration are registered separately.

7. Output Devices

The detector response can be indicated in simple or complex ways. In general, complexity is associated with a more elaborate detector, greater convenience and greater cost. The simple colorimeters with a barrier layer cell produce electrical signals proportional to the light intensity reaching the detector which are not easily amplified. The output device is a galvanometer whose scale is necessarily linear with respect to %T. Absorbance values must be read from a logarithmic scale (Fig. 7.1, p. 130).

With a phototube or photomultiplier, the signal can be amplified electronically before operating the output device. Earlier instruments with DC amplifiers gave final signals still proportional to light intensity making some form of logarithmic scale necessary for absorbance readings. In the *'null-point' method* for measurement, the detector output with the blank solution in the light beam is opposed to an adjustable reference voltage which is altered until balance is achieved as indicated by a milliammeter with central zero calibration. With the test solution in the beam, any absorption of light alters the balance which is restored by adjusting a potentiometer on the reference side of the balance. The resistance change is proportional to light intensity change and hence transmission. A logarithmic scale on the potentiometer enables absorbance to be read. Such manual balancing of signals is slow.

Most modern instruments are of the *direct reading type* where the amplified detector signal operates a galvanometer, servo-potentiometer recorder or digital display. With a linear amplifier the deflection of the galvanometer or recorder is proportional to transmission so the galvanometer scale or chart paper must be calibrated logarithmically if absorbance is to be read. The servo-recorders work on the null-point principle but this is achieved automatically. Any out of balance signal is made to adjust the potentiometer in the direction required to improve the balance and once this is achieved, movement ceases. The mechanical movement also affects the position of a pen on the recorder.

With double beam instruments (p. 137) the ratio of the signals derived from both beams is directly related to %T. The output can operate various devices as before. The type of double beam instrument in which a single detector responds to the two beams alternately produces an AC signal which can be amplified linearly or logarithmically. In the latter case, the signal is directly related to absorbance and if this operates a voltmeter or servo-recorder, the deflection can be adjusted by altering the amplifier gain. The deflection is then a measure of absorbance times a factor. If Beer's law is obeyed this represents concentration, i.e. we have a *direct read-out instrument*. In instruments used for studying enzyme kinetics, the recorder is used to display absorbance against time and hence the rate of change which is related to enzyme activity (Chapter 22, p. 483). If, however, an instrument is used in such a way that the wavelength setting is changed continuously at a steady rate then the servo-recorder will produce a curve relating absorbance to wavelength, i.e. the absorption spectrum.

By passing the output signal through an analogue to digital converter the resultant voltage can operate a printer, typewriter, paper tape, card punch, or visual digital display. The result is thus available either for direct issue as a report, for visual inspection, or in a form suitable for electronic data processing. The latter permits calculation of rate of change of the signal with time in some enzyme-rate analysers or in fast centrifugal analysers (Chapter 8).

Types of Instruments

A variety of instruments is available each possessing a combination of the features previously discussed but there is no rigid classification of types. In broad terms *colorimeters, absorptiometers, photometers* using spectral isolation by means of absorption filters, interference filters, interference wedges, small diffraction gratings or prisms with bandwidths of 20 to 50 nm, can be separated from *spectrophotometers* using better prisms or diffraction gratings with bandwidths of less than 10 nm and in which absorbances can be read at continuously varying wavelengths. Spectrophotometers can be subdivided into single or double beam instruments and when the latter have a wavelength drive coupled with a recorder chart they are usually referred to as *recording spectrophotometers*. Most colorimeters fall into the single beam category although the Technicon colorimeter of the AutoAnalyzer II is a double beam instrument.

Photoelectric Colorimeters

The first colorimeters were simple devices incorporating a low level of illumi-nation, a simple lens and filter system, a barrier layer cell and a galvanometer. Newer developments arising from the need to speed up the final reading operation involve the use of direct reading instruments often linked with a flow-through cuvette. The light source and wavelength selection remain simple but the detector and output systems benefit from the application of electronics. In particular, a relatively simple photomultiplier linked to a logarithmic amplifier provides a signal suitable for digital display in concentration units.

Spectrophotometers

Many instruments are now available covering a wide price range; they tend to fall into three broad groups.

[1]. *Manually-operated single beam spectrophotometers.* Just the visible region is covered by the simplest instruments but operation in the ultraviolet is available at extra cost. The simplest output device is a meter linear in %T but this becomes a meter or simple electronic digital display, linear with absorbance in the more expensive instruments. Facilities for easy multiplication by a factor then give the output in concentration units. The output signal may be capable of operating a digital printer, which is an integral part of the equipment in the most expensive models. Most instruments are only calibrated up to 2 absorbance (A) units although a few go up to 3A and there may be a facility to measure negative A values.

Current instruments have wavelength scales accurate to 0·5 to 2 nm with a reproducibility of wavelength setting of 0·2 to 0·5 nm. Absorbance scales are accurate to 0·3 to 0·5 % at 1 A with a reproducibility of reading of 0·2 to 0·5 %. The bandpass of the emerging radiation from the monochromator is usually 4 to 8 nm so that measurements of sharp peaks may be subject to distortion. The stability of the output signal in modern instruments has improved and the short term variation (noise) usually lies in the range 0·0002 to 0·001 A, while longer term variation (drift) in most of these instruments varies from 0·001 to 0·003 A/h.

[2]. *Single beam spectrophotometers capable of spectral scanning.* These operate in the ultraviolet and visible regions and their average cost is about five times that of instruments in the first group. Developments in instrumental design have produced much more stable single beam instruments than before, and it is now possible to scan a blank solution over the desired wavelength range and to store information on the detector (photomultiplier) response at predetermined increments of wavelength. This involves conversion of the analogue output of the detector into digital form and storage in the memory of a built-in microprocessor. After repeating the scan on the test solution with minimum delay, a second set of data points is obtained. The instrument can then compare the digital results for blank and test at each wavelength and can calculate the absorbance in the same way as an electronic digital calculator operates. The result is displayed either on a simple digital device, but more often on the screen of a video display unit (VDU) incorporated in the equipment. By attaching a printer-plotter, permanent digital information or a graphical record of absorbance against wavelength can be produced. In some cases, the absorption spectrum can be displayed directly on the VDU screen. Alternatively, some instruments operate at constant wavelength to measure the change of absorbance with time after initial zero setting with a blank solution. Such information is useful for kinetic studies.

The more sophisticated uses of such an instrument are critically dependent on the stability of the light beam over the time period of use. Careful control of the lamp power supply and the detector voltage is required and the optical systems have been refined to include optimum lamp alignment, sealing of the optical system and location of optical components far from any heat source. The performance figures of these instruments show improvement over those in the first group. Absorbance scales extend from negative values up to at least 2·5 A and often up to 3 A or even beyond. Wavelength scales are accurate to 0·5 nm with a reproducibility of wavelength setting of 0·1 to 0·2 nm. Absorbance scales are accurate to 0·3 to 0·5% at 1 A with a reproducibility of the reading of 0·1 to 0·25%. The bandpass of the emerging radiation is often adjustable down to 0·2 nm but may be fixed in the range 0·5 to 2 nm. Noise and drift vary somewhat and are not always much better than the figures quoted for the first group of instruments. Noise figures are usually 0·0004 to 0·0005 A and drift, 0·0003 to 0·006 A/h.

[3] *Double beam spectrophotometers capable of spectral scanning.* Their cost varies widely depending on the degree of sophistication but virtually all double beam instruments are intended for continuous monitoring of the change of A with wavelength or with time. The absorbances of test and blank solutions are determined simultaneously so that the responses of the photomultiplier detector for both samples can be compared simultaneously. The output in the simpler instruments is a digital display with the option of linking an external recorder to produce permanent records of absorption spectra or kinetic changes. As in the last group, more costly instruments utilise digitisation of the detector signal, storage of information in a microprocessor memory and its display on a VDU which may also provide direct graphical representation of changes. Other instruments can be linked to an independent microcomputer. Calculations can be performed on the digitised information stored and permanent records are available using a printer/plotter.

Performance figures are generally best in this group. Wavelength scales have an accuracy of 0·2 to 0·5 nm and reproducibility of setting of 0·05 to 0·2 nm. Absorbance scales often extend from negative figures to 4 A with an accuracy of 0·2 to 0·4% and reproducibility of reading of 0·1 to 0·2%. Adjustable bandpasses are usual with figures down to 0·5 nm or less. Noise and drift are, as might be expected, rather better than for the 'stable' single beam instruments. Typical figures for noise are 0·0001 to 0·0003 A with drift reduced to 0·0003 to 0·0005 A/h.

In the last two groups those instruments under microprocessor control have the potential for further data manipulation. Thus derivative spectra can be obtained. The first derivative is the rate of change of absorbance with wavelength; the second derivative is the rate of change of the first derivative with wavelength, etc. Such calculations may be available up to the fourth or even higher derivatives and are helpful in the proper characterisation of inflections or shoulders on peaks and may aid resolution of difficult analytical problems. The microprocessor memory may also be capable of storing reference spectra or the last few spectra examined for comparison purposes. Scanning speeds are frequently adjustable. Fast scanning loses some spectral detail but is sometimes convenient. Coverage from 200 to 800 nm in less than one minute is possible in about one-third of the models. The diode-array instruments (p. 139) allow the whole spectrum to be examined in one second or less. Other rates of change of absorbance can be calculated. The change with time at constant wavelength is the basis of various investigations of enzyme kinetics.

Other variations are seen with cuvettes and their holders. Flow cells, thermostatted cuvette holders for enzyme work, and the automatic changing of cuvette position in a 4 or 6 cell carrier are available as options on many models.

The Use of Photoelectric Instruments

Certain general principles are worth discussion.

Calibration Curves. Since the formula given on p. 131 only holds when Beer's law is obeyed, a calibration curve should be prepared for the range of concentrations to be covered in practice. If this calibration is linear, only one standard and a blank need to be included with each batch of tests; otherwise several standards must be used to define the curve. Standards should be included with each batch of determinations as variations in chemical reactions and instrument behaviour cause variability in the absorbance produced from one batch to another. It is useful to document the successive absorbance readings of the standard for quality control purposes (Chapter 12, p. 291). This gives information about instrumental changes and deterioration of standards and allows corrective action to be taken early. Only rarely, e.g. when a standard substance is difficult to obtain, should it be necessary to rely on a previously prepared calibration curve.

Absorbance Range. Satisfactory results are only obtained when the absorbance (A) lies within a certain range. Twyman and Lothian (1933) produced a theoretical error curve for photometric measurements (Fig. 7.3) which is derived as follows using the symbols on p. 130.

$$A = \log I_O / I_E \text{ or } I_E = I_O / 10^A$$

differentiating with respect to I_E

$$\frac{dA}{dI_E} = \frac{-0.434}{I_E}$$

This gives the relative error in A as

$$\frac{dA}{A} = \frac{-0.434 \cdot dI_E}{A \cdot I_E} = \frac{-0.434 \cdot 10^A \cdot dI_E}{A \cdot I_O}$$

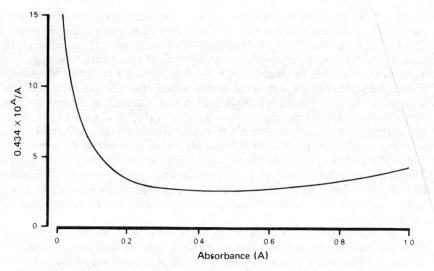

Fig. 7.3. Theoretical Error Curve for Photometric Measurements.

The error in the scale reading (dx) should be proportional to the error in measuring the light intensity (dI_E) and thus

$$\frac{dA}{A} = \frac{-0.434 \cdot 10^A}{A} \times \frac{k \cdot dx}{I_O} \text{ where k is a constant}$$

The value of $k \cdot dx/I_O$ should be constant for a particular instrument and the relative error is least when $10^A/A$ is minimal. This is the case when A is 0·434 but the expression only increases by up to 25% above this minimal value over the absorbance range 0·2 to 0·8. The assumption that $dI_E = k \cdot dx$ may be invalid for some instruments. The error curve then departs from that predicted by the simpler theory. In general, however, it is desirable to adjust the sensitivity of the determination so that the range of concentrations to be measured gives absorbances between 0·15 and 1·0.

Use of Blanks. In order to measure the absorbance of samples it is first necessary to adjust the reading of the meter or other output device at each end of its range. The %T is adjusted to 100 and 0, corresponding to absorbances of 0 and infinity respectively.

The infinity setting is important as the correct value of I_O depends on correct settings at *both* ends of the scale but the adjustment is often overlooked. Variations in infinity setting depend on variations in dark current of the detector and electrical or mechanical bias of the output device. In a single beam instrument the setting is made following complete occlusion of the beam; in double beam instruments, the sample beam is occluded.

The setting to zero absorbance is made with a suitable reference solution in the light path for a single beam instrument or in both beams if two are used. The choice of the reference fluid will usually lie between water and one or more types of blank solution. When reading a series of unknowns it is essential to check the zero reading at intervals and to readjust if any drift has occurred. Drift has to be differentiated from changes in the reference solution itself. If water is used as reference fluid the only change likely to occur is the development of air bubbles, which can obstruct the light beam, if the reference sample heats up during its sojourn in the instrument. This should not happen in a well-designed system. If a chemical blank is prepared this may be a *reagent blank* if the whole analytical procedure has been carried out on a water sample. In those methods in which primary aqueous standards, or water for the blank are introduced into the analysis at a point following preliminary protein precipitation of serum samples, this blank is often referred to as a *standard blank*. The difference in absorbance between the unknown and the reagent blank, or between standard and standard blank where appropriate, is required.

If water is used as the reference solution, the blank reading is subtracted from that of the test solution. This is time-consuming and the difference will have a total error compounded from the errors of two separate readings. It is probably the best method when each sample requires an individual blank as in some enzyme determinations. If the reading of the blank is small compared to water, is applicable to all samples, and is stable over the period of all the readings, it is convenient to use the solution to adjust to zero absorbance. The arithmetic is then simplified. A sufficient volume of blank should be prepared to check the zero setting at intervals using an aliquot and taking care to avoid contamination of the blank aliquot by residues in the cuvette sample measured immediately before the checking step, i.e. carry-over (p. 190) should be kept to a minimum. The cuvette can be rinsed with some of the blank solution before refilling to check the zero. After checking, the blank aliquot should preferably be discarded. In cases where the absorbance of the blank solution against water is a significant fraction of that of the samples, or if the blank is unstable, the use of such a solution to zero the instrument needs consideration. Instability requires careful timing of the measurement of blank and test samples and separate preparation of each blank used for checking the zero. If the blank absorbance is significant, the value will probably vary between replicate blanks and the use of a single blank for zero adjustment may introduce a systematic error. Furthermore, in such a case any systematic difference in path lengths between the reference and sample cuvettes in a double beam instrument will produce further bias.

These considerations should be borne in mind when choosing the best reference solution.

Choice of Filter or Wavelength. In selecting an appropriate filter two conditions should, if possible, be fulfilled. The wavelength of maximum transmission of the filter which is chosen should be such that there is a linear relationship between absorbance and concentration, and secondly the sensitivity, that is the gradient of this line, should be such as to cover the desirable absorbance range for the range of concentrations to be measured.

Although there are occasional exceptions the filter used is generally that which allows maximum absorption for the complementary colour as shown in Table 7.1. Thus for red to orange solutions, blue to blue-green filters are used, etc. Initially the filter which gives the maximum absorbance reading for a given solution should be used to assess the linearity and sensitivity of the calibration curve for concentrations covering the desired range.

When using a spectrophotometer or a colorimeter with a continuously variable wavelength setting the absorption curve of the reaction product (Fig. 7.4) is prepared by measuring absorbance at wavelength intervals the size of which is reduced near absorption peaks in order to define the peak wavelength more carefully. This is usually selected as optimal and the linearity and sensitivity can be assessed as before.

Volume of Reaction Mixture. In most instruments the light path in the cuvette is 1 cm. Cuvettes of longer path length are available for increased

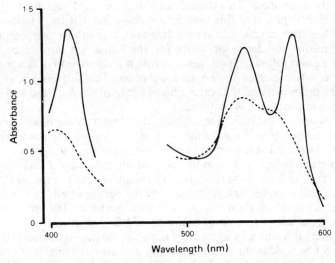

Fig. 7.4. Absorption Curve of Oxyhaemoglobin as Determined by a Spectrophotometer (——) and a Filter Colorimeter (– – – –); after Broughton and Riley (1965).

sensitivity. The volume of fluid needed to fill the 1 cm cuvette varies from a few μl to about 10 ml, and in most cases the techniques described in this book can be scaled appropriately to give the volume required for a particular instrument without loss in sensitivity.

TABLE 7.1
Complementary Colours

Wavelength (nm)	Colour	Wavelength (nm)	Colour
400–435	violet	555–575	yellow-green
435–480	blue	575–600	yellow
480–490	green-blue	600–620	orange
490–500	blue-green	620–700	red
500–555	green	620–700 400–480	purple (red + blue)

The two columns indicate complementary colours. For a given colour of solution the choice of filter is indicated in the opposite column.

Sources of Error in Photometric Measurements

Photometric measurements involve finding the absorbance at a particular wavelength and the calculation of concentration from this measurement. If the calibration curve is linear the concentration is obtained by multiplying the absorbance by a factor which depends on the sensitivity of the method and instrument. Whereas many analytical methods involve direct comparison of the absorbance of test samples and standards, in some cases the absorbance is compared directly with that predicted for the relevant pure substance when the molar absorption coefficient is known. This is the case, e.g. with enzyme determinations linked to NADH or to *p*-nitrophenol, in the standardisation of thyroxine or bilirubin solutions, and for the determination of proteins. The requirements for accuracy are more stringent in this second type. Those aspects which need consideration are the accuracy of the measurement of wavelength and absorbance, the linearity of the calibration curve and the effect of stray light.

Measurements are normally made at the wavelength of the absorption peak of the substance under investigation. The absorbance readings obtained using light of different bandwidths but the same mean wavelength are likely to differ and this is especially so when the absorption peak for that substance is narrow (Fig. 7.4). With monochromatic light the wavelength can be made to coincide exactly with peak absorption but with a wide bandwidth an appreciable fraction of the light will consist of wavelengths which are absorbed less strongly making the mean absorbance lower (Rand, 1969). The different sensitivity of the detector at the limits of the bandwidth may distort the readings further. A narrow bandwidth is thus needed for high sensitivity and Beer's law is more likely to be obeyed over a wider range in monochromatic light.

When an accurate determination of absorbance is essential, the narrow bandwidth and continuous wavelength selection of the spectrophotometer are mandatory. The necessity for accurate wavelength setting is most demanding when the absorption peak is sharp. If the bandwidth, wavelength and light path of the solution are fixed with sufficient accuracy, a given solution should give identical absorbance readings on any instrument with these same characteristics. That instruments do not always do this is clearly shown in several surveys in which reference solutions have been circulated (Beeler, 1974; Stevens, 1980). Both wavelength setting and absorbance can be at fault. Procedures for assessment of their accuracy are necessary. Rand (1969), Burgess and Knowles (1981) and Eldridge and Beetham (1985) summarise methods for evaluating linearity, sensitivity, wavelength calibration, stray light and photometric accuracy.

Calibration Materials for Checking Wavelengths and Absorbance

A variety of methods is available to check wavelength and absorbance accuracy.

1. Wavelength Checks Using Spectral Lamp Sources

These are most easily used with single beam instruments. Although any of the hollow cathode lamps used for atomic absorption flame photometry could be used for this purpose, the low pressure mercury arc is particularly useful as it produces a characteristic pattern of sharp and relatively intense emission lines from the ultraviolet to the visible region. The major lines are at 253·65, 313·16, 365·01, 404·66, 435·84 and 546·94 nm with minor ones at 269·73, 302·15, 334·15, 407·78, 576·96 and 579·07 nm. Such lamps are commercially available and allow the calibration to be checked over a wide range. The deuterium lamp has one useful emission line at 486 to 487 nm which can be used as a single initial check.

2. Wavelength Checks Using Glass Filters Containing Holmium Oxide or Didymium

These glass filters containing rare earth elements show peaks of varying intensity and sharpness (Table 7.2). The holmium oxide glass is useful in the ultraviolet and

TABLE 7.2

*Wavelengths of Absorption Peaks of
Holmium (H) and Didymium (D)
Glasses*

Glass	Wavelength (nm)
H	$241 \cdot 5 \pm 0 \cdot 20$
H	$279 \cdot 4 \pm 0 \cdot 30$
H	$287 \cdot 5 \pm 0 \cdot 35$
H	$333 \cdot 7 \pm 0 \cdot 55$
H	$360 \cdot 9 \pm 0 \cdot 75$
H	$418 \cdot 4 \pm 1 \cdot 1$
H	$453 \cdot 2 \pm 1 \cdot 4*$
H	$536 \cdot 2 \pm 2 \cdot 3$
D	$573 \quad \pm 3 \cdot 0$
D	$586 \quad \pm 3 \cdot 0$
H	$637 \cdot 5 \pm 3 \cdot 8$
D	$685 \quad \pm 4 \cdot 5$
D	$741 \quad \pm 5 \cdot 5$
D	$803 \quad \pm 6 \cdot 3$

* Centre peak of a triplet with other
peaks at 446 and 460 nm.

visible regions while didymium extends into the infrared. These commercially available filters easily fit into rectangular cuvette holders. Fig. 7.5 shows some holmium oxide peaks. The error in assigned wavelengths increases with wavelength, the peaks being less critically defined than the spectral lines of mercury. Calibration should always be checked at at least two wavelengths and preferably as many peaks as possible should be shown to lie within limits simultaneously. Alternatively, a solution of holmium oxide in perchloric acid can be used (Rand, 1969).

3. Wavelength and Photometric Checks Using Liquid Solutions of Substances with Known Absorption Characteristics

The above checks for wavelength are inapplicable for photometric accuracy. The need for reference materials was clearly shown by the studies of Rand (1969). Substances of known purity can be used to prepare stable solutions giving reproducible readings for absorption maxima and peak absorbance values.

Using Acid Potassium Dichromate

Reagents.
1. Potassium dichromate; the analytical grade treated as below is satisfactory. The National Bureau of Standards supplies a specially pure brand: NBS (SRM 136b) but this is not essential.
2. Sulphuric acid, 5 mmol/l. Dilute 10 ml standard sulphuric acid, 500 mmol/l, to 1 litre with water.

Technique. Dry a portion of potassium dichromate in a hot air oven at 80 to 90 °C for 3 to 4 h and then cool in a desiccator. Carefully weigh out 50·0 mg and transfer quantitatively with sulphuric acid to a well-washed 1 l volumetric flask.

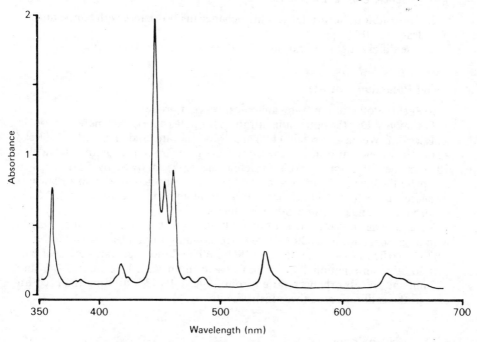

Fig. 7.5. Absorption Spectrum of Holmium Oxide Glass Filter.
See also Table 7.2, opposite.

Make up to the mark with sulphuric acid and mix thoroughly. This solution is stable for at least a year but may show layering. Therefore mix thoroughly before use if it has been standing for a time. Thoroughly wash two silica cuvettes and check that they are matched when filled with sulphuric acid. If not, it is best to check further cuvettes and obtain a matching pair. If this is not possible it will not affect the wavelength check. An accurate absorbance assessment is then obtained by reversing the solutions in the cuvettes and repeating the readings.

Wavelength Check. Rinse one cuvette with the dichromate solution, refill and read against the acid blank at 5 nm intervals from 370 nm downwards changing to 1 nm intervals from 355 nm to define the flat peak stretching from 352 to 348 nm. Extend the interval until 260 nm is reached and then again read at 1 nm intervals to 255 nm to identify the second peak.

Absorbance Check. If the wavelength characteristics are correct, take three absorbance readings against the blank at each peak wavelength, zeroing the instrument each time with the acid solution. If a null-point reading is made, move the absorbance setting away from its previous position initially. Rinse the cells and reverse the solutions, repeat the readings in triplicate and take the mean of the six readings for each peak. This eliminates errors due to unmatched cuvettes.

Results. This solution shows peaks at 350 and 257 nm. The mean absorbance should be 0.535 ± 0.005 at 350 nm, an absorptivity index of 10.7 ± 0.11 $g^{-1}cm^{-1}$ $(1.07 \pm 0.01 \ m^2/g)$. At 257 nm the corresponding figures are 0.720 and 14.4 (1.44) (Rand, 1969).

Notes.

1. Standard solutions at several stated concentrations are available commercially.

2. The solution shows relatively little change in absorbance with temperature—less than 0.1 % per °C.
3. Use different concentrations of dichromate to check linearity.

Using Potassium Nitrate

Reagent. Potassium nitrate, analytical reagent grade.

Technique. Dry the potassium nitrate as for potassium dichromate and cool in a desiccator. Weigh accurately 11·90 g, dissolve in water and make up to 1 l. Read against a water blank in matched cuvettes from 325 nm in 5 nm intervals to 305 nm, then at 1 nm intervals to define the peak, followed by 5 nm steps to complete the curve. Having established the peak wavelength the absorbance is measured as before. Check that the solution temperature is 22 to 25 °C as absorbance changes significantly with temperature.

Results. The characteristics for this solution are a peak wavelength of 302 nm with an absorbance of 0.820 ± 0.006 corresponding to an absorptivity index of 0·070 3 to 0·070 5 $l\,g^{-1}\,cm^{-1}$ (Rand, 1969). When Rand circulated sealed vials of this solution internationally, the peak wavelength varied between 297·5 and 312 nm and the absorbances varied from 0·742 to 0·873 indicating the need for care in the calibration of these instruments.

Using p-Nitrophenol

Reagents.
1. p-Nitrophenol.
2. Sodium hydroxide solution, 10 mmol/l.

Technique. Recrystallise p-nitrophenol from hot water by boiling 300 to 400 ml deionised water in a litre beaker and stirring in the nitrophenol. Allow to cool slightly. If oily droplets appear wait for these to settle and then pour off the solution into a clean beaker and leave overnight, when p-nitrophenol crystallises as near colourless needles. Separate under suction using a sintered glass filter, rinse with cold water and suck dry. Spread on filter paper for 30 to 60 min before storing overnight in a vacuum desiccator containing silica gel. Prepare a stock solution of p-nitrophenol, 1 mmol/l, by dissolving 139·1 mg in water and making up to 1 l. Transfer 20 ml of this stock solution to a 500 ml volumetric flask using a class A pipette and make up to volume with sodium hydroxide solution at 25 ± 1 °C. Read against a blank of the sodium hydroxide solution, as outlined for the two previous solutions using 1 nm intervals from 395 to 405 nm. Record the absorbance at the peak wavelength.

Results. Bowers and McComb (1975) reported a wavelength maximum of 401 nm and an absorbance of 0·736.

Other Materials for Wavelength and Absorbance Checks

Another solution recommended by Rand (1969) is cobalt(ous) ammonium sulphate which has an absorption peak at 512 nm. Two solutions of this material are sold by Oxford Laboratories as part of their Spectro-Chek kit and also allow a check of linearity. The same company also provides solutions of potassium chromate in sodium hydroxide with an absorption peak at 373 nm.

The National Bureau of Standards provides a series of coloured glasses (SRM-930) to check absorbance accuracy. They are open to the criticism that the absorbance changes with time even under conditions which avoid surface scratching.

Stray Light

Stray light can cause significant departures from Beer's law, with resultant loss of photometric accuracy particularly with high absorbance values in the ultraviolet region. It is defined as unwanted radiation energy sensed by the detector. It usually arises from scattering from optical components or other internal surfaces; it can also result from light leaks from outside the instrument. It includes light of the desired wavelength which has not passed through the sample and of other wavelengths, some of which passes through the sample but is only partly absorbed.

If the stray light is not absorbed by the sample for either reason and causes a detector signal corresponding to x %T, then for an apparent %T of t the true figure will be $(t - x)$. The apparent absorbance of $\log(100/t)$ will be less than the true absorbance of $\log[(100 - x)/(t - x)]$. Table 7.3 gives the apparent and true absorbances calculated for different degrees of stray light. The error increases with increase in true absorbance as the stray light becomes more marked. If the detector signal due to stray light remains constant its effect will be more important when the detector is relatively insensitive to the wavelength set. Thus the effects are worst at the lower end of the ultraviolet range. The reduction in absorbance at the lower limit of the spectrophotometer's range distorts absorption peaks in this region. If stray light is significant, the measured absorption peak moves to higher wavelengths.

TABLE 7.3
Effect of Stray Light on Absorbance Readings

Apparent Readings*		True absorbance† with stray light (%T)						
Absorbance	%T	0	0·02	0·05	0·1	0·2	0·5	1·0
0·301	50	0·301	0·301	0·301	0·301	0·302	0·303	0·305
0·699	20	0·699	0·699	0·700	0·701	0·702	0·708	0·717
1·000	10	1·000	1·001	1·002	1·004	1·008	1·020	1·041
1·301	·5	1·301	1·303	1·305	1·309	1·318	1·345	1·394
1·699	2	1·699	1·703	1·710	1·721	1·744	1·822	1·996
2·000	1	2·000	2·009	2·022	2·045	2·096	2·299	∞
2·301	0·5	2·301	2·319	2·347	2·398	2·522	∞	—

* Absorbance calculated from $\log(100/t)$—see text.
† Absorbance calculated from $\log[(100 - x)/(t - x)]$—see text.

Current instruments have much improved stray light characteristics than formerly; this is partly attributable to the greater use of holographic gratings. With a new instrument stray light figures of 0·02 to 0·04 %T are common at 220 and 340 nm but the performance deteriorates as optical surfaces become dirty or tarnished. It will be apparent that when very high absorbances are to be measured, the stray light characteristics must be still lower and in the best instruments stray light may be reduced to as low as 0·001 %T making possible absorbance readings up to 6.

There is no agreed method for measuring stray light. Corning Vycor 7910 glass, 3·0 to 3·6 mm thick transmits no light at 205 nm so that any reading at this wavelength is due to stray light of a longer wavelength. A suitable solution is sodium iodide in water $(10{\cdot}0 \pm 0{\cdot}1$ g/l) which has a %T of much less than 1 at 210 to 260 nm. It was used by Beeler and Lancaster (1975) who circulated ampoules of sodium iodide, alkaline chromate and acid potassium dichromate. The iodide solution was read at 240 nm and the other solutions at specified wavelengths. At 240 nm the iodide absorbance should be much greater than 2·00, or less than 1 %T. Of 159 laboratories, 15 % found lower values and the effects of this stray light were reflected in the readings for the other solutions at 240 nm. Fig. 7.6 shows the results for laboratories with no stray light problem (Group A) and the others (Group B), compared with the mean values for the reference laboratories. The median value for the Group B laboratories is close to the mean for the reference and Group A laboratories but the scatter is obviously much wider.

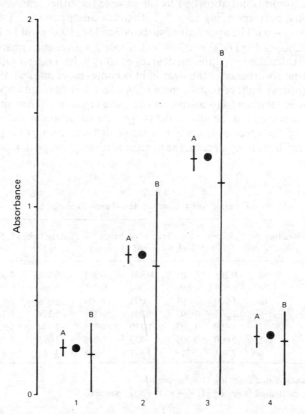

Fig. 7.6. The Effect of Stray Light on Absorbance Measurements at 240 nm (after Beeler and Lancaster, 1975).
The vertical line shows the mean ± 2 standard deviations; the horizontal line is the median value and the circle is the reference mean. For the meaning of A and B, see text above. Comparisons 1 to 3 are for a dichromate solution; 4 is for a chromate solution.

In some instruments a filter excluding visible light is incorporated for use at low wavelengths to reduce the effect of stray light. This should be used in accordance with the manufacturer's instructions when working in the relevant range. Fog (1962) has shown that absorptivity indices determined in the presence of stray light vary with concentration but extrapolation back to zero concentration gives a result similar to that obtained in the absence of stray light.

FLUORIMETRY

Although fluorimetry is less widely used than absorptiometric methods a number of fluorimetric techniques are current. These permit an increase in sensitivity by as much as 3 to 4 orders of magnitude and in suitable cases allow measurement of concentrations as low as one part in 10^{12} or 1 ng/l. For a full study of the subject see Udenfriend (1962, 1969) and for a useful review, Bridges (1978).

The emission of electromagnetic radiation is shared by the processes of *fluorescence, phosphorescence and luminescence.* In luminescence the energy of the emitted radiation, usually visible light, originates from energy in various other forms and the light continues for as long as the stimulating energy continues. In fluorescence and phosphorescence the exciting radiation is electromagnetic, usually within the range 200 to 800 nm. The absorption of such radiation has already been discussed under photometric measurements (p. 129). The energy absorbed causes molecules of the substance involved to pass into an excited state. In many cases this is dissipated in molecular collisions but in some cases after part of the energy has been lost, the molecule returns to its ground state by re-emission of a quantum of energy smaller than that absorbed. Thus the emitted radiation is of a lower frequency, and hence longer wavelength. If the excited state persists for less than 10 ns the process is called *fluorescence* but for excited states with longer survival times, the term *phosphorescence* is used. In some cases, phosphorescent light may be emitted for several minutes as is seen in the markings and hands of clock dials which glow for a short time in the dark following exposure to light. Studies of phosphorescence have given useful information on short-lived molecular species formed in chemical reactions but have found little place in routine clinical biochemical work. Only fluorimetry will therefore be considered further.

The fundamental equation (p. 130) for light absorption is

$$\log(I_O/I_E) = \varepsilon ct \quad \text{or} \quad I_O/I_E = 10^{\varepsilon ct} = e^{2 \cdot 303 \varepsilon ct}$$

Thus the light absorbed is given by

$$I_O - I_E = I_O(1 - e^{-2 \cdot 303 \varepsilon ct})$$

and if the solution is very dilute so that the fraction of light absorbed is very low, this approximates to

$$I_O - I_E = I_O(2 \cdot 303 \varepsilon ct)$$

The intensity of the fluorescent light, F, depends on the quantum efficiency, ϕ, the ratio of the number of fluorescent photons emitted to the number of photons absorbed.

$$F = (I_O - I_E)\phi = 2 \cdot 303 \phi \cdot I_O \cdot \varepsilon ct$$

The meter reading will depend on the amplification of the detector signal which is proportional to F and thus

$$\text{Meter reading} = K \cdot \phi \cdot I_O \cdot \varepsilon ct$$

where K is a factor incorporating the figure $2 \cdot 303$ and allowing for the facts that only part of the emitted fluorescence reaches the detector and that the amplifier gain can be adjusted. For a particular compound in a given cuvette excited at a fixed wavelength, ϕ, ε, t will be constant and

$$\text{Meter reading} = K' \cdot I_O \cdot c$$

Thus if the amplifier gain and I_O are fixed, the meter reading is linearly related to the concentration, a different relationship from that appertaining to the absorption of light. The linearity is not maintained at higher concentrations where a significant fraction of light is absorbed and the above approximation is no longer valid. Provided the detector is sensitive enough and the amplifier is stable, very low concentrations can be measured satisfactorily and the linearity is maintained over a concentration range of 1000-fold, a range much wider than is feasible with light absorption measurements which are prone to considerable error at very low or high absorbances (p. 144).

Fig. 7.7 indicates in diagrammatic form the optical arrangements in most fluorimeters. The appropriate wavelength for the exciting or primary radiation is selected from the light source and then falls on to a solution of the substance under study in a cuvette. The fluorescent light is emitted in all directions but it is usual to select that part emerging at right angles to the incident beam, the unabsorbed part of which passes directly through the cuvette and enters a light trap. The appropriate wavelength is selected from the emitted light and this secondary beam then falls on to the detector. The output from this is amplified and displayed. Fluorimeters may be divided into *filter fluorimeters* and *spectrofluorimeters* depending on the method of wavelength selection. In the former, the primary wavelength selection is made by one or more filters but interference wedges are often used for the secondary beam. Wavelength selection in spectrofluorimeters is by monochromators, usually using diffraction gratings.

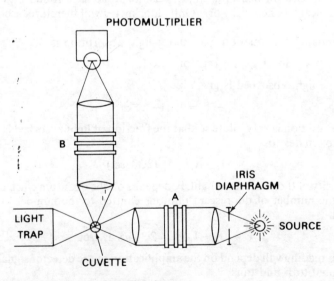

Fig. 7.7. Optical Pathway in Most Fluorimeters.

   Light from the source passes through a wavelength selector A, a combination of filters or a monochromator. Emitted fluorescent radiation passes through a similar selector, B, to reach the photomultiplier.

Light Sources

The equation relating meter reading to concentration indicates that greater sensitivity is obtained if I_O is increased. There is no such advantage in absorption measurements. A high radiation intensity, especially in the ultraviolet region, is obtained from an arc lamp. The mercury vapour lamp has its energy concentrated in a small number of sharply defined lines (p. 147) and allows intense relatively monochromatic light to be selected using filters. This imposes limitations on the choice of wavelength for excitation and precludes scanning of the excitation spectrum. Lamps using other elements are available: zinc emitting at 472 nm and thallium at 538 nm.

A high intensity source with a very nearly continuous spectrum extending down to 220 nm is the xenon arc, used in spectrofluorimeters. It allows both excitation and emission spectra to be investigated and the choice of wavelengths for optimal performance is unrestricted. Any instability of such a source leads to instrumental noise at higher amplification.

Wavelength Selection

Filter instruments with a mercury arc source require further attenuation of the exciting radiation to minimise the effect of other spectral lines. This and the restricted choice of wavelengths reduce the sensitivity of the instrument compared with a spectrofluorimeter. However, the sensitivity is still considerable and the relatively monochromatic exciting beam is satisfactory for many purposes.

When a monochromator is used, a low f-number (p. 135) is needed. Large diffraction gratings are usually used to achieve the light intensity and their constant dispersion allows a constant slit width to be used during a scan. Usually the primary grating is blazed at about 300 nm and the secondary one at 500 nm to provide maximum energy in the most useful ranges. Such instruments often use simple interchangeable slits of varying width. Both slits are usually equal to obtain maximal passage of radiant energy. This energy varies with the square of the width while the bandwidth varies directly with it. Resolution and sensitivity are thus in conflict but testing with several slit widths allows selection of the best compromise. Under good conditions, the bandwidth may be as low as 0·5 nm but this may need to be increased to 20 nm when much more energy transmission is needed. Blocking filters may be necessary to exclude overlap of higher order spectra.

Cuvettes

These should not fluoresce especially at high sensitivity. Quartz or synthetic silica is required below 320 nm but above this wavelength glass cells can be employed. As light has to pass through the cuvette in all directions, all faces are optically clear. The cuvette should be large enough to avoid exciting radiation, scattered within the plane of the cuvette wall, especially from small scratches, reaching the slit of the secondary monochromator. The cuvette temperature should be kept constant, if necessary by a circulating fluid. Fluorescence decreases to a varying degree with rise in temperature and can amount to a several per cent decrease for each °C rise.

Detector

A high sensitivity photomultiplier is needed to maintain the overall sensitivity of the instrument, especially for the spectrofluorimeter which is therefore sometimes described as a *spectrophotofluorimeter*. The output from the photomultiplier is passed through a linear amplifier. Many instruments incorporate a switch to allow amplification to be adjusted precisely thereby covering different ranges of sensitivity and allowing proper comparison of readings of different samples covering differences of two or three orders of magnitude in the output from the photomultiplier.

Output Devices

Simpler instruments have an analogue display using a meter scale. Digital displays are possible and the output can be fed to an external recorder. In spectrofluorimeters the chart paper movement is linked to scanning of the wavelength of the primary or secondary beam to record the excitation or emission 'spectrum'. The recording is distorted by the different sensitivity of the detector and the energy distribution of the diffraction grating as the wavelength alters. However, the final curve is of considerable practical use as it indicates the wavelength settings which give maximal sensitivity or the best discrimination between two different fluorescent materials.

Additional Modifications. Fluorimeters are available with *double beam* operation with the advantages described for absorptiometric methods (p. 137). Part of the light from the exciting beam is directed to another detector allowing the ratio of the primary and secondary beam signals to be examined. The effects of lamp instability are reduced thereby.

Accessories for use with fluorimeters include scanners of electrophoretic strips and thin-layer chromatography plates. Thermostatted cuvette holders taking several cells are available for enzyme studies. Flow-through cuvettes allow their incorporation in continuous flow systems. It is possible to arrange for automatic blank subtraction and for print out of results.

The incorporation of a polariser in the primary and secondary beams allows a study of fluorescence polarisation which can give information on the size and shape of macromolecules.

Use of Fluorimeters

The high sensitivity of fluorimetry allows the use of small samples of serum and often more dilute reagents thus avoiding, in many cases, the need for deproteinisation of the sample and the interfering effects of haemolysis or jaundice. Although the method is directly applicable to naturally fluorescent compounds, in other cases it is possible to form a fluorescent derivative from a non-fluorescent substance. The high sensitivity may avoid the need for tedious purification steps if the contaminants are non-fluorescent.

The number of fluorescent substances is much fewer than the number of light absorbing substances. An additional aid to specificity is that the fluorescent spectra of two substances which absorb at the same wavelength can show quite different maxima with separation up to 250 nm. Even when two substances have similar excitation and emission spectra it may be possible to choose reaction conditions which suppress the fluorescence of one. Thus pH changes may profoundly affect fluorescence by altering the ionisation of groups within the molecule and some substances only fluoresce over a small pH range.

When making fluorimetric measurements it is essential to use a blank solution (p. 144). The reading of this is subtracted from the sample reading and should be relatively low. At high sensitivity it may be necessary to purify the reagents, including solvents, to achieve this. Other interfering fluorescent substances can occur in biological samples and although they may be revealed by various blanks, omitting different reagents in turn but including the sample, it is advisable to scan the excitation and emission spectra and to compare these with the spectra obtained for the pure substance. Any distortion will indicate the need for further investigation. If such interference occurs or blanks are high, it is sometimes possible to modify the exciting and emission wavelengths to improve the discrimination. It will be appreciated that the intensity of emitted fluorescent light is proportional to ε, the molar absorption coefficient. This is greatest at the peak wavelength of the absorption spectrum of the substance to be measured. The choice of exciting wavelength is therefore best restricted to peak absorption wavelengths initially. At wavelengths other than these, ε is lower as is the sensitivity. However, when an interfering compound is present the relative responses of the test substance and interfering substance may result in the use of an excitation wavelength somewhat removed from the absorption peak. Note however, that the spectrum of the emitted fluorescent light is only altered by such changes in excitation wavelength in respect of its intensity and not in its wavelength distribution or quantum efficiency. If the substance under study has more than one peak in its excitation spectrum, another peak wavelength should be investigated. Spillage of fluorescent material in the sample chamber should be avoided and all glassware and cuvettes should be rigorously cleaned.

An important phenomenon in fluorimetry is *quenching*, a reduction in the amount of emitted light reaching the detector. This can occur in a number of ways. Other substances in the solution or the solvent itself may absorb some of the exciting radiation or the emitted radiation or even both. The presence of buffer ions can also affect the energy state of excited molecules and may reduce it sufficiently to abolish fluorescence. Thus chloride and phosphate ions quench quinine and indole fluorescence respectively. The effect of the buffer concentration and type may thus need study even if the pH is correct. The phenomenon of self-quenching occurs at higher concentrations of the fluorescing substance when the absorption of the primary beam becomes significant making the approximation in the equation predicting linearity (p. 153) no longer valid.

Checking of Performance

This can be done by using a set of fluorescent glass standards or by testing a known concentration of quinine sulphate. This gives information on the accuracy of wavelength calibration in both beams and allows the sensitivity and linearity of response to be checked.

LUMINOMETRY

Luminescence is the emission of light from a chemical reaction below the temperature of incandescence. It is usually an oxidative reaction occurring in solution to produce molecules in an excited state. A proportion of these release energy in the form of photons, the others lose energy as heat. Many luminescent substances are known but those most often used are luciferin, luminol and certain acridinium salts. *Chemiluminescence* is luminescence produced by simple chemical means such as oxidation with hydrogen peroxide, sometimes in the presence of a simple catalyst such as a metallic ion. If the catalyst is an enzyme, the phenomenon is usually called *bioluminescence*. In bioluminescent systems, a higher proportion of energy is emitted as photons. The photon yield, this proportion, in such systems is in the range of 10 to 90 %; lower figures are seen in most chemiluminescent reactions.

Luminescent measurements have the advantage of high sensitivity compared to spectrophotometry. Under ideal circumstances it should be possible to measure as little as one attomole (10^{-18} mol) of the analyte but in practice, this limit is not achieved. As the result of a specific reaction, luminescent light is virtually monochromatic so that elaborate wavelength selection is not needed in a luminometer. The essential features of such an instrument are: (1) A light-tight, thermostatically-controlled chamber in which the sample in its cuvette is placed. (2) A method of adding luminescent reagents to the cuvette without letting in light but achieving adequate and rapid mixing. (3) A photomultiplier detector with amplifier and timer which are linked to a small microprocessor to allow the light signal to be analysed in the most appropriate manner before information is displayed on an output device. Some instruments allow a batch of samples to be loaded following which individual samples enter the light-tight chamber sequentially under automatic control. The light emitted in the reaction may be measured as a peak value for a short-lived reaction, as an integrated value for a relatively steady signal, or as the rate of change of a varying signal. The first two are suitable for end-point measurements of concentration, the last is useful for studying enzyme activity. In addition to sensitivity, another advantage shared with fluorimetry is that the dynamic range of the response may be linear over 4 or 5 orders of magnitude.

Use of Luminometers

The availability of commercial luminometers, standardised purified reagents, and simple sample preparation methods offers a technique which has high sensitivity, specificity and speed combined with simplicity and the possibility of automation. Three widely used systems are firefly and bacterial luminescence and luminol chemiluminescence. Their principles and applications are outlined below.

1. ATP Measurement Using Firefly Luminescence

The reaction sequence is catalysed by luciferase in the presence of magnesium ions.

$$\text{Luciferin} + \text{ATP} + \text{O}_2 \xrightarrow{\text{luciferase}} \text{Oxyluciferin} + \text{AMP} + \text{CO}_2 + \text{photon}$$

Nearly one photon, of maximal intensity at 562 nm, is emitted for each molecule of ATP reacting, making this the most sensitive bioluminescent method. Luminometers are available which can measure less than one fmol (10^{-15} mol) of ATP. With purified reagents the system is specific for ATP. As this substance is only found in nature in living cells, the method has been used to detect such cells in various types of biological material. By linkage to another reaction, the method has been used to measure ATP-specific enzymes and their substrates, e.g. creatine kinase, creatine phosphate and triglycerides.

2. Measurement of Coenzymes Using Bacterial Bioluminescence

The coenzymes are NADH and NADPH and the system uses a purified oxidoreductase, specific for one or other of the coenzymes, obtained from the bacterium *Beneckea harveyi*. In a coupled reaction, bacterial luciferase catalyses the oxidation of an aldehyde by oxygen.

$$NAD(P)H + H^+ + \text{Flavine mononucleotide (FMN)} \xrightarrow{\text{oxidoreductase}}$$

$$NAD(P)^+ + FMNH_2$$

$$FMNH_2 + R \cdot CHO + O_2 \xrightarrow{\text{luciferase}} FMN + R \cdot COOH + H_2O + \text{photon}$$

The photon has maximal intensity at 495 nm but the photon efficiency is only about 10% reducing the theoretical sensitivity by a factor of 10. In practice, 100 fmol of NADH can be measured. The system is applicable to the assay of the large number of specific oxidoreductases using NADH or NADPH or both, or to the substrates of such enzymes, by measuring the coenzyme produced by the particular oxidoreductase as the first stage of a series of linked reactions. It can also be used to measure such enzymes if they are used as labels in enzyme immunoassays.

It is possible to select operating conditions such that a constant light signal is emitted which is proportional to the concentration of NAD(P)H allowing easy calibration by adding known amounts of coenzyme to the system. In enzyme kinetic studies, such additions produce stepwise increments in the steady time-progress curve for calibration purposes.

3. Chemiluminescent Measurements Using Luminol

Of several substances used, luminol has been the most popular. It is oxidised at pH 10 to 11 by hydrogen peroxide when catalysed by chromium, copper, iron or haemin compounds. At neutral pH, peroxidase and various oxidases act as catalysts.

Luminol

The photon with maximal intensity at 430 nm is produced with a photon efficiency of only 1%. The sensitivity is of the order of 1 pg of hydrogen peroxide or 0·1 pg of peroxidase per ml of solution. This system is potentially applicable to the measurement of hydrogen peroxide produced by specific enzyme methods from, e.g. glucose or urate, or to the measurement of peroxidase and other oxidases. Peroxidase is used as a marker in enzyme immunoassays and luminol itself is a marker in luminescent immunoassays.

For a review of the applications in clinical biochemistry see Whitehead *et al.* (1979) and Campbell *et al.* (1985).

TURBIDIMETRY AND NEPHELOMETRY

Some analytical methods give an insoluble product in finely divided form so that the particles remain in suspension. If a beam of light passes through, some is scattered—the Tyndall effect. Although the intensity of the original light beam is always reduced, the variation in the intensity of the scattered light in different directions is a complex matter not fully understood. It depends on the size and shape of the scattering particles, the wavelength of the light and the refractive indices of the particle and solvent. If the ratio, particle radius/wavelength is less than 0·1, light scattering is relatively symmetrical but as the ratio increases, especially as it exceeds 1, there is concentration of scattered light in a forward direction at angles of 45° or less, away from the light beam. *Turbidimetry* measures the reduction of intensity of the incident beam and is thus similar to the study of light absorption in spectrophotometry. *Nephelometry* measures the intensity of the scattered light and thus bears a similarity to the measurement of emitted light in fluorimetry.

Turbidimetric measurements are made with the usual types of photometer. The absorbance, and therefore the sensitivity, increases as wavelength decreases. However, the selection of the most appropriate wavelength is influenced by the absorption peaks of other substances present. If a small, stable and reproducible particle can be obtained without any tendency to sediment, the absorbance is proportional to the concentration of the insoluble material—sometimes over a surprisingly wide range.

Nephelometric measurements are often made arbitrarily at right angles to the incident beam. A fluorimeter is conveniently used if the wavelength setting is the same for primary and secondary beams. Instruments allowing variation of the angle of the scattered light under examination are uncommon and more costly. Recent developments in nephelometer design include a laser beam as an intense, monochromatic light source and the collection of forward scattered light after ensuring that the main emergent beam has entered a light trap. One instrument uses a scattering angle of 31°.

Just as fluorimetry offers advantages over spectrophotometry in sensitivity and a wide range of concentrations measured, so nephelometry has similar advantages over turbidimetry. The light scattering effect may be invisible to the human eye. With such sensitivity it is important that errors are not introduced due to suspended dust in the reagents. Examples of turbidimetric procedures are the determination of protein content of urine and cerebrospinal fluid. Nephelometric procedures are used for the determination of specific proteins by immunological methods.

FLAME PHOTOMETRY

In flame photometry a solution containing the substance to be determined is passed under carefully controlled conditions as a very fine spray into the air supply of a burner. In the flame the solution evaporates and the substance is first converted to the atomic state or to its constituent radicles, in which the electrons in the outermost shell are in their lowest energy state closest to the nucleus—the ground state. As the temperature rises the thermal energy of the flame excites these electrons so that they are able to absorb one or more quanta of thermal energy and move into higher energy orbits further from the nucleus. If the energy supplied increases it can become great enough for the electrons to escape from the atom to form an ion. This is the ionisation potential at which atomic characteristics are lost. At the temperature used in flame photometry this degree of energy is not reached. The electrons in the higher energy orbits are in a metastable state and are prone to return to lower energy orbits including the ground state. In doing so the energy previously absorbed is released as quanta of light the wavelengths of which, being dependent on the energy levels the electrons can assume, are characteristic of the substance, thus giving rise to the emission spectrum. The more energy supplied the more complex the spectrum, since more orbital transitions take place, each producing its distinctive line. In *emission flame photometry*, the relatively low energy flame only excites a few elements, mainly the alkali metals. Part of the light, which is emitted in all directions, is collected by a reflector and falls on a detector. The light intensity and hence the detector output is directly proportional to the concentration of the substance in the flame. Under the usual conditions only a small proportion of the atoms present in the flame are excited into emission: 1 to 5 % in the case of alkali metals and less for the other elements. Most atoms therefore remain in the ground state. The technique has been used to determine sodium, potassium and lithium.

As atoms in the ground state are excited by quanta of identical energy to those re-emitted on return to the ground state, light of wavelengths corresponding to the lines of the emission spectrum, if passed through the flame, are absorbed by the ground state atoms. These are in the majority and represent those which have not been thermally excited. If a beam of such light is focused on the slit of a photoelectric instrument the fall in intensity can be measured. The physical law governing the fall in intensity is the Beer–Lambert law and the absorbance measures the concentration of the absorbing atoms in *atomic absorption flame photometry*. The strongest absorption usually takes place at the wavelength which corresponds to the transition from the ground state to the lowest excited state. The width of the resonance wavelength band is such that if light from a continuous source of radiation were used, as in spectrophotometry, a bandwidth about 0·05 nm would be required, a resolution beyond the capability of most monochromators. The source is thus one generating the line spectrum of the relevant element. As this technique depends on the number of atoms in the ground state it is up to 100 times more sensitive than emission flame photometry which depends on the number of excited atoms. The relative sensitivity depends on the particular element being estimated and it has proved useful for elements such as calcium and magnesium which are poorly excited by thermal energy. Its greater sensitivity makes it useful for the biologically important trace metals. As the light used is specific for the element being determined, there is less trouble from spectral interference from other substances than with emission flame photometry.

In absorption flame photometry the excited electrons continuously fall back to the ground state, re-emitting light of the characteristic wavelength in all directions. The instrument is so designed that only the minute fraction emerging in the same direction as the main light beam reaches the detector. The effect on the detector is virtually identical with that occurring in the absorption of light by coloured substances when the absorbed energy is converted to other forms and not released as light. More recently it has been possible to measure the light emitted from the flame in a direction at right angles to that of the beam. This is similar to the technique of fluorimetry so that the technique is termed *atomic fluorescence flame photometry*. This technique, which is still being developed, offers the advantage of greater sensitivity than atomic absorption flame photometry. The difference is similar to that between fluorimetric and absorptiometric measurements (p. 154). The technique is advantageous in the determination of trace elements, several of which can be measured simultaneously. For a review of atomic fluorescence methods see Kirkbright and West (1972) and of flame photometry in general see Dawson (1978).

Emission Flame Photometry

This technique is also known as *flame emission spectroscopy*. The sample in the form of fine droplets is sprayed into the flame where light emission occurs. This light passes through a wavelength selector to reach a detector connected to an output device. In *direct reading instruments* the emitted light intensity is compared directly with that obtained from standards similarly treated. In *internal standard instruments* the light intensity emitted from the element under investigation is compared with that from an element which acts as an internal standard. This second element is one which is normally absent from serum and lithium is commonly used.

The Nebuliser

This most important part of the apparatus produces a steady fine spray of droplets of uniform size necessary for constant emission of light. Only if the rate of delivery of particles is constant is the detector output proportional to concentration. The nebuliser works by directing a jet of air or oxygen under pressure across the end of a capillary tube which dips into the sample. Liquid rises up the capillary and is blown off as a spray from its upper end. Further liquid is sucked up the tube by the Venturi effect. When the droplets pass into the flame, the water evaporates and the residue is decomposed thermally so that atomisation is achieved. Two systems are available, *direct atomisation with turbulent flow burners* and *indirect atomisation with laminar flow or pre-mix burners*. In the former the nebuliser and burner form one unit in a similar manner to an oxyacetylene torch and all the droplets pass into the flame so that it is economical of material. The air or oxygen stream mixes with a burning cone of hydrocarbon at its surface, and as the hydrocarbon enters the flame separately from the air, the flame cannot flash back. A high solid content in the solution can be tolerated, the burner is easy to clean and it can be used with a variety of gas mixtures. The variability in size of the solvent particles causes some variability of light output and the flame can be excessively noisy. In indirect atomisation, which is more common, a series of baffles in a spray chamber lie between the nebuliser jet and the flame. Most of the larger droplets fall out of the air stream before they reach the flame making the light emission much steadier. The flame is also less noisy, but indirect atomisation is less sensitive as only 5 to 10% of the sample reaches the flame. The burner jets may be more difficult to keep clean. Both gases enter the spray chamber and mix before ignition at the burner making the danger of flash-back greater so that the choice of fuel and oxidant mixture is more limited.

Whichever system is employed it is essential that the sample capillary should not clog up and should be easily cleaned. Serum, even when diluted, has a different viscosity from aqueous standards and the rate of flow up the sample capillary and disintegration into droplets can be reduced sufficiently to make the rate of spraying of a protein-containing test solution less than that of aqueous standards, with consequent reduction in apparent concentration.

Burner and Flame

When supplied with fuel and air or oxygen at constant pressure the burner should produce a steady flame. Most burners for low temperature flames have a series of holes where the gas burns in the presence of adequate air to produce a series of blue cones without yellow streaks. This appearance is used to set the flame correctly. It is important that the physical form of the flame and its temperature remain constant. Table 7.4 lists the gas mixtures in use. The propane-air flame is commonly used for the determination of sodium, potassium and lithium. The development of higher flame temperatures for atomic absorption flame photometry improved the use of flame emission for measuring other elements. It is now a competitive technique for some elements and complementary for others mainly due to the use of the nitrous oxide—acetylene flame whose temperature approaches that of the oxyacetylene flame, 3060 °C. It has the advantage of a relatively safe flame speed of 160 cm/s, almost the same as air-acetylene, compared with 1130 cm/s for oxygen-acetylene. This reduces the danger of flashback. The flame head design is much more critical than for other mixtures and the higher temperatures lead to increased interference (p. 165).

TABLE 7.4

Gas Mixtures for Flame Photometry

	Mixture	*Approximate temperature* (°C)
Town gas	air	1700
Butane	air	1900
Propane	air	1925
Acetylene	air	2200
Town gas	oxygen	2700
Propane	oxygen	2800
Butane	oxygen	2900
Acetylene	nitrous oxide	2955

Wavelength Selection

Instrument design has developed depending on the need for either a fast-reading instrument with limited capability, or for more sophisticated equipment with wider detection functions. In the former category comes equipment for measuring sodium, potassium, lithium and possibly calcium where wavelength selection is not critical, the principal lines being: sodium, 589 nm; potassium, 766 nm; lithium, 671 nm; calcium, 554 nm. These are conveniently isolated using interference filters or a diffraction grating. Problems of spectral interference arise with more elaborate instruments using higher flame temperatures requiring the use of monochromators with bandwidths comparable to the better spectrophotometers. Many can be used both for flame emission and for atomic absorption modes.

Detectors

Simple instruments use barrier layer photocells; selenium cells sensitive in the near infrared are available for the 766 nm line of potassium. The more expensive instruments employ photomultipliers.

Output Devices

Initially galvanometers were used but the fluctuating signal made reading troublesome unless damped by an integrating circuit. In many instruments the amplified signal from the photomultiplier operates a digital display or an external recorder. Most instruments for clinical biochemistry are at least dual channel, that is they give simultaneous outputs for sodium and potassium using two independent light paths, detectors and displays. As the dilution needed for sodium is greater than for potassium, the detector response in the potassium channel needs greater amplification. Such dual channel operation has to be distinguished from the true double beam type of instrument described in the next section.

Internal Standard Instruments

In this type of instrument, a fixed amount of an element not normally present in the specimen is introduced and by using a double beam method the ratio of the intensities of the light emitted by the element being determined and by the added element is measured. By using an internal standard in this way several sources of error in the direct reading instrument can be removed. Thus fluctuations due to variations in the nebuliser and flame are almost eliminated since they affect both substances equally. Lithium has been mainly used as the internal standard being closely related to sodium and potassium, and normally absent from blood. Changing conditions tend to affect the emission of these three elements similarly. As a double beam instrument is used, one beam recording lithium, the other sodium or potassium, the difference between the two outputs, the error signal, can be used to drive the servomotor of a recorder or to operate a digital display. In order to measure sodium and potassium simultaneously, three detectors are required and the ratios of the sodium or potassium signal to that of the lithium signal are measured independently. Some instruments can be adapted to measure lithium in the serum of patients receiving this element by using potassium as the internal standard.

This ratio method reduces the effects of variation in the nebuliser and burner system. Its validity depends on a proper choice of internal standard, available in a high state of purity. The element chosen should have an excitation potential of the same order as that of the elements being determined, and as a result the wavelengths of the emitted radiation should be similar. This avoids errors due to differences in the flame background spectrum. Thus the lithium line at 671 nm is convenient for potassium, 766 nm and sodium, 589 nm but is less satisfactory for the main calcium line at 423 nm. It is also desirable that the internal standard and analytical elements should have similar ionisation potentials. The ratio of the light intensity of the analytical and reference elements should not be affected by changes in concentration of the other ions in the sample (see ionic interference, below).

The intensity of the emission from the reference element should be similar to that from the analytical element. The lithium concentration is usually 15 mmol/l in solutions containing sodium and potassium up to 4 mmol/l. If the intensity of the internal standard is too high, the greater amplification needed to measure the analytical element leads to instability. If the reference signal is too weak it is necessary to reduce the amplification and this leads to lowered sensitivity. Most internal standard instruments display the reference signal which should remain within certain limits. Any obstruction in the sampling capillary for example, will reduce the signal and give a warning of unsatisfactory operating conditions.

Interference in Emission Flame Photometry

In determining the amount of a particular element present, other elements can affect the result. Such interference may be of three kinds: *spectral*, which occurs either when the emission lines of two elements cannot be resolved or arises from the general background of the flame itself; *ionic*, due to the fact that in the presence of each other, two elements each emit more light than they would separately (Foster and Hume, 1959); *formation of compounds of low volatility* as in the case of phosphorus which halves the calcium emission.

Spectral interference due to poor resolution is uncommon in clinical chemistry determinations as relatively few elements occur in sufficient concentration. The main problem is with the 586 nm calcium line when there is some interference by the more intense 589 nm sodium line. This has been overcome by precipitating the calcium. Interference due to the flame background can be overcome by using internal standards or an external standard solution containing the same elements in approximately the same proportions as in the test solution. The latter procedure also reduces ionic interference which increases with flame temperature. As there is approximately 30 times as much sodium as potassium in serum, the sodium may increase the amount of light produced by the potassium although the latter has a negligible effect on sodium emission. This ionic interference is overcome by using a potassium standard containing sodium in a proportion equal to that found in serum or urine as appropriate. Internal standards such as lithium do not correct for ionic interference since the internal standard enhances the emission of the elements of interest and is itself enhanced to a degree which varies with their concentration. For methods of overcoming the low volatility of calcium phosphate see p. 170.

A further type of interference occurs from *self absorption*. The effect is due to the excessive concentration of an element reducing its own emitted radiation whereas the interferences described above relate to other elements. When the concentration rises beyond a critical level, the concentration of unexcited atoms in the flame is such as to absorb some of the light originating from excited atoms in the flame. The principle is the same as that exploited in atomic absorption methods but is inconvenient in this case as it leads to a non-linear relationship between concentration and detector signal. The effect is most likely to be seen with sodium in biological samples as this is present in high concentration. Dilution of these to a sufficient degree to avoid self-absorption increases the need for sensitive detectors to measure the potassium radiation.

Use of Emission Flame Photometers

In principle, a dilution of the sample is sprayed into the flame and the response compared with those obtained from standards. The dilution used for serum or urine is often 1 in 200 and is either made manually or by an automatic dilutor which is an integral part of the flame photometer. If manual dilution is performed, the solution must be made homogeneous taking care not to contaminate it with the fingers. The diluent is either water or a solution of the internal standard.

Practice varies with regard to the standards. It is desirable that these contain both sodium and potassium together in a range covering the concentrations to be measured. The earlier practice of using prediluted standards when manual dilution of samples is performed is not satisfactory as contamination from the storage container is proportionately more significant and any variability in the operation of the dilutor is not allowed for. In instruments with automatic dilutors, the samples and standards are treated similarly. After adjusting the zero reading when aspirating water and adjusting the sensitivity to the internal standard when such is employed, the linearity should be checked. Most modern instruments operate under conditions where linearity is satisfactory over the whole analytical range of concentration. If this performance can be shown to be maintained, calibration using a single standard is possible.

Protein interference is much less with the higher dilutions usually used for sodium and potassium but may be significant with lower dilutions. Several possibilities then arise. It may be convenient to use a serum sample as a secondary standard for calibration purposes. The concentration of the element in question in this material is determined independently. It may be possible to add a known quantity of the substance to be analysed to a serum which has previously been dialysed until free from the naturally occurring substance. In some cases, purified protein free from the element in question can be added to the aqueous standard. In all cases it is important to check the linearity of response.

Flame photometers are liable to show 'drift'. This may be either a change in the zero, a change in sensitivity, or both. It is therefore advisable to check the instrumental performance at regular intervals during an analytical run. Zero drift may arise from changes in temperature of electronic components, changes in external light near the instrument or the accumulation of light-emitting material on the burner. These effects can be monitored by sampling water at intervals. Variations in sensitivity arise from a change in flow rate through the sample capillary, variations in flame temperature and alterations in the sample chamber particularly if drainage of condensed droplets is impeded or solid matter accumulates on its walls. The effects are monitored by sampling a standard after zero checking. The sample capillary is vulnerable to partial blockage by particulate matter in the samples. The flame temperature may change if the gas flows alter and it tends to rise if the sample capillary is not immersed in liquid apart from the necessary period during change of samples. Rapid fluctuations in sensitivity lead to instability of the output signal and require investigation of the cause and its correction before valid readings are obtainable.

Atomic Absorption Spectroscopy

Although atomic absorption flame photometry originally arose as a modification of flame photometry, later developments including flameless atomisation make the broader term desirable. The technique has a wider application than emission flame photometry and the general principles are described here.

The elements of clinical biochemical interest which can be determined by the technique are sodium, potassium, calcium, magnesium and lithium; such essential trace elements as copper, zinc, iron, manganese, chromium and cobalt; toxic or non-essential trace elements including cadmium, mercury, lead, beryllium, tantalum, gold, molybdenum and arsenic. Flame emission techniques are more sensitive than atomic absorption for sodium, potassium and lithium. For the first two, emission methods are preferable.

The major advantages of the method are its specificity and sensitivity. The specificity arises from the specific radiation used although various types of interference (p. 170) may impair performance. Sensitivity is attributable partly to the high specificity and to the amplification of the detector response and may be quoted as the concentration in the sample which absorbs 1 % of the light intensity, corresponding to an absorbance of 0·0044. The term 'limit of detection' which depends on the background 'noise' is the minimum amount detectable with 95 % certainty and may be calculated as twice the standard deviation of replicates of a blank solution. The precision of the method can be high, the coefficient of variation being 0·2 to 1·0 % at best, but falling to 20 % near to the detection limit.

With the modern high sensitivity instrument it is possible either to use very small sample volumes as in the flameless atomiser techniques, or to dilute the sample considerably to reduce interference from other biological substances such as protein.

The proportion of atoms which are in an excited state at various temperatures is given by the equation

$$N_1/N_0 = (g_1/g_0)e^{-E/kT}$$

where N_1 = number in excited state, N_0 = number in ground state, g_1 and g_0 are the statistical weights of these two states, E = energy difference of excited and ground states, k = Boltzmann's constant and T is the absolute temperature. The number of atoms available for determination by absorption methods is given by N_0. The results of the calculation for several elements (Table 7.5) indicate that only a small proportion is excited. The proportion is greater with increasing temperature and with increasing wavelength of the resonance line. The emission which depends on N_1, is poor for wavelengths less than 270 nm and is exponentially related to flame temperature. The number of atoms in the basal state is virtually unaffected by flame temperature provided vaporisation has occurred. Fluctuations in flame gas supplies are thus less important for atomic absorption than for flame emission. The former is also especially suitable for the shorter wavelengths.

The basic equipment needed is similar to that used for emission flame photometry with the addition of a suitable light source for the resonance wavelength. The effect of various types of interference can be overcome by instrumental methods and by chemical modifications.

TABLE 7.5

Proportion of Atoms in Excited State at Different Temperatures

Element	g_1/g_0	Temperature (K) 2000	2500	3000	Wavelength (nm)
Na	2	0.10×10^{-4}	1.14×10^{-4}	5.83×10^{-4}	589
Ca	3	0.12×10^{-6}	3.67×10^{-6}	35.5×10^{-6}	423
Cu	2	4.82×10^{-10}	4.04×10^{-8}	66.5×10^{-8}	325
Mg	3	3.35×10^{-11}	0.52×10^{-8}	15.0×10^{-8}	285
Zn	3	7.45×10^{-15}	0.67×10^{-11}	55.0×10^{-11}	214

Light Source

This is the critical component. It is necessary to generate sufficient energy in a narrow band of radiation and a stable power supply is needed for constant intensity. The narrow absorption band of the element being determined makes it extremely difficult to measure the extinction if a continuous spectral source is used making a line source essential.

Vapour discharge lamps are useful for obtaining pure spectra of the alkali metals and mercury.

Hollow cathode lamps are frequently used. The cylindrical cathode contains the required element either in pure metallic form or as an alloy or coating. The cathode and anode are sealed in a gas-tight chamber filled with helium, argon or neon at a pressure of 1 to 3 mmHg to act as carrier gas. Application of an electrical potential produces positive ions of the carrier gas. Their acceleration and impact on the cathode dislodges small quantities of the required element which is excited to emission following collision with other carrier gas ions. Earlier lamps filled with argon had several disadvantages but the 'high spectral output' variant with a shielded cathode and better choice of carrier gas and pressure gives satisfactory results with relatively simple equipment. Such lamps are available for all elements that can be determined by atomic absorption spectroscopy. They are easy to change and their output, which is fully stabilised in 7 to 15 minutes, depends only on the current supplied. They give sharp lines of moderately high intensity, the half bandwidth being only 1 to 2 pm in the most favourable cases. They are expensive to manufacture and their life is limited. Some deteriorate on storage, making it advisable to check the lamp emission periodically and thereby prolong the shelf life. With elements such as nickel, the collision process may cause unsuitable radiation from the ionic form of the metal and thus the *high intensity hollow cathode lamp* was introduced to overcome this. The metal atoms are excited by a low energy electric discharge across two auxiliary electrodes rather than by the high energy carrier gas ions. This enhances by some 50 to 100 times the radiation from the easily excited ground state of the metal atom at the expense of radiation from the metal ion and carrier gas. Their disadvantages of extra power supply, cost, short life and limited range of elements have prevented their wider use particularly with improvements in the traditional hollow cathode lamps. Increases in light output in either case allow the use of narrower slits in the monochromator or less amplification with consequent better linearity and sensitivity.

The microwave-excited electrodeless discharge tube is a later development. A quartz tube contains the element, usually as its volatile iodide, and an inert gas at a pressure of 1 to 3 mmHg. Energy of the characteristic wavelength is emitted when the tube is placed in a high frequency electrostatic field produced by a microwave generator. They produce emission lines up to 1000 times as intense as those from a hollow cathode lamp, are cheaper and have a long life. Against this are the disadvantages: the cost of the generator, the more critical optical alignment needed, the warm-up time increased to as long as two hours, the increased number of operating parameters and the restricted range of elements available.

Formation of Atomic Vapour

Although originally introduced as a variant of flame spectroscopy, the technique now includes other ways of producing an atomic vapour.

Nebuliser and Flame System. *Direct atomisation* with turbulent flow burners and *indirect atomisation* with laminar flow or pre-mix burners are used as in emission flame photometry (p. 162). Pre-mix burners give better results but differ from those used in emission flame instruments in that the multiple holes are replaced by a single long slot so that the light beam traverses the length of the flame. The burner heads for air-acetylene and similar flames are usually of stainless steel with a slot of 0.5×100 mm, but with the higher temperature nitrous oxide-acetylene flame the slot length is reduced to 50 mm and aluminium cooling fins may be added to reduce any tendency to flash back. Other designs include multislot burners and those specifically intended for use with solutions containing a high concentration of dissolved solids.

Those fine droplets produced by the nebuliser which enter the flame are evaporated and the solid particles then melt and volatilise. In oxygen-supported flames the element is usually converted to its oxide and some oxides, particularly that of aluminium, volatilise with difficulty. The dissociation of the oxide is increased at higher temperatures and with a reduced oxygen content of the flame. The latter can be varied by the relative flow of oxygen and acetylene and is low in a fuel-rich flame. For elements forming refractory oxides and for other involatile particles there are advantages in using the hotter, reducing nitrous oxide-acetylene flame. In certain special cases, hydrogen-oxygen, hydrogen-air and hydrogen-argon flames may be employed. For many elements the proportion of atoms which are in the excited state is only altered slightly at higher temperatures (p. 167) which are mainly needed to increase the total number of atoms in the flame. With sodium, potassium, copper and zinc, atomisation is satisfactory in the air-acetylene flame and hotter flames increase the number of ions formed as the ionisation potential may be exceeded.

The absorbance is directly proportional to the flame length. Irregularities in droplet concentration are less important with a long path but in general a definite part of the flame will contain the highest concentration of the absorbing species depending on the variation of temperature and oxygen content. Provision is usually made to adjust the height of the burner in relation to the light beam to maximise the absorbance.

Direct atomisation in the flame has been used for such volatile elements as lead, zinc, mercury and arsenic. Kahn *et al.* (1968) placed the sample in a small tantalum boat which is moved towards the flame. The sample is dried, ashed and finally inserted directly into the flame to produce a transient cloud of atomic vapour and consequent response of the detector. This increases the sensitivity 100-fold. Delves (1970) used a nickel cup in the same way but the vapour was passed directly into a horizontal nickel tube heated in the flame. The method has been especially used for the determination of lead in blood with a sensitivity of 0·1 ng. A further technique involves preparation of the volatile hydrides of selected elements. These are passed directly into a silica tube heated in the flame thus increasing the sensitivity 100 times over the conventional flame technique. In each case matrix interference effects are important (p. 171).

Electrothermal Atomisation. This technique employs no flame but the element is atomised by heating electrically. The various methods (Kirkbright, 1971) have much higher sensitivity than indirect flame atomisation, sometimes for as little as 1 pg. Small samples can be used without preliminary dilution or extraction but the effects of molecular absorption and matrix interference are worse as is the precision. Various devices are available commercially. The graphite or tantalum rod atomiser incorporates a small recess in the rod into which the sample is placed. The rod is heated electrically to increasing temperatures to produce drying, ashing, and finally vaporisation into a laminar flow of nitrogen or argon passed immediately above the rod. In the graphite furnace, the sample is placed in a graphite tube through which the light beam and nitrogen or argon pass. The three stages of heating are performed as before. In each case the final heating is to about 3000 °C for 1 s.

A similar technique is the *cold vaporisation method* for mercury which is volatile at ambient temperature and can be carried by a stream of gas into the absorption tube through which the light beam passes.

Wavelength Selection

The resolution needed is achieved using a grating or prism monochromator to separate the resonance line from those of the carrier gas in the lamp and the other lines of the element under investigation. When an instrument is used for both emission and absorption modes, a higher resolution monochromator is needed. In use, the slit width is reduced to the minimum compatible with an acceptable signal.

In most cases the half width of the absorption line, usually about 5 pm, is greater than that of the source line and both are much less than the bandwidth of the monochromator. Under such circumstances Beer's law is obeyed up to absorbance values of 0·5 to 1. Above this, the absorption may vary across the line width causing a lower absorbance than predicted by Beer's law but for most biological applications high absorbance values are not reached.

Detector and Output Devices

A photomultiplier is used in conjunction with an amplifier and if this is logarithmic the signal is proportional to absorbance and can operate a recorder or digital display. In instruments also used in the emission mode an alternative linear amplifier provides the appropriate signal. In atomic absorption spectroscopy two sources of light pass through the monochromator to the detector, the resonance line from the lamp and the emission from the flame. By modulating the lamp output, at 350 to 400 Hz, either by a mechanical chopper or an AC supply (Fig. 7.8, p. 171) an alternating signal reaches the detector which is electronically separated from the continuous signal of the flame background.

Interferences

The various types of interference are similar to those in emission flame photometry (p. 164) as any factor which alters the behaviour of the atom population in the ground state affects both absorption and emission.

Spectral interference. This is almost entirely eliminated, the only line measured being the resonance line from the lamp. In multi-element lamps, two elements may emit lines of closely similar wavelength making a good monochromator desirable. Selection of a secondary line for the element required may also eliminate the effect.

Ionic Interference. If ionisation occurs, loss of atomic properties reduces the absorbance. Electrons resulting from the partial ionisation of sodium or potassium in acetylene flames suppress ionisation of other elements. This is exploited by deliberately adding potassium to the final sample in a concentration of 1 g/l. When analysing biological samples, sodium and potassium should be included in the standard solutions at a similar concentration to that of the samples. Other ions are added if they also affect ionisation of the analyte and are present in the sample.

Chemical Interference. Formation of poorly volatile compounds reduces the atomic population. Phosphate interference in the determination of calcium occurs with the air-acetylene flame which is not hot enough to volatilise calcium phosphate. The hotter nitrous oxide-acetylene flame eliminates this interference but some calcium atoms are ionised. At lower temperatures the interference is reduced by adding lanthanum or strontium salts which have a greater affinity for phosphate than does calcium. Alternatively, EDTA is added to form a calcium complex which readily dissociates in the flame.

Other Interferences. These occur when trace elements are determined with minimal pre-processing of the sample and are particularly troublesome when working near the sensitivity limit. *Molecular absorption* by components of the flame increases background noise. In the air-acetylene flame, peaks occur between

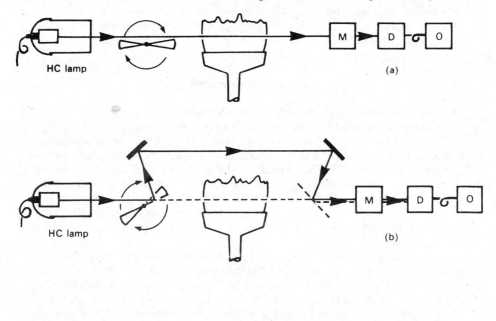

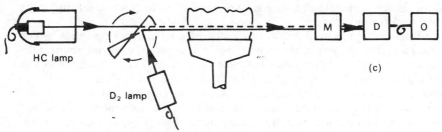

Fig. 7.8. Optical Pathways in Atomic Absorption Spectrophotometers.
(a) Single beam instrument with mechanical modulation of light from a hollow cathode lamp. (b) Double beam instrument with mechanical chopping device producing the beams alternately. A half-silvered mirror (⟍) recombines the beams. (c) Dual-channel arrangement with a deuterium lamp as the second light source used for flame background correction. In each diagram, M = monochromator, D = detector and O = output device.

420 and 570 nm; in the nitrous oxide-acetylene flame, between 350 and 440 nm. If the principal line of an analyte falls in such a zone and interference is marked, a secondary line may be used. Light scattering by particulate matter is one form of *matrix interference*. It occurs if solids are released into the light path from untreated samples and is particularly apparent in the flameless techniques and at wavelengths below 300 nm. Background correction by optical methods (see p. 172) can correct for this effect or a nearby resonance line can be measured as a blank. Careful control of heating with equilibration of the temperatures of the inert gas and sample in the furnace before final vaporisation occurs is claimed to reduce matrix interference. Extraction of a complex of the element by an organic solvent also removes interfering solids and may achieve some increase in concentration in addition.

Another form of matrix interference arises from changes in the viscosity of the sample which affects nebulisation. Organic extracts may show a higher efficiency of nebulisation which can be exploited to increase the sensitivity. An example is the use of methyl isobutyl ketone (4-methyl-pentan-2-one) to extract ammonium pyrrolidine dithiocarbamate (APDC) complexes of trace elements.

Types of Instruments

Modifications have been introduced to overcome interference, to reduce background noise and to simplify the measuring operations.

There are single and double beam instruments. In the latter the light from the source lamp is mechanically chopped into two beams, only one of which passes through the flame (Fig. 7.8). The recombined beams fall on the detector alternately to produce an alternating signal the size of which increases with greater absorption in the flame. Dual channel instruments differ in that two beams of light originating from two sources combine to pass through the flame and fall on the detector (Fig. 7.8). The most expensive instruments employ double beam/dual channel operation.

The advantages of double beam operation are that the lamp emission does not need to have reached a stable output, the base line is steadier and there is little or no zero drift. However, the lower light intensity of each beam requires either a wider slit setting on the monochromator with some loss of sensitivity or the use of a larger, more costly monochromator with smaller f-number. Such instruments can be slower to operate and there is no correction for light scattering due to the flame background.

Such correction is available in one mode of dual channel operation which utilises a deuterium lamp as the second source. This produces a continuum in the relevant part of the spectrum allowing the flame background to be measured. The difference in the detector responses to the two sources is then attributed to specific absorption of the resonance line. A more specific method of background correction which relies on the Zeeman effect permits the resonance line to be used for the measurement of atomic and background absorption. The Zeeman effect occurs when an atomic spectral line is subjected to a strong magnetic field. In the simplest case the line splits into three components: one, the π component is situated at the original wavelength and two σ components ($\sigma+$ and $\sigma-$) appear equidistant from it, one to each side. Their combined intensities equal the original intensity. The π component is polarised in the plane of the magnetic field and the σ components at right angles to it. Some elements show more complex patterns. Under normal operating conditions only atomic spectral lines are split; other absorption bands and particulate absorption are unaffected. With the magnetic field off, the attenuation of the beam from the specific lamp is due to both atomic and background absorption. If the magnetic field is applied to the atomic vapour in the furnace, the σ components are shifted away from the resonance line and no longer attenuate the beam. If that beam is also polarised at right angles to the π component, this will also no longer absorb the radiation leaving only background absorption to be measured specifically. In practice an alternating magnetic field is applied and the two signals are analysed electronically.

Some double beam instruments can be converted to work in this dual beam mode but are then effectively operating under single beam conditions regarding changing emission from lamps, etc. With dual channel/double beam operation both light sources operate under double beam conditions. A single detector receives modulated signals from both sources and the responses to the separate sources are sorted electronically. Such instruments may be used in several ways.

1. by using two different hollow cathode lamps, two different elements may be determined simultaneously, thus saving sample volume and time;
2. under similar conditions the second element may be an internal standard added to the sample with potential improvements in accuracy and precision;
3. by using a deuterium lamp as the second source, background correction is made under true double-beam operating conditions.

Other features may simplify operation. For low absorbances, scale expansion is advantageous particularly if any part of the range can be expanded so that full scale deflection of the output device represents the expanded portion. Such expansion increases the background noise but instability of the output can either be corrected visually or by integration of the signal over a suitable time period. The variable amplification of the output also allows direct display in concentration mode. Some instruments include electrical correction for deviations from Beer's law to widen the range of concentration handled. Other convenient features are an automatic zero setting, operated while sampling a blank solution, and automatic calibration to a pre-set concentration, operated while sampling a standard solution. Several instruments allow a number of hollow cathode lamps to be held in a turret on standby to speed up the change from one element to another.

The choice of instrument depends on the elements to be determined, their concentration in the samples encountered, the amount of sample available and the desirability of introducing time-consuming preliminary purification and concentration steps as against direct determination in the presence of interfering materials. Thus for the elements and samples of clinical biochemical interest, magnesium and calcium determinations and probably copper and zinc may be performed satisfactorily with the simpler instruments. With the moderately sophisticated instruments a wide range of elements can be determined by flame methods particularly if chemical extraction and concentration procedures are employed. Flameless atomisation techniques used with such equipment increase the sensitivity and avoid the need for preliminary processing but the precision may suffer. The most elaborate, and hence most expensive, instruments offer the advantages of better precision and virtually no pre-processing even for those elements which are almost unassayable with the simpler instruments.

Operation of Atomic Absorption Flame Photometers

After igniting the flame and switching on the lamp(s) allow the instrument to warm up while aspirating water into the flame. After reaching stable operating conditions check the zero transmission setting, adjust to zero absorbance and then aspirate a standard. Maximise the signal from this after setting the monochromator to the nominal wavelength by further adjustments of the flame and wavelength setting. Follow the manufacturer's instructions to alter the proportion of fuel and other gas flows and adjust the burner height to achieve optimal flame conditions. Then make minor adjustments to the wavelength setting to ensure that the peak of the absorption line is centred on the monochromator slit. Reduce the slit width sufficiently to obtain high selectivity of wavelength without introducing signal instability. Repeat the setting of the zero absorbance for the blank and then recheck the standard. If several standards are used, prepare a standard curve and then aspirate the samples. At regular intervals check the zero setting using the blank and the reading of a suitable standard in order to assess any drift either of zero setting or of sensitivity.

When making up standards and reagents, particularly for trace element work, use high purity chemicals and good quality distilled water. Check the reagent blank carefully against the latter. Certain points are important in relation to standards in order to allow for interferences appropriately. If a serum sample is diluted little, viscosity effects will be important and the standards should have a similar viscosity. Include in the standards those elements which can interfere, in similar concentration to that in the samples. If a suppressant is added to the sample, add it also to the standard, e.g., lanthanum salts or EDTA in calcium methods or sodium or potassium as a suppressor of ionisation. If an organic solvent is employed to increase the sensitivity, add it to the standard in the same final concentration. If chelation and organic extraction are employed, treat standards similarly.

Certain precautions are generally advisable. Keep the burner clean by removing any accumulated deposits regularly and check that the sampling capillary is not obstructed. Check the wavelength calibration at intervals by noting the peaks in detector response on scanning the output of several different hollow cathode lamps so as to cover the whole wavelength range needed. When working with organic solvents keep them away from the instrument until ready for sampling. Avoid leaving the flame unattended so that unexpected changes in gas flows do not go unheeded. Avoid looking at the flame or source directly to reduce ultraviolet damage to the eye.

General precautions concerning the use of gas cylinders have been described earlier (p. 7). Acetylene which is frequently used in atomic absorption spectroscopy is supplied in cylinders in which the gas is dissolved in acetone. Under these conditions the pressure registered on the high pressure side of the outlet reduction valve is not directly proportional to the amount of acetylene remaining and is affected by the storage temperature. Keep and use such cylinders, preferably in a special gas store area, in the upright position to avoid liquid acetone reaching the outlet. Some acetone vapour is removed with the acetylene and the proportion increases as the cylinder contents are used. It is advisable to discontinue use once the pressure falls below 100 lb/in^2 (690 kPa) at room temperature or somewhat lower if stored outside the laboratory. Otherwise the increasing proportion of acetone affects the flame luminosity and a sudden fall as the last of the acetylene leaves the cylinder may cause the flame to blow back. Acetylene may explode spontaneously in tubing at high pressure. The piped acetylene supply from the cylinder to the instrument should not be at a pressure greater than 9 lb/in^2 (62 kPa), according to Home Office Regulations Statutory Rules and Orders (1937) No. 54, amended No. 805, unless special Home Office approval is obtained. Some instruments require pressures slightly in excess of this figure for proper operation but rarely more than 15 lb/in^2 (103 kPa). The Home Office Regulations also require the tubing to be made from steel. Copper forms an explosive acetylide and is best avoided although some authorities allow the use of brass containing less than 65% copper.

Atomic Fluorescence Flame Photometry

Only general principles are considered here. The method is essentially an emission technique. Atoms are excited by absorption of radiation from a source which is not seen by the detector. Light emitted from the excited atoms is viewed at right angles to the exciting beam as in a fluorimeter.

Although some of the excited atoms emit the resonance wavelength by simply returning to the ground state other changes are permissible which include the possibility of assuming metastable states and the loss or gain of energy by collision with gas molecules in the flame. The consequence is that quanta of sizes larger or smaller than the resonance quantum are emitted so that other wavelengths, shorter or longer than the resonance one, are emitted. In general, the intensity of the fluorescent light, I_f, emitted is given by

$$I_f = \phi I_0 \varepsilon l k c$$

where c = concentration of the element in the sample, k = a constant to allow for the efficiency of nebulisation and atomisation, l = flame length, ε = atomic absorption coefficient, I_0 = intensity of the original source and ϕ = the ratio of the number of atoms emitting fluorescence when in the excited state to the number being excited during a given period of time.

Advantages of the technique are several. The fluorescent intensity is directly proportional to I_0 and the sensitivity is increased by using a high energy source, often a microwave discharge lamp although a continuum may be employed in suitable cases. The sensitivity is also increased by further direct amplification of the detector signal. Both these advantages are shared by fluorimeters (p. 153). Burners may be simpler and optical alignment of the beam with the flame length is easier. The greater choice of fluorescent wavelengths may avoid some interference problems.

However, the sensitivity varies with small changes in light source intensity, I_0, and with ϕ making it important to keep these factors stable. Scattering of light by particles in the flame increases the background noise more than in atomic absorption methods. Despite this, the technique offers the same advantages in selected cases as does fluorimetry over light absorption methods.

REFERENCES

Beeler M. F. (1974). *Amer. J. Clin. Pathol*; **61**: 789.

Beeler M. F., Lancaster R. G. (1975).*Amer. J. Clin. Pathol*; **63**: 953.

Bowers G. N., McComb R. B. (1975). *Clin. Chem*; **21**: 1988.

Bridges J. W. (1978). In *Scientific Foundations of Clinical Biochemistry, Vol. 1, Analytical Aspects.* (Williams D. L., Nunn R. F., Marks V., eds) p. 72. London: William Heinemann Medical Books.

Broughton P. M. G., Riley C. (1965). *Colorimeters with Flow Through Cells, Scientific Report No. 1.* London: Association of Clinical Biochemists.

Brown S. S., Gowenlock A. H. (1971) *Ann. Clin. Biochem*; **8**: 171.

Burgess C., Knowles A. eds (1981). *Techniques in Ultraviolet Spectrometry. Vol. 1. Standards in Absorption Spectrometry.* London: Chapman and Hall.

Campbell A. K., Holt M. E, Patel A. (1985). In *Recent Advances in Clinical Biochemistry, Vol. 3, p. 1.* Edinburgh: Churchill Livingstone.

Dawson J. B. (1978). In *Scientific Foundations of Clinical Biochemistry, Vol. 1, Analytical Aspects.* (Williams D. L., Nunn R. F., Marks V., eds) p. 95. London: William Heinemann Medical Books.

Delves H. T. (1970). *Analyst*; **95**: 431.

Eldridge P. H., Beetham R. (1985). *News Sheet, Association of Clinical Biochemists*; **271**: 15.

Fog J. (1962). See Rand R. N. (1969). *Clin. Chem*; **15**: 839.

Foster W. H., Hume D. N. (1959). *Anal. Chem*; **31**: 2033.

Home Office Regulations, Statutory Rules and Orders No. 54. (1937). *An Order in Council on Acetylene.* London: HMSO.

Home Office Regulations, Statutory Rules and Orders No. 805. (1947). *Compressed Acetylene Order.* London: HMSO.

Kahn H. L., Peterson G. E:, Schallis J. E. (1968). *Atomic Absorption Newsletter*; **7**: 35.

Kirkbright G. F. (1971). *Analyst*; **96**: 609.

Kirkbright G. F., West T. S. (1972). *Chemistry in Britain*; **8**: 428.

Lee L. W., Schmidt L. M. (1983). *Elementary Principles of Laboratory Instruments*, 5th ed. St. Louis: Mosby.

Parlett G. R. (1978). In *Scientific Foundations of Clinical Biochemistry, Vol.* 1, *Analytical Aspects.* (Williams D. L., Nunn R. F., Marks V., eds) p. 55. London: William Heinemann Medical Books.

Rand R. N. (1969). *Clin. Chem*; **15**: 839.

Stevens J. F. (1980). *Ann. Clin. Biochem*; **17**: 87.

Twyman F., Lothian G. F. (1933). *Proc. Phys. Soc*; **45**: 643.

Udenfriend S. *Fluorescence Assay in Biology and Medicine*, Vol. 1 (1962) and Vol. 2 (1969). London and New York: Academic Press.

Whitehead T. P., Kricka L. J., Carter T. J. N., Thorpe G. H. G. (1979). *Clin. Chem*; **25**: 1531.

8

WORK SIMPLIFICATION— AUTOMATED PROCEDURES

As clinical biochemistry has evolved, the demand for laboratory investigations has increased. A wider range of tests has developed to assist in the diagnosis of disease and to monitor progress. Within this spectrum of investigations there is a smaller group, so frequently requested that large batches of samples require processing daily. The trend for many years has been for the number of such requests to increase logarithmically and hence in any laboratory there will come a stage when the extra workload requires either proportionately more staff or equipment to allow the existing staff to work more efficiently.

When the volume of work is not great this can be achieved by mechanical aids supplementing traditional analytical methods. This approach, sometimes referred to as *work simplification*, involves a change in equipment and reappraisal of the organisation of the analytical bench and method to improve the efficiency of practices no longer adequate. Automatic pipettes and diluters increase the efficiency of performing these traditional analytical steps and modified light-measuring instruments allow, e.g., automatic aspiration of the final solution into the cuvette, simple standardisation and direct output in concentration units in visual or printed form (see Chapter 7, p. 140).

An alternative approach has been the development of *dry chemistry systems* (see Steinhausen and Price, 1985 for a review). Here all reagents are held in dry form on a solid matrix in the form of a film or strip. All stages of the reaction occur in this matrix after direct addition of the analytical sample.

For the more common tests, however, such approaches are still inadequate to deal with a large workload and instruments designed to handle the whole analytical process mechanically have become commonplace. The practice has become known as *automation*, a term which strictly implies a self-regulating process with an element of feed-back which detects any tendency to malfunction and readjusts the equipment so that it continues to function correctly. Such desirable equipment is, as yet, not available and the current processes are more correctly termed mechanisation. As the term 'automated equipment' is widely used to describe the present instruments in which the feed-back element is the human supervisor, it is used in that sense in this book.

AUTOMATIC DISPENSERS AND DILUTERS

The term *dispenser* indicates a device which performs the same function as a pipette, delivering a stipulated volume of fluid, be this serum, aqueous reagent or organic solvent. Most dispensers use a syringe as the measuring device. In a *diluter*, two syringes measure two separate volumes; the patient's sample requiring analysis and the diluent. Other reagents may then be added by dispensers thus reproducing the usual manual procedure.

Dispensers

A range of dispensers is available but the majority fall into one of three main categories:

1. The Hand-held Mechanical Pipette (Fig. 8.1). Several are available sharing the common features of a disposable plastic tip and a push-button at the opposite end operated by the thumb. Depressing the button displaces air from the enclosed syringe so that on releasing the pressure, liquid enters the tip from which it can later be displaced by repressing the button, often to a greater extent, to expel all liquid from the non-wettable tip. Liquid does not enter the syringe section. The tip can be changed between samples to reduce carryover and for safety purposes if hazardous specimens are being handled. In the different positive displacement method, the liquid to be dispensed is sucked into a glass or plastic capillary tube by a stainless steel plunger usually fitted with a Teflon tip. The method is particularly suitable for small volumes and such dispensers are available down to 1 μl.

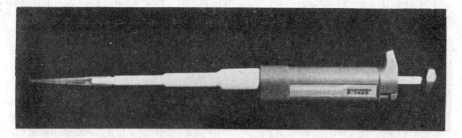

Fig. 8.1. A Hand-held Mechanical Pipette. (Oxford Laboratories).

Instruments available are either fixed volume, adjustable in defined increments, or adjustable to any volume within defined limits. The volume range covered by the range of dispensers is 1 μl to 10 ml. In general the performance is better than the traditional pipetting methods. The accuracy lies on average within 0·5 to 2% of the nominal volume but in some pipettes the degree of warming by being held in the hand reduces the volume delivered. Most measurements of accuracy are made using water, and the volume dispensed may vary when serum is used. Some pipettes allow for minor adjustments to be made to overcome these defects. In those pipettes which can be adjusted to deliver a range of volumes, the precision of resetting is usually satisfactory provided the scale markings allow for fine adjustments. The precision of these pipettes varies with sample volume and in the case of variable volume pipettes is usually worse than average at the lower end of the volume range. The average achievable coefficient of variation (CV) in per cent for aqueous solutions is better than 0·2 for volumes of 500 μl or more, better than 0·3 for 100 and 200 μl, but then deteriorates with smaller volumes: 0·4 (50 μl), 0·5 (20 μl), 0·9 (10 μl), 1·4 (5 μl). As the error of measuring a small sample volume may be an important part of the total error of an analytical method, these figures should be borne in mind when selecting the sample volume.

For all such pipettes the performance deteriorates if the internal mechanism is not regularly inspected and serviced or if the instrument is not used in the recommended fashion.

2. The Integral Syringe and Reagent Bottle (Fig. 8.2). These pipettes are syringes mounted on top of a reagent bottle and are intended for adding the

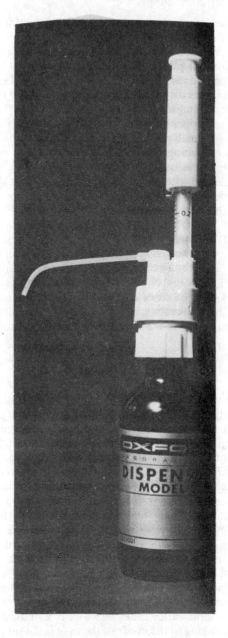

Fig. 8.2. Dispenser Syringe on Reagent Bottle (Dispenser M, Oxford Laboratories).

reagent to the analytical mixture in a series of tubes. The syringe is filled from the bottle through a tube dipping into the reagent and is expelled through the delivery jet. The syringe plunger is depressed by hand to dispense the reagent and the syringe refills by a spring mechanism. The syringe is usually adjustable to any selected volume within the range of syringe calibration but the precision is again less satisfactory at the lower end of the volume range. A valve mechanism allows fluid to be aspirated from the bottle during filling without air entering the dispenser tip and allows later expulsion through the tip without back-flow into the bottle. The syringe and tip are either of glass or plastic construction. Glass gives better precision but plastic syringes are more robust.

The volumes dispensed vary with syringe size but cover the range from 40 μl to 50 ml. The usual volumes dispensed are greater than those for which hand-held pipettes are commonly employed. The accuracy of delivery is within 2% of the nominal volume at the upper range of the syringe capacity but is affected by wear of the syringe plunger, small particles of dust in the valve system and also by the force with which the plunger is depressed. Too rapid expulsion, although convenient for saving time, usually results in poorer accuracy and precision and should be avoided. Readjustment of syringe setting is usually less precise than with hand-held pipettes. The precision of the glass syringe type is comparable with the hand-held pipettes of similar volume but the more robust plastic syringe dispensers have a CV of 0·5% at their maximum volume.

3. **Mechanical Dispensers** (Fig. 8.3). These operate in a similar manner to the latter group, except that the syringe plunger is driven by an electric motor. This offers more control over the ejection step and is less tiring for repetitive use. The dispenser tip is often at the end of a flexible tube allowing easy addition of reagent to test tubes in racks at the rate of around 50 volumes per minute. The errors of syringe wear and faulty operation of valves are still potential problems and the CV is usually of the order of 0·5% at the maximum volume of the syringe.

Diluters

Although dilution of a serum sample can be achieved by using two separate dispensers consecutively, there are advantages in combining the operations in a single instrument, the diluter. Most diluters utilise two syringes, a smaller one for the sample volume and a larger one for the diluent volume. The syringes are either operated by hand or by mechanical means (Fig. 8.4). Unlike most dispensers the syringes are both filled with fluid, the diluent, and both syringes are linked to a common outlet jet. During operation the sample syringe plunger is first withdrawn to aspirate the serum sample into the outlet jet. Both syringes then discharge their contents through the outlet jet washing out the serum sample into a receptacle. Finally, the larger (diluent) syringe is refilled. A valve mechanism ensures that during the sampling step fluid is only drawn in from the tip, during the expulsion step fluid passes only through the tip, and during the refilling of the larger syringe fluid is only withdrawn from a reservoir.

The efficiency of washing out the sample from the tip depends on its design and on the relative volumes of sample and diluent. The most efficient wash occurs with a high diluent to sample ratio. Efficient washing avoids the problem of small droplets of serum clinging to the inside of the tip when a simple dispenser is used. This error becomes more important as the sample volume lessens. In the diluter, the proper functioning of valves is critical in aspirating the correct sample volume. The shape and composition of the tip is important in avoiding the formation of an adherent droplet. If this is diluent, it may dilute the sample significantly before aspiration, and if a drop of serum clings to the tip after withdrawal from the sample, this produces an erroneously large sample volume. Non-wettable capillary tips such as PTFE are used for small sample volumes.

The accuracy of dilution is dependent on the accuracy of measurement of both sample and diluent volumes but is not critical if standards are put through the

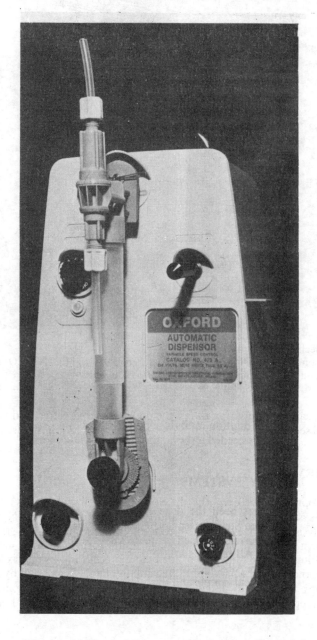

Fig. 8.3. Mechanical Dispenser (Oxford Laboratories).

whole procedure. The precision of dilution is more important and is greatly influenced by the precision of the sample syringe and by the efficiency of washing out if low dilution ratios are used. The performance of diluters can thus vary considerably but a CV of 1 to 1·5% with dilution ratios of 1:10 to 1:100 using a sample volume in the range 20 to 100 μl should be achievable. With smaller

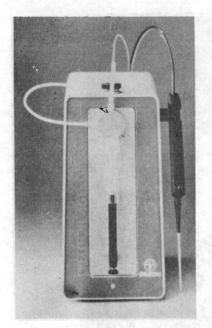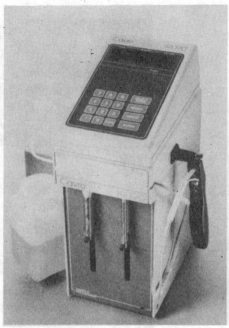

Fig. 8.4. Mechanical Diluter.
   Left: Gilson Diluter 401 (courtesy of Anachem Ltd), right: Cavro IQ 190 Sample Processor (courtesy of Scientific & Medical Products Ltd).

volumes of sample or dilution ratios, the performance of different diluters varies and careful selection is needed if the analytical method requires these conditions.

'DRY CHEMISTRY' SYSTEMS

A novel approach has been the development of 'dry chemistry' or 'bedside chemistry' systems (see Steinhausen and Price, 1985 for a review). Now used for serum analysis, they have developed from the earlier technology of stick tests for urinary constituents. All reagents are held in dry form on a solid matrix in the form of a film or strip. All stages of the reaction occur in this matrix after direct addition of the analytical sample and the colour change is assessed by reflectance spectroscopy (p. 131) in a dedicated instrument. Such developments allow analytical methods to be located outside the main laboratory and close to the patient.

Matrix Construction

The details vary with the manufacturer but discrete layers with different functions can be identified. The *support layer* is usually of thick plastic, white in colour if it is also to be reflective. The *reflective layer* reflects incident light onto the optical sphere system which focuses it onto the detector. The *reagent layer* contains all the necessary reagent chemicals in dry form. These dissolve in the fluid to be tested and the reaction then occurs. Sometimes a true reaction layer is divided from an *indicator layer*, in which the final colour develops, by a semi-permeable *separating layer* which allows the reaction product formed in the reagent layer to be purified before the final colour reaction occurs. In more elaborate matrices, a *plasma separation layer* ensures that when a whole blood sample is applied, only plasma reaches the reagent layer. A *spreading layer* may be incorporated to ensure uniform penetration of sample to the reagent layer.

Analytical Systems

Three main systems are current and are described briefly.

The *Ames Seralyser* system is the simplest and uses prediluted serum as the sample (30 μl). The strip construction (Fig. 8.5A) embraces a paper, reagent/ indicator layer held on a foil reflective layer. After adding the sample, the strip is inserted in a reflectance photometer, stabilised at 37 °C. It is irradiated with polychromatic light and the reflected light passes through an interference filter to the detector. Both end-point and kinetic methods are available and reaction times vary from 0.5 to 4 min. Two-point calibration is used with the Kubelka–Munk function (p. 131) and methods are available for a range of analytes including enzymes.

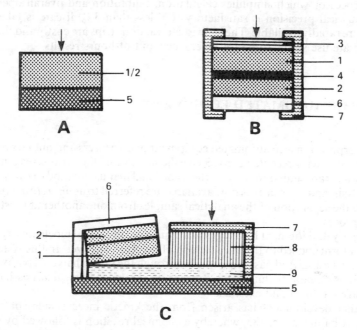

Fig. 8.5. 'Dry Chemistry' Systems.
  A. Ames Seralyser System.
  B. Kodak Ektachem System.
  C. Boehringer Reflotron System.
  The systems are shown in diagrammatic cross section. The arrow indicates the point of sample application. In each case the layer figures refer to: 1. reagent layer, 2. indicator layer, 3. spreading layer, 4. semi-permeable membrane, 5. reflecting support layer, 6. transparent support layer, 7. cover, 8. plasma separation layer, 9. plasma reservoir.

The *Kodak Ektachem* system is more complex and uses undiluted serum (10 μl). This may be added automatically to the matrix in the larger, automated Ektachem 400 and 700 systems but a simpler instrument (Ektachem DT60) allows manual addition of sample. There are several layers in the system (Fig. 8.5B). The sample passes through a spreading and reflective (white) layer to reach the reagent layer. Reaction products pass through a separative layer to reach the indicator layer which can be irradiated through the transparent supporting layer. Reactions take about 5 min at 37 °C and two-point calibration is again used. Although most reactions are colorimetric, it is also possible to use a potentiometric detector to measure electrolytes.

The *Boehringer Reflotron* system is more complex but allows the use of whole undiluted blood as well as undiluted serum as a 30 μl sample. The matrix design (Fig. 8.5C) incorporates plasma separation and reaction parts. The sample is applied to a protective layer but cells and plasma are separated by a glass fibre filter layer, the plasma entering a reservoir held on a reflective support. The reaction commences when the reagent section is pressed into contact with the plasma reservoir. Plasma enters a reagent layer, the products passing to an indicator layer which is irradiated through a transparent protective layer, using monochromatic light. The nature of the mathematical function relating concentration to reflected light (p. 132) is determined by a coded strip on each matrix.

In each of these systems, the dedicated optical instrument includes a small microprocessor which simplifies calculation, calibration and overall operation. The analytical precision is satisfactory (CV less than 5%) if care is taken and results are rapidly available. The individual reaction strips are costly and the most appropriate use seems to be for emergency, out-of-hours results.

TYPES OF AUTOMATED EQUIPMENT

The incorporation into automated equipment of dispensers and diluters requires a system of moving receptacles to receive the sample and the various reagents. The various steps are similar to those in the traditional manual method of carrying out the analysis, and instruments now available are referred to as *discrete analysers* to indicate the separation of the analytical samples from one another at most stages of the process.

The early development by Skeggs of automation in clinical biochemistry took a different form and led to the introduction of the AutoAnalyzer. In this system, the samples to be analysed pass sequentially through the same analytical pathway in a continuous stream of fluid. This concept of *continuous flow analysis* has been successively refined and extended.

Another development has arisen from the kinetic measurement of enzyme activity (Chapter 22, p. 483) whereby a chemical reaction is followed by optical means. Such kinetic methods are not restricted to enzyme measurements. The reaction may either be followed to completion or the rate of change of absorbance in the early stages of a chemical reaction may be related to the concentration of the analyte. This approach is used in the *centrifugal analyser* in which the component reagents and sample are mixed in the rotor of a centrifuge and the optical changes are measured at virtually the same time in each of a number of reaction vessels arranged around the periphery of the rotor.

CONTINUOUS FLOW ANALYSERS

All samples and reagents pass along plastic or glass tubes. The reagents flow continuously but the samples are introduced serially at intervals, usually separated by a wash fluid. The relative proportions of sample and reagents are determined by their individual flow rates down tubes which are initially separate. Mixing occurs when tubes join to form a common pathway and, when all components of the reaction mixture have been added, this passes along a single tube. Chemical reactions take place as the fluid traverses the system.

The physics of flow of liquid along tubes is complex but flow rates diminish from the highest rate in the axial stream to a very slow flow where the liquid is retarded by the tube wall. Also when two streams of liquid merge, the degree of mixing is influenced by the different velocities of flow across the cross-section of the combined stream. In the AutoAnalyzer, unlike flow injection analysis (p. 196), a series of air bubbles is introduced into the liquid stream to segment this in small lengths. Mixing within segments is achieved by repeatedly inverting them and the differential flow rate is greatly modified by the 'purging' effect of the air bubble as it passes over the tube surface.

The system permits a wide range of analyses to be performed. Various separation steps are possible, those used most often being the separation of small molecules from protein by dialysis, and extraction of the aqueous reaction mixture by an organic solvent with later phase separation by relative density. Although originally used with colorimetric methods, the colorimeter can be replaced by such devices as a spectrophotometer, fluorimeter, nephelometer, flame photometer or radioactivity counter where appropriate.

The different specific functions are carried out by *modules* and several such modules involved in one analytical method are linked together to form an *analytical channel*. The analytical *system* is a collection of linked modules arranged in such a way that analysis of a series of specimens for one or more constituents may be performed. A single channel system will analyse for one substance in each specimen. Multi-channel systems carry out two or more analyses concurrently on each specimen. The development of the AutoAnalyzer over the years has improved analytical performance and sensitivity while making available multi-channel analysis with automatic preparation of printed reports. For detailed discussion of these developments see the 5th edition of this book.

The Proportioning Pump

This module determines the relative flow rates of sample and all reagents, replacing the use of pipettes of different sizes in manual methods. The pumping technique involves the peristaltic action produced by a series of rollers passing along an array of parallel plastic 'pump tubes'. Each roller compresses all tubes so that the rate of flow in each tube depends on the square of the pump tube diameter. Tubes with a range of diameters and nominal pumping rates are available in three materials: Tygon, suitable for most reagents; Acidflex for reagents containing corrosive acid; Solvaflex, for certain organic reagents. The array of tubes under moderate tension and firmly held at each end is referred to as the manifold.

Pump design has changed over the years but a common system is to have a series of rollers on a continuous belt drive. As each roller moves along the manifold it forces liquid forward ahead of it in each tube but when it eventually loses contact with the manifold, back flow is prevented by one or more other rollers behind, already forcing liquid forward. Originally air was similarly pumped along one of the tubes and entered the system in a relatively uncontrolled fashion to create the bubble pattern. Later pumps incorporate a block in this tube on the outlet side of the pump, the block being temporarily released every 2 s to give a regular entry of bubbles. Other variations in pump design have been claimed to improve the slight pulsatile nature of the peristaltic flow.

A diagrammatic form of the pump and manifold (Fig. 8.6) is used in flow diagrams throughout this book.

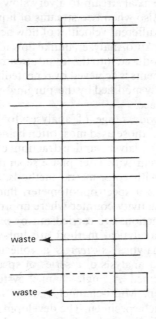

waste ◄

waste ◄

Fig. 8.6. Diagrammatic Representation of Proportioning Pump and Manifold.
The pumping direction is to the left with the arrows indicating liquids going to waste. The dotted lines represent tubing from other parts of the system, not passing through the pump rollers. Otherwise tubes at the right are connected to reagents, while tubes at the left join the continuous set of tubes in the rest of the system.

The Sampler

This module holds the batch of samples awaiting analysis in separate cups on a circular tray which is moved at intervals. A probe connected by plastic tubing to the manifold enters the samples serially. The volume of sample aspirated is determined by the pumping rate and the dwell time of the probe in the sample.

Initially, air was allowed to enter the sample line during the period the probe was not immersed in the sample but this gave rather poor carryover (p. 190) characteristics. These improve if the sampler design is altered so that the probe now passes directly from the sample into a wash reservoir between samples. The relative times the probe spends in the sample and the wash fluid and the number of samples consumed per minute are adjustable by timing devices, initially mechanical cams, later superseded by electrical timers which give more precise control. The ratio of sampling to wash times is usually adjustable up to 9:1.

A diagrammatic form of the sampler (Fig. 8.7) is used in flow diagrams throughout this book.

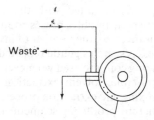

Fig. 8.7. Diagrammatic Representation of the Sampler Unit.
The upper tube delivers fluid to the wash reservoir and excess goes to waste.

The Dialyser

This module separates small and large molecules by allowing the former to pass through a semi-permeable membrane from the donor (sample) stream of liquid and air bubbles to a recipient stream again segmented by air bubbles. The dialysis rate depends on temperature but complete passage of small molecules into the recipient stream is rarely achieved and may be only a few per cent of the total. The analytical process then requires that a constant fraction should dialyse but this is not always the case when simple aqueous and protein-containing solutions are compared. The ability to carry out the analysis on a small proportion of the original sample arose from improvements in the sensitivity of the whole analytical system.

The dialyser consists of two rectangular Perspex plates each having a groove cut into one surface. The U-shaped grooves vary in length from 75 to 600 mm. The grooved surfaces of the plates are mirror images and can be located precisely one over the other so that when a sheet of semi-permeable membrane is clamped between the plates, a tube is produced of circular cross section with a diameter of 0·8 mm, divided longitudinally by the membrane. Nipples at the end of each plate allow the sample and recipient streams to enter and leave, each stream traversing one side of the dialyser. The two streams flow in the same direction; operation in counter-current mode gives poor separation of one sample from the next and the benefit of the wash phase between samples is greatly reduced.

A diagrammatic form of the dialyser (Fig. 8.8) is used in flow diagrams throughout this book.

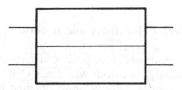

Fig. 8.8. The Dialyser Unit.

Mixing Coils

These coils bring about adequate mixing when two streams of fluid join. They are multi-turn glass coils (Fig. 8.9) mounted with the coil axis horizontal. As a segment of liquid between two air bubbles passes round a turn of the coil in the vertical plane, the segment is inverted, the number of inversions depending on the number of turns. The process resembles gentle repeated inversion of a stoppered tube to mix its contents. Mixing coils are used whenever two or more streams join. If the two liquids are immiscible, solvent extraction occurs while the liquids traverse the coil. Both the mixing and extraction processes are more efficient if the bubble pattern is regular thereby producing segments of constant length. This is more important the smaller the coil diameter.

Fig. 8.9. The Mixing Coil.
   A typical coil is shown to the left and the diagrammatic form to the right. SMC = small mixing coil.

Some mixing coils are water-jacketed to allow rapid cooling of the reaction mixture. Heating for longer times is dealt with in the next section. In some analytical methods it is necessary to introduce a time delay. Short delays are achieved by inserting one or more mixing coils in the circuit but longer delays are better achieved using a delay coil. This is either of glass or polythene tubing with a much larger diameter per turn. It is arranged so that the plane of the turns is horizontal and the coil may be immersed in a water bath. Mixing is not a function of this coil.

The Heating or Incubator Bath

This module maintains the reaction mixture at a constant temperature for a defined time to bring about the required chemical change under controlled conditions. It consists of a glass delay coil mounted in a thermostatically controlled, sealed oil bath. Most baths are set at 37 or 95 °C but some are adjustable to 120 °C or even higher. No mixing occurs on passing through the coil but the transit time depends on the coil volume and the flow rate. The standard length is 1·5 m and the coil is usually located with the dialyser and all mixing coils in a 'reaction cartridge'. The input streams from the pump are connected to one end of this compact unit and the colorimeter is connected to its outlet giving a readily interchangeable unit.
   A diagrammatic form of the heating bath (Fig. 8.10) is used in flow diagrams throughout this book.

The Colorimeter and Recorder

This unit measures the intensity of colour produced in the reaction and provides a graphical display of the change in colour with time. Other detectors can replace the colorimeter and the recorder may be supplemented by a printer.

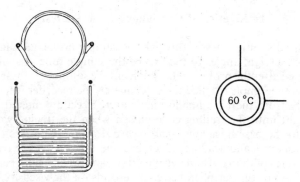

Fig. 8.10. The Heating Bath.
A typical glass coil which lies within the bath is shown on the left. The diagrammatic form is on the right.

A continuous flow channel is operated with a measuring device fitted with a flow-through cuvette. Several of the instruments discussed in Chapter 7 (p. 141) can be used but the choice is limited by considerations of cost and stability. A double beam spectrophotometer is costly and rarely justified by analytical requirements. On the other hand many single beam colorimeters have insufficient stability for long term operation. In the simpler AutoAnalyzer II systems the colorimeter, linked to a recorder, is a double beam instrument with phototube detectors and employs two cuvettes if an additional analytical channel produces individual sample blanks. The ratio of the detector outputs is amplified logarithmically giving a signal proportional to absorbance, and hence concentration, if Beer's law is obeyed. The amplification increases the sensitivity of the system and its degree is adjustable so that the recorder deflection can be set to a scale reading equal to concentration.

In such a system the fluid reaching the colorimeter is still segmented by air bubbles but these must be excluded from the cuvette as they occlude the light beam. Air bubble removal is achieved by using a glass junction situated immediately before the cuvette which allows bubbles to rise vertically and leave with some of the liquid by one route while the remainder of the liquid is pumped through the cuvette at a constant rate. Once the debubbler has been passed the analytical stream is again unsegmented like the fluid in the sample line (see p. 192). Although this unsegmented length is kept as short as possible there will be differences in flow rates between axial and peripheral streams and these may be exaggerated with poor design of the cuvette or with increased viscosity of the reaction mixture.

A diagrammatic form of the colorimeter and recorder (Fig. 8.11) is used in flow diagrams throughout this book.

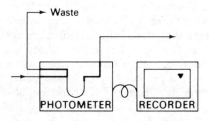

Fig. 8.11. Diagrammatic Representation of the Colorimeter and Recorder.

The Kinetics of Continuous Flow Analysis

When a coloured solution passes through the sample probe, its leading edge is sharply defined at right angles to the axis of the sample tube. A similar trailing edge is produced after the probe is removed from the solution. If these edges were to persist until the sample reached the colorimeter, the recorder response would move abruptly from the base line as the coloured section entered and would remain constant until the trailing edge passed when the tracing would return immediately to the base line. This *square wave response* is not seen in practice because the forward and trailing edges become distorted as a result of the different flow rates of the axial and peripheral streams when a fluid passes along a tube. Retardation of the peripheral stream depends on the viscosity of the fluid and on the nature of the tube wall. The effect is considerably reduced by the regular segmentation of the fluid by air bubbles which purge most of the fluid from the walls leaving a thin film to mix with the following segment. The rates of change at the start and end of the square wave response are both reduced to give a curved peak. Analysis of the factors determining its shape has improved the performance of continuous flow systems.

Contamination of a segment of fluid by the fluid left on the tube wall is called *sample interaction*. Each segment interacts with the following one resulting in *carryover* which occurs in any system where one sample can contaminate a later one. Carryover increases the peak produced by a sample of low concentration when preceded by a sample of higher concentration. It will reduce the peak size if this is preceded by a sample of lower concentration. Carryover is used here in the way described by Broughton *et al.* (1969) based on a method of measuring it in practice. If three samples of specimen A (A_1, A_2, A_3) are followed by three samples of specimen B (B_1, B_2, B_3), and the apparent concentrations of A_3, B_1 and B_3 are a, b and b' respectively, then the *fractional carryover*, K, is defined as

$$K = \frac{b - b'}{a - b'}$$

The *percentage carryover* is $K \times 100\%$. K is always positive and independent of the actual concentrations of A and B in practice. The error in calculating K increases if the concentrations of A and B are either similar, making $(b - b')$ and $(a - b')$ small, or so different that one is measured at an absorbance value which has poor precision (p. 143).

Analysis as Lag and Exponential Phases

If a sample is sampled continuously, the recorder tracing eventually reaches a plateau. If the probe is then removed from the specimen the tracing eventually returns to the base line. Thiers *et al.* (1967) and Walker *et al.* (1970), investigating the rise curve and fall curve (Fig. 8.12) in detail found them to be approximately exponential in character although their initial slopes are not as steep as expected. In true exponential decay the logarithm of the reading is linearly and inversely related to time. If log absorbance at points on the fall curve is plotted against time, the linear part of the curve is preceded by a less steep, curved section. There can thus be defined an initial lag time and an exponential decay (Fig. 8.13). An identical result is obtained for the rise curve if the logarithm of the difference between the absorbance and the plateau absorbance is used. The curve of Fig. 8.13 is unaffected by the actual plateau absorbance.

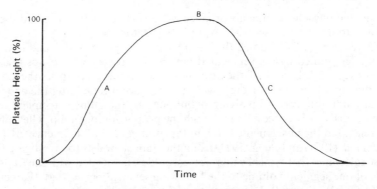

Fig. 8.12. Expanded AutoAnalyzer Peak Showing a Plateau.
A, B, C are the rise curve, plateau phase and fall curve respectively.

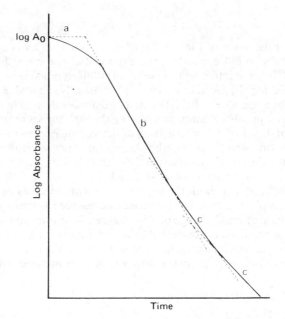

Fig. 8.13. Lag and Exponential Phases of an AutoAnalyzer Peak.
   The curve is derived from that of Fig. 8.12. The lag phase, a, and the exponential phase, b, of Walker *et al.* (1970) are shown with the later exponential contributions to the c phase of Spencer *et al.* (1977). A_0 = plateau absorbance (A in text).

   The lag phase, a, in a number of AutoAnalyzer I methods varied from 4 to 32 s. Walker *et al.* used the symbol, b, to characterise the exponential decay phase. If the absorbance, y, falls exponentially from an initial value, A, then the value at time t is given by the equation:

$$y = A \cdot \exp(-t/b) \text{ and } t = b \cdot \ln 2 \text{ when } y = 0 \cdot 5\, A$$

For various AutoAnalyzer I methods b varied from 6 to 39 s. Carlyle *et al.* (1973), Spencer (1976) and Spencer *et al.* (1977) found other later components of the exponential phase when the absorbance values fell below 0·1 and used the term 'c phase' to describe these other exponential factors.

Walker *et al.* (1970) studied the AutoAnalyzer I system and found that *a* was mainly determined by the segmented part of the stream while *b* was related to such unsegmented parts of the stream as the sample line up to the point of introduction of air bubbles, the flow cell and adjacent tubes after the debubbler, and any dilution circuit involving debubbling of the effluent recipient stream from the dialyser with recycling through the proportioning pump. The *c* phase is also related to the unsegmented stream (Spencer *et al.*, 1977). Thiers *et al.* (1971), Fleck *et al.* (1971) and Begg (1971) using theoretical models to investigate the lag phase calculated that typical values for *a* would be associated with the transfer of 0·8% of one segment volume to the following segment per second. Walker *et al.* (1970) and Walker (1971) suggest that the exponential factor *b* is the more important. If this were the only factor, the plateau absorbance *A* could be predicted from the absorbance, *h*, at any point on the rise curve from the equation

$$A = h + b\frac{dy}{dt}$$

where dy/dt is the slope of the rise curve at the point under consideration.

This equation would convert a true exponential rise curve followed by an exponential fall curve into a square wave form but in practice produces a curve with a flattened top. Its ascending part is symmetrically sigmoid in shape and can be described by a mean time, *D*, and its standard deviation, σ_D. They interpret *D* as the mean *dwell time* of the sample on passing through the segmented stream and regard σ_D as an index of the deformation of the leading edge of the sample due to interaction in this stream, i.e. another lag factor. They used these concepts to develop a theoretical model to describe the overall flow through the system which is similar to that of Thiers *et al.* (1971) and Begg (1971) for the unsegmented stream but indicates that both the lag and exponential factors operate continuously in the complete system. The lag phase *a* is then seen as the exponential effect acting on a phase of rapid change of absorbance whose duration is controlled by σ_D. The exponential phase represents the continuing effect of *b* acting on a segmented stream which has reached a steady state at the debubbler. In practice σ_D can be measured more precisely than *a* which has an indeterminate starting point.

Factors Influencing a, σ_D, b and c.

The study of the factors affecting the shape of the recorder peak has been important in the development of AutoAnalyzer systems.

The lag phase *a* was shown by Walker *et al.* (1970) in the AutoAnalyzer I to depend on the volume of the system, particularly that of any delay coils. The effect is to increase *a* by 0·36 s/ml coil volume for glass coils or 0·12 s/ml for polyethylene coils. The presence of a dialyser also increases *a* by 4 to 24 s depending on the method, and the effect is more marked still if there is a serious imbalance in the flow rates of the two streams in the dialyser. Provided the bubble size is constant, the value of *a* rises as the length of fluid between bubbles diminishes. Walker and Andrew (1974) found that σ_D is proportional to the volume of the system and the bore of the tubing, the time interval between bubbles and the ratio of air to pumping rates. A minor component is the flow rate through the flow cell to which σ_D is inversely related; the effect vanishes if this flow rate exceeds 2 ml/min. They derived the expression:

$$\sigma_D^2 = k V_B t_D (1 + a/l)$$

where k = a constant, V_B = mean volume of an air bubble, t_D = dwell time of a sample in the system, a = air pumping rate and l = liquid pumping rate. The practical consequences are the reduction of a/l. Dwell time is reduced by using a smaller system volume and a more sensitive photometer to measure the smaller quantity of reaction product. The air pumping rate is fixed after adjusting the time interval between bubbles to below $0.5 \sigma_D$ but the increase in l is limited by the poorer stability of the longer fluid segment, increase in reagent consumption and either reduced sensitivity of the method or increased sample volume. Most of these points were incorporated when developing the AutoAnalyzer II system.

The exponential factor b is inversely related to the flow rate through the cuvette which is limited by the total liquid flow rate, l, in the segmented stream. Also b increases with the sample line length (0.06 s/cm) and the length of fluid separating the debubbler and flow cell. In the AutoAnalyzer II, b is considerably reduced by using an integral debubbler and flow cell. Spencer (1976) used the 'stopped flow' method of Walker *et al.* (1970) to separate the flow cell contribution from the total value of b and found residual components due to the dialyser and the rest of the system. Fleck *et al.* (1971) found b decreased as the manifold aged, possibly due to increased pumping rate through the flow cell.

The c phase delays still further the attainment of plateau or baseline levels and Spencer *et al.* (1977) found that part of the c phase was attributable to flow cell design. The first of the extra components of the c phase was removed by using a 'pecking' probe (p. 195) to aspirate the sample. The probe pecks twice at the sample initially to generate two additional air bubbles in the first part of the sample segment. These remove droplets of water adhering to the sample line after the previous wash suggesting that most of c is attributable to the unsegmented streams. The advantage of reducing c by this probe action is offset by an increase of a on the rise curve only.

Sample Wash Ratios and Carryover in Relation to a and b

Walker *et al.* (1970) showed that if only b is operative the height reached by the peak is determined by the sampling time, s, and is 95 % of the plateau value if $s = 3b$ and 98 % if $s = 4b$. If a is comparable with b these figures are reduced in practice to 92 and 97 %, and if a is twice b they are only reduced to 86 and 93 %. The peak height should approach the plateau level both for ease of measurement and so that minor variations in s do not greatly affect the peak height as they would when the recorder pen is tracing its maximum slope.

The wash time, w, is important in separating one peak from another. The fall curve from a peak of absorbance A_1, will just be differentiated from the next peak of absorbance A_2 if

$$A_2 = A_1 \cdot \exp(-w/b)$$

This is related to carryover, K, and is approximated by the expression

$$K = \exp(-p/b)$$

where p = peak interval ($w + s$). K is 0.01 if $p = 4.5 b$ and 0.0025 if $p = 7 b$. If s is kept at $3 b$ to obtain a reasonable peak height, the wash times to achieve these carryovers will be $1.5 b$ and $3 b$ respectively giving sample/wash ratios of $2:1$ and $1:1$. If the sampling time is much longer in relation to b as happens with the low figures for *b* achieved in the AutoAnalyzer II, plateau levels are reached at sampling rates of 60/h. It follows that the base line is reached during the fall curve, carryover is very low and the wash time can be reduced to a small fraction of *p* to produce flushing of the sample line. Sample/wash ratios of 8 : 1 are then often used.

An important source of carryover is the debubbled stream passing through the flow cell. In the AutoAnalyzer II the integral flow cell and debubbler is efficient but the flow rate through the cell is often greater than desirable for sensitivity and reagent economy. This is improved if the total flow passes through the cell without debubbling. Neeley *et al.* (1974) introduced the *signal comparator*, an electronic device which detects the presence of a bubble and only makes measurements between bubbles. They were able to develop a miniaturised glucose oxidase system for blood glucose working at 150 samples/h with a 3 : 1 sample to wash ratio using an 18 μl sample and 128 μl reagent volume per test. The peaks were over 99 % of plateau level and the system compared favourably with a conventional one operating at 60/h. A similar reduction in carryover and conservation of reagents is seen in the Technicon SMAC system (p. 195) which uses a similar device.

Factors Affecting Accuracy and Precision

Various factors which influence carryover have been discussed above, as has the importance of precise measurement of sampling times at fast speeds of sampling and the need to work with peak heights above 80 % of plateau level. Spencer (1976) described an inter-sample effect impairing the precision of the peak height measurement, attributing this to compression of the air bubble in the sample pump tube separating the end of the sample from the water wash. After the air bubble passes the last roller of the proportioning pump, it is compressed by the following column of liquid and alters the resistance at the junction of the sample, diluent and air lines. Less serum enters the system for about 10 s, producing a notch on the tracing, the position of which varies with the distance between the pump and the junction. By adjusting this, the notch can be displaced from the peak. At high sampling rates the length should be as short as possible.

An important factor is *drift*, a slow change in performance during an analytical run. Drift takes two forms. *Baseline drift* is a gradual change in the absorbance of the reagent blank. It is often present when the reagent flow is started initially but persists to a lesser degree in some cases. The drift can be in either direction and is best detected if the recorder baseline can move to slightly negative values and, if necessary, by introducing one or more water samples at intervals between the serum samples. If the base line drifts upwards and the sensitivity is unchanged, the peak position moves upwards similarly so that the apparent peak heights are erroneously high. *Sensitivity drift* may occur with baseline drift or independently. It results from a change in reaction conditions and is detected by incorporating a repeating sample, the drift control, at regular intervals. The peak heights of this will vary a little due to interaction with differing preceding samples and to other random errors but by examining the general trend of the drift control peaks, the presence of sensitivity drift is shown by a change in their distance from the base line. Occasionally when the base line cannot be measured, the two types of drift can be differentiated by using two different drift controls. An example of sensitivity drift is the change in the temperature of the dialyser block as ambient temperature alters.

The AutoAnalyzer II is intended for single point calibration but the extent to which Beer's law is obeyed should be studied by running a series of aqueous standards or a series of known mixtures of two sera, one with a high concentration of the analyte and the other with a low one. If a non-linear response is found this is sometimes correctable by altering details of the analytical method. Otherwise multi-point standardisation is needed if errors are to be avoided.

Multi-channel Continuous Flow Analysers

The combination of several analytical channels separately linked to a single sampler saves equipment and laboratory time. Although originally done on an *ad hoc* basis, manufacturers now provide multi-channel equipment as a matter of policy.

The systems use similar components to those of the AutoAnalyzer II including short path dialysers and integral flow debubblers. The colorimeter has a single light source with separate detectors for each channel and the output from each is sampled in turn. Steady state is achieved for each channel resulting in a flat-topped signal. It can be arranged that the peak values are displayed on a single recorder as a series of horizontal lines crossing the scales of pre-calibrated chart paper appropriate to the analyses being performed. Calibration is single point using a calibration serum, and assumes linearity of response over the range required. Drift is monitored by introducing a drift control serum at every tenth sample position. The operator adjusts the calibration manually as required after checking that the base line is correct in the simpler instruments. Reliance on single point calibration with a serum assumes that the assigned values are correct and are maintained during storage in the lyophilised state and after reconstitution during subsequent use.

In the discussion of the factors controlling the optimum performance of continuous flow systems, emphasis was placed on reducing the exponential factor b and the total system volume. This has reached its peak in the Sequential Multiple Analyzer plus Computer (SMAC) which operates at up to 200 samples/h, performing 20 tests on less than 400 μl of sample. Unsegmented lengths of fluid are completely eliminated. A pecking probe sampler introduces four intrasample air bubbles which are removed before dilution. The sample is prediluted 1 in 6, and mixed with four large air bubbles and pumped at a high flow rate before resampling by individual peristaltic pumps into the reaction cartridges. The bubbles are large enough to be sampled by all analytical cartridges so that no length of tube is free from bubbles. An electronic signal comparator (p. 194) in the colorimeter allows the whole segmented stream to pass through the flow cell without debubbling. The total volume of the system is reduced to a minimum by using tubing of 1 mm diameter, placing the predilution circuit close to the reaction cartridges and reducing the groove dimensions on the dialyser plates. The flow cell with a volume of only 2 μl is located close to the analytical cartridge to reduce the liquid pathway length and wash characteristics are improved by increasing the injected bubble rate to 90/min.

These developments improve the rate of analysis to a degree which requires a computer to carry out the necessary monitoring and adjustments to a degree of refinement not possible manually. This checks the energy levels with water flowing through the system, the reagent blank signals, base line drift and noise. Checks on the system dwell time and sensitivity follow and then the individual channels are calibrated. Checks are made to verify that the machine operation remains within specification. The computer automatically checks the base line, recalibration is performed every 25th sample or on request, or whenever the computer recognises the need, producing an instrument with an element of feedback much more like true automation than the simple mechanisation of the earlier continuous flow systems. The results of such checks are collated in a printed report for quality control records.

When samples enter the system their dwell time is checked individually and the shape of the peak is compared with an experimentally determined ideal peak. If these checks are acceptable the results are calculated, stored, added to other information on the same patient and issued as a printed report.

Flow Injection Analysis

Increasing interest has been focused on flow injection analysis (FIA) as a general analytical technique but its use in clinical biochemistry is, so far, limited. As with continuous flow analysis, the sample enters a continuous stream of reagent but the details of the approach to reaction conditions and measurement are quite different.

In FIA a small, precisely measured volume of sample is injected into a flowing reagent stream and at a precisely controlled time, reaches a flow through detector which measures the reaction product. No air bubbles enter the stream and the reaction product is measured before steady state reaction conditions are reached. This makes for a simpler system and rapid production of the detector signal, often only a few seconds after sample injection. Sample and reagent volumes are low and a sample throughput of 150/h or more is possible, with similar accuracy and precision to those of traditional continuous flow methods.

Basic Principles. Sample introduction in FIA is by injection rather than timed aspiration as used by the AutoAnalyzer. Injection methods are similar to those used for HPLC (p. 60) and result in a slug of sample in the carrier fluid. As this is carried along the system, the front of the slug assumes a parabolic shape as the flow rate falls on moving from the axial stream towards the wall of the tube containing the fluid. A parabolic tail with its longest part in contact with the wall also occurs. Radial diffusion of molecules from higher to lower concentration at the head and tail diminishes the sharpness of the parabolic shape and, under carefully selected conditions, greatly reduces the carryover previously thought unavoidable in flow systems unpurged by air bubbles. In particular, a high flow rate through a narrow bore *coiled* rigid tube introduces centrifugal forces across the radius of the tube and further reduces carryover.

Theoretical and practical investigations of the various processes operating during FIA indicate that:

1. Mean transit time, $t = \text{constant.}\ a^2 \cdot l^{1 \cdot 025} \cdot q^{-1 \cdot 025}$
2. Width of detector response, $\Delta t = \text{constant.}\ a^2 \cdot l^{0 \cdot 64} \cdot q^{-0 \cdot 64}$

where a = tubing internal diameter, l = tube length and q = flow rate. Thus t and Δt are similar to the retention time and peak width encountered in column chromatography (Chapter 3, p. 46). If Δt is kept small, the sensitivity and rate of sample throughput improve. Typical conditions may be flow rates of 0·5 to 5 ml/min; tube internal diameter, 0·5 to 0·8 mm; length of tube 1 or 2 m.

Practical Systems. Two main types of FIA system have developed. In the low-pressure system, peristaltic pumps are combined with manual or automated sample injection. The high-pressure system uses similar high-pressure pumps and injection techniques to HPLC (p. 59). Provided that the flow rate is kept constant, the lack of compressible gas bubbles means that the transit time between injection site and detector can be controlled precisely so that reactions which have only been partially completed can be used satisfactorily. Indeed, it is possible as a variant to employ precisely controlled intermittent pumping, either to halt the reaction mixture for a period of time in a heated reaction coil or to stop it in the detector cuvette for kinetic studies. This is the *stop flow technique.*

Almost any type of flow-through detector can be adapted for FIA so that reaction products may be measured by colorimetric, fluorimetric, atomic absorption, flame emission and ion-specific electrode techniques among others.

For a fuller account of this technique see Rocks and Riley (1982) and Růžička and Hansen (1981).

DISCRETE ANALYSERS

Unlike the continuous flow systems which bear a strong resemblance to one another despite refinement of detail, the discrete analysers comprise a hetero-geneous set of instruments. As with the AutoAnalyzer there has been a progression from simple mechanised instruments to more elaborate equipment controlled by its own computer. No simple method of classification is apparent and whichever is employed some instruments can be placed in more than one category. The number of instruments on the market is relatively large and the type of instrumentation is changing. In this account it will neither be possible nor desirable to cover all instruments which have been produced but the authors have excluded those discrete analysers which are dedicated to one analysis only, e.g. glucose or urea analyser or those which only perform two or more fixed analyses already selected by the manufacturer.

The instruments may be single or multi-channel. By the former we imply that each sample is analysed for one selected constituent only. Although in some instruments a batch of samples may be loaded and the change from one analysis to another may be rapidly achieved to allow the batch to be processed for the different individual analyses requested, we prefer to regard these as single channel analysers. Some discrete analysers lend themselves to performing analyses on a small batch or even a single sample making them useful for the emergency laboratory. The multi-channel analysers may be able to select which of a total battery of tests should be performed on an individual sample. Finally the method of analysis may be a traditional end-point colorimetric method but some instruments are particularly suited to study the rate of the reaction under consideration. Bearing these points in mind the authors have used the idiosyncratic classification outlined in Table 8.1.

Certain problems beset all these analysers and most are common to continuous flow systems also. Many traditional chemical methods work poorly in the presence of protein but its removal by the common manual technique of precipitation followed by filtration or centrifugation is difficult to achieve mechanically without human intervention. As a consequence there has been increasing interest in developing chemical methods which work in the presence of protein. Frequently detergents are used to keep the protein in solution. A second consideration is the method of measuring the volumes of sample and reagents and arranging their orderly addition to the reaction vessel. This is usually achieved by using mechanised diluters (p. 180) and dispensers (p. 178). The proper mixing of the reaction mixture after each addition is not always easy to bring about.

TABLE 8.1
A Classification of Discrete Analysers

A. *Single Channel Instruments*
 1. Discontinuous operation
    (a) For batch processing
    (b) For single or few specimens
 2. Continuous operation
    (a) For batch processing
    (b) For single or few specimens
 3. Reaction rate analysis
    (a) For batch processing
    (b) For single or few specimens

B. *Multi-channel Instruments*
 1. Small instruments, up to six channels
 2. Large instruments
    (a) Non-discretionary – all tests performed on each sample
    (b) Discretionary – tests selected for each sample

C. *Centrifugal Fast Analysers*

Common methods are to use the force of the jet of reagent to bring about stirring or to employ convection currents when the reaction vessel is heated to a temperature above that of the reagents. The use of a stirrer produces adequate mixing but can make carryover (p. 190) worse if adherent fluid is transferred to the next reaction vessel. Carryover also occurs during the aspiration of the sample and in the colorimeter cuvette. Incubation at different temperatures may be necessary, the reaction tubes are heated in an air or water bath or in a metal block. The final measurement in most cases uses a flow-cell colorimeter preferably with a linearised, adjustable output to give the result in concentration units in visual or printed form. Another general problem is the correct identification of the sample in the analytical system. This is often done by consideration of the order of loading of the specimens but more elaborate instruments involve labels readable by a computer. The efficiency of these various processes affects the accuracy and precision of the system. Although instruments differ, certain general principles allow objective testing of the performance of most of these analysers (Broughton *et al.*, 1969 and 1974).

Discrete analysers have parts of the complete instrument which perform specific functions. Sometimes they are physically separate and are then similar to the modular arrangement of continuous flow systems. Again classification is difficult in view of the wide range of instruments but the following functions can often be defined. Firstly there is a *sampler* which aspirates the sample and transfers it with diluents to a tube held in a reaction unit. The *reaction unit* may have an integral *incubator* to produce the required temperature. Other reagents are added to it as the reaction proceeds. The *measuring unit* is usually a colorimeter but other detectors such as a flame photometer are available. At this point the samples traverse a common flow path consecutively so carryover may occur. Often the cuvette is first rinsed with the reaction mixture and then filled. The absorbance is read with the fluid stationary in the cuvette before final emptying. The colorimeter response is then of the square wave pattern (p. 190) and operates some form of *display unit* (p. 140) to produce a result in digital or analogue form.

Different Types of Analyser

Single Channel Instruments. In the single channel instruments for discontinuous operation, manual intervention is needed at some stage in the process. Some instruments of this type lend themselves to the analysis of small batches or single samples in the emergency laboratory. In the single channel instruments intended for continuous operation, once the sample has been loaded, all processes are performed automatically and a result is produced without the need for further intervention by the operator. Some are convenient for handling the work of the smaller laboratory and can be changed easily from one analyte to the next. Other more elaborate equipment is more appropriate for the emergency laboratory, allowing any one out of a group of 30 or more analyses to be carried out with prepackaged reagents with little or no instrumental preparation time before the analysis starts.

Reaction Rate Analysers. Many of these instruments were originally developed for the determination of enzymes by kinetic methods under zero-order reaction conditions (Chapter 22, p. 483) when the rate of change of absorbance is proportional to the enzyme activity. Determination of substances which are not enzymes is, however, possible using initial reaction rate methods. These have the advantage of speed in that the reaction does not go to completion as in end-point methods. Also interfering substances may react at a slower rate so that the kinetic method then offers greater specificity.

Some of the instruments considered earlier are capable of working in a reaction rate mode and some of the instruments in this section can also work with end-point methods so that the distinction in classification is not clear-cut. The earlier instruments often had a graphical output of change in absorbance with time and thus resemble a recording spectrophotometer added to automatic handling of a series of specimens. More recently, a small process computer controls the operation of the equipment and performs the calculations to give a printed result in appropriate units. The separate stages in the analysis are sample measurement and dilution, preincubation, reaction initiation followed by mixing, transfer to the photometer light path, serial measurement of the absorbance over a period of time and either graphical recording or calculation by the computer with production of the printed result. In the case of enzyme determinations, the diluent contains most of the components of the reaction mixture. Side reactions go to completion during any preincubation stage before the required reaction is initiated by adding the remaining component(s) of the reaction mixture. Even then there is sometimes a lag phase before the enzyme reaction proceeds according to zero-order kinetics. Various temperatures have been proposed for enzyme reactions, e.g. 25, 30, 35, 37°C and some reaction rate analysers permit a choice. This is also useful for work with non-enzymic materials either in the kinetic or end-point modes. For such work the ability to add additional reagents at points during the analyses is useful as is the facility for measuring individual blanks.

Many instruments have been produced and their method of operation and degree of elaboration of processing of the kinetic measurements vary considerably. In some, the reaction rate produced by each sample is measured sequentially but in others the reactions proceed simultaneously in several samples which are all examined at regular intervals allowing parallel assessment of enzyme activity to be made with some saving in time. The output varies from a simple graphical time-progress curve to computer fitting of observed points to those predicted for zero- or first-order kinetics, with a printed report of enzyme activity and an estimate of the goodness of fit with the theoretical time progress curve. Such 'kinetic packages' are also available for the more sophisticated spectrophotometers (p. 143).

Multi-channel Analysers. Some are relatively small machines analysing samples for 2 to 6 different constituents simultaneously. Others are larger and permit simultaneous analysis for up to 30 or more constituents after making a preliminary dilution of the sample before presenting it to each channel. In the larger instruments it is possible to select the appropriate analyses to be done for each specimen instead of always operating on all channels as is usual with multi-channel continuous flow equipment. Such discretionary working is possible because each analytical channel does not depend on a continuous flow of reagents but can be activated when necessary to dispense the diluted sample and the reagents into the reaction vessel. This conserves reagents and avoids the production of unnecessary results.

The larger instruments are necessarily complex and their operation is under computer control. Data processing facilities which may be present in such equipment include patient identification, sample identification, selection of analytical channels for each sample individually, calibration checks, computation of the results and their collation in the form of a composite report, preparation of quality control information from the analysis of various quality control materials and by the computation of daily means of patients' results after truncation, the alerting of the operator to the need for re-analysis of batches giving unsatisfactory quality control results, and the possibility of limited storage of information on the results of patients and control materials in the computer's memory.

Centrifugal Fast Analysers. These micro-analytical systems arose from the initial work of Anderson (1969, 1970) and are sometimes referred to as parallel fast analysers.

The reaction takes place in the rotor of a centrifuge and usually the photometer is mounted near the rotor circumference with its light path parallel to the axis of rotation (Fig. 8.14). A series of cuvettes is located at the rotor periphery and each passes through the photometer beam as the rotor spins. A flow channel containing two or three discrete wells is located along the radius from each cuvette to the centre of the rotor (Fig. 8.15). The diluted sample is placed in one well and reagents in the other(s). The details of the design vary from one instrument to another but when the rotor spins, the reagents and sample pass along the flow channel into the cuvette by centrifugal force. Mixing is aided by various methods depending on the instrument. The photometer detector then generates a series of pulses corresponding to the light transmitted by each cuvette as it enters the beam sequentially. The signals from each cuvette are stored and analysed further. As each cuvette generates several hundred pulses per minute, the average of several successive readings gives a virtually instantaneous result with less error than a single reading. Repetition of such mean readings at defined intervals allows kinetic studies to be made simply on all samples in the rotor simultaneously. Usually one of these is a blank and standards may be included. Electronic blank correction and automatic calibration is then straightforward. If desired, end-point methods can be used. The degree of elaboration of data handling depends on the particular instrument and its constituent computer.

The sample volumes (5 to 40 μl) allow paediatric samples to be used and the reagent volumes, usually less than 500 μl, reduce running costs. As all the samples in a batch are treated identically and measured simultaneously a high replicate precision is to be expected.

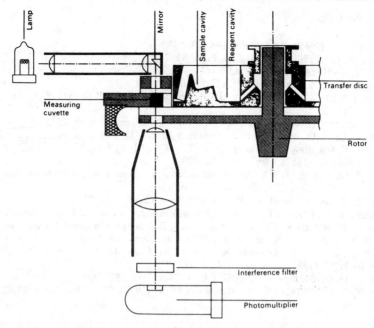

Fig. 8.14. The Optical System of a Centrifugal Analyser During Operation (Union-Carbide Centrifichem).

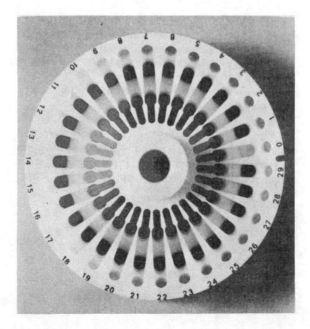

Fig. 8.15. The Rotor of a Centrifugal Analyser (Union-Carbide Centrifichem). Flow channel 0 is for a reagent blank, the others are for samples.

REFERENCES

Anderson N. G. (1969). *Analyt. Biochem*; **28**: 545.
Anderson N. G. (1970). *Amer. J. Clin. Path*; **52**: 778.
Begg R. D. (1971). *Analyt. Chem*; **43**: 854.
Broughton P. M. G. *et al.* (1969). *J. Clin. Path*; **22**: 278.
Broughton P. M. G., Gowenlock A. H., McCormack J. J., Neill D. W. (1974). *Ann. Clin Biochem*; **11**: 207.
Carlyle J. E., McLelland A. S., Fleck A. (1973). *Clin. Chim. Acta*; **46**: 235.
Fleck A., Begg R. D., Williams P. I., Racionzer D. (1971). *Ann. Clin. Biochem*; **8**: 13.
Neeley W. E., Wardlaw S., Swinnen M. E. T. (1974). *Clin. Chem*; **20**: 78.
Rocks B., Riley C. (1982). *Clin. Chem*; **28**: 409.
Růžička J., Hansen E. (1981). *Flow Injection Analysis*. New York: Wiley-Interscience.
Spencer K. (1976). *Ann. Clin. Biochem*; **13**: 438.
Spencer K., Dixon K., Northam B. E. (1977). *Clin. Chim. Acta*; **77**: 189.
Steinhausen R. L., Price C. P. (1985). In *Recent Advances in Clinical Biochemistry*, Vol. 3. (Price C. P., Alberti K. G. M. M. eds) p. 273. Edinburgh: Churchill Livingstone.
Thiers R. E., Cole R. R., Kirsch W. J. (1967). *Clin. Chem*; **13**: 451.
Thiers R. E., Reed A. H., Delander K. (1971). *Clin. Chem*; **17**: 42.
Walker W. H. C. (1971). *Clin. Chim. Acta*; **32**: 305.
Walker W. H. C., Andrew K. R. (1974). *Clin. Chim. Acta*; **57**: 181.
Walker W. H. C., Pennock C. A., McGowan G. K. (1970). *Clin. Chim. Acta*; **27**: 421.

9
RADIOISOTOPIC TECHNIQUES

Various aspects of the use of radioisotopes are discussed in other parts of this book, e.g. the safety aspects of handling radioisotopes and the use of radioisotopes in hormone determinations by radioimmunoassay. This chapter is mainly concerned with the nature of radioactivity and the methods used to measure radioisotopes.

NUCLEAR STRUCTURE

Radioactivity is a property of the positively charged atomic nucleus where virtually all the mass of the atom is concentrated. Estimates of the nuclear diameter indicate that it is related to the atomic weight (A) as $1\cdot4 \times A^{\frac{1}{3}}$ fm. This is about 10^{-5} times the atomic diameter so that only 10^{-15} of the atomic volume is occupied by the nucleus. It follows that its density is high, probably of the order 10^{17} kg/m^3. The nucleus is composed only of protons and neutrons. The *proton* (p) bears a unit positive charge and has a mass of $1\cdot007\ 277$ atomic mass units (amu). One amu is 1/12th the mass of a single atom of ^{12}C and is approximately $1\cdot66 \times 10^{-24}$ g. The *neutron* (n), as its name implies, bears no electrical charge and is slightly heavier than the proton, $1\cdot008\ 665$ amu. The term *nucleon* embraces both types of nuclear particles. The number of protons in a nucleus defines the *atomic number* (Z) and determines the total number of electrons in the various orbits around the nucleus. The chemical properties thus depend on Z. The *atomic weight* (A) is determined by the total number of nucleons (p + n). In the description of atomic reactions it may be necessary to describe both parameters of any atom X, namely $^A_Z X$, for example $^{12}_6 C$ is the usual carbon atom.

The word *nuclide* embraces all possible variations of $^A_Z X$. Most naturally occurring nuclides are stable but a few are unstable and constitute the naturally radioactive nuclides. Nuclides which have the same value of Z but varying A are referred to as *isotopes* indicating that they are to be found in the same place in the periodic table. They have identical chemical properties but varying atomic weights. The term *isobars* is sometimes used to describe those nuclides of the same mass but with differing Z values. For any nuclide the number of protons equals Z and the number of neutrons equals A − Z. The atomic mass of a particular nuclide can be determined in the mass spectrometer with a high degree of precision. This observed mass is less than that calculated from the numbers and individual masses of the protons and neutrons. According to the theory of relativity, mass (m) and energy (E) are interchangeable and related by the expression

$$E = mc^2 \quad \text{where } c = \text{velocity of light.}$$

The loss of mass of 1 amu is equivalent to an energy of 931 MeV (see below). Energy originating in this way provides the *binding energy* of the nucleus. The average binding energy per nucleon for the stable nuclides is 8·4 MeV, a figure which is about one million times greater than the binding energy of an electron in the outer shells of the atom.

Only in two stable nuclides does the nucleus contain more protons than neutrons, $^1_1$H and $^3_2$He. The n:p ratio is approximately 1:1 for nuclides up to $^{40}_{20}$Ca and then becomes progressively larger to reach 1·59 :1 in $^{238}_{92}$U. The nuclei of large atomic mass have progressively lower binding energies per nucleon and show rather slow spontaneous disintegration. These *natural radioisotopes* have very long half-lives (p. 212), e.g. $^{238}_{92}$U, 4·5 × 10^9 years; $^{235}_{92}$U, 7·1 × 10^8 years; $^{232}_{90}$Th, 1·39 × 10^{10} years. Their disintegration products are also radioactive with shorter half-lives, and a series of products is produced until eventually a stable isotope of lead is reached in each case. A few other naturally occurring radioisotopes of smaller Z are known. Those of medical interest are ^{40}K (half-life 1·27 × 10^9 years) and ^{14}C (half-life 5730 years).

It is possible to produce artificial nuclides and these have an n:p ratio deviating from that of the stable nuclides. Many are unstable and constitute the *artificial radioisotopes*, some of which are used in medical investigations. Most of these have relatively short half-lives.

UNITS IN RADIOACTIVITY MEASUREMENTS

There are units in use to express the amount of radioactivity and the energy of radiations.

The SI unit of radioactivity is the *becquerel* (Bq) and corresponds to one disintegration per second. Traditionally, radioactivity was measured in terms of the *curie* (Ci), originally defined as the activity of 1 g of radium and later expressed more precisely as 3·7 × 10^{10} disintegrations per second. The curie is still sometimes used, often as its subdivisions mCi and μCi. One mCi equals 37 MBq and 1 MBq equals 27 μCi.

The *electron volt* is the energy gained by moving a charge equal to that of one electron through a potential difference of one volt. If one coulomb moves through this potential difference the energy is one joule. As the charge on the electron is 1·6 × 10^{-19} C it follows that 1 eV equals 1·6 × 10^{-19} J. This is inconveniently small for many nuclear energy uses and the practical unit is 10^6 times larger, the MeV (1·6 × 10^{-13} J).

RADIOACTIVE EMANATIONS

Following the initial discovery by Becquerel in 1896 that uranium salts blacken a photographic plate it was realised that uranium emitted a radiation later shown by Rutherford to be of two types, alpha and beta. Later a more penetrating component, gamma radiation, was identified. These three types continue to form the basis of the classification of radioactive emanations.

α-Particles

These were shown to be positively-charged particles identical with the nuclei of helium, $^4_2$He. They have a mass of four amu and a charge equal but opposite to that of two electrons. Elements emitting α-particles are virtually confined to the natural heavy radioisotopes, $^{238}_{92}$U, $^{235}_{92}$U, $^{232}_{90}$Th and their disintegration products with Z greater than 82. The artificial transuranic elements with Z equal to 93 to 103 are also α-emitters. For any particular nuclide the energy of all α-particles is the same and lies in the range 4·1 to 8·8 MeV.

Alpha particles are easily absorbed by solids, a thin sheet of card absorbing the most energetic. In their passage through matter they collide with atoms and dislodge electrons producing a dense trail of ionisation before their energy is finally expended by multiple collisions. Even in air they have a range of only a few centimetres depending upon their initial energy.

β-Particles

These were originally recognised as electrons ($β^-$) but it was later observed that some radioisotopes emit positrons ($β^+$) or anti-electrons and both are considered as β-particles. The positron has a mean life-time of only 0·1 $μs$ owing to combination with its anti-particle, an electron. The two masses are both annihilated with the formation of two γ-photons (quanta) of energy 0·511 MeV, equivalent to the mass loss.

The β-particles are rather more penetrating than α-particles but produce less ionisation. The maximal energy varies considerably depending on the isotope: ^{3}H, 0·018 MeV; ^{14}C, 0·156 MeV; ^{32}P, 1·71 MeV (Table 9.1). For a given nuclide however, there is a considerable variation in the energy of its β-particles with the commonest (modal) energy perhaps only one-fifth of the maximal energy. This is unlike the situation with α-particles and is attributable to the simultaneous emission of another particle with the total energy (constant) variably distributed between the two particles. The origin of the two types of β-particle and their associated particles is the disintegration of a neutron or proton:

$$n \to p + β^- + \bar{v}$$

or

$$p \to n + β^+ + v$$

where v and $\bar{v}$ are the neutrino and anti-neutrino respectively. These have negligible mass and no charge and are not detected by any of the usual methods for β-particles.

Although more penetrating than α-particles, the β-particles are easily absorbed by thin metal sheets and even the more energetic are stopped by a 5 mm thickness of aluminium. Even with thick sheets, however, some radiation appears on the side remote from the source of β-particles. This is X-radiation of short wavelength arising from the sudden arrest of the β-particle. It is referred to as *bremsstrahlung* or 'braking radiation'.

γ-Radiation

Unlike the other two emanations this is not particulate but is high energy electromagnetic radiation with a wavelength of the order of 1 pm. It has similar properties to X-radiation which does not originate from the nucleus but from changes in the energy of electrons. Quanta of γ-radiation penetrate matter much more readily than α- and β-particles but produce less dense ionisation than β-particles. As they pass through matter they are attenuated by three processes. In *photoelectric absorption* the γ-photon is completely absorbed and its energy is used to displace an electron from an inner orbital (usually K shell) of an atom and to give it kinetic energy. This secondary electron, usually called a photo-electron, behaves like a β-particle, producing ionisation.

In the *Compton effect* the γ-photon is scattered by collision with a free electron and loses some, but not all, of its energy. The energy lost is converted into the kinetic energy of the Compton or recoil electron. This second type of secondary electron is again like a β-particle with ionising properties. The third process is only found with γ-photons with energy greater than 1·022 MeV. This amount of energy is lost in *pair production*, the creation of an electron and positron, the opposite process to positron loss (p. 205). Each has an energy of 0·511 MeV. The positron is destroyed rapidly but the electron produces ionisation. Low energy γ-radiation is mainly attenuated by photoelectric absorption while over the range from 0·05 to 5 MeV, Compton scattering predominates. Pair production is an important component only with energies above 5 MeV. The relative proportion depends on the atomic number of the medium through which the radiation passes so that for higher Z values, the greater is the photoelectric absorption.

The total attenuation of γ-rays follows the usual exponential law of absorption (compare p. 129):

$$I = I_0 e^{-\mu x}$$

where μ is the absorption coefficient and x is the thickness of the absorber. Different media are compared by their half-value thickness, $x_{\frac{1}{2}}$, which reduces the intensity by half.
Thus:

$$e^{-\mu x_{\frac{1}{2}}} = 1/2 \quad \text{or} \quad x_{\frac{1}{2}} = \ln 2/\mu$$

and $x_{\frac{1}{2}}$ is related to μ as the half-life is to the fractional disintegration rate (p. 212). For γ-rays of energy 1 MeV, $x_{\frac{1}{2}}$ is 9 mm in lead.

When radioactive decay occurs with emission of an α- or β-particle from the nucleus, the latter may be left in an excited state. Another way in which the nucleus becomes excited is by *K electron capture* whereby an electron from the innermost orbit (K shell) is captured by the nucleus. The energy levels of the excited nucleus are quantised and the ground state is reached by the emission of γ-radiation of defined energies. Some nuclides emit only a few energies but others produce a complex spectrum of γ-radiation (see Table 9.1). The energy of the main γ-radiations from isotopes of medical interest varies from 0·014 MeV for [57]Co to 2·75 MeV for [24]Na. In a few nuclides the daughter atom exists for a period in a metastable state before the γ-radiation is eventually emitted. The process is referred to as *isomeric transition*. An important example is ^{99m}Tc with a half-life of 6·03 h produced by the decay of [99]Mo.

Other emanations from radionuclides should be mentioned. Following K electron capture an electron is transferred from one of the higher shells to the K shell to fill the gap. The energy lost is emitted either as X-radiation in the form of a spectrum of energies up to about 0·1 MeV, or as kinetic energy of an electron removed from the atom. This *Auger electron* has a definite but low energy in the range up to 0·08 MeV, which is weaker than the β-particles from [14]C. Examples of isotopes with electron capture decay are [22]Na, ^{51}Cr, [57]Co and [125]I (Table 9.1). Sometimes the excited nucleus may transfer its energy to a K shell electron which is then emitted from the atom with a defined kinetic energy as an *internal conversion electron*. Finally, two photons of electromagnetic radiation of energy 0·511 MeV each are produced when a positron and electron collide and are annihilated. Isotopes of medical interest in which this occurs are [22]Na and [58]Co.

TABLE 9.1
Principal Emanations of Selected Radionuclides

Nuclide	Half-life	Type of decay	β-Radiation %[a]	Energy Maximum & (mean) (MeV)	γ- & X-Radiation %[a]	Energy (MeV)	Specific activity (MCi/mol)
^{3}H	12·26 a	β^-	100	0·018 6 (0·006)			29·1 × 10⁻³
^{14}C	5730 a	β^-	100	0·156 (0·049)			64·2 × 10⁻⁶
^{22}Na	2·60 a	β^+, EC, γ	90·6	0·546 (0·216)	100 / 181[b]	1·27 / 0·511[b]	0·138
^{24}Na	15·0 h	β^-, γ	99·9	1·392 (0·555)	99·9 / 100	2·75 / 1·37	212
^{32}P	14·3 d	β^-	100	1·710 (0·695)			9·09
^{35}S	87·0 d	β^-	100	0·167 (0·049)			1·50
^{42}K	12·4 h	β^-, γ	82·0 / 18·0	3·520 (1·563) / 2·000 (0·824)	18·0	1·52	250
^{47}Ca	4·53 d	β^-, γ	17·9 / 82·0	1·985 (0·816) / 0·688 (0·240)	75·1 / 6·8 / 6·8	1·30 / 0·81 / 0·49	27·8
^{51}Cr	27·7 d	EC, γ	68·5[c]	0·005[c]	10·2 / 21·7[d]	0·32 / 0·005[d]	4·68
^{59}Fe	45·0 d	β^-, γ	52·3 / 46·1	0·467 (0·150) / 0·273 (0·081)	44·1 / 55·5	1·29 / 1·10	2·86
^{57}Co	270 d	EC, γ	69·8[e] / 110[c]	0·007[e] / 0·006[c]	12·0 / 87·9 / 88·0 / 51·3[d]	0·136 / 0·122 / 0·014 / 0·007[d]	0·483
^{58}Co	71·3 d	β^+, EC, γ	15·5 / 52·1[c]	0·474 (0·201) / 0·006[c]	99·5 / 31·0[b] / 21·7[d]	0·81 / 0·511[b] / 0·006[d]	1·84

TABLE 9.1 (Continued)

Nuclide	Half-life	Type of decay	β-Radiation %	β-Radiation Energy Maximum & (mean) (MeV)	γ- & X-Radiation %	γ- & X-Radiation Energy (MeV)	Specific activity (MCi/mol)
^{67}Ga	78·1 h	EC, γ	33·5[e]	0·09[e]	16·1	0·30	40·1
			66·7[c]	0·008[c]	23·9	0·18	
					38·0	0·093[d]	
					51·6[d]	0·009[d]	
^{75}Se	120 d	EC, γ	44·6[c]	0·010[c]	11·7	0·40	1·08
					24·1	0·28	
					57·5	0·26	
					55·7	0·14	
					164	0·12	
					53·8[d]	0·011[d]	
^{90}Y	64·0 h	β$^-$	100	2·273 (0·931)			48·4
^{99m}Tc	6·03 h	γ	12·0[e]	0·13[e]	100	0·14	520
					98·6	0·002	
^{111}In	2·81 d	EC, γ	10·4[e]	0·16[e]	100	0·25	46·7
			16·1[c]	0·02[c]	100	0·17	
					84·6[d]	0·025[d]	
^{113m}In	99·4 min	γ	37·9[e]	0·37[e]	100	0·39	1890
^{123}I	13·0 h	EC, γ	15·1[e]	0·13[e]	22·6[d]	0·026[d]	241
			13·1[c]	0·026[c]	83·6	0·16	
^{125}I	60·2 d	EC, γ	13·3[e]	0·03[e]	100[d]	0·025[d]	2·19
			21·1[c]	0·025[c]	100	0·035	
^{131}I	8·06 d	β$^-$, γ	89·8	0·606 (0·192)	63·9[d]	0·03[d]	16·2
					83·8	0·36	

132I	2·38 h	β⁻, γ	19·7	2·120	(0·836)	18·3	0·95	1390
			12·7	1·597	(0·601)	77·2	0·77	
			10·8	1·450	(0·536)	99·0	0·67	
			18·4	1·165	(0·414)	13·9	0·63	
			14·1	0·721	(0·235)	16·3	0·52	
133Xe	5·31 d	β⁻, γ	98·3	0·346	(0·101)	100	0·081	24·7
			11·4[e]	0·076[e]		21·8[d]	0·034[d]	
			53·4[e]	0·045[e]				
198Au	2·69 d	β⁻, γ	98·6	0·961	(0·316)	99·7	0·41	48·3
203Hg	46·5 d	β⁻, γ	100	0·212	(0·058)	100	0·28	2·77
201Tl	73·1 h	EC, γ	18·3[e]	0·24[e]		10·2	0·17	42·9

Minor components (less than 10 per cent) and weak radiations have been omitted. For X-radiation, Auger and internal conversion electrons an average figure is given with a total percentage. For full details see Dillman and Von der Lage (1975).

[a] Percentage of disintegrations emitting the radiation.
[b] Annihilation energy, two photons per positron.
[c] Auger electrons.
[d] X-radiation.
[e] Internal conversion electrons
For half-life data: a = years, d = days, h = hours.

DISINTEGRATION SCHEMES

Nuclear disintegration may not always proceed in the same way. Thus β-particles may be emitted with several different maximal energies thereby leaving the nucleus in different energy states. A nucleus may disintegrate either by β-particle emission or by electron capture in a ratio (branching ratio) characteristic of the nuclide. Some nuclides emit β^+-particles and undergo electron capture (Table 9.1, p. 208) but with ^{40}K, the naturally occurring radioisotope, it is a β^- particle which is associated with electron capture. Some radioisotopes emit both β^+ and β^- particles and undergo electron capture, e.g. ^{64}Cu, ^{74}As, ^{84}Rb, ^{126}I. Apart from these particle variations several γ-rays can be emitted depending on the energy levels in the excited nucleus. The various possibilities are conveniently indicated in diagrammatic form indicating the various radiations and energy levels (Fig. 9.1). The latter are indicated by horizontal lines with vertical arrows between them indicating γ-radiation of energy equal to the difference between the energies linked by the arrow ends. Diagonal lines indicate particle emission or electron capture as appropriate. A daughter nuclide of higher Z is shown to the right and one with lower Z to the left.

Fig. 9.1(a) indicates emission of β^- particles with one maximal energy leaving a nucleus in the ground state so that no γ-radiation occurs, e.g. ^{3}H, ^{14}C, ^{32}P, ^{35}S and ^{90}Y. Fig. 9.1(b) shows γ-emission as well. As only one γ-ray is emitted its energy is found in all nuclear disintegrations. The emission of two β^- energies, followed by γ-radiation is seen in Fig. 9.1(c). For ^{42}K the single γ-ray occurs in the same percentage of nuclear disintegrations as lead to the higher energy level following β^- emission. The three γ-rays from ^{198}Au will have energies of 1·088, 0·676 and 0·412 MeV. That of the lowest energy occurs in 99·7% of disintegrations (Table 9.1) corresponding to 99% following emission of the higher energy β^- particle and 0·7% following emission of the lower energy one followed by γ-decay to the 0·412 MeV level. The 0·676 MeV γ-ray (1·088–0·412) will thus also occur in 0·7% of disintegrations leaving 0·3% for the 1·088 MeV γ-rays. When several β^- particle energies are present the final γ-pattern is more complex as seen, e.g. in ^{132}I (Table 9.1) but the same principles apply. Fig. 9.1(d) shows disintegration by electron capture followed by γ-emission and Fig. 9.1(e) is an example of a branched decay scheme. Further details of the radiations for medically useful isotopes are given in Table 9.1. For detailed disintegration schemes of 120 radionuclides see Dillman and Von der Lage (1975).

NUCLEAR CHANGES

It is a feature of radioactive changes that the sum of the masses of the products is less than the mass of the original nuclide. This can be used to investigate the possibility of a postulated radioactive disintegration. Thus calculations for most nuclides show that loss of an α-particle would give products of total mass greater than that of the nuclide itself indicating that the emission of this particle will not occur spontaneously. For those few nuclides which emit an α-particle the product has an atomic weight (A) four less than the parent nuclide and an atomic number (Z) two less.

Thus:

$$\alpha\text{-emission: } A \to A - 4; \ Z \to Z - 2$$

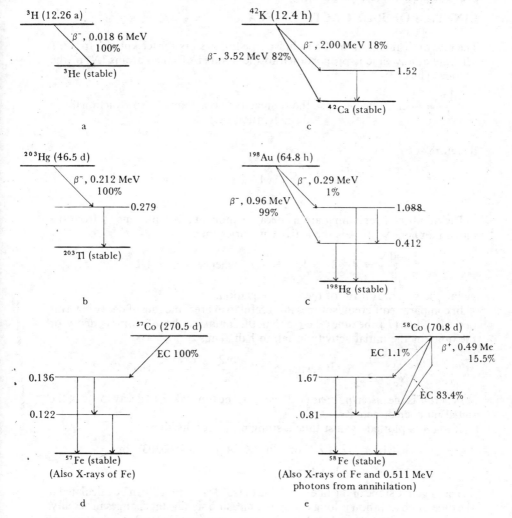

Fig. 9.1. Nuclear Disintegration Schemes.

(a) Simple β^--emission, (b) single β^--emission followed by γ-ray emission, (c) two types of β^--emission with subsequent γ-emission, (d) electron capture followed by γ-ray emission, (e) branched decay, partly electron capture and partly positron emission with subsequent γ-ray emission.

In each case the energy of a γ-ray is indicated by the start and end of vertical arrows linking two energy levels of which the difference is the γ-ray energy in MeV.

If a β^- particle is emitted the nuclide will change only in Z as a neutron changes to a proton. Thus:

$$\beta^- \text{ emission: A, unchanged; } Z \to Z+1$$

If a β^+ particle is emitted or if electron capture occurs, a proton is changed to a neutron and hence:

$$\beta^+ \text{ emission, electron capture: A, unchanged; } Z \to Z-1$$

Any emission of a γ-ray will not alter A or Z.

KINETICS OF RADIOACTIVE DECAY

The rate of disintegration of a radioisotope follows first-order kinetics (p. 483). The rate at any time is proportional to the number of intact atoms (N) of the isotope. Thus:

$$\frac{dN}{dt} = -\lambda N \quad \text{where} \quad \lambda = \text{the radioactive decay constant or fractional disintegration rate}$$

therefore

$$\int_{N_o}^{N_t} \frac{dN}{N} = -\lambda \int_0^t dt \quad \text{whence} \quad N_t = N_o . e^{-\lambda t}$$

The number of remaining atoms decays exponentially with time (t) from the initial number, N_o. If A is the activity in curies then

$$\frac{-dN}{dt} = A \times 3.7 \times 10^{10} = \lambda N \quad \text{whence} \quad A_t = A_o e^{-\lambda t}$$

giving the practical form of the decay equation.

In comparing different isotopes it is useful to express the rate of decay in terms of the *half-life*, (T), the time taken for half the initial number of atoms to decay, or the time for the initial activity to fall to half, Thus

$$\frac{N_t}{N_o} = \frac{1}{2} = e^{-\lambda T} \quad \text{whence} \quad T = \frac{\ln 2}{\lambda} = \frac{0.693}{\lambda} = 0.693 \hat{T}$$

Where $\hat{T}$ is the *mean life-time* ($1/\lambda$) which is the time taken to decay to $1/e$ of the initial number or activity.

If $\log A$ is plotted against time a straight line results since

$$\ln (A_t/A_o) = -\lambda t \quad \text{or} \quad \log (A_t/A_o) = -\lambda t/2.303 \quad \text{or}$$

$$\log A_t = \log A_o - \lambda t/2.303$$

The negative slope of the line is $\lambda/2.303$ or $0.301/T$ so that T can be calculated if the time of observation is long enough to measure significant changes in activity. For isotopes with a long half-life a different approach is needed and the total number of disintegrations per second is measured directly for a known mass of isotope. Thus for the isotope ${}_Z^A X$ (p. 203) let there be n disintegrations per second for g grams. The number of atoms of the nuclide in this mass is

$$N = \frac{g}{A} \times 6.02 \times 10^{23} \quad \text{where} \quad 6.02 \times 10^{23} = \text{Avogadro's number and}$$

$$A = \text{atomic weight}$$

Then as $-\dfrac{dN}{dt} = n = \lambda N \quad n = \dfrac{\lambda g}{A} \times 6.02 \times 10^{23}$

and

$$T = \frac{0.693}{\lambda} = \frac{g}{A n} \times 4.17 \times 10^{23} \text{ seconds}$$

In this way it is possible to measure a half-life of the order of 10^6 years. The half-lives of isotopes of medical interest are given in Table 9.1 (p. 208).

It is also possible to calculate the maximum *specific activity* of a nuclide. This is the activity of a particular mass of the nuclide and is often quoted in units of Ci/mol or multiples thereof. If the specific activity is S Ci/mol then considering 1 mol of nuclide:

$$\text{as} \quad -\frac{dN}{dt} = \lambda N \qquad S \times 3\cdot 7 \times 10^{10} = \lambda \times 6\cdot 02 \times 10^{23}$$

and

$$S = \lambda \times 1\cdot 63 \times 10^{13} \quad \text{or} \quad 1\cdot 13 \times 10^{13}/T \quad \text{where} \quad T \text{ is in seconds}$$

The specific activity of the pure nuclide is thus inversely related to the half-life and the values for isotopes of medical interest are shown in Table 9.1 (p. 208). Radioisotopes which are pure are usually referred to as 'carrier-free' and may be employed in chemical reactions to produce labelled derivatives, e.g. the radio-iodination of hormones in radioimmunoassay (p. 114). If one radioisotope atom is introduced into each molecule of the hormone, the product will have the same specific activity as the original radioisotope. The measurement of the actual specific activity achieved then indicates the extent of labelling. Alternatively if the specific activity is known then the amount of the radioactive substance corresponding to a given amount of radioactivity can be calculated.

PRODUCTION OF RADIOISOTOPES

Artificial radioisotopes are produced by irradiation of target materials, usually in a nuclear reactor where there is a high neutron flux. Neutrons collide with the nuclei of the target and are captured. The new nucleus which is in an unstable state may then emit a γ-photon or another particle, usually a proton or an α-particle. The changes will thus be:

$$^A_Z X + ^1_0 n \rightarrow ^{A+1}_Z X + \gamma \qquad \text{e.g.} \quad ^{23}_{11}Na \, (n, \gamma)^{24}_{11}Na$$

$$^A_Z X + ^1_0 n \rightarrow ^A_{Z-1} X + ^1_1 p \qquad \text{e.g.} \quad ^{58}_{28}Ni \, (n, p)^{58}_{27}Co$$

$$^A_Z X + ^1_0 n \rightarrow ^{A-3}_{Z-2} X + ^4_2 \alpha \qquad \text{e.g.} \quad ^6_3 Li(n, \alpha)^3_1 H$$

Of these reactions, (n, γ) is the one most frequently used. The nuclear reactor obtains its neutron flux from nuclear fission of uranium. The fission products are the nuclides which have the highest nuclear binding energy and cover the range of Z from 50 to 70 predominantly. The isotopes $^{131}_{53}I$, $^{132}_{52}Te$ and $^{133}_{54}Xe$ are medically useful products obtained by such fission.

Other radioisotopes are produced by bombardment with high energy protons, α-particles or deuterons (d, ^2H nuclei) in the cyclotron. Capture of one of these particles produces an unstable nucleus with later emission of a γ-photon or another particle. Some examples are:

$$^A_Z X + ^1_1 p \rightarrow ^{A-3}_{Z-1} X + ^4_2 \alpha \qquad \text{e.g.} \quad ^{60}_{28}Ni \, (p, \alpha)^{57}_{27}Co$$

$$^A_Z X + ^4_2 \alpha \rightarrow ^{A+4}_{Z+2} X + \gamma \qquad \text{e.g.} \quad ^{63}_{29}Cu \, (\alpha, \gamma)^{67}_{31}Ga$$

$$^A_Z X + ^4_2 \alpha \rightarrow ^{A+2}_{Z+2} X + 2^1_0 n \qquad \text{e.g.} \quad ^{109}_{47}Ag(\alpha, 2n)^{111}_{49}In$$

$$^A_Z X + ^2_1 d \rightarrow ^{A-2}_{Z-1} X + ^4_2 \alpha \qquad \text{e.g.} \quad ^{24}_{12}Mg(d, \alpha)^{22}_{11}Na$$

$$^A_Z X + ^2_1 d \rightarrow ^A_{Z+1} X + 2^1_0 n \qquad \text{e.g.} \quad ^{51}_{23}V \, (d, 2n)^{51}_{24}Cr$$

Some short-lived radionuclides are prepared in the laboratory from a precursor. The use of such a generator or 'cow' allows the product to be removed as required and used at once. Such generators are available for the following isotopes:

$$\ce{^{99}_{42}Mo} \xrightarrow[67\,h]{\beta^-} \ce{^{99m}_{43}Tc}$$

$$\ce{^{113}_{50}Sn} \xrightarrow[118\,d]{EC} \ce{^{113m}_{49}In}$$

$$\ce{^{132}_{52}Te} \xrightarrow[78\,h]{\beta^-} \ce{^{132}_{53}I}$$

GENERAL CONSIDERATIONS IN RADIOACTIVITY MEASUREMENTS

In clinical biochemistry most measurements of radioactivity are made on samples removed from the patient, e.g. serum, urine or faeces. Counting *in vivo* is common in departments of nuclear medicine and involves the measurement of the concentration and distribution of an isotope in the body, sometimes in a situation where this is changing rapidly. Most of the following account refers to *in vitro* counting.

It is rare to need to determine the absolute radioactivity of a sample and the count rate of samples relative to standards under defined conditions is usually measured. Even then several factors determine the choice of method. Thus the radioisotope is important particularly the nature and energy of its emanations. In general γ-emitters are most convenient and require little sample preparation before counting. However, the isotopes of the common elements carbon, hydrogen, sulphur and phosphorus are only β-emitters. Many nuclides emit β- and γ-radiation; it is then usual to choose the latter. Nuclides with short half-lives decay appreciably during a protracted study but standards behave similarly so that direct comparison with standards will allow for this. If for any reason such standards cannot be used, all count rates must be corrected to a fixed arbitrary time by using the equations of radioactivity decay. If other radioisotopes are present some method must be used to distinguish the isotope of interest either by selection of a characteristic energy of its γ-radiation or by a choice between β- and γ-counting. Self-absorption by the sample is also important in relation to the radioisotope used. This is usually trivial with γ-rays as they are able to penetrate most biological samples easily but with β-particles particularly with those of low energy as emitted by ^{32}S, ^{14}C and especially ^{3}H, self-absorption is very marked requiring either a very thin layer of sample or conversion into a gas or, as is most often done, the incorporation of the sample into the detector itself as in liquid scintillation counting.

Other considerations apply to the samples requiring measurement. The size, nature and number of the samples and their activity determine the choice of method partly by imposing restrictions on the nature of the detector and the time available for counting each sample. The efficiency of the counting system varies with the size of the sample. Other factors concerning the sample include the time required to prepare this in a form suitable for counting or the need to re-use the sample for other analyses. Again γ-emitters lend themselves to minimal pre-processing of samples and hence easier application to further analyses.

Available apparatus varies from simple manually operated counters to elaborate automatic equipment with facilities for counting more than one isotope at the same time, automatic sample changing and print-out of results. The costs vary accordingly. In any equipment, an important consideration is the *background* counting rate, the rate present with no sample in the counter. It is analogous to a reagent blank in colorimetry and is deducted from the sample counting rate. Background counts arise partly within the instrument and partly by the influence of external radiation on the counting equipment. Various aspects of the background are discussed later in relation to individual methods. Examples of background arising within the equipment are the dark current pulses of photomultipliers, chemiluminescence in liquid scintillators, and radionuclides present in the glass of photomultipliers or sample vials, in steel covering of counters and in lead used for shielding. External γ-radiation may pass into the detector and contribute to the background. This arises from natural terrestrial radioactivity and radioactive components of building materials as well as from any radioactive materials stored in the laboratory. It is reduced by shielding the detector and sample with lead and by placing the counter remote from the main isotope stores in the laboratory. Cosmic radiation is a constant component of the background and arises from showers of high energy particles which pass through the shielding to affect the detector. This component of the background is generally proportional to the volume of the sensitive part of the detector.

Counting Errors

Nuclear distintegrations occur in a random fashion and at low count rates the irregularity of pulses is obvious making the number of counts in a defined time subject to variation. The number varies according to the Poisson distribution (p. 269) and for this the standard deviation (p. 270) of the number of counts, N, is given by $\sqrt{N}$. Thus if there are N counts in a time t, the count rate, n, is given by

$$n = N/t$$

and hence the standard error, SE (p. 269), of n, σ_n and its coefficient of variation, CV (p. 238), will be given by

$$\sigma_n = \frac{\sqrt{N}}{t} = \sqrt{\frac{n}{t}} \quad \text{and} \quad CV_n = \frac{100 \sqrt{n/t}}{n} = \frac{100}{\sqrt{nt}} = \frac{100}{\sqrt{N}}$$

Thus for 100 counts the CV is 10% and is reduced to 1% by making 10 000 counts. Below this level, equipment errors become as important as statistical errors of counting and the former can be assessed if the observed CV is larger than predicted from the simple equation above.

Very often it is necessary to measure the ratio between two count rates, n_1 and n_2 as in the comparison of a sample with a standard. The error of the ratio is related to the CV of the separate counts (p. 271) as follows:

$$CV \text{ ratio} = \sqrt{CV_1^2 + CV_2^2} = 100 \sqrt{\frac{1}{n_1 t_1} + \frac{1}{n_2 t_2}}$$

If the total counting time is restricted, this is minimal when

$$\frac{t_1}{t_2} = \sqrt{\frac{n_2}{n_1}}$$

It is also necessary to measure the difference between two count rates as for example in deducting background counts. As discussed later (p. 250) the SE of the difference is

$$\sigma \, \text{diff} = \sqrt{\frac{n_1}{t_1} + \frac{n_2}{t_2}}; \quad \text{minimal when} \quad \frac{t_1}{t_2} = \sqrt{\frac{n_1}{n_2}}$$

if the total counting time, $t_1 + t_2$, is restricted.

It is then important to apportion this in the most efficient way. If $c =$ the observed count rate of a sample and b is the background count rate, the corrected count rate of the sample, s is given by $(c - b)$ and the errors in measurement are minimised if the total time, t, available for counting is divided between t_c, the time for the sample and t_b, the time for the background so that

$$t_c = \frac{t\sqrt{c}}{\sqrt{c} + \sqrt{b}} \quad \text{and} \quad t_b = \frac{t\sqrt{b}}{\sqrt{c} + \sqrt{b}} \quad \text{i.e.} \quad \frac{t_c}{t_b} = \sqrt{\frac{c}{b}} \quad \text{as before}$$

Thus if b is approx. 100 counts/min and c is approx. 1600 counts/min then t_c should be $4t/5$ and t_b should be $t/5$. Thus if the actual counts are:

background, 96 counts in 1 min; sample, 6360 in 4 min

then
$$b = 96 \pm \sqrt{96}/1 = 96 \pm 9 \cdot 80$$

and
$$c = 6360/4 \pm \sqrt{6360}/4 = 1590 \pm 19 \cdot 94$$

and hence
$$s = 1590 - 96 \pm \sqrt{19 \cdot 94^2 + 9 \cdot 80^2}$$
$$= 1394 \pm 22 \cdot 21 \ (CV = 1 \cdot 59\%)$$

The effect of background on the counting error is obviously more important as s approaches b. If s is $10 \times b$, variations in the latter have little importance but if s equals b the SE is more than twice as great as would be the case if there were no background and hence a counting time more than 4 times as long would be needed to eliminate the background effect. In practice it is desirable to work with samples having a count rate of at least $10b$ and counters of high efficiency and low background aid this. The limit of detection of a radioisotope is that giving a count rate of about $0 \cdot 1b$ but the error in measurement is very high.

A practical example of the errors of counting is given below:

background, 120 counts in 5 min, i.e. $b = 24$ counts/min
sample, 12 405 counts in 15 min, i.e. $c = 827$ counts/min
standard, 13 240 counts in 1 min
then

$$b = 24 \pm \sqrt{120/5} = 24 \pm 2 \cdot 19$$

$$c = 827 \pm \sqrt{12405}/15 = 827 \pm 7 \cdot 43$$

$$\text{std} = 13240 \pm \sqrt{13240}/1 = 13240 \pm 115 \cdot 07$$

$$s = c - b = 803 \pm \sqrt{7 \cdot 43^2 + 2 \cdot 19^2} = 803 \pm 7 \cdot 75 \ (0 \cdot 965\%)$$

$$\text{std} - b = 13216 \pm \sqrt{115 \cdot 07^2 + 2 \cdot 19^2} = 13216 \pm 115 \cdot 09 \ (0 \cdot 871\%)$$

$$\text{ratio} \frac{\text{sample}}{\text{standard}} = \frac{803}{13216} \pm \sqrt{0 \cdot 965^2 + 0 \cdot 871^2} = 0 \cdot 06076 \pm 1 \cdot 300\%$$

or
$$= 0 \cdot 06076 \pm 0 \cdot 00079$$

In many counters it is possible to make adjustments which affect the counting efficiency and the background to different degrees, allowing the best counting conditions to be selected. For low activity samples maximal sensitivity is obtained when s^2/b is maximal and the adjustment is made to achieve this. Alternatively, if two types of counter are available the choice between them can be made on these grounds. For samples of higher activity it is better to consider a figure of merit, Q, for the instrument such that

$$Q = \sqrt{c} - \sqrt{b}$$

Thus if one compares two counters for 1 nCi of ^{14}C (2220 disintegrations/min) a liquid scintillation counter might offer 85% counting efficiency (1887 counts/min) at a background of 60 counts/min while a sophisticated Geiger-Müller counter might have an efficiency of 18% (400 counts/min) but with a background of only 1 count/min. The formula s^2/b would give results of 5·93 $\times 10^4$ and 16 $\times 10^4$ respectively indicating that the Geiger-Müller arrangement is preferable but Q is 36·4 and 19·0 suggesting that the liquid scintillation counter is better for this amount of activity. At amounts of ^{14}C less than 7·8 pCi the advantage swings to the Geiger-Müller arrangement.

Another useful index is the minimum time t taken to achieve a given CV, x, for the result. It can be shown that

$$t = \frac{1}{x^2 Q^2}$$

allowing two equipments to be compared to see whether the time is reasonable or not. If the time available is fixed then the formula gives Q for any specified value of x.

When using a ratemeter (p. 228) the time constant, τ, can be varied. If the mean count rate is $\bar{n}$ then the signal will fluctuate with a CV defined by

$$CV = 100/\sqrt{2\bar{n}\tau}\,\%$$

In order to follow rapid changes in activity τ must be short and hence $\bar{n}$ needs to be high for an acceptable CV. If a sample is being counted, its activity will change slowly and τ can be longer although the correct reading will not be obtained until after about 5τ. This allows lower activity samples to be measured with greater precision.

INSTRUMENTS FOR THE DETECTION AND MEASUREMENT OF RADIOACTIVITY

Various devices used to measure radiation rely on swift charged particles affecting the material within the detector. For the purposes of clinical biochemistry such swift particles are electrons. These may be β-particles or electrons produced by the interaction of γ- or X-rays and bremsstrahlung with atoms within the detector. These fast moving electrons can excite or ionise other atoms in the detector. In excitation the atom is temporarily in an unstable state and its return to its resting state may be detected by emission of light as in scintillation counters or by a chemical change as in photographic emulsion detectors. When ionisation occurs the electrons and positive ions produced are responsible for the operation of Geiger-Müller counters, proportional counters and ionisation chambers.

Most detectors produce a small electrical pulse which requires further electronic manipulation such as amplification, sorting of different pulses and their recording. Sometimes individual pulses, after sorting if necessary, are counted by the recording system during a defined time period–the *scaler* method. In other instruments the average number of pulses per time interval is displayed by the recording system–the *ratemeter* method.

Scintillation Counters

The photons emitted by the excited atoms in the detector proper are picked up by a photomultiplier (p. 139) and thereby converted into an electrical pulse the size of which is proportional to the number of photons. The latter is related to the energy deposited in the scintillator. There are two main types of scintillator in general use. Solid inorganic iodide crystals are employed mainly for γ-ray or X-ray measurement but have limited application for β-particles. Organic scintillators are used in solution or are incorporated into plastic materials composed of carbon, hydrogen and oxygen, i.e. of atoms of relatively low atomic number. Liquid scintillators are mainly used for β-particles but occasionally large plastic scintillators are used for detecting γ-rays. Small plastic scintillators are used for β-particles of moderate or high energy.

It is more convenient to use γ-emitters as counting procedures are simpler.

Crystal Scintillation Counters

The scintillator is a clear crystal of sodium iodide containing a trace of thallium iodide. Thallium-activated sodium iodide crystals are of high density (3·7 g/ml) and as iodine has a high atomic number ($Z = 53$) γ-radiation is detected by its photoelectric effect rather than the Compton effect (p. 205). The thallium atoms in the crystal lattice alter the electron energy bands locally. When these electrons are excited they emit the scintillations on returning to a lower level. The conversion of γ-energy to light is approximately 10 % efficient so that a 1 MeV γ-ray produces about 30 000 photons of light. This permits the detection of low energy radiation and aids the discrimination of scintillations of different intensity, arising from γ- or X-rays of different energy.

As the crystal is hygroscopic it is enclosed in a watertight cover. This has a clear optical window on one face which is applied to the photomultiplier tube with a thin intervening layer of silicone fluid as an optical coupler; the rest of the crystal is covered with aluminium of thickness 0·5 to 1·5 mm lined with alumina as an optical reflector. Such crystals are available in sealed form in various shapes and sizes up to a length or diameter of 76 cm (30 in). The aluminium/alumina covering prevents all but the more energetic β-particles from reaching the crystal although some bremsstrahlung may be detected. The behaviour to different energies of γ- or X-radiation is also important. High energy γ-rays pass easily through the aluminium cover and may also pass straight through the crystal unless this is large. Low energy γ-radiation and most X-radiation is captured by the crystal more readily but for the weakest energies the aluminium covering may itself absorb the radiation. Crystals with thinner aluminium coverings down to 0·025 mm or beryllium down to 0·2 mm thickness are produced. Optical efficiency is greater if the crystal is permanently linked through an optical liquid coupler to the photomultiplier without any intervening optical window but neither element of the crystal/photomultiplier combination is re-usable if one fails.

Most sodium iodide (Tl) crystals are grown singly. A more expensive polycrystalline form has the advantages of greater mechanical strength and availability in the form of very large scintillators with a better scintillation performance. Single caesium iodide crystals activated by sodium or thallium have also been used. They have even higher γ-absorption than sodium iodide crystals and are only slightly hygroscopic so do not need an air-tight container. In all cases the decay time of the scintillation is very short allowing counting rates of up to 10 000 counts/s to be handled.

Photomultiplier. This converts light energy to an electrical pulse. Photons striking the photocathode eject electrons from it and these are converted into progressively larger numbers of electrons by the successive amplification steps in the photomultiplier. The final pulse size at a fixed amplification depends on the number of electrons ejected from the photocathode. The conversion of light energy from photons into electrons is about 10 to 25 % efficient so that the 30 000 photons produced from a 1 MeV γ-ray (see p. 218) may produce 3000 to 7500 electrons assuming all reach the photocathode. As the number of photons produced is approximately proportional to the γ-ray energy the sizes of the final pulses will depend on the γ-ray spectrum of the nuclide.

Electrons are also emitted spontaneously from the photocathode and dynodes usually as single electrons due to thermionic processes. They constitute the dark current of the photomultiplier and are a component of the background (p. 215) count rate. The dark current is highest with the most efficient photocathodes but is reduced by cooling the photomultiplier. The pulses resulting from the dark current are of low intensity and their effect is considerably reduced by coincidence circuitry (p. 224).

Scintillation Spectra. The pulse from the photomultiplier is passed through a pre-amplifier and amplifier producing a final pulse of several volts in magnitude. The frequency with which pulses of different magnitude occur defines the scintillation spectrum. If a source of γ-rays is placed over the scintillator the spectrum shows peaks corresponding to the main energies of the various γ-rays emitted and other zones due to reduced energies produced by Compton scattering. The spectra are characteristic of the γ-source and the details of the detector. If two radioisotopes are present together their spectra may be such that characteristic peaks for the two isotopes are clearly separated. The isotope with the more energetic radiation can then be measured if some method is available to count only pulses whose magnitudes fall within its characteristic peak. Compton scattering from the higher energy radiation may interfere with a lower peak from the second isotope. This interference has to be allowed for if this second isotope is counted simultaneously.

The simplest device, a _discriminator_, suppresses all pulses below a preset size. If the two isotope peaks are very different, the larger pulse can be selected. Alternatively, if only one isotope is present the discriminator can suppress the small peaks resulting from the dark current background. A more useful device, the _pulse height analyser_, allows only pulses between two selected sizes (the 'window') to reach the counting system. The window can be set to define the peak of interest. More elaborate instruments incorporate a _multichannel pulse-height analyser_ whereby the pulses falling in different 'windows' of constant width can be separated and counted at the same time. By careful selection of the discriminator bias or the window settings the most satisfactory operating conditions can be chosen.

Different types of crystal scintillator. The effectiveness of a crystal scintillator in creating a pulse from a γ-ray depends on the size and shape of the crystal and its position relative to the source.

The *geometrical efficiency* is the fraction of the rays emitted from a source which can enter the crystal volume. If a point source is placed on the plane face of a cylindrical crystal, the geometrical efficiency is 0·5. The efficiency in the frequently used well crystal (Fig. 9.2a) approaches 1·0 for samples at the bottom of the well.

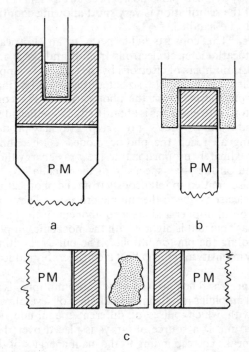

Fig. 9.2. Crystal Scintillators.
   (a) Well type with sample in tube, (b) pillar type with surrounding sample container, (c) flat crystal type with solid sample in container between two detectors.
PM = photomultiplier tube.

The *intrinsic efficiency* is the probability that a γ-ray entering the crystal will undergo an interaction before it would otherwise leave it. The efficiency is larger for γ-rays of lower energy and for larger crystal thicknesses. It can be 1·0 but falls to 0·30 for a 2·6 MeV γ-ray and a crystal thickness of 25 mm.

The *total absorption fraction* is the probability that a γ-ray interacting in the crystal will be totally absorbed therein. It is highest for large crystals and low γ-energies. The total probability that a γ-ray gives up its maximum energy within the crystal is obtained by multiplication of the three probabilities. In addition there will be the effect of any absorption by matter such as the crystal covering or source container interposed between the crystal and the source.

In general, larger crystals have greater efficiency, greater cost and greater background. The relationship of the sample to the crystal is usually one of three types shown in Fig. 9.2. The well crystal (a) allows small samples (5 to 15 ml) to be placed within the crystal and to be detected with relatively high geometrical efficiency. This varies from near 1 at the bottom of the well to 0·5 near the top. If the sample volume is kept constant the mean efficiency is similar for standards and unknowns. This type of crystal is used in many automatic gamma counters. Larger volumes can be placed in a container surrounding a pillar-type crystal (Fig. 9.2b) which gives a geometrical efficiency falling progressively from 0·5 near to the crystal surface on moving to the edge of the container. The reduced efficiency may be compensated for by the use of a larger sample if, e.g. urine is to be counted. The flat crystal (Fig. 9.2c) is used in some cases for larger samples by placing the sample between two such crystals, thereby increasing the geometrical efficiency. Several photomultipliers may be needed to cover the crystal area. Large flat crystals with several photomultipliers on one face are used in the gamma camera for organ scanning using γ-emitting isotopes. The radiation from the patient passes through a grid of holes in a lead block which effectively exposes different parts of the crystal to the radiation from different areas of the organ. The distribution of scintillations in the crystal is displayed on a cathode ray tube.

Automated Gamma Counters

Automated counters can handle a batch of samples either in serial or parallel mode. In the serial counter, up to several hundred samples are loaded in a transport system which moves them one by one to a counting position comprising a well-screened, relatively large, crystal scintillator with a photomultiplier tube. Each sample is counted for a preset time or number of counts, whichever is reached first, and the individual results are recorded serially in printed form. If necessary, the counting circuits can be automatically readjusted for a different isotope once a batch of the first isotope has been processed.

In the parallel counter, up to 12 samples loaded manually are counted simultaneously for a defined period before the results for each are processed. Manual intervention is needed to load the next batch or to alter the counting characteristics. In this system each sample is in contact with a separate, relatively small crystal scintillator with its photomultiplier tube. The screening of each crystal is less heavy than in the serial type so that each detector may respond to a varying degree to a single sample placed over one of them. This is referred to as *cross-talk* and is minimised if a relatively weak γ-emitter such as ^{125}I is used. This also allows much of the radiation to be captured in a smaller crystal. Such equipment uses an inbuilt computer which first assesses cross-talk between the various detectors using a single standard placed in each counting position in turn. The relative sensitivity of each counting position can also be measured for later correction to a standard sensitivity. When all the samples are being counted simultaneously, the computer records the number of counts at each position and at the end recalculates the count rate having corrected for the effects of cross-talk and relative sensitivity.

Such parallel counters are cheaper than the large serial counters and are very convenient for a moderate workload of ^{125}I-labelled samples where repeated manual intervention is possible. The serial counters offer the possibility of counting 24 h daily and are more suitable for a wider range of isotopes.

Organic Scintillation Counters

The crystal scintillator is an inefficient detector of β-particles as they are mainly absorbed by the crystal covering. In *liquid scintillation counting* the β-emitter is dissolved or suspended in the fluid medium and the energy of the β-particles excites the solvent molecules with a geometrical efficiency of 1·0. This energy is then transferred to a primary solute which emits it as a scintillation of characteristic wavelength. Sometimes a secondary solute is added to absorb the light and re-emit it at a longer wavelength, if this corresponds to the peak spectral response of the photomultiplier. The molecules of the solvents and solutes are composed of atoms with low atomic numbers and are relatively poor absorbers of γ-rays.

Scintillator chemicals incorporated into a solid plastic give detectors of varying size and shape used for measurement of radiation from the whole human body. A thin disc of such a *plastic scintillator* may be mounted on the window of a photomultiplier for the detection of β-particles of medium energy. It need not be covered by metal if operated in the dark and its geometrical efficiency approaches 0·5 for samples placed in contact with it. A thin tube of plastic scintillator may also be used as a well-type counter with higher geometrical efficiency. Some β-particles are absorbed within the sample (self-absorption) and this is important for weak β-emitters such as ^{14}C, ^{35}S and, especially, ^{3}H. The following discussion relates to liquid scintillation counting.

Counting medium. The best solvents for transformation of the energy of β-particles into excited molecules are alkylbenzenes, particularly toluene and xylene. Despite the high geometrical efficiency for the capture of β-particles, conversion into light by the primary scintillation solute is only 3% efficient at best. A β-particle of energy 0·010 MeV produces about 80 photons some of which may not reach the photomultiplier due to absorption. As the conversion of photons into electrons at the photocathode is 10 to 25% efficient, such a β-particle might release only 6 to 15 electrons. The situation is very different from that of crystal scintillation counting with γ-rays (p. 219). The β-particles from ^{3}H have a mean energy of only 0·006 MeV and thus produce only weak electrical pulses from the photomultiplier, some of which will be difficult to distinguish from those arising from its dark current (p. 219). The situation is better for the weak β-emitter ^{14}C whose mean particle energy is almost 10 times greater.

Various primary solutes have been used (Table 9.2) of which PPO is perhaps the most popular. The wavelength of light emitted is a good spectral fit for the newer bi-alkali photomultipliers. With the older types a secondary solute is needed (Table 9.2). Such a wavelength shifter is not necessary with the newer tubes for ^{14}C but it may be advantageous with ^{3}H. Although toluene is the best energy transducer, aqueous samples do not mix with it and it is somewhat toxic; *p*-dioxane is more miscible with water but its efficiency is only 70 to 80% that of toluene and it needs more careful purification as it forms a peroxide which diminishes the counting efficiency by chemical *quenching*. Polar solvents such as ethanol or methanol added to toluene or dioxane-based media improve miscibility with water but also cause some quenching. Naphthalene added to dioxane-based solutions assists transfer of energy to the primary scintillant and reduces quenching. Two types of quenching are recognised. *Chemical quenching* occurs if a substance interferes with the energy transfer processes leading to emission of light along the particle track. *Optical quenching* is the absorption of emitted light by the solution. Both reduce the intensity of the scintillation.

The choice of scintillator depends on the nature of the sample and its miscibility with toluene or dioxane. The optimal concentration of the scintillator depends on the solvent, being lower for a higher efficiency of energy transfer as in toluene. It is higher for any solvent if quenching is present. The best concentration is determined empirically by finding the lowest concentration giving maximal

TABLE 9.2
Scintillation Solutes for Liquid Scintillation Counting

Substance	Abbreviation	Optimal wavelength (nm)	Comments
Primary Solutes			
p-Terphenyl	TP	350	Limited solubility at low temperatures or in presence of water.
2,5-Diphenyloxazole	PPO	365	Often used. Solubility in toluene 240–410 g/l depending on temperature.
2,(4'-Biphenyl)-5-phenyl-1,3,4-oxadiazole	PBD	365	As p-terphenyl. Solubility in toluene at 0 °C, 10 g/l.
2,(4'-t-Butylphenyl-5,(4"-biphenyl))-1,3,4-oxadiazole	Butyl PBD	365	Solubility in toluene, 57–120 g/l. Less affected by quenching. More expensive than PPO.
5-Bis-2,(5'-t-butyl-benzoxazolyl)-thiophene	BBOT	435	Poor match for photomultipliers other than S20 trialkali type.
Secondary Solutes			
1,4-Bis(5'-phenyloxazol-2'-yl)-benzene	POPOP	420	Often used.
1,4-Bis(4'-methyl-5'-phenyloxazol-2'-yl)-benzene	Dimethyl POPOP	430	More soluble in toluene than POPOP.
p-Bis(o-methylstyryl)-benzene	bis MSB	420	Higher concentration needed than with POPOP. Good quenching resistance.
2(4'-Biphenyl-benzoxazole)	PBBO	396	Often used with butyl PBD.

pulses from the detector. For toluene the usual concentration ranges (g/l) for the commoner scintillants are: PPO, 4 to 7; BBOT, 6 to 16; butyl PBD, 6 to 20. The effect of quenching on the count rate of a standard can be tested by adding increasing amounts of carbon tetrachloride.

Non-polar samples are added to a toluene- or xylene-based medium avoiding halogenated hydrocarbons if possible as they cause quenching. With slightly quenched samples and a bi-alkali photomultiplier the primary scintillants alone in concentrations at the lower end of the above ranges are satisfactory. For moderately quenched samples 6 to 8 g/l PPO + 0·6 g/l dimethyl POPOP is preferable. With the old photomultipliers for slightly quenched samples it is necessary to add 0·1 to 0·25 g/l of POPOP or dimethyl POPOP to PPO (4 to 6 g/l), butyl PBD (4 to 10 g/l) or BBOT (4 to 10 g/l).

For aqueous samples many mixtures have been advocated which will hold up to 40 % of water by volume. They are based on toluene, xylene or dioxane and in general the counting efficiency falls as the amount of water increases. One such mixture is toluene/Triton X-100 which holds up to 40 % water but also mixes with non-polar materials. The usual mixture is PPO (4 g), POPOP (0·2 g), toluene (667 ml), Triton X-100 (Rohm and Haas, 333 ml). The counting efficiency (%) is 74 (^{14}C) and 29 (^{3}H) at 5 % water falling to 66 (^{14}C) and 19 (^{3}H) at 40 % water. For a water content of 12 to 23 % the mixture tends to separate into two phases with detrimental effects on the counting rate. Below 12 % a stable clear solution exists and above 23 % a translucent stable gel occurs. Several ready prepared scintillation mixtures based on xylene are commercially available for a variety of specimens.

Biological fluids such as urine or serum may be added direct to such mixtures, but for blood or soft tissues addition of a strong base may be necessary before the sample can be incorporated. Common solubilisers are Hyamine 10-X (Rohm and Haas), Soluene-30 (Packard Instruments), NCS (Nuclear Chicago Limited) or BBS-3 (Beckman Instruments). Decolorisation may be required for which benzoyl peroxide added before digestion is helpful. Chemiluminescence is suppressed by adding butylated hydroxytoluene or glacial acetic acid after solubilisation. Samples such as plasma can be added directly to the toluene/Triton X-100 system. Solid samples such as scrapings from thin-layer chromatograms may also be counted in suspension in this system or by adding to Cab-O-Sil (Godfrey L. Cabot Inc), a thixotropic silica gel. Electrophoresis strips can be counted if the dried strip is cut into sections and immersed in the scintillation fluid. Orientation of the strip may be critical for weak β-emitters especially ^{3}H.

Interferences in Liquid Scintillation Counting. Background pulses from the counter arise other than by irradiation of the scintillant by external sources such as cosmic rays. The dark current of the photomultiplier (p. 219) contributes as does chemiluminescence (p. 158) in the sample from other chemical interactions and phosphorescence (p. 153) from the walls of the vial in which the liquid scintillant is placed. The last three sources of interference are mainly attributable to the emission of single photons from the vial or single electrons from the photomultiplier cathode. The small pulses produced are similar to those caused by weak energy β-particles from ^{3}H making discrimination by pulse height methods difficult. The dark current is reduced by cooling the photomultiplier, sometimes to as low as $-20\,^\circ$C, but this may produce solubility problems for the sample. Phosphorescence is reduced by choosing special glass or plastic vials and not exposing them to intense light. Chemiluminescence is reduced by altering the pH or adding suppressants. The use of a coincidence counter makes these interferences much less important.

Counting Equipment Arrangements. The simplest arrangement uses a single photomultiplier sited close to the sample vial. Its output is passed through a pre-amplifier to a linear amplifier. The final pulse is sorted by a single channel pulse height analyser (p. 219) before passing to a scaler. The pulses arising from ^{14}C can usually be separated from background and this isotope can be counted at $10\,^\circ$C with an efficiency of 60 % with a typical background figure of 30 counts/min. For ^{3}H, however, discrimination is more difficult and even on cooling to $-10\,^\circ$C the background may be 300 counts/min and the counting efficiency only 20 %.

As a considerable part of the background is attributable to single photon events this is reduced in the more complex instruments by placing the vial between two photomultipliers. Genuine scintillations are likely to produce sufficient photons to reach both detectors simultaneously but for single photon events and dark current electrons both photomultipliers are unlikely to respond at the same instant as only one is affected by a particular event. The outputs of the two detectors are passed through a coincidence circuit which only transfers a pulse to the rest of the system if both react simultaneously. Usually the transferred pulse is amplified and sorted by a pulse height analyser into three 'windows' within which the counts are separately recorded by scalers. This permits separation from some residual background and allows, e.g. ^{3}H and ^{14}C to be counted at the same time. Alternatively, two channels can be used to correct for quenching. This type of counter is often operated at ambient temperature but cooling may reduce the background still further. Typical counting efficiencies for ^{14}C and ^{3}H are 95 and 60% respectively with background reduced to 20 counts/min.

Quenching Corrections. Quenching reduces the average pulse height of scintillations for a particular radioisotope thereby altering the number of pulses accepted by the window setting of the pulse height analyser. Several methods have been used to correct for the effect.

1. If quenching is constant in all samples and standards the window setting can be optimised for the reduced peak heights. This situation is uncommon.
2. After counting the sample (Cs) an *internal standard* of known unquenched count rate is added and the sample is re-counted to find the increment in count rate. Then:

$$\text{Corrected sample count rate} = (Cs - \text{background}) \times \frac{\text{standard count rate}}{\text{increment}}$$

   There is the possibility of a pipetting error for the standard, two counts are needed and the final sample is contaminated by the standard.
3. A γ-source in the instrument is used in the *external standard* method. The sample is counted before and after placing the source near the vial to determine the increment in count rate. A series of standards is prepared with increasing quantities of a quenching agent such as acetone or chloroform to provide measurable quenching. The increments from the γ-source for these standards is plotted against the degree of quenching and this calibration curve is used to measure the quenching in other samples. Again two counts are needed and the system may not be valid for counting suspensions.
4. In the *channels ratio* method for one isotope, two adjacent channel windows are set so that the count rate is similar in both for unquenched samples. Quenching reduces the pulse height and the number of counts in the upper window while increasing that in the lower window. The ratio for the two channels alters and this can be investigated for standards of known quenching as in 3. Each sample need only be counted once. A disadvantage is that with low activity samples the counting errors in each channel increase and the ratio is subject t an even greater error.
5. A frequently used approach is to combine methods 3. and 4. above. After counting each sample the external standard is brought into position and counts are measured in two channels. The *external standard channels ratio* is used to measure the extent of quenching.
6. Some systems attempt to compensate automatically for quenching by sensing the spectral shift and making electronic adjustments so that each sample is counted under optimal conditions.

Ionisation Counters

Unlike scintillation methods, ionisation counters rely on detecting the ions produced by fast moving electrons interacting with the contents of the counter. In the *ionisation chamber* the positive ions and electrons produced from the air within it are separated by attraction to a cathode and anode at a potential difference of up to a few hundred volts. A small current of the order of 10^{-14} A flows proportionate to the rate of production of the ions and is measured by an electrometer. Such devices are useful for the determination of radioactive doses but are little used in clinical biochemistry laboratories. In *proportional counters* and *Geiger-Müller counters* the cylindrical counter chamber is filled with argon, the chamber wall is the cathode and a central axial very fine wire is the anode held at a higher voltage than in the ionisation chamber. The electrical field around the anode is therefore high and electrons are accelerated towards the anode to reach sufficient energy to cause further ionisation by collision with argon molecules and the process is repeated. Unlike the ionisation chamber there is an amplification step resulting in an avalanche of electrons and positive ions moving towards their respective electrodes and a pulse of current is produced. In proportional counters the voltage is such that the avalanche is confined to the region of generation of the original ion pair. The pulse size is rather small and depends on the number of ion pairs produced by a particle so that discrimination between α- and β-particles is possible. In practice it is more usual to increase the anode voltage still further to operate in the Geiger-Müller (GM) region.

Geiger-Müller Counters

Here the field is such that any ion pair produces ionisation along the whole length of the anode resulting in a larger pulse of constant size lasting about 1 μs as the electrons are discharged. The positive argon ions move more slowly to the cathode and during this period, 100 to 300 μs, the GM tube is insensitive to further ionising radiation. This is the *dead-time* and is much longer than that found with the smaller shower of ions in the proportional counter. As the positive ions are converted to neutral atoms at the cathode they emit photons which are able to ionise other argon atoms in the gas thereby prolonging the discharge still further. This is prevented by adding a quenching agent to absorb the photons. This may be an organic compound such as ethanol or ethyl formate which is slowly destroyed by the photons giving the tube a life of 10^8 to 10^9 counts or a halogen such as bromine may be used which is dissociated by the photons but re-forms again later to prolong the life at least a hundred-fold.

If the dead-time, t seconds, is known then if there are apparently n counts/s the counter will be unresponsive for nt seconds and the true count rate, n' will be given by:

$$n' = n/(1 - nt)$$

This correction is usually satisfactory provided n' is less than $(10t)^{-1}$. In practice it is often difficult to determine the dead time for a particular counter and it is usual to connect this to a *quenching unit* which imposes an electronic dead-time of, say 400 μs, a time longer than the range of counter dead-time encountered. In this case the correction is satisfactory if n' is less than 250 counts/s or 15 000 counts/min.

The relationship between the count rate and anode voltage for a particular source in a GM tube is shown in Fig. 9.3. Up to a threshold voltage, A, no pulses are recorded and then the rate increases up to B. At voltages between A and B it behaves as a proportional counter. As the voltage is increased to C the count rate increases only slowly. This plateau region extends over several hundred volts before the count rate increases rapidly and the quenching mechanism is unable to prevent continuous discharge occurring. Usually GM tubes are operated at 50 to 100 V above B. The actual voltage may be 500 V for halogen quenching and 1000 V or more for an organic-quenched tube. Over this plateau or GM range the pulse size is independent of the energy of the exciting radiation so that pulse height analysers are redundant but a discriminator reduces unwanted electronic

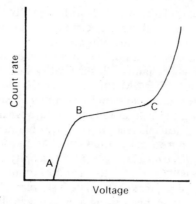

Fig. 9.3. Operating Characteristics of a Geiger-Müller Tube.
A—Threshold voltage, B–C—plateau region.

noise. The pulse size is such that little or no further amplification is needed before a scaler or ratemeter is operated.

GM tubes are relatively inefficient detectors of γ-rays as these pass through the counter gas filling without absorption and any effect is mainly due to interaction with the walls of the counter. For a 1 MeV γ-ray the efficiency may be only 1%. For β-rays, any particle entering the counter gas is almost certain to be detected and the efficiency depends on the ease with which the β-particles can penetrate into this sensitive volume. In the end-window GM tube (Fig. 9.4) with metal body the window material is mica with a thickness corresponding to 2 mg/cm² which absorbs half of any β-particles from ^{14}C that strike it. If the ^{14}C source is a very thin film on a planchet close to the window, self-absorption is low and the geometrical efficiency is 30 to 40% so that the overall efficiency is 15 to 20%. For ^3H the mica window absorbs virtually all the β-particles. For GM tubes shielded by lead the background is mainly attributable to cosmic radiation and depends on the area presented to the direction of the radiation. Background rates are usually around 1·5 counts min^{-1} cm^{-2} The more energetic β-particles can also be

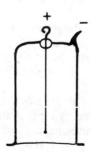

Fig. 9.4. Geiger-Müller End Window Counter.

measured by plastic scintillators (p. 222) with virtually no dead-time and low background but with more elaborate electronic equipment.

For ^3H the sample has to be introduced into the gas-filled volume of the counter itself. The sample is spread thinly on a planchet to avoid self-absorption and after passing through a chamber flushed with a helium-butane mixture it is introduced into the base of a GM tube in a similar position to the planchet beneath the mica window of an end-window counter. The windowless counter is continually flushed with the helium-butane mixture when counting efficiencies approaching the geometrical efficiency of 40 % are obtained. These counters have been replaced for many purposes by liquid scintillation counters but are the basis of *chromatogram and electrophoretic strip radioactivity scanners* with weak β-emitters. If the isotope is ^{14}C or ^{35}S a thin window of mica or, preferably, Mylar (window weight 0·1 mg/cm^2) makes the system simpler. Chromatograms with γ-emitting markers are best scanned using a crystal scintillator. In each case the detector is linked to a ratemeter. End-window GM tubes are also employed in *radiation monitors* where they are usually linked to a ratemeter.

The Ratemeter. Both analogue and digital devices are in use. They integrate the pulses over a period of time and display the mean rate either on a meter or chart recorder (analogue system) or in digital form.

In the *analogue ratemeter* each pulse adds a charge to a capacitor linked in parallel to a resistor. The charge leaks through the resistor and the current is recorded. In the steady state the rate of charging of the capacitor is balanced by the leakage current. The values of the capacitor and resistor determine the time-constant, τ, of the combination. If the detector is exposed suddenly to radiation, the maximal response occurs after a time of 5τ. With small τ and a low activity source, the random nature of radioactive disintegration is shown by a fluctuating response which is smoothed as τ increases. If the source exposed to the detector changes with time as in chromatogram scanning, τ is adjusted by altering the value of the capacitor or resistor to allow the activity change to be followed satisfactorily without too much noise in the tracing. Ratemeters also incorporate various shunts to adjust the full-scale sensitivity of the instrument for different source activities.

Digital ratemeters are recycling scalers in which the display is held while a new count is accumulated over a pre-selected short time period. The new count then replaces the old one automatically and the process is repeated.

Other Detectors of Radioactivity

Ionising radiations activate the silver ions of *photographic emulsions* in the same way as light photons. Development in the normal fashion then reveals the effect. Photographic film will record spots of activity on chromatograms but it is slow. Emulsions are exploited in autoradiography for β-emitting isotopes such as ^3H or ^{14}C combined with microscopic examination to make use of the high resolution achievable. Radioactivity in individual cells of a tissue section can then be investigated semi-quantitatively by noting the number of silver granules produced.

In the *liquid emulsion technique* the photographic emulsion in gel form is melted and the specimen is coated by dipping in the dark. The dried emulsion is developed after a suitable exposure time in the dark and the underlying tissue can be stained by the usual histological methods. Alternatively, the *stripping film technique* is used whereby a very thin photographic emulsion film is floated on water and transferred to the specimen on a microscope slide before processing as before. As the thickness is controlled more carefully than in the liquid emulsion film, it is preferable for semi-quantitative methods.

Examples of the Use of Radioisotopes

There are several uses of radioisotopes in clinical biochemistry. A nuclide may be produced from a trace element in a sample removed from the patient or may be used as a radioactive reagent in analysing such a sample. A radioisotope may be administered to a patient before examining a sample removed later. Finally the localisation of the isotope within the patient may be studied.

1. **Activation Analysis.** If an element is irradiated in a nuclear reactor it may be converted to a measurable nuclide (p. 213). If this product can be measured selectively, the high sensitivity of radiochemical methods permits the determination of small quantities of the original element. The method has been used to determine arsenic in small biological samples with a sensitivity of about 1 ng of the element.

2. **Radioactive Reagents.** The high sensitivity of radioactive methods is made use of in the determination of small quantities of biochemically important substances as with the use of ^{125}I- or ^{131}I-labelled hormones in radio-immunoassay methods.

3. *In vitro* **Measurements and Administration of Radioisotopes to Patients.** Here, the isotope is usually measured in a sample of blood, urine or faeces collected some time after its intravenous or oral administration.

Dilution studies are used to measure the volume of distribution of a selected substance or its amount. A dose of the substance in labelled form is given and after adequate mixing a sample of blood, or occasionally urine, is examined to determine the extent of its dilution. The ratio r of the dose to that of a standard solution is measured, e.g. by weighing, and the standard is then diluted considerably to v litres before counting. If the diluted standard activity is s counts $min^{-1} l^{-1}$, the patient's sample activity p counts $min^{-1} l^{-1}$ and during equilibration w litres of urine are excreted with a mean activity of u counts $min^{-1} l^{-1}$, then:

$$s.v.r = u.w + p.D \quad \text{where} \quad D = \text{distribution volume (l)}$$

and thus

$$D = (s.v.r - u.w)/p$$

Depending on the biological behaviour of the substance administered, the method can be used to measure physiologically important spaces. Thus ^{125}I- or ^{131}I-labelled human serum albumin (HSA) will measure the plasma volume and the patient's own red blood cells (RBCs) labelled with sodium $[^{51}Cr]$ chromate will allow the red cell volume to be estimated. The important body fluid volumes (Chapter 23, p. 550) are measured by using tritiated water for total body water and sodium $[^{35}S]$ sulphate or $[^{77}Br$ or $^{82}Br]$ bromide for extracellular fluid.

If the total concentration (mmol/l) of the substance under consideration is measured in the patient's sample, the total quantity in the distribution volume can be found. Thus if ^{22}Na, ^{24}Na, ^{42}K or ^{43}K are given as their chlorides the exchangeable sodium or potassium content of the body can be measured. This simple one-compartment distribution model can be refined to study the distribution of labelled substances between several compartments in dynamic equilibrium.

Metabolic studies use the behaviour of a trace amount of a labelled substance to show the way in which the body handles the unlabelled material. For detailed studies of biochemical metabolic pathways, most organic substances have to be followed using the isotopes ^{14}C or ^3H with the consequent difficulties of counting. For molecules containing phosphorus and sulphur, their β-emitting isotopes can also be used. Clinical studies employing other isotopes, preferably γ-emitters for counting convenience, include calcium metabolism ($[^{47}Ca]$ calcium chloride), iron metabolism ($[^{59}Fe]$ ferric citrate) and vitamin B_{12} metabolism using the vitamin labelled with ^{57}Co or ^{58}Co. The rate of disappearance of red cells or albumin from the plasma can be studied using ^{51}Cr-RBCs or ^{125}I- or ^{131}I-HSA respectively. Such labelled red cells have also been used to measure faecal blood loss. Loss of protein through the gut wall, protein-losing enteropathy, is investigated using polyvinylpyrrolidone labelled with radioiodine or using ^{51}Cr injected as its chloride to combine with serum proteins *in vivo*.

4. *In vivo* Measurements of Radioisotopes for Diagnostic Purposes. This use is virtually restricted to γ-emitters as they have to affect detectors external to the body. An exception is the use of ^{32}P as sodium phosphate to detect superficial tumours by its relatively energetic β-emission. The longest established use is that of radioiodide uptake by the thyroid as an index of thyroid function but considerable progress has been made in devising suitably labelled substances with similar organ specificity. Such radiopharmaceuticals are now widely used in

TABLE 9.3

Radiopharmaceuticals Used for Organ Studies
(Used for scintigraphy of the organ unless stated otherwise)

Organ	Substance
Adrenal	6-Methyl-$[^{75}Se]$-selenomethyl-19-norcholest-5(10)-en-3β-ol (for cortex)
Bone	^{99m}Tc, as polyphosphate and related compounds
Brain	^{113m}In, in chelated form
	^{99m}Tc, as pertechnetate
Cerebrospinal	^{111}In, in chelated form
fluid	^{169}Yb, in chelated form
Heart and	$[^{113m}In]$-labelled transferrin
blood vessels	^{99m}Tc, as pertechnetate or labelled albumin } (Blood pool and dynamic
	or erythrocytes } functional studies)
	$[^{201}Tl]$-thallous chloride (for myocardium)
	$[^{125}I]$-human fibrinogen (for thrombus formation)
Kidney	^{113m}In, in chelated form
	^{99m}Tc, as gluconate, dimercaptosuccinate or in chelated form
	$[^{123}I, {}^{125}I$ or $^{131}I]$-iodohippurate (also for renal plasma flow)
	$[^{51}Cr]$-EDTA (for measuring glomerular filtration rate)
Liver and	$[^{51}Cr]$-labelled damaged erythrocytes (for spleen)
spleen	$[^{99m}Tc]$-labelled colloid or as complexes with N-substituted imino diacetic acids (for biliary tract)
Lung	^{113m}In, in particulate form
	$[^{99m}Tc]$-labelled macroaggregated albumin or microspheres
	^{81m}Kr or ^{133}Xe (for lung ventilation studies)
Pancreas	$[^{75}Se]$-selenomethionine
Parathyroid	$[^{201}Tl]$-thallous chloride
Thyroid	^{99m}Tc, as pertechnetate
	^{123}I or ^{131}I as iodide (for uptake studies)
Tumours	$[^{67}Ga]$-gallium citrate (for lymphoid tissue tumours)

nuclear medicine and allow organ imaging studies to be carried out with the gamma camera (p. 221). Some examples are collected in Table 9.3.

Radioisotopes are also used for therapeutic purposes. Examples are the use of ^{131}I for treating thyrotoxicosis and some types of thyroid carcinoma, of ^{32}P-phosphate for polycythaemia vera and the injection of ^{90}Y as its silicate for local treatment of peritoneal or pleural metastatic tumours or synovitis of the knee joint.

REFERENCES AND FURTHER READING

Belcher E. H., Vetter H. eds. (1971). *Radioisotopes in Medical Diagnosis.* London: Butterworths.

Dillman L. T., Von der Lage F. C. (1975). *Radionuclide Decay Schemes and Nuclear Parameters for Use in Radiation Dose Estimation.* NM/MIRD Pamphlet No. 10. Society of Nuclear Medicine, 475 Park Avenue S., New York.

McAlister J M. (1979). *Radionuclide Techniques in Medicine.* London: Cambridge University Press.

10
STATISTICS

In clinical biochemistry, as in other sciences, experimental observations are usually determined by certain basic laws or are used to examine particular hypotheses. Such observations are, however, subject to random factors obscuring agreement with the law or hypothesis. Statistical methods are important in that they subject observations liable to chance variation, the *stochastic variables*, to mathematical criteria thereby providing an objective appraisal of experimental results where the issue is in doubt, rather than relying on subjective impressions. The subject is a large one and here only those aspects most commonly used in daily laboratory practice are discussed; numerical examples are included. Many laboratory workers now have access to electronic calculators of varying degrees of sophistication. They ease the tedium of arithmetical computation but it is often possible to speed up calculations by modification of mathematical formulae and this is especially useful if a calculator is not available.

Certain terms are in common use. The attribute which is being measured is the *random variable* (or *variate*) and is usually given the symbol x. If x can take all possible values within some interval it is a *continuous variable*, e.g. the serum sodium concentration which can, in principle, be measured to any degree of precision so that no values within the wide pathological range are prohibited. A *discontinuous variable* can only assume selected values which differ from one another by discrete amounts. Thus the number of patients on whom a serum sodium has been measured is a discrete variable as it must be an integer value. *A ranked variable* may be used and is helpful when the values are not known but individual observations can be put in order of magnitude. A set of 24 h urine samples can be ranked visually by volume without actual measurement. The total number of all the different values of a variable is the *population*. In practice the *parent population* is large, e.g. the serum sodium values of all persons in the British Isles, and cannot be examined fully. Accordingly, we have to rely on testing a *sample* randomly selected from the population. If a series of samples is taken they comprise the *sampling population*. The frequency with which the different values of the variable occur in the parent population is the frequency distribution or *distribution* for short. With a discrete variable the distribution will also be discrete while a continuous variable produces a continuous distribution. A particular distribution may take a recognised form but, if unknown, reliance will have to be made on examination of the variation in samples as it is rarely possible to examine the whole population. The distribution of the sampling population is the *sampling distribution*. Thus the distribution of the serum sodium in normal healthy people can be investigated by measuring the variable in one or more samples of such people. Certain distributions have been widely studied and are described by mathematical formulae employing one or more variable factors which are referred to as *parameters*. If the parameters are known, they define the distribution exactly. In practice they have usually to be estimated from a sample and may then be described as *statistics* of the sample to indicate the difference.

A frequency distribution can be described in terms of the *absolute frequency*, the relative frequency, or the percentile frequency. The first is the actual number of occasions on which a particular value or range of values of the variable occurs. The *relative frequency* is the actual number divided by the total number of times the variable is measured while the *percentage frequency* is 100 times the relative frequency. *Probability*, a term regularly used in statistics, is the relative frequency of a variable in the population and its numerical value will vary from zero to one. An impossible event has a probability (P) of zero while an absolutely certain event has a probability of one. Most probabilities lie between these limits. If two or more mutually exclusive events comprise all possible events then the sum of the separate probabilities is one. Thus if in a particular population the relative frequency or probability of a serum sodium concentration of 138 mmol/l or less is 0·55, then the probability of a value above 138 mmol/l is 0·45. For many purposes in clinical biochemistry we are concerned with a continuous probability distribution as the variable is also continuous. Such a distribution can be represented by a continuous curve when the variable x is plotted on the horizontal axis with the *probability density function y* on the ordinate. In general the curve will be represented by the equation

$$y = f(x)$$

and the area beneath the curve between the two values of x, x_1 and x_2, will be determined by integration as

$$\text{Area} = \int_{x_1}^{x_2} f(x)\,dx$$

If the total area under the curve is made equal to one then smaller areas will represent values between 0 and 1 and are probabilities. Thus the total area under the curve gives the probability of any value of x occurring as equal to 1, that is, a certainty. The integral expression above then gives the probability that the value of x falls between x_1 and x_2. For certain well-recognised distributions as, e.g. the normal distribution, the mathematical expression for $f(x)$ is known and the areas between values of x can be found from tables. A common statistical problem is to decide whether a result is a significant one or not. The problem usually reduces to deciding whether a result, x, calculated from a sample is likely to belong to a known or hypothetical distribution. In the distribution of Fig. 10.1 it is obvious that if the result corresponds to a value near to the peak of the curve it is highly likely to belong to the distribution but if it corresponds to a value towards either tail of the curve, this is less likely. In Fig. 10.1, two values x_l and x_r, are marked

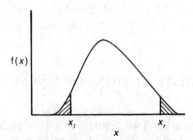

Fig 10.1. Continuous Probability Distribution of the Variable x.
The values x_l and x_r define the shaded areas in the tails, each equal to 0·025 of the total area.

such that the areas to the left of x_l and to the right of x_r each represent 0·025 of the total area. Then the probability that a true member of the distribution population lies to the left of x_l is 0·025, to the right of x_r is 0·025, and in one or other of these tails is 0·05. Also, the probability that a true member of the population lies between x_l and x_r is 0·95. In practice it is often accepted that a result occurring with a probability of 0·05 or less is sufficiently unlikely to occur by chance that it can be accepted as likely to be significantly different from the distribution under consideration. The statement is usually put in the form 'the result is significant (P < 0·05)'. The two limits x_l and x_r, in this description are referred to as *two-sided or two-tailed significance limits or confidence limits* (CL) and the range between them is the *confidence interval*. A statement about such limits is accompanied by the probability level to which it applies.

In some cases it may be necessary to decide whether a result lies in only one tail of the distribution. If the left tail is under consideration, then if the area to the left of x_l is 0·05 of the total area and a result falls within it, it is regarded as significantly different from the population (P < 0·05). The *one-sided or one-tail significance limits* are then x_l and ∞ and the confidence interval includes all values greater than x_l. A similar argument applies to a one-sided limit at the right tail when the significance limits are $-\infty$ and x_r.

The general concept of a *significance test* has just been described. Although there are many such tests, all are based on the same principle. In each case the *null hypothesis* is that there is no difference between the sample and the population with which it is compared. The result of the test is the probability that the null hypothesis is correct. Thus the statement, P = 0·05, implies that the null hypothesis has only a 1 in 20 chance of being correct. It will never be possible to be absolutely sure that the null hypothesis is wrong and P is the chance of rejecting it when it is true. The value of P at which the hypothesis is rejected depends on the circumstances. If the consequences of rejecting the null hypothesis erroneously are of great practical importance it is prudent to require a much lower probability before presuming that it can be rejected. Statistical statements are therefore accompanied by a P value. If a test of significance fails to show a significant difference one is uncertain of identity of the sample result and the population with which it is compared. It is not possible to say 'there is *no* difference' but the null hypothesis is provisionally accepted until further results become available for testing a larger sample. Small differences are more likely to be demonstrated with larger numbers of observations.

In making tests of significance, a powerful test or one which discloses a genuine difference is desirable but only possible if the nature of the distribution from which the sample was drawn is known. Tests which require this distribution to be of a certain form are likely to give misleading results if this is not in fact the case. A more reliable but less powerful test would then be one making fewer assumptions. In later sections the nature of the assumptions needed before the test can be used validly is noted.

PARAMETERS OF DISTRIBUTIONS OF UNKNOWN FORM

This section deals with *distributions of any form* while the extension to particular distributions is discussed later. Two features of a distribution of general interest are the central tendency and the degree of variation around this. The former is defined by the *mean*, μ, and the latter by the *variance* or mean square deviation, σ^2. The square root of the variance is the *standard deviation* (SD), σ. The smaller σ, the closer most values of the variable x will be to μ. The probability that a particular value of x falls at a certain distance from μ will thus depend on σ. For *any* distribution the probability that x lies at $k\sigma$ from μ is $1/k^2$. This is the Chebyshev Inequality and may be formally expressed as

$$\text{Probability } (|x - \mu| \geqslant k\sigma) \leqslant 1/k^2$$

Thus if μ is 100 and σ is 20 then the probability that a member of the population lies outside the range $100 \pm 2 \times 20$ $(\mu \pm k\sigma)$ is $1/2^2$ or 0·25. This is equivalent to saying that 75 % of the values of x lie within the range 60 to 140. If the 95 % range is required k will be $\approx 4\cdot5$ giving the figures 10 to 190. Thus $P < 0\cdot05$ that a value of x is less than 10 or more than 190. This degree of uncertainty can be greatly improved if the form of the distribution is known.

Sometimes it is convenient to use a *transformation* of a variable. Common transformations are addition or subtraction of a constant value or multiplication by a constant. In the first case the transformed variable, t, will be

$$t = x \pm a \tag{1}$$

and it can be shown that

$$\mu_t = \mu_x \pm a \tag{2}$$

and

$$\sigma_t = \sigma_x \tag{3}$$

If μ_t has been found, then

$$\mu_x = \mu_t \mp a \tag{4}$$

Alternatively, if

$$t = b \cdot x \tag{5}$$

then

$$\mu_t = b \cdot \mu_x \tag{6}$$

and

$$\sigma_t = b \cdot \sigma_x \tag{7}$$

while

$$\mu_x = \mu_t/b \tag{8}$$

and

$$\sigma_x = \sigma_t/b \tag{9}$$

The two transformations may be combined as

$$t = b \cdot x \pm a \tag{10}$$

$$\mu_t = b \cdot \mu_x \pm a \tag{11}$$

$$\sigma_t = b \cdot \sigma_x \tag{12}$$

and

$$\mu_x = (\mu_t \mp a)/b \tag{13}$$

and

$$\sigma_x = \sigma_t/b \tag{14}$$

Standardised Variables. A common transformation in statistical tests is to use a variable c which has a mean of zero and a variance of one. Such a variable is called a standardised variable and is obtained by the transformation

$$c_x = (x - \mu_x)/\sigma_x \tag{15}$$

and in accordance with the above equations

$$\mu_c = \mu_x/\sigma - \mu_x/\sigma = 0 \qquad \text{from (11)}$$

and

$$\sigma_c = \sigma_x/\sigma_x = 1 \qquad \text{from (12)}$$

Estimate of the Mean

The population mean is often unknown and is estimated from a sample taken from the population. If the values of x are $x_1, x_2, \ldots x_n$, for n items constituting the sample, then the estimate of μ will be called $\bar{x}$ and

$$\bar{x} = \Sigma x/n \qquad \text{where} \qquad \Sigma x = x_1 + x_2 + \ldots x_n \qquad (16)$$

Example 1. If the serum sodium results in a sample of 5 sera are 142, 138, 139, 140, and 139 mmol/l then $\bar{x} = 698/5 = 139.60$ mmol/l.

It is sometimes convenient to use a transformation to simplify calculation if this has to be done by hand.

Example 2. The table shows 10 results for serum calcium (x) transformed to t by multiplying by 100 and deducting 247.

Serum Calcium Results (mmol/l)

x	t	t^2	
2·51	4	16	
2·49	2	4	
2·38	−9	81	Then $\bar{t} = 3/10 = 0.3$ from (16) and hence from (13)
2·52	5	25	
2·47	0	0	$\bar{x} = \dfrac{0\cdot3 + 247}{100} = 2\cdot473$ mmol/l
2·45	−2	4	
2·50	3	9	
2·46	−1	1	
2·48	1	1	
2·47	0	0	

$$\Sigma t = 3 \quad \Sigma t^2 = 141$$

(Note that $\bar{x}$ and $\bar{t}$ can be used like μ_x and μ_t in (2), (8) and (13) above.)

No approximations are introduced by such a calculation. However, for large samples it is convenient to group the results into a number of separate classes each comprising a range of results, d, in magnitude, to reduce the computational labour. The mid-point value of each class is then taken as the average of all results within the class. The labour is reduced further if this mid-point value is suitably transformed.

Example 3. In the table the results of measuring serum alkaline phosphatase in U/l are classified so that x is the mid-point of a class each of which is of width d equal to 5 U/l, and the first class covers results between 20·5 and 25·5 U/l, mid-point 23. For convenience t is the transformed variable obtained by subtracting the mid-point value of the commonest class (43) and dividing by d. The frequency in each class, f, is listed and the computation is described opposite to the table using the expression

$$\bar{t} = \Sigma(ft)/\Sigma f \qquad (17)$$

Serum Alkaline Phosphatase Results
(U/l)

x	t	f	ft	ft^2	
23	−4	5	−20	80	
28	−3	8	−24	72	From (17), $\bar{t} = \dfrac{99}{169} = 0\cdot585\,8$
33	−2	15	−30	60	
38	−1	24	−24	24	
43	0	33	0	0	then as $t = \dfrac{x-43}{5}$,
48	1	29	29	29	
53	2	21	42	84	$\bar{x} = 5\bar{t} + 43 = 45\cdot929$ from (13)
58	3	17	51	153	
63	4	10	40	160	
68	5	7	35	175	

$$\Sigma f\,169 \quad \Sigma(ft)\,99 \quad \Sigma(ft^2)\,837$$

Estimate of the Variance and Standard Deviation

The population variance σ^2 is also often unknown and has to be estimated from a sample of n items for which the values of x are as before, $x_1, x_2, \ldots x_n$. If the population mean, μ, is known then the sample variance, designated s^2, is defined as

$$s^2 = \frac{\Sigma(x - \mu)^2}{n} \tag{18}$$

that is the variance is the mean square deviation from the mean. When, as is often the case, μ is not known, $\bar{x}$ is used instead and the expression is altered to allow for the fact that $\bar{x}$ has had to be calculated from the same sample as follows

$$s^2 = \frac{\Sigma(x - \bar{x})^2}{n - 1} = \frac{S_x}{n - 1} \tag{19}$$

In each case the SD, s, is the square root of s^2. Although this is the formal definition, the formula is inconvenient for practical use. An equivalent form for S_x not involving any approximation is

$$S_x = \Sigma x^2 - (\Sigma x)^2/n \tag{20}$$

The values of x can be transformed by adding or subtracting a constant without affecting the variance (3).

Example 4. For the serum sodium figures of Example 1 the calculation is set out after deducting 139 ($t = x - 139$) as follows:

Serum Sodium Results
   (mmol/l)

x	t	t^2
142	3	9
138	-1	1
139	0	0
140	1	1
139	0	0

$\Sigma t = 3$ $\Sigma t^2 = 11$

Then $s_x^2 = s_t^2 = \dfrac{S_t}{n-1} = \dfrac{11 - 3^2/5}{5 - 1}$ from (19) and (20)

$= 9 \cdot 2/4$
$= 2 \cdot 300$

thus the SD $s_x = 1 \cdot 517$ mmol/l

If a constant multiplier or divider is used in the transformation the SD has to be adjusted as in (7), (9), (12), (14).

Example 5. The variance of the serum calcium figures of Example 2 will then be calculated as

$$s_t^2 = \frac{S_t}{n-1} = \frac{141 - 3^2/10}{9} = 15 \cdot 566 \qquad \text{from (19) and (20)}$$

Thus $s_t = \sqrt{15 \cdot 566} = 3 \cdot 945$ and as from (9)

$$s_x = s_t/100, \quad \text{hence } s_x = 0 \cdot 039\ 5 \text{ mmol/l}$$

For a grouped frequency table as in Example 3 the formula for the variance is modified as was that for the mean (see (17)). The expression is

$$s_t^2 = \frac{\Sigma(ft^2) - \Sigma(ft)^2/\Sigma f}{(\Sigma f) - 1} \tag{21}$$

Example 6. Hence for the figures in Example 3

$$s_t^2 = \frac{837 - 99^2/169}{168} = 4.6369$$

and so

$$s_t = \sqrt{4.6369} = 2.1533$$

From the transformation,

$$s_x = d \cdot s_t \ (d = 5)$$

hence

$$s_x = 5 \times 2.1533 = 10.766 \text{ U/l}$$

In grouping the original results into classes a small error arises. The mean is unaffected but the variance is slightly higher than expected and it is usual to correct for this. *Shepherd's correction* is

$$s_t^2 \text{ (corrected)} = s_t^2 - 1/12 \qquad (22)$$

Thus in the above example

$$s_t^2 \text{ (corrected)} = 4.6369 - 1/12 = 4.5535$$

and the corrected value of s_t is 2.1399 making $s_x = 10.670$ U/l.

Variance and Standard Deviation of the Mean. The sample mean $\bar{x}$ will vary randomly as successive samples are drawn from the parent population. If the sample size is n and the variance of the sample is s^2 then the variance and SD of the mean are:

$$\text{Variance of the mean} = s^2/n \qquad (23)$$

$$\text{and SD of the mean} = s/\sqrt{n} \qquad (24)$$

The latter is often referred to as the *standard error of the mean* (SE) and gives an indication of the variability and reliability of the mean.

Example 7. For the previous examples:

Serum sodium (mmol/l), Examples 1 and 4:

$$\text{Mean} = 139.60, \ \text{SE} = 1.517/\sqrt{5} = 0.68$$

Serum calcium (mmol/l), Examples 2 and 5:

$$\text{Mean} = 2.473, \ \text{SE} = 0.0395/\sqrt{10} = 0.012$$

Serum alkaline phosphatase (U/l), Examples 3 and 6:

$$\text{Mean} = 45.929, \ \text{SE} = 10.670/\sqrt{169} = 0.821$$

Such calculations help in deciding how many significant figures to quote for results such as the mean and for the above cases some final rounding off is desirable to give the results in the form:

Mean serum sodium (mmol/l) = 139.6 ± 0.7 (SE)

Mean serum calcium (mmol/l) = 2.47 ± 0.01 (SE)

Mean serum alkaline phosphatase (U/l) = 45.9 ± 0.8 (SE)

Coefficient of Variation. This estimate of variability is independent of the units used in the calculation. Thus the mean serum calcium above and its SD could be written as:

Serum calcium (mmol/l) = 2.473   SD = 0.0395

or
$$\text{Serum calcium (mg/100 ml)} = 9.892 \quad SD = 0.158\,0$$

but both have the same relative variability. This is conveniently expressed as the coefficient of variation (CV) or *relative SD*, defined in terms of the mean, $\bar{x}$, and SD, s, as:

$$CV = 100 \cdot s/\bar{x} \text{ per cent} \tag{25}$$

In the serum calcium example the CV in both cases will be 1.597%. This expression is occasionally also referred to as the '*percentage error*'.

Quantiles and Percentiles

In any continuous distribution the members of the population or of a sample drawn from the population can be ranked in ascending order of magnitude. The *quantile* is the general term for a parameter describing position in the rank order. A *percentile* is a particular form of quantile and if one takes the pth percentile then $p\%$ of the sample will lie below this point in the rank order and $(100 - p)\%$ will lie above it. The 50th percentile is usually called the *median* which describes the mid-point of the ordered sample. Occasionally the median and the 25th and 75th percentiles are used as *quartiles* to divide the sample into four equal groups. The interquartile range between the 25th and 75th percentiles then embraces the central half of the population or sample and is used as an estimate of its dispersion. In clinical biochemistry it is often helpful to consider the '95% range' of a set of results taken, e.g. from apparently healthy people. This excludes the most extreme 5% of results and is defined by the 2·5th and 97·5th percentiles.

If the n numbers of a sample or population are ranked then the rank number r closest to the pth percentile is calculated from

$$r = n \cdot p/100 + 0.5 \tag{26}$$

If r is a whole number the value of the rth member of the ordered sample is taken as the pth percentile. If it is a fraction then the pth percentile lies somewhere between the two values corresponding to the two order integer numbers either side of the fraction.

Example 8. If 77 people were examined for their serum iron concentration the median (50th percentile) would be calculated from

$$r = \frac{77 \times 50}{100} + 0.5 = 39$$

and the median serum iron would correspond to the value for the 39th member of the sample when the results were arranged in increasing order. If, however, there were 78 people then $r = 39.5$ and the median would lie between the values shown by the 39th and 40th members.

If many readings are made they are often grouped as in Example 3. Then using the abbreviations d, x and f as in that Example the mean values in successive classes will be $x_1, x_2, \ldots x_i, \ldots x_n$ with corresponding frequencies $f_1, f_2, \ldots f_i, \ldots f_n$. The cumulative frequency $F(i)$ corresponding to class x_i is then defined as $f_1 + f_2 + \ldots + f_i$, or Σf_i. The procedure for finding the pth percentile is then as follows:

1. Calculate $\dfrac{p \cdot \Sigma f}{100}$ and compare with $F(i)$ for different values of i.

2. If this corresponds exactly with $F(i)$ the required percentile is $x_i + 0.5 d$, the class upper boundary of the ith class as d is the class width.

3. If it lies between two values $F(i)$ and $F(i + 1)$ the percentile lies between $x_i + 0.5 d$ and $x_i + 1.5 d$.

Example 9. In Example 3 it is required to calculate the 2·5th and 97·5th percentiles. For the first step the results are:

For the 2·5th percentile $\dfrac{p \cdot \Sigma f}{100} = \dfrac{2.5 \times 169}{100} = 4.23$

For the 97·5th percentile $\dfrac{p \cdot \Sigma f}{100} = \dfrac{97.5 \times 169}{100} = 164.77$

For the latter $F(9) = 162$, $F(10) = 169$ (see also Example 10) so that the 97·5th percentile lies between $63 + 0.5 \times 5$ and $63 + 1.5 \times 5$ or 65·5 and 70·5. An approximation would be that as there are 7 observations in the top class, the required figure lies $(164.77 - 162)/7$ above 65·5, i.e. is 65·9. A similar argument for the 2.5th percentile gives the figure $20.5 + 4.23/5$ or 21·3. The '95 % range' is then 21·3 to 65·9 U/l. The median value, 45·48, can be calculated similarly.

Relationship between Mean, Median and Mode. The *mode* is the value of the variable x which occurs most frequently. For *symmetrical continuous distributions* the mean, median and mode are identical but they diverge as the distribution becomes more *asymmetrical*. They are related according to the following approximation:

median $\approx$ (2/3) mean + (1/3) mode   or   mode $\approx$ 3 × median − 2 × mean

In practice it is the degree of agreement between the median and the mean (45·48 and 45·93 for the data in Examples 9 and 3) which is useful in deciding whether a distribution is symmetrical or not. The mode could be calculated as 44·58.

Tests of Significance

When the form of the distribution is unknown it is still possible to perform tests to assess, e.g. the differences between two groups of results by using the methods of *non-parametric statistics*. Such tests make no assumptions about distribution forms but are less powerful than the appropriate tests for distributions where the form is known, e.g. a number of tests used for the normal distribution below. The details of non-parametric methods cannot be given here but they can be used, e.g. to provide confidence limits for the estimates of quantiles including the median and hence to compare the median with the mean as a test of symmetry of a distribution. The reader is referred to Siegel (1956) for a full account and to Example 29 (p. 266).

THE NORMAL DISTRIBUTION

This bell-shaped symmetrical distribution, also known as the Gaussian distribution, is often encountered in biological measurements and also describes random errors in analytical methods. For variables which are not normally distributed it is sometimes possible to apply a transformation which brings this about. Thus the variable x may be replaced by the transformation *log x* and if this is normally distributed the variable is said to have a log-normal distribution.

Other transformations have been used in an effort to reach the required 'normal' form. A main reason for this aim is that the properties of the normal distribution are well defined and tests of significance are more powerful than for other distributions. A useful property is that the means of samples drawn randomly from a population of *any* distribution become distributed in a 'normal' fashion as the size of the sample increases (central limit theorem).

The equation for the probability density function (p. 233) for the variable *x* in a normal distribution is:

$$y = \frac{1}{\sigma\sqrt{2\pi}}\exp[-\tfrac{1}{2}((x-\mu)/\sigma)^2] \tag{27}$$

It is apparent that two parameters only, the mean, μ, and the standard deviation, σ, define the curve fully. In some cases it is helpful to use the standardised variable *c* (see (**15**)) when the equation simplifies to:

$$y = f(c) = \frac{1}{\sqrt{2\pi}}\cdot\exp(-c^2/2) \tag{28}$$

The properties of this probability density function are tabulated in standard statistical works (p. 272). They give, e.g. the height of the curve for any value of *c*. This is maximal at $0\cdot3989$ when *c* is zero, or when *x* equals μ. This is equivalent to the statement that the mean equals the mode. The heights will also be identical for any value of *c* and $-c$, that is the curve is symmetrical. Other tables list the areas under the curve defined by different vertical lines (Fig. 10.2) and these will correspond to the probabilities of the occurrence of values of *c* between the limits defined by the vertical lines. As an example the area lying between *c* values one unit either side of zero is $0\cdot683$ of the whole area (Fig. 10.2b). Since

$$c = (x-\mu)/\sigma \quad \text{then} \quad x = \mu + c\sigma$$

and the probability that values of *x* lie within one SD of the mean is $0\cdot683$. This may also be stated in the form: $68\cdot3\%$ of all values of *x* lie within one SD of the mean. For $c = 2$ the probability is $0\cdot955$, or $95\cdot5\%$ lie within 2 SD of the mean while only $4\cdot5\%$ lie further than 2 SDs from the mean in the two tails of the curve,

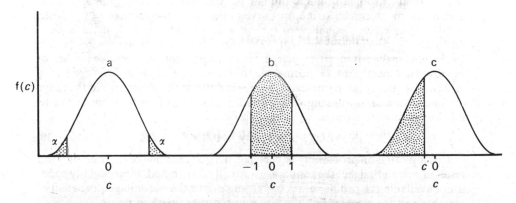

Fig 10.2. The Probability Density Function of *c*.
    The curve is symmetrical about $c = 0$. (a) Area in two tails, each of fractional area α. (b) Area lying within equal distances either side of 0; in this case ± 1. (c) Area enclosed between the limits of *c* from $-\infty$ to c'. These areas are tabulated in standard texts.

2·25% in each. If the form of the distribution is unknown, the Chebyshev inequality predicts that this could be as high as 25% (p. 235). Knowledge of the form of the distribution allows more definite statements to be made.

If the fractional area in one tail is α the probability of a value occurring in equal areas in both tails is 2α. The relation between 2α and c is shown in Table 10.1.

Table 10.1 is applicable to a number of significance tests. Many of these are two-tail tests applied to a null hypothesis (p. 234) in which 2α is the probability that the hypothesis is true. In selected cases a one-tail test is used and the probability associated with a particular value of c is α which is half the value in the Table. Thus the probability that a null hypothesis is true on a one-tail test when c is 1·96 will be 0·025.

TABLE 10.1
*Relation Between Probability (2α) and Number of
SDs from the Mean (c)*

c	2α	2α	c
1	0·317 31	0·100	1·64
2	0·045 50	0·050	1·96
3	0·002 70	0·025	2·24
4	0·000 06	0·010	2·58
		0·001	3·29
		0·000 1	3·89

Use of Probability Paper and the Probit Transformation

Using the standardised variable c as above, the *probit* is defined as $c + 5$. If this is plotted on the ordinate against x on the abscissa the equation

$$\text{Probit} = c + 5 = \frac{x}{\sigma} - \frac{\mu}{\sigma} + 5 \qquad (29)$$

shows that this is a straight line and that when the probit equals 5, then x corresponds to the mean, μ. As values of c less than -5 occur with a very low probability, virtually all probits are positive.

Probability paper has on the ordinate the probability α corresponding to the area below the normal distribution curve to the left of the value of c (Fig. 10.2c, p. 241). Thus when c equals zero (probit = 5) α is 0·50 or 50% if the scale is calibrated in percentage probability. The variable x is on the abscissa as before. Probability paper is used to give a visual impression of how well a set of experimental results fits a normal distribution. The data are arranged as a grouped frequency table (see Example 3). Then if x_i is the *upper limit* of the range of values of the variable in the ith line and Σf_i is the sum of the frequencies f up to this line (cumulative frequency), then:

$$\text{Percentage probability} = 100 \times \Sigma f_i / \Sigma f \% \qquad (30)$$

This is plotted on probability paper against x_i for each line of the table and will result in a straight line if the results are normally distributed. If probability paper is not available the probit values corresponding to the percentage probabilities are obtained from tables and are plotted on ordinary graph paper.

If the results conform to a normal distribution then the mean of the sample plotted, $\bar{x}$, corresponds to the value of x linked to 50% probability as read from the best straight line fitting the observed points. As 1·645 SDs each side of the mean extend from 5 to 95% probability, the difference in the values of x corresponding to these probabilities is equal to 3·29 times the SD, s. If probits have been used, the mean is opposite the probit value 5 and one SD is the change in x for a change in probit of one unit.

Example 10. For the data on alkaline phosphatase listed in Example 3 the results of the calculation are shown below and in Fig. 10.3. The plot is consistent with a normal distribution for this sample. The mean is read as 45·9 U/l and s as 11·1 U/l corresponding to the previous calculation of 45·93 (Example 3) and 10·67 (Example 6).

x_i	Σf_i	$(F(i))$ *Percentage probability*
25.5	5	3.0 (100 × 5/169)
30.5	13	7.7
35.5	28	16.6
40.5	52	30.8
45.5	85	50.3
50.5	114	67.5
55.5	135	79.9
60.5	152	89.9
65.5	162	95.9
70.5	169	100

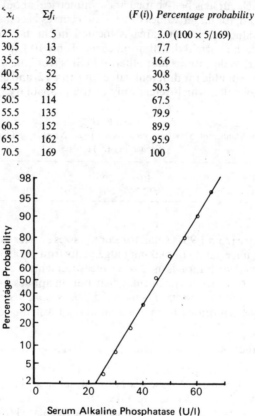

Fig 10.3. Plot of Data on Serum Alkaline Phosphatase for Examples 3 and 10 on Probability Paper.
The best straight line has been fitted by eye.

Other Distributions Associated with the Normal Distribution

Three other continuous distributions used in statistical calculations in clinical biochemistry are the Student, t, distribution, the chi-squared, χ^2, distribution, and the variance ratio, F, distribution.

The t Distribution

The standardised normal distribution of c has already been discussed where c was defined by (15). If the population parameters μ and σ are unknown they are estimated from a sample as $\bar{x}$ and s respectively. Then t is defined as:

$$t = (x - \bar{x})/s \tag{31}$$

The estimate of t depends on the reliability of $\bar{x}$ and s which will be less satisfactory for smaller samples. An important number is the number of degrees of freedom (df), v, for t, which is one less than the number of items, n, in the sample, i.e. $(n - 1)$. The complex formula describing the shape of the distribution curve depends only on v and a family of curves results corresponding to different values of v. Each curve is bell-shaped and symmetrical about zero as is the curve for c and, indeed, for larger values of v the two curves become virtually identical. For smaller values of v more area is located in the tails than in the centre, compared with the normal distribution curve. Table 10.1 (p. 242) shows that the probability (2α) of deviations more than 1·96 SDs from the mean is 0·05. Similar tables for t are available for different values of v (p. 272) and an extract from these is given in Table 10.2 which refers only to the probability (2α) of 0·05.

TABLE 10.2

Relation Between Number of SDs from the Mean (t) *and Number of Degrees of Freedom* (v) *for Probability* (2α) *of* 0·05

v	1	2	5	10	20	30	50	100	200	∞
t	12·71	4·30	2·57	2·23	2·09	2·04	2·01	1·98	1·97	1·96

The difference from 1·96 is small for sample sizes greater than, say 30 to 50, but the increasing uncertainty of making judgements from small samples is apparent. In practice the t distribution is used when measurements are made on sample sizes of less than 30 or so while the normal distribution applies for larger samples. In each case, however, the *results are only valid if the sample distribution is* consistent with it having been drawn from a parent *normal* distribution.

The χ^2 Distribution

This continuous distribution is of great theoretical importance in statistics but its practical use in clinical biochemistry is rather restricted. If v independent measurements x_1, x_2, ... x_v are taken from the same *normally distributed population* with mean μ and SD, σ, then c can be calculated for each from (15) and χ^2 is defined as

$$\chi^2 = c_1^2 + c_2^2 + \ldots c_v^2 \tag{32}$$

where v is the number of df of χ^2. The formula for its distribution curve depends only on v and a family of curves results as for t. For small values of v the curves are asymmetrical and for no value of v is χ^2 less than zero. However, for large values of v the curve approaches that of a normal distribution quite closely with the peak corresponding to $(v - 2)$.

In its practical use the χ^2 distribution is applied to situations where results are classified into n subgroups as a grouped frequency table (see Example 3) arising either from exact measurement, or from semi-quantitative measurement (e.g. 0, +, + +, + + +) or even from some attribute which cannot be quantified (e.g. male, female). The frequency, O, observed in each compartment from such a table is then compared with the frequency, E, which would be expected from some hypothesis to be tested. Then the value of χ^2 is calculated by summation from all table compartments according to the formula

$$\chi^2 = \sum_1^n \frac{(O-E)^2}{E} \tag{33}$$

It is applicable to samples taken from *any form of population* and divided in any convenient way. The only limitation is that E should not be too small, usually 4 being taken as the lowest limit. Subgroups can be combined into larger groups if this occurs. The usual use of the χ^2 distribution is to test for the association between two variables when these are grouped in a contingency table. If the variables can be quantified then correlation and regression methods (p. 257) can also be used but the χ^2 method may be shorter if the results are grouped and is essential if one or both variables cannot be quantified.

Example 11. A particular test has been carried out on 150 patients to see whether the results are affected by the colour of the patient's hair. Here the test results are coded semi-quantitatively but the method would also be suitable for quantitative measurements which were subdivided into four classes. The contingency table below lists the number of occasions on which a particular test result was found with a particular hair colour.

Hair Colour	Test Result −	+	+ +	+ + +	Totals
Fair	7	10	14	8	39
Dark	10	9	12	7	38
Red	6	5	8	6	25
Grey/white	15	17	12	4	48
Totals	38	41	46	25	150

The observed number O of fair-haired patients with a negative test is 7. The expected number is calculated from the *null hypothesis* that there is no connection between hair colour and test result. As 38 out of 150 tests are negative it would then be expected that out of 39 fair-haired patients $39 \times 38/150$ would have a negative test. This is the value for E and the contribution towards χ^2 for the first compartment is

$$\frac{(7 - 39 \times 38/150)^2}{39 \times 38/150} \text{ or } \left(\frac{7 \times 150}{39 \times 38} - 1\right)^2 \times \frac{39 \times 38}{150} = 0 \cdot 839\,5$$

If this procedure is followed for each compartment the result of adding the separate contributions gives χ^2 as 7·498. It can also be checked that the lowest value for E is 25/6 for red-haired patients with a + + + result. As this is greater than 4 no further action is needed. The *df* are calculated for such a table from the expression

$$v = (\text{rows} - 1)(\text{columns} - 1) \tag{34}$$

which gives $(4 - 1)(4 - 1)$ or 9 *df*. Tables of values of χ^2 in relation to probability are given for each value of v (p. 272). For 9 *df* P = 0·60 for $\chi^2 = 7\cdot357$ and χ^2 increases as P falls becoming 16·919 when P = 0·05. This probability is that of the null hypothesis being true, and the result indicates that this is likely (P $\approx$ 0·6). There is no reason to abandon the hypothesis and we conclude that the results show there is no relation between test result and hair colour.

It is possible to examine the contribution of each compartment to the total value of χ^2. If this is done for the above table two compartments account for over 40 % of the total. They both concern grey/white-haired patients who have more + and fewer + + + results than might be expected. This could be followed up by comparing this hair colour with all the other colours combined. The table will have two rows only and hence v becomes 3. Recalculation of χ^2 then gives a figure of 6·343 (0·05 < P < 0·10). This is approaching the conventional limit of 0·05 for rejection of the null hypothesis. It appears possible that grey/white-haired patients give a different result. More patients could be tested to see if the situation became clearer or alternatively as grey/white hair is more often seen in older patients, the original data could be re-examined after re-classification by age rather than hair colour.

This trivial example has shown the usefulness of the χ^2 test and other examples will probably occur to the reader. The smallest contingency table in which the results can be classified will have two rows and two columns and hence only one *df*. The calculation can then be simplified. If the four entries in the table are a, b, c, and d, while n is the grand total, then

$$\chi^2 = \frac{n\{|ad-bc|-n/2\}^2}{(a+b)(c+d)(a+c)(b+d)}; \quad v = 1 \tag{35}$$

where $|ad-bc|$ means that the sign of this difference is always to be taken as positive. The correction factor, $-n/2$, in the formula is usually incorporated to allow for bias arising from the use of only four classes.

The *F* Distribution

This describes the distribution of the ratio of the variances of two samples drawn from the *same normal distribution*. If the greater variance is s_1^2 and the lesser is s_2^2 then the variance ratio F is defined by

$$F = s_1^2/s_2^2; \quad s_1 > s_2. \tag{36}$$

If there are n_1 members of the first sample and n_2 of the second then the *df* v_1 and v_2 of the two samples are (n_1-1) and (n_2-1) respectively. The formula describing the distribution of F depends only on v_1 and v_2 so that like the distributions of t and χ^2 a family of curves results. Like χ^2 the F distribution is asymmetrical and negative values of F are precluded. The mean value is $v_2/(v_2-2)$ and approaches one as v_2 becomes larger, that is the two samples will tend to have the same variance the larger they are provided both are from the same normal distribution. The more they differ the greater is F. Each table of F (p. 272) applies for one probability level and lists the value of F for each pair (v_1, v_2). If the value of F found is greater than the one in the table for P = 0·05 then P < 0·05, that the null hypothesis—both variances are drawn from the same normal distribution—is true. In other words the two variances are significantly different. In different circumstances a two-tail or one-tail test is required (p. 234). *The probability associated with each table is for the one-tail test* and applies where the variance of a sample is only to be tested to see if it is *greater* than the variance of the other sample. The opposite case is not of interest. If, however, it is required to assess *any* difference between the variances of two samples, then a two-tail test is appropriate and the table headed P = 0·025 applies for a two-tail test at P = 0·05.

The test is based on a parent *normal* distribution for the two samples which should have distributions compatible with the supposition that they are normal. With small samples this is difficult to check but it is advisable to see that they are roughly symmetrical and peaked.

Example 12. Two analytical methods for serum urea are compared by analysing the same serum repeatedly over a similar period of time in order to compare their precision. As discussed in Chapter 12 (p. 286) the precision is measured by the SD of the method under consideration. The results (mmol/l) for each method are thus combined to give the mean and SD as follows:

$$\text{Method A} \quad \bar{x}_A = 10\cdot20, \quad s_A = 1\cdot75, \quad n_A = 15$$
$$\text{Method B} \quad \bar{x}_B = 10\cdot31, \quad s_B = 1\cdot09, \quad n_B = 16$$

If the experiment was designed to test two proposed methods of general interest then there is no preconceived idea which is likely to be better and a two-tail test is needed. The calculation, from (36), is:

$$F = \frac{1\cdot75^2}{1\cdot09^2} = 2\cdot58 \text{ for } (14, 15)\,df.$$

The value of F in the table (P = 0·05) is 2·42 and in the table (P = 0·01) is 3·56. As the two-tail test is appropriate these probabilities have to be multiplied by 2 and we conclude that the probability that there is a difference in precision is just less than 0·10 and has not reached the conventional level of significance. No difference has therefore been established although further testing may alter the situation. If, however, Method A is a new method which is being assessed against method B, which has been in regular use in the laboratory, with a view to replacing it if definitely better, then a one-tail test is appropriate and A is clearly not better than B. If the situation were reversed so that A was the established method and B was the new contender then the calculation would proceed as before to give $F = 2\cdot58$. The probability that the SD of method A is greater than that of method B by chance is then just less than 0·05 on the one-tail test and the difference is therefore significant. This could be expressed also as 'the precision of the new method, B, is better than that of the established method, A'. Although the difference is 'significant', there is a chance of almost 0·05 that there is no real difference. The decision on a change in method is likely to be affected by many factors and this level of probability may be insufficient to justify a change; it would be prudent to continue testing. If after twice as many measurements for each method, F is still 2·58, this applies to (29, 31) df and P < 0·01. The statistical grounds for change are more certain but other factors such as cost, equipment, or analysis time may still delay the change-over.

Examples of the Use of the Normal Distribution

The following examples require that *the samples tested must be normally distributed.* If there is doubt about this a rapid classification of the figures in the form of a grouped frequency table (see Example 3) is helpful. If the distribution is obviously asymmetrical with a bias towards high values (positively skewed) the transformation to the logarithm of the readings often produces a more symmetrical pattern and the transformed values should be used for the calculations. If the distributions of the initial figures or various transformations remain quite unlike a normal distribution the tests described in the next sections are likely to give misleading results. Less powerful but more reliable non-parametric tests are then preferable.

Rejection of Discrepant Results

When a group of results supposedly all drawn from one population is examined, one of them sometimes seems to be different from the rest. The difficulty is to decide whether to exclude it or not. Sometimes the reason for the 'outlier' is a transcription error as, e.g. one figure of 39 mmol/l among a group of results from healthy males for serum sodium. Other reasons may be transient serious malfunction of a measuring instrument or accidental contamination of one reaction tube. Rejection of very deviant outliers is then justifiable but the mean and SD of the remaining results represents variation attributable to other random factors and is not to be taken as the variation under all circumstances.

With less distant outliers it is less easy to decide if this represents the effect of such an unusual error or whether it is a chance finding of a genuine result lying in the tail of the normal distribution curve. Some objective criterion is desirable to decide on exclusion. If the mean and SD of the sample are calculated the mean will be biassed in the direction of the outlier and the SD will be increased, the effects being greater the fewer observations in the sample. *Chauvenet's criterion* is based on the number of sample SDs the outlier lies from the sample mean. If this is greater than a prescribed figure (Table 10.3) the outlier can be rejected and the sample mean and SD are recalculated to give better estimates of the population parameters. The figures in Table 10.3 vary with sample size as expected.

TABLE 10.3
Chauvenet's Criterion for Exclusion of Outliers

No. in sample	No. of SDs from Mean
6	1·73
8	1·86
10	1·96
15	2·13
20	2·24
30	2·39
50	2·58
100	2·80
500	3·29

Example 13. The serum potassium results obtained from 11 apparently healthy males are: 3·9, 4·2, 4·6, 4·3, 4·1, 5·2, 4·3, 4·5, 4·8, 4·3 and 4·4 mmol/l. The figure of 5·2 looks suspiciously high. Calculation of the mean and SD gives 4·418 and 0·354 mmol/l indicating that 5·2 lies 2·21 SDs from the mean and should therefore be excluded. Recalculation of the mean and SD then gives 4·340 and 0·255 mmol/l. The next most discrepant figures, 3·9 and 4·8 are respectively 1·73 and 1·81 SDs from the mean and cannot be rejected from the remaining 10 figures. Our best estimate of the serum potassium in normal healthy males would be $4·34 \pm 0·26$ (SD) mmol/l. The figure of 5.2 mmol/l lies 3·37 new SDs from the new mean and a '*t* test' shows that the probability that it belongs to the residual group of 10 is less than 0·01. It may represent a haemolysed or old specimen.

Determination of 'Normal Ranges'

In this context 'normal range' indicates the 95 or 99% ranges of results in a normally distributed population. If a large sample (200 or more) is investigated, this range is calculated as $\bar{x} \pm c \cdot s$ where $\bar{x}$ and s are the mean and SD and c is taken from Table 10.1 (p. 242) for values of 2α of 0·05 or 0·01 for the 95 or 99% ranges respectively. For smaller samples c is replaced by t for the correct number of df.

Example 14. A normally distributed variable in a large sample gives the figures

$$\bar{x} = 99·52; \quad s = 5·18$$

then, 95% range $= 99·52 \pm 1·96 \times 5·18$ or 89·4 to 109·7
and, 99% range $= 99·52 \pm 2·58 \times 5·18$ or 86·2 to 112·9

If the same figures for $\bar{x}$ and s were obtained for 11 readings (10 df), then 95% range $= 99·52 \pm 2·23 \times 5·18$ or 88·0 to 111·1.

Strictly the use of t is restricted to cases where the true mean μ is known and a slightly larger tolerance factor can be obtained from special statistical tables. The difference is small, however, and in the above case 2·23 would be replaced by 2·33.

If the original sample figures have been transformed into logarithms, then the calculations are performed on these.

Example 15. Following logarithmic transformation $\bar{x}$ is 1·997 9 and s is 0·071 4 for 11 observations, then as in the last Example

$$95\% \text{ range} = 1·9979 \pm 2·23 \times 0·0714$$

or $\quad$ 1·838 6 to 2·157 1

These limits are symmetrical about the mean but when the logarithms are transformed back to the original units the results become

$$\text{Mean} = 99·52 \quad 95\% \text{ range} = 69·0 \text{ to } 143·6$$

The upper limit lies further from the mean than does the lower one as befits the original asymmetrical distribution.

In all cases the calculated limits should be compared with the original data. For the 95 % range, approximately 1 in 40 results should lie below the lower limit and a similar number beyond the upper limit. If this is not the case then the original assumptions of a normal or log-normal distribution may be unwarranted.

Confidence Limits (CL) of the Mean

The SE of the mean indicates the uncertainty attached to this measurement. The means of a series of samples drawn from a population will vary and the SE indicates the scatter about their grand mean. This is likely to be closer to the population mean than a single sample mean. However, the latter can be used to estimate the probable range in which the true mean, μ, will lie. The CL are calculated from its SE (24) as

$$\text{CL of the mean} = \bar{x} \pm c \cdot s/\sqrt{n} \text{ or } \bar{x} \pm t \cdot s/\sqrt{n} \tag{37}$$

depending on the size of n. The appropriate value of c or t is selected for the required confidence level as in the last section using $(n-1)$ df for t. The smaller is s and the larger n, the narrower the range will be, or in order to be sure of the result a reasonable number of replicates must be measured as carefully as possible.

Example 16. The results of measuring the calcium concentration (mmol/l) in an unassayed control serum on 31 occasions have a mean of 2·122 and SD of 0·046.

$$\text{Then: } 95\% \text{ CL of the mean} = 2·122 \pm 2·04 \times 0·046/\sqrt{31}$$
$$= 2·11 \text{ to } 2·14 \text{ mmol/l}$$

taking t from Table 10.2 (p. 244) for 30 df and probability level 0·05. Although no certain value can be attributed to the control serum it is unlikely to be outside the above range.

Confidence Limits of the SD

In a similar way the CL of the SD, s, of a sample of size n taken from a population can be used to obtain an indication of σ, the SD of the population. The appropriate range for a certainty of $(1 - 2\alpha)$ 100 % is calculated from:

$$\text{Lower limit} = s\sqrt{v/\chi^2_\alpha}; \quad \text{upper limit} = s\sqrt{v/\chi^2_{1-\alpha}} \tag{38}$$

where $v = (n-1)$ df and χ^2 is obtained for v df for $P = \alpha$ and $1 - \alpha$ from tables of χ^2 values.

Example 17. In Example 16 the value of s was 0.046 from 31 measurements. In order to calculate the 95 % CL ($\alpha = 0.025$) the limits are:

$$\text{Lower limit} = 0.046\sqrt{30/46.98} = 0.036\,8 \text{ mmol/l};$$
$$\text{Upper limit} = 0.046\sqrt{30/16.79} = 0.061\,5 \text{ mmol/l}.$$

The limits are not symmetrical about s and there is considerable uncertainty about the true SD, that is about the precision of the calcium method under investigation.

Comparison of Sample Mean with a Hypothetical Value

It is sometimes necessary to compare the results of a number of analyses with a figure μ predicted from some theoretical considerations or provided as a reference value. This is equivalent to testing whether the hypothetical value differs from the likely range of sample means as judged by the mean and SD of the analytical results. The null hypothesis is that there is no difference and the appropriate formulae are:

$$c = \frac{|\bar{x} - \mu|\sqrt{n}}{s} \quad \text{or} \quad t = \frac{|\bar{x} - \mu|\sqrt{n}}{s} \text{ (for } (n-1)\,df) \tag{39}$$

where $\bar{x}$, s, n, t, and c have the usual meaning. The probability attached to the calculated value of c or t is read from tables and is the probability that the null hypothesis is correct. As before (p. 249) c is used for large samples and t for small ones. If a difference proves to be statistically significant its absolute value should be considered in the practical context. The difference may be too small to be of much practical importance.

Example 18. If the calcium results for the control serum of Example 16 refer to an assayed product with a manufacturer's figure of 2.135 mmol/l, we can test the probability that the results agree with this figure from **(39)** as follows:

$$t = \frac{|2.122 - 2.135|\sqrt{31}}{0.046} = 1.573$$

The table of values of t for 30 df shows the probability to lie between 0.10 and 0.20. There is a reasonable probability that the null hypothesis is true and that the results agree with the manufacturer's figure. If we are anxious to establish a genuine difference then many more analyses would be needed as t is proportional to $\sqrt{n}$. If the mean and SD remained exactly the same after 60 analyses then t becomes 2.189 and is just significant in that $P < 0.05$. A small difference from the manufacturer's figure seems likely and if the latter is to be replaced, the laboratory 95 % CL can be recalculated as 2.110 to 2.134 mmol/l.

Comparison of Two Samples

If, e.g. two laboratories each analyse the same material a number of times it is unlikely that their mean results and SDs will be identical even if there is no true difference between the laboratories. The problem is investigated by making the null hypothesis that no difference exists and calculating the probability that this is true by comparing the mean difference with the SE of the difference.

An important fact is that the variance of the sums or differences of pairs of results drawn from two different samples A and B of sizes n_A and n_B is equal to the sum of the variances of the two samples, s_A^2 and s_B^2. Thus

$$\text{SD difference (or sum)} = \sqrt{s_A^2 + s_B^2} \tag{40}$$

The mean difference is easily calculated from the two sample means, $\bar{x}_A$ and $\bar{x}_B$ as

$$\text{Mean difference} = \bar{x}_A - \bar{x}_B \qquad (41)$$

Like any other mean this has its own SE and by analogy with the formula for SE of a simple mean (**24**) the SE of the difference in means is

$$\text{SE of difference} = \sqrt{s_A^2/n_A + s_B^2/n_B} \qquad (42)$$

The appropriate probability for the null hypothesis by analogy with (**39**) is then obtained by calculating c, provided n_A and n_B exceed 30, as

$$c = |\bar{x}_A - \bar{x}_B| / \sqrt{s_A^2/n_A + s_B^2/n_B} \qquad (43)$$

The probability level associated with the value for c is obtained from the usual tables.

Example 19. When the same freeze-dried serum was circulated to many laboratories for the determination of serum albumin and outliers had been excluded, two main groups were defined using an automated BCG method (A) and a manual BCG method (B). The main results (g/l) listed below are to be analysed for any systematic difference:

$$\text{Method A:} \quad \bar{x}_A = 36\cdot60, \quad s_A = 1\cdot58, \quad n_A = 76$$
$$\text{Method B:} \quad \bar{x}_B = 35\cdot94, \quad s_B = 2\cdot31, \quad n_B = 75$$

Then the calculation of c is:

$$c = \frac{36\cdot60 - 35\cdot94}{\sqrt{\dfrac{1\cdot58^2}{76} + \dfrac{2\cdot31^2}{75}}} = \frac{0\cdot66}{0\cdot322\,5} = 2\cdot047 \quad \text{hence } 0\cdot04 < P < 0\cdot05$$

The difference is statistically significant but small, $0\cdot66$ g/l. Whether this significant difference is of practical importance is a different matter and has to be assessed in the light of other experience.

If small samples have to be compared, a t test is usually employed. Firstly the sample variances are examined by the variance ratio test (p. 246) to see if they are significantly different as further testing depends on the outcome. In most cases the variances will not differ and the procedure is then to calculate a common SD (compare (**40**)) from which is derived the SE of the difference (compare (**42**)) which is then compared with the mean difference (**41**) as in (**42**). The appropriate steps are:

$$\text{Common SD} = s = \sqrt{\frac{S_A + S_B}{n_A + n_B - 2}} \quad \text{where } S_A, S_B \text{ are calculated as in (20)} \qquad (44)$$

$$\text{SE of difference} = \sqrt{s^2/n_A + s^2/n_B} = s\sqrt{1/n_A + 1/n_B} \qquad (45)$$

and hence

$$t = |\bar{x}_A - \bar{x}_B| / s\sqrt{1/n_A + 1/n_B} \quad \text{for } (n_A + n_B - 2)\, df \qquad (46)$$

The probability attached to the value of t is the probability that the null hypothesis is true.

Example 20. Laboratories A and B analysed the same sample several times on the same day and reported the results for serum iron (μmol/l) as follows:

$$\text{Laboratory A:} \quad 50\cdot5, \ 52\cdot0, \ 52\cdot5, \ 54\cdot0.$$
$$\text{Laboratory B:} \quad 53\cdot0, \ 55\cdot5, \ 56\cdot0, \ 57\cdot5, \ 59\cdot0.$$

The comparison of results involves the following calculations:

	A	B
$\Sigma x_{A,B}$ (16)	209	281
$\Sigma x_{A,B}^2$	10926·50	15812·50
$\bar{x}_{A,B}$ (16)	52·25	56·20
$n_{A,B}$	4	5
$S_{A,B}$ (20)	6·25	20·3
$s_{A,B}^2$	2·083	5·075

$$F = \frac{5 \cdot 075}{2 \cdot 083}$$
$$= 2 \cdot 44 \ (P > 0 \cdot 05)$$

$$s = \sqrt{\frac{6 \cdot 25 + 20 \cdot 3}{4 + 5 - 2}} = \qquad 1 \cdot 947\,5$$

$$t = \frac{|52 \cdot 25 - 56 \cdot 20|}{1 \cdot 947\,5 \sqrt{\frac{1}{4} + \frac{1}{5}}} = \qquad 3 \cdot 023 \qquad \text{for} \quad 7 \quad df \quad (0 \cdot 01 < P < 0 \cdot 02)$$

There is a low probability that the null hypothesis is true and we conclude that laboratory B produces significantly higher results than laboratory A.

In the case where two small samples have significantly different variances by the F test the procedure is to calculate t in the same way as c in (43). If sample 1 has the larger variance the value of t applies for v df where

$$v = \left(\frac{k^2}{n_1 - 1} + \frac{(1 - k)^2}{n_2 - 1} \right)^{-1} \tag{47}$$

having calculated k as

$$k = \frac{n_2 s_1^2}{n_2 s_1^2 + n_1 s_2^2} \tag{48}$$

Example 21. If in a similar comparison of serum iron results to that of Example 20 the figures for laboratory A are unchanged but laboratory B using an unreliable method gives $\bar{x}_B = 59 \cdot 20$ and $s_B^2 = 39 \cdot 50$ for 5 results as before, the calculation will be:

$$F = \frac{s_B^2}{s_A^2} = \frac{39 \cdot 50}{2 \cdot 083} = 18 \cdot 96 \quad P < 0 \cdot 05 \quad \text{for (4, 3) } df \text{ and two-tail test.}$$

$$t = \frac{|52 \cdot 25 - 59 \cdot 20|}{\sqrt{\dfrac{2 \cdot 083}{4} + \dfrac{39 \cdot 50}{5}}} = \frac{6 \cdot 95}{2 \cdot 902} = 2 \cdot 40 \qquad \text{from (43)}$$

$$k = \frac{4 \times 39 \cdot 50}{4 \times 39 \cdot 50 + 5 \times 2 \cdot 083} = 0 \cdot 938\,2 \qquad \text{from (48)}$$

$$v = \left(\frac{0 \cdot 938\,2^2}{4} + \frac{0 \cdot 061\,8^2}{3} \right)^{-1} = 0 \cdot 221\,3^{-1} = 4 \cdot 52 \qquad \text{from (47)}$$

The table of t values gives 2·776 and 2·571 for 4 and 5 df respectively for $P = 0·05$. It is concluded that the null hypothesis cannot be confidently rejected ($P > 0·05$) and that it would be unwise to accept the rather large difference in the mean results, 52·25 and 59·20 μmol/l as a genuine one. Further progress would depend on the situation but if laboratory A wishes to be sure that it gets lower results than B, then more chemical analyses will have to be completed.

Comparison of Paired Samples

In the last section the same material was analysed several times in each of two samples. If several different specimens covering a wide range were each analysed once in each laboratory, the SD would naturally be much higher in each sample and any difference would be harder to demonstrate. In such a case the power of the test is much greater if the two results for the *same* specimen x_A and x_B are linked as a pair enabling the difference d, to be calculated as $(x_A - x_B)$. If there is no real difference between the two samples, the values of d will be scattered either side of zero so that the mean difference $\bar{d}$ should not differ significantly from 0. The appropriate test is therefore as shown in (39) where $\mu = 0$. If the t test is used this is usually referred to as the *paired t test*. It should be noted that *the sample results should be normally distributed* and that the paired results must refer to two measurements on the *same* material; it is not legitimate to put results in rank order and then to compare pairs.

Example 22. Ten sera were analysed for sodium using different flame photometers and standard solutions (A and B). The results were:

Sample	Method A	Method B	$(A - B) = x$	x^2	
1	132	134	-2	4	$\bar{x} = -5/10 = -0.5$
					from (16)
2	141	140	1	1	$s^2 = \dfrac{25 - (-5)^2/10}{9}$
3	128	130	-2	4	
4	138	135	3	9	
5	137	138	-1	1	$= 2.50$ from (19) and (20)
6	139	139	0	0	
7	135	136	-1	1	$t = \dfrac{|-0.5 - 0|\sqrt{10}}{\sqrt{2.5}}$
8	140	140	0	0	
9	137	138	-1	1	$= 1.00$ from (39)
10	136	138	-2	4	for $(10 - 1) = 9$ *df.*

$$\Sigma x = -5 \qquad \Sigma x^2 = 25$$

57

The probability attached to t is read from tables as $0.30 < P < 0.40$ from which it is concluded that the null hypothesis is likely to be true or that no significant difference has been established between the two instruments and standards at the time the measurements were made.

Comparison of Several Samples and the Analysis of Variance

Sometimes the situation arises that several samples require comparison of their variances or means. The samples may have been taken under different circumstances and the comparison then allows the variability between circumstances to be assessed despite the innate variability of individual samples. Several factors may influence the results and by a careful design of the experimental method of collecting such results it is possible to assess the relative importance or significance of the different factors. This analysis of variance is a large subject and only selected aspects are treated here. The example is of the 'completely randomised design' which is perhaps the simplest variant and one of some interest in clinical biochemistry.

The results are first analysed to assess whether there is any significant difference in the variances of the different samples. This is an extension of the comparison of two variances (p. 246). If the variances are not significantly different then the means of the different samples are compared, an extension of the comparison of the means of two samples (p. 251).

Comparison of Variances

Let there be n samples with variances $s_1^2, s_2^2, \ldots s_i^2, \ldots s_n^2$ and numbers in each sample of $n_1, n_2, \ldots n_i, \ldots n_n$, with a grand total N. The null hypothesis is that the variances of the populations from which the samples are drawn are all identical and equal to a common variance (σ^2), or

$$\sigma_1^2 = \sigma_2^2 = \ldots \sigma_i^2 = \ldots \sigma_n^2 = \sigma^2 \tag{49}$$

The best estimate of σ^2 is s^2 based on compilation of the sample variances in a manner analogous to (44)

$$s^2 = S/(N - n) \tag{50}$$

where

$$S = S_1 + S_2 + \ldots + S_i \ldots + S_n. \quad (S_1 \text{ etc. calculated as } (20)) \tag{51}$$

the *df* are $(n_1 - 1) + (n_2 - 1) + \ldots + (n_i - 1) \ldots + (n_n - 1) = N - n$.

Bartlett's test is then performed by calculating the complex expression:

$$\chi^2 = 2\cdot302\,6\left\{(N - n)\log s^2 - \sum_1^n (n_i - 1)\log s_i^2\right\}/k; \quad \text{for } (n - 1)\,df \tag{52}$$

where

$$k = 1 + \left\{\sum_1^n \left(\frac{1}{(n_i - 1)} - \frac{1}{(N - n)}\right)\right\}/3\,(n - 1) \tag{53}$$

The probability associated with the value of χ^2 is the probability that the null hypothesis is correct. A typical application in clinical biochemistry is the use of repeated analyses of a quality control serum in one analytical run, with repetition of the procedure on successive days. The number of results per day may vary but the test considers whether the variability within the day changes significantly or not, that is whether the within-run precision is altering.

Example 23. The results of such a protocol for serum albumin are set out below.

Serum albumin (g/l)
(Results to nearest 0·5 g/l

Day	in serial order)	n_i	S_i	s_i^2
Monday	40·5, 41, 40, 42, 39, 41	6	5·208 3	1·041 7
Tuesday	41·5, 40, 41, 39·5, 41, 42	6	4·333 3	0·866 7
Wednesday	39·5, 41, 40, 39, 41·5	5	4·300 0	1·075 0
Thursday	40, 40, 40·5, 38·5	4	2·250 0	0·750 0
Friday	40·5, 42, 40, 40·5	4	2·250 0	0·750 0
Monday	42, 43, 41, 39·5, 42, 40·5	6	7·833 3	1·566 7
Tuesday	41, 42·5, 41, 39, 40, 41·5	6	7·333 3	1·466 7
Wednesday	42·5, 39·5, 41·5, 41, 42	5	5·300 0	1·325 0
Thursday	40, 41, 40·5, 41	4	0·687 5	0·229 2
Friday	40, 42, 41, 42·5	4	3·687 5	1·229 2
	Totals $N = 50$		$S = 43\cdot183\,2$	

Then from **(50)** $s^2 = 43.183\,2/(50-10) = 1.079\,6$

and from **(53)** $k = 1 + \left\{ \left(\dfrac{1}{5} - \dfrac{1}{40} \right) + \left(\dfrac{1}{5} - \dfrac{1}{40} \right) \cdots \right.$

$$\left. \cdots + \left(\dfrac{1}{3} - \dfrac{1}{40} \right) \right\} \Big/ 3(10-1) = 1.088\,3$$

and from **(52)** $\chi^2 = \dfrac{2.302\,6}{1.088\,3} \{ 40 \log 1.079\,6$

$$- (5 \log 1.041\,7 + 5 \log 0.866\,7 \ldots + 3 \log 1.229\,2) \}$$

$$= \dfrac{2.302\,6}{1.088\,3} \times 1.531\,4 = 3.240$$

Examination of the χ^2 tables for 9 *df* gives $0.95 < P < 0.975$ so that the null hypothesis cannot be rejected and the variability of the variances noted in the table is acceptable as all having been drawn from a population with common variance $1.079\,6$. In fact the P value is so high as to give rise to suspicion that the figures have been adjusted slightly during recording!

Comparison of Means

Once no difference in variances has been established the means can be compared. The total variability of the individual figures is divided into the variability between samples and a residue representing the inherent variability within samples which is similar in all samples.

Let $\bar{x}_1, \bar{x}_2, \ldots \bar{x}_i, \ldots \bar{x}_n$, be the means of samples 1 to n and let $\bar{\bar{x}}$ be the grand mean of all the observations, each of which is represented by the symbol x. Let $T_i =$ total of n_i results in sample i

Then $$\bar{\bar{x}} = (\Sigma x)/N; \quad T_i = \Sigma x_i; \quad \bar{x}_i = T_i/n_i \tag{54}$$

The sums of squares (see **(20)**) which are later divided by *df* to obtain variances are then calculated as follows:

Sum of squares of all results about the grand mean

$$= \Sigma (x - \bar{\bar{x}})^2 = \Sigma x^2 - (\Sigma x)^2/N \quad \text{see (20)}$$

$$= \Sigma x^2 - C \quad \text{(where } C = (\Sigma x)^2/N) \tag{55}$$

The sum of squares *between* samples is obtained by replacing each result in a sample by the sample mean to abolish within-sample variation and then proceeding as before, hence:

Sum of squares between samples

$$= \Sigma \{ n_i (\bar{x}_i - \bar{\bar{x}})^2 \}$$

$$= \Sigma (T_i^2/n_i) - (\Sigma x)^2/N = \Sigma (T_i^2/n_i) - C \tag{56}$$

The sum of squares attributable to variation *within* the samples is then the difference between the two, namely:

$$\Sigma x^2 - \Sigma (T_i^2/n_i) \tag{57}$$

The *df* for each sum of squares will be $(N-1)$ for the total, $(n-1)$ for between samples and hence $(N-n)$ for within samples. We can then draw up a table as follows:

	Sum of squares	df	Variance
Between samples	$\Sigma(T_i^2/n_i) - C$	$n-1$	$\{\Sigma(T_i^2/n_i) - C\}/(n-1)$
Within samples	$\Sigma x^2 - \Sigma(T_i^2/n_i)$	$N-n$	$\{\Sigma x^2 - \Sigma(T_i^2/n_i)\}/(N-n)$
Total	$\Sigma x^2 - C$	$N-1$	

It is then possible to test whether the variance between samples is greater than within samples by the variance ratio or F test (p. 246) in its one-tail form. If this ratio gives a P value of < 0.05 the null hypothesis that the means of samples were identical is unlikely to be true and the separate sample means and their SEs can be calculated in the usual way and examined. If however the P value is > 0.05 it is concluded that no difference between means has been established. In the results for Example 24, the clinical biochemist will interpret the within-days variance (s_W^2) in terms of the within-day precision. The between-days variance is the sum of s_W^2 and another variance, s_B^2, attributable to *additional* imprecision between days, multiplied by the average number of samples per day. In practice we usually consider the *total* variance $(s_W^2 + s_B^2)$ when considering the between-day precision. All the calculated variances (and SDs) are estimates and subject to sampling error.

Example 24. Taking the results in the table in Example 23, the means and totals for the samples become:

	Total (T_i)	Mean $(\bar{x}_i)$	Total (T_i)	Mean $(\bar{x}_i)$
Monday	243·5	40·583 3	248·0	41·333 3
Tuesday	245·0	40·833 3	245·0	40·833 3
Wednesday	201·0	40·200 0	206·5	41·300 0
Thursday	159·0	39·750 0	162·5	40·625 0
Friday	163·0	40·750 0	165·5	41·375 0

Grand total $= 2039$; grand mean $(\bar{\bar{x}}) = 2039/50 = 40.780$

We calculate $C = 2039^2/50 = 83\,150.420\,0$

$$\Sigma T_i^2/n_i = (243.5^2/6 + 245^2/6 + \ldots + 165.5^2/4) = 83\,161.316\,7$$

$$\Sigma x^2 = (39^2 + 40^2 + 40.5^2 + \ldots + 42.5^2) = 83\,204.500\,0$$

and then as $N = 50$ and $n = 10$ the variance table becomes:

	Sum of squares	df	Variance	
Between days	10·896 7	9	1·210 7	$s_W^2 + s_B^2 \cdot (N/n)$
Within days	43·183 3	40	1·079 6	s_W^2
Total	54·080 0	49	$F = 1.122$	

The F value of 1·122 corresponds to a P value of > 0.05 for (9, 40) *df*, indicating no significant increase in variance between days. The best estimate of the serum albumin concentration in the control serum is 40·78 g/l and the within-day SD is $\sqrt{1.079\,6}$ or 1·039 g/l giving a CV of 2·55%.

The between-day variance may be calculated if wished as follows:

$s_W^2 + s_B^2 \cdot (N/n) = 1.079\,6 + s_B^2 \cdot (50/10) = 1.210\,7$, and thus $s_B^2 = 0.026\,2$
Total between-day variance $= 1.079\,6 + 0.026\,2 = 1.105\,8$
This corresponds to a between-day SD of 1·052 giving a CV of 2·58%.

In the special case when there are two observations for each of n samples, that is when duplicate analyses are performed, the expression for the within-sample SD simplifies to

$$\text{Within-sample SD} = \sqrt{\frac{\Sigma d^2}{2n}} \tag{58}$$

where d is the difference between duplicates. This SD is the estimated common SD of all samples (see **49**) and is often used as a means of measuring precision. If the duplicates for all samples are determined on the same day the result is the average SD for that particular day. If duplicates for any one sample are performed on the same day but different samples are analysed on different days, then the calculated SD is the average within-day SD over the time period studied. If duplicates for each sample are performed on different days, then the SD will be the average between-day SD over the time studied.

It should be realised that the SD applies to the whole range of concentrations covered by the samples analysed. The assumption is that the variance is the same for all samples but it is well recognised in practice that the precision of a method varies with concentration. Hence it is desirable that when the SD is calculated from duplicates, the samples should be grouped to cover separate rather limited concentration ranges. The SD can then be considered as applying to the mean concentration of the relevant group and the CV can be calculated separately for each group by (25).

Regression and Correlation Methods

In clinical biochemistry the general nature of the relationship between two variables is often studied graphically. One variable, x, is plotted on the abscissa and the other, y, on the ordinate so that for a particular value of x the result of y can be recorded as a point on the graph. Two rather different examples are (1) a calibration curve in which the concentration of standard solutions is taken as x and the absorbance readings as y, and (2) a comparison of the results of two methods during the analysis of many different sera where the selection of the method to call x is less obvious although usually it will be either a reference or a well-established method. The statistical methods and assumptions differ in the two cases.

In this discussion the nature of the relationship is taken to be linear. If inspection of the plotted points shows that this is not valid either more elaborate curve fitting methods are needed or the original variables may be subjected to a transformation (p. 235) which will give an acceptably linear relationship. Once a linear plot has been accepted the relationship between y and x can be expressed in terms of the equation of a straight line:

$$y = a + bx$$

where b is a parameter defining the slope of the line, the average amount y changes with unit increase in x, and a is a parameter of position of the line, the intercept on the vertical axis or the value of y when x is zero. Thus if a and b are known the expected value of y can be calculated for any value of x. The line is the *regression line* and b is the *regression coefficient*.

Regressions of the First Kind

In regressions of the first kind exemplified by the calibration curve, the values of x are chosen arbitrarily and are often equally spaced over the required range. For the statistical analysis two requirements must be met for the values of y. *For any value of* x *the values of* y *must be normally distributed and the variance must be independent of* x. The equation of the line is calculated so as to minimise the sum of the square of the deviation of each value of y from the value Y predicted for its associated x value from the expression $(a + bx)$. This is done as follows, having obtained n pairs of x and y results as $(x_1, y_1), (x_2, y_2) \ldots (x_i, y_i) \ldots (x_n, y_n)$.

Calculate Σx, Σx^2, Σy, Σy^2, and Σxy where the last is obtained by multiplying x_i by y_i and summing for all values of i. Calculate $\bar{x}$ and $\bar{y}$ (16).

Calculate S_x and S_y (see (20)) and also calculate S_{xy} defined similarly as

$$S_{xy} = \Sigma(xy) - \Sigma x \cdot \Sigma y/n \tag{59}$$

Then

$$b = S_{xy}/S_x \quad \text{and} \quad a = \bar{y} - b\bar{x} \tag{60}$$

The total variance of y is partly attributable to the fact that y changes with x but there is also a component due to the variability around the regression line. This is the common variance which was a condition of the analysis and is calculated as:

$$s_{y.x}^2 = \frac{1}{n-2}(S_y - b \cdot S_{xy}) \quad \text{or} \quad \frac{1}{n-2}(S_y - (S_{xy})^2/S_x)$$

$$\text{or} \quad \frac{1}{n-2}(S_y - b^2 \cdot S_x) \tag{61}$$

The regression coefficient b is an estimate based on the sample of n pairs and has its own SE, s_b, related to this common variance by the expression

$$s_b^2 = s_{y.x}^2/S_x \tag{62}$$

Thus depending on the size of n the value of b can be compared with some hypothetical value β in the usual way by calculating

$$t \text{ or } c = |b - \beta|/s_b \quad \text{where } t \text{ has } (n-2) \, df. \tag{63}$$

Alternatively the CL of b can be expressed as

$$CL = b \pm c \cdot s_b \quad \text{or} \quad CL = b \pm t \cdot s_b \tag{64}$$

where the values of c or t are appropriate for the probability level desired.

In a similar way the SE of the intercept, s_a, is calculated as

$$s_a^2 = s_b^2 \sqrt{(\Sigma x^2)/n}. \tag{65}$$

Finally, the uncertainty in the calculation of Y predicted from a given value of x will be affected by the variability about the regression line and the variability of the slope. The regression line always passes through the point $(\bar{x}, \bar{y})$ and the

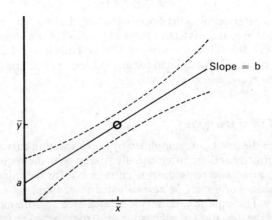

Fig 10.4. Parabolic Confidence Limits for Y Equidistant from a Regression Line of the First Kind.

They approach the line most closely near the point $\bar{x}, \bar{y}$ shown by o. The intercept a and the slope b refer to the regression equation $y = a + bx$.

uncertainty in Y becomes greater the further x is from $\bar{x}$. The CL for Y are defined by two parabolas lying one on each side of the regression line (Fig. 10.4). These are calculated from the overall variance about the regression line, s_Y^2 for the appropriate probability as:

$$s_Y^2 = s_b^2 (S_x/n + (x - \bar{x})^2) \tag{66}$$

CL on estimate of $y = \bar{y} + b(x - \bar{x}) \pm t \cdot s_Y$ with $(n - 2)\, df$ for t. (67)

Example 25. In setting up a manual method for serum urea four standards were processed in quadruplicate and read against a blank. The results were:

x	y			
Urea (mmol/l)	Absorbance $\times$ 1000			
10	90	95	110	120
20	195	210	210	230
30	300	315	320	330
40	400	415	420	435

The variances can be checked and shown not to differ and so far as can be ascertained they are compatible with a normal distribution. We can then calculate

$$\Sigma x = 400 \quad \Sigma x^2 = 12\,000 \quad \Sigma y = 4195 \quad \Sigma y^2 = 1\,321\,125$$

$$\Sigma xy = (10 \times 90 + 10 \times 95 + \ldots\, 40 \times 435) = 125\,800 \quad n = 16$$

From which: $\quad \bar{x} = 25 \cdot 000\,0 \quad \bar{y} = 262 \cdot 187\,5$

$S_x = 2000, \quad S_y = 221\,248$ from (20); $\quad S_{xy} = 20\,925$ from (59)

$b = 20\,925/2000 = 10 \cdot 462\,5$ from (60)

$a = 262 \cdot 187\,5 - 25 \times 10 \cdot 462\,5 = 0 \cdot 625\,0$ from (60)

$s_{y.x}^2 = \frac{1}{14} (221\,248 - 10 \cdot 462\,5 \times 20\,925) = 165 \cdot 727\,7$,

$s_{y.x} = 12 \cdot 873\,5$ from (61)

$s_b^2 = 165 \cdot 727\,7/2000 = 0 \cdot 082\,863\,8 \quad s_b = 0 \cdot 287\,9$ from (62)

$s_a^2 = 0 \cdot 082\,863\,8 \sqrt{12\,000/16} = 2 \cdot 269\,3 \quad s_a = 1 \cdot 506$ from (65)

The regression equation will be

$$y = 10 \cdot 46 x + 0 \cdot 63$$

where y is absorbance $\times$ 1000. If actual absorbance figures are used, the equation becomes

$$y = 0 \cdot 010\,46 x + 0 \cdot 000\,63$$

The line can be drawn by defining two points, the intercept, $+0 \cdot 000\,63$ on the y axis, and the value of $y = 0 \cdot 262\,2$ for a serum urea of 25 mmol/l; the latter pair being $\bar{y}$ and $\bar{x}$.

The 95 % CL of the regression coefficient can be calculated using $t = 2 \cdot 145$ for 14 df as follows:

$$95\% \text{ CL} = 10 \cdot 462\,5 \pm 2 \cdot 145 \times 0 \cdot 287\,9 \qquad \text{from (64)}$$

corresponding in absorbance units to $0 \cdot 009\,84$ to $0 \cdot 011\,08$.

It is obvious that b is very significantly different from zero, a figure which would indicate no significant colour increase over the urea concentration studied. The slope b is a measure of the sensitivity of the method and if it was necessary to select a method in which the sensitivity corresponded to $0 \cdot 02$ absorbance units per mmol/l the slope found would be compared with this figure. It is clear that $0 \cdot 02$ lies well outside the 95 % CL of the slope and the desired sensitivity has not been achieved.

The intercept a is $+0 \cdot 000\,63$ absorbance units and its SE is $0 \cdot 001\,51$ indicating that it is not significantly different from zero.

Finally the 95 % CL for the estimates of urea concentrations of 25 and 60 mmol/l are calculated from $t = 2\cdot145$ for 14 df and s_Y as:

at 25 mmol/l $s_Y^2 = 0\cdot082\,864\,(2000/16 + (25 - 25)^2) = 10\cdot358\,00$

at 60 mmol/l $s_Y^2 = 0\cdot082\,864\,(2000/16 + (60 - 25)^2) = 111\cdot866\,40$

both from **(66)**

Hence at 25 mmol/l

$95\% \text{ CL} = 262\cdot187\,5 \pm 2\cdot145 \times \sqrt{10\cdot358\,00}$ or $255\cdot284$ to $269\cdot091$

and at 60 mmol/l
$95\% \text{ CL} = 262\cdot187\,5 \pm 10\cdot462\,5(60 - 25) \pm 2\cdot145 \times \sqrt{111\cdot866\,40}$

or $605\cdot688$ to $651\cdot062$

from **(67)**

These figures are to be divided by 1000 to obtain the actual absorbance figures; at 25 mmol/l, CL $= 0\cdot255$ to $0\cdot269$ and at 60 mmol/l, CL $= 0\cdot606$ to $0\cdot651$.

In regressions of the first kind the single regression equation is used to calculate y from x or to calculate x from y.

Regressions of the Second Kind

In dealing with regressions of the second kind as in the comparison of two methods applied to the same sera, the requirements are different although many calculations are similar. The first requirement is that *both x and y must be random normally distributed variables.* It is less easy to achieve this in practice than to meet the requirements for regressions of the first kind. Deliberate selection of sera to include a good number of high and low results is unlikely to produce a bivariate normal distribution, and calculations based on the second type of regression may give misleading information.

Traditional Method of Calculating Regression Lines. When these requirements are met it has been customary to calculate two separate regression lines by minimising the sum of the squares of the deviations of the points from the regression line. *It is a requirement that the analytical error of one of the methods is very small in relation to that of the other method and that the variance of this other method is constant at all concentrations covered.* The first requirement may be met if one method is a definitive method (Chapter 13, p. 300). Then if the results from this method are plotted on the x axis, the regression line of y on x is calculated by minimising the sum of the squares of the *vertical* deviations from the line. This regression of y on x is used to calculate y from a knowledge of x. The appropriate equation is

$$y = a_{y \cdot x} + b_{y \cdot x} \cdot x \tag{68}$$

and $a_{y \cdot x}$ and $b_{y \cdot x}$ are calculated exactly as in **(59)**. Alternatively, if the results of the method with minimal analytical error are plotted on the y axis, the minimal sum of the squares of the *horizontal* deviations from the line is needed. Then the regression of x on y is used to calculate x from a knowledge of y and the related equation is

$$x = a_{x \cdot y} + b_{x \cdot y} \cdot y \tag{69}$$

where

$$b_{x \cdot y} = S_{xy}/S_y \quad \text{and} \quad a_{x \cdot y} = \bar{x} - b_{x \cdot y} \cdot \bar{y} \tag{70}$$

Note that $a_{x \cdot y}$ is the intercept on the x axis and the slope $b_{x \cdot y}$ is in relation to the

y axis. Both lines pass through the point $\bar{x}$, $\bar{y}$. The second line can be drawn from this point to the intercept on the x axis.

In clinical biochemistry it is often necessary to compare two analytical methods, A and B, which have similar analytical errors. It has been customary to calculate the two separate regression lines and to use the 'appropriate' one to calculate the predicted result by method B from a result obtained by method A, and *vice versa*.

Example 26. Two methods for serum calcium (mmol/l) were compared on 30 randomly selected sera showing a normal distribution. Results from an AutoAnalyzer cresolphthalein complexone method were plotted on the x axis and those from an automatic compleximetric titrator on the y axis. The results were summarised as

$$\bar{x} = 2\cdot4010 \quad S_x = 1\cdot183\,316 \quad S_{xy} = 1\cdot180\,697$$
$$\bar{y} = 2\cdot3592 \quad S_y = 1\cdot827\,029$$

Thus

$$b_{y\cdot x} = \frac{1\cdot180\,697}{1\cdot183\,316} = 0\cdot997\,787 \quad a_{y\cdot x} = -0\cdot036 \qquad \text{from (60)}$$

and

$$b_{x\cdot y} = \frac{1\cdot180\,697}{1\cdot827\,029} = 0\cdot646\,239 \quad a_{x\cdot y} = 0\cdot876 \qquad \text{from (70)}$$

In order to calculate an expected titrimetric result from an AutoAnalyzer result the equation is:

Titrimetric result $= -0\cdot036 + 0\cdot998 \times$ AutoAnalyzer result

For the opposite conversion the appropriate equation is

AutoAnalyzer result $= 0\cdot876 + 0\cdot646 \times$ Titrimetric result

The slope, $0\cdot646$ is relative to the y axis but the equation can be rewritten

Titrimetric result $= -1\cdot356 + 1\cdot547 \times$ AutoAnalyzer result

where the slope is in relation to the x axis as shown by the steeper, broken line in Fig. 10.5. Each of the equations is satisfied by $\bar{x}$ and $\bar{y}$.

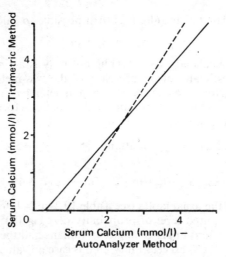

Fig 10.5. The Two Regression Lines for Example 26.
The continuous line is the regression of y on x. The lines cross at $\bar{x}$, $\bar{y}$.

The SEs of the two slopes are calculated as before using the equations (61) and (62) for the SE of $b_{y.x}$ and similar equations with y and x transposed for the SE of $b_{x.y}$. The tolerance limits for points scattered about the regression lines are no longer defined by two parabolas as in a first type regression as extreme values of both x and y will be uncommon and most observations will be scattered about the point $\bar{x}$, $\bar{y}$. The population of points is enclosed by an ellipse with its axis corresponding approximately to the mean slope of the two regression lines. The limits of this ellipse may be calculated (for details see 5th edition of this book). The existence of two regression lines makes it difficult to gain a clear idea of the agreement between the two methods and this arises from transgression of the original requirement that one method should have minimal analytical error. It is usual for both methods to have appreciable imprecision.

Deming's Method of Calculating One Regression Line. A full mathematical treatment is given by Deming (1943) and a simpler account appears in Mandel (1964). It is assumed that the ratio (λ) of the analytical variances $(s_x^2$ and $s_y^2)$ of the two methods is known but the absolute figures are not required. The calculations also assume that these variances apply to all concentrations covered in the comparison. A single regression line is calculated by minimising the sum of the squares of deviations of points from the line. When λ equals one, the deviations are measured *perpendicular* to the line but in other cases deviate progressively from the perpendicular depending on λ (see Deming, 1943; Mandel, 1964).

If x and y are again normally distributed variables with n pairs of results $(x_1, y_1), (x_2, y_2) \ldots (x_n, y_n)$ and if the (constant) precision (p. 286) of the method giving the x results is s_x and that of the method giving the y results is s_y, then λ the ratio of the variances is defined as

$$\lambda = s_y^2 / s_x^2 \tag{71}$$

Then using the usual linear regression equation $y = a + bx$ and the previously used symbols S_x, S_y, S_{xy} calculated by (20) and (59), the slope, b, of the regression line can be calculated as

$$b = \frac{(S_y - \lambda \cdot S_x) + \sqrt{(S_y - \lambda \cdot S_x)^2 + 4 \cdot \lambda \cdot S_{xy}^2}}{2 \cdot S_{xy}} \tag{72}$$

and a can be calculated as in (60). It is then possible to calculate s_y^2 as

$$s_y^2 = (S_y - b \cdot S_{xy})/(n - 2) \tag{73}$$

from which s_x^2 is calculated as s_y^2/λ. Thus not only is a single regression line obtained but also estimates of the precision of the two methods.

Confidence limits for the slope are discussed in detail by Creasy (1956) and are expressed in a convenient, if complicated, practical formula (Davies and Goldsmith, 1972) as follows

$$\text{Confidence limits} = \sqrt{\lambda} \cdot \tan(\tan^{-1}\{b/\sqrt{\lambda}\} \pm 0.5 \times \sin^{-1}\{2t\theta\}) \tag{74}$$

where

$$\theta^2 = \lambda (S_x \cdot S_y - S_{xy}^2)/(n - 2)\{(S_y - \lambda S_x)^2 + 4 \cdot \lambda \cdot S_{xy}^2\} \tag{75}$$

and t is taken from the usual tables (see Table 10.2, p. 244) for $(n - 2)$ degrees of freedom and the required level of probability (2α), e.g. 0.05 for 95 % CL. The trigonometrical functions apply to angles in radians and the calculation breaks down if the value of $\{2t\theta\}$ exceeds unity. In this case no value of the slope can be excluded from the CL at that value of t.

An example will help to clarify the calculation.

Example 27. Using the same data as in Example 26 taking the value of λ as 2, we can also look up t for $(30-2)$ df and $P = 0.05$ as 2.0484. The regression coefficient, b, is first calculated from (72) as

$$b = \frac{(1.827\,029 - 2 \times 1.183\,316) + \sqrt{(1.827\,029 - 2 \times 1.183\,316)^2 + 4 \times 2 \times 1.180\,697^2}}{2 \times 1.180\,697}$$

$$= 1.204\,046$$

Hence

$$a = 2.359\,2 - 1.204\,046 \times 2.401\,0 = -0.531\,7 \qquad \text{from (60)}$$

The equation for the regression line is thus

$$\text{Titrimetric result} = -0.532 + 1.204 \times \text{AutoAnalyzer result}$$

the line lying between the two traditional regression lines.

We calculate θ from (75) and then the 95 % CL from (74) as follows

$$\theta^2 = 2(1.183\,316 \times 1.827\,029 - 1.180\,697^2)/(30-2)\,\{(1.827\,029$$

$$-2 \times 1.183\,316)^2 + 4 \times 2 \times 1.180\,697^2\}$$

$$= 0.004\,793\,145 \text{ whence } \theta = 0.069\,232\,54$$

$$2t\theta = 2 \times 2.0484 \times 0.069\,232\,54 = 0.283\,631\,87$$

as this is less than 1 further calculations can proceed.

$$95\,\% \text{ CL} = \sqrt{2} \times \tan\,(\tan^{-1}\,(1.204\,045\,74/\sqrt{2}) \pm 0.5 \times \sin^{-1}\,\{0.283\,631\,87\})$$

$$= \sqrt{2} \times \tan\,(0.705\,299\,64 \pm 0.143\,789\,75)$$

$$= 0.890 \text{ to } 1.607$$

In these calculations rounding off should be left to the end and as many significant figures as possible should be carried through the calculation. It is obviously an advantage if a program written for a small computer can be used.

Note that the limits are not symmetrical about the best estimate of the slope, 1.204. Further calculations of the SDs of the two methods using (73) are

$$s_y^2 = (1.827\,029 - 1.204\,046 \times 1.180\,697)/(30-2) = 0.014\,479$$

Hence

$$s_x^2 = 0.014\,479/2 \quad \text{and} \quad s_y = 0.1203 \quad \text{and} \quad s_x = 0.0851$$

The slope will vary with λ. Similar calculations for Example 27 show that when the methods have the same SD ($\lambda = 1$), b is 1.309 and b lies within 8 % of this result for λ values between 0.45 and 2.0 corresponding to a ratio of the SDs of the methods from 0.67 to 1.41, a not unrealistic range in practical terms. When λ is very large, i.e. when s_x^2 is very small, the slope becomes 0.998, the value obtained by the traditional method for the regression of y on x which requires that there is no error in the x measurements. Similarly if λ is very small, i.e. s_y^2 is very small, the slope becomes 1.547, the slope in relation to the x axis when the regression of x on y is calculated as was done earlier (p. 261).

Furthermore, Cornbleet and Gochman (1979) have shown that the Deming regression coefficient is little affected by other changes in the data base. If instead of x and y being normally distributed, their distribution is log-normal, there is little change in b. Also if the errors of the two analytical methods are not constant over the concentration range studied but instead the CV is constant, which is more likely in practice, this also has little effect on b.

Correlation

A further parameter of the second type of regression is the *correlation coefficient*, r, which is a measure of the dependence of x on y and varies from -1 to $+1$. If r is 1 the two variables are totally dependent on one another and y increases as x increases, while if r is -1 although they are still totally dependent, y falls as x rises. The points describing pairs of x, y values in each case lie exactly on a straight line but this line can have any slope and it does *not* follow that because $r = 1$ then $x = y$ for all values of x and y. If $r = 0$ there is no correlation at all and x and y are totally independent of one another. The two regression lines are at right angles to each other and parallel to the x and y axes. In many cases r will have a value between 0 and either $+1$ or -1, and the plotted points lie either side of the regression lines. The closer r approaches 1 (or -1) the closer the two regression lines agree and the closer the points fit to the lines.

The definition of the correlation coefficient is

$$r = \frac{S_{xy}}{s_x \cdot s_y} = \frac{S_{xy}}{\sqrt{S_x \cdot S_y}} = \sqrt{b_{y.x} \times b_{x.y}} \tag{76}$$

If r is positive, both bs are positive. If r is negative, so are both bs. If r is zero so are both bs. If r is 1 then $b_{y.x} = 1/b_{x.y}$.

The significance of the value of r can also be tested. The simplest case is to test whether r is different from zero. The appropriate test is

$$t = r\sqrt{n-2}/\sqrt{1-r^2} \quad \text{for} \quad (n-2)\, df \tag{77}$$

The P value corresponding to t is the probability of the truth of the null hypothesis of no difference between r and zero. In general, however, the distribution of r from repeated samples is not normal and simple significance tests are only feasible after transforming r into z which is approximately normally distributed. The relationships are

$$z = \tanh^{-1} r = \tfrac{1}{2}\left\{ \ln \frac{(1+r)}{(1-r)} \right\} \tag{78}$$

$$r = \tanh z = \frac{e^{2z}-1}{e^{2z}+1} \tag{79}$$

but standard statistical tables (p. 272) are available to allow the appropriate conversions to be read off directly. The variance of z is simply related to n

$$s_z^2 \approx 1/(n-3) \tag{80}$$

so that the usual tests of significance can be carried out. Thus in order to compare r from n pairs with a hypothetical value ρ the two values are transformed into z and ζ and the test is then similar to (**39**) used for comparing a mean with a hypothetical value

$$c = |z - \zeta|/s_z = |z - \zeta|\sqrt{(n-3)} \tag{81}$$

Similarly when comparing two correlation coefficients r_1 and r_2 based on n_1 and n_2 pairs we transform to z_1 and z_2 and calculate

$$c = |z_1 - z_2|/\sqrt{s_1^2 + s_2^2} = |z_1 - z_2|/\sqrt{1/(n_1-3) + 1/(n_2-3)} \tag{82}$$

We can also calculate the CL on our estimate of r by converting to z and calculating first the CL on z as

$$\text{CL for } z = z \pm c/\sqrt{n-3} \tag{83}$$

where c is taken from Table 10.1 (p. 242) for $100\,(1-2\alpha)\,\%$ CL, that is c is 1·96 for 95 % CL. The two limiting z values are then retransformed into r values which are not equidistant from the original value of r.

Example 28. For the figures in Example 26 for 30 pairs, r is $\sqrt{0\cdot998 \times 0\cdot646}$ or 0·803. To test the significance of the difference from zero

$$t = \frac{0\cdot803\sqrt{28}}{\sqrt{1-0\cdot803^2}} = 7\cdot13 \quad \text{for } (30-2)\,df \tag{from (77)}$$

The P value is $< 0\cdot001$ so r is very significantly different from zero.
From tables the z value corresponding to $r = 0\cdot803$ is 1·107 00.
Hence from **(83)**

$$95\,\% \text{ CL for } z = 1\cdot107\,00 \pm \frac{1\cdot96}{\sqrt{30-3}} = 0\cdot729\,80 \text{ to } 1\cdot484\,20$$

and from tables 95 % CL for r will vary from 0·623 to 0·902.
If r is to be compared with a reference value selected from other considerations as 0·850 any possible difference will be calculated after z transformations to 1·107 00 (as before) and 1·256 15.
Hence

$$c = |1\cdot107\,00 - 1\cdot256\,15|\sqrt{(30-3)} = 0\cdot775 \tag{from (81)}$$

and from tables $P = 0\cdot44$ indicating that the observed r is definitely not lower than 0·850.
Finally, if a similar comparison on 40 other sera were done in another laboratory with a resultant correlation coefficient of 0·885 the two can be compared after z transformation of the second r to 1·398 38 as follows:

$$c = |1\cdot107\,00 - 1\cdot398\,38|/\sqrt{1/(30-3) + 1/(40-3)} = 1\cdot151 \tag{from (82)}$$

The P value is 0·25 indicating that the null hypothesis cannot be rejected and hence no difference in correlation coefficient has been established.

There are several reservations about the use of correlation coefficients, particularly in the comparison of methods. The interpretation of r is likely to be misleading if the two variables are not normally distributed. In such cases it is better to use Spearman's coefficient of rank correlation (p. 266). If x and y have a legitimate, highly significant correlation it does not follow that x and y are causally related; both x and y may be influenced similarly by a third factor. The use of the correlation coefficient to compare methods has been severely criticised by Altman and Bland (1983). It gives information about the measure of association between the results from two methods but it is not a measure of the agreement between the methods themselves. They show that if the measurement errors of the methods are small in comparison to the variation between the actual measurements (e.g. serum concentrations), then r will always be high and very significantly different from zero even if the methods agree poorly. Also if the measurement errors are similar to the variation in serum concentrations studied, r will inevitably be small no matter how good the agreement between the methods.

More elaborate statistical techniques, outside the scope of this chapter, may be employed to study the effect of several factors operating simultaneously. If, e.g. three factors A, B and C influence the variable x it is possible to calculate partial correlation coefficients between any two factors having eliminated the effect of the third. If regression analysis is used it is possible to calculate a multiple linear regression equation for example of the form

$$y = a + bx_1 + cx_2 + dx_3$$

where the variables x_1, x_2, x_3 all affect y. Multiple regression equations of this type may be extended to Discriminant Function Analysis in which, e.g. the mean results of three different biochemical tests x_1, x_2, and x_3, suitably weighted by the factors b, c and d can be added to produce the result y. If the mean results are derived from different groups of patients with different diseases the value of y may differ markedly with disease. Similar combination of the results x_1, x_2, and x_3 from an individual patient could then be of greater diagnostic value than a single observation. For all these extensions of regression and correlation studies, more elaborate statistical texts should be consulted.

If paired results from *distributions of any form* are to be compared then Spearman's coefficient of rank correlation is useful. The values of x are ranked in ascending order as $X_1 \ldots X_i \ldots X_n$. The same procedure is done independently for y to give the ascending order $Y_1 \ldots Y_i \ldots Y_n$. For each of the n pairs of original results the rank orders (i, j) are noted and for each pair the difference in rank order d is found. Then Spearman's coefficient, R, is calculated as

$$R = 1 - (6 \cdot \Sigma d^2 / n(n^2 - 1)) \tag{84}$$

For values of n of 20 or more R is approximately normally distributed between the values -1 to $+1$ with a mode of zero. Its SD is given by

$$s_R \approx 1/\sqrt{n-1} \tag{85}$$

allowing the deviation of R from zero to be tested for significance in the usual way.

Example 29. The following pairs of results for serum urea were obtained on 20 different sera by two methods x and y:

Serum Urea (mmol/l)

Method x	Method y	Rank Order X_i	Rank Order Y_j
6·3	9·5	2	8
16·6	12·3	16	10
8·6	14·0	5	15
20·5	13·8	20	13
9·2	8·3	8	2
10·5	8·8	11	4
9·0	8·0	7	1
16·3	16·3	15	18
6·6	12·6	3	12
18·7	13·9	18	14
7·8	12·5	4	11
12·1	9·0	13	5
6·1	9·7	1	9
20·1	20·0	19	20
10·1	9·1	10	6
18·4	18·4	17	19
8·9	14·1	6	16
15·7	15·7	14	17
11·2	9·3	12	7
9·6	8·6	9	3

$$\Sigma d^2 = ((2-8)^2 + (16-10)^2 + \ldots + (9-3)^2)$$
$$= 816$$

$$R = 1 - \frac{6 \times 816}{20 \times (400 - 1)} \quad \text{from (84)}$$
$$= 0.386\ 5$$

$$s_R = \frac{1}{\sqrt{20-1}} = 0.229\ 4 \quad \text{from (85)}$$

Therefore

$$R \text{ is } 0.386\,5/0.229\,4 = 1.685 \text{ SDs from } 0$$

and this corresponds to P = 0·092. Calculating the correlation coefficient r gives a figure of 0·672 2. When tested from the difference from zero

$$t = 0.672\,2\sqrt{20-2}/\sqrt{1-0.672\,2^2} = 3.852 \qquad \text{from (77)}$$

corresponding for 18 df to 0·001 < P < 0·005.

The correlation coefficient r is apparently very significant but Spearman's R is not significantly different from zero. The use of r is misleading as inspection shows that the results for each method are not normally distributed, perhaps because of deliberate selection of the 20 sera to cover a wide range fairly evenly. The non-parametric method for R gives a better impression of the poor correlation between the results of the two methods.

THE BINOMIAL DISTRIBUTION

Most of the statistical methods described so far have been applicable to continuous variables. The binomial distribution applies to discontinuous variables. If there are only two mutually exclusive outcomes of making a test on a single observation and if the probability of the first outcome is p while that of the second is q then $p + q$ equals 1. If n independent tests are carried out then the discontinuous variable a will describe the number of times the first outcome occurred in the n tests and the value of a will be an integer in the range from 0 to n. The probabilities of the different outcomes corresponding to different values of a are given by the terms of the binomial expansion

$$(p+q)^n \qquad \qquad (86)$$

in which the general expression for each term is

$$\text{Probability} = \frac{n!}{a!\,(n-a)!}\,p^a q^{n-a} \qquad (87)$$

This is the probability that a individual tests will have the outcome of probability p. The distribution is determined by two parameters only, namely p and n since q is $(1-p)$. It is possible to show that the mean value of a is given by

$$\bar{a} = np \qquad \qquad (88)$$

and the variance of a is given by

$$s_a^2 = npq \qquad \qquad (89)$$

Example 30. Sensitivity to the muscle relaxant scoline is an inherited and recessive abnormality. If two heterozygotes marry then the probability p that a child will be homozygous for the abnormal gene is $\frac{1}{4}$ and the probability that a child will be clinically unaffected (normal or heterozygote) will be $\frac{3}{4}$. The binomial distribution will then give the chances of different numbers of affected children in a family with four children from (87) as follows:

No. children affected (a)		Probability	

0	$\dfrac{4!}{0!\,4!}\left(\dfrac{1}{4}\right)^0\left(\dfrac{3}{4}\right)^4 = \dfrac{81}{256}$	
1	$\dfrac{4!}{1!\,3!}\left(\dfrac{1}{4}\right)\left(\dfrac{3}{4}\right)^3 = \dfrac{108}{256}$	
2	$\dfrac{4!}{2!\,2!}\left(\dfrac{1}{4}\right)^2\left(\dfrac{3}{4}\right)^2 = \dfrac{54}{256}$	Total $= \dfrac{256}{256}$
3	$\dfrac{4!}{3!\,1!}\left(\dfrac{1}{4}\right)^3\left(\dfrac{3}{4}\right) = \dfrac{12}{256}$	
4	$\dfrac{4!}{4!\,0!}\left(\dfrac{1}{4}\right)^4\left(\dfrac{3}{4}\right)^0 = \dfrac{1}{256}$	

The most probable result is one child affected and either one or no affected child will occur in almost 74% (189/256) of such families on average. The mean number of affected children per family is $4 \times \frac{1}{4}$ or 1 (from **88**) and the SD is $\sqrt{4 \times \frac{1}{4} \times \frac{3}{4}}$ or 0·866 (from **89**).

It often happens that p is not known and has to be estimated from the sample. If from n observations a have the desired property then the estimate of p is a/n and its SE is given by

$$\text{SE of } p = \sqrt{\frac{pq}{n}} = \sqrt{\frac{\dfrac{a}{n}\left(1-\dfrac{a}{n}\right)}{n}} = \frac{1}{n}\sqrt{\frac{a\,(n-a)}{n}} \tag{90}$$

Provided that p or q is not very small and n is above 30 the binomial distribution becomes similar to the normal distribution and the SE can be treated as for such a distribution. This is convenient when comparing two percentages which are expressed in fractional form (a/n). Then the significance of the difference between such fractions is calculated as

$$c = \frac{\left|\dfrac{a_1}{n_1} - \dfrac{a_2}{n_2}\right|}{\sqrt{p(1-p)\left(\dfrac{1}{n_1} + \dfrac{1}{n_2}\right)}} \quad \text{where} \quad p = \frac{a_1 + a_2}{n_1 + n_2} \tag{91}$$

The CL on the difference (if established) will be

$$\text{CL} = \left|\frac{a_1}{n_1} - \frac{a_2}{n_2}\right| \pm c\sqrt{\frac{\dfrac{a_1}{n_1}\left(1-\dfrac{a_1}{n_1}\right)}{n_1} + \frac{\dfrac{a_2}{n_2}\left(1-\dfrac{a_2}{n_2}\right)}{n_2}} \tag{92}$$

where c is selected from Table 10.1 (p. 242) for CL of $100\,(1-2\alpha)\%$.

Example 31. Glucose tolerance tests were carried out on a group of elderly people, 60 of whom had been noted to have post-prandial glycosuria while 50 others had none. The blood glucose was measured 2 h after 50 g glucose was given orally and a note was made if this exceeded 7 mmol/l. This occurred in 31 of those with post-prandial glycosuria and in only 17 of the others. In order to test whether this is a significant increase we calculate from **(91)**

$$c = \frac{\left|\dfrac{31}{60} - \dfrac{17}{50}\right|}{\sqrt{\dfrac{48}{110} \times \dfrac{62}{110}\left(\dfrac{1}{60} + \dfrac{1}{50}\right)}} = \frac{0\cdot176\,67}{0\cdot094\,964} = 1\cdot860$$

using

$$p = \frac{31 + 17}{60 + 50} = \frac{48}{110}$$

The value of c gives P just $> 0\cdot05$ and the null hypothesis of no difference cannot be rejected. It is not established that post-prandial glycosuria gives a greater number of abnormally high blood glucose levels at 2 h.

If the 95 % CL on the difference was required then $c = 1\cdot96$ and from **(92)**

$$95\,\%\,\text{CL} = 0\cdot176\,7 \pm 1\cdot96 \sqrt{\frac{\dfrac{31}{60} \times \dfrac{29}{60}}{60} + \frac{\dfrac{17}{50} \times \dfrac{33}{50}}{50}} = 0\cdot176\,7 \pm 0\cdot182\,3$$

or the percentage difference for glycosurics compared with non-glycosurics is $-0\cdot6$ to $35\cdot9$.

Finally if in a binomial distribution p is very small, the distribution instead of tending to become normal, approaches the Poisson distribution (see below) and np corresponds to λ of this distribution.

THE POISSON DISTRIBUTION

This also applies to a discontinuous variable in the situation where a rarely occurring random event is taking place in a particular time, area, volume, etc. under observation. Then the probability that the event will occur exactly 0, 1, 2, ... x times during such observation is given by:

$$\text{Probability} = \frac{e^{-\lambda}\lambda^x}{x!} \tag{93}$$

where λ is the single parameter which determines the Poisson distribution and x can be zero or any positive integer, however large. An example encountered in clinical biochemistry is radioactive disintegration where the probability that any particular nuclide atom will disintegrate during the observation period is small but the actual number of disintegrations x occurring during successive equal time periods is likely to vary. It does so according to the Poisson distribution.

A feature of such a distribution is that the mean value of x is λ and that the variance of x is also λ. It is usually necessary to estimate λ from the observational data. Thus from n observational periods the mean value of x can be found and set equal to λ and this will also be the variance of x. Although special tables are available to give the exact probability values determined by the Poisson expression **(93)** it is fortunate that if $n\bar{x}$ is greater than 30 or so then the distribution approximates to a normal one and familiar significance tests can be employed. Thus as the variance of $\bar{x}$ is also $\bar{x}$ the SD is $\sqrt{\bar{x}}$ and

$$\text{SE of } \bar{x} = \sqrt{\bar{x}/n} \tag{94}$$

Example 32. The count rate of a radioactive solution was found on one measurement only to be 400 counts/min. Thus we estimate

$$\bar{x} = 400 \qquad \text{SE of } \bar{x} = \sqrt{400/1} = 20$$

and as $n\bar{x} = 400$ the distribution will be normal and the 95 % CL of the count rate will be calculated as usual as $\pm 1.96 \times$ SE.

Thus

$$95\% \text{ CL} = 400 \pm (1.96 \times 20) \quad \text{or} \quad 361 \text{ to } 439 \text{ counts/min.}$$

In a similar way the difference between two values of $\bar{x}$ can be calculated in the same way as (**43**) as follows:

$$c = |\bar{x}_1 - \bar{x}_2|/\sqrt{\bar{x}_1/n_1 + \bar{x}_2/n_2} \tag{95}$$

and the CL will be given by:

$$\text{CL} = |\bar{x}_1 - \bar{x}_2| \pm c\sqrt{\bar{x}_1/n_1 + \bar{x}_2/n_2} \tag{96}$$

where c is selected from Table 10.1 (p. 242) for CL of 100 $(1 - 2\alpha)\%$.

Example 33. A radioactive solution was counted for four successive one minute periods followed by four successive measurements of the counter background for one minute each. The results have to be analysed to see if the count rate is significantly greater than background.

$$\text{Solution counts } (x_1) = 80, 72, 76, 64 \qquad \bar{x}_1 = 73.00$$
$$\text{Background counts } (x_2) = 60, 58, 66, 56 \qquad \bar{x}_2 = 60.00$$

Hence from (**95**)

$$c = 73.00 - 60.00/\sqrt{73/4 + 60/4} = 2.254$$

Thus $0.01 < P < 0.025$ and the difference is significant. The actual increase above background has 95 % CL calculated using $c = 1.96$ as

$$95\% \text{ CL} = 73 - 60 \pm 1.96\sqrt{73/4 + 60/4} = 13.00 \pm 11.30$$

That is, we are 95 % certain that the count rate is between 1.7 and 24.3 counts/min above background!

Further examples of the use of Poisson statistics appear on pp. 215 to 216.

Calculation of the Cumulative Effect of Several Errors

Most analytical methods involve a number of different steps each with its own error, e.g. the measurement of sample, standard, and reagent volumes. In calculating the final answer, the results from separate measurements each with its own error have to be combined in some way. It is sometimes instructive to study the relative importance of the various individual errors in their contribution to the total final error of the measurement. Two different methods of error combination arise. In the first case the total error produced by adding or subtracting two measurements each with its own error is required but in the second case one measurement is either multiplied or divided by the second. In many cases both types of error combination will be present.

In the first case we can consider the two readings as means obtained from replicates. If these are $\bar{x}_A$ and $\bar{x}_B$ with variances s_A^2, s_B^2 and number of replicates n_A, n_B, then as indicated in (**42**),

$$\text{SE of } (\bar{x}_A + \bar{x}_B) \quad \text{or} \quad (\bar{x}_A - \bar{x}_B) = \sqrt{s_A^2/n_A + s_B^2/n_B}$$

In the case of multiplication or division it is percentage errors of the means expressed as CV which have to be combined rather than absolute SEs as before. Then if $\bar{x}_A$, $\bar{x}_B$ are the two means and CV_A and CV_B are the CVs of the means:

$$\text{CV of } (\bar{x}_A \times \bar{x}_B) \quad \text{or} \quad (\bar{x}_A / \bar{x}_B) = \sqrt{CV_A^2 + CV_B^2} \tag{97}$$

Both types of calculation require that the replicates be compatible with a normal distribution although this may be basically a binomial or Poisson distribution with sufficient observations to normalise the distribution. If necessary, transformation of the data (p. 235) should be done. An example of both types of error calculation in combination is the determination of the concentration of an analyte in a test sample from a knowledge of the concentration of a standard and the colorimeter readings for the test sample (T), the reagent blank (B), the standard (S) and the standard blank (SB) as discussed on p. 145. The appropriate formula for the calculation is

$$\text{Concentration of test} = \text{concentration of standard} \times \frac{(T - B)}{(S - SB)}$$

Whichever type of error combination is used it follows from the above formulae that if one CV or SE is very much less than the other, the total error (CV or SE) is very little different from the larger CV or SE. If the smaller error is less than one-third of the larger then the total error is increased by less than 5% over the larger error. There is therefore little point in devoting much attention to the relatively small errors until the major errors have been improved.

Example 34. The following figures for absorbance were obtained in measuring the plasma glucose concentration using a standard of 10 mmol/l

	Absorbance × 1000	Mean	Variance	SD
Plasma (T)	120, 123, 127, 124	123·500	8·333 33	2·886 8
Reagent blank (B)	8, 5, 6	6·333	2·333 33	1·527 5
Standard (S)	605, 608, 604	605·667	4·333 33	2·081 7
Standard blank (SB)	1, 2	1·500	0·500 00	0·707 1

Then

$$(T - B) = 117 \cdot 167 \qquad SE = \sqrt{\frac{8 \cdot 3}{4} + \frac{2 \cdot 3}{3}} = 1 \cdot 691 \, 5 \qquad CV = 1 \cdot 443 \, 7\% \text{ from } (42)$$

and

$$(S - SB) = 604 \cdot 167 \qquad SE = \sqrt{\frac{4 \cdot 3}{3} + \frac{0 \cdot 5}{2}} = 1 \cdot 301 \, 8 \qquad CV = 0 \cdot 215 \, 5\% \text{ from } (42)$$

thus

$$\text{CV of } \frac{(T - B)}{(S - SB)} = \sqrt{1 \cdot 443 \, 7^2 + 0 \cdot 215 \, 5^2} = 1 \cdot 459 \, 6 \qquad \text{from } (97)$$

$$\text{and mean ratio} = 0 \cdot 193 \, 93$$

and the ratio is expressed with its SE as $0 \cdot 193 \, 93 \pm 0 \cdot 002 \, 83$ (SE), calculating SE as CV × mean ratio/100. Assuming that the error in making up the standard can be ignored, then

$$\text{Plasma glucose} = 1 \cdot 94 \pm 0 \cdot 03 \text{ (SE)}$$

Several points in the example are worthy of comment. The SEs of $(T - B)$ and $(S - SB)$ are of similar magnitude and are less than the SD of T or S as expected as they indicate the variability of the mean figures whereas the SDs indicate the variability of the individual readings. In the case of this plasma with a low glucose the CV of the corrected test sample is almost 7 times greater than that of the corrected standard and the latter error contributes little to the total CV. The error in making up the standard has been ignored. This is justified if the CV is less than one-third of 1·460, the total CV of the ratio. If this is not the case, the CV of the standard must be combined with that of the ratio according to (97) to give the total CV, convertible to the SE if needed. Finally, if only one reading for T, B, S, SB was made, selection of single readings from the above list would give a test sample concentration of 1·85 to 2·03 mmol/1, a considerably wider range than that found from the replicate measurements and the total error as would be expected.

REFERENCES AND FURTHER READING

Shorter simpler texts recommended for further reading are indicated by*.

Altman D. G., Bland J. M. (1983). *The Statistician*; **32**: 307.

*Bailey N. T. J. ed. (1981). *Statistical Methods in Biology*, 2nd ed. London: Unibooks.

Cornbleet P. J., Gochman N. (1979). *Clin. Chem*; **25**: 432.

Creasy M. A. (1956). *J. Roy. Statist. Soc*; Sect. B, **18**: 65.

Davies O. L., Goldsmith P. L. eds. (1972). *Statistical Methods in Research and Production*, 4th ed. p. 209. Edinburgh: Oliver and Boyd.

Deming W. E. (1943). *The Statistical Adjustment of Data*. New York: John Wiley & Sons.

Documenta Geigy (1982). *Scientific Tables*, 8th ed., Vol. 2. Basle: Ciba-Geigy.

Fisher R. A., Yates F. (1963). *Statistical Tables for Biological, Agricultural and Medical Research*, 6th ed. Edinburgh: Oliver and Boyd.

*Lindley D. V., Scott W. F. (1984). *New Cambridge Elementary Statistical Tables*. Cambridge: Cambridge University Press.

Mandel J. (1964). *The Statistical Analysis of Experimental Data*. pp. 288–292. New York: John Wiley & Sons.

*Moroney M. J. (1972). *Facts from Figures*, 2nd ed. Harmondsworth: Penguin Books.

Pearson E. S., Hartley H. O. (1966). *Biometrika Tables for Statisticians, Vol.* 1, 3rd ed. Cambridge: Cambridge University Press.

*Siegel S. (1956). *Nonparametric Statistics for the Behavioural Sciences*, International Student Edition. London, Tokyo, etc: McGraw Hill Kogakusha Ltd.

*Sprent P. (1977). *Statistics in Action*. Harmondsworth: Penguin Books.

11

THE 'NORMAL RANGE'
REFERENCE VALUES

It was customary to quote 'normal' ranges for the concentration of constituents in body fluids to indicate the values found in persons who are in good health and, by inference, to define results which indicate that some abnormality is present. The term 'normal' is ambiguous as it may be used to mean healthy, but also ideal, habitually found, or distributed in a Gaussian fashion. There are also difficulties in deciding when a result indicates abnormality. Some results may be excluded from the normal range because they are at the limit of the observed range. False reasoning then implies that 'normals' are those free from disease, but the presence of disease is deduced by difference from 'normals'. The changes in many constituents with increasing age are also difficult to reconcile with the concept of 'normal' as there is an increasing chance of death (i.e. abnormality) in elderly subjects. In many, the changes may antedate death for some time, even though the individual appears to be in 'normal' health for an old person. Finally, the 'normal' range concept carries the implication that results outside it are 'abnormal' and potentially harmful despite the convention that the normal range includes only 95% of normal people. These difficulties in defining a normal range in a useful way have led to the concept of *reference values* (Gräsbeck *et al.*, 1978). This is the first of several reports of the International Federation of Clinical Chemistry's Expert Panel on the Theory of Reference Values (EP-TRV).

Reference values are the values of a particular quantity obtained from individuals in defined states of health. The observed value obtained by measuring this quantity on material obtained from a particular individual under study is compared with the reference values for interpretative purposes. Reference values include *all* results from individuals in the defined state. The criteria used for the selection of these individuals must be stated together with the specimen collection conditions (EP-TRV, 1984b). Thus data reported should include information on whether the screening procedure for the state of health was subjective or objective, details of sex, age, race, posture, fasting, time of day, exercise, menstrual cycle etc., whether a tourniquet was used and for how long, treatment of specimen following collection, analytical method used and its performance. Martin *et al.* (1975a) give a useful review of early work on some of these variables. For geriatric populations it has been suggested that only individuals surviving for a stated period after sampling should be included. If the total data are subjected to statistical treatment to exclude results at one or both ends of the reference range, e.g. between the 2·5th and 97·5th percentiles, the appropriate term is a *reference interval* but the statistical procedure should be stated and if a parametric method is used, e.g. mean ± 2 standard deviations, it should be justified (EP-TRV, 1983; 1984a). It is also possible to define *individual reference values* for repeated measurements on a particular individual.

This concept does not lack clarity but the formidable tasks in assembling suitable reference values are only just being tackled. However, much work has been done in defining the relative importance of various factors which determine the reference values. It is clear that the appropriate reference values for an ambulant, apparently healthy person may well differ from those for a hospital patient confined to bed and under treatment with various drugs. Alström *et al.* (1975) have described standardised conditions for collection of specimens for the two reference values.

INTRA-INDIVIDUAL AND INTER-INDIVIDUAL VARIATION

If a time series of measurements is made on an individual, the range of results for some analytes covers a relatively narrow part of the reference interval. The total observed variance (s_{P1}^2) is the sum of the intra-individual variance (s_P^2) due to biological variations in the individual and the analytical variance (s_A^2) which includes both within-day and day-to-day components. Thus, $s_{P1}^2 = s_P^2 + s_A^2$.

Knowledge of the intra-individual variation is required to evaluate changes in serial results from patients, to judge the usefulness of conventional reference intervals and to set desirable standards of analytical performance. Several approaches have been used to obtain this information (see e.g. Pickup *et al.*, 1977 and Cotlove *et al.*, 1970). The intra-individual variance obtained in such studies depends not only on the population of individuals observed and the analytical procedures used, but also on the time intervals between successive measurements (Harris and Yasaka, 1983). Despite this, several studies have yielded similar results for the average intra-individual variation for commonly determined plasma constituents (Table 11.1). An investigation of the biological variation of analytes in urine has also been undertaken (Shepherd *et al.*, 1981).

TABLE 11.1
Average Intra-Individual Variation of Plasma Constituents. (After Pickup et al., 1977)

Constituent	Average CV (%)
Sodium	0·5–1·4
Calcium	1·1–1·7
Total protein	2·0–3·0
Albumin	2·8–3·8
Potassium	3·2–6·2
Creatinine	4·2–4·4
Alkaline phosphatase	4·8–10·1
Inorganic phosphate	5·8–9·6
Urea	11·1–14·2
Bilirubin	22·0–26·0

The size of s_P relative to s_A is important in deciding whether changes in the observed readings for an individual are attributable to real biological change or to laboratory error. For several substances s_A is greater than s_P, namely magnesium, creatinine, thyroxine and LD. For others, s_A is greater than half s_P producing an 11 to 40% increase of $s_{P'}$ over s_P; such substances include albumin, alkaline phosphatase, AST, bilirubin, calcium, creatinine and sodium. Knowledge of the average intra-individual variance should help to decide whether an observed change in consecutive results is likely to arise solely from normal biological variation. This would be particularly useful if it could be applied to the results from patients who are ill. Fraser *et al.* (1982, 1983) have shown that for a number of plasma constituents, the average intra-individual variation found in patients with myocardial infarction or renal disease is similar to that found in healthy adults.

Use of the average intra-individual variance overlooks the differing intra-individual variation among the individuals of the same reference group over the same length of time. The population of intra-individual variances describes an approximately log-normal distribution for some analytes. Once such a distribution has been defined for a reference group, it would be possible to state the probability of an observed change in serial results being due to biological variation alone. For specific clinical needs, a *reference change* could be defined as the difference between two consecutive test results in an individual that is statistically significant in a given proportion of similar persons (Harris and Yasaka, 1983).

The reference values for the whole group of individuals will depend on the apparent group variance $(s_{G'}^2)$ which is a sum of separate variances as before.

$$s_{G'}^2 = s_G^2 + s_P^2 + s_A^2$$

where s_G^2 is the inter-individual variance describing the variability of the 'true' means of the different individuals in the group. The ratio $R = s_P/s_G$ has been used by Harris (1974, 1975) to assess the appropriateness of group reference values for interpreting changes in measurements on an individual. If $R < 0.6$ the usual reference interval will almost always be insensitive to significant alterations of an individual's results. As R increases the likelihood of the individual's results lying outside the reference interval when significant change has occurred increases until when $R = 1.4$ the reference interval and the average individual reference interval give identical information.

Those substances which have an R value less than 0.6, and are therefore very 'individual' to a particular person, are alkaline phosphatase, cholesterol, cortisol, creatinine, GGT, IgG, IgA, IgM, complement fraction C3 and several other specific serum proteins, thyroxine, triglycerides and urate. Values of R between 0.6 and 1.0 are seen for ALT, AST, bilirubin, glucose, LD, magnesium, phosphate, total protein, and urea. Substances with R values between 1.0 and 1.4 include albumin, calcium, chloride, CK and potassium, while R for sodium exceeds 1.4 (Butts *et al.*, 1977; Harris, 1974; Pickup *et al.*, 1977; Statland *et al.*, 1976; Williams *et al.*, 1978).

For those substances for which the group reference interval is insensitive, the detection of significant individual change does not seem to be improved by taking reference ranges from sub-groups divided by age and sex (Butts *et al.*, 1977; Williams *et al.*, 1978). If early detection of abnormality is to be made in an individual, repeated readings over a period of time will be needed to define the individual reference interval but this will be impracticable for most members of the population. More marked changes might be expected with more obvious disease and then the group or sub-group reference intervals would be more appropriate for the detection of an individual change.

FACTORS AFFECTING REFERENCE VALUES

In addition to errors of instrumental analysis several factors have been shown to affect reference values. Often several of these are acting simultaneously and carefully designed experimental protocols are required, followed by analysis of variance (p. 253), before their relative importance can be assessed. Earlier work in this field has been summarised by Martin *et al.* (1975a).

There is reasonable agreement between different authors regarding the effects of age and sex (Table 11.2). Although statistically significant, some of the differences are relatively small in clinical terms. The effects of body weight are usually less important but a positive correlation has been found for alkaline phosphatase and CK and for ALT (mainly males) and AST (Goldberg and Winfield, 1974; Siest *et al.*, 1975) for GGT (Schiele *et al.*, 1977) and for urate (Goldberg *et al.*, 1973). The effects of smoking, blood pressure and social class have usually been small when investigated (see the last four authors).

TABLE 11.2

The Effect of Sex and Age on Various Plasma Constituents

Constituent	Sex Difference	Effect of Increasing Age
Albumin	M > F	Falls
Alkaline phosphatase	M > F (adults)	Marked rise in puberty, adult levels when growth ceases. Rises in adults; especially in F after menopause.
ALT	M > F	Varies in different reports.
AST	M > F	Falls to minimum at 30; later rise, especially F.
Bilirubin	M > F	Little change apart from post-menopausal rise.
Calcium	M > F	Falls, especially M.
Cholesterol	M > F	Rises, especially in post-menopausal F.
CK	M > F	Falls in M; rises in F.
Creatinine	M > F	Slight rise.
Glucose	M > F	Rises.
GGT	M > F	Falls in M; rises in F.
HBD	None	Rises in F.
Iron	M > F	Falls.
β-Lipoproteins	M > F	Little change.
Magnesium	M > F	Rises, especially F.
5′-Nucleotidase	None	Rises in F.
Phosphate	F > M	Little change apart from post-menopausal rise.
Potassium	None	Rises.
Sodium	None	Rises, especially F at menopause.
Thyroxine	F > M	Little change.
Total proteins	M > F	Little change.
Triglycerides	M > F	Rises.
Urate	M > F	Rises in F; steady or falls in M.
Urea	M > F	Rises.

See especially: Goldberg *et al.* (1973); Goldberg and Winfield (1974); Roberts (1967); Wilding *et al.* (1972); Williams *et al.* (1978). Also: Penttilä *et al.* (1975); Schiele *et al.* (1977); Siest *et al.* (1975).

The effect of variations in the state of the subject and the method of blood collection may be more important. Careful studies by Bokelund *et al.* (1974) showed significant differences in results attributable to the collection of specimens, centrifugation, separation and storage. Those most affected were sodium, potassium, and protein-bound substances such as AST, ALT, bilirubin, iron, LD and total lipids. The effect of venous occlusion by tourniquet (Statland *et al.*, 1974) even for periods as short as 3 min is significant. The percentage changes for affected constituents were potassium (-6), AST ($+9$), bilirubin ($+8$), cholesterol ($+5$), iron ($+7$), total lipids ($+5$), total protein ($+5$), while albumin and alkaline phosphatase showed smaller increases. The changes can be rapid, occurring within 40 s of occluding the vein and this has led Alström *et al.* (1975) to recommend that the tourniquet should be avoided if possible. Preparation of the patient to avoid the stress of venepuncture is recommended for the collection of several analytes including ACTH, cortisol, human growth hormone and prolactin.

Changes in posture are also important factors. Statland *et al.* (1974) found percentage changes for this factor when isolated from analytical, tourniquet, and diurnal effects to be significant. After lying supine for 30 min the main effects (as percentage change) were for acid phosphatase (-6), albumin (-7), AST (-12), calcium (-5), potassium (-5) and total protein (-7). Such changes are in relation to samples taken with the subject seated for 15 min. If the subject stands for 30 min, the changes are less marked and in the opposite direction: albumin ($+3$), alkaline phosphatase ($+5$), cholesterol ($+4$), phosphate ($+3$), total lipids ($+5$), total protein ($+2$).

Mild exercise produces significant changes in albumin, ALT, calcium, creatinine, glucose, phosphate, potassium, total protein, urate and urea (Galteau *et al.*, 1974; Statland *et al.*, 1973b). The taking of a meal also produces significant changes in alkaline phosphatase, iron, LD, phosphate, sodium, total lipids and urate (Statland *et al.*, 1973b).

The diet has a significant effect on the plasma levels of glucose, lipoproteins, urea, urate and protein while less marked effects on the concentrations of LD, alkaline phosphatase, and growth hormone have been recorded. Racial differences in plasma lipids are largely due to preferences in the habitual diet.

Many biochemical changes occur during pregnancy. These include increases in the plasma concentration of alkaline phosphatase, thyroxine-binding globulin, ceruloplasmin, transferrin, cholesterol, triglycerides and a number of hormones. Decreases in the concentration of albumin, urea and osmolality also occur. These changes can lead to diagnostic confusion if not understood and may warrant the use of separate reference intervals during pregnancy.

While variations in sampling procedures are an important fraction of the total intra-individual variation, other short term and long term variations occur without changes in the health of the subject. Changes occurring within the hour are probably attributable to tourniquet variations (Winkel *et al.*, 1974) but changes over 6 h (diurnal variations) are well-documented for acid phosphatase, albumin, bilirubin, chloride, cortisol, iron, lipids, sodium, phosphate, potassium, total protein and urea (Roberts, 1967; Statland *et al.*, 1973a; Winkel *et al.*, 1975). Changes over a few months for samples taken at the same time of day having excluded analytical variation are also significant for most constituents investigated with the possible exception of albumin, calcium and sodium (Williams *et al.*, 1970; Winkel *et al.*, 1974, 1975; Young *et al.*, 1971). This between-day variability is usually greater than within-day variation but its origin is uncertain. It may represent dietary or climatic changes or be attributable to biological rhythms of longer duration.

Genetic factors are difficult to demonstrate in the face of these other variables but Havlik *et al.* (1977), studying 11 plasma constituents in monozygotic and dizygotic twins, found that genetic factors were important for bilirubin, glucose (1 h post-prandial), urate and urea. Reference values for some analytes may differ among ethnic groups. The influence of different socio-economic conditions may be difficult to separate from that due to racial, genetic factors. A study of three ethnic groups in England showed that total serum amylase activity is significantly different in Britons, Asians and West Indians (Tsianos *et al.*, 1982).

The relative importance of the various factors determining the reference values of a few enzymes has been studied in some detail. For the transaminases, ALT and AST, see Goldberg and Winfield (1974) and Siest *et al.* (1975) and for GGT see Schiele *et al.* (1977). The changes in childhood and later life for alkaline phosphatase have been reported for an optimised *p*-nitrophenyl-phosphate method at 30 °C (Fleisher *et al.*, 1977) or at 37 °C (Penttilä *et al.*, 1975) and for the Kind and King phenylphosphate method at 37 °C (Round, 1973).

POPULATIONS STUDIED IN DERIVING REFERENCE VALUES

There has been no uniformity in the choice of population on which measurements should be made. In order to obtain reasonably large numbers so that the sub-groups divided by age and sex can have sufficient members, blood donors have been selected as they have already passed a limited health screen (Flynn *et al.*, 1974; Roberts, 1967). Others have used small numbers of young healthy adults, carefully selected, in order to study the factors influencing the reference values (see the studies of Bokelund, Statland, Winkel and colleagues quoted in the last section), or results from many laboratories each of whom has studied about 20 selected healthy volunteers may be combined (Schauble *et al.*, 1977). Several studies have used people attending well-population screening clinics (Goldberg *et al.*, 1973; Goldberg and Winfield, 1974; Hohnadel, 1972; Schiele *et al.*, 1977; Siest *et al.*, 1975; Wilding *et al.*, 1972; Williams *et al.*, 1970, 1978). Depending on the conditions attached to attendance the population studied may be biased by social class but there is reasonably good agreement between the results of different studies and those of blood donors.

Most hospital laboratories find it difficult to obtain sufficient specimens from 'healthy' people but handle large numbers of samples from hospital in-patients and out-patients. Many of the results fall within the conventional 'normal' ranges and attempts have been made to use such data in order to define reference values which might be more appropriate for hospital patients as their posture, diet, collection of specimens and their later handling, may all differ appreciably from those of ambulant, apparently healthy persons. Thus Payne and Levell (1968) discussed the non-specific effects of illness on serum sodium in the majority of hospital patients who showed a wider range and lower mean than healthy ambulant volunteers. The crude data from the whole range of hospital patients must contain an unknown proportion of abnormal results which form other populations superimposed on a central major population representing the 'usual' hospital patient for which reference values might be useful. These other populations may be found at either or both ends of the 'usual' population (Fig. 11.1) and their mean and scatter are uncertain. Sometimes the presence of a second population to the right of the 'usual' mean will merely be visible as a skew distribution (Fig. 11.2). Various statistical methods have been proposed to dissect the 'usual' from other 'abnormal' distributions.

The application of such methods to crude hospital data (Hofmann, 1963) often results in reference intervals which are wider than those found on 'healthy' populations (Amador and Hsi, 1969). It is possible that more careful selection of a sub-group of hospital patients will give more satisfactory results. Exclusion may be based on the appearance of the specimen, abnormal results for other biochemical investigations or the reason for the referral of the patient.

Cord blood specimens have been used in an attempt to overcome the considerable difficulties in establishing reference intervals for neonates. There are

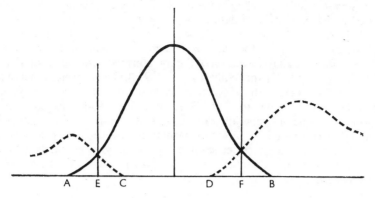

Fig. 11.1. Mixed Population of Hospital Patients.

The continuous line represents the 'usual' hospital patients for whom the reference values vary from A to B. The reference interval has been selected as from E to F. Two abnormal populations are also present, shown by the broken lines. They include individuals whose results may be as high as C or as low as D; those between E and C, and between D and F fall inside the reference interval.

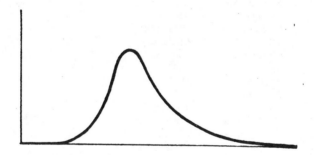

Fig. 11.2. Positively Skewed Distribution Curve.

This could arise if the major 'usual' population is normally distributed and is contaminated with a smaller population having abnormally high results.

shortcomings to this approach since cord blood is a mixture of arterial and venous blood, and the concentration of some analytes changes in the few days following delivery.

Statistical Methods

When apparently healthy populations have been selected, the results for certain substances are not distributed in a Gaussian fashion although others are. Opinion is divided as to whether to apply a transformation (p. 235) so that the distribution curve will become Gaussian thereby allowing the more efficient parametric methods to be used to define a reference interval or whether to apply the simpler but less efficient non-parametric methods, making no assumption as to the form of the distribution.

There is moderately good agreement as to which variables are normally distributed and which approximate to a log-normal, positively skewed distribution (Table 11.3). Martin *et al.* (1975b) describe many transformations for normalising data and prefer the parametric method of defining a 95 % range by the mean ± 1·96 × standard deviation of the transformed variables as do Flynn *et al.* (1974), Hohnadel (1972) and Williams *et al.* (1978). Others prefer to use a non-parametric method, taking the 95 % reference interval as that lying between the 2·5th and 97·5th percentiles (p. 239). Reed and Wu (1974) used a computer simulation technique to generate random results from various distribution shapes and then compared various transformation-parametric methods with the percentile method for the generated sample. Only with symmetrical distributions did the former have any advantage; for some distributions the non-parametric method was clearly preferable.

TABLE 11.3

Distributions of Different Substances in Plasma in Apparently Healthy Subjects. (Names in brackets indicate some uncertainty in the literature)

Gaussian (Normal)	Log normal or positively skewed
Albumin	(Alkaline phosphatase)
Bicarbonate	ALT
Calcium	AST
Chloride	(Bilirubin)
CK	Cholesterol
(Creatinine)	(Glucose)
Magnesium	GGT
Phosphate	Iron
Potassium	(LD)
Sodium	Total lipids
Total protein	Triglycerides
	(Urate)
	(Urea)

The calculation of reference intervals from data which include values below the minimum detectable value presents a problem. Two methods have been used to overcome this difficulty. The 'undetectable' observations may be allotted a value midway between zero and the minimum detectable value. Alternatively, the latter may be used to represent all 'undetectable' readings. In both cases the lower limit of the reference interval is taken to be zero or is regarded as approximate. The maximum-likelihood estimation method has been proposed as a more appropriate statistical method for the determination of reference intervals with such data (Tsay *et al.*, 1979). Using this method for TSH assays, they were able to calculate a lower limit for the reference interval containing 95% of the population and could predict the percentage of 'undetectable' results lying within this interval.

If reference intervals are calculated from a mixed population, the various sub-populations must be removed to allow the main 'normal' population to be examined. Martin *et al.* (1975c) discuss various graphical and numerical methods which purport to achieve this. Hofmann (1963) used a graphical method by plotting cumulative frequencies on probability paper (p. 242). The best straight line fit to the majority of the points defined a central Gaussian distribution and permitted removal of results distorting the curve. Successive approximations to the straight line plot were made after such removal and were believed to isolate the central normal distribution. The approach has met with criticism and is not generally accepted (Amador and Hsi, 1969; Elveback, 1972). It may be more reliable when the contaminating populations are small. A more sophisticated graphical method, proposed by Bhattacharya (1967), has been applied by Gindler (1970) to resolve three overlapping Gaussian distributions with rather greater success.

Numerical methods have been used when the contaminating population produces a skewed distribution with an obvious tail at one side only. It is then possible to truncate the distribution by removing the distorting tail and to use numerical methods to reconstitute the theoretical normal distribution curve (see Bliss, 1967). The method works reasonably well if there is only one contaminating population which is not large and has a reasonable separation from the main population. A somewhat simpler method was proposed by Becktel (1970) and has been investigated for clinical biochemical use with moderate success by Best et al. (1970).

These methods imply that the central distribution is Gaussian but as Table 11.3 indicates this assumption is not always warranted. In such cases it may be possible to work with logarithms of the original figures but this transformation may not be valid if the nature of the central distribution in a mixed population is not known *a priori*.

Multi-variate 'Normality'

Often a battery of biochemical tests is performed on hospital patients or on persons attending a well-population screening clinic. The results are then examined for evidence of 'abnormality'. If the various substances measured change independently in disease, then for each one the probability of a result falling within the conventional reference interval is 0·95 and of falling outside 0·05. If n different substances are investigated then the incidence of $0, 1, 2, \ldots n$ results falling outside the appropriate reference interval will be described by the binomial distribution (p. 267) according to the formula $(0·95 + 0·05)^n$. Thus for 12 substances it can easily be calculated that the probabilities of obtaining 0, 1, 2, and 3, 'abnormal' results are 0·540, 0·341, 0·099 and 0·017 (see Sunderman, 1970). Thus nearly half a group of healthy subjects would be expected to produce one or more 'abnormal' results.

Various suggestions have been made to overcome this dilemma. Schoen and Brooks (1970) suggested the use of wider reference intervals chosen so that if P is the probability of one result falling within the reference interval the P should be selected so that P^n, which defines the probability of *all* results being within the reference interval, should equal 0·95. For 12 tests this implies the use of a 99.5 % reference interval. Grams et al. (1972) have used a different approach requiring computer facilities. If two variables are plotted on the x and y axes, the two reference intervals will define a rectangular area in which the 'normal' results might be expected to lie. Examination of the actual results from healthy subjects will usually show that these form a circular or elliptical grouping and methods are available to define the area in the two-dimensional plot which encompasses 95 % of all results. The process can be extended to three or more dimensions, so that eventually any result can be imagined as plotted in n-dimensional 'space' in order to be compared with the cluster of results which defines the location of 95 % (or any selected figure) of results from healthy subjects. The distance of the patient's point in *n*-dimensional space from the edge of the 95 % region can be calculated and used as an index of 'normality' or 'abnormality' of the patient's multiple test profile. Such statistical analysis can sensitively detect minor multiple abnormalities in the profile but may be insensitive to one very abnormal result (Boyd and Lacher, 1982).

The Diagnostic Use of Reference Intervals

It is usual to use the reference interval in the same way as the normal range was used in order to decide whether the result from an individual indicates the presence of some abnormality, e.g. a disease process. Reference to the right hand side of Fig. 11.1 (p. 279) indicates the problem of deciding whether the observed value belongs to the reference population or the diseased population shown by the broken line. The further the reference interval is terminated to the right the fewer members of the reference population will be beyond it but this will be at the expense of including more members of the diseased population within the reference interval. The position of the end of the reference interval has been given such names as *discrimination value* (Sunderman, 1975), decisive, critical, border-line or cut-off value, screening level and operating position. If a result falling beyond the discrimination value is described as 'positive', and one falling within the reference interval is 'negative', then the positive results can be divided into 'true positives' in which the disease is found to be present, and the 'false positives' in which no disease can be demonstrated. Similarly, there will be 'true negatives' in which the disease is absent and 'false negatives' in which the disease is present.

In an ideal situation the selected discrimination value should result in no false positives or false negatives but this is rarely encountered in practice. Some method is needed whereby the discrimination value is chosen to optimise the detection of patients with a disease and the exclusion of subjects without it. This is the province of Bayesian statistics and six basic facts must be known before the selection can be made:

1. The disease sought must be clearly defined using criteria other than the result of the test under consideration.
2. The stage of the disease process being sought should be defined.
3. The prevalence of the disease at this stage or beyond in the population studied should be known. This will differ for the hospital patient population and a supposedly healthy general population.
4. The clinical *sensitivity* of the test must be known. This is the incidence of true positive results in persons with the defined disease. It is calculated by dividing the number of true positives by the sum of the true positives and the false negatives.
5. The clinical *specificity* of the test must be known. This is the incidence of true negative results in persons without the disease and is calculated by dividing the number of true negatives by the sum of the true negatives and the false positives.
6. The clinical consequences and social costs of positive and negative misdiagnoses should be assessed in order to decide what is an acceptable figure for such misdiagnoses.

As an example let us take a disease which has a prevalence of 0·01 (or 1 %) in the population under study, say patients attending their family doctor. If the discrimination value has been selected so that the sensitivity is 0·90 and the specificity is 0·98 (i.e. false positives reduced to 0·02) then the following calculations can be made simply.

(a) Probability that the disease is present when the test is positive.

$$= \frac{\text{True positives in total population}}{\text{Total positives (true and false)}} = \frac{0\cdot01 \times 0\cdot90}{0\cdot01 \times 0\cdot90 + 0\cdot99\,(1 - 0\cdot98)} = 0\cdot313.$$

(b) Probability that the disease is absent when the test is negative.

$$= \frac{\text{True negatives in total population}}{\text{Total negatives (true and false)}} = \frac{0\cdot99 \times 0\cdot98}{0\cdot99 \times 0\cdot98 + 0\cdot01 \times (1 - 0\cdot90)}$$
$$= 0\cdot9990.$$

If the same conditions were used for a population with a disease incidence of 10% (0·10) as might happen for a selected hospital in-patient group, the two probabilities become 0·833 and 0·9888 but if a healthy population is being screened the disease incidence may only be 0·002 and the two probabilities then become 0·083 and 0·9998.

The same discrimination value has very different interpretations depending on the disease incidence. Whether any of the above outcomes is acceptable will depend on criterion (6) above. Changing the discrimination value will alter the sensitivity and specificity but the same type of calculation can again be done. The best compromise will depend on all factors under consideration.

For further accounts of this approach see Martin *et al.* (1975d), McNeil *et al.* (1975), Schwartz *et al.* (1973), Sunderman and van Soestbergen (1971) and Galen and Gambino (1975).

REFERENCES

Alström T., Gräsbeck R., Hjelm M., Skandsen S. (1975). *Scand. J. Clin. Lab. Invest*; **35**, Suppl. **144**: 3.
Amador E., Hsi B. P. (1969). *Amer. J. Clin. Path*; **52**: 538.
Becktel J. M. (1970). *Clin. Chim. Acta*; **28**: 119.
Best W. R., Mason C. C., Barron S. S., Shepherd H. G. (1970). *Clin. Chim. Acta*; **28**: 127.
Bhattacharya C. G. (1967). *Biometrics*; **23**: 115.
Bliss C. I. (1967). *Statistics in Biology*, Vol. 1, Chap. 7. New York: McGraw-Hill.
Bokelund H., Winkel P., Statland B. E. (1974). *Clin. Chem*; **20**: 1507.
Boyd J. C., Lacher D. A. (1982). *Clin. Chem*; **28**: 1735.
Butts W. C., James G. E., Keuhnemann M. (1977). *Clin. Chem*; **23**: 511.
Cotlove E., Harris E. K., Williams G. Z. (1970). *Clin. Chem*; **16**: 1028.
Elveback L. (1972). In *Clinically Orientated Documentation of Laboratory Data* (Gabrieli E. R. ed.) p. 117. London and New York: Academic Press.
EP-TRV. (1983). *Clin. Chim. Acta*; **127**: 441 F.
EP-TRV. (1984 a, b). *Clin. Chim. Acta*; **137**: 97 F; **139**: 205 F.
Fleisher G. A., Eickelberg E. S., Elveback L. R. (1977). *Clin. Chem*; **23**: 469.
Flynn F. V. *et al.* (1974). *Clin. Chim. Acta*; **52**: 163.
Fraser C. G., Hearne C. R. (1982). *Ann. Clin. Biochem*; **19**: 431.
Fraser C. G., Williams P. (1983). *Clin. Chem*; **29**: 508.
Galen R. S., Gambino S. R. (1975). *Beyond Normality: The Predictive Value and Efficiency of Medical Diagnosis*. New York: Wiley and Sons.
Galteau M. M., Siest G., Boura M. (1974). *Clin. Chim. Acta*; **55**: 353.
Gindler E. M. (1970). *Clin. Chem*; **16**: 124.
Goldberg D. M., Handyside A. J., Winfield D. A. (1973). *Clin. Chem*; **19**: 395.

Goldberg D. M., Winfield D. A. (1974). *Clin. Chim. Acta*; **54**: 357.

Grams R. R., Johnson E. A., Benson E. S. (1972). *Amer. J. Clin. Path*; **58**: 188.

Gräsbeck R. *et al.* (1978). *Clin. Chim. Acta*; **87**: 459 F.

Harris E. K. (1974). *Clin. Chem*; **20**: 1535.

Harris E. K. (1975). *Clin. Chem*; **21**: 1457.

Harris E. K., Yasaka T. (1983). *Clin. Chem*; **29**: 25.

Havlik R., Garrison R., Fabsitz R., Feinleib M. (1977). *Clin. Chem*; **23**: 659.

Hofmann R. G. (1963). *J. Amer. Med. Ass*; **185**: 864.

Hohnadel D. C. (1972). In *Clinically Orientated Documentation of Laboratory Data*; (Gabrieli E. R. ed.) p. 83. London and New York: Academic Press.

Martin H. F., Gudzinowicz B. J., Fanger H. (1975). In *Normal Values in Clinical Chemistry, A Guide to Statistical Analysis of Laboratory Data*; (a) Chap. 2; (b) Chap. 3; (c) Chap. 5; (d) Chap. 6. New York: Dekker.

McNeil B. J., Keeler E., Adelstein S. J. (1975). *New Eng. J. Med*; **293**: 212.

Payne R. B., Levell M. J. (1968). *Clin. Chem*; **14**: 172.

Penttilä I. M. *et al.* (1975). *Scand. J. Clin. Lab. Invest*; **35**: 275.

Pickup J. F., Harris E. K., Kearns M., Brown S. S. (1977). *Clin. Chem*; **23**: 842.

Reed A. H., Wu G. T. (1974). *Clin. Chem*; **20**: 576.

Roberts L. B. (1967). *Clin. Chim. Acta*; **16**: 69.

Round J. M. (1973). *Brit. Med. J*; **3**: 137.

Schauble M. K., Becktel J. M., Gullick H. D., Kaplow L. S. (1977). *Amer. J. Clin. Path*; **67**: 386.

Schiele F., Guilmin A. M., Detienne H., Siest G. (1977). *Clin. Chem*; **23**: 1023.

Schoen I., Brooks S. H. (1970). *Amer. J. Clin. Path*; **53**: 190.

Schwartz W. B., Gorry G. A., Kassirer J. P., Essig A. (1973). *Amer. J. Med*; **55**: 459.

Shepherd M. D. S., Penberthy L. A., Fraser G. C. (1981). *Clin. Chem*; **27**: 569.

Siest G. *et al.* (1975). *Clin. Chem*; **21**: 1077.

Statland B. E., Bokelund H., Winkel P. (1974). *Clin. Chem*; **20**: 1513.

Statland B. E., Winkel P., Bokelund H. (1973a). *Clin. Chem*; **19**: 1374.

Statland B. E., Winkel P., Bokelund H. (1973b). *Clin. Chem*; **19**: 1380.

Statland B. E., Winkel P., Killingsworth L. M. (1976). *Clin. Chem*; **22**: 1635.

Sunderman F. W. Jr. (1970). *Amer. J. Clin. Path*; **53**: 288.

Sunderman F. W. Jr. (1975). *Clin. Chem*; **21**: 1873.

Sunderman F. W. Jr., van Soestbergen A. A. (1971). *Amer. J. Clin. Path*; **55**: 105.

Tsay Y., Chen I., Maxon H. R., Heminger L. (1979). *Clin. Chem*; **25**: 2011.

Tsianos E. B., Jalali M. T., Gowenlock A. H., Braganza J. M. (1982). *Clin. Chim. Acta*; **124**: 13.

Wilding P., Rollason J. G., Robinson D. (1972). *Clin. Chim. Acta*; **41**: 375.

Williams G. Z., Widdowson G. M., Penton J. (1978). *Clin. Chem*; **24**: 313.

Williams G. Z., Young D. S., Stein M. R., Cotlove E. (1970). *Clin. Chem*; **16**: 1016, 1022, 1028.

Winkel P., Statland B. E., Bokelund H. (1974). *Clin. Chem*; **20**: 1520.

Winkel P., Statland B. E., Bokelund H. (1975). *Amer. J. Clin. Path*; **64**: 433.

Young D. S., Harris E. K., Cotlove E. (1971). *Clin. Chem*; **17**: 403.

12

QUALITY CONTROL

A major role of the clinical biochemistry laboratory is the measurement of substances in body fluids or tissues for the purpose of diagnosis, treatment or prevention of disease, and for the greater understanding of disease processes. Modern medicine increasingly relies on the provision of analytical results and if these are to play their proper role, they must be trustworthy. Experience has shown that all analytical results are subject to errors arising from several sources and it is necessary that these should be minimised. Other laboratory disciplines also produce errors and the problem is one which bedevils all human endeavour. For an account of the errors of clinical examination see Koran (1975).

The International Federation of Clinical Chemistry's Expert Panel on Nomenclature and Principles of Quality Control in Clinical Chemistry (IFCC-EP) has published a series of Recommendations (Büttner et al., 1978, 1979a, b, 1980, 1981a, b). These include a glossary of recommended terms and their definitions. Quality control (QC) in clinical biochemistry is defined (Büttner et al., 1979a) as 'the study of those sources of variation which are the responsibility of the laboratory, and of the procedures used to recognise and minimise them, including all sources (such as random variation and bias) which arise within the laboratory between the receipt of the specimen and the despatch of the report. The responsibility of the laboratory may extend to the collection of the specimen from the patient, and the provision of a suitable container. Crude errors or mistakes (e.g. wrong sample identification, incorrect transcription), although they cannot be controlled by the usual statistical QC methods, are nevertheless the concern of the laboratory.'

The subject involves consideration of a reliable analytical method (Chapter 13, p. 305). Important reliability criteria of the selected method are its accuracy, precision, specificity and sensitivity. The main emphasis of QC is to monitor the precision and accuracy of the performance of analytical methods. Besides being important for patient care, QC is designed to give the laboratory staff confidence in their methods. It is not intended to find scapegoats or to punish mistakes, but should lead to defined actions and responsibilities for remedial action if analytical performance deteriorates.

TERMINOLOGY

In this section the authors have used the IFCC-EP terminology (Büttner et al., 1979a). The basic assumptions on which consideration of QC is based are: concentration and other types of quantity are continuous variables (p. 232); specimen concentrations or other quantities have true values and measurements obtain useful estimates of these; precision and accuracy refer to a set of results obtained under stated conditions, not to single results.

An *analytical method* is a set of instructions which describes the procedure, materials and equipment necessary to obtain a *result*, the final value obtained for a measured quantity. Methods require *calibration*, the process of relating the value indicated on the scale of an instrument or analytical device to the quantity required to be measured. This requires a *standard*, the material or solution with which the sample is compared in order to determine the result. The term *calibration standard* is used if it is necessary to avoid confusion with other meanings of 'standard'. Various types of standard are defined:

Arbitrary standard. Calibration standard containing an unknown quantity of the specified substance. The content is assigned by convention and expressed in arbitrary units, e.g. international biological standards, immunoglobulin standards.

Internal standard. A substance, not normally present in the specimen and clearly distinguishable from the substance to be analysed, which is added in known amount to the sample, or to both the standard and sample, for the purpose of correcting results for inaccuracy.

Primary standard material. Substance of known chemical composition and sufficient purity to be used in preparing a *primary standard solution* in which the concentration is determined solely by dissolving a weighed amount of primary standard material in an appropriate solvent and making up to a stated volume or weight.

Secondary standard solution. Solution used as a calibration standard in which the concentration or other quantity has been determined by an analytical method of stated reliability.

The reliability criteria of an analytical method are defined as:

Accuracy. Agreement between the best estimate of a quantity and its true value. It has no numerical value but this is expressed by the term *inaccuracy*, the numerical difference between the mean of a set of replicate measurements and the true value. This difference (positive or negative) may be expressed in the units in which the quantity is measured, or as a percentage of the true value. Other words synonymous with inaccuracy are *bias* and *systematic error*.

Precision. Agreement between replicate measurements. It has no numerical value but this is expressed by the term *imprecision*, the standard deviation (SD) or coefficient of variation (CV) of the results in a set of replicate measurements. The mean value and number of measurements must be stated, and the design used must be described in such a way that other workers can repeat it. This is particularly important whenever a specific term is used to denote a particular type of imprecision, such as between-laboratory, within-day, or between-day. The phrase *random error* is sometimes used for imprecision.

Specificity. The ability of an analytical method to determine solely the component(s) it purports to measure. It has no numerical value. It is assessed on the evidence available on the components which contribute to the result, and on the extent to which they do. A related term is *interference*, the effect of a component, which does not by itself produce a reading, on the accuracy of measurement of another component.

Sensitivity. The ability of an analytical method to detect small quantities of the measured component. It has no numerical value but this is expressed by the term *detection limit*, the smallest single result which, with a stated probability (commonly 95 %), can be distinguished from a suitable blank. The limit may be a concentration or an amount and defines the point at which the analysis becomes just feasible.

These criteria help to define the *analytical range* of a method, the range of concentration or other quantity in the specimen over which the method is applicable without modification. Analytical methods have different reliability criteria and have been categorised as follows:

Definitive method. A method which after exhaustive investigation is found to have no known source of inaccuracy or ambiguity.

Reference method. A method which after exhaustive investigation has negligible inaccuracy in comparison with its imprecision.

Method of known bias. An analytical method in which the amount of bias has been established (the amount may be zero).

Method of unknown bias. An analytical method of unknown accuracy.

The application of analytical methods of various types gives a value for the concentration of the *analyte*, the component being measured, in a standard or specimen. The reliability of this value will vary so that different terms have been defined as follows:

True value. A term of self-evident meaning. True values are estimated from other values, the best being the definitive value.

Definitive value. A value given by a definitive method.

Reference method value. Next best available estimate of the true value; most probable value derived from a set of results obtained by the most reliable reference methods available.

Assigned value. Value assigned either arbitrarily (e.g. by convention), or from preliminary evidence as, e.g. in the absence of a recognised reference method. This corresponds to the value given by a method with known or unknown bias.

Certified value. Value certified by some official body subject to conditions established by that body.

Stated value. Value without official certification.

Finally, a group of terms applies to the materials and methods of quality control.

Control material is material used for QC purposes. It takes the form of a *control specimen* or *control solution*, a specimen or solution which is analysed solely for QC purposes, not for calibration. These are usually inserted into an analytical *run*, a set of consecutive assays performed without interruption. The results are usually calculated from the same set of calibration standard readings. However, this definition may not be universally applicable, and in these cases the word *series* should be used after defining it.

Quality control has been divided into *internal quality control*, the procedure of utilising the results of only one laboratory for quality control purposes, and into *external quality assessment* in which the results of several laboratories which analyse the same specimen(s) are utilised.

Calibration and Control Materials

The fundamental difference between the use of samples of these two materials must be clearly understood. No sample can be used simultaneously for calibration and control purposes. With a calibration sample the analytical value attached to the sample is accepted and the analytical samples, be they from patients' specimens or control specimens, are compared with that value. The results from control samples are accepted as they arise and are then analysed statistically for a totally different purpose—the assessment of accuracy and precision as part of the monitoring of an analytical method. Control materials must go through all stages of the assay whereas, with some complex assays, calibration material can only be used in the final stages. Although different preparations are used for calibration and control purposes, a number of general points applies to both types of material.

For calibration standards the composition should be considered in relation to the analytical method and the type of specimens to be analysed. Thus a primary standard solution in water may be satisfactory for some analyses whereas for others, as in multi-channel automated analysis of sera, a secondary standard which is also serum is usually necessary. Control materials should normally be similar in composition to the samples being analysed. For many purposes control sera will be employed. Both types of material should be homogeneous and stable. The stated value must be accurate for calibration material and for control material if this is to be used to assess accuracy. Control material with unstated values is used for the study of precision and of changes in accuracy. Preparation details for control materials are more difficult to obtain than for calibration materials as they are often commercial secrets but the method of arriving at a stated value should be quoted. Finally, other calibration and control materials than sera may be used for part of an analytical process, e.g. didymium and holmium glass filters for checking the wavelength calibration of spectrophotometers (p. 147).

Composition. They are prepared from pure substances, partially purified materials such as enzymes and protein fractions and from natural products, often in combination. Marked variations in the physical and chemical characteristics of the standard, control materials and patients' specimens can affect the validity of analytical results by matrix effects although the ideal analytical method should be insensitive to these. Most clinical biochemical methods applied to biological materials show matrix effects: physical (e.g. viscosity, surface tension effects) and chemical (non-specificity, interference). Matrix effects can produce differences in calibration between aqueous and serum standards and differences in precision using aqueous and serum control materials.

Classification. This depends on the use, the methods used to assign values, and the composition. A primary standard solution has its composition defined by its method of preparation and the purity of the material used, not by analysis. Where conditions permit, it is the most direct method of assessing accuracy. It is used always with reference methods. Repeated preparation of fresh primary standard allows the stability of other materials and reagents to be checked and the effects of interference to be studied.

With many analytical methods, matrix effects require the standards and control specimens to simulate patients' specimens. This is sometimes done by dissolving pure analyte in a suitable matrix of zero or insignificant analyte concentration. More often, biological material such as serum, modified if necessary by depletion or additions, is used as a secondary standard or control specimen. Its composition has then to be determined by analysis.

Calibration standards require the uncertainty of the assigned value to be small in relation to the precision of the analytical method for which they are used. Precision control material should resemble patients' specimens and should be available in several concentrations of the analyte including the upper end of the reference interval and near the limit of the analytical range. It should also possess small between-sample variability. Accuracy control material can either be precision control material with an assigned value or can be a primary calibration standard. The latter may be advantageous in detecting changes in accuracy when a biological standard is used.

Specifications. Many control materials and some calibration standards are supplied in vials either in liquid or lyophilised form. It is important that vial to vial variability is low. This requires homogeneity of the bulk preparation before dispensing into vials and control of the volume dispensed if lyophilisation follows. Attention to the composition and volume of the reconstituting fluid is necessary in that case and it is often better to reconstitute several vials and to mix the contents if the stability of the analyte permits. With care, the total variation between reconstituted vials should have a CV of less than 0·25 % which will affect overall analytical precision only slightly. Turbidity or opalescence in reconstituted lyophilised control materials can cause poor precision.

Stability is important and varies with the analyte and specimen (Lawson *et al.*, 1977). Most materials have a recommended shelf-life as normally stored and after any reconstitution, but this will vary between analytes.

The assignment of values in primary calibration standards usually has an error of less than 0·2 % but with secondary standards there is greater uncertainty depending on the performance of the analytical method. The assigned value is often derived from analyses in several different laboratories but differences in accuracy, precision and methods can make the result uncertain.

Methods of Preparation. The starting materials are of varying purity and the base material chosen to dissolve the analyte is a matter of judgement. Often human serum is employed and is obtained from donors, following plasmapheresis, or by careful pooling of surplus patients' samples (see Bowers *et al.*, 1975). Human serum can not be recommended for this purpose because of the hazards of human immunodeficiency virus and should only be used where animal-based products are unsuitable. The regulations for the use of human material are set out in Health Notice HN(86) 25 (DHSS, 1986). Animal serum has the advantages of availability and freedom from human immunodeficiency virus but some components differ in composition or concentration from human sera and matrix effects may cause errors in assays designed for human material. Thus ox serum is unsuitable for assessment of analytical control of some thyroxine radioimmunoassay methods (Ratcliffe *et al.*, 1978). Sera may be modified by selective filtration, enzyme treatment or by the addition of analytes preferably in liquid form. Difficulties arise when adding enzymes which are usually of animal origin and may give final products with different kinetic properties from human sera. Addition of lipids, particularly cholesterol, creates problems but bovine lipoprotein fractions (Proksch and Bonderman, 1976) or soluble esters (Steel, 1977) have been used. Prevention of bacterial contamination by filtration or antibiotic addition aids stability as does lyophilisation. Division of material into small fractions in bottles or vials increases the chance of chemical or bacterial contamination. Quality control materials can be tested for their ability to mimic the analytical characteristics of human samples (Bretaudiere *et al.*, 1981).

Lyophilised materials only match the original composition if the reconstituting water volume is selected to allow for the partial specific volume of the solids in the original material. Different concentrations of analyte can be achieved by reconstitution with varying volumes of diluent and by correcting for the volume of solid material present. If the final volume is significantly different from the original volume, there will be a greater matrix effect. With some analytes the time after reconstitution is critical, e.g. the activity of alkaline phosphatase increases for 12 h or more and depends on the storage temperature. Stabilised liquid control materials are being used to overcome some of the problems of lyophilised products.

For further details of calibration and control materials see Büttner *et al.* (1981a). and DHSS (1986).

INTERNAL QUALITY CONTROL PROCEDURES

The various factors involved in the assessment and selection of an analytical method are discussed in the next chapter. The final choice of a method for routine use will be a matter of individual judgement but once a method has been brought into regular use, its performance must be monitored continuously by QC techniques so that changes in accuracy or precision can be recognised and corrective action taken. The results of replicate analyses of QC sera and, in some cases, of patients' specimens are often displayed in graphical form.

Levey-Jennings Charts

The use of simple charting procedures in clinical biochemistry was popularised by Levey and Jennings (1950). Fig. 12.1 shows such a chart for 20 consecutive daily

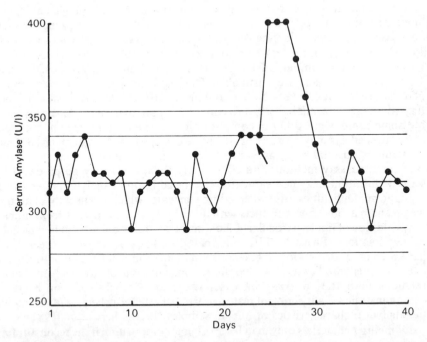

Fig. 12.1. Levey-Jennings Chart for Serum Amylase Results.

The horizontal lines are derived from the results of the first 20 days. The mean figure was 315 U/l and the 2 SD and 3 SD limits above and below this value are drawn. At the arrow, 3 successive points are seen at the upper warning limit which should have caused further investigation before the serious lapse in accuracy during the following 5 days. This was traced to a faulty thermostat in the incubator bath. Replacement is followed by regaining analytical control.

measurements on a QC serum. The points are joined and a horizontal line is drawn through the mean value. Following calculation of the SD, other lines are drawn at 2 and 3 SDs above and below the line. The mean line is related to accuracy and the other lines are measures of imprecision at the time the method was introduced. Provided that the accuracy and precision are regarded by other criteria as satisfactory, the plotting of further points allows detection of changes of accuracy or precision. Such extended plotting in time is likely to show changes in both indices. The worsening of precision over longer time periods is mainly attributable to changes in accuracy (Broughton and Annan, 1971). The 2 and 3 SD lines may therefore require revision in the light of a longer experience than the first 20 analytical days but any widening of the limits should be accompanied by consideration of whether the poorer precision implied is still acceptable.

Several features are examined to see whether the method is performing satisfactorily. If the performance of the analytical method remains unchanged then succeeding points will be evenly scattered on either side of the mid-line indicating no change in accuracy. Provided the precision is maintained the points will only fall outside the 2 SD limits, sometimes called *warning limits*, on average one in 20 occasions and outside the 3 SD limits, sometimes called *action limits*, on average three times in 1000, assuming that the results are normally distributed around the mean. *Changes in accuracy* should be detectable before the graph passes beyond the warning limits. As an arbitrary rule, six consecutive points lying on the same side of the mid-line should arouse suspicion and prompt examination of such aspects as a possible new batch of standards or reagents or a deterioration in the same, a change of pipette or in an instrument, or even a change in operator. Sometimes such a change is attributable to evaporation of samples when placed in sample cups some time before an analysis. It is revealed if standards are not similarly treated but are added to the sample tray just before analysis. The effects can be quite marked (Burtis *et al.*, 1975; Glenn and Hathaway, 1976). *Changes in precision* are indicated by greater variability about the mean with a more frequent transgression beyond the warning limits. If the warning limits are exceeded on consecutive occasions this is unlikely to occur by chance and suggests a significant and sudden change in accuracy (Fig. 12.1). For this reason a result falling outside the warning limit should at least prompt some appraisal of the possible reason and a reanalysis of the control serum. A further result beyond the warning limit almost certainly implies a change in accuracy whereas if this result falls much nearer the mid-line the method remains under suspicion pending further points being plotted. If a result falls beyond the action limits, the chances of true error are much higher and there is a real danger that all the results are erroneous.

The performance of the control procedure can be improved by devising a combination of rules which can be applied to QC results as they are produced, preferably with computer assistance. The operator can then be alerted when the results do not conform to the set of rules (Westgard *et al.*, 1981). The performance of a method should be monitored at different concentrations, selected so as to cover the reference interval and perhaps two suitable pathological levels. The choice of level will depend on the analyte but for many, pathologically high readings are more common than low ones and in that case one level might be selected at the clinically important zone just beyond the upper end of the reference interval and a second at a higher level. As the same control sera are often used for different analytes, the combination of three desirable levels for each into three different sera may introduce incompatibility and some compromises may be needed. In many cases it is possible to plot all three lines on the same chart paper thereby aiding interpretation of any changes.

It should be emphasised that control samples should be randomly inserted amongst patients' samples to include the effects of carryover. It is also established (Gowenlock and Broughton, 1968) that when the analyst knows that the sample is a control serum, the results are often unconsciously biassed in such a way as to improve apparent precision once the previous trends of results have been established. This is more likely for manual methods. For this reason it is advisable to include the same control serum at intervals disguised as a sample from a patient and to plot this result on the chart in a distinguishable way.

Other Charts Using Control Sera

The availability of commercial control sera with stated values is useful in the investigation of apparent changes in accuracy. However, such sera can be inserted into analytical runs in such a manner that the analyst is unaware of the expected result. This might be done by disguising the serum as a patient's sample or by reconstitution with a different amount of water, unknown to the analyst. The results for the various materials are plotted as percentage deviation from the expected figure in date order on a single chart. The information is useful for detecting changes in accuracy (Whitehead, 1977).

If replicate analyses of the same material are performed in one run then an additional estimate of within-run precision is available. If many replicates are used their SD can be plotted daily as in a Levey-Jennings chart. If duplicates only are measured the error in SD will be high but can be estimated from $\bar{d}$, the mean difference between duplicates on 20 days, by the simple formula $0.89 \times \bar{d}$. The difference between duplicates is plotted daily and will vary between zero and defined warning and action limits. These are set at $2.81 \times \bar{d}$ and $4.12 \times \bar{d}$ respectively.

When two quality control sera are in use for the same analyte it is sometimes helpful to display the results on a two-dimensional chart (Youden plot). The simple system proposed by Tonks (1963) is essentially two Levey-Jennings charts at right angles (Fig. 12.2a). The results for the two sera are plotted as one point defined by the two axes. These are marked off in 'standardised' (p. 235) fashion, zero in each case representing the mean result for replicate analyses and the units are the *average* SD of the two sera. The square defined by 2 SDs either side of each zero line would be expected to enclose 95% of all results. Skendzel and Youden (1969) prefer to use a central circular area of radius 3 SD; this will enclose 99% of results. It is claimed that this charting technique discriminates between systematic and random errors. A systematic error (bias) affecting both sera would be expected to result in the point plotted lying close to the 45° diagonal (or diameter) but displaced from the centre of the square. A series of such points lying consistently to one side of the centre would indicate bias, even if the points still lie within the 2 SD limits. More marked bias would result in the point lying outside the square but still near the 45° line. Random errors are likely to affect only one serum and will produce points lying at various distances from the 45° line although if the precision has not worsened, 95% should lie within the square or circle.

This interpretation has been challenged by Elion-Gerritzen (1977) who points out that if the two sera have very different means, their SDs may not be similar. If they are, the above interpretation holds but when SDs are proportional to concentration as often happens it is then better to draw the 2 SD limits separately to define a central rectangle (Fig. 12.2b) whose diagonal will not lie at 45°.

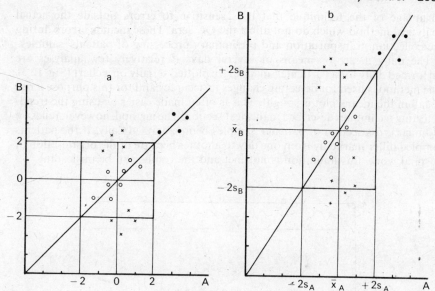

Fig. 12.2. Two-dimensional (Youden) Plots for Two Control Sera A and B.

(a) The mean results for A and B are marked as zero and their combined SD is used to graduate the axes; the central square defines ± 2 SD limits for both sera.

(b) The situation when A and B have different means and SDs. The axes are calibrated separately for the two sera; the mean values $(\bar{x}_A, \bar{x}_B)$ and deviations from these in the appropriate SD units (s_A, s_B) are shown. The rectangle encloses the ± 2 SD limits for the two sera.

Points, O, show the expected plot when the method is in control. Points, ●, indicate deterioration in accuracy (systematic error) for *both* sera. Both O and ● lie close to the diagonal lines. Points, ×, indicate random errors affecting only serum B, suggesting a deterioration in precision.

The systematic errors will be close to this new diagonal while random errors are scattered either side. Thus misunderstandings as to the type of error could occur if the 45° line is always used.

Use of Results from Patients' Samples

Selected patients' samples can be reanalysed on the following day preferably in disguised form to produce repeat results and give information about between-run precision. The charting techniques of the previous section are applicable.

An alternative approach is to utilise the majority of the patients' results in a single day to calculate the daily mean for each analyte. In order to avoid bias by very deviant results, it is usual to truncate the total collection of results by exclusion of those lying beyond selected limits. The selection of the truncation limits is important as it affects the sensitivity of the later applications of the technique (Dixon and Northam, 1970). If the daily analytical results are always a random sample drawn from a 'constant' patient population, the means of such daily random samples should be relatively constant, varying only by virtue of the errors of sampling and these will be smaller, the larger the number in the sample (p. 238). Such daily means will be affected by laboratory or other errors and it is an advantage of the technique that it is sensitive to errors outside the actual analytical method which do not affect the QC sera. These include errors during the collection, transportation and preliminary processing of patients' samples.

The daily mean, or means of several days if relatively few analyses are performed daily for a particular analyte, are plotted serially on a chart (Fig. 12.3). The method is used for detecting changes in accuracy and for this purpose a rise or fall in the means plot is sought. This is often made easier by using the trend-detecting techniques described in the next section. The method, however, relies on a similar cross section of patients' samples being analysed daily. If the patients sampled differ markedly from one day to another because of the organisation of hospital work, this limitation is not met and the results can be misleading.

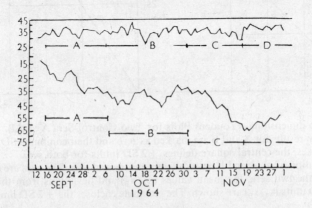

Fig. 12.3. Control Chart of Daily Means. (After Whitehead, 1977.)

The upper part of the chart shows the daily mean plotted as in the Levey-Jennings' chart; the lower part shows the cusum plot. Small changes in accuracy are shown more clearly in the cusum line. This has four zones—A, B, C, D—of different slope corresponding to the periods of service of four different staff members who prepared and read the calibration curves for the AutoAnalyzer used for the analysis. Individual differences in techniques have led to slight but detectable systematic errors between operators.

A patient's results can be compared with a previous set to determine the possibility of error. This is the basis of the Delta Check method (Nosanchuk and Gottman, 1974). The difference between the results for each analyte should fall within given limits and if the upper limit is exceeded the most recent result is suspected of being erroneous. This method is particularly useful for detecting transposed specimens and transcription errors, but any source of analytical error may cause the limit to be exceeded. Some correct results will cause the delta check to fail if the clinical state of the patient has altered appreciably and large changes in results are appropriate. Thus, optimal performance of delta check methods requires careful selection of limits to maximise the detection of errors without causing excessive numbers of false positives.

Ideally a QC scheme should cover all events from the taking of the specimen to the delivery of the report to the correct clinician. Duplicate specimens taken from the same patient can be monitored during their progress through the analytical process. With the cooperation of clinical staff, such specimens can form the basis of a low cost QC scheme which is sensitive to errors at all stages in the process (Zarembski *et al.*, 1980).

Further Methods of Handling Quality Control Results

A few methods for the further mathematical manipulation of the results obtained from the procedures of the last two sections have been described. They offer better identification of significant changes in quality control but add to the labour of maintaining adequate records of performance. In some cases they have been implemented by using a laboratory computer with the advantage that the print-out can summarise only the significant alterations allowing easy detection of problems. Mostly they are trend detection methods which detect changes in accuracy more readily than the simple plots already described allow.

The *cumulative sum technique* (Woodward and Goldsmith, 1964) can be applied to the results from QC sera or to daily means. The principle is simple: each day a constant value close to the expected result is deducted from the result under consideration and the residue is added algebraically to the previous day's cumulative sum (cusum) to produce the current cusum value. The calculation is set out below for a series of daily results for serum sodium for which the constant to be deducted has been selected as 139 mmol/l.

Daily result	Less 139	Cusum
138	−1	−1
139	0	−1
138	−1	−2
140	1	−1
139	0	−1
139	0	−1
138	−1	−2
140	1	−1
139	0	−1
141	2	1
140	1	2
139	0	2
141	2	4
140	1	5

The cusum values plotted daily will tend to lie on a straight line so long as accuracy is unchanged but any change, as after the 9th result above, is reflected as change in the line *slope*. The absolute slope is unimportant but changes are easily seen and may allow definition of the day on which the accuracy changed (Fig. 12.3, opposite), in retrospect.

Trigg's technique for trend analysis has been applied to clinical biochemistry by Cembrowski *et al.* (1975). This uses exponential smoothing to derive a 'tracking signal' which is plotted in a similar way to the cusum but the technique provides limits which the tracking signal should not exceed. The method has the advantage that it provides good estimates of the current result (related to accuracy) and the current SD of the method (related to precision) although it does not seem to give any earlier warning than the cusum method. It lends itself well to computer analysis. As the method is rather complex, the reader is referred to the original authors for details.

Indices of Precision and Accuracy. Whitehead (1977) describes two other indices which can be calculated, by computer if necessary, from QC data.

The *precision index* compares the absolute percentage change in two consecutive QC results with the between-run CV of the analytical method, determined without the analyst knowing the nature of the samples analysed. Thus if x_a and x_b

are successive QC results and the true value is also known, then we calculate each day

$$\frac{(100 \times |x_a - x_b|/\text{true value})}{CV} \times 100$$

This figure is calculated for ten days and the average result is noted as the precision index. A running ten day mean is then plotted daily. The expected result is 66 and figures usually fall in the range 0–200. The chart is examined for changes in slope and these indicate the point of change in precision.

The *accuracy index* is related but each day the observed result is compared with the true value and its percentage deviation is calculated in relation to the method CV paying due regard to the direction of the deviation. Thus if x_a is the result for one day, we calculate

$$\frac{(100 \times (x_a - \text{true value})/\text{true value})}{CV} \times 100$$

This is averaged over ten days as before and the resultant accuracy index is then plotted daily as a running mean. If the method remains accurate the index varies little around zero but changes in accuracy result in a rise or fall of the index, the magnitude of which indicates the direction and size of the bias.

EXTERNAL QUALITY ASSESSMENT PROCEDURES

These procedures use the results of many laboratories analysing samples of the same specimens in order to supplement the information derived from internal QC (Büttner *et al.*,1978; Whitehead, 1977; Whitehead *et al.*, 1973). They do not supplant the latter but assess the performance of the internal QC of the participating laboratories. Many different schemes are in operation and vary in the analytes covered and in the number of participating laboratories.

The overall SD between laboratories for results on the same specimen shows the 'state of the art' in progress towards the goal where all laboratories get closely similar results. Although the SD is diminishing, variation between laboratories using different methods, standards, and QC materials for the same analyte is undesirably great. Careful standardisation between participating laboratories greatly reduces inter-laboratory variation (Lippel *et al.*, 1977). If the true value of the specimens circulated is known, information on accuracy is produced. This is rarely known, however, so the results are used to derive a consensus value to allow comparison of accuracy of laboratories or methods. Depending on the design of the external quality assessment scheme it may be possible to obtain estimates of individual laboratory precision, linearity and accuracy with similar information about methods (see, e.g. Jansen *et al.*, 1977; de Leenheer *et al.*, 1976; Grannis, 1976 and the Wellcome Group Quality Control Programme (Wellcome Diagnostics Limited, Dartford, Kent)). Further information, not obtainable from internal QC methods, can be sought, e.g. the effects on laboratory performance of work load, staff numbers, various calibration standards and reagents and the extent of blank errors. The scope of external schemes can be extended by asking the participants for clinical interpretation of the results obtained. This is not widely used but has yielded valuable information on several assays, including human growth hormone.

As the composition of the material circulated is unknown to the analyst, external quality assessment is a more objective test of laboratory performance.

Not all laboratories treat the sample in the same way but it should preferably be treated exactly like a patient's sample and not be subject to replicate analysis. Although most schemes are voluntary and often anonymous, laboratories with poor performance may not participate. Both these factors can lead to an over-optimistic view of the 'state of the art'. Adequate comparison depends on good stability of the analytical specimen so that samples reaching each laboratory are indeed comparable. Liquid serum is less suitable for this purpose if delays occur between despatch from the central organisation and receipt by the laboratory. Lyophilised material is more stable but reconstitution errors are then added to the other variables. If a small local scheme is used, some of these limitations disappear as in the use of tonometered whole blood, chilled in ice, for external quality assessment of blood gas analysis (Delaney *et al.*, 1976; Minty and Nunn, 1977). For a large scheme when laboratories are grouped by analytical method, there are sufficient numbers in different groups to enable valid comparisons of their mean results to be made—that is, the comparative accuracy of the methods can be assessed. In order to be informative, specimens should be circulated frequently and a digest of results returned rapidly, requiring a central organis-ation with data-processing facilities. The United Kingdom has two major schemes which circulate samples at approximately fortnightly intervals: the National External Quality Assessment Scheme and the Wellcome Group Quality Control Programme. Other, smaller schemes for other analytes also operate.

The results of the individual analyses are usually compared with some consensus value. Alternatively, if the scheme has relatively few participants, a number of reference laboratories can be used to obtain a target value. The degree of agreement is often related to some measure of 'satisfactory' performance. Laboratories using very similar methods can have their results combined so that the means and SD of their results can be calculated, usually after deletion of very deviant results. 'Satisfactory' performance is a matter of professional judgement and criteria change as performance improves generally. Whitehead *et al.* (1973) and Whitehead (1977) use a 'variance index' to give a general impression of a laboratory's performance for a range of different analytes in the National External Quality Assessment Scheme. Such performance is better in larger laboratories and is gradually improving. The Wellcome Scheme is designed so that each laboratory's precision and relative accuracy for each analyte can be assessed.

An invaluable aspect of the larger schemes is that information is available about the performance of different methods in a wide range of laboratories. It is obvious from the results that some methods give a mean value which differs markedly from that of several other methods. Some methods also show a much wider scatter of results between participants. It is reasonable to regard such methods with suspicion and not to recommend their continued use. Where the mean figures for different methods lie closely together, particularly if the methods are based on different principles, it seems likely that their average result will lie very close to the true value. This hypothesis can be tested if a reference method is available (Pickup *et al.*, 1975) but such methods are relatively few. Information is also available about the average precision of the different methods and about the percentage of laboratories using a particular method who achieve 'satisfactory' precision, a higher percentage indicating a more 'robust' method.

Action may be needed as a consequence of participating in external schemes. A very deviant result should prompt a check for an error of clerical or arithmetical type—sometimes two samples have been transposed but occasionally contami-nation may have to be invoked as an explanation if internal QC was satisfactory for that batch. Widely scattered but less deviant results falling either side of the method mean value indicate poor precision and should prompt reappraisal of the analytical method, the staff performing it and the instruments used. Continuing poor precision is sometimes attributable to outmoded equipment. Re-equipment or the use of a different, more robust method should be considered. Consistent deviation from the target value indicates bias. Depending on the selection of the target value, this may only reflect the fact that all methods agree with one another poorly; however this is unusual. If the current method as a whole gives results different from the majority of other methods which agree with one another, replacement of the method on the grounds of bias should be considered. If the 'target' is the method mean and consistent bias is observed, this should lead to a reappraisal of calibration standards, pipettes and other measuring equipment, and inspection of reagents for evidence of deterioration.

REFERENCES

Bowers G. N., Burnett R. W., McComb R. B. (1975). *Clin. Chem*; **21**: 1830.

Bretaudiere J-P., Dumont G., Rej R., Bailly M. (1981). *Clin. Chem*; **27**: 798.

Broughton P. M. G., Annan W. (1971). *Clin. Chim. Acta*; **32**: 433.

Burtis C. A., Begovich J. M., Watson J. S. (1975). *Clin. Chem*; **21**: 1907.

Büttner J. *et al.* (1978). *Clin. Chim. Acta*; **83**: 189F.

Büttner J., Borth R., Boutwell J. H., Broughton P. M. G. (1979a). *Clin. Chim. Acta*; **98**: 129F.

Büttner J. *et al.* (1979b). *Clin. Chim. Acta*; **98**: 145F.

Büttner J., Borth R., Broughton P. M. G., Bowyer R. C. (1980). *Clin. Chim. Acta*; **106**: 109F.

Büttner J. *et al.* (1981a). *Clin. Chim. Acta*; **109**: 105F.

Büttner J. *et al.* (1981b). *Clin. Chim. Acta*; **109**: 115F.

Cembrowski G. S., Westgard J. O., Eggert A. A., Toren E. C. Jr. (1975). *Clin. Chem*; **21**: 1396.

Delaney C. J., Leary E. T., Raisys V. A., Kenny, M. A. (1976). *Clin. Chem*; **22**: 1675.

DHSS Health Notice HN(86)25. (1986). *HIV LAV/HTLV III—'AIDS' virus Antibody in Diagnostic Reagents and Quality Control and Calibration Materials.* Health Services Management. London: HMSO.

Dixon K., Northam B. E. (1970). *Clin. Chim. Acta*; **30**: 453.

Elion-Gerritzen W. E. (1977). *Amer. J. Clin. Path*; **67**: 91.

Glenn G. C., Hathaway T. K. (1976). *Amer. J. Clin. Path*; **66**: 645.

Gowenlock A. H., Broughton P. M. G. (1968). *Z. Anal. Chem*; **243**: 774.

Grannis G. F. (1976). *Amer. J. Clin. Path*; **66**: 206.

Jansen A. P. *et al.* (1977). *Clin. Chim. Acta*; **74**: 191.

Koran L. M. (1975). *New Engl. J. Med*; **293**: 642, 695.

Lawson N. S., Haven G. T., Moore T. D. (1977). *Amer. J. Clin. Path*; **68**: 117.

de Leenheer A. P., de Ruyter M. G. M., Steyaert H. L. C. (1976). *Clin. Chim. Acta*; **71**: 229.

Levey S., Jennings E. R. (1950). *Amer. J. Clin. Path*; **20**: 1059.

Lippel K. *et al.* (1977). *Clin. Chem*; **23**: 1744.

Minty B. D., Nunn J. F. (1977). *Ann. Clin. Biochem*; **14**: 245.

Nosanchuk J. S., Gottman A. W. (1974). *Amer. J. Clin. Path*; **62**: 707.

Pickup J. F. *et al.* (1975). *Clin. Chem*; **21**: 1416.

Proksch G. J., Bonderman D. P. (1976). *Clin. Chem*; **22**: 1302.

Ratcliffe W. A., Logue F. C., Ratcliffe J. G. (1978). *Ann. Clin. Biochem*; **15**: 203.

Skendzel L. P., Youden W. J. (1969). *Amer. J. Clin. Path*; **51**: 161.

Steel A. E. (1977). *Clin. Chem*; **23**: 2350.

Tonks D. B. (1963). *Clin. Chem*; **9**: 127.

Westgard J. O., Barry P. L., Hunt M. R., Groth T. (1981). *Clin. Chem*; **27**: 493.

Whitehead T. P. (1977). *Adv. Clin. Chem*; **19**: 175.

Whitehead T. P., Browning D. H., Gregory A. (1973). *J. Clin. Path*; **26**: 435.

Woodward R. H., Goldsmith P. L. (1964). *Cumulative Sum Techniques*, ICI Monograph No. 3. Edinburgh: Oliver and Boyd.

Zarembski P. M., Bateson M. C., Griffiths P. D. (1980). *Ann. Clin. Biochem*; **17**: 61.

13
SELECTION OF ANALYTICAL METHODS

Many of the methods currently in use in clinical biochemistry laboratories are acknowledged as being unreliable. This is probably the most important reason why the standard of performance of many laboratory tests is inadequate. Other reasons include poor equipment, staff deficiences, overwork and overcrowded laboratories (Broughton, 1978). Many methods in use were chosen because they were convenient or popular at the time they were selected rather than because of evaluated merit. Often the choice has been dictated by the available instrumentation, but in many cases there is no simple or clear reason why a particular method was chosen.

The evidence about methods is often conflicting, but in many cases the information available is not used. As Broughton says, 'Selection of a method for routine use is a complex process, and pragmatism and intuition often play as large a part as scientific considerations.' He suggests that psychological factors also play a part. These include: (1) the need for simplicity, convenience and ease of use, (2) faith in the reputation of the author or manufacturer, (3) fashion and the elegance of a new technique, (4) the glamour associated with a new instrument, (5) resistance to change and (6) constant search for improvement.

An analytical method (p. 287) may be of three types: definitive method, reference method and methods of known or unknown bias, sometimes called field methods (Tietz, 1979). *Definitive methods* are 'analytical methods that are capable of providing the highest accuracy among all methods for determining specific analytes and that are of sufficient accuracy for the stated end purpose of such methods.' These methods have negligible systematic error, and usually require sophisticated instrumentation, a high level of skill and high quality reagents. *Reference methods* are 'analytical methods with a thoroughly documented accuracy, precision and low susceptibility to interfering substances, sufficient to achieve the stated end purpose.' These methods are not intended for routine day-to-day use, but should be of the type which many different laboratories can use to test the performance of routine and proposed methods. They may be used to assess bias and interference. *Field methods* are 'routinely used analytical methods', which hopefully have been shown to have 'adequate precision, accuracy, and specificity for their intended use.' Some field methods have received the endorsement of a qualified body, such as a national association, and have become *recommended or selected methods*. Rodgerson and Tietz (1975) suggested that recommended methods should be developed urgently in an attempt to deal with the situation where many unsatisfactory methods are in use. This Chapter is concerned with the selection of field methods.

INITIAL SPECIFICATIONS—FIRST STAGE

The selection of a method requires information about the quality of each method and the knowledge and experience to judge which factors are important, so that the laboratory's ideal requirements can be balanced against a realistic assessment of what is available (Broughton, 1978). Previously there were few guidelines but Broughton (1978), Büttner *et al.* (1979) and White and Fraser (1984) have all made significant attempts to rectify this. They and Westgard *et al.* (1974) insist that laboratories should evaluate methods before adopting them, no matter how well documented or recommended they are. The same criteria should be applied to commercially prepared kit methods (Lloyd, 1978; Percy-Robb *et al.*, 1980). 'An evaluation kit for clinical chemistry' produced by White and Fraser (1984) emphasises that evaluation is necessary to characterise the method fully and produce a foundation on which to base quality control and assurance programmes.

The first stage in method selection is to define carefully the needs of the laboratory and its users who have certain requirements if the test results are to be medically useful (Westgard *et al.*, 1974). The function, performance characteristics and other factors that are ideally required should be listed. In order to define a specification, various questions must be answered:

1. *What are the service requirements?* These include details of the workload, limitations of cost and instrumentation, required performance characteristics and staffing.
2. *Is the method required to provide an urgent, on-demand service, or a routine batch service or some combination of these?* A method which has a one-hour 'start-up' procedure is clearly unsuitable for the former but may be well suited to a large batch once or twice a week.
3. *What are the sample limitations and from what kind of patients will the specimens be derived?* If the major patient population comprises children or neonates, this will give extra weight to limitations on sample volume. If the samples are likely to include a significant proportion with a high infection risk, specimen handling techniques and cleaning of instruments may assume more importance than otherwise.

Further Consideration of Service Requirements

Workload estimates help to select the type of method. Will a manual method be able to handle present and projected workloads, or will an automated system be required? Will a kit method, either manual or automated, best meet the needs of the laboratory? If automated equipment is to be chosen, the selection might be influenced by the inclusion of other tests or the potential for development and introduction of other methods later. However, this should not have undue influence to the detriment of the method primarily under consideration.

Target costs are important at this stage if budget limitations are likely. If the method is replacing an existing method, it is essential to know the effect on revenue expenditure. Some increase may be tolerated in order to provide an improved service. Limitations on capital expenditure have obvious importance.

Analytical performance required of a method is an important, but often neglected, part of the specification. The laboratory should have tolerance limits for the imprecision of a method based upon clinical usefulness (Büttner *et al.*, 1981).

Various yardsticks have been proposed for determining the target precision of methods for the more common analytes and the subject has been reviewed by Fraser (1983). One approach is to calculate the analytical precision which would be necessary to have an acceptably low effect on inter-individual variation

(p. 275). Figures have been suggested by Cotlove *et al.* (1970) and Young *et al.* (1971). Alternatively, one can consider the precision needed in order to detect changes which are medically significant (Tonks, 1963; Barnett, 1968; Glick, 1976), or survey the perceived requirements of clinicians (Campbell and Owen, 1967; Barnett, 1968; Skendzel 1978; Barrett *et al.*, 1979; Elion-Gerritzen, 1980a). Others suggest using 'state of the art' criteria and various reports have appeared. Stevens and Hjelm (1985) have updated earlier reports derived from the Wellcome Quality Control Programme, as have Ross and Fraser (1982) with similar data collected by the College of American Pathologists. More recently, various groups or individuals have suggested analytical goals for a number of analytes (Gilbert, 1975; World Assoc. of Soc. of Path., 1979; Fraser, 1980; Ross and Fraser, 1982) but different goals may be desirable for different clinical situations (Elion-Gerritzen, 1980a, b; Büttner *et al.*, 1981). For example, the detection of a single abnormal result poses the question 'is this result sufficiently deviant from the reference range to warrant further investigation or treatment?'. The analytical performance required will depend on the reference range for the analyte and the clinical significance of a high or low value. This is a different question from 'is this result different from the previous ones?' when changes in an individual with treatment or time are being monitored to aid judgements about efficacy of treatment or progression of disease.

Comparison of various goals and achievements are shown in Table 13.1. It would seem that at least half of laboratories using automated methods can achieve even the most rigorous criteria for cholesterol, glucose, phosphate, potassium, total protein, urate, urea and, perhaps, albumin and bilirubin. The situation is less satisfactory for bicarbonate, calcium, chloride, creatinine, magnesium and sodium.

Further aspects of performance characteristics include information about the requirements for specificity, detection limit and analytical range. Specificity requirements should be clarified by knowledge of the clinical situations in which the method will be used. Where particular drugs may be frequently prescribed it is important to show that these do not interact.

INITIAL SPECIFICATIONS—SECOND STAGE

When the test requirements and constraints have been defined, a list of candidate methods can be constructed from which the final selection is to be made. This list should preferably include no more than three options which will later be reduced to one warranting fuller evaluation. The objective of this pre-evaluation assessment (White and Fraser, 1984) is to indicate which candidate method is likely to perform all or part of the clinical tasks required and harmonise with the current laboratory organisation and philosophy, while being economic without becoming outdated quickly.

Published Information

The first stage in selection is a careful reading of the candidate methods in the light of the requirements (Büttner *et al.*, 1979) that the published instructions which comprise an analytical method should include the following items: (1) the principle of the method in outline; (2) the specifications of the reagents, instruments and other equipment needed; (3) the method of preparing the calibration standard and deriving its stated value; (4) requirements for the specimen—volume, preservatives, anticoagulants, storage; (5) full description of steps, especially critical ones, with tolerances of measurements; (6) calibration procedure and calculation of results; (7) analytical range intended; (8) safety precautions.

This information can be supplemented from studies of the literature, or by canvassing the opinions of others and will suggest what further investigation is required.

In proposing a commercial method or equipment as a candidate for further evaluation, much must be gleaned from the sales literature and it will usually be necessary to supplement this from other available sources such as published evaluations, or the views of other laboratories using the method. It should be possible to assemble information about analytical performance and capabilities in this way and White and Fraser (1984) have designed a useful check-list to facilitate this.

Comparative Information

Much useful information regarding the analytical performance of various methods comes from external quality assessment programmes such as the Wellcome Group Quality Control Programme and the National External Quality Assessment Schemes, NEQAS (p. 297). The former publishes an end-of-period report which gives the mean bias of methods from an 'all-method' zero reference as well as the median precision of the methods currently in use together with some indication of the performance and number of users of the different methods. This can help to exclude certain methods which have a consistently poor performance. The various NEQAS schemes often make recommendations about methods in use for particular analytes, and this information should be consulted before any final decisions are made.

EVALUATION OF A CANDIDATE METHOD

When a candidate method has been chosen for further evaluation, a familiarisation period should be allowed (White and Fraser, 1984) before this begins. This will allow performance data to be collected under routine conditions (Broughton, 1978).

The purpose of the evaluation is to measure the performance characteristics of the method experimentally for comparison with target performance figures. Performance characteristics (Büttner *et al.*, 1979) listed by the IFCC-EP (p. 286) are of two kinds, practicability and reliability criteria. Testing of these can be performed in any order and it is often possible to gather different types of information simultaneously.

Practicability Criteria

Several aspects require assessment.

Speed. This involves the assessment of two different characteristics, the number of specimens which can be processed in a given time and the time taken before a result is available from a particular specimen. This requires three measurements: (1) the number of specimens which can be analysed per hour or other convenient period, (2) the time taken to produce a result from one specimen when the analyst is unprepared for it, and (3) the time taken to produce a result from one specimen when the analyst has had time to prepare for it.

TABLE 13.1

Desirable and Achievable Precision of Analytical Methods. (Figures in parentheses are CV as %.)

Columns under **Desirable Precision***: Cotlove (1970), Young (1971), Barnett (1968), Tonks (1963), Barrett (1979). Columns under **Achievable Precision+**: Individual labs, USA labs (50%, 90%), European labs (50%, 90%).

Analyte	Approx. Conc.	Cotlove (1970)	Young (1971)	Barnett (1968)	Tonks (1963)	Barrett (1979)	Individual labs	USA 50%	USA 90%	European 50%	European 90%
Albumin	40 g/l	1.5 (3.8)	0.9 (2.3)	2.5 (7.1)		1.1 (3.7)	(3.1)	(5.0)	(8.2)	1.1	2.3
Bicarbonate	25 mmol/l	0.8 (3.2)	0.9 (3.6)		(8.8)	1.8 (9.0)		(3.4)	(5.9)	0.9	1.3
Bilirubin	20 µmol/l			4.0 (20.0)	(10.0)	2.1 (10.5)	(3.3)	(12.2)	(20.6)	2.6	5.3
	400 µmol/l			30.0 (7.5)		17.9 (6.0)		(9.3)	(15.8)		
Calcium	2.5 mmol/l	0.040 (1.6)	0.046 (1.8)	0.062 (2.5)	(5.0)	0.021 (0.81)	0.044 (1.2)	(3.0)	(5.3)	0.055	0.110
								(2.2)	(3.5)		
Chloride	100 mmol/l	0.09 (0.9)	1.2 (1.2)	2.0 (2.0)	(2.4)	1.8 (1.6)		(1.9)	(3.1)	1.5	2.5
								(1.6)	(2.5)		
Cholesterol	6.5 mmol/l	0.44 (6.8)	0.39 (6.0)	0.52 (8.0)	(10.0)	0.18 (2.8)	0.13 (4.0)	(4.9)	(8.7)	0.14	0.30
								(3.9)	(6.7)		
Creatinine	130 µmol/l		3.9 (3.0)		(10.0)	20 (15.4)	4.9	(7.9)	(13.9)	7.2	19.0
	450 µmol/l							(5.7)	(10.0)		
								(5.1)	(8.9)		
								(2.9)	(5.2)		
Glucose	5.5 mmol/l	0.25 (4.5)	0.18 (4.0)	0.28 (5.0)	(10.0)	0.18 (2.7)	0.10 (2.1)	(3.7)	(5.9)	0.19	0.35
	8.8 mmol/l							(3.3)	(5.2)		
								(3.3)	(5.3)		
								(2.7)	(4.3)		
Magnesium	1.0 mmol/l	0.030 (3.0)	0.027 (2.7)				0.03	(4.9)	(9.4)	0.05	0.110
Phosphate	1.5 mmol/l	0.075 (4.9)	0.090 (6.0)	0.081 (5.4)	(10.0)	0.05 (4.0)	0.036	(3.1)	(5.5)	0.040	0.097

Potassium	3·0 mmol/l	0·14	(4·7)	0·16	(5·3)	0·25	(8·3)	(8·8)	0·11	(3·7)	(1·1)	(2·4)	(3·6)	0·07
	6·0 mmol/l	0·14	(2·3)	0·16	(2·7)	0·25	(4·2)		0·11	(2·2)		(2·6)	(4·0)	0·12
T. Protein	70 g/l	2·2	(3·1)	1·3	(1·9)	3·0	(4·3)	(7·0)	1·8	(2·9)	0·84	(2·6)	(1·8)	(2·7)
												(2·2)	(4·5)	1·5 2·4
Sodium	140 mmol/l	0·5	(0·4)	1·3	(1·0)	2·0	(1·4)	(2·3)	1·8	(1·3)	(0·7)	(1·1)	(1·8)	(2·7)
												(2·2)	(3·7)	1·3 2·3
Urate	0·35 mmol/l	0·034	(9·7)	0·023	(6·6)	0·030	(8·5)	(10·0)	0·018	(5·1)	0·007	(2·2)	(1·1)	(5·7)
													(9·9)	0·014 0·036
	0·53 mmol/l								0·018	(3·1)			(3·0)	(5·6)
													(8·7)	
Urea	9·6 mmol/l	0·54	(5·6)	0·61	(6·3)	0·71	(7·4)	(12·0)	0·89	(9·9)	0·18	(2·3)	(5·1)	(6·6)
													(11·0)	0·33 0·70
	17·8 mmol/l												(2·9)	(3·5)
													(6·0)	
													(8·9)	
													(5·0)	

* The figures of Cotlove et al. (1970) and Young et al. (1971) are based on knowledge of intra-individual variation. Those of Barnett (1968), of Tonks (1963) and of Barrett et al. (1979) are based on what is medically desirable.

+ The individual laboratories are two large ones. The figures in parentheses are taken from Whitehead (1977), the others are from Williams et al. (1978). Figures for US laboratories (Ross and Fraser, 1982) show the CV achieved by 50% and 90% of them, the upper figures refer to manual methods, the lower to automated methods. The figures for European laboratories are as SDs and refer to all methods. They have been derived from consideration of results in the Wellcome Group Quality Control Programme (Stevens and Hjelm, 1985).

If the speed of sampling can be varied this can affect the accuracy and precision of the method and any effect should be assessed. For example, faster speeds often impair precision, usually by increasing carryover.

Cost. There is no standard way of describing the costs of a method, so it is important that the method of calculating them is fully described to enable comparisons to be made. The true cost includes such *indirect costs* as heating, lighting and staff not involved in the assay. It is difficult to measure and apportion these. *Direct costs* include capital and labour costs, maintenance and costs of reagents and such consumables as specimen containers, calibration standards, control sera and equipment consumables—tubes, membranes and stationery. Unless the instrument is a dedicated analyser it may be difficult to allocate a proportion of the capital and maintenance costs to a particular method.

The cost per specimen will vary with the batch size and it is essential to calculate this for different workloads. Direct labour costs may be fixed if the analyst is dedicated to the method or may vary in relation to the batch size. Information about consumable and labour costs for different workloads will help to decide the most economical batch size. This can be compared with that calculated from the desired frequency of performing the method.

Skill Requirements. According to Broughton (1978), although the amount of skill required to obtain reliable results is an important factor in selecting a method, it is usually only judged intuitively. It is difficult to define skill requirements, but they include manual dexterity, knowledge and experience. All are difficult to measure but have an approximate relationship to the type or grade of analyst. As an example, studies have shown that although a senior analyst obtained better precision than a junior one with a particular manual method for AST, simplification of the procedures resulted in each being able to achieve a consistently good performance. It is thus important that the performance of a method is assessed by the type of staff who will normally operate it. This may be overlooked if new methods are evaluated and introduced by more senior staff. If a method is intended for use by different staff members, e.g. in an out-of-hours situation, it should be assessed under these conditions. If the method is insufficiently robust to be used by a particular grade of staff it will be necessary to determine what level of skill is required, how performance changes with a change of operator and whether the limitations imposed by this are acceptable.

Dependability. This includes the mechanical and electrical reliability of equipment and the risk and frequency of breakdowns and method failure. A log is kept during evaluation and similar information is collected, if possible, from other laboratories. Items which should be logged include unscheduled down-time and the times when it has been necessary to reject batches. This aspect of the robustness of the method may be independent of the skill of the analyst.

Safety. This includes assessment of electrical, mechanical, chemical and microbiological hazards. Chemical hazards include the use of poisonous, carcinogenic or radioactive materials. Hazards which may be caused by accidents such as spillage, and actions required to deal with them, should be assessed and described.

Reliability Criteria

Four aspects require assessment.

Imprecision. Its determination involves the analysis of replicates under defined conditions. In addition to random errors, imprecision is affected by the use of different specimens, concentrations, runs and days, as well as different reagent batches, standards, instruments and analysts. All these factors will be relevant to the overall quality of performance, but when assessing method imprecision, the second group should preferably be kept constant, at least for the initial study of within-run imprecision.

When designing a study of imprecision, consideration must be given to the choice of specimen. The decision to be made is between patients' samples and control specimens or a combination of both. Aqueous solutions are not suitable because they do not resemble patients' specimens. Patients' samples are preferable but should come from a wide variety of patients, typical of those for whom the method would be routinely used. However, patients' specimens are rather unstable, and must be used over a short time interval. In this way they could be used to assess within-run and between-day imprecision from duplicate measurements, although this between-day estimate would give no indication of imprecision caused by progressive changes with time.

Control specimens are frequently used, but many are of bovine or equine origin. The material is usually lyophilised and thus requires reconstitution, making it even more different from patients' samples while introducing an extra procedure. However, despite these reservations, control specimens enable replicate samples to be measured over longer time periods, such as 20 consecutive days.

Within-day imprecision is suitable for a rapid assessment of precision and for comparing two methods. About 100 patients' samples are analysed in duplicate in random order by both methods. The concentrations should cover the whole analytical range and, if several runs are needed, duplicates should be kept in the same run. Calculate the standard deviation (or CV) from duplicates with the proviso that several concentration ranges may need to be calculated separately (p. 257). Alternatively, one or more control sera are analysed so that at least 20 results are obtained in the usual way.

Between-day imprecision requires analysis of replicates over a period of time, usually using three specimens whose concentrations span the analytical range of the method. One sample of each of these is analysed for 20 consecutive days in a random position in the batch. The results are first plotted to check that there has been no change in accuracy over this period as they will only be of use if produced during a period of constant accuracy. When satisfactory results have been collected, the SD is calculated to give an estimate of the between-day imprecision. This should not be greater than twice the within-run precision determined under optimal conditions (Whitehead, 1977). If the same control material is used for both measures, the mean value of the results for the two conditions should not alter significantly (p. 250).

Lyophilised control specimens are commonly used for this assessment and some workers suggest sufficient material for the whole experiment should be reconstituted, pooled, divided into aliquots and frozen. One of each concentration is then analysed daily after careful thawing and mixing to ensure homogeneity. If this method is employed, the results must be examined for significant regression with time, which may indicate instability of the stored sample rather than changing accuracy.

By measuring several replicates from several control samples for several days, an estimate of the within-batch and between-batch imprecision can be evaluated by a one way analysis of variance (p. 256).

Accuracy. The assessment of accuracy is more difficult than that of precision because the true values of samples analysed are not usually known. Accuracy can be assessed initially by comparison of results from the candidate method with those obtained by a method of known accuracy. This comparison method is unlikely to be a definitive method since these exist for only a few analytes and are only available in a few special laboratories. It may occasionally be a reference method which is being used specifically for the purpose of comparison with the candidate method. These methods are more suitable for assigning values to reference materials. The most likely situation is that the candidate method will be compared with a method of known inaccuracy, often the existing method. This may well raise questions about whether differences reflect fundamental differences between the methods. Other procedures involving linearity checks, recovery and the investigation of poor specificity may need to be used.

It is desirable to analyse several different control samples to assess accuracy but the validity of this approach depends on the accuracy of their stated values. In many cases these have been obtained from replicate analyses made in a few laboratories. Also it is not uncommon to find that control samples give different values for different methods when this is not the case with patients' samples. It is now possible to obtain control material which has been used in large external quality assessment schemes and for which, consequently, method-specific consensus values are available. These are particularly useful. If several different control samples from various manufacturers agree with their assigned values, the accuracy of the method is not seriously in question. However, if some results are different the procedure may be regarded as testing the reliability of the manufacturer's stated value.

Comparison of Two Methods. Having chosen the comparison method, often the method in current use, perform replicate analyses by both methods of at least 100 patients' specimens. Do this over several days, selecting specimens with values covering the whole analytical range. This is important where the population results are distributed in a markedly skewed fashion making some values less common. Note any lipaemic, haemolysed or jaundiced samples, and any which are likely to contain drugs. If individual results by the two methods disagree, it will then be necessary to study interference. If it is not possible to use the same calibration standards for both methods, use each method to analyse the standards of the other method.

Evaluation of the results of this kind of study often causes problems, and statistical tests are often applied inappropriately (Westgard and Hunt, 1973). It is essential to plot the paired patients' results with the candidate method on the ordinate. Simple observation of this plot yields more valid information than many statistical tests. A curvilinear relationship shows unsatisfactory accuracy. A wide scatter shows poor precision of one or both methods, and this may be concentration-dependent. Compare the precision of both methods, possibly at different concentrations, using the F test (p. 246). If the relationship appears linear, plot the absolute difference between the two methods, $|y - x|$, against their mean, $(x + y)/2$. Repeat this with logarithms of the data, plotting $|\log y - \log x|$ against $(\log x + \log y)/2$. Examine these plots to see if the arithmetical differences increase with mean values, which indicates that the variance is not constant over the range. In this case, see if the plot of data after logarithmic transformation shows little change, suggesting that this has made the variance reasonably constant. Using the original or transformed data, whichever has the more consistent variance, the relationship of y to x can be validly calculated. This is often done using least-squares linear regression, but this may be incorrect if the underlying assumptions (p. 260) of this approach are not met (Cornbleet and Gochman, 1979). The most important assumption made is that the x values are measured without error. In method comparison studies this is almost always never the case. Other, more complicated, methods of analysis have been proposed which take into account the errors associated with the x and y results. Visual examination of plots of the data in relation to a line of identity ($y = x$) is often much more informative (Altman and Bland, 1983). The purpose of this procedure is to determine whether the methods agree, and if not, to indicate whether any disagreement is largely due to proportional bias (slope differing from 1) or constant bias (non-zero intercept) or a combination of both. Proportional bias may be caused by errors associated with the calibration standards, and constant bias with interference or non-specificity of one of the methods. If bias exists, but is acceptable, a regression equation can be used to calculate the confidence limits of the value of x corresponding to different y values (the candidate method) and see if they are acceptable. In this case use of the Deming regression equation would be more appropriate (p. 262).

Linearity. Information on linearity is often forthcoming by comparing methods. If the relationship is non-linear, the linearity of the candidate method should be assessed by comparing the results of replicate measurements on a series of samples whose relative concentrations are known. These may be aqueous primary standards but sera should also be investigated, and in those cases where the protein matrix affects the reaction, they are the only appropriate material. A convenient approach is to mix two sera with high and low analyte concentrations in several known proportions.

Recovery. Useful for studying proportional bias, this is insensitive to constant bias (Kemp, 1984). It is convenient for studying different stages of a method (extraction, hydrolysis or precipitation) to assess losses. Two analyses are carried out, before and after addition of a known amount of analyte to a specimen. It is not always possible to add the correct biological material for recovery, e.g. conjugated bilirubin. The apparent increase in concentration is compared with that predicted from the amount added. Recovery is expressed either as a percentage or as the percentage difference from the theoretical value of 100%.

The two concentrations should be in the analytical range, but the estimate involves the summation of the errors of the two measurements (p. 270). Use several different concentrations and specimens to see whether interfering substances are present in some but not others. Even then, the confidence limits on the mean recovery can be rather wide.

Specificity and Interference. Most analytical methods show some lack of specificity or interference if a sufficiently wide range of investigations is made, so testing depends on the intended use. Comparison of two methods may show particularly discrepant results for certain samples and these should be examined for interference or non-specificity. Interference may arise from bilirubin, haemoglobin or turbidity in the sample. Non-specificity may arise from drugs in the sample or the use of too wide a bandwidth in the spectrophotometer. In some cases selected substances can be added to human serum for testing.

Blanks (p. 144) are often used to correct for non-specificity and their appropriateness can be tested. The *reagent blank* corrects for contributions from the reagents to the final reading, and should normally be small. In some cases *sample blanks* are used to correct for other substances in the sample. Their effect may sometimes be studied by using samples free from the analyte. This is easily done with methods for measuring drugs, and can be done with hormone methods if a sample from a patient deficient in the hormone is available. If such sera are unavailable, the usual procedure is to omit one of the reagents at a key stage and, if possible, add it later. The residual variation in the final result is noted. Sample blanks too should give only small readings, particularly in relation to the readings for samples with values near the lower end of the analytical range. Experience will show whether variation between different sample blanks is sufficiently great to require an individual blank to be run with each test sample.

Awareness of the effects of drugs on test results is developing, aided by the use of computer compiled lists (Young *et al.*, 1975), and an IFCC-EP has prepared guidance on the evaluation of analytical interference (Galteau and Siest, 1984). The literature on the subject is growing rapidly (Salway, 1978) and the computerised data banks which are required to handle the vast amount of data (Siest and Dawkins, 1984) are being developed.

Sensitivity. This is best measured by the *detection limit*, the smallest result which can be distinguished from the blank. The analytical range of a method should encompass the concentrations most commonly encountered. At low concentrations, variations in sample blank may have a disproportionate effect. Variation of the sample volume may allow adjustment of the sensitivity. The detection limit can be measured by analysing 20 replicates of a blank sample or samples and calculating the mean (M) and standard deviation (S) of the readings. The standard deviation at the lower end of the analytical range will usually be similar. For most purposes, the lowest concentration which can be confidently (P > 0·99) distinguished from the blank is M + 2·6 S and results below this should be reported as 'less than' this value.

ASSESSMENT OF THE EVALUATION

This is probably the most difficult part. The results must be assessed and compared with the overall requirements. The perfect analytical method is an illusion, because requirements depend on local and on clinical circumstances (Broughton, 1978). Requirements may be conflicting and good precision may have to give way to speed. Precision may be improved by measurements in duplicate, but this will increase the cost. The selection of a method, therefore, requires value judgements made on the basis of all relevant information. This is the responsibility of the scientist, who must judge which method to select with full knowledge of its strengths and deficiencies so that it will meet the laboratory and clinical requirements.

REFERENCES

Altman D. G., Bland J. M. (1983). *The Statistician*; **32**: 307.
Barnett R. N. (1968). *Amer. J. Clin. Pathol*; **50**: 671.
Barrett A. E. *et al.* (1979). *J. Clin. Pathol*; **32**: 893.
Broughton P. M. G. (1978). *Prog. Clin. Pathol*; **7**: 1.
Büttner J. *et al.* (1979). *Clin. Chim. Acta*; **98**: 145F.
Büttner J. *et al.* (1981). *Clin. Chim. Acta*; **109**: 115F.
Campbell D. G., Owen J. A. (1967). *Clin. Biochem*; **1**: 3.
Cornbleet P. J., Gochman N. (1979). *Clin. Chem*; **25**: 432.
Cotlove E., Harris E. K., Williams G. Z. (1970). *Clin. Chem*; **16**: 1028.
Elion-Gerritzen W. E. (1980a). *Amer. J. Clin. Pathol*; **73**: 183.
Elion-Gerritzen W. E. (1980b). *J. Clin. Pathol*; **33**: 902.
Fraser C. G. (1980). *Pathology*; **12**: 209.
Fraser C. G. (1983). *Adv. Clin. Chem*; **23**: 299.
Galteau M. M., Siest G. (1984). *Clin. Chim. Acta*; **139**: 223F.

Gilbert R. K. (1975). *Amer. J. Clin. Pathol*; **63**: 960.

Glick J. H. (1976). *Clin. Chem*; **22**: 475.

Kemp G. J. (1984). *Clin. Chem*; **30**: 1168.

Lloyd P. H. (1978). *Ann. Clin. Biochem*; **15**: 136.

Percy-Robb I. W. *et al.* (1980). *Ann. Clin. Biochem*; **17**: 217.

Ross J. W., Fraser M. D. (1982). *Amer J. Clin. Pathol*; **78**: 578.

Rodgerson D. O., Tietz N. W. (1975). *Clin. Chem*; **21**: 1057.

Salway J. G. (1978). *Ann. Clin. Biochem*; **15**: 44.

Siest G., Dawkins S. G. (1984). *Clin. Chim. Acta*; **139**: 215F.

Skendzel L. P. (1978). *J. Amer. Med. Assoc*; **239**: 1077.

Stevens J. F., Hjelm, G. C. E. (1985). *News Sheet (Assoc. Clin. Biochem.)*; **182**: 14.

Tietz N. W. (1979). *Clin. Chem*; **25**: 833.

Tonks D. B. (1963). *Clin. Chem*; **9**: 217.

Westgard J. O., Carey R. N., Wold S. (1974). *Clin. Chem*; **20**: 825.

Westgard J. O., Hunt M. R. (1973). *Clin. Chem*; **19**: 49.

White G. H., Fraser C. G. (1984). *J. Automat. Chem*; **6**: 122.

Whitehead, T. P. (1977). *Adv. Clin. Chem*; **19**: 175.

Williams G. Z., Widdowson G. M., Penton J. (1978). *Clin. Chem*; **24**: 313.

World Assoc. of Soc. of Path., Subcommittee on Analytical Goals in Clinical Chemistry (1979). *Amer. J. Clin. Pathol*; **71**: 624.

Young D. S., Harris E. K., Cotlove E. (1971). *Clin. Chem*; **17**: 403.

Young D. S., Pestaner L. C., Gibberman V. (1975). *Clin. Chem*; **21**: 1D.

14

COLLECTION OF SPECIMENS

BLOOD

Collection of Blood Specimens

Capillary or venous blood is used for most determinations made on blood.

Capillary Blood. This is usually obtained from a finger or thumb. The most convenient place is on the thumb about 5 mm from the nail edge but a finger tip can also be used. Clean the skin with isopropyl alcohol and allow to dry. Individually wrapped swabs soaked with isopropyl alcohol are available commercially. Prick the skin with a disposable sterile blood lancet or an automatic spring-loaded lancet. A better flow of blood is obtained if the hand is warm and if, firstly, the arm is allowed to hang limply and is then gently swung for a short time. After pricking, apply gentle pressure to the thumb and let the blood run directly into a capillary tube held inclined at an angle slightly downwards from the horizontal. When the operator is familiar with the technique, the tube fills easily and quickly. If, however, the blood ceases to flow before the tube is filled, do not exert undue pressure since this may alter the concentration of some constituents, but allow the arm to swing loosely and exercise the thumb for a moment or two to restore the circulation before applying pressure again. The blood begins to clot in about 2 to 3 min. The tube can be sealed with plasticine or a special plastic cap. Both heparinised and plain capillary tubes are manufactured and they can be centrifuged to obtain plasma or serum. This method is usually employed to collect volumes up to 200 μl. Alternatively the blood can be allowed to drop into a small tube with or without anticoagulant. Some workers use the lobe of an ear but the technique is more difficult to acquire. The heel is convenient for collecting blood from infants. The ankle is grasped to congest the foot and a prick made in the heel after applying a very thin film of a silicone oil or grease to the skin to form a non-wettable surface.

Venous Blood. This is collected most often. While the blood may be taken from any convenient vein, one on the front of the elbow or forearm is usually used. The arm should be warm to improve the circulation and distend the vein. Extend the arm and apply a tourniquet a few centimetres above the elbow to obstruct the venous return. Sterilise the skin over the vein. Insert a disposable sterile needle fixed to a disposable syringe of appropriate capacity into the vein, which can be held steady by the thumb of the operator's other hand. When the needle enters the vein withdraw the plunger slightly. If blood appears, release the tourniquet when minimal congestion is required. Otherwise release the tourniquet when the desired amount of blood has been collected. Place a swab over the puncture site and withdraw the needle. Press on the swab firmly to arrest bleeding. Remove the needle carefully avoiding contamination of the fingers and slowly transfer the blood to an appropriate container, preferably with the syringe nozzle touching the side of the container and using minimal force. If the tourniquet is applied very tightly or for long periods, water and small molecules (but not proteins or cells) pass through the vein wall to raise the plasma concentration of all protein fractions and those substances such as calcium which are wholly or partly bound to protein. It may also cause some haemolysis of red cells.

If the blood is collected in a plain container and allowed to clot, the clot shrinks and expresses serum which can be removed after centrifuging at 2000 to 3000 rpm. Clotting can be prevented by using a receptacle containing an anticoagulant (p. 314). Centrifugation then separates the red cells from the supernatant plasma. Plasma differs from serum in containing fibrinogen and anticoagulant. Some tests require serum, others plasma, while many can be carried out on either. For some tests whole blood is used (p. 316). The clotting process takes much longer in plastic than in glass containers but siliconised plastic tubes speed clotting. Some tubes are supplied containing plastic granules the density of which is such that they form a layer between the red cells and serum or plasma after centrifugation. This simplifies removal of the upper layer.

Arterial Blood. This is less frequently examined. It is used for blood gas determinations and when studying arterio-venous differences of, e.g. blood glucose. It is usually obtained by inserting a needle into the radial, brachial or femoral artery. Much firmer pressure on the puncture site after removal of the needle is needed than for venepuncture and this should be maintained for several minutes. The composition of capillary blood is closer to that of arterial blood than to venous blood.

For safety precautions in the collection of all blood specimens see p. 13.

Time of Collection of Blood Specimens

Since the most satisfactory specimen is a post-absorptive one, the best time for taking blood is after fasting overnight. This also helps the laboratory as regards planning the day's work. Specimens should reach the laboratory without undue delay. However, conditions in many hospitals make it difficult to organise a collection system satisfying these requirements. For some determinations it is advisable to minimise lipaemia, so specimens are taken mid-morning after a light breakfast with a low fat content. Some blood constituents such as iron and cortisol show a diurnal variation with highest concentrations during the morning, so the best time of collection will be determined by this.

All specimens should be clearly labelled with the date, and preferably time, of collection. Also it is important that the concentration of the analyte or the technique used for its determination should not be affected by any procedures carried out on the patient. For example, prostatic examination may raise the serum acid phosphatase. Many drugs interfere with assays either by physiological action or by direct interference with the assay (Salway, 1978; Young *et al.*, 1975). It may therefore be important to know what drugs the patient is receiving.

Avoiding Haemolysis

Plasma or serum should not be haemolysed. Even when haemolysis is not visible, many specimens will show it on spectroscopic examination. Any appreciable haemolysis, certainly visible haemolysis, makes the sample unsuitable for some determinations, e.g. potassium. Haemolysis is minimised by avoiding mechanical breakdown of red cells and movement of water out of or into the cells. When taking blood, constrict the arm minimally, draw the blood slowly and steadily into the syringe and expel it slowly and gently into the container with the syringe tip touching the side so that the blood runs slowly down. Do not expel blood through the needle. Avoid an excessive amount of anticoagulant and mix gently. If plasma is to be separated, centrifuge at moderate speeds, 2000 to 3000 rpm. When obtaining serum allow to clot in a capped container and centrifuge as for plasma. At room temperature clotting may take 15 to 30 min. The longer the time allowed, the more the clot retracts and the more serum is obtained. If it is necessary to loosen the clot do this as gently as possible using a dry, thin rod. On standing, changes in distribution of substances between blood cells and serum occur so if these might influence the results, separate the serum within 30 to 45 min.

Anticoagulants

Heparin. A mucoitin polysulphate that inhibits thrombin formation from prothrombin, heparin is the most satisfactory anticoagulant since it does not produce a change in red cell volume or interfere with subsequent determinations. It is available as the sodium, potassium, ammonium and lithium salts. About 2 mg/10 ml of blood is used. As heparin does not dissolve easily it is often used as a film prepared from a solution dried on the walls of the container. However, it is more costly than other anticoagulants.

Ethylene diamine tetra-acetates (EDTA). EDTAs chelate calcium ions. The dipotassium and dilithium salts are used most; the disodium salt is less soluble. They do not alter the red cell volume and are used for blood collected for haematological examination. Use 10 to 20 mg/10 ml of blood.

Oxalates and Citrates. *Oxalates* act by precipitating calcium. *Potassium oxalate* is the most commonly used oxalate as it is the most soluble. Although 10 to 20 mg/10 ml blood are needed to prevent clotting, 20 to 30 mg of finely powdered salt is preferable. *Sodium citrate* converts calcium into a soluble non-ionised form. Nevertheless, citrated plasma is unsatisfactory for the determination of calcium. About 30 mg sodium citrate per 10 ml of blood will prevent clotting, but twice this amount is usually used. Appreciable withdrawal of water from cells results with both oxalate and nitrate, rather more with the latter as more is used. With oxalate the plasma can be diluted by several per cent.

Sodium Fluoride. This is also an anticoagulant but larger amounts are required than of either oxalate or citrate, as much as 10 mg/ml being needed. It is used more as a preservative as it inhibits red cell metabolism and bacterial action. It is used mixed with potassium oxalate, three parts oxalate to one of fluoride, but is better mixed with EDTA, one part of the disodium salt to two parts of fluoride, using 30 mg/10 ml blood.

Changes in Blood on Keeping

Several changes may take place.

1. *Loss of carbon dioxide.* As the carbon dioxide content of plasma exceeds that of air, it diffuses from the plasma to the atmosphere and from the cells to the plasma. This loss makes the blood more alkaline. The pH change is lessened by the conversion of bicarbonate ions to carbon dioxide and water using hydrogen ions derived from other blood buffer systems. This takes place mainly in the cells as the buffer concentration is higher and carbonic anhydrase is available. The fall in intracellular bicarbonate concentration is offset by diffusion from the plasma into the red cells, while chloride ions move in the reverse direction to preserve electrical neutrality.

To avoid these changes, blood collected in a heparinised syringe is kept cooled in ice with the needle sealed until it can be analysed. Smaller quantities collected in heparinised capillaries are sealed with plasticine and are similarly cooled. These are essential precautions for the measurement of blood gases.

2. *Conversion of glucose to lactic acid*. This is glycolysis (see p. 321).
3. *Increase in plasma inorganic phosphate* due to hydrolysis of organic phosphates present in the red cells. To avoid this, serum or plasma should be separated shortly after collection.
4. *Formation of ammonia from nitrogenous substances*, of which urea is the chief, may occur quickly. It is increased if the blood has been contaminated with bacteria. The blood should be chilled immediately after collection with sterile precautions.
5. *Passage of substances through the red cell membrane*. Potassium and phosphate, for example, are present in much higher concentration in the cells than in the plasma. Serum or heparinised plasma should be separated shortly after collection. Diffusion of potassium occurs more rapidly in blood at 4 °C than at room temperature as the sodium pump is less active. Separated samples show no further changes in potassium or phosphate on storage at 4 °C.
6. *Conversion of pyruvate to lactate*. The blood should be mixed with a protein precipitant to prevent this conversion immediately after collection.
7. *Other conversions*. Many hormones, particularly peptides, are affected by proteases in the blood making them unstable. Special handling such as collection into ice-chilled tubes and immediate centrifugation in a refrigerated centrifuge followed by freezing of the plasma may be required.

If blood is to be stored it should be collected under aseptic conditions. In general, serum or plasma should be separated as soon as possible after taking the blood and stored at 4 °C for up to 24 h or frozen for longer periods.

Type of Blood to be Used

The reasons for the choice of whole blood, serum or plasma for a particular determination are discussed under each substance later. There are, however, some general points of importance.

As the plasma rather than the red cells is in equilibrium with the interstitial fluid it is the change in plasma concentration which is significant so plasma or serum should usually be used. This is obligatory when the concentrations in the plasma and cells differ markedly, e.g. inorganic ions and some enzymes. Although the concentrations in the cell water may be the same as in the plasma water, the water content of cells is less than that of plasma making the concentration in the plasma several per cent higher than in whole blood. This occurs with glucose and urea. Some cell constituents may interfere in certain determinations, again favouring the use of serum or plasma.

Plasma and serum are almost interchangeable. Clearly, plasma must be used for fibrinogen. Otherwise two factors are relevant to the choice. If it is essential to separate the cells immediately, plasma is used. Where it is essential to minimise haemolysis and the release of other substances from the cells where their concentration is higher than in the plasma, e.g. some enzymes, it is claimed that it is easier to obtain serum free from haemolysis than plasma. This may be true for oxalate or citrate anticoagulants but it is much less important with heparin if sufficient care is taken. Serum or heparinised plasma are thus the specimens of choice for most substances. If plasma is not used within a few hours, fibrin clots can form which cause problems in automatic sampling devices by blocking narrow-bore tubing.

Whole blood is used immediately when very rapid changes occur, as with ammonia, lactate, pyruvate and pH, or when the substance is mainly in the cells as with lead and blood pigments. In a few instances it may be desirable to carry out a determination on the separated cells when the substance is normally only present in the red cells.

It may be necessary to precipitate the proteins from whole blood immediately after collection to preserve the analyte and details are given in the appropriate sections of the book. Many modern methods for plasma or serum constituents do not require the removal of protein other than by dialysis in continuous flow automated techniques. Early manual methods employed various ways of removing proteins and details will be found in the 5th edition of this book.

Measuring Blood

For safety reasons mouth pipetting of biological fluids including blood should not be performed. Automatic pipettes with disposable tips, described in Chapter 8, can be used satisfactorily. With the piston type of pipette the 'reverse' technique is recommended to ensure that the correct volume is delivered. If the liquid is expelled to the tip of the pipette, care must be taken that the last drop is expelled. As blood is more viscous than aqueous solutions this is best achieved by placing the pipette tip below the surface of the recipient solution. Alternatively, a mechanical diluter may be employed in which the blood sample taken into the tip is washed out with the diluent.

URINE

Collection of Urine Specimens

Single specimens of urine are used for ward examinations and qualitative tests, but for quantitative work 24 h collections are preferable. Since great variations of concentration occur during the day and there are diurnal variations in the excretion of some substances, it is the daily output of a substance which is usually significant. It is most convenient to collect the specimen from one morning to the next. At some suitable time, such as 0800 h, the patient empties his bladder and the urine is discarded. All specimens passed during the following 24 h are saved, and the specimen obtained by emptying the bladder at the same time (0800 h) the following morning is added to them. If the patient wishes to defaecate, the bladder should be emptied first to avoid loss of urine. There are several sources of error in the collection of 24 h specimens. Thus the first 0800 h specimen may not be discarded. The most likely error, however, is from specimens being thrown away inadvertently during the collection period. The creatinine content of the specimen can be used as a rough check on the reliability of the collection (p. 354).

Changes on Storage

The chief changes on storage arise from bacterial action. Urine for chemical examination is not usually collected aseptically and easily becomes infected.

However, if the urine is passed into, and kept in, clean well-washed receptacles and containers, little change will take place in a 24 h specimen by the time it reaches the laboratory, particularly if it has been kept in a cool place, preferably in a refrigerator, and is covered or stoppered. Such specimens should be sent to the laboratory as soon as possible after collection is completed.

The most important effect of bacteria is to convert urea into ammonium carbonate accounting for the ammoniacal odour and alkalinity of grossly contaminated urine. Such urines are obviously unsuitable for the determination of urea, ammonium, pH and total nitrogen. Micro-organisms may also act on glucose. If the urine becomes alkaline, phosphates may be precipitated. On standing, even in an uninfected urine, uric acid and urates may be deposited since they are less soluble in cool urine. Before carrying out analyses, any deposit must be well mixed with the urine before sampling. Uric acid and urates dissolve on moderate warming, phosphates after adding a little acid. Other changes which may occur are the oxidation of urobilinogen to urobilin and the rapid oxidation of ascorbic acid.

Preservatives for Urine

If urines are to be stored these changes should be prevented. The choice of preservative depends on the purpose for which the urine is being collected.

Acid is often satisfactory; 10 ml concentrated *hydrochloric acid* is adequate for a 24 h specimen but 50 ml of 2 mol/l acid is preferable. Such urines are particularly suitable for the determination of urea, ammonium, oxalate and calcium. Uric acid may be precipitated so the deposit must be well mixed before taking a sample. Acid should not be used for steroid determinations. For urobilinogen and porphobilinogen determinations the urine is made alkaline with 5 g sodium bicarbonate and covered with light petroleum.

Chloroform, toluene, light petroleum, thymol and formalin have been used but have disadvantages. *Toluene* and *light petroleum* form a thin layer on the surface and this contaminates pipettes unless the urine is placed in a separating funnel and the lower layer of urine run off. Moreover, these substances only prevent further surface contamination with bacteria, rather than stopping the growth of bacteria already introduced during the passage and collection of urine. *Chloroform* is more satisfactory in both respects. Since it settles to the bottom, it mixes with any deposit. Sufficient chloroform is used to give a saturated solution in the urine. *Thymol*, either a few crystals or 5 ml of a 100 g/l solution in isopropanol, is satisfactory for a wide range of substances including inorganic ions, urea, amino acids, creatinine, proteins, reducing substances, ketones and amylase. *Formalin*, 3 to 4 drops to 100 ml, can be used but greater amounts may give positive results with reducing tests for glucose. To preserve urine for the determination of ascorbic acid, add either *acetic acid* (10 ml) or *metaphosphoric acid* (5 g) to each 100 ml urine.

It is satisfactory in most cases to use specimens collected in cool, clean containers. Otherwise thymol, acid or chloroform should be used if possible. Any further points are dealt with under individual methods.

Volume of Urine

The daily output of urine on an average diet and normal fluid intake is between 1200 and 1500 ml but may vary widely both physiologically and for pathological reasons. While greatly influenced by the volume of fluids taken, the type of diet also has an effect. A high protein diet increases the volume because of the diuretic effect of the increased amount of urea formed. If the ambient temperature is high, volume is diminished and exercise has a similar effect. The minimum volume of urine needed to remove the daily osmolar load is about 500 ml. The ratio of day urine (0800 to 2000 h) to night urine (2000 to 0800 h) is at least 2 : 1 and sometimes 3 : 1 in health. In renal disease this ratio is reduced or even reversed.

An increased volume of urine, *polyuria*, is found in a number of conditions, particularly in diabetes insipidus when 10 to 20 l may be passed. In diabetes mellitus up to 5 or 6 l may be excreted daily. In chronic renal failure the volume is somewhat increased to 2 to 3 l daily. A reduced volume, *oliguria*, is found in pyrexia, acute nephritis, acute liver disorders, diarrhoea and in cardiac and renal failure. Total suppression of urine, *anuria*, may occur after a period in shock and in acute nephritis, for example.

FAECES

Faeces are partly of dietary origin: products of digestion which have not been absorbed, undigested parts of the food, particularly cellulose and other fibres, derivatives of foodstuffs as a result of bacterial action, such as indole, skatole, gases and fatty acids. Other components come from secretions entering the intestine and include enzymes, altered bile pigments, mucus and debris from intestinal wall cells. Bacteria and occasionally parasites are also present with a variable amount of water.

Collection of Faeces

Faeces are often collected in a bed pan but it is more convenient when the whole stool is to be sent to the laboratory for it to be passed directly into a large disposable container. For such examinations as occult blood it is convenient to send a representative portion of the stool in a small sealed carton. For quantitative determinations the whole stool should be sent within a short time after completing the collection. It is preferable to avoid using stools containing liquid paraffin or barium salts, or which have been collected after an enema has been given.

Admixture with urine should not occur. Usually simple inspection is sufficient to check but a good indication is given by the presence of considerable amounts of chloride as this is only excreted in small amounts in normal stools. A simple qualitative test will suffice.

Preservation of Faeces

Usually fresh specimens should be used to avoid the need for preservation. If they have to be kept, they are best stored in a refrigerator. If faecal nitrogen is to be measured, mix the faeces with about 200 ml water and homogenise. To an aliquot of this add carefully, with constant stirring, an equal volume of concentrated sulphuric acid and store until a convenient time for the analysis.

Marking Faeces

In balance studies it may be necessary to collect all the urine and faeces passed over a period of time. While collection of the urine is straightforward, that of the faeces is more difficult. Several substances, particularly charcoal, carmine and gentian violet have been used to mark the start and end of the experimental period. The dyes are the more successful. Give 0·5 to 1 g in capsules before breakfast on the first morning of the test, when collection of urine begins, and again before breakfast on the last day of the test, the point at which urine collection ceases. The faecal collection commences with the first specimen to contain the dye and includes all specimens up to but excluding that which contains the second dose of the dye. Such marking is often unsatisfactory and little better than collecting for the same period as used for the urine. Whitby and Lang (1960) used chromium sesquioxide, Cr_2O_3, given as three 500 mg capsules, one with each main meal. The stools are homogenised and the Cr_2O_3 determined in an aliquot after oxidation to dichromate, or by atomic absorption spectrophotometry. The volume of the homogenate corresponding to 1·5 g of the oxide corresponds to one day's output of faeces. Chromium sesquioxide obtained commercially must be purified by removal of dichromate with acid (Fisher *et al.*, 1972).

The Amount of Faeces

Daily Quantity. The daily quantity of faeces varies with the fibre content of the diet, the amount of water taken and the transit time through the gut. The weight of a day's faeces ranges from 60 to 400 g for an adult, the highest figures being found with a high fibre diet and the low ones with a low fibre diet rich in protein. A greatly increased bulk is found in steatorrhoea, when 500 to 1000 g may be passed daily. Such an increase is obvious on inspection.

Water Content. On a typical mixed diet the faeces contain 70 to 80% water but the amount is lower on a high protein diet and higher with a high fibre intake. The higher the fat content of the faeces the higher the water content. In diarrhoea the water content exceeds 90%.

Total Solids. The daily excretion of faeces expressed as dry weight is 25 to 45 g. It is higher on a high fibre diet but on fasting falls to 2 to 3 g.

Faecal pH. The pH varies from 5 to 9, again being influenced by the diet. There are also considerable variations in a single stool. Usually the pH is slightly alkaline but its wide variation makes the determination of little value except when acid stools with a pH of less than 5 are passed by infants with disaccharidase deficiencies. Freshly passed specimens must be used. The simplest method is to use a moistened indicator paper and apply it to the stool.

Odour. The odour of normal faeces is mainly due to the action of bacteria on proteins to produce indole and skatole, the quantity depending on the amount of meat in the diet. Substances such as organic sulphur compounds and hydrogen sulphide contribute to the odour of faeces with a more disagreeable smell.

REFERENCES

Fisher M. T., Atkins P. R., Joplin C. F. (1972). *Clin. Chim. Acta*; **41**: 109.
Salway J. G. (1978). *Ann. Clin. Biochem*; **15**: 44.
Whitby L. G., Lang D. (1960). *J. Clin. Invest*; **39**: 854.
Young D. S., Estaner L. C., Gibberman V. (1975). *Clin. Chem*; **21**: 1–432D.

15

GLUCOSE, OTHER SUGARS AND KETONES

Since the introduction of insulin for the treatment of diabetes mellitus, the determination of blood 'sugar' has been one of the tests most frequently carried out in the biochemical laboratory. Early techniques involved the precipitation of blood proteins, reduction of either alkaline solutions containing Cu^{2+} to cuprous oxide or of alkaline ferricyanide to ferrocyanide, followed by measurement of such reduction iodometrically or colorimetrically. Other reducing substances in blood, particularly in the red cells, affect these reactions. Glutathione is one of the most important but glucuronates, threonine, urate and ascorbate contribute to a lesser degree. The reagents used for protein precipitation and variations in the composition of the alkaline copper or ferricyanide reagents influence the degree of interference. Details can be found in earlier editions of this book.

With the introduction of techniques using glucose oxidase, which oxidises glucose to gluconic acid and hydrogen peroxide with relatively little effect on other sugars present in blood, it was expected that true glucose values would be obtained. However, both positive and negative errors can arise. Fluoride, protein precipitants, urate, bilirubin, glutathione and ascorbate may influence the action of the enzymes used in this technique and such effects should be minimised if the desired specificity is to be achieved.

A totally different technique (Hultmann, 1959) uses the colour given by aldoses with o-toluidine in glacial acetic acid. This base reacts quantitatively with the aldehyde group of an aldohexose to form a glycosylamine and then a Schiff base.

Glycosylamine   Schiff base

In the absence of such aldoses as galactose and lactose, procedures using this reaction give very similar results to those using glucose oxidase. Sample deproteinisation is unnecessary but may overcome errors due to haemoglobin and bilirubin, both of which significantly increase the glucose result. Important disadvantages of the original method included instability of the colour produced and of the o-toluidine reagent, poor between-batch precision and the problems of using glacial acetic acid. Later modifications overcame some of these drawbacks by the addition of thiourea or borate to improve colour stability or by the use of a less acidic reagent. The o-toluidine method was adapted as a simple, reliable, specific and inexpensive method for the AutoAnalyzer but it lost favour and is now used mainly as an ancillary method.

The hexokinase/glucose-6-phosphate dehydrogenase method is virtually specific for glucose and has been proposed as a 'reference' method (Passey et al., 1977). The method is unaffected by haemolysis, lipaemia, or the presence of increased amounts of urate, ascorbate or bilirubin. The reagents are expensive but since only small volumes are used in the current generation of analysers, this method is being increasingly used.

More recently, the successful purification of glucose dehydrogenase has led to its use in the development of new blood glucose methods. Glucose dehydrogenase reacts with β-D-glucose converting it to D-gluconolactone with reduction of NAD^+ to NADH. Glucose dehydrogenase also catalyses the dehydrogenation of xylose but this only becomes significant after oral xylose loading. There is no interference by ascorbate, urate, bilirubin, fluoride or heparin.

Any technique chosen for routine use should preferably give results near to the true glucose concentration since other reducing substances may vary appreciably in the same individual even over short periods. When controlling the therapy of diabetic patients such variations may not affect the usefulness of the results obtained with non-specific methods, but for glucose tolerance tests and when the glucose concentration is abnormally low it is necessary to use a specific technique. Accordingly, enzymatic methods are preferred for the clinical laboratory.

Glucose determinations are done in batches, as emergency requests, or sporadically as patients arrive at an out-patient clinic. These needs are served by the combination of a fast automated system and a semi-automated glucose analyser.

Glycolysis. Glucose disappears fairly rapidly from whole blood on standing, so that up to 0·5 mmol/l may be lost hourly at room temperature. This is due to its conversion to lactate by glycolysis which results from cell metabolism. There is no loss of glucose from serum or plasma free from cells. The rate of glycolysis can be decreased by adding sodium fluoride to the anticoagulant. A mixture of sodium fluoride and potassium oxalate in the proportion of one part to three prevents significant loss of glucose for two to three days, so that the blood can be sent through the post. Excess fluoride should not be used as it can interfere with some glucose oxidase techniques. Addition of 20 mg of the mixture to 5 ml blood is adequate. Disposable containers incorporating such a mixture are available labelled for blood glucose estimation. Alternatively, a mixture of EDTA and fluoride can be used. If capillary blood is collected, this may be added directl ᵗ⌐ the protein-precipitating solution, thereby preventing glycolysis.

DETERMINATION OF BLOOD AND PLASMA GLUCOSE

Choice of Blood Specimen

Because of the large number of determinations on individual diabetic patie: capillary blood has often been used. This avoids frequent venepunctu automatically measures the volume of blood required at the time of collecti avoids a centrifugation step, while glycolysis can be avoided by putting the blood directly into protein precipitant or diluent containing preservative. However, there has been an increasing tendency to use plasma or serum which gives a more accurate measurement of the glucose concentration of extracellular fluid. The glucose concentration in the water of cells and plasma is the same but the water content of cells, 73 %, is less than that of plasma, 93 %. Plasma glucose is thus higher than the concentration in whole blood. This may be corrected for by multiplying the whole blood glucose concentration by 1·15 and adding 0·33 mmol/l to derive the plasma or serum glucose. This correction is reasonably accurate if the haematocrit is normal. If it is low as in anaemia, the whole blood concentration is closer to that of plasma and is more divergent in polycythaemia.

Plasma is preferred to serum as the blood can be added directly to the mixture of anticoagulant and preservative and then separated immediately. This gives a larger sample for analysis than serum from the same volume of blood and there is less glycolysis. If serum is used it must be separated as soon as possible, but not later than 30 to 40 min after blood collection. In summary, whole blood is more convenient but plasma gives a better measure of the glucose content of ECF.

A further choice is between capillary (arterialised) blood and venous blood. The glucose content differs little in the fasting state but after glucose intake, the venous glucose concentration is lower than the capillary figure by up to 2 mmol/l as a consequence of cell utilisation of glucose.

I. Glucose Oxidase Methods

In these methods, the aldehyde group of β-D-glucose is oxidised by glucose oxidase to give gluconic acid and hydrogen peroxide.

$$\beta\text{-D-Glucose} + H_2O + O_2 \rightarrow \text{gluconic acid} + H_2O_2$$

The hydrogen peroxide may be broken down to water and oxygen by a peroxidase and if an oxygen acceptor is present, it will be converted to a coloured compound which can be measured. Initially, o-dianisidine and o-tolidine were used but were potentially carcinogenic and other oxygen acceptors have replaced them. Morley *et al.* (1968) used guaiacum while Trinder (1969) used phenol and condensed its oxidation product with 4-aminophenazone to give a coloured product as in the determination of alkaline phosphatase.

The reagents used by Trinder have a high affinity for oxygen and the reaction is nearly instantaneous. Some oxygen acceptors of lesser affinity are susceptible to interference from drugs possessing a greater affinity for oxygen, resulting in underestimation of glucose. One such oxygen acceptor gives low glucose figures in the presence of the anti-diabetic drug, tolazamide (Sharp *et al.*, 1972), isoniazid, hydrallazine and iproniazid (Sharp, 1972) and paracetamol (Kaufmann-Raab *et al.*, 1976). None of the first four drugs interfere with the 4-aminophenazone method and paracetamol is unlikely to interfere as it affects other methods by virtue of its phenol group. Such groups are in excess in the Trinder method. This is the colorimetric method of choice and is given below. Only two reagents are required: the protein precipitant (a phosphotungstate reagent containing phenol) and a colour reagent (glucose oxidase, peroxidase and 4-aminophenazone).

The glucose oxidase/peroxidase colorimetric methods used currently are relatively free from interference compared to earlier techniques. There is no interference by urate, creatinine, glutathione or haemoglobin and only minor interference from xylose, galactose and levodopa. Ascorbate may however significantly decrease results by retarding colour development. The delay becomes most significant in the kinetic modifications of these assays. Fast-reacting oxygen-acceptors are more resistant to ascorbate interference.

The oxygen consumed in the reaction has also been determined polarographically as in the glucose analysers introduced by Beckman and Analox Instruments (Alpha Laboratories). By monitoring the rate of glucose oxidation directly, interference due to secondary enzyme systems or low affinity chromogens is avoided. In a comparison of ten glucose methods, the Beckman Glucose Analyser was found to have analytical performance characteristics closest to those of the Proposed Product Class Standard Hexokinase Method (US Department of

Health Education and Welfare, Food and Drug Administration, 1974). Whole blood is usually unsuitable for use with these analysers due to interference by oxygen exchange with haemoglobin. However, whole blood can be used with the Analox GM7 Oxidase Analyser if it is collected into special anticoagulant tubes containing fluoride, heparin and sodium nitrite.

Yellow Springs Instruments also produce manual and automated glucose analysers capable of measuring glucose concentration in whole blood. These analysers employ immobilised glucose oxidase on a resin sandwiched between polycarbonate and cellulose acetate membranes. A hydrogen peroxide electrode detects the oxidation of glucose by the glucose oxidase. Only substances with a molecular weight of less than 100 should reach the electrode so that interference by drugs should not occur. However, the original membranes did not prevent gross interference by paracetamol (Farah *et al.*, 1982) although this has been greatly reduced by the introduction of a modified membrane (Townsend, 1983).

Hydrogen peroxide produced by the action of glucose oxidase can also be measured by its oxidation of luminol in strongly alkaline conditions. This chemiluminescent method is very sensitive, has been used in continuous flow systems and is linear over a wide range of concentrations. Potential interferences in biological materials have not been fully investigated (Williams *et al.*, 1976).

Glucose Oxidase Method Using Phenol and 4-Aminophenazone

1. *Manual Technique* (*Trinder*, 1969)
   Reagents.
   1. Protein precipitant. Dissolve $10 \cdot 0$ g sodium tungstate (Na_2WO_4, $2H_2O$), $9 \cdot 0$ g sodium chloride and $10 \cdot 0$ g disodium hydrogen phosphate (Na_2HPO_4) in about 800 ml water. Add about 125 ml $1 \cdot 0$ mol/l hydrochloric acid to bring the pH to $3 \cdot 0$ using narrow range indicator paper. Add $1 \cdot 0$ g phenol and make to 1 litre with water. This reagent is stable indefinitely.
   2. Colour reagent. Mix 75 ml disodium hydrogen phosphate solution (40 g Na_2HPO_4/l), 215 ml water, 5 ml Fermcozyme 653 AM Glucose Oxidase (Hughes & Hughes Limited, Romford, Essex) and 5 ml Peroxidase RZ $0 \cdot 6$ ($1 \cdot 0$ g/l, Sigma). Add 300 mg sodium azide and 100 mg 4-aminophenazone. The reagent is stable for up to 8 weeks at 4°C. (See p. 6 for azide hazard.)
   3. Standard glucose solution, 10 mmol/l ($1 \cdot 80$ g/l) in benzoic acid (10 g/l). Prepare 24 h before use to allow for equilibration of the α- and β-forms.

Technique. Add 100 μl plasma to $2 \cdot 9$ ml protein precipitant, mix well, centrifuge and pipette $1 \cdot 0$ ml clear supernatant into a $1 \cdot 6$ cm test tube. For the blank take $1 \cdot 0$ ml protein precipitant and for the standard, $1 \cdot 0$ ml of a mixture containing 100 μl glucose standard and $2 \cdot 9$ ml protein precipitant. To each add $3 \cdot 0$ ml colour reagent and incubate at 37°C for 10 min, shaking briefly two or three times. Read tests and standard against the blank at 515 nm.
   Calculation.

$$\text{Plasma glucose (mmol/l)} = \frac{\text{Reading of unknown}}{\text{Reading of standard}} \times 10$$

To check linearity, prepare a standard curve as follows

Plasma glucose (mmol/l)	0	5·0	10·0	15·0	20·0	25·0
Standard solution (ml)	0	0·1	0·2	0·3	0·4	0·5
Protein precipitant (ml)	6·0	5·9	5·8	5·7	5·6	5·5

To $1 \cdot 0$ ml of each, add $3 \cdot 0$ ml colour reagent and proceed as above.

Note. Glucose oxidase reacts only with β-D-glucose. Since the α- and β-forms are in equilibrium in plasma, the glucose standard solutions must reach equilibrium after preparation. This may take up to 24 h at room temperature.

2. Manual Technique without Protein Precipitation (*Trinder*, 1969; *modified*)

Reagents. These are identical to those for the manual method above except that the sodium tungstate is omitted from the protein precipitant to give the diluent.

Technique. Add 25 μl plasma, standard or distilled water to 1·0 ml diluent to prepare the test, standard or blank. To each add 3·0 ml colour reagent, mix and incubate at 37° C for 15 min shaking briefly two or three times. Read the test and standard against the blank at 515 nm.

Calculation. As above. For the assay of glucose concentrations greater than 20 mmol/l, use 10 μl plasma and modify the calculation appropriately. Glucose concentrations in CSF or in hypoglycaemic plasma can be measured more accurately by using 50 or 100 μl of sample.

3. Technique for the Technicon AutoAnalyzer (*Richardson*, 1977)

When Pennock *et al.* (1973) reviewed the methods for glucose estimation then available, they concluded that the Trinder (1969) macro and micro methods were the best AutoAnalyzer methods for accurate and precise estimation of plasma or blood glucose even in the hypoglycaemic range. However, the sample rates were only 40/h and the micro method used five times as much enzyme as the macro method. Richardson (1977) used the increased sensitivity of the sulphonated 2,4-dichlorophenol reagent to develop a method for AAII systems in which the micro samples of Barham and Trinder (1972) are retained but sample rates are increased to 90/h. Enzyme consumption is reduced to a third.

Reagents.
1. Sample diluent, 'Floxsal'. Dissolve 1 g sodium fluoride, 2 g potassium oxalate $(COOK)_2$, $2H_2O$, and 9 g sodium chloride in water, make to 1 litre, mix well and store at room temperature.
2. 4-Aminophenazone solution (25 mmol/l). Dissolve 5 g 4-aminophenazone in water and make to 1 litre. Store at 4° C.
3. Stock solution of sulphonated 2,4-dichlorophenol, 20 g/l. To 10 g 2,4-dichlorophenol add 20 ml concentrated sulphuric acid and heat for 5 h on a water bath at 100° C. (The quality of commercially supplied 2,4-dichlorophenol varies. If the solid is not white, distil it in an all-glass apparatus fitted with an air condenser.) Cool, add carefully 400 ml water, neutralise with 10 mol/l sodium hydroxide, add 10 ml sulphuric acid, 1 mol/l, and make to 500 ml with water. Filter if not quite clear. This reagent keeps indefinitely. The reagent is also available commercially as '2,4-Dichlorophenol (sulphonate), 0·123 mol/l' from BDH Chemicals Limited.
4. Phosphate buffer. Dissolve 20 g Na_2HPO_4, 20 g KH_2PO_4 and 4 g sodium azide in water and make to 1 litre. The pH should be $6·8 \pm 0·1$. Store at room temperature. (For hazards of disposal see p. 6.)
5. Sodium chloride solution, 180 g/l. Store at room temperature.
6. Diluent. Mix 25 ml reagent (3) and 50 ml reagent (5) and dilute to 1 litre with water. Store at 4° C.
7. Colour reagent. To 50 ml reagent (2) and 250 ml reagent (4) add 20 ml Fermcozyme 653AM and 20 mg Peroxidase RZ 0·6. Dissolve, mix well and dilute to 1 litre. Store at 4° C.
8. Saturated benzoic acid solution. Dissolve 40 g benzoic acid in about 800 ml water with heating, make up to 1 litre and allow to cool. Decant the solution

from the crystals and use as the diluting solution for the glucose standards.

9. Stock standard glucose solution, 50 mmol/l. Dissolve 9·0 g pure anhydrous glucose in saturated benzoic acid solution and dilute to 1 litre with the same. Allow to stand at room temperature for 24 h before use. Alternatively, use the BDH Glucose Standard Solution, 50 mmol/l.

10. Intermediate stock standard solution, 5 mmol/l. Dilute 10 ml stock standard to 100 ml with saturated benzoic acid solution.

11. Working standard glucose solutions. Dilute 2, 5, 10, 15, 20, 25 ml volumes of the intermediate stock standard to 100 ml to give solutions containing 0·1, 0·25, 0·50, 0·75, 1·00 and 1·25 mmol/l respectively, equivalent to 2, 5, 10, 15, 20 and 25 mmol/l for test samples diluted 1 in 20. Store at 4°C. Alternatively, dilute the stock solution directly to solutions containing 2, 5, 10, 15, 20 and 25 mmol/l which can be diluted 1 in 20 like the plasma samples using the same dilutor. Any discrepancies in the behaviour of the dilutor can then be checked by comparing the standard curves prepared in the two ways.

Technique. The manifold required is shown in Fig. 15.1. The sampling rate is 90/h with a 6 s wash cycle and a printer range setting from 0 to 30 mmol/l. Load the sample tray with two low standards and then the rest of the standard curve; follow the top standard with a low standard before introducing the diluted samples. This checks the degree of carry-over and ensures minimal contamination of the first sample. Prepare samples by diluting 100 μl plasma with 1·9 ml Floxsal diluent. Capillary or fluoride samples can be used, as can whole blood if preferred.

To maintain sensitivity and precision, at weekly intervals remove the dialyzer and flush the system with dilute hypochlorite solution.

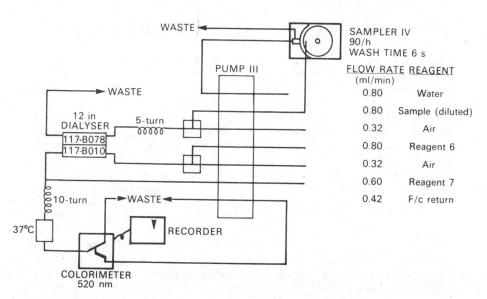

Fig. 15.1. AutoAnalyzer Flow Diagram for Plasma Glucose Using Glucose Oxidase (Richardson, 1977).

II. Hexokinase Method

The hexokinase method is virtually specific for glucose. This enzyme in the presence of ATP converts glucose into its 6-phosphate:

$$\text{D-Glucose} + \text{ATP} \rightarrow \text{Glucose-6-phosphate} + \text{ADP}$$

Other hexoses react but have no significant effect at concentrations encountered in biological fluids. The glucose-6-phosphate is specifically converted by its dehydrogenase (G-6-PD) in the presence of NAD^+ into 6-phosphogluconate:

$$\text{Glucose-6-phosphate} + \text{OH}^- + \text{NAD}^+ \rightarrow \text{6-Phosphogluconate}^- + \text{NADH} + \text{H}^+$$

The NADH produced is proportional to the glucose present and can be measured by the increased absorbance at 340 nm or by fluorescence with emission at 456 nm. Both end-point and kinetic methods have been used (Widdowson and Penton, 1972; Lloyd et al., 1978; Mieling et al., 1979).

The method is unaffected by haemolysis, lipaemia, or the presence of increased amounts of urate, ascorbate or bilirubin. Drugs affecting some of the oxidase methods do not interfere but high levels of anticoagulants may affect the reactions and the organic mercurial preservative, thiomersal, interferes. This is added to some control sera and glucose standards and is an enzyme inhibitor.

Most methods use commercially prepared reagents and have been modified for use on centrifugal fast analysers and other discrete analysers. These methods use plasma or serum without deproteinisation and may have a high blank reading for which correction should be made. These direct assays also show some interference by lipid and haemoglobin (Passey et al., 1977).

Technicon Corporation Limited have introduced a hexokinase method for the SMAC which uses hexokinase immobilised in a coiled nylon tube 30 cm long with a bore of 1 mm. A dialysis step decreases interference. It is claimed that the enzyme in the coil is stable for one month and that this time period is unaffected by the number of assays performed.

SOLID PHASE TESTS FOR GLUCOSE IN BLOOD AND PLASMA

The need for the rapid production of glucose results in laboratories and clinics has led to the development of several solid phase, or dry chemistry, tests for the determination of glucose in blood and plasma. All such tests are based on variations of the glucose oxidase/peroxidase linked assays.

In the earlier strip tests (e.g. Dextrostix, Ames) a large drop of blood was placed on the test area of the strip and was later removed with a fine jet of water after a timed interval. The colour produced was compared with a colour chart or read on a meter (e.g. Glucometer, Ames), which removed the subjective visual comparison but required calibration. Opinions varied concerning the value of these strips beyond distinguishing hypo- and hyperglycaemia. Despite this, Dextrostix was found to be clinically useful for monitoring diabetic ketoacidosis and for detecting hypoglycaemia, if used and stored correctly. Dextrostix has a working range up to 22 mmol/l using the Glucometer. This range was too narrow for some purposes and was widened by the introduction of BM Test Glycemie 1–44 (originally 20–800) (Boehringer Corporation). Whole blood placed on the test area is gently wiped off with a cotton wool pad after 1 min. The strip develops two colours simultaneously which improves the accuracy of the visual comparison with a colour chart which shows colours corresponding to glucose concentrations of 1·1, 2·2, 4·4, 6·7, 10·0, 13·3, 22·2 and 44·4 mmol/l. The colour can also be read on the Reflolux meter, which decreases errors in reading while restricting the working range to 2·0 to 22·0 mmol/l. The instrument is calibrated with a special strip. Experience confirms that the BM 1–44 test gives a good estimate of the blood glucose concentration. The strips are easy to read and are stable when stored at room temperature.

A similar two-colour test area is used with Visidex II strips (Ames) which also have a working range up to 44 mmol/l and are read against a colour chart. This is claimed to be facilitated by the provision of a holed colour comparator. Several studies have shown that both BM 1–44 and Visidex II produce results correlating well with those from conventional analysers.

Further simplification came with the introduction of the Reflocheck System (Boehringer Corporation), based on a microprocessor-controlled instrument. This uses bar-coded test strips which give automatic calibration. The working range with the meter is 1·1 to 25 mmol/l and the strips can be read visually between 3·5 and 44 mmol/l. The results correlate well with those from the Beckman Analyser when correction is made for the difference between whole blood and plasma glucose.

Glucose can be measured on a few dry chemistry analysers (p. 182). The Ames Seralyser uses glucose oxidase coupled to peroxidase and 3,3',5,5'-tetramethyl-benzidine. The rate of colour development is measured at 640 nm. Thomas *et al.* (1982) found a within-batch CV of less than 2·5 % in the range 4·1 to 19·6 mmol/l, for which the between-batch CV was better than 5 %. The results correlate well with the hexokinase method. Bilirubin interferes and icteric samples cannot be assayed. The manufacturer recommends that the assay should not be used for monitoring diabetic ketoacidosis or neonatal hypoglycaemia. The Kodak Ektachem analysers use a modified Trinder method, replacing the phenol by 1,7-dihydroxynaphthalene. A between-batch CV of less than 3 % and acceptable correlation with hexokinase and glucose oxidase assays is claimed.

For a review of blood glucose assays see Burrin and Price (1985).

TESTS FOR GLUCOSE AND OTHER REDUCING SUBSTANCES IN URINE

Earlier tests for reducing substances in urine were those of Benedict and Fehling in which alkaline Cu^{2+} reagents are reduced to cuprous oxide. The amounts of reducing substances in normal urine are insufficient to give a positive reaction with such tests. Although intended to detect glucose, other reducing substances also react. These include other sugars—pentoses, fructose, galactose and lactose—glucuronates, salicyluric acid, homogentisic acid and, in concentrated urine, urate and creatinine. Benedict's reagent is less likely to react with the last two and is more sensitive for detecting glucose.

Tests for reducing substances are now mostly used in a tablet or stick form, and a positive test may require further investigation to identify the reducing substance. More specific stick tests based on glucose oxidase are available.

Test for Reducing Substances

Clinitest

This convenient form of Benedict's test (Ames Company) is an alkaline copper reagent made up in tablets containing copper sulphate, sodium hydroxide (38·5 %), sodium bicarbonate and citric acid. A small test tube and dropper are provided. Measure 5 drops of urine and 10 drops of water into the tube and add one tablet. Owing to the large amount of sodium hydroxide present, sufficient heat is generated to give rapid reduction. To obtain the correct result it is essential to follow the instructions exactly, particularly to observe the reaction until complete and not to shake the tube until 15 s after boiling ceases. A colour chart allows a rough assessment of the sugar concentration up to 20 g/l.

Identification of the Reducing Substances

Any urine giving a positive test for reducing substances should be tested using a specific method for glucose if there is the possibility that some substance other than glucose may be present. Failure to detect glucose requires further investigation of the nature of the reducing substance. For carbohydrates, earlier tests such as yeast fermentation and osazone preparation have been superseded by chromatographic techniques. Although paper chromatography can give satisfactory results, thin-layer techniques are quicker and more sensitive.

Thin-layer Chromatography

Reagents.
1. Silica gel G (Merck or Camlab), 250 μm on 10 × 20 cm plates. Prepared plates on glass or plastic are convenient.
2. Solvent mixture: *n*-butanol–acetic acid–water, 75/25/6 v/v. The water content is important—if less than 5 parts the run tails, if more than 10 there is bearding.
3. Visualising agent, aniline-diphenylamine. Dissolve 10 ml aniline and 10 g diphenylamine in 1 litre of acetone. Mix 10 volumes of this with 1 volume of orthophosphoric acid (sp. gr. 1·75).
4. Standards. Mix equal volumes of 10 g/l solutions of glucose, galactose and lactose in isopropanol; 1·5 μl then contains 5 μg of each of these sugars.

Technique. A suitable amount of each sugar is 2·5 to 7·5 μg. Determine the concentration of reducing substances and calculate the volume containing this quantity, diluting the urine if necessary so that 2 to 5 μl can be used. Apply samples along a line 2 cm from the short edge at 1 cm intervals with standards on either side of the urine spots. Run until the solvent front has risen about 15 cm. This takes 2 to 3 h. Dry under hot air, spray with visualising agent and heat for 5 min at 110° C in an oven.

R_f values are approximately: lactose, 0·14; galactose, 0·35; fructose, 0·39; glucose, 0·42; pentoses, 0·5–0·9. Glucose, galactose and lactose give a grey colour, fructose a pinkish one. The separation of glucose and galactose is as good as the best obtained on paper and the run is much quicker. Some methods include borate in the solvent but this makes little difference to the separation of simple sugars.

The use of kieselguhr layers with ethyl acetate–isopropanol–water, 18/1/1, gives quicker development (14 cm in 35 min) but the spots are less discrete and the separation of glucose and galactose is less good.

Tests for Individual Reducing Substances

Colour tests for sugars other than glucose include Seliwanoff's test for fructose, Bial's test for pentoses and the methylamine test for lactose. They have become obsolete and details can be found in earlier editions of this book. Homogentisic acid (p. 764) and salicyluric acid (p. 385) are discussed elsewhere.

Specific Tests for Glucose

These tests like those for plasma glucose determination employ glucose oxidase, a vegetable peroxidase and a detector reaction, but in stick form.

Clinistix. This stick (Ames Company) has an area impregnated with *o*-tolidine, the enzymes and a pink dye. The *o*-tolidine is oxidised to a blue substance thereby producing various shades of purple. The colour is noted 10 s after dipping the stick in the urine. Positive results can be obtained with glucose concentrations above 1·1 to 5·5 mmol/l (0·2 to 1·0 g/l), the sensitivity varying with pH, temperature and the concentration of other urinary inhibitory constituents including ascorbate. Because of this the test cannot be used quantitatively but is useful as a screening test to exclude the presence of a significant amount of glucose.

Diastix. An area in this stick (Ames Company) is impregnated with the usual enzymes, potassium iodide and a blue background dye. The iodine liberated in the final reaction blends with the blue colour to produce a series of colour changes 30 s after wetting the stick with urine. A greenish colour may be given with as little as 0·6 to 5·5 mmol/l (0·1 to 1·0 g/l), depending on the amount of urinary constituents which inhibit the reaction. The colour changes vary through shades of green to varying intensities of brown giving some semi-quantitative information up to a glucose concentration of 110 mmol/l (20 g/l). This test now provides the glucose-detecting zone in the multiple test sticks: Keto-diastix, N-Multistix-SG, Multistix-SG, Bili-Labstix, Labstix and N-Labstix.

BM-Test Glucose. This stick (Boehringer Corporation) has an area impregnated with the enzymes, an unstated indicator and a yellow background dye. The reaction product is green-blue in colour giving a gradation in shade, 30 to 60 s after dipping in the urine, varying from a faint green to a deep blue-green. The reaction is independent of pH over the range 4 to 9 but inhibitors, particularly ascorbate, affect the lower limit of detection. This is 1·6 mmol/l (0·3 g/l) under good conditions and corresponds to the upper limit of glycosuria in normal random urine specimens.

The test when combined with other tests in various multiple stick tests (BM 3, 4, 4S, 5, 6, 6 Bili, and 8) uses a different indicator giving colours ranging from orange to red-brown as the glucose concentration increases.

Diabur-Test 5000. This stick (Boehringer Corporation) is based on the same reaction as above but has two areas with different sensitivities to glucose. The more sensitive, pale yellow area changes to pale green at glucose concentrations around 3·3 mmol/l (0·6 g/l) and reaches full colour intensity at 110 mmol/l (20 g/l). The less sensitive, white area turns light blue at 28 mmol/l (5 g/l) reaching dark blue at 280 mmol/l (50 g/l). This combination permits semi-quantitative determination of urinary glucose concentration over the range 3·3 to 280 mmol/l. The results agree with those measured by a hexokinase method (Kattemann *et al.*, 1982). The test is unaffected by the pH of the specimen but high levels of ascorbate diminish the colour.

Note. With all these specific stick tests, it is possible to detect traces of glucose in the urine undetected by the Clinitest or Benedict's test. False positive results occur if there are residues of hydrogen peroxide, hypochlorite or detergents containing perborate in the urine container. All oxidise the detector substance.

Investigation of a Positive Test for a Reducing Substance in Urine

With rare exceptions such as galactose and fructose, only glucose of the many possible reducing substances in urine has pathological significance. Having found glycosuria, one must decide whether the patient has diabetes mellitus. If the symptoms of diabetes are present, the diagnosis is confirmed by plasma glucose estimation, or by a glucose tolerance test in those cases where the fasting plasma glucose is not diagnostic (see p. 335).

An important group of cases is that without symptoms suggesting diabetes, in which a positive test has been obtained during routine medical examination, as in pregnancy, for life insurance, etc. In the majority of such cases the reducing substance is glucose but clinical diabetes is uncommon.

In an adult, the important point is to exclude diabetes so it is usual to perform a glucose tolerance test. If that is normal, the positive reduction test can be regarded as of little clinical significance. If it is desired to determine the nature of a non-glucose reducing substance, the most useful procedure is thin-layer chromatography to identify the sugar present. *In a neonate or infant*, the presence of a reducing substance in the urine should always be further investigated to determine its nature.

Quantitative Determination of Glucose in Urine

For many purposes, a sufficiently good estimate of the amount of glucose can be obtained from Clinitest. The precipitate is greenish at a glucose concentration of 14 mmol/l, greenish yellow at about 28 mmol/l and yellowish orange at around 56 mmol/l. An estimate of daily excretion is sometimes required. A 24 h specimen is collected and the glucose concentration is measured quantitatively. Any of the plasma glucose methods can be applied to urine after dilution to bring the glucose concentration within the range of the method used. In most cases this means to below about 22 mmol/l. The dilution necessary can be gauged from the qualitative test.

KETOSIS

The most important consequence of the increased metabolism of fat in diabetes mellitus is the accumulation in the blood of acetoacetate, $CH_3.CO.CH_2.COO^-$, 3-hydroxybutyrate, $CH_3.CH(OH).CH_2.COO^-$, its reduction product, and of acetone, $CH_3.CO.CH_3$, formed by decarboxylation of acetoacetic acid.

Unless adequate intracellular glucose is available, free fatty acids released from adipose tissue are oxidised to acetyl CoA by all tissues except the brain. Much of the acetyl CoA is condensed to acetoacetate which is in turn reduced to 3-hydroxybutyrate. The liver is the main site of ketogenesis. When the ketones begin to accumulate in the blood they also appear in the urine. Although diabetics are able to metabolise ketones normally, their increased production may exceed the capacity for catabolism. Testing of the urine for these substances is an important part of the routine examination of diabetic patients.

Ketosis following starvation or vomiting occurs in the same way as the ketosis of diabetes and small amounts of ketones may occasionally be detectable in the early morning urine specimens of normal persons.

Qualitative Tests for Ketone Bodies in Urine

Earlier tests for ketone bodies in urine included Gerhardt's ferric chloride test and Rothera's nitroprusside test. The former is non-specific, reacting with phenolic groups, e g. salicylate, to give a variety of colours, some similar to the red-brown colour produced by acetoacetate. Rothera's test is negative with phenols, but is positive with both acetoacetate and acetone. It is now available in tablet or stick form.

Acetest. This is in tablet form (Ames Company). One drop of urine is applied to the tablet containing sodium nitroprusside, glycine and disodium phosphate. A purple colour is given by acetoacetate and acetone and is compared with a colour chart after 30 s.

Stick Tests. *Ketostix* (Ames Company) and *BM-Test Keton* (Boehringer Corporation) are plastic strips, one end of which is impregnated with a buffered mixture of sodium nitroprusside and glycine. The test end is dipped into a fresh specimen of urine, serum or plasma and removed immediately, briefly touching the tip on the side of the container to remove excess liquid. The colour produced is compared with the colour chart, 15 s (Ketostix) or 30 to 60 s (BM-Test) later. The test is positive if a lavender or purple colour develops. The test area may be combined with others in a range of multiple stick tests.

These tests are best done on fresh specimens passed into clean containers free from disinfectants and detergents to avoid decomposition of acetoacetic acid. The sensitivity is less for acetone. According to the manufacturers, Acetest, Ketostix and the BM-Test are sensitive to 1.0 mmol/l (0.1 g/l) of acetoacetate and to 4, 13 and 7 mmol/l (0.25, 0.8 and 0.4 g/l) respectively of acetone. Rickers and Miall (1958) found Ketostix was negative in 8 out of 100 cases in which Acetest was positive; in these the Acetest was only weakly positive. No reaction inhibitors have been described. Phenyl ketones give an orange-red colour, 8-hydroxy-quinoline a greyish colour and some indicators, bromsulphthalein, phenol red and phenolphthalein, may give a red-purple colour under the alkaline conditions on the stick or tablet. The same colours will be obtained with these indicators on making the urine alkaline.

None of these commonly used tests detects 3-hydroxybutyrate, for which there is no test in routine use. This substance almost always occurs together with acetoacetate. If it is desired to test for 3-hydroxybutyrate, it must first be oxidised to acetoacetate by hydrogen peroxide. Add a few drops of acetic acid to some urine diluted 1 in 2 with water. Boil for a few minutes to remove acetone and acetoacetic acid. Add 1 ml hydrogen peroxide, '10 volumes strength', warm gently, cool and apply to an Acetest tablet. A positive reaction indicates that 3-hydroxybutyrate was originally present in the urine.

Determination of Ketones in Blood and Urine

This determination in blood and urine is not often required. Earlier methods were based on a semi-quantitative Rothera's test or on the production of a red colour by the reaction of acetone with salicylaldehyde. Details can be found in earlier editions of this book. Such methods have been superseded by enzymatic techniques.

Fluorimetric Enzymatic Method for 3-Hydroxybutyrate and Acetoacetate

Gibbard and Watkins (1968) devised a fluorimetric enzymatic assay using D-3-hydroxybutyrate dehydrogenase to catalyse the interconversion of the two acids. Because of its greater stability, it is more convenient to determine 3-hydroxybutyrate, particularly as its ratio to acetoacetate is relatively constant, between 2·2 and 2·9 according to Bergmeyer and Bernt (1965). D-3-Hydroxybutyrate is determined at pH 8·5, while hydrazine is included to remove acetoacetate as it is formed. Acetoacetate is almost quantitatively reduced at pH 8·5 when excess NADH is present.

Spectrophotometric Enzymatic Method for Acetoacetate

A continuously monitored spectrophotometric assay of acetoacetate in blood was developed for use with the LKB 8600 Reaction Rate Analyser (Price *et al.*, 1977) but can be modified for use with any analyser capable of recording reaction rates over short periods. The conversion of NADH to NAD$^+$ in the D-3-hydroxybutyrate dehydrogenase reaction is monitored and first-order conditions are used so that the initial rate of reaction is proportional to acetoacetate concentration. The method allows even low concentrations of acetoacetate to be measured with a CV of less than 10%.

Acetoacetate is unstable at room temperature. According to Salway (1969), 10 to 15% is lost within one hour, but it is reasonably stable at 4° C for several hours. Price *et al.* (1977) studied acetoacetate stability in plasma and in perchloric acid extracts and recommended that if the analysis is not done at once, the plasma or acid extract should be stored at − 20° C. The plasma should be analysed within 24 h, the acid extract within 48 h. Neutralising the perchloric acid extract decreased the stability of the acetoacetate at − 20° C.

REFERENCES

Barham D., Trinder P. (1972). *Analyst*; **97**: 142.
Bergmeyer H. U., Bernt E. (1965). *Enzymol. Biol. Clin*; **5**: 65.
Burrin J. M., Price C. P. (1985). *Ann. Clin. Biochem*; **22**: 327.
Farah D. A., Boag D., Moran F., McIntosh S. (1982). *Brit. Med J*; **2**: 172.
Gibbard S., Watkins P. J. (1968). *Clin. Chim. Acta*; **19**: 511.
Hultmann E. (1959). *Nature*; **183**: 108.
Katteman R. *et al.* (1982). *Dtsch. Med. Wschr*; **107**: 97.
Kaufmann-Raab I. *et al.* (1976). *Clin. Chem*; **22**: 1729.
Lloyd B. *et al.* (1978). *Clin Chem*; **24**: 1724.
Mieling G. E. *et al.* (1979). *Clin. Chem*; **25**: 1581.
Morley G., Dawson A., Marks V. (1968). *Ann. Clin. Biochem*; **5**: 42.
Passey R. B. *et al.* (1977). *Clin. Chem*; **23**: 131.
Pennock C. A., Murphy D., Sellers J., Longdon K. J. (1973). *Clin. Chim. Acta*; **40**: 193.
Price C. P., Lloyd B., Alberti K. G. M. M. (1977). *Clin. Chem*; **23**: 1893.
Richardson T. (1977). *Ann. Clin. Biochem*; **14**: 223.
Rickers H., Miall J. B. (1958). *Amer. J. Clin. Pathol*; **30**: 530.
Salway J. G. (1969). *Clin. Chim. Acta*; **25**: 109.
Sharp P. (1972). *Clin. Chim. Acta*; **40**: 115.
Sharp P., Riley C., Cook J. G. H., Pink P. J. F. (1972). *Clin. Chim. Acta*; **36**: 93.
Thomas L., Plischke W., Storz G. (1982). *Ann. Clin. Biochem*; **19**: 214.
Townsend J. C. (1983). *Clin. Chem*; **29**: 2119.
Trinder P. (1969). *Ann. Clin. Biochem*; **6**: 24.
US Department of Health Education and Welfare, Food and Drug Administration (1974). *Fed. Regist*; **39**: 126, 24136.
Widdowson G. M., Penton G. R. (1972). *Clin. Chem*; **18**: 295.
Williams D. C., Huff G., Seitz W. R. (1976). *Clin. Chem*; **22**: 372.

16

TESTS IN DISORDERS OF GLUCOSE METABOLISM

INSULIN

Insulin is the major hormone influencing glucose metabolism and is produced in the pancreas by the β (or B)-cells of the islets of Langerhans. It is synthesised via precursor molecules, preproinsulin and proinsulin. The latter is a single-chain polypeptide folded in such a way that two disulphide bridges form between cysteine residues at different points in the chain. The active hormone is formed by the middle section of the proinsulin chain being split off to leave the insulin molecule, which consists of two peptide chains A and B, of 21 and 30 amino acid residues respectively, linked by the two disulphide bridges. The portion of the molecule split off is known as the connecting peptide or C-peptide. Hence, β-granules of the pancreatic islets contain insulin, an equivalent amount of C-peptide and a small amount of unconverted proinsulin. Stimuli to insulin secretion cause release of the three components in these proportions and, although insulin is metabolised more rapidly than C-peptide, concentrations of the two in peripheral blood do correlate.

Proinsulin has a much slower metabolism than insulin, but will cross-react immunologically and can account for up to about 20% of immunoreactive 'insulin' in the peripheral plasma of normal subjects. In cases of pancreatic islet cell tumour, it may constitute most of the circulating insulin-like peptide. Some cases of diabetes mellitus have been shown to have higher than normal proinsulin levels, but this is not a consistent finding.

Insulin secretion is influenced by a number of factors including the plasma glucose concentration perfusing the pancreas. A rise in this concentration stimulates release and synthesis of insulin, probably mediated in part through stimulation of glucagon release from the pancreatic α (or A)-cells. Glucagon has a direct effect on the β-cells, stimulating insulin release. Certain gut hormones, such as gastric inhibitory polypeptide (GIP), released into the circulation when glucose is present in the gut, also stimulate insulin secretion and account for the enhanced insulin response to an oral glucose load compared with an intravenous one. Ingestion of certain amino acids, such as arginine, has a similar effect via gut hormones. Normal potassium concentrations are also necessary for optimal insulin secretion. Hypokalaemia or potassium depletion can result in reduced glucose tolerance.

Insulin has both anti-catabolic and anabolic effects on the liver, adipose tissue and muscle. It inhibits production of glucose and ketone bodies by the liver and stimulates glycogen and fatty acid synthesis. It inhibits adipose tissue lipolysis and stimulates glucose uptake and lipid synthesis. In muscle, it inhibits protein catabolism and stimulates glucose and amino acid uptake for glycogen and protein synthesis. (For a more detailed review of insulin action see Cherrington and Steiner, 1982.)

In absolute or relative insulin deficiency, such as occurs in diabetes mellitus, fuel accumulation is hindered and excessive mobilisation of tissue stores occurs.

In fact, the above processes are reversed aided by other hormones present such as glucagon, cortisol, catecholamines, growth hormone and thyroid hormones, which have actions opposing those of insulin.

In normal, healthy individuals under 50 years of age, insulin secretion maintains plasma glucose concentrations within the range 3·0 to about 8·0 mmol/l, even after a meal. Whole blood glucose concentrations are about 15 % lower. In people over the age of 60 years, higher levels up to 10·0 mmol/l may be found after a meal.

Despite the central role of insulin in glucose metabolism, insulin assays find virtually no application in the routine diagnosis and management of diabetes mellitus; however, they may be important in diabetes research and are often employed in the investigation of hypoglycaemia.

DIABETES MELLITUS

Diabetes mellitus is a clinical syndrome associated with an abnormally high plasma glucose concentration, either when fasting or after ingestion of carbohydrate, and is often accompanied by the presence of glucose in the urine, from which the name of the condition is derived. It may result from diminished insulin production by the β-cells of the islets of Langerhans, but this is not always the case and hence diabetes is of heterogeneous origin. It occurs with differing degrees of severity and in its severest form causes ketoacidosis, coma and ultimately death if not treated. At the other extreme, it may be present without clinical symptoms. However, for most diabetic patients, the long term sequelae are the greatest problem and include nephropathy, retinopathy, neuropathy and arteriosclerosis.

The prevalence of diabetes mellitus varies in different populations of the world, but in the United Kingdom is considered to affect about 2 % of the population and is, therefore, a major health problem. Each patient requires medical supervision for the rest of his life to maintain metabolic control and examination and treatment for any associated morbidity, such as retinopathy. Of course, prevalence figures depend on the methods and criteria used to assess the presence or absence of the disease and an attempt to standardise these has been made by the World Health Organisation (WHO, 1980; 1985).

The classification of diabetes mellitus and related conditions has also been rationalised (Table 16.1). The old terms, juvenile-onset diabetes and maturity-onset diabetes, have been discarded in favour of *Type I* or *insulin-dependent*

TABLE 16.1
Classification of Diabetes Mellitus

A. '*Idiopathic*'
   Type I (Insulin-dependent)
   Type II (Non-insulin-dependent)
B. *Secondary to other conditions*
   Pancreatic disease, damage or surgery
   Various endocrine diseases
   Drugs or chemicals
   Insulin receptor abnormalities
   Certain genetic syndromes
C. *Gestational*

diabetes mellitus (IDDM) and *Type II* or *non-insulin-dependent diabetes mellitus* (NIDDM), respectively. These are the two main types, which may be further subdivided and there are other minor categories. A new term, *impaired glucose tolerance*, identifies a group of individuals whose response to the ingestion of a glucose load lies between normal and diabetic responses. A proportion of subjects in this intermediate group eventually become diabetic but some remain stable and a few revert to normal. For example, pregnancy can produce temporarily impaired glucose tolerance. Also, impaired glucose tolerance or even diabetes can result from elevated levels of hormones that are antagonistic to the actions of insulin, e.g. in Cushing's syndrome.

The Diagnosis of Diabetes Mellitus

The definitive diagnostic test for diabetes mellitus is the oral glucose tolerance test (GTT), which is conventionally performed by assaying blood glucose levels at 30 min intervals for at least 2 h after ingestion of a glucose load. Urine samples may also be collected during the test for qualitative assessment of urine glucose. However, it is not usually necessary to carry out a full conventional GTT to make a diagnosis. The WHO Report (1985) suggests that in the presence of suggestive symptoms, a random venous plasma glucose above 11·1 mmol/l is sufficient to establish a diagnosis of diabetes, while a value less than 5·5 mmol/l virtually excludes it. In asymptomatic patients at least one other figure in the diabetic range is needed on another occasion to confirm the diagnosis. Only if values lie in the 'uncertain' range between these two figures is it necessary to perform an oral GTT using the procedure below.

The upper figure for capillary blood plasma becomes 12·2 mmol/l. For whole blood the lower figure is 4·4 mmol/l and the upper is 10·0 mmol/l for venous blood and 11·1 mmol/l for capillary blood.

Oral Glucose Tolerance Test

Measure the blood glucose concentration two hours after a load of 75 g of glucose has been taken orally in the morning after an overnight fast lasting 10 to 16 h, during which water is permitted. In children the dose of glucose should be 1·75 g/kg body weight up to a maximum of 75 g. For patients on a low carbohydrate diet, i.e. less than 125 g per day, at least three days preparation on a less restrictive diet is advisable, but it may be limited to 150 g per day. Otherwise, formal dietary preparation is not usually necessary. The patient should sit quietly during the test and avoid undue exercise, and smoking is not allowed as there is some evidence that it can raise glucose levels. Potential effects of drug therapy must also be borne in mind (National Diabetes Data Group, 1979).

At the start of the test, collect a fasting blood sample for glucose estimation then give 75 g of glucose orally, dissolved in 250 to 300 ml water. The patient should be allowed up to 15 min to drink this. As alternatives, flavoured glucose solutions or partial hydrolysates of corn starch can be used. They have the advantage that they are less likely to cause nausea, but are more expensive. Vomiting, of course, but also severe nausea, render the test unreliable.

Collect a further blood sample 2 h after administering the glucose. Additional intermediate blood samples may be taken but only the 1 h specimen is likely to be of assistance in diagnosis. Urine samples are only of value if an estimate of the patient's renal threshold is required, which may be of interest if urine sugar is to be used for monitoring control.

INTERPRETATION

Two-hour venous plasma glucose values of 11·1 mmol/l or more are diagnostic of diabetes mellitus (Table 16.2). Values below 7·8 mmol/l are normal and those in the range 7·8 to 11·1 mmol/l are classified as impaired glucose tolerance. However, in the absence of symptoms of diabetes, at least one additional abnormal glucose value is considered to be necessary to confirm a clinical diagnosis of diabetes, e.g. a 1 h post glucose value of 11 mmol/l or more during the first GTT, or an elevated 2 h or fasting value on a subsequent occasion.

TABLE 16.2
Diagnostic Criteria for the Oral Glucose Tolerance Test Using a 75 g Load (WHO, 1985)

	Glucose concentration (mmol/l)			
	Venous whole blood	Capillary whole blood	Venous plasma	Capillary plasma
Diabetes Mellitus				
Fasting	≥ 6·7	≥ 6·7	≥ 7·8	≥ 7·8
and/or 2 h after glucose	≥ 10·0	≥ 11·1	≥ 11·1	≥ 12·2
Impaired Glucose Tolerance				
Fasting	< 6·7	< 6·7	< 7·8	< 7·8
and 2 h after glucose load	≥ 6·7– < 10·0	≥ 7·8– < 11·1	≥ 7·8 – < 11·1	≥ 8·9– < 12·2

The WHO also regards these criteria as suitable for use during pregnancy but accepts that different clinical action may be needed in this situation. It is also recognised that the criteria may not be universally applicable. Factors such as age may have a bearing on the way in which the results are interpreted and acted upon, as there is a tendency for glucose tolerance to worsen with increasing age. The choice of the 2 h 'cut-off' value was made on the basis of experience suggesting that subjects with 2 h glucose values below that point rarely develop specific complications attributable to diabetes.

The responsibility that falls upon both laboratory worker and clinician for correct performance and interpretation of GTTs is considerable, because they may be responsible for condemning an individual to the lifelong social, financial and legal restrictions associated with the diabetic condition, e.g. increased insurance risk, driving licence restrictions. On the other hand, subjects with impaired glucose tolerance should not be regarded as normal, as they are at increased risk of developing diabetes and should be reinvestigated at a later date to check for any deterioration. It is, therefore, important that the patient should be correctly classified and the laboratory has an obligation to ensure that correct interpretations, or at least the correct criteria for interpretation, are provided for the clinician. Especially noteworthy in this context is the fact that different laboratories measure glucose in different ways. The WHO figures assume a specific enzymatic method for glucose estimation, but it is also necessary to take account of the type of specimen (i.e. venous or capillary, plasma or whole blood) and to adjust the criteria accordingly (Table 16.2, above). Whole blood glucose values are about 15% lower than plasma values except in anaemia or polycythaemia, and capillary values are, on average, 7 to 8% higher than venous values.

The 75 g glucose load was chosen by the WHO because it was considered that a greater challenge than 50 g was needed, but that 100 g would cause problems of nausea and vomiting. However, there are some laboratories still using 50 g and with this dose, the 2 h values in the GTT would be expected to be about 1 mmol/l lower than after 75 g. The fasting criteria would, of course, be unaffected by the size of the glucose load.

Increased Glucose Tolerance. In normal subjects given a glucose load, blood glucose levels rise to a peak at 30 or 60 min and then fall to near-fasting levels at 2 h but some individuals show very little rise. Flat curves are seen in patients with hypoactivity of other endocrine organs, e.g. in hypopituitarism and Addison's disease but also in malabsorption and in a proportion of normal subjects.

Lag Curve. Some otherwise normal individuals show an exaggerated rise in blood glucose following an oral load but the level quickly falls and the 2 h concentration is within normal limits. Transient glycosuria usually occurs. This phenomenon probably results from an increased rate of glucose absorption from the gut, following rapid emptying of the stomach and occurs in some hyperthyroid patients.

A similar type of curve can occur in patients who have had a partial gastrectomy and may be associated with a temporary swing back to hypoglycaemic levels at about 2 to 3 h after ingestion. This is called *reactive hypoglycaemia*. The patient may experience symptoms of hypoglycaemia (dizziness, sweating, weakness, nausea, palpitations, etc.) which are relieved by taking rapidly absorbed carbohydrate. Occasionally, an extended GTT, up to 4 to 5 h, may be performed to identify this as the cause of the symptoms (see p. 348).

Comment. The standard oral GTT is primarily a diagnostic test for diabetes mellitus whatever its cause, and although abnormal responses, e.g. flat curves, may occur in other diseases, the test is superfluous in the investigation of these conditions. Once a diagnosis of diabetes has been made in a patient, further GTTs are not normally helpful in the management of the disease, but in impaired glucose tolerance, the test should be repeated at intervals of one or two years until the prognosis becomes clearer.

Urine Testing

Renal Threshold

Glucose is not normally detectable in urine by routine qualitative testing methods, but if plasma glucose exceeds about 10 mmol/l, glycosuria usually occurs. This level is referred to as the *renal threshold* and varies somewhat from person to person. Some non-diabetic individuals exhibit glycosuria owing to a lowered renal threshold caused by reduced renal tubular reabsorption of glucose. This is termed *renal glycosuria* and may also occur in late pregnancy. In some cases, there is a genetic basis for the disorder with the defect affecting only glucose, but otherwise the finding is usually of no great pathological significance. However, in some cases there may be a wider defect of tubular reabsorption, as in the Fanconi syndrome and in Wilson's disease (p. 632).

The renal threshold can also be raised, especially in elderly subjects, possibly related to a reduced glomerular filtration rate, which would allow the plasma glucose to attain a higher concentration before the reabsorptive capacity of the tubules is exceeded. Diabetics of long standing also often have elevated renal thresholds and, as mentioned earlier, this may have implications in monitoring the efficacy of treatment.

Reducing Substances in Urine

In normal urine, reducing substances including glucose are present in quantities too small to give positive results with the common qualitative tests, but may be detectable by chromatography. Glycosuria may be considered to be present when urine contains more glucose than 0·8 mmol/l and, as well as in diabetes and cases of lowered renal threshold, it can occur transiently during infection, anaesthesia and in certain other situations. Severe liver disease can also produce glycosuria.

Lactose. After glucose, lactose is the most commonly found carbohydrate in urine, occurring in female urine during lactation and sometimes being detectable towards the end of pregnancy. It is also common in neonates and the condition is harmless. However, it needs to be distinguished from glycosuria, which may arise from diabetes mellitus. Tests for reducing substances measure both, but glucose can be detected specifically using appropriate 'dipstick' tests (p. 329) and these should always be employed if reducing substances are found in the urine of a pregnant or lactating woman, e.g. during a GTT.

Galactose. Galactose is found in the urine only very rarely. It may be excreted after eating considerable amounts of galactose or lactose and it has been said to occur occasionally in lactation. Normally, galactose is converted to glucose by the actions of the enzymes galactokinase and hexose-1-phosphate uridylyltransferase, but a hereditary deficiency of the latter enzyme occurs in certain individuals producing an accumulation of galactose-1-phosphate in various tissues with associated galactosuria. Urine, therefore, gives a positive test for reducing substances but a negative test for glucose. Chromatography is required for positive identification of increased urine galactose levels, but examination of red cells permits detection of the enzyme deficiency, both in this condition and in a milder form of galactosaemia resulting from galactokinase deficiency.

Fructose. Fructosuria may be found after ingestion of fructose-rich foods such as fruit, honey, syrup and jams. It may also occur in liver disease and, along with glycosuria, in diabetes mellitus. Two hereditary deficiencies of enzymes can also produce fructosuria (Froesch, 1976). These are *essential fructosuria*, a benign condition occurring mainly in certain Jewish families owing to a lack of fructokinase, and *hereditary fructose intolerance*, a more serious condition caused by a deficiency of fructose-1-phosphate aldolase in the liver, which leads to accumulation of fructose-1-phosphate with development of hypoglycaemia, nausea and vomiting after fructose ingestion.

Pentoses. Pentosuria is rare, but may occur as *alimentary pentosuria* following excessive ingestion of such fruits as grapes, cherries and plums, when the pentoses excreted are L-arabinose and L-xylose. There is a recessive hereditary deficiency of xylitol dehydrogenase, called *essential pentosuria*, which results in L-xylulose excretion and occurs mainly in Jews. Neither condition is harmful.

Galactose, fructose and pentoses have no renal threshold and so are excreted as soon as there is an appreciable plasma level.

Glucuronates. Glucuronic acid from glucuronates has a reducing activity and may be present in urine in increased amounts during therapy with drugs that are excreted in this form, e.g. salicylate.

Homogentisic acid. Homogentisic acid occurs in the urine in the rare condition *alkaptonuria* (p. 764) and has a reducing activity. The urine also shows characteristic darkening on standing, owing to oxidation.

Uric acid and creatinine. When present in high concentrations, these substances may give slight reduction.

Ketone Bodies in Urine

Ketone bodies are excreted in the urine of diabetics during periods of metabolic imbalance and periodic qualitative testing for these can be helpful for management of the patient, especially in insulin-dependent cases.

Urinary Protein

While positive qualitative tests for albumin in the urine of a diabetic patient may indicate significant nephropathy, there is now increasing evidence that so-called 'microalbuminuria' (small, but abnormal quantities of albumin at concentrations below those detectable by the usual qualitative tests) in diabetes is a reliable prognostic index for the development of nephropathy (Viberti *et al.*, 1982; Mogensen, 1984). Tests for this are becoming available and it may be that better control of diabetes will delay or prevent the development of microalbuminuria and nephropathy.

TESTS IN THE TREATMENT OF DIABETES

Home Monitoring

Diabetes mellitus is unusual in that after an initial period of stabilisation, subsequent monitoring and treatment may rest partially in the hands of the patient. This is usually encouraged by diabetologists, who feel that greater involvement of the patient makes for better control.

A few years ago, urine testing was the mainstay of monitoring, but the improvement in dry chemistry strip tests for blood glucose has made it possible for many patients to estimate their own blood levels, either by simple visual inspection of a test strip or by quantitating the colour change of the strip using a reflectance meter. This type of testing, combined with occasional urine checks for glucose and ketones, enables the patient to become more independent of the hospital laboratory. However, it has to be said that such methods are less accurate and precise than most laboratory-based procedures and may also be adversely affected by the patient's technique. It is, therefore, still necessary for periodic checks to be made by the hospital.

Glucose Profiles

Blood glucose measurements are performed in most diabetic clinics in such a way that the physician has the result and can adjust treatment accordingly when he sees the patient. However, tests done in these circumstances are not always representative of blood levels throughout a normal day in the patient's life, and in order to get a more realistic picture some diabetologists ask their patients to collect blood samples by finger prick at intervals of perhaps 4 h throughout a 24 h period. These samples may be collected into tubes containing a fluoride/oxalate preservative and returned to the laboratory for estimation. This should be done as soon as possible after the final collection because some deterioration of this type of specimen has been reported (De Pasqua *et al.*, 1984). An alternative method of collection is as blood spots on filter paper which has been previously treated with boric acid as preservative (Wakelin *et al.*, 1978; Taylor and Pennock, 1982).

As a diabetic subject's insulin requirements usually diminish with increased physical activity, it is more realistic to monitor his glucose levels while he is going about his normal daily routine, rather than when he is in hospital in relatively sedentary circumstances and not governing his own diet. The purpose of doing a glucose profile is to detect unwanted troughs and peaks, such as hypoglycaemic episodes during the night, which may be followed in the morning by grossly elevated levels (Gale and Tattersall, 1979). This type of rebound hyperglycaemia is sometimes called the 'Somogyi effect' after the person who first described it, and paradoxically, it is corrected by a reduction in the insulin dose rather than by an increase.

Measurement of the cortisol/creatinine ratio in an overnight collection of urine has been proposed as an alternative means of detecting nocturnal hypoglycaemia avoiding the need for multiple blood samples (Moore *et al.*, 1979; Asplin *et al.*, 1980). The test is based on the well-known response of the hypothalamic-pituitary-adrenal axis to hypoglycaemia. Although it is subject to interference from other forms of stress and to deficiencies in urine collection and variability of creatinine excretion, this test is considered useful by some workers (Ohworiole *et al.*, 1983) but has not found universal application.

Glycosylated Haemoglobin and Other Glycosylated Proteins

As a single glucose measurement in an out-patient clinic is not necessarily representative of a patient's control over any length of time, other tests have been introduced. These are based on the fact that an increased blood glucose concentration leads to an increased rate of glycosylation of various blood proteins, i.e. glucose residues become attached to the protein molecules. Haemoglobin is the protein most extensively studied in this way.

Glycosylated Haemoglobin

Several other terms are used for this entity, including glycated haemoglobin, HbA_{1c}, HbA_1 and 'fast-fraction' haemoglobin. There are slight differences between them, some of which relate to the method of estimation or its specificity, but all depend on glucose in the blood becoming bound to haemoglobin in the red cells.

In the normal adult, about 90 % of the haemoglobin is HbA and glucose is able to combine fairly rapidly, but reversibly, with the α-amino group of the valine residue at the N-terminus of the β-globin chains to form an aldimine (Schiff base) intermediate, which is labile but can undergo a slow, irreversible Amadori rearrangement to form a stable ketoamine derivative known as HbA_{1c}. This chemical reaction is not under the influence of enzymes.

β-Globin-Val-NH$_2$ +

$$
\begin{array}{ccc}
\text{HC=O} & \text{HC = N-Val-}\beta\text{-Globin} & \text{H}_2\text{C-NH-Val-}\beta\text{-Globin} \\
| & | & | \\
\text{HCOH} & \text{HCOH} & \text{C=O} \\
| & | & | \\
\text{HOCH} & \text{HOCH} & \text{HOCH} \\
| \quad \rightleftharpoons & | \quad \longrightarrow & | \\
\text{HCOH} \quad \text{Rapid} & \text{HCOH} \quad \text{Slow} & \text{HCOH} \\
| & | \quad \text{Amadori} & | \\
\text{HCOH} & \text{HCOH} \quad \text{rearrangement} & \text{HCOH} \\
| & | & | \\
\text{CH}_2\text{OH} & \text{CH}_2\text{OH} & \text{CH}_2\text{OH} \\
\\
\text{Glucose} & \text{Labile} & \text{Stable} \\
& \text{aldimine} & \text{ketoamine}
\end{array}
$$

Other sites of glycosylation occur on the α-chain and at ε-amino groups on lysine residues within the chains, but only the combination at the N-terminus of the β-globin chain produces physical changes in the haemoglobin molecule that result in altered electrophoretic mobility and different behaviour on ion-exchange chromatography.

In addition to HbA$_{1c}$, there are several other subspecies of HbA$_1$ (HbA$_{1a1}$, HbA$_{1a2}$, HbA$_{1b}$), which differ in the type of carbohydrate bound. Also, glycosylation is not restricted to HbA. If other haemoglobins are present, they too may be glycosylated, and whether they are or not, may produce anomalous results in some of the assay methods.

Glycosylation proceeds slowly throughout the 120-day life span of the average red cell, and therefore, a measure of glycosylated haemoglobin reflects the average blood glucose concentration over the preceding several weeks and a sudden fall from high to low glucose concentrations will not produce a corresponding rapid fall in glycosylated haemoglobin. However, it has been shown that a fairly rapid rise in glycosylated haemoglobin can occur during poor diabetic control (Brooks, Nairn *et al.*, 1980). This is attributed to the rapid reversible formation of so-called 'labile HbA$_1$', the intermediate Schiff base, which is measured by some of the assay techniques. (For more detailed reviews of glycosylated haemoglobin, see Mayer and Freedman, 1983; Peacock, 1984.)

Analytical Methods for Glycosylated Haemoglobin

Sample Collection and Preparation. A sample of anticoagulated whole blood is required. The favoured anticoagulant may depend on the assay method, but the time of sampling is unimportant and whole blood samples will usually store satisfactorily for up to one week at 4 °C. Longer storage as a deep-frozen haemolysate is possible, but the maximum duration varies with the assay method. All methods require lysis of red cells before analysis. Some simply use an aliquot of whole blood, others specify removal of plasma and washing of red cells first. Removal of plasma becomes essential in some methods if lipaemia is present. 'Labile HbA$_1$' may be removed by incubating erythrocytes in isotonic saline for 5 to 6 h at 37 °C before lysing them. Alternatively, some methods include a borate treatment to achieve this.

Cation-Exchange Chromatography. The original methods for glycosylated haemoglobin were slow, long-column chromatographic techniques capable of separating HbA$_{1c}$ (Allen *et al.*, 1958; Trivelli *et al.*, 1971). In 1977, a short-column technique was described by Kynoch and Lehmann, but was suitable only for total HbA$_1$ as the components were not fully resolved. The separation was performed on BioRex 70 cation-exchange resin. Subsequently, other modifications have been published and a number of commercial versions are available as test kits, one of which is now capable of greater resolution to separate HbA_{1c}. In these methods, haemolysate is added to the column followed by an eluting buffer, which washes off the HbA_1, leaving the HbA_0 on the column. The HbA_1 is measured colorimetrically in the eluate and expressed as a percentage of the total haemoglobin, the latter being determined either by the use of a second elution buffer to wash the retained HbA_0 off the column or by colorimetric measurement of a dilution of the original haemolysate.

There are disadvantages with the cation-exchange method. It is sensitive to variations in pH and ionic strength of the buffers and to changes in ambient temperature. Results must therefore be expressed at a standard temperature, either by correction to it or by performing the assay in a temperature-controlled environment. 'Labile HbA_1' will be included unless steps are taken to remove it.

Colorimetric Method. Flückiger and Winterhalter (1976) described a method for measuring ketoamine-linked hexoses which are hydrolysed to 5-hydroxy-methylfurfuraldehyde (HMF) when heated with oxalic acid. Reaction with 2-thiobarbituric acid yields a coloured product. Both terminal hexose groups and those at other points in the globin chains are measured, but aldimines do not react, eliminating interference from labile intermediates. The technique is laborious manually but can be automated. However, reaction conditions must be carefully controlled and standardisation is somewhat arbitrary. The method has been investigated in detail by Standefer and Eaton (1983).

Electrophoresis and Electroendosmosis. As the isoelectric point of HbA_1 differs only slightly from that of HbA_0, conventional electrophoresis is not suitable for its separation. Menard et al. (1980) used agar gel, which is negatively charged and helps to separate HbA_1 from HbA_0 by virtue of the latter's more positive charge. This is called electroendosmosis and a commercial kit is available for HbA_1 assay by this method. It includes labile intermediates unless the specimen is pre-treated. Quantitation is by scanning densitometry.

Affinity Chromatography. The diol groups on glycosylated haemoglobin are able to bind to a phenylboronic acid affinity gel, facilitating separation from unglycosylated haemoglobin. A haemolysate is applied to a column of the affinity gel and the glycosylated haemoglobin is retained on the column. A sorbitol solution is then applied to displace the glycosylated fraction and the eluate quantitated colorimetrically. This technique is less sensitive to temperature and pH changes and appears to give fairly good results (Gould et al., 1982) but there have been reports of variation in performance between different batches of the gel. This method measures glycosylation at various sites in the haemoglobin molecule and can also be used for other glycosylated proteins. Results are therefore not necessarily comparable with those of cation-exchange chromatography.

Other Methods. High pressure liquid chromatography (HPLC), isoelectric focusing, immunoassay and batch chromatography using cation-exchange resin in a slurry have also been employed to measure glycosylated haemoglobin. HPLC and isoelectric focusing both offer good specificity but are not ideally suited to routine use.

INTERPRETATION

It is not possible to suggest reference ranges here as these vary even with modifications of the same method. The aim of the diabetologist is usually to keep a patient's glycosylated haemoglobin in the top half of the range or a little above it. Lower values in insulin-treated diabetics may mean that periods of hypoglycaemia are occurring and this should be avoided.

It must be remembered that anything altering the red cell life will also affect the glycosylated haemoglobin, so that haemolytic anaemia will produce lower levels than appropriate for the prevailing glucose concentrations. Increased HbA_1 concentrations have been found in iron-deficiency anaemia (Brooks *et al.*, 1980). In uraemia, shortened red cell life tends to lower HbA_1, but an opposing effect occurs owing to carbamylation of haemoglobin to give a product eluting with HbA_1 from cation-exchange columns. This product does not appear to affect the colorimetric method. High doses of aspirin produce an acetylated haemoglobin which can interfere positively with column and electroendosmosis techniques.

Haemoglobin variants can give erroneous results (Table 16.3). Haemoglobins F and H co-elute from the short columns with HbA_1 giving high values, whereas haemoglobins S, C and D do not, even when glycosylated; hence, their presence gives rise to falsely low results with cation-exchange methods.

TABLE 16.3
The Influence of Some Haemoglobin Variants on Glycosylated Haemoglobin Results

Hb type	Cation-exchange short column method	Agar gel electrophoresis
HbC	↓	Separates glycosylated and unglycosylated HbC
HbD	↓	—
HbF	↑	↑
HbH	↑	—
HbS	↓	Separates glycosylated and unglycosylated HbS

↓—Falsely low results. ↑—Falsely high results.
The colorimetric and affinity chromatography methods are not susceptible to this type of interference.

Interpretation of glycosylated haemoglobin results in pregnancy needs to take into account observations that there is normally a decrease in HbA_{1c} in the second half of pregnancy. This may be related to the higher proportion of young red cells in the circulation.

There have been suggestions that glycosylated haemoglobin measurement could be used instead of the GTT to diagnose diabetes, but a study by Lester *et al.* (1985) shows that the test is not sufficiently discriminatory.

Other Glycosylated Proteins

Other proteins also become glycosylated when subjected to higher than normal glucose concentrations (Day *et al.*, 1979). Glycosylated albumin has been measured (Guthrow *et al.*, 1979). Affinity chromatography or the thiobarbituric acid reaction can be used. A simpler method, avoiding the separation of albumin, measures glycosylated total serum protein by the thiobarbituric acid reaction (McFarland *et al.*, 1979) and an alternative method using nitroblue tetrazolium has been described (Johnson *et al.*, 1982) in which the ketoamine, termed '*fructosamine*', reduces the nitroblue tetrazolium in alkaline solution to form a coloured product that can be measured at 530 nm. The method involves measuring the rate of the reaction between 10 and 15 min after mixing the colour reagent and sample, by which time the earlier non-specific colour development has subsided. Automated versions of the method have been published (Lloyd and Marples, 1984; Hindle *et al.*, 1985), but the pH of the reaction is critical and the original authors of the manual method have since amended the reaction pH stated in their first paper. The correct pH is now said to be 10·35. Unfortunately, the reference data obtained with the automated techniques above are for a different pH.

Albumin has been shown to have an effect on the fructosamine method and so the standards, consisting of 1-deoxy-1-morpholino-fructose (DMF) are made up in albumin/saline. However, the source of the albumin also influences colour development and there is even some variation from batch to batch of the same albumin making standardisation difficult. Advantages of the method are its cheapness, ease of automation, speed of analysis and good precision, but there is considerable difficulty in comparing results from one laboratory with those of another. Each laboratory must, therefore, establish its own reference ranges very carefully.

As albumin has a half-life of only 17 days, glycosylated albumin reflects glucose control over a much shorter period than glycosylated haemoglobin and so the two measurements are not strictly comparable, although good correlation has been reported between fructosamine and glycosylated haemoglobin (Lloyd and Marples, 1984; Hindle *et al.*, 1985).

Summary of Tests in the Treatment of Diabetes

The monitoring and control of diabetes mellitus may now be approached in several different ways and may include active involvement of the patient, although the age, intelligence and physical aptitude of the individual must be taken into account. Different tests provide different information and should be used selectively, bearing in mind the cost.

Diabetic Hyperglycaemic Coma

In untreated or inadequately treated diabetes mellitus, blood glucose levels rise and ketosis may develop owing to the increased catabolism of fats with production of acetoacetic and β-hydroxybutyric acids. Some of the acetoacetic acid is decarboxylated to acetone. The urine contains considerable amounts of glucose and ketone bodies and may contain albumin and granular casts. Plasma glucose is usually higher than 25 mmol/l and may occasionally exceed 55 mmol/l.

The accumulated acids produce a metabolic acidosis with low plasma bicarbonate and low blood pH, which may fall below pH 7·0 in severe cases. Measurements of blood gas and acid–base balance are therefore of value. Large volumes of acid urine are produced and together with the vomiting which may occur, result in a state of dehydration. Sodium and chloride are lost in the urine and the reduction in plasma volume reduces cardiac output and blood pressure. In turn, this affects renal blood flow and is partly responsible for the rise in plasma urea which often occurs, but increased protein breakdown may also contribute. Plasma creatinine results in diabetic coma may be unreliable because acetoacetic acid and, to a lesser extent, high glucose concentrations produce a positive interference in many versions of the Jaffé technique. As renal impairment becomes more marked, the urine volume may fall to subnormal levels.

During development of the acidosis, potassium moves out of the cells in exchange for hydrogen ions, leading to hyperkalaemia and increased urinary potassium loss. The patient's breath may smell of acetone, while the typical acidotic breathing found in diabetic ketoacidosis known as Kussmaul breathing, is of a deep, sighing nature caused by stimulation of the respiratory centre by the low plasma pH.

Diabetic ketoacidosis may develop over several days and is frequently precipitated by an infection, but may also be consequent upon reduced insulin therapy, trauma or myocardial infarction. In as many as 45 % of cases, no reason can be found.

Treatment

Treatment consists of correcting the above abnormalities, firstly by giving insulin to increase glucose utilisation and inhibit keto-acid formation. Intravenous isotonic saline is needed to correct dehydration, but intravenous bicarbonate is not normally employed unless the blood pH is below 7·0, because the acidosis usually corrects itself naturally as the patient's metabolism returns to normal. Plasma inorganic phosphate concentrations may fall to very low levels at this point as carbohydrate metabolism resumes, and some workers advocate phosphate replacement therapy to correct the deficit. The return of normal cellular metabolism and correction of the acidosis also results in redistribution of potassium back into the cells, revealing the underlying deficiency in the form of hypokalaemia, which can be dangerous if not carefully controlled. A fall in plasma magnesium also occurs.

Hyperosmolar Non-Ketotic Diabetic Coma

This form of diabetic coma occurs mostly in elderly or middle-aged patients and is associated with very high glucose concentrations, and consequently, high plasma osmolality (over 350 mmol/l) but no evidence of ketoacidosis. Plasma sodium levels are often above 145 mmol/l and clinical dehydration is present.

Lactic Acidosis

In some cases of diabetic coma, lactate makes a contribution to the acidosis. It may result from poor tissue perfusion, hence falling into the 'Type A' category of lactic acidosis. In the past, the more serious 'Type B' form has occurred, carrying a high mortality, with large accumulations of lactate despite normal circulation. This has been particularly associated with diabetic therapy using phenformin, a biguanide which also appears to hinder the liver's ability to metabolise lactate, thus causing lactic acidosis. Phenformin has now been withdrawn from routine use in both the United Kingdom and the USA. Other biguanides, such as metformin, are considered to be safer and are still available for prescription.

Treatment of lactic acidosis has traditionally been by infusion of large quantities of sodium bicarbonate, but the value of this has recently been questioned and dichloracetate suggested as a possible alternative (Park and Arieff, 1983).

TESTS FOR INVESTIGATING HYPOGLYCAEMIA

Hypoglycaemia may be defined as a whole blood glucose concentration of less than 2·2 mmol/l or a plasma glucose concentration of less than 2·5 mmol/l. It is a biochemical state that may give rise to the clinical syndrome of *neuroglycopenia*, which varies considerably in severity but may include light-headedness, weakness, hunger, facial flushing, cold sweats, unsteadiness, palpitations and tachycardia, anxiety, and behavioural changes including aggressiveness, somnolence, or even coma.

Some of the causes of hypoglycaemia can be broadly classified according to Table 16.4. The subject is reviewed in detail by Marks and Rose (1981a) and more briefly by Gale (1985). The most common cause of hypoglycaemia is inappropriate insulin therapy in diabetes and, less frequently, treatment with oral hypoglycaemic agents, especially when normal meals have not been taken. Factitious hypoglycaemia is sometimes seen, where deliberate inappropriate use of insulin is the cause. Reactive hypoglycaemia may occur in some subjects after meals, especially following partial gastrectomy, where rapid transit and absorption of carbohydrate stimulates a rapid rise in insulin release. Addison's disease and hypopituitarism may be associated with hypoglycaemia because of the reduced insulin antagonism resulting from lowered levels of other hormones. In the rare cases of insulinoma, insulin secretion is inappropriately high for the prevailing blood glucose concentrations.

TABLE 16.4
Some Causes of Hypoglycaemia

Pancreatic lesions, e.g. insulinoma, islet cell hyperplasia
Endocrine disease, e.g. hypopituitarism, hypoadrenalism
Extra-pancreatic tumours
Some forms of liver and kidney disease
Essential reactive
Factitious
Drugs, alcohol etc.
Starvation
Excessive exercise
Congenital disorders, e.g. certain glycogenoses, hereditary fructose intolerance

---

In the investigation of suspected hypoglycaemia, the first priority is demonstration of a low blood glucose when symptoms occur. A specific method should be used for glucose assay (e.g. glucose oxidase, hexokinase) and the sample should be collected into an appropriate preservative and analysed without undue delay. Blood should also be collected for possible insulin assay later. The time and site of blood collection should be recorded together with the patient's clinical condition, drug therapy and the time since food was last taken. The patient's response to administration of rapidly absorbed carbohydrate should also be observed and noted. In adults, a random plasma glucose of less than 2·8 mmol/l merits further attention, especially if hypoglycaemic symptoms have been observed. A plasma glucose greater than 2·8 mmol/l in a symptomatic subject virtually excludes neuroglycopenia due to hypoglycaemia, providing that collection of blood has not occurred too late.

The second priority in the investigation is to identify the cause of the documented hypoglycaemia and to make the distinction between hypoglycaemia during fasting and that provoked by stimuli such as meals, sugars, drugs or alcohol. The following dynamic function tests may help in this.

Dynamic Function Tests

Prolonged Fasting

The aim of the prolonged fast is to demonstrate *Whipple's triad*, which is the name given to the following set of conditions:

1. Symptoms of hypoglycaemia during fasting.
2. Proven hypoglycaemia in association with symptoms.
3. Relief of symptoms when glucose is administered.

Because of the potential danger, the test should be carried out in hospital under medical supervision with glucose solution for intravenous administration at hand. The patient is allowed unsweetened, non-caloric beverages and water, but no food. The patient should be encouraged to take exercise during the test. Blood samples for immediate glucose estimation and subsequent insulin assay are collected every 6 h or whenever symptoms occur. Symptoms due to neuroglycopenia can be confirmed by an EEG. The test is terminated at 72 h or earlier by glucose administration if marked symptoms occur. In the latter situation, some authorities recommend giving intravenous saline before glucose, the purpose of this being to ensure that symptomatic relief is not simply related to fluid administration.

INTERPRETATION

Insulinoma is extremely unlikely, but not impossible, in individuals who fail to show symptomatic hypoglycaemia in this test. The vast majority of people with a disease characterised by fasting hypoglycaemia demonstrate Whipple's triad during the first 12 to 36 hours. In those associated with hyperinsulinism, immunoreactive insulin and C-peptide levels are inappropriately high at the time of hypoglycaemia, i.e. greater than 10 mU/l and 1 μg/l, respectively. This permits the distinction between insulin-dependent causes of fasting hypoglycaemia (e.g. insulinoma, nesidioblastosis) and non-insulin-dependent causes, e.g. liver disease, non-pancreatic endocrine disease, glycogen storage diseases, in which insulin and C-peptide levels are low.

It must be stressed that many healthy people, especially women and children, become biochemically hypoglycaemic on fasting for 48 to 72 h, but do not experience symptoms and therefore do not fulfil Whipple's criteria.

Insulin Hypoglycaemia With C-Peptide Assays

In centres where C-peptide assay is available, this test can be performed more rapidly than the prolonged fast, but is contra-indicated in cases of ischaemic heart disease, epilepsy or clinical evidence of hypopituitarism or hypoadrenalism. The patient should fast overnight and can come to hospital as a day patient.

Insert an indwelling cannula into a peripheral vein and keep patent with heparinised saline. Take specimens for blood glucose and C-peptide. Two sets should be collected 15 min apart and these are the baseline samples. Provided that plasma glucose is greater than 2·5 mmol/l, inject soluble insulin intravenously through the cannula (0·10 U/kg body weight up to a maximum of 10 U). Collect blood at 20, 30, 60, 90, 120 and 180 min for glucose and C-peptide measurements. Cortisol and growth hormone measurements are also performed by some workers as part of this test. Close medical supervision must be maintained, and if symptoms become severe, stopped by giving intravenous glucose (50 ml of 50 % w/v solution). Intravenous hydrocortisone (100 mg) should also be available in case glucose fails to produce rapid alleviation of symptoms. For the test to be valid, plasma glucose must fall below 2·5 mmol/l.

INTERPRETATION

Normal individuals become neuroglycopenic at 20 to 30 min after the insulin and this lasts for 20 to 30 min. If plasma glucose falls below 2·5 mmol/l, plasma cortisol should rise by at least 220 nmol/l to a peak greater than 550 nmol/l and growth hormone should rise to above 20 mU/l. Plasma C-peptide concentration should fall below 1·5 µg/l. Failure to do so is strong evidence for hyperinsulinism, providing that adequate hypoglycaemia was achieved. However, exceptions do occur and hyperinsulinism should be confirmed by the prolonged fast test. False negative C-peptide suppression tests may occur in hyperinsulinism associated with predominant proinsulin secretion and in cases of intermittent or partially suppressible insulin secretion by tumours.

Stimulation Tests

Several stimulation tests have been used in the investigation of spontaneous hypoglycaemia and all depend on provoking an exaggerated response from islet cell tumours. Most of them are now considered unreliable. The intravenous tolbutamide test is still used occasionally and was described in the 5th edition of this book. The C-peptide suppression test is now regarded as superior. The glucagon test still has a place when a prolonged fast or insulin hypoglycaemia is contra-indicated. Glucagon has a glycogenolytic effect and does not depress blood glucose.

Glucagon Test. Collect bloods for glucose and insulin measurements, then give glucagon intravenously (30 µg/kg body weight up to a maximum of 1 mg) through an indwelling cannula over 2 to 3 min. Collect further blood at 5 min intervals for 30 min.

Normal subjects show a transient rise in plasma insulin of 30 to 100 mU/l above the baseline and a rise in plasma glucose of 1·5 to 4·0 mmol/l, returning to basal levels in 2 to 3 h. In over 70 % of insulinoma cases, an early and exaggerated rise of plasma insulin occurs to above 150 mU/l within 5 to 10 min followed by a rapid fall. Conditions associated with insulin resistance are also characterised by an exaggerated insulin response to glucagon, e.g. obesity, acromegaly, Cushing's syndrome.

Extended Glucose Tolerance Test. This is not useful in fasting hypoglycaemia, but may be helpful in support of a tentative diagnosis of essential reactive hypoglycaemia. However, results can be difficult to interpret (Marks and Rose, 1981b).

Fast the patient overnight, then insert an indwelling cannula into a peripheral vein. Give orally, over 10 to 15 min, 100 g glucose dissolved in 300 to 500 ml flavoured water. Collect blood for glucose, plasma cortisol and growth hormone at 30 min intervals for 5 h. The patient should be closely observed and any symptoms and their time of occurrence noted. Mild physical activity may be allowed. If symptoms develop, the effect of intravenous saline may be worth observing before giving glucose.

Most normal subjects show a rise in blood glucose followed by a fall to a nadir at 2 to 5 h. A venous plasma glucose of 2·5 mmol/l or less together with hypoglycaemic symptoms and a post-nadir rise in plasma cortisol of at least 220 nmol/l and growth hormone levels of greater than 20 mU/l are consistent with, but not proof of, reactive hypoglycaemia. The rise in plasma cortisol is considered essential for clinical significance to be attached to the other findings.

Despite the apparent good control of conditions that can be achieved in the extended glucose tolerance test, current opinion is that demonstration of a plasma glucose of less than 2·5 mmol/l concurrent with spontaneous clinical symptoms of hypoglycaemia is better evidence for reactive hypoglycaemia.

REFERENCES

Allen D. W., Schroeder W. A., Balog J. (1958). *J. Amer. Chem. Soc*; **80**: 1628.
Asplin C. M., Hockaday T. D. R., Smith R. F., Moore R. A. (1980). *Brit. Med. J*; **280**: 357.
Brooks A. P., Metcalfe J., Day J. L., Edwards M. S. (1980). *Lancet*; **2**: 141.
Brooks A. P., Nairn I. M., Baird J. D. (1980). *Brit. Med. J*; **281**: 707.
Cherrington A. D., Steiner K. E. (1982). *Clinics in Endocrinol. Metab*; **11**: 307.
Day J. F., Thorpe S. P., Baynes J. W. (1979). *J. Biol. Chem*; **254**: 595.
De Pasqua A., Mattock M. B., Phillips R., Keen H. (1984). *Lancet*; **2**: 341.
Flückiger R., Winterhalter K. H. (1976). *FEBS Letters*; **71**: 356.
Froesch E. R. (1976). *Clinics in Endocrinol. Metab*; **5**: 599.
Gale E. (1985). *Brit. J. Hosp. Med*; **33**: 159.
Gale E. A. M., Tattersall R. B. (1979). *Lancet*; **1**: 1049.
Gould B. J., Hall P. M., Cook J. G. H. (1982). *Clin. Chim. Acta*; **125**: 41.
Guthrow C. E. *et al.* (1979). *Proc. Nat. Acad. Sci. USA*; **76**: 4258.
Hindle E. J., Rostron G. M., Gatt J. A. (1985). *Ann. Clin. Biochem*; **22**: 84.
Johnson R. N., Metcalf P. A., Baker J. R. (1982). *Clin. Chim. Acta*; **127**: 87.
Kynoch P. A. M., Lehmann H. (1977). *Lancet*; **2**: 16.
Lester E., Frazer A. D., Shepherd C. A., Woodroffe F. J. (1985). *Ann. Clin. Biochem*; **22**: 74.
Lloyd D., Marples J. (1984). *Clin. Chem*; **30**: 1686.
McFarland K. F. *et al.* (1979). *Diabetes*; **28**: 1011.
Marks V., Rose F. C. (1981). *Hypoglycaemia*. Oxford: Blackwell Scientific Publications. (a) p. 110; (b) p. 441.
Mayer T. K., Freedman Z. R. (1983). *Clin. Chim. Acta*; **127**: 147.
Menard L. *et al.* (1980). *Clin. Chem*; **26**: 1598.
Mogensen C. E. (1984). *New Engl. J. Med*; **310**: 356.
Moore R. A., Smith R. F., Asplin C. M. (1979). *Lancet*; **1**: 409.
National Diabetes Data Group (1979). *Diabetes*; **28**: 1039.
Ohworiole A. E., Nairn I. M., Baird J. D. (1983). *Ann. Clin. Biochem*; **20**: 136.
Park R., Arieff A. (1983). *Clinics in Endocrinol. Metab*; **12**: 339.
Peacock I. (1984). *J. Clin. Pathol*; **37**: 841.
Standefer J. C., Eaton R. P. (1983). *Clin. Chem*; **29**: 135.
Taylor R. P., Pennock C. A. (1982). *Ann. Clin. Biochem*; **19**: 22.
Trivelli L. A., Ranney H. M., Lai H. T. (1971). *New Engl. J. Med*; **284**: 353.
Viberti G. C. *et al.* (1982). *Lancet*; **1**: 1430.
Wakelin K., Goldie D. J., Hartog M., Robinson A. P. (1978). *Brit. Med. J*; **2**: 468.
WHO Expert Committee on Diabetes Mellitus. Second Report. (1980). Technical Report Series 646. WHO, Geneva.
WHO. (1985). Technical Report Series 727. WHO, Geneva.

17

CREATININE, URATE AND UREA

These three low molecular weight nitrogenous substances are considered together in this chapter for convenience.

CREATININE

Creatine, methyl guanidoacetic acid, is synthesised in the liver, passes into the circulation and is taken up almost entirely by skeletal muscle for conversion to creatine phosphate. During muscle contraction, energy is supplied by the conversion of ATP to ADP. Creatine phosphate is the source of a high energy phosphate bond for the immediate reformation of ATP by the action of creatine kinase (p. 510). Otherwise, resynthesis of ATP occurs during aerobic glycolysis and requires oxygen. Creatine phosphate thus provides additional ATP during anaerobic muscular activity. Following aerobic glycolysis, some ATP is used to rephosphorylate creatine.

Creatine (and its phosphate) are converted spontaneously into the internal anhydride, creatinine.

$$
\begin{array}{ccc}
\mathrm{NH} & \mathrm{CH_3} & \\
\parallel & | & \\
\mathrm{C} & -\mathrm{N} - \mathrm{CH_2} \\
| & & | \\
\mathrm{NH_2} & & \mathrm{COOH} \\
& \text{creatine} &
\end{array}
\rightarrow
\begin{array}{ccc}
\mathrm{NH} & \mathrm{CH_3} & \\
\parallel & | & \\
\mathrm{C} & -\mathrm{N} - \mathrm{CH_2} \\
| & & | \\
\mathrm{NH} & --- & \mathrm{CO} \\
& \text{creatinine} &
\end{array}
$$

About 2% of the total creatine is converted daily so that the amount of creatinine produced is related to the total muscle mass and remains approximately the same from day to day unless the muscle mass changes. Conversion of creatine to creatinine also occurs readily on warming in acid solution, but in neutral solutions creatinine is slowly hydrolysed to creatine.

The two substances are handled differently by the kidney. Both are filtered at the glomerulus but whereas tnere may be some additional tubular secretion of creatinine, creatine is reabsorbed by the tubules and at low plasma concentration this ensures that there is little or no creatine in the urine.

The Determination of Serum Creatinine

The methods most commonly used for this determination are based on the *Jaffé reaction*, the production of a red colour with an alkaline picrate solution. The chemistry of this reaction has been extensively studied. The formation of a 1:1 Janovsky complex by the reaction of the methylene group of creatinine with the meta position on the picrate anion has been proposed (Butler, 1975). More recent nuclear magnetic resonance studies suggest a complex involving both meta positions in the picrate anion and attack by either the methylene group or the enolised carbonyl group of creatinine (Vasiliades, 1976).

Many factors affect the results obtained with this apparently simple method and the more pertinent are discussed here. For fuller reviews see Cook (1975), Narayanan and Appleton (1980) and Spencer (1986).

The maximal absorbance of the creatinine-picrate complex is at 490 nm, which is close to that of the alkaline picrate reagent itself. Accordingly, only instruments with a narrow bandwidth should be used. This avoids measuring the decrease in yellow colour as the picrate is consumed in the reaction. If the wavelength selected is increased from 490 to 520 nm, linearity improves but the absorbance decreases. The balance of opinion favours wavelengths greater than 505 nm. The absorbances of the reagent and the reaction product increase with temperature, but not to the same extent. Thus temperature changes during the analysis may cause errors, although the effect is less marked at higher wavelengths such as 520 nm. Instruments capable of maintaining a constant temperature are essential for reaction rate methods.

The intensity of the colour produced in the Jaffé reaction is little affected by picrate concentration over the range 5 to 37 mmol/l. The rate of colour development, however, increases with picrate concentration and the time taken to reach the maximal absorbance must be determined for end-point assays.

The pH of the reaction mixture profoundly affects the reaction rate and maximal absorbance. No reaction occurs below pH 7, but increasing the sodium hydroxide concentration accelerates the colour development although eventually the maximal absorbance begins to fall. Failure to control the pH of the reaction mixture inevitably leads to errors. The use of acid aqueous creatinine standards influences the results in reaction rate methods or assays where measurements are made before colour development is complete. The effect depends on the initial pH of the alkaline picrate reagent (Cook, 1975).

The Jaffé reaction is not specific for creatinine. In serum, up to 20 % of the total chromogens can be other substances but this falls to less than 5 % for urine. In whole blood the figure is much higher than in serum, the preferred blood component for this assay. Proteins give a positive Jaffé reaction and protein removal is usual before adding the alkaline picrate. This is not considered necessary with the small sample volumes used in reaction rate methods but even then haemolysis may cause errors.

Interferences with the Jaffé reaction take different forms. Substances reacting like creatinine and contributing to the total colour produced include acetone, acetoacetate, pyruvate and some cephalosporin antibiotics. Blood constituents such as glucose, ascorbate, histidine and adrenaline may cause fading or enhancement of the colour or modify the kinetics of the reaction. The magnitude and direction of these interferences depend on the concentration of the interfering substances, their rate of reaction and the assay conditions. For example, acetoacetate has been reported to show positive, negligible and negative interference (Cook, 1975). Many modifications are alleged to improve the specificity of the Jaffé reaction. These include adsorption of the creatinine, dialysis, use of different pH, extraction of interfering substances and reaction rate measurement.

The most commonly used adsorbent is Lloyd's reagent, a hydrated aluminium silicate. Protein is precipitated with tungstic acid and the supernatant fluid is mixed with Lloyd's reagent which adsorbs creatinine in acid conditions. After centrifugation, the pellet is resuspended in alkaline picrate to elute the creatinine and give the colour reaction. Lloyd's reagent adsorbs some Jaffé-positive keto acids such as pyruvate so not all interference is removed. Despite this shortcoming, the use of Lloyd's reagent provides an accurate if laborious manual method and has been proposed as a Selected Method (Haeckel, 1981). In continuous flow systems some non-creatinine chromogens are removed by dialysis.

Slot (1965) reported that the colour given by creatinine fades rapidly after acidification whereas that from non-creatinine chromogens remains. He used this to determine the creatinine by difference, reading the absorbance before and 5 min after adding sulphuric acid. Grafnetter *et al.* (1967) modified the assay further to give better performance at low creatinine levels. An alternative manipulation of pH (Yatzidis, 1974) measured the difference in absorbance at 500 nm in two alkaline picrate reagents of pH 9·65 and 11·50 as an index of the 'true' creatinine. Deproteinisation was not necessary. Such methods based on differential pH measurements have not become popular, possibly due to the need for two measurements with different reagents making the methods less suitable for automated analysis.

Some of the interfering substances react more quickly than creatinine (e.g. acetoacetate) and others more slowly (e.g. glucose). Depending on the reaction conditions it is possible to select a time interval during which the predominant reactant is creatinine (Spencer, 1986). Even then, reaction rate assays are not fully specific and the degree and type of interference depend on the conditions of the assay (Kroll and Elin, 1983; Lebel *et al.*, 1984; Mori and Jarvie, 1983; Spencer, 1986). High levels of bilirubin significantly decrease the creatinine result, possibly as a result of conversion to biliverdin by the alkaline picrate. Despite these difficulties, kinetic methods performed on a discrete analyser are currently the most popular and their precision and bias are, in general, satisfactory.

Several methods have been based on the ability of creatinine to yield coloured products in reactions with various organic compounds. They do not appear to have any particular advantages over the Jaffé reaction but details are given by Cook (1975), Narayanan and Appleton (1980), Parekh and Sims (1977) and Spencer (1986).

Enzymatic methods are being developed. The conversion of creatinine to creatine by creatininase (EC 3.5.2.10, creatinine amidohydrolase) can be combined with the Jaffé reaction. The difference between the apparent creatinine concentration before and after the enzyme action is a measure of the creatinine content (Miller and Dubos, 1937; Masson *et al.*, 1981). This enzyme from *Pseudomonas* species may be used in fully enzymatic methods with other enzymes including creatinine deaminase (EC 3.5.4.21, creatinine iminohydrolase) from *Flavobacterium filamentosum* and creatinase (EC 3.5.3.3, creatine amidinohydrolase). The first converts creatinine to N-methylhydantoin and ammonia and the second hydrolyses creatine to sarcosine and urea.

Creatininase has been used in an enzyme-linked system as follows:

creatinine + H_2O → creatine   (creatininase)
creatine + ATP → creatine phosphate + ADP   (creatine kinase)
ADP + phosphoenolpyruvate → ATP + pyruvate   (pyruvate kinase)
pyruvate + NADH + H^+ → lactate + NAD^+ (lactate dehydrogenase)

Creatininase and creatinase have been linked to sarcosine oxidase and a peroxidase system for measuring the hydrogen peroxide produced:

creatinine + H_2O → creatine   (creatininase)
creatine + H_2O → sarcosine + urea   (creatinase)
sarcosine + O_2 + H_2O → glycine + CH_2O + H_2O_2 (sarcosine oxidase)
H_2O_2 → H_2O + O^- (peroxidase)

An example of the use of *creatinine deaminase* involves the measurement of ammonia formed in the reaction:

creatinine → *N*-methylhydantoin + NH_3 (creatinine deaminase)
NH_4^+ + NADPH + 2-oxoglutarate →   (glutamate
glutamate + $NADP^+$ + H_2O dehydrogenase)

Alternatively the ammonia can be measured by the change in colour of a pH indicator, a method used in the Kodak Ektachem Analyser.

Although these techniques look promising, none has had sufficient use for proper assessment of performance. They are claimed to be more specific than the Jaffé reaction methods and show no interference by ketones, glucose, bilirubin and the cephalosporin antibiotics (Fossati *et al.*, 1983; Jaynes *et al.*, 1982; Sundberg *et al.*, 1983; Tanganelli *et al.*, 1982).

Reverse phase HPLC has been used to improve specificity by performing the Jaffé reaction 'on-line' on the column effluent (Brown *et al.*, 1977). Later, ultraviolet absorption has been used to measure creatinine separated by HPLC using either reverse phase (Ambrose *et al.*, 1983; Okuda *et al.*, 1983) or cation-exchange columns (Ambrose *et al.*, 1983; Spierto *et al.*, 1980). Lim *et al.* (1978) attempted to establish a definitive assay of creatinine in serum and urine using HPLC initially, followed by conversion to *O*-trifluoroacetylcreatinine and its quantitation by gas chromatography/mass spectrometry. All these procedures are useful for comparison with new methods but are unsuitable for batch analysis.

The authors have no longer included in the methods section the single-channel AutoAnalyzer methods (see 5th edition) as they are being replaced by either continuous flow methods of the Jaffé type on multi-channel analysers or kinetic Jaffé methods tailored to specific discrete analysers. For their practical details, the relevant manufacturers' literature should be consulted. A traditional manual method, perhaps the best of its class, has been retained.

The methods for serum creatinine can be used for urine if this is first diluted appropriately.

Determination of 'True Creatinine' (Method of Owen *et al.*, 1954; Ralston, 1955)

After precipitating proteins the creatinine is adsorbed on to Lloyd's reagent, a hydrated aluminium silicate, and the colour then developed with alkaline picrate.

Reagents.
1. Sodium tungstate solution, 100 g Na_2WO_4, $2H_2O$/l.
2. Sulphuric acid, 0·33 mol/l.
3. Lloyd's reagent. This is obtainable from BDH Chemicals, Limited. Test each fresh batch to show that it adsorbs satisfactorily.
4. Oxalic acid, saturated solution.
5. Sodium hydroxide, 2·5 mol/l.
6. Picric acid, saturated solution. Owen *et al.* recrystallised the solid twice from water, made up freshly every few days and kept in a dark bottle.
7. Alkaline picrate solution. Prepare freshly before use. Add 5·5 ml of sodium hydroxide to 27·5 ml of picric acid solution and dilute to 100 ml with water.
8. Standard creatinine solution 10 mmol/l. Prepare a stock solution containing 113 mg per 100 ml in hydrochloric acid, 100 mmol/l. Keep at 0 °C for not more than four weeks.
9. Standard solutions for use. Dilute 0·5 and 1·0 ml of the stock solution to 200 ml to give solutions containing 25 and 50 μmol/l respectively.

Technique. Measure 1 ml serum (or plasma) into a suitable test tube 150 × 25 mm (6 × 1 inch) and add 1·5 ml water, 0·5 ml sodium tungstate, and 1 ml sulphuric acid. Mix thoroughly, stand 30 min and filter through a Whatman No. 1 paper. Add 3 ml filtrate (= 0·75 ml serum) and 0·3 ml saturated oxalic acid to 60 mg Lloyd's reagent in a conical centrifuge tube and shake at intervals for 10 min. At the same time treat 3 ml water (as blank) and 3 ml of the two standards in the same way. Centrifuge at high speed for 10 min. Decant the supernatant fluid and stand inverted on a filter paper to drain as completely as possible. Add 5 ml alkaline picrate solution to the centrifuge tube, loosen the deposit with a fine glass rod, stopper and shake at intervals for 10 min. Again centrifuge at high speed for 10 min. Place in a water bath at 20 °C until this temperature is reached, then read test and standards against the blank at 520 nm.

Calculation. For the weaker standard:

Serum creatinine (μmol/l)

$$= \frac{\text{Reading of unknown}}{\text{Reading of standard}} \times \frac{4}{1} \times 25$$

$$= \frac{\text{Reading of unknown}}{\text{Reading of standard}} \times 100$$

For the stronger standard the factor is 200. A standard curve can be prepared as follows:

Serum creatinine (μmol/l)	0	100	200	300	400	500
Stock standard diluted to 200 ml (ml)	0	0·5	1·0	1·5	2·0	2·5

Take 3 ml of each standard and carry through as with the supernatant in the text.

For values above 500 μmol/l use less serum, making up the initial volume with water.

Note. Urine samples can be subjected directly to the Jaffé reaction after dilution but without deproteinisation or adsorption on to Fuller's earth. In this case the standards used should cover the expected range for urinary creatinine and should be diluted similarly to the urine.

INTERPRETATION

Because of the variable non-specific nature of the Jaffé reaction there has been uncertainty as to how much of the Jaffé chromogen is creatinine. In normal serum, at least 80 % of the colour is due to creatinine and for good Jaffé methods the reference range is 70 to 130 μmol/l, being a little higher on average for men than for women since it is related to muscle size. For more specific methods of measurement the range is 60 to 115 μmol/l.

There is little non-creatinine chromogen in urine and the normal daily excretion ranges from 9 to 18 mmol. Again for men, values are in the upper part of the range and for women in the lower part. On a normal diet almost all the urinary creatinine is derived endogenously. An appreciable exogenous component is only present when considerable amounts of foods rich in creatine and creatinine (meats) are consumed. The excretion of endogenous creatinine, being related to the amount of body creatine, i.e. the muscle mass, is fairly constant from day to day and has been used to check the accuracy of successive 24 h urine collections. Scott and Hurley (1968) and others have, however, reported rather wide variations in creatinine output in such collections made under carefully controlled conditions.

Serum creatinine is increased in renal failure. There is conflicting evidence about the proportion of non-creatinine chromogens as renal function deteriorates, but Roscoe (1953) found it to decrease as the serum creatinine rose. Values up to 1800 μmol/l are not uncommon in the later stages of renal failure when they may reach or even exceed 2700 μmol/l. The pre-renal factors which can increase serum urea have less influence on the creatinine result.

For the use of creatinine clearance see p. 771. For a comprehensive review of the early literature on creatinine see Peters and Van Slyke (1946).

URATE

In man, urate is the end product of the metabolism of purines, two of which, adenine (6-aminopurine) and guanine (2-amino-6-hydroxypurine) occur in nucleotide form in RNA and DNA. Addition of a ribose residue at position nine converts these two purines to the nucleosides, adenosine and guanosine and phosphorylation of the ribose moiety gives the nucleotides, adenylic acid and guanylic acid respectively. In DNA, the ribose is replaced by deoxyribose.

In purine biosynthesis the first purine produced is inosinic acid, the 5-phosphate ester of inosine, in which hypoxanthine (6-hydroxypurine) is condensed with ribose. Adenylic and guanylic acids are produced from inosinic acid. The course of purine metabolism is shown in Fig. 17.1 with the more relevant enzymes involved. Most mammals have the enzyme uricase which oxidises urate to the much more soluble allantoin. Man and the apes are exceptions, so for them the metabolism ends at urate, which is thus the excretion product of nucleic acid metabolism. Hypoxanthine, one of the intermediate

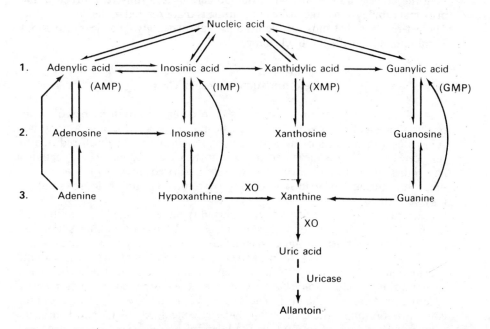

Fig. 17.1. The Course of Purine Metabolism.
* = hypoxanthine guanine ribosylphosphate transferase (HGPRT); XO = xanthine oxidase

products, however, is in part recycled by the action of the enzyme hypoxanthine guanine ribosylphosphate transferase (HGPRT), which converts hypoxanthine and guanine in the presence of ribosyl phosphate into inosinic acid and guanylic acid respectively.

Uric Acid   Allantoin

Uric acid is 2,6,8-trihydroxypurine and like other hydroxypurines can exist in keto and enol forms. From the formula it can be seen why it forms salts, though it is dibasic not tribasic, only monosodium and disodium salts being known. It is present as the monosodium salt in plasma. The miscible pool of urate in the body is about 7·2 mmol (1200 mg) of which there is a turnover of about half daily, i.e. about 3·6 mmol (600 mg) is formed daily and about the same amount lost, of which about 75 % is excreted in the urine and about 25 % destroyed by bacteria in the colon. In addition to this endogenous source, urate is also formed from purine-containing compounds present in food. The largest amount of these is in foods rich in cell nuclei, i.e. in nucleoproteins. Richest are organ meats such as sweetbreads, liver, heart and kidneys, next come flesh meats, poultry and fish, especially sardines. There are only small amounts in vegetables and cereals, little or none in fruits and milk products.

In the kidney urate is filtered at the glomerulus and fully reabsorbed in the proximal tubule so that the urate in the urine is that excreted in the distal tubule. The net result is that most of the urate is reabsorbed giving a clearance about 10 ml/min, 8 % of the inulin clearance.

Determination of Serum Urate

One of the most common methods used to determine urate is based on its reaction in alkaline solution with a phosphotungstate (or arsenophospho-tungstate) reagent. This oxidises the urate to allantoin and is itself reduced to tungsten blue which is measured by its absorbance at 700 nm. These methods have inherent sources of error. Some urate is carried down with the protein precipitate during deproteinisation giving low results. The final coloured solution may be turbid.

Attempts to avoid the formation of turbidity have included the addition of lithium salts to the phosphotungstate reagent, the use of sodium silicate or glycerine-sodium silicate solutions as the alkali and the addition of urea to the alkaline reagent. Several alkaline reagents have been used of which sodium cyanide and sodium carbonate have been the most popular. Carbonate gives lesser sensitivity than cyanide but the colour is more reproducible and the reagent is non-toxic. Another difficulty is that Beer's law may not be obeyed over the urate concentration range found in serum. Patel (1968) added EDTA and hydrazine sulphate to the reagent to improve the linearity.

Substances in blood and urine other than urate may react to give falsely high results. They include ascorbate, thiols such as cysteine and glutathione, methylated purines (e.g. caffeine, theobromine and theophylline), gentisic acid (a metabolite of salicylate), paracetamol and very high concentrations of glucose. Early attempts to overcome this non-specificity involved preliminary precipitation of urate as an insoluble salt (e.g. silver). Several of these salts are however slightly soluble leading to under-estimation. Specificity can also be improved by using a blank containing the sample pre-incubated with uricase (EC 1.7.3.3, urate: oxygen oxidoreductase) to destroy the urate.

The ability of urate to reduce other metal complexes has been used to measure it in serum. Thus urate converts the pale blue cupric ion in the presence of 2,2'-bicinchoninate to form the lavender-coloured cuprous 2,2'-bicinchoninate complex, a method available as a commercial kit. Such methods are subject to similar interferences as the phosphotungstate methods and are rarely used.

Currently popular methods of measuring urate involve the use of the highly specific enzyme, uricase. The earliest methods of this type involved differential spectrophotometry. The urate ion has a characteristic absorption peak in the ultraviolet at 293 nm. The reaction products, allantoin, carbon dioxide and hydrogen peroxide have little absorption at this wavelength so that the decrement in absorbance after uricase activity is a specific measure of the urate concentration. However, proteins and other substances account for most of the absorbance at 280 to 293 nm so that in methods which avoid deproteinisation, the absorbance change after uricase activity may be difficult to measure precisely when the sample blank absorbance is so high. Protein removal with trichloracetic acid is recommended, in which case the absorbance maximum is shifted to 283 nm. A manual uricase method using such deproteinisation and measurement in Tris buffer, pH 8·5, has been proposed as a candidate reference method for the determination of serum urate (Duncan *et al.*, 1982). The recovery of added urate is good, the precision satisfactory and only xanthine interferes. If the Tris buffer is replaced by borate buffer, EDTA also interferes. In routine use, the precision of the direct spectrophotometric methods has been rather worse than that of the manual or automated phosphotungstate methods. This probably reflects the increased error inherent in measuring the difference between two readings, each with its own error.

Alternatively, the hydrogen peroxide produced by the action of uricase on urate can be measured by means of catalase- or peroxidase-linked reactions. Kageyama (1971) used methanol and catalase and measured the formaldehyde formed using the Hantzsch reaction.

$$\text{uric acid} + 2H_2O + O_2 \rightarrow \text{allantoin} + H_2O_2 + CO_2 \qquad \text{(uricase)}$$

$$H_2O_2 + CH_3OH \rightarrow HCHO + 2H_2O \qquad \text{(catalase)}$$

$$HCHO + 2 \text{ acetylacetone} + NH_3 \rightarrow 3,5\text{-diacetyl-1,4-dihydrolutidine} + 3H_2O$$

Deproteinisation was unnecessary and glucose, ascorbate, haemoglobin and bilirubin did not interfere. The method showed good correlation with a direct spectrophotometric method but was more precise and was linear up to 1200 μmol/l at 405 nm.

In Kageyama's method, colour-forming reactions take 70 min to reach completion. Alternative methods were developed for the newer discrete analysers. Catalase and hydrogen peroxide oxidise ethanol to acetaldehyde which can either be oxidised further to acetate by aldehyde dehydrogenase (Haeckel, 1976) or reduced to ethanol by alcohol dehydrogenase (Trivedi *et al.*, 1978). As the first method involves the conversion of $NADP^+$ to NADPH and the second one the conversion of NADH to NAD^+, the reactions can be followed at 340 nm, either by end-point or reaction rate methods. Ethanol-converting enzymes in a specimen produce acetaldehyde continuously from ethanol and give falsely high values in the aldehyde dehydrogenase method. This occurs in patients with acute liver or renal disease and can be prevented by the inclusion of oxalate and pyrazole in the assay (Bartl *et al.*, 1979). The addition of xanthine to inhibit uricase competitively makes this enzymic step the rate-determining one and allows the method to be used in reaction rate mode.

The measurement of hydrogen peroxide using a peroxidase system analogous to that used in the measurement of glucose using glucose oxidase (p. 322) is exploited in the Peridochrom Uric Acid kit (Boehringer Corporation). Klose *et al.* (1978) used a uricase-peroxidase coupled reaction with 4-aminophenazone and dichlorophenol. The method did not require deproteinisation or a sample blank and was suitable for continuous flow analysis. Ascorbate oxidase was added to eliminate ascorbate interference and the method gave good agreement with a direct spectrophotometric assay.

In all uricase methods, azide present as a preservative in some quality control materials may inhibit the enzyme. Xanthine is also a potent inhibitor of uricase and can cause serious errors (Duncan *et al.*, 1982). Such interference has occurred in a patient on cyclophosphamide and allopurinol (Hande *et al.*, 1979).

Data from external quality assurance schemes indicate that the phosphotungstate methods have a slight positive bias compared with the all-method mean. Precision appears to be more dependent on the instrument used than on the type of assay. As a group, continuous flow systems have better precision than discrete and centrifugal analysers but there is a wide range of performance in each method group. The precision of manual methods is less satisfactory. The authors have not included a manual method in this edition for this reason, but details of three such methods can be found in the 5th edition if needed. The newer uricase techniques are usually tailored to a specific instrument and the manufacturer's literature should be consulted for these. We have retained a continuous flow method in which hydroxylamine is used as the colour intensifier.

AutoAnalyzer II Method (Technicon AAII–13a)

Reagents.
1. Saline-Brij. Add 0.5 ml Brij 35, 300 g/l, to 1 litre of sodium chloride solution, 9 g/l. Mix and filter.
2. Phosphotungstate reagent. Dissolve 80 ml orthophosphoric acid (sp. gr. 1·75) in approximately 500 ml water in a litre flask containing several glass beads and having a ground glass joint. Add 100 g sodium tungstate ($Na_2WO_4, 2H_2O$), attach a reflux condenser and boil gently for 4 h. Cool and transfer quantitatively to a litre volumetric flask and make to the mark with water.
3. Sodium tungstate solution, 400 g/l. Filter and add 1 ml of wetting agent FC-134, 2 g/l.
4. Hydroxylamine hydrochloride solution, 2 g/l.
5. Stock standard urate solution, 5 mmol/l. Dissolve 0·6 g lithium carbonate in 150 ml water and shake to dissolve. Filter if necessary and warm to 60°C. Pour the warm solution into a litre volumetric flask into which 840 mg uric acid has been placed. Warm the flask under running water from a hot tap while swirling the contents. Solution should be complete in 5 min. Run cold water over the flask, add 20 ml formalin, half fill the flask with water, add 25 ml sulphuric acid, 500 mmol/l, slowly while shaking, make to the mark with water and store in an amber bottle.

6. Working standard, 500 µmol/l. Dilute 10 ml of the stock standard to 100 ml with water. To check linearity prepare similarly standards covering the range 100 to 700 µmol/l in 100 µmol/l steps. Store at 4°C.

Technique. The flow diagram is shown in Fig. 17.2. The sample rate is 60/h. For values greater than 700 µmol/l, dilute the sample with sodium chloride solution, 9 g/l. Check the noise level by running the standard. The trace should not vary by more than 0·5 transmission lines from the mean. Greater variation is usually due to a poor bubble pattern or worn pump tubes. A precipitate may form in the lines; if so it is advantageous to include filters in the reagent lines. At the end of a run wash with distilled water for 20 min.

Serum and aqueous standards may not agree. If so, use a reliable reference serum as standard.

The average between-batch CV for the method is 4·6 % at a urate concentration of 400 µmol/l.

INTERPRETATION

The reference interval of urate in serum has been variously quoted. There is general agreement that the range for men has an upper limit of about 420 µmol/l with a mean of 300 µmol/l, and that the range for women is lower with an upper limit of 355 µmol/l and a mean of 240 µmol/l. The range for men alters little with age but that for women after the menopause rises towards that for men. Levels are somewhat higher towards the end of pregnancy and in the first year of life.

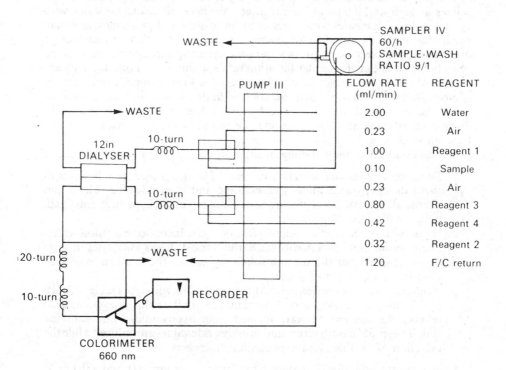

Fig. 17.2. Determination of Serum Urate Using the AutoAnalyzer II.

The main disease of interest is *gout* in which there is an increased urate pool in the body. Urate deposits occur in and about the joints and the blood level is often raised although not invariably so. Neither is the serum urate closely related to the severity of symptoms. Many cases of gout have serum urate concentrations in the range 420–720 μmol/l, though higher figures have been reported. The determination may have some diagnostic value in differentiating gouty from non-gouty arthritis.

Cases of gout are classified as primary or secondary. In *primary gout*, some stage in the synthesis or excretion of urate is defective. The mechanisms causing urate overproduction centre on three enzymes which have 5-phosphoribosyl-1-pyrophosphate (PRPP) as one of their substrates. In some patients, PRPP synthetase activity is increased producing high levels of PRPP which stimulates the next enzyme in the pathway, PRPP amidotransferase. In other cases, excess purine synthesis occurs because both enzymes are insensitive to feed-back inhibition. Partial or total absence of HGPRT (Fig. 17.1, p. 355) decreases utilisation of PRPP by this enzyme, giving the potential for excessive purine production. Complete deficiency of HGPRT occurs in the Lesch–Nyhan syndrome, a rare sex-linked recessive inherited disorder found only in men. All the symptoms of gout are present with other characteristic neurological signs and symptoms. In some cases of primary gout, urate production is normal but impaired renal tubular handling of urate is the cause of the hyperuricaemia. The defect appears to be in tubular secretion (Levinson and Sorensen, 1980).

In *secondary gout* increased production or impaired excretion of urate occurs as the result of some other disease. There is increased turnover from increased cell breakdown in polycythaemia, leukaemia (greater in myeloid than in lympho-cytic), pernicious anaemia, chronic haemolytic anaemia and lymphosarcoma. Values as high as 1200 μmol/l occur after treatment of leukaemic states with cytotoxic drugs. Increases sometimes occur in toxaemia of pregnancy, and may reach 600 μmol/l unrelated to any increase in serum urea. Similar increases of uncertain cause are seen in psoriasis and in hypertriglyceridaemia. In chronic renal failure, a fall in glomerular filtration rate and diminished tubular mass are associated with hyperuricaemia, but clinical gout is a rare complication. There is competitive inhibition of tubular excretion of urate by increased blood levels of lactate (as in Types I and VI glycogen storage disease) or acetoacetate (as in diabetes or starvation). Low values may be found in Wilson's disease and the Fanconi syndrome.

Several *drugs* affect the handling of urate by the body in one of three ways.

1. *Impairment of tubular secretion of urate.* The drugs include salicylates in small doses, pyrazinamide, guanethidine and acetazolamide. These and almost all diuretics, except spironolactone, can cause hyperuricaemia and, occasionally, clinical gout.
2. *Impairment of the tubular reabsorption of urate.* Increased excretion with a fall in serum urate occurs with such uricosuric drugs as salicylates in large doses, benemid, benzfurane and sulphinpyrazone. The first two have been used in the treatment of gout.
3. *Xanthine oxidase inhibition.* Allopurinol (4-hydroxypyrazole (3,4d)-pyrimidine), an analogue of hypoxanthine, inhibits this enzyme and so reduces the amount of urate formed from hypoxanthine and xanthine (Fig. 17.1, p. 355). Both serum and urinary urate values are reduced while the excretion of xanthine and hypoxanthine increases.

Urinary urate excretion is reduced by drugs in groups (1) and (3) but is increased by those in group (2).

For further discussion of purine metabolism and of gout see Bywaters and Glynn (1970), Wyngaarden and Kelley (1978), Balis (1967, 1976) and Cameron and Simmonds (1981).

Determination of Urate in Urine

Methods similar to those for serum have been applied to urine. With phosphotungstate and arsenophosphotungstate methods, substances other than urate contribute to the colour. Interference by thiols is particularly important and can be avoided by the addition of 0·2 g phenylmercuric acetate per litre of urine. Only 80 to 90 % of the colour is normally due to urate and the proportion may be lower still. Thus chemical methods are inaccurate and uricase methods are preferable for urine.

Store the urine at 4 °C, avoiding the uricase-inhibitor azide if a preservative is to be added. Mix the urine well and warm for a few minutes at 60 °C to dissolve any urates in the deposit before diluting and proceeding immediately with the determination. Most uricase methods are suitable provided the urine is diluted 1 in 10 before assay.

INTERPRETATION

The urinary urate is made up of an exogenous part, the amount of which depends on the quantity of nucleoprotein-rich foods in the diet, and of an endogenous part resulting from the breakdown of nucleoprotein. On a nucleoprotein-free diet this latter ranges from 1·8 to 3·0 mmol/24 h, but increases when nucleoprotein-containing foods are being taken, a typical figure on an average diet being 3·5 to 4·2 mmol/24 h. On a high purine diet urate excretion may exceed 6·0 mmol daily.

Urate clearance averages about 10 ml/min. Urinary urate follows a characteristic course in gout, being low before an attack and increasing during the attack. The output varies in some cases with administration of those substances which alter renal tubular handling of urate. A consistently high excretion is found in leukaemia especially during cytotoxic drug therapy and in conditions in which there is increased metabolism of nucleoprotein without impairment of renal function. Administration of cortisone or ACTH increases urate excretion.

Urate Crystals from Material in Joints

Such material often contains masses of needle-shaped crystals of sodium acid urate of characteristic microscopic appearance. The murexide test (p. 759) or phosphotungstate reduction can be used to confirm the presence of urate. Confusion may occasionally occur in the condition of *pseudo-gout* where the crystals are calcium pyrophosphate. The chemical tests for urate are negative, the serum urate is normal and the crystals behave differently in polarised light.

UREA

Urea is the main end product of protein catabolism. Deamination of amino acids takes place in the liver which is also the site of the urea cycle whereby the ammonia released is converted into urea.

Determination of Serum Urea

Some techniques use the formation of ammonia from urea by the action of urease (EC 3.5.1.5, urea amidohydrolase) found in soya and jack beans. The ammonia formed has been determined by aeration into acid, colorimetrically by nesslerisation or by the Berthelot reaction, and by using coupled enzyme assays. For many years the urease-nesslerisation method was commonly used despite problems with turbidity, colour instability and non-linear calibration. The reaction of ammonia with phenol and hypochlorite first noted by Berthelot in 1859 was later introduced to give a more sensitive technique with a stable colour which obeys Beer's law. More recently the Berthelot method has been superseded by the glutamate dehydrogenase method, currently one of the most commonly used urea methods.

Alternatively, urea may be measured without conversion to ammonia by making use of its ability to react with diacetyl monoxime or *o*-phthalaldehyde direct.

Urease Methods. Urease is completely specific for urea which it hydrolyses to carbamic acid and ammonia, the former then decomposing to give carbon dioxide and a second molecule of ammonia:

$$NH_2 . CO . NH_2 + H_2O \rightarrow NH_3 + NH_2 . COOH \rightarrow 2 NH_3 + CO_2$$

The enzyme acts optimally at $55°$ C and pH 7·0 to 8·0 and is inhibited by ammonia and fluoride. It is important that sufficient urease activity is present to convert all the urea under the test conditions when selecting an end-point method and to make the urease reaction the rate-determining step in a reaction-rate assay. If this is not checked, non-linearity is likely to occur, particularly in end-point methods at high urea concentrations.

All urease methods are susceptible to contamination with ammonia from the atmosphere of the laboratory, from small amounts in the reagents and from the presence of endogenous ammonia in the specimen. The problem is decreased by the use of blanks, and this is usually done. A blank was included in the original glutamate dehydrogenase method (Talke and Shubert, 1965) but some kit and analyser manufacturers have omitted this precaution, assuming that the endogenous ammonia concentration in the sample is much lower than that of urea and that the potential for contamination is decreased because of the shorter incubation times. Kits or instruments omitting blanks in such assays may be unsuitable for the determination of urinary urea.

In the Berthelot reaction, ammonia reacts with phenol in the presence of hypochlorite to form an indophenol which gives a blue coloured compound in alkali. Nitroprusside acts as a catalyst, increasing the rate of the reaction, the intensity of the colour obtained and its reproducibility. Chaney and Marbach (1962) reduced the number of reagents for colour production to two by combining some of them. The reactions (Martinek, 1969) are:

$$NH_3 + HOCl \rightarrow NH_2Cl + H_2O$$

$$NH_2Cl + C_6H_5OH \rightarrow O=C_6H_4=NCl$$

$$O=C_6H_4=NCl + C_6H_5OH \rightarrow O=C_6H_4 =N-C_6H_4O^-$$

The Berthelot reaction has been adapted for use with the AutoAnalyzer by Wilcox *et al.* (1966) and Wilson (1966). It is used in discrete analysers and is available in kit form. Its sensitivity makes it very suitable for paediatric work. For emergency work, the total time taken for the test can be cut by increasing the amount of urease used so that the incubation period is decreased. The working range can be increased by working at a less sensitive wavelength (Napier and Lines, 1969), and the time taken for the colour development step can be cut by incubating at a higher temperature. Gordon *et al.* (1978) have investigated optimal conditions for this reaction.

In the urease/glutamate dehydrogenase method, glutamate production from ammonia and 2-oxoglutarate is measured by the absorbance change at 340 nm owing to the concomitant conversion of NADH to NAD^+. Each molecule of urea hydrolysed causes the production of two molecules of NAD^+. On discrete and centrifugal analysers this method is more commonly used as a reaction rate method since this means shorter analysis times and decreased effects of potential interfering substances thus removing the need for sample blanks. Sampson and Baird (1979) described an optimised reaction rate method for serum urea which agrees well with the Berthelot method and is subject to interference only by very high levels of bilirubin and gross haemolysis. The candidate reference method for urea in serum is also based on the glutamate dehydrogenase method (Sampson *et al.*, 1980).

The products of urease activity have also been measured by the associated increase in conductivity of the ammonium and carbonate ions produced from the non-ionic urea. This is the basis of the method on the Beckman Astra analyser and gives good precision and a high degree of accuracy. On the Kodak Ektachem, the thin film technique allows ammonia formed in the reaction to pass through a layer of cellulose acetate butyrate which retards hydroxyl ions in the specimen. The ammonia then diffuses into an indicator layer.

Direct Colorimetric Methods. Urea reacts with diacetyl in hot acid solution at nearly $100°C$ to give a coloured product (Fearon, 1939) but Beer's law is not obeyed and the reaction was not investigated further until continuous flow analysers were developed. When urea is heated with compounds containing two adjacent carbonyl groups, such as diacetyl $CH_3CO.CO.CH_3$, coloured products are formed. Diacetyl monoxime, $CH_3.CO.C=NOH.CH_3$, has usually been used because of its greater stability. On heating it decomposes to give hydroxylamine and diacetyl which then condenses with the urea. The chemistry of the reaction has been studied in detail (Butler *et al.*, 1981).

$$CH_3.CO.CO.CH_3 + CO(NH_2)_2 \longrightarrow \underset{\underset{\underset{CO}{\diagdown\diagup}}{N\quad N}}{CH_3.C-C.CH_3} + 2H_2O$$

In earlier versions of the technique, unpleasant reagents containing strong sulphuric and phosphoric acids were used. Subsequent modifications reduced the strength of the acid and substituted nitric acid for phosphoric. Thiosemicarbazide and Fe^{3+} ions were added to catalyse the reaction and to restore colour intensity lost by the use of weaker acids. The reaction is not fully specific for urea and the results with this method are higher than those from the urease methods especially in uraemic patients. The method does not detect ammonia.

Another direct colorimetric method involves the condensation of urea with *o*-phthalaldehyde to form an isoindoline derivative which is then reacted with 8-(4-amino-1-methylbutylamino)-6-methoxyquinoline to produce a coloured product with intense absorption at 510 nm. This method has a consistent positive bias compared to urease methods, and is adapted for use on the American Monitor Parallel Analytical System and on the Ames Seralyser.

Method Choice. The manual diacetyl monoxime method of Marsh *et al*. (1965) is given for those laboratories needing a manual method for emergency purposes or for small work loads. An alternative would be a manual Berthelot technique for which a number of suitable kits are available. For automated methods the single channel AutoAnalyzer methods are now largely replaced either by dedicated discrete analysers or by multi-channel continuous flow systems. For details of these the manufacturers' literature should be consulted. A single-channel method appears in the 5th edition of this book.

Manual Diacetyl Monoxime Method (Marsh *et al.*, 1965).

Reagents.
1. Trichloracetic acid, 100 g/l.
2. Stock diacetyl monoxime, 25 g/l in water.
3. Stock thiosemicarbazide, 2·5 g/l in water.
4. Acid ferric chloride solution. Add 1 ml sulphuric acid to 100 ml of a ferric chloride solution containing 50 g/l in water.
5. Acid reagent. Add 10 ml orthophosphoric acid (sp. gr. 1·75), 80 ml sulphuric acid and 10 ml acid ferric chloride solution to 1 litre of water and mix.
6. Colour reagent. To 300 ml acid reagent add 200 ml water, 10 ml stock diacetyl monoxime and 2·5 ml stock thiosemicarbazide.
7. Urea standards containing 5, 10, 15, 20, 30, 40 and 50 mmol/l.

Technique. Add 1 ml water and 1 ml trichloracetic acid to 0·2 ml serum. Mix well, centrifuge, take 0·2 ml supernatant and add 3 ml colour reagent. At the same time put up a reagent blank and an appropriate standard (say 10 mmol/l) by replacing the serum with water or the standard for the first step above. Heat in a boiling water bath for 20 min, cool to room temperature in cold water, and read test and standard against the blank at 520 nm within 15 min. It is advisable to prepare a standard curve using the range of standards given, since Beer's law may not be obeyed.

Calculation.

$$\text{Serum urea} = \frac{\text{Reading of unknown}}{\text{Reading of standard}} \times \text{concentration of standard.}$$

Stick Tests

These have traditionally been semi-quantitative tests for use with whole blood, plasma or serum. An example is *Azostix* (Ames Company) which employs urease and bromothymol blue as indicator for the assay of urea in whole blood. The sample must be free from fluoride and added ammonium salts, and should be at room temperature. The test area at one end of the stick is impregnated with urease and indicator and is covered by a semi-permeable membrane. The whole membrane surface is covered with blood for 60 s, during which time urea diffuses through the membrane, is converted to ammonia and alters the colour of the indicator from yellow to various shades of green or greenish-blue. After rinsing off the blood for 2 s with a jet of water, the colour is immediately compared with a colour test chart corresponding to approximately 3, 7·5, 14 and 22 mmol/l.

A quantitative stick test based on the *o*-phthalaldehyde method has been developed for use with the Ames Seralyser.

INTERPRETATION

Although urea diffuses readily into all body fluids, the concentration in the red cells is greater than in the plasma, possibly because some is bound to haemoglobin. The concentration in cell and plasma water is similar and this combination of factors, bearing in mind the lower water content of the cells, results in the plasma (or serum) concentration being only slightly greater than in whole blood. The use of plasma or serum is preferable however.

The generally accepted reference range for the serum urea on a normal diet is 2·3 to 8·3 mmol/l. It is somewhat higher in men than women, particularly in the young, and there is a slow rise with age from a mean of 4·0 mmol/l in young adults to 6·6 mmol/l in the elderly. The urea concentration depends on the protein content of the diet. The concentration does not vary greatly during one day but can fall in normal persons and in patients with renal disease on a low protein intake. Thus a fall in urea is not always reflected in improvement in other renal function tests in the latter group. In pregnancy, serum urea is lower than in the non-pregnant state due to haemodilution. It is commonly between 2·5 and 3·3 mmol/l and rarely above 4·0 mmol/l.

Increases in urea are seen in renal disorders and in non-renal conditions. A three-part classification is often used.

1. **Pre-renal Uraemia.** An important cause is reduction of plasma volume, usually the result of salt and water depletion. This diminishes the blood pressure and cardiac output with consequent reduction in renal blood flow and glomerular filtration rate. Urea retention is a consequence. It is seen in severe, protracted vomiting as in pyloric and intestinal obstruction; in paralytic ileus with the accumulation of a large volume of intestinal contents; in external loss of intestinal contents as in severe, prolonged diarrhoea. Very high values for urea are found in these conditions particularly if they are prolonged before treatment is instituted. Figures in the range 33 to 50 mmol/l occur but rapidly return to normal with fluid replacement. Smaller increases are seen in the fluid depletion associated with diabetic ketoacidosis or Addisonian crises. Similar values occur in shock due to haemorrhage, burns or toxaemia.

Increased protein catabolism associated with pyrexial and toxic states or the metabolic response to injury may cause moderate increases. If haemorrhage into the alimentary tract occurs, digestion of the protein passing along the intestine and the later deamination of the absorbed amino acids is an additional factor to the circulatory impairment associated with this condition.

2. **Renal Uraemia.** Intrinsic renal disease which diminishes the glomerular filtration rate leads to urea retention and an increase in plasma concentration until the higher concentration in the glomerular filtrate compensates for its diminished volume in slowly progressive, chronic renal diseases. In acute renal failure with anuria, the rate of increase in the plasma concentration is much more rapid as little or none is excreted. For consideration of the changes in different renal diseases, see Chapter 29 (pp. 782–788).

3. **Post-renal Uraemia.** Obstruction to the flow of urine after it leaves the kidney leads to back pressure on the renal pelvis and diminished glomerular filtration of urea. If prolonged, secondary renal damage occurs and an element of renal uraemia is added. A common cause is benign prostatic hypertrophy, and the determination of serum urea is helpful in this condition. Other causes include urinary calculi, urethral stricture and malignant tumours involving both ureters.

Decreases in serum urea, other than those mediated by haemodilution or low protein intake, are seen in severe liver disease with destruction of cells leading to impairment of the urea cycle.

Determination of Urinary Urea

It is often useful and sometimes essential to know the urea concentration in the urine and to calculate the daily excretion. Analytical methods for serum urea can be adapted for urine and it will usually be most convenient to select the method already in use in the laboratory. Because of the wide variations in concentration, dilution with water or isotonic saline, usually to 1 in 10 to 1 in 20, is needed to bring the urea concentration into the satisfactory range for the method. With the diacetyl monoxime method, conversion of urea to ammonia by bacterial action on standing leads to low values. In urease techniques this is less important although some is lost to the atmosphere if decomposition is marked and the urine is allowed to stand for a long time. In urease methods on fresh urine, the ammonium content can be determined separately by excluding urease from one sample if the true urea content is required.

INTERPRETATION

A high urea concentration in the urine reflects the concentrating power of the kidney and is progressively diminished as renal impairment proceeds. In pre-renal uraemia, urinary urea concentration is often quite high. The average concentration over the day is about 330 mmol/l but depends also on the fluid intake. The total daily excretion, about 500 mmol on average, is much less affected by water intake and reflects protein catabolism, either of dietary protein in excess of synthetic needs or of endogenous protein. On an ordinary diet, urea nitrogen forms about 80 to 90% of the total urinary nitrogen excretion but falls towards 60% on a low protein diet.

Provided endogenous protein catabolism is within the usual limits, the daily urea excretion reflects the dietary intake of protein both in the normal person and in slowly progressive renal disease. In acute renal impairment, urea excretion falls and the serum concentration rises rapidly. Determination of daily urea excretion is helpful in the management of cases of acute renal failure and in assessing the ability of a transplanted kidney to handle an increasing dietary protein intake.

Note. Fluids thought to be urine, or to be contaminated with urine, can often be recognised by measuring their urea concentration. It may be necessary to determine the serum urea at the same time.

REFERENCES

Ambrose R. T., Ketchum D. F., Smith J. W. (1983) *Clin. Chem*; **29**: 256.
Balis M. E. (1967). In *Advances in Clinical Chemistry*. (Bodansky O., Stewart C. P. eds) London and New York: Academic Press. **10**: 157.
Balis M. E. (1976) In *Advances in Clinical Chemistry*. (Bodansky O., Latner A. L. eds) London and New York: Academic Press. **18**: 213.
Bartl K., Brandhuber M., Ziegenhorn J. (1979). *Clin. Chem*; **25**: 619.
Brown N. D. *et al.* (1977). *Clin. Chem*; **23**: 1281.
Butler A. R. (1975). *Clin. Chim. Acta*; **59**: 227.
Butler A. R., Hussain I., Leitch E. (1981). *Clin. Chim. Acta*; **112**: 357.
Bywaters E. G. L., Glynn L. E. (1970). In *Biochemical Disorders in Human Disease*, 3rd ed (Thompson R. H. S., Wootton I. D. P. eds) p. 273. London: Churchill Livingstone.
Cameron J. S., Simmonds H. A. (1981) *J. Clin. Pathol*; **34**: 1245.
Chaney A. L., Marbach E. P. (1962). *Clin. Chem*; **8**: 130.
Cook J. G. H. (1975). *Ann. Clin. Biochem*; **12**: 255.
Duncan P. H. *et al.* (1982). *Clin. Chem*; **28**: 284.
Fearon W. R. (1939). *Biochem. J*; **33**: 902.

Fossati P., Prencipe L., Bertl G. (1983). *Clin. Chem*; **29**: 1494.
Gordon S. A., Fleck A., Bell J. (1978). *Ann. Clin. Biochem*; **15**: 270.
Grafnetter D., Janošová Z., Červinková I. (1967). *Clin. Chim. Acta*; **17**: 493.
Haeckel R. (1976). *J. Clin. Chem. Clin. Biochem*; **14**: 101.
Haeckel R. (1981). *Clin. Chem*; **27**: 179.
Hande K. R., Perini F., Putterman G., Elin R. (1979). *Clin. Chem*; **25**: 1492.
Jaynes P. K., Feld R. D., Johnson G. F. (1982). *Clin Chem*; **28**: 114.
Kageyama N. (1971). *Clin. Chim. Acta*; **31**: 421.
Klose S., Stoltz M., Munz E., Portenhauser R. (1978). *Clin. Chem*; **24**: 250.
Kroll M. H., Elin R. J. (1983). *Clin. Chem*; **29**: 2044.
Lebel R. R., Gutmann F. D., Mazumdar D. C., Grzys M. (1984). *New Engl. J. Med*; **310**: 1671.
Levinson D. J., Sorensen L. B. (1980). *Ann. Rheum. Dis*; **39**: 173.
Lim C. K., Richmond W., Robinson D. P., Brown S. S. (1978). *J. Chromatogr*; **145**: 41.
Marsh W. H., Fingerhut B., Miller H. (1965). *Clin. Chem*; **11**: 624.
Martinek R. G. (1969). *J. Amer. Med. Technol*; **31**: 678.
Masson P., Ohlsson P., Björkhem I. (1981). *Clin. Chem*; **27**: 18.
Miller B. F., Dubos R. (1937). *J. Biol. Chem*; **121**: 457.
Mori L., Jarvie T. (1983). *Clin. Chem*; **29**: 733.
Napier J. A. F., Lines J. G. (1969). *Ann. Clin. Biochem*; **6**: 59.
Narayanan S., Appleton H. D. (1980). *Clin. Chem*; **26**: 1119.
Okuda T., Oie T., Nishida M. (1983). *Clin. Chem*; **29**: 851.
Owen J. A., Iggo B., Scandrett F. J., Stewart C. P. (1954). *Biochem. J*; **58**: 426.
Parekh A. C., Sims C. (1977). *Clin. Chem*; **23**: 2066.
Patel C. P. (1968). *Clin. Chem*; **14**: 764.
Peters J. P., Van Slyke D. D. (1946). In *Quantitative Clinical Chemistry*, Vol. 1, 2nd ed. pp. 897–936. London: Ballière, Tindall and Cox.
Ralston M. (1955). *J. Clin. Pathol*; **8**: 160.
Roscoe M. H. (1953). *J. Clin. Pathol*; **6**: 207.
Sampson E. J., Baird M. A. (1979). *Clin. Chem*; **25**: 1721.
Sampson E. J. *et al.* (1980). *Clin. Chem*; **26**: 816.
Scott P. J., Hurley P. J. (1968). *Clin. Chim. Acta*; **21**: 441.
Slot C. (1965). *Scand. J. Clin. Lab. Invest*; **17**: 381.
Spencer K. (1986). *Ann. Clin. Biochem*; **23**: 1.
Spierto F. W. *et al.* (1980). *Clin. Chem*; **26**: 286.
Sundberg M. W. *et al.* (1983). *Clin. Chem*; **29**: 645.
Talke H., Shubert G. A. (1965). *Klin. Wochenschr*; **43**: 174.
Tanganelli E. *et al.* (1982). *Clin. Chem*; **28**: 1461.
Trivedi R. C., Rebar L., Desai K., Strong L. J. (1978). *Clin. Chem*; **24**: 562.
Vasiliades J. (1976). *Clin. Chem*; **22**: 1664.
Wilcox A. A. *et al.* (1966). *Clin. Chem*; **12**: 360.
Wilson B. W. (1966). *Clin. Chem*; **12**: 151.
Wyngaarden J. B., Kelley W. H. (1983). In *The Metabolic Basis of Inherited Disease*, 5th ed. (Stanbury J. B., Wyngaarden J. B., Frederickson D. S. eds.) p. 1043. New York: McGraw-Hill Inc.
Yatzidis H. (1974). *Clin. Chem*; **20**: 1131.

18

AMINO ACIDS

There are 21 amino acids which are commonly found in proteins, (L-stereoisomer of those with an asymmetrical C atom). They are linked by peptide bonds and differ in the structure of their side chains which vary considerably. They can be classified as follows

1. *Monoamino monocarboxylic acids*
   (a) Aliphatic
      (i) Unsubstituted—glycine, alanine, valine, leucine, isoleucine
      (ii) With a hydroxyl group—serine and threonine
   (b) Aromatic—phenylalanine and tyrosine
   (c) Heterocyclic—tryptophan and histidine.
2. *Monamino dicarboxylic acids*—glutamic acid and aspartic acid, also present as their amides, glutamine and asparagine.
3. *Diamino monocarboxylic acids*—lysine and arginine.
4. *Sulphur-containing amino acids*—methionine and cysteine (–SH), two molecules of which can combine to form cystine (–S–S), thereby yielding a bridge between polypeptide chains in proteins.
5. *Acids containing an imino group*—This is instead of an amino group, as in proline and hydroxyproline.

The nature of the side chains influences greatly the properties of a protein, particularly the tertiary structure and the specific molecular form, e.g. of an active site of an enzyme. Thus a mutation causing replacement of a single amino acid by another can radically alter the structure and function of a protein, often causing disease.

Many non-protein amino acids are known, some present in the diet others formed by intermediary metabolism of amino acids, e.g. ornithine, β-amino-isobutyric acid, taurine and homocystine. (See Meister, 1965a for a review of amino acid structure and properties.)

In humans, extracellular and intracellular amino acid pools are maintained by a number of processes. In the diet, protein and non-protein sources provide amino acids which are absorbed by active transport into the portal blood. Protein as such must be hydrolysed in the intestine prior to absorption as free amino acids or small peptides which are further hydrolysed in mucosal cells (Matthews, 1971). Those amino acids which cannot be synthesised in sufficient amounts to meet the need of the body are classed as *essential* (i.e. isoleucine, leucine, lysine, methionine, phenylalanine, threonine, tryptophan, valine and, in early infancy, histidine) and must be obtained in the diet (Rose, 1938; Snyderman *et al.*, 1963). The others, classed as *non-essential*, can be synthesised endogenously provided sufficient nitrogen and other nutritional components are available. Further, there is continual turn-over of body proteins which replenishes the pools of amino acids. For example, the half-life of plasma albumin is 15 days, that of muscle proteins is 160 days.

Free amino acids are utilised as the synthetic precursors of numerous vital proteins of the body, e.g. structural, carrier proteins and enzymes (Szekely, 1980). Some are incorporated into peptide hormones, others have a well documented physiological function, e.g. the neurotransmitter, γ-aminobutyric acid, while some have a suspected but unproven function, e.g. cystathionine in human brain (Tudball and Beaumont, 1979). Excess amino acids are degraded by complicated metabolic pathways, sometimes involving the synthesis of other amino acids, resulting in a loss of nitrogen either by deamination or transamination. This nitrogen acts as a precursor for the many diverse nitrogen-containing compounds synthesised in the body, e.g. purines, pyrimidines, polyamines, adrenaline and creatine. Excess nitrogen is converted to urea which is excreted. The carbon skeletons of amino acids are further degraded by energy-producing pathways.

Protein amino acids tend to be efficiently conserved by the kidney. Reabsorption of the filtered load by the renal tubule is greater than 98 % for most, and more than 90% for all of them. Some non-protein amino acids have a similarly high renal threshold, e.g. ornithine, while others have a much lower threshold, e.g. homocystine and argininosuccinic acid.

The sum of all these physiological processes of amino acid turn-over is reflected by the nitrogen balance. In a healthy adult receiving adequate protein, intake of nitrogen will equal excretion (nitrogen equilibrium). In active growth, intake exceeds excretion and so the balance is positive, while in disease, there may be a negative balance particularly because of increased tissue breakdown (see Scriver and Rosenberg, 1973a for a review of physiology and general metabolism of amino acids).

It is evident that normal homeostasis of amino acids requires proper functioning of digestion, absorption, transport, metabolism and excretion. All of these can be deranged either due to a primary genetic disorder or secondary to some other disease process. Perturbation of amino acid homeostasis will be reflected in blood or urine levels of single or groups of amino acids or closely related metabolites. In this chapter, methods for detection of amino acid disorders are described. The main features of the more important disorders are summarised.

GENERAL METHODS FOR ANALYSIS OF AMINO ACIDS

The most widely used techniques for amino acid analysis are chromatographic. Reliable interpretation requires careful standardisation of techniques and construction of maps using standard amino acid solutions. Importantly, much experience is required to recognise normal and abnormal patterns. Clinical, dietary and therapeutic details of patients can be invaluable. For example, amino acid excretion is influenced by dietary intake of certain proteins, foods or intravenous alimentation. Drugs or antibiotics can yield ninhydrin-positive compounds. Some patients with an inherited disorder may exceptionally show abnormalities only after loading tests. Intermittent forms of inherited disorders may only be detected by analysis of several samples, especially collected during an episode of illness.

The most suitable reagent for measurement or detection of amino acids is ninhydrin (1,2,3-triketohydrindene hydrate). This reacts with alpha-substituted amino acids to form a coloured product in the following overall reaction.

$$2\ \text{(indanetrione structure)} + RCH(NH_2)COOH \rightarrow \text{(coloured product structure)} + RCHO + CO_2$$

coloured product

The complex obtained with most alpha-amino acids has maximum absorbance at 570 nm, with others at a lower wavelength, e.g. 440 nm for proline and hydroxyproline.

Due to low specificity many other nitrogenous compounds also react, although often to a much lower degree. These include amines, acids with the amino group substituted at other than the alpha carbon atom and amino sugars (Schonberg and Singer, 1978). This has important implications for the clinical application of amino acid analysis. Ninhydrin has been used for staining of chromatograms, for quantitative analysis of amino acids by column chromatography and for determination of total amino acids with measurement of either colour intensity or carbon dioxide liberation (see the 5th edition of this book, p. 491).

1. Total Amino Acid Nitrogen Determination

Methods of amino acid analysis based on separation of amino acids in plasma or urine also provide a semi-quantitative or quantitative estimate of total amino acid content and, as such, are the methods of choice for investigation of amino acid levels in disease states. However several methods have been described for direct determination of total amino acids (Frame *et al.*, 1943; Russell, 1944; Albanese and Irby, 1944; Sobel *et al.*, 1957; Dubin, 1960; Wells, 1969; Lorentz and Flatter, 1974). Goodwin (1968, 1970) described a method based on the reaction of 2,4-dinitrofluorobenzene with amino groups, applied to blood and urine (see 5th edition of this book, pp. 491, 493). All of these methods suffer to a varying degree from lack of specificity. Also, an increase of a single amino acid may not be evident by this method.

A simple alternative method based on separation of the amino acid fraction of urine or deproteinised blood, using cation-exchange resin with measurement of total amino acids by one of the above methods, has the advantage of also providing a desalted fraction for subsequent chromatography.

Reagents.
1. Cation exchange resin. Zeokarb (Duolite) 225, 100–200 mesh, is converted to the H^+ form with excess 4 mol/l hydrochloric acid followed by washing with water until the supernatant is neutral.
2. Ammonium hydroxide, 2 mol/l.

Technique. Prepare a 20×6 mm column of the resin using a glass pasteur pipette plugged with glass wool. Apply 1·0 ml urine to the column. Allow to drain and wash column with 4×1 ml distilled water, discarding eluate and washings. Elute amino acids with 2 mol/l ammonium hydroxide, discarding the first 0·5 ml and collecting until the effluent is alkaline. This can be assessed by darkening of the resin as it becomes alkaline but should be checked with a pH indicator paper. The sample is dried *in vacuo* (40 °C) and redissolved in 1 ml distilled water.

2. Paper Chromatography

This powerful method has been widely applied for separation of amino acids but has now been largely superseded by thin-layer chromatography (see p. 375). A typical two-dimensional paper system with a standard map is described by Parry (1957), (see 5th edition, p. 496). However, one-dimensional paper chromatography of amino acids in plasma or urine is a simple method for analysis of large numbers of samples. Indeed, this method is used by a number of centres in the UK for newborn population screening for phenylketonuria and other amino acid disorders (Scriver *et al.*, 1964; Komrower *et al.*, 1968) using liquid plasma from heel-prick blood samples. Ascending chromatography can be conveniently performed on 250 × 250 mm sheets in plastic frames using glass tanks (Shandon, Universal Frame Chromatank) and is particularly useful for large numbers of samples, while there are several proprietary glass tanks suitable for the descending method. Plasma can be directly applied since potentially interfering proteins are precipitated by the acidic solvent. The volume of urine applied is based on the creatinine content.

Reagents.
1. Solvent system. Butan-1-ol–glacial acetic acid–water (12/3/5 v/v).
2. Ninhydrin reagent. Dissolve 250 mg ninhydrin in 100 ml acetone. Isatin, 10 mg can also be included, if required, to enhance the colour produced with the iminoacids.

Technique. Plasma, 10 μl, or urine (not desalted) containing 4 μg creatinine (see p. 384 for different loading required for Pauly reagent or iodoplatinate staining) is applied as a small spot at the origin, drawn 25 mm from the bottom of a 250 × 250 mm sheet of Whatman 3MM paper ('A' pattern) for ascending chromatography, or 10 cm from the bottom of a length of 3 MM paper for descending chromatography. Develop overnight in freshly prepared solvent. Dry the papers at room temperature and locate amino acids by dipping in the ninhydrin reagent followed by heating at 75 °C for 5 min. Most amino acids produce red–purple spots, proline and hydroxyproline stain yellow, or blue if isatin is used in the ninhydrin reagent. Secondary staining of chromatograms can be used to detect histidine (Pauly reagent, see p. 384) or citrulline and tryptophan (Ehrlich's reagent, see p. 384). Standard amino acid mixtures can be run as markers and to allow semi-quantitative estimation of concentration. This method gives good separation of some amino acids, particularly those which are found in the more common inherited disorders, but poorer separation of others. Fig. 18.1 shows a map of the relative mobilities of amino acids found in plasma and chromatograms of plasma samples including ones from patients with phenylketonuria and branched-chain amino acidaemia. Fig. 18.2 shows chromatograms with abnormal urine samples.

3. High Voltage Electrophoresis—One-dimensional

This technique allows rapid analysis of amino acids and is useful for urine since salts do not interfere. It can be used to confirm findings obtained by chromatography, especially identification of basic amino acids or cystine and homocystine after oxidation. In addition methylmalonic acid can be detected by staining with the indicator, Fast blue. (Gutteridge and Wright, 1970). Using a buffer of pH 2, most amino acids migrate towards the cathode, although oxidation products of sulphur amino acids move towards the anode.

Reagents.
1. Buffer. Make 66 ml glacial acetic acid and 33 ml formic acid 900 g/l to 1 litre with distilled water.
2. Ninhydrin reagent. Dissolve 250 mg ninhydrin and 0·5 ml lutidine in 100 ml acetone.

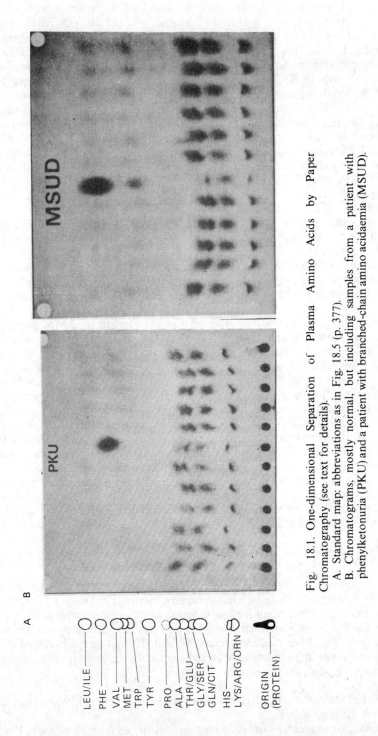

Fig. 18.1. One-dimensional Separation of Plasma Amino Acids by Paper Chromatography (see text for details).

A. Standard map: abbreviations as in Fig. 18.5 (p. 377).

B. Chromatograms, mostly normal, but including samples from a patient with phenylketonuria (PKU) and a patient with branched-chain amino acidaemia (MSUD).

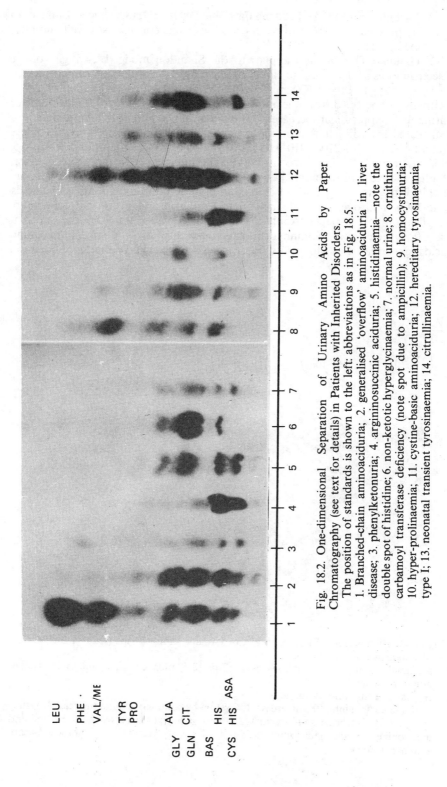

Fig. 18.2. One-dimensional Separation of Urinary Amino Acids by Paper Chromatography (see text for details) in Patients with Inherited Disorders. The position of standards is shown to the left: abbreviations as in Fig. 18.5.

1. Branched-chain aminoaciduria; 2. generalised 'overflow' aminoaciduria in liver disease; 3. phenylketonuria; 4. argininosuccinic aciduria; 5. histidinaemia—note the double spot of histidine; 6. non-ketotic hyperglycinaemia; 7. normal urine; 8. ornithine carbamoyl transferase deficiency (note spot due to ampicillin); 9. homocystinuria; 10. hyper-prolinaemia; 11. cystine-basic aminoaciduria; 12. hereditary tyrosinaemia, type I; 13. neonatal transient tyrosinaemia; 14. citrullinaemia.

3. Fast blue reagent. Add 100 mg Fast blue B salt (BDH Chemicals Limited) to 15 ml ethanol, 5 ml water and 0·9 ml glacial acetic acid, stir well and filter before use.

Technique. This method applies to the Shandon model L 24 high voltage electrophoresis apparatus but can be easily adapted for other instruments which have a cooling facility. A 600 mm length of Whatman No. 3 MM paper is marked with a line one-third from the anode for application of samples. The volume of urine to be applied can be based on the creatinine content (8 μg creatinine) or calculated according to the specific gravity as follows: for specific gravities of less than 1·005, 1·005–1·010, 1·010–1·015, 1·015–1·02, or greater than 1·02, use 45, 22·5, 15, 10, or 5 μl of urine respectively. Dip the filter paper in the electrophoresis buffer, blot to remove excess liquid and place on the cooling plate. Samples are applied in 2 cm long streaks. For oxidation of sulphur-containing amino acids add 100 μl hydrogen peroxide (300 g/l) to 1 ml urine and leave for 10 min before application to the paper. Apply a voltage of 3 kV for 1 h. Dry the paper at 40–50 °C then dip in the ninhydrin reagent and heat at 75 °C for 5 min. Amino acids are revealed as blue spots. See Fig. 18.3 for a map of the more common

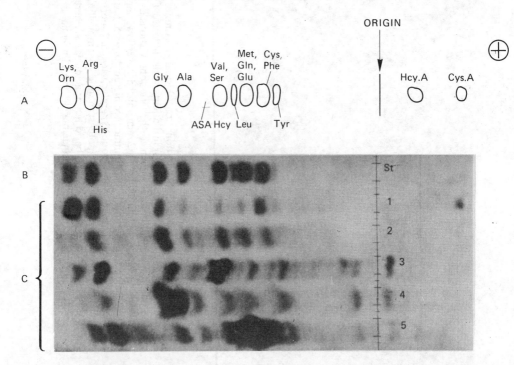

Fig. 18.3. High Voltage Electrophoresis of Urinary Amino Acids (see text for details). + = anode and − = cathode.

A. Standard map: abbreviations as in Fig. 18.5, plus Cys.A, cysteic acid; Hcy.A, homocysteic acid.

B. Standard mixture of amino acids.

C. Patients with inherited disorders. 1. Cystine-basic aminoaciduria (increased cystine, cysteic acid and basic amino acids); 2. homocystinuria (increased homocystine and methionine); 3. argininosuccinic aciduria; 4. hyperglycinaemia; 5. branched-chain aminoacidaemia.

amino acids and the patterns obtained with some abnormal urines. For detection of methylmalonic acid cut the paper at a line 5 cm towards the cathode from the origin. Stain the anodic portion by dipping in the Fast blue reagent. On drying in air, methylmalonic acid reacts to give a magenta colour. Similarly, other organic acids may be detected, e.g. acetoacetic acid, phenylpyruvic acid or *p*-hydroxyphenylpyruvic acid.

4. Thin-layer Chromatography

Chromatography on thin-layers of microcrystalline cellulose has largely super-seded the use of paper due to the advantages of improved resolution and smaller spot size giving increased sensitivity. Smaller quantities of reagents are required and analysis times are considerably shorter. For urine a disadvantage is the need for desalting.

One-dimensional Chromatography for Plasma Amino Acids. This can be used for liquid plasma or for dried blood on filter paper after elution of amino acids (modified from Ireland and Read, 1972).

Reagents.
1. Solvent. Butan-1-ol–acetone–glacial acetic acid–water (35/35/10/20 v/v).
2. Eluant. Ethanol/water (70:30 v/v).
3. Ninhydrin reagent. As for paper chromatography.

Technique. Prepare a 100 mm long piece of thin-layer plate (cellulose tlc aluminium sheet without indicator, Merck type 5552 or equivalent) by drawing a line 20 mm from the bottom for the origin, scoring a line 5 mm from the top and scraping the edges to give a 2 mm wide border free from cellulose. Liquid plasma (1 μl) can be applied directly as a spot. Dried blood spots on filter paper must first be treated with eluant by placing a punched out 6 mm disc in a tube containing 100 μl eluant. Allow to stand at least 30 min with intermittent vortex-mixing, then apply 25 μl eluate to the tlc plate with air drying between applications to prevent the spot size exceeding 6 mm. Develop the chromatograms twice in freshly mixed solvent with air-drying between runs and stain by dipping in the ninhydrin reagent and heating at 75 °C for 3 min. Fig. 18.4 illustrates chromatograms obtained with liquid plasma for monitoring of phenylalanine levels in treated phenylketonuric patients. The separation is similar to that obtained by paper chromatography (see p. 370) but resolution, particularly of phenylalanine is improved.

Two-dimensional Chromatography for Urinary Amino Acids. A suitable combination of solvents provides remarkably good resolution of amino acids in urine. The presence and, to some extent, quantity of amino acids in a sample can be determined in a single test. Several combinations of solvents (e.g., Wadman *et al.*, 1969, Von Arx and Neher, 1963) produce adequate separations, but one system should be selected and used consistently to obtain maximum experience of normal and abnormal patterns of amino acids. The volume of sample applied has been based on amino nitrogen content by some workers (e.g. Wadman *et al.*, 1969) but is more commonly based on creatinine or total nitrogen. The more extensive the desalting achieved, the better the separation obtained, but against this the potential loss of components must be considered, e.g. loss of acidic or basic compounds by ion-exchange desalting.

Desalting. The ion-exchange method for determining amino nitrogen, de-scribed above, provides desalted samples suitable for chromatography. An

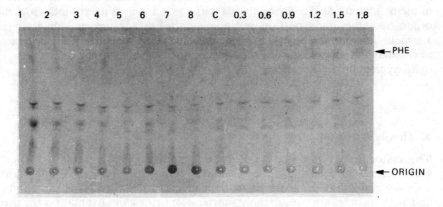

Fig. 18.4. One-Dimensional Thin-layer Chromatography of Plasma Amino Acids. Monitoring of Treatment of Patients with Phenylketonuria.
Phe—phenylalanine. 1–8: plasma samples from patients with phenylketonuria. 0·3, 0·6, 0·9, 1·2, 1·5, 1·8 = plasma phenylalanine standards (mmol/l) obtained by applying 1 μl control plasma together with 0·5, 1·0, 1·5, 2·0, 2·5 and 3·0 μl respectively of 0·6 mmol/l phenylalanine solution.

alternative simpler technique is partial desalting with an organic solvent. Add 0·25 ml urine to 1 ml propan-2-ol, keep at 4° C for 30 min (preferably overnight), centrifuge at 2000 g for 5 min, and use the supernatant for chromatography.
Reagents.
1. Solvent system 1. Pyridine–acetone–ammonia (sp. gr. 0·88)–water (90/60/10/35 v/v).
2. Solvent system 2. Butan-1-ol–acetone–glacial acetic acid–water (35/35/10/20 v/v).
3. Ninhydrin reagent. Dissolve 250 mg ninhydrin in 100 ml acetone.
4. Reference amino acid mixture. Dissolve the following in 100 ml distilled water: 40 mg of glycine, histidine, proline and hydroxyproline, 20 mg of glutamic acid, aspartic acid, serine and alanine, 10 mg of phenylalanine, tyrosine, tryptophan, valine, leucine, isoleucine, methionine, β-aminoisobutyric acid, cystine, homocystine, glutamine, asparagine, taurine, threonine, lysine, arginine and ornithine. Store − 20 °C.

Technique. Prepare 100 mm square sheets of cellulose on aluminium tlc plates by scraping cellulose from the edges to give a 2 mm wide border. Mark the origin 20 mm from each edge at the right hand bottom corner and apply desalted urine containing 2 μg of creatinine in a compact spot with hot air drying. Include the reference mixture (1 μl) with each batch of samples. Solvent development can be performed in any suitably sized glass tank with the tlc plates 'sandwiched' between glass plates but prevented from touching by bending slightly the top corners. Alternatively, use spring-type holders to suspend the plates in the correct orientation. Develop twice in each solvent with thorough drying in air at room temperature between runs (taking about 1 h for each development). Locate amino acids by dipping in ninhydrin and leaving at room temperature or heating at 75 °C for 3 min. As a rough indication of concentration, the intensity of individual amino acids can be scored relative to that of an amino acid on the standard chromatogram, e.g. glycine.

INTERPRETATION

As with other separation methods reliable interpretation requires a good deal of experience and knowledge of normal and abnormal patterns. Fig. 18.5 shows a reference map of amino acids and normal and abnormal chromatograms. The normal pattern of amino acid excretion varies with age and the general state of

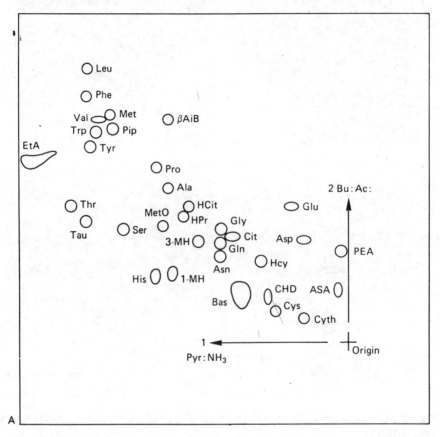

Fig. 18.5. Two-Dimensional Separation of Amino Acids by Thin-layer Chromatography. (see text for details).

+ = origin; 1 = first solvent—pyridine, acetone, ammonia, water; 2 = second solvent—butan-1-ol, acetone, water, acetic acid.

1—Ala, alanine; 2—ASA, argininosuccinic acid; 3—Asn, asparagine; 4—Asp, aspartic acid; 5—βAiB, β-aminoisobutyric acid; 6—Bas, basic amino acids, lysine, arginine, ornithine; 7—Cit, citrulline; 8—Cyth, cystathionine; 9—CHD, cysteine-homocysteine disulphide; 10—Cys, cystine; 11—EtA, ethanolamine; 12—Gln, glutamine; 13—Glu, glutamic acid; 14—Gly, glycine; 15—His, histidine; 16—HCit, homocitrulline; 17—HCy, homocystine; 18—HPr, hydroxyproline; 19—Leu, leucine and isoleucine; 20—Met, methionine; 21—MetO, methionine sulphoxide; 22—1-MH, 1-methylhistidine; 23—3-MH, 3-methylhistidine; 24—Phe, phenylalanine; 25—PEA, phosphoethanolamine; 26—Pip, pipecolic acid; 27—Pro, proline; 28—Ser, serine; 29—Tau, taurine; 30—Thr, threonine; 31—Trp, tryptophan; 32—Tyr, tyrosine; 33—Val, valine; X—ampicillin.

A: Map of Standards. Although the basic amino acids are shown as a single spot, on some occasions they may separate due to minor variations in chromatographic conditions.

B: Urines from Patients with Various Inherited Disorders.

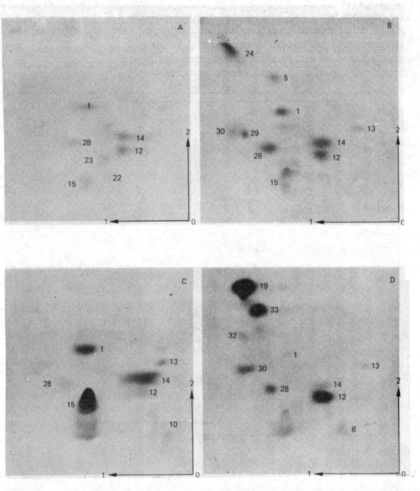

Fig. 18.5B (i). A—normal; B—phenylketonuria; C—histidinaemia; D—branched-chain aminoaciduria.

nutrition. In adults and older children relatively few amino acids are excreted reflecting conservation of the filtered load by active reabsorption in the renal tubule. Glycine (strongest), glutamine, alanine, serine, taurine, histidine and methylhistidines (both related to protein intake) are often clearly detected. There can be trace amounts of tyrosine, cystine and glutamate with other amino acids usually not detectable. In younger children, up to the age of about 2 years, the pattern is similar but often more marked, with tyrosine a little more prominent. Branched-chain amino acids, threonine and basic amino acids are sometimes present in small quantities but taurine is rarely present. In the first few weeks of life the overall excretion of amino acids is highest, with a more intense pattern than is found in later life. In addition to those amino acids listed above, traces of phenylalanine and asparagine may be found. More specifically glycine, proline and hydroxyproline can be increased reflecting immature development of the

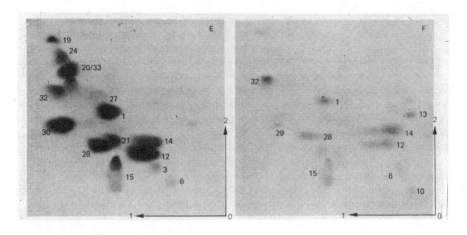

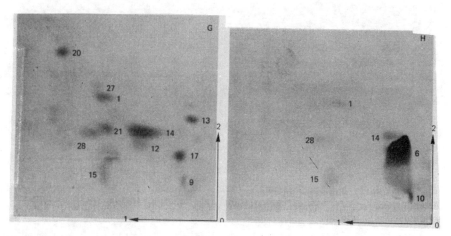

Fig. 18.5B (ii). E—hereditary tyrosinaemia, type I; F—neonatal transient tyrosinaemia; G—homocystininuria (newborn); H—cystine-basic aminoaciduria.

renal tubular reabsorption system for these amino acids (Brodehl and Gellissen, 1968). Cystine and basic amino acid excretion can be increased. Taurine is often present in clearly detectable amounts in the first few days of life.

Dietary influences on amino acid excretion can be considerable, e.g. glycine, proline and hydroxyproline increase after intake of gelatin. Homocitrulline is found after intake of sterilised milk preparations (Gerritsen *et al.*, 1963). Histidine and methylhistidine reflect meat intake. β-Aminoisobutyric acid excretion is high in a small proportion of the population. It may have no known pathological effect or it can reflect tissue breakdown (Scriver and Rosenberg, 1973b). Ninhydrin-positive compounds can be found in urine following antibiotic therapy (Potter, 1974) or drug intake (e.g. Brandt and Christensen, 1984). All these factors must be considered in interpretation of urinary amino acid analysis although generalised or specific amino acid increases usually stand out clearly.

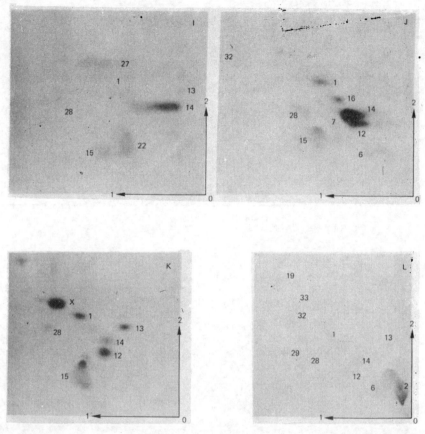

Fig. 18.5B (iii). I—hyperprolinaemia, (note increased glycine excretion); J—citrullinaemia; K—ornithine carbamoyl transferase deficiency (patient on ampicillin); L—argininosuccinic aciduria.

5. Quantitative Amino Acid Analysis—Column Chromatography

Modern equipment allows quantitative determination of amino acids in physiological fluids in a single analysis with a high degree of specificity, sensitivity and accuracy. Systems are fully automated with computer or microprocessor control and data acquisition. Either stepwise or gradient buffer changes elute amino acids from a micro-spherical cation-exchange resin. Amino acid detection is by ninhydrin monitored at 570 nm and 440 nm (for proline and hydroxy-proline), or more recently by orthophthaldialdehyde monitored fluorimetrically. Fluorimetry has the advantages of linearity with a much wider range of amino acid concentrations, greater sensitivity and the use of more stable reagents. Disadvantages are the need for oxidation of the column effluent to detect cystine and the imino acids and low sensitivity for homocystine even following oxidation. Analysis times range from 2 to 4 h for a complete amino acid profile to 30 to 45 min for single or groups of amino acids, e.g. phenylalanine and tyrosine. The application of this method to studies of amino acids in health and disease has been widely reported (e.g. Rattenbury, 1981). A typical separation of plasma amino

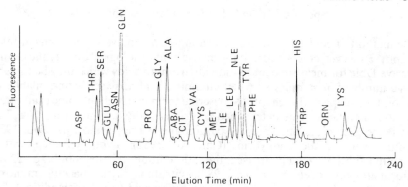

Fig. 18.6. Quantitative Amino Acid Analysis by Ion-exchange Chromatography.
This typical separation of amino acids in normal plasma was obtained using the Hilger
J180 amino acid analyser. Gradient elution with lithium citrate-borate buffers and
fluorimetric detection were employed. See legend to Fig. 18.5 for key to abbreviations
but additional ones are: ABA—α-aminobutyric acid; ILE—isoleucine; NLE—
norleucine (internal standard); ORN—ornithine; LYS—lysine.

acids is shown in Fig. 18.6. Although many laboratories may not have access to an
amino acid analyser, correct sample preparation is important before sending to a
reference laboratory for analysis.

Other methods have been described for quantitative amino acid analysis.
Gas–liquid chromatography has been tried (Adams, 1974) but its wider use has
been precluded by problems associated with formation and stability of volatile
derivatives of amino acids. More promising, but still to be established, is high
performance liquid chromatography with either pre-column derivatisation and
reverse phase separation (Turnell and Cooper, 1982; Bidlingmeyer *et al.*, 1984) or
ion-exchange and post-column detection with ninhydrin or orthophthaldialdehyde (Drescher *et al.*, 1981). See also Chapter 3, p. 66.

Sample Preparation. There are several possible pitfalls in the preparation of
blood samples for amino acid analysis (Perry and Hansen, 1969). For example,
plasma must be obtained free of leucocytes, platelets or erythrocytes after
centrifugation to prevent false elevation of levels of taurine, aspartic acid and
glutamic acid. Delay in deproteinising must be avoided to prevent loss of
disulphide amino acids by binding to plasma proteins. Perry and Hansen (1969)
found a complete loss of cystine in plasma stored for one week at − 20 °C before
deproteinising. The choice of protein precipitant is important, e.g. losses of
tryptophan observed with picric acid are much less when sulphosalicylic acid is
used.

Reagent. Sulphosalicylic acid solution. Dissolve 12·5 g in 100 ml water. Store
at 4 °C.

Technique. Collect blood with lithium heparin as anticoagulant and centrifuge
at 2000*g* for 5 min (preferably at 4 °C). Remove plasma taking care not to disturb
or take up the buffy coat and deproteinise within 30 min. Add one volume of
sulphosalicylic acid solution to 2 volumes of plasma (1 ml is adequate) and mix
thoroughly. Use the supernatant obtained after centrifugation at 6000*g* for
amino acid analysis.

Specific Methods for Individual Amino Acids

The method of choice for quantitative amino acid analysis is column chromatography. However, colorimetric, fluorimetric, microbiological or enzymic methods are available for measurement of individual amino acids which may be useful for large numbers of samples or when an amino acid analyser is unavailable. It is beyond the scope of this chapter to describe them in detail but some examples are listed. A number can be determined colorimetrically; arginine with 1-naphthol (Rosenberg *et al.*, 1956) or hydroxyquinoline (Ceriotti and Spandrio, 1957a); proline with acidic ninhydrin (Chinard, 1952); hydroxyproline with *p*-dimethylaminobenzaldehyde (see the 5th edition of this book, p. 525) or fluorimetrically (Bellon *et al.*, 1983); citrulline with diacetyl monoxime (Archibald, 1944); cystine with phosphotungstic acid (see the 5th edition of this book, p. 521); cysteine with 2,6-dichloro-*p*-benzoquinone (Fernandez and Henry, 1965); serine (Frisell and Mackenzie, 1958) and threonine (Neidig and Hess, 1952) with periodate; tyrosine using 1-nitroso-2-naphthol (Ceriotti and Spandrio, 1957b). Tryptophan can be measured fluorimetrically (Duggan and Udenfriend, 1956). Several enzymatic methods are available using commercially available enzymes, e.g. arginine, using octopine dehydrogenase (Gade, 1985); glutamic acid using glutamate dehydrogenase (Beutler, 1985); glutamine with glutamine synthetase (Mecke, 1985); lysine with lysine decarboxylase (Romette, 1985); phenylalanine and tyrosine with phenylalanine ammonia lyase (Shen and Abell, 1985); asparagine and aspartic acid with asparaginase and aspartate amino transferase (Mollering, 1985).

Particularly useful is the fluorimetric determination of phenylalanine and tyrosine (Wong *et al.*, 1964) which has a wide application for screening in automated systems (Hill *et al.*, 1965) and for monitoring of treatment in patients with phenylketonuria.

Fluorimetric Method for Phenylalanine (McCaman and Robins, 1962; Wong *et al.*, 1964; Faulkner, 1965)

This technique uses the enhancement of the fluorescence of a phenylalanine ninhydrin reaction produced by a peptide L-leucyl-L-alanine. This allows phenylalanine to be measured quantitatively in a final concentration of 100 nmol/l in the presence of other amino acids.

Reagents.
1. Succinate buffer, 300 mmol/l, pH 5·8. Dissolve 3·54 g succinic acid in about 80 ml water, bring to pH 5·8 with sodium hydroxide and make up to 100 ml with water.
2. Ninhydrin solution, 30 mmol/l. Dissolve 0·534 g in 100 ml water.
3. L-Leucyl-L-alanine, 5 mmol/l. Dissolve 10·1 mg in 10 ml water, and keep frozen in small amounts.
4. Copper reagent. Dissolve separately in about 300 ml water, 1·6 g anhydrous sodium carbonate, 65 mg sodium potassium tartrate and 60 mg copper sulphate ($CuSO_4$, $5H_2O$); add in that order and make to a litre with water.
5. Trichloracetic acid, 600 mmol/l (98 g/l), and 300 mmol/l (49 g/l).
6. Phenylalanine standard. Dissolve 41·25 mg L-phenylalanine in 50 ml trichloracetic acid, 600 mmol/l. Make to 100 ml with water. Dilute 1 to 10 with trichloracetic acid, 300 mmol/l, for use. This contains 250 μmol/l.

Technique. To 1 volume of serum (5 to 100 μl) add 1 volume of trichloracetic acid, 600 mmol/l, mix, stand for about 10 min and then centrifuge. Mix 20 μl supernatant (test) or 20 μl phenylalanine standard with 200 μl succinate buffer, 80 μl ninhydrin and 40 μl dipeptide. For the test blank replace the dipeptide with water. For the standard blank replace phenylalanine with trichloracetic acid (300 mmol/l).

To each add 2 ml copper reagent, heat at 60 °C for 2 h and measure the fluorescence. (Excitation wavelength, 365 nm; emission 505 to 530 nm).

Calculation. Serum phenylalanine (μmol/l)

$$= \frac{(\text{Reading of unknown} - \text{reading of blank})}{(\text{Reading of standard} - \text{reading of standard blank})} \times 500$$

Fluorimetric Method for Tyrosine (Udenfriend, 1962; Wong *et al.*, 1964)

The reaction of tyrosine with a 1-nitroso-2-naphthol reagent also containing sodium nitrite and nitric acid is used. Excess reagent is removed with dichloroethane.

Reagents.
1. Nitrosonaphthol reagent. Dissolve 2 g 1-nitroso-2-naphthol in 1 litre ethanol (950 ml absolute ethanol made to a litre with water). Before use mix 2 volumes with 3 volumes of 3 mol/l nitric acid and 2 volumes of 100 mmol/l sodium nitrite solution.
2. Dichloroethane.
3. Trichloracetic acid, 600 mmol/l.
4. Tyrosine standards, 150, 300, and 600 μmol/l in water. Keep at 4 °C.

Technique. To each of 100 μl serum or plasma (the test), 100 μl standard, or 100 μl water (the blank), add 100 μl trichloracetic acid. Stand 10 min and centrifuge. Add 500 μl nitrosonaphthol reagent to 50 μl supernatant, incubate at 33 °C for 20 min, then add 2·5 ml water and 7·5 ml dichloroethane to each, mix and centrifuge. Transfer the aqueous upper layer to other test tubes and allow to stand for about 40 min at about 25 °C. Read the fluorescence within 30 min. (Excitation wavelength 460 nm; emission 570 nm.)

Calculation. Serum tyrosine (μmol/l)

$$= \frac{\text{Reading of unknown}}{\text{Reading of standard}} \times 150, 300 \text{ or } 600.$$

SPECIFIC METHODS FOR DETECTION OF AMINO ACIDS AND THEIR DERIVATIVES

There are many alternative detection reagents which can be used either to confirm the identity of amino acids detected with ninhydrin or to detect ninhydrin-negative metabolites related to particular amino acids. Some of the more useful reagents for studying inherited diseases are described in detail. Also see Smith and Seakins (1976a) for a more extensive list.

1. Iodoplatinate Reagent for Sulphur-containing Amino Acids

This reagent can be used to stain paper and thin-layer chromatograms (Toennies and Kolb, 1951) or with column chromatography for quantitative amino acid analysis (Fowler and Robins, 1972).

Reagents.
1. Chloroplatinic acid, stock solution. Dissolve 1 g chloroplatinic acid (40%
Pt; BDH Chemicals Limited) in 100 ml water. This stock solution is stable at
room temperature. Dilute 1 in 10 with water for use.
Iodoplatinate stain reagent. Mix freshly, 5 ml chloroplatinic acid (1 g/l),
⌡0 mg potassium iodide, 0·5 ml 2 mol/l hydrochloric acid, then add 25 ml
acetone (analytical grade).

Technique. Papers or tlc plates are dipped in the reagent. On drying in air,
compounds containing sulphur in oxidation state II or IV react to give white or
cream spots on a magenta background, taking up to 1 h to develop. Thus cystine,
homocystine, cysteine-homocysteine mixed disulphide, cystathionine and
methionine react, whereas cysteic acid and methionine sulphone (oxidation
state VI) do not. Several antibiotics, e.g. ampicillin, yield sulphur-containing
metabolites which will be detected. This stain can be used after one-dimensional
paper chromatography of urine (volume containing 16 μg creatinine) to screen for
sulphur-containing amino acids and allows easy distinction of cystine and
homocystine.

2. Pauly Reagent for Phenolic Acids and Imidazoles

Pauly's diazotised sulphanilic acid reagent can be used as a secondary stain for
histidine after one-dimensional paper chromatography of plasma, or directly on
urine chromatograms for phenolic acids and imidazoles.

Reagents.
1. Sulphanilic acid solution. Dissolve 9 g sulphanilic acid and 90 ml concentrated hydrochloric acid in 900 ml water.
2. Sodium nitrite solution, 50 g/l in water.
3. Sodium carbonate solution, 100 g/l in water.

Immediately before use mix one volume of (1) with one volume of (2), stand at
room temperature for 5 min in a fume cupboard then add two volumes of (3).

Technique. Chromatograms can be dipped or sprayed with the reagent.
Histidine and imidazoles produce vivid red spots on a light yellow background.
p-Hydroxyphenylpyruvate (fleeting orange), *p*-hydroxyphenyllactate and
p-hydroxyphenylacetate (blue/grey) react as does *o*-hydroxyphenylacetate which
gives an orange colour. Due to the low specificity of this reagent many drug
metabolites and other compounds can interfere (e.g. salicylate).

Use of this stain in conjunction with one-dimensional paper chromatography
of urine (volume containing 8 μg creatinine loaded) allows simple screening for
this class of compounds.

3. Ultraviolet Absorbance and Fluorescence

Viewing of chromatograms under ultraviolet light of wavelength 280 nm,
sometimes provides valuable information. For example, tryptophan metabolites,
particularly those of the kynurenine pathway, are highly fluorescent and purines
and pyrimidines are revealed as absorbent spots. It should be noted that normal
urine constituents may also fluoresce, e.g. riboflavin.

4. Ehrlich's Reagent for Tryptophan, its Derivatives and Citrulline

This can be used as a secondary stain with one-dimensional paper chromatography of plasma or directly with urine chromatograms (Smith and Seakins,
1976b).

Reagent. Dissolve 1 g *p*-dimethylaminobenzaldehyde in 10 ml concentrated hydrochloric acid and 40 ml acetone. Use immediately.

Technique. Dip or spray chromatograms and leave to dry at room temperature. Tryptophan and indoles produce grey-blue coloured spots and several kynurenine pathway metabolites react, e.g. kynurenine produces an orange colour. Citrulline is detected by its pink colour. Staining of one-dimensional paper chromatograms of urine (4 μg creatinine loaded) with this reagent is a useful screening method. Normal urine contains a trace of tryptophan, urea (yellow) and indoxyl sulphate (orange).

5. Chemical Spot Tests

There are several chemical spot tests which can be used as an initial screen for some amino acids or metabolites in urine. They suffer from lack of specificity and sensitivity especially with dilute urine. The following examples can be useful in screening for amino acid disorders.

1. *Cyanide/nitroprusside for disulphide compounds*. Add 0·5 ml sodium cyanide solution (50 g/l) to 1 ml urine. Stand for 10 min then add (dropwise) freshly prepared sodium nitroprusside solution (0·5 g in 10 ml water). Cystine and homocystine produce a pink-purple colour.

2. *Ferric chloride reagent for phenylpyruvic acid*. Add 2 drops ferric chloride solution (50 g/l water) to 1 ml urine. Add sulphuric acid (50 ml/l in water) dropwise to dissolve any precipitate. Phenylpyruvic acid gives an immediate green colour. Several other compounds also react, e.g. *p*-hydroxyphenylpyruvic acid, homogentisic acid and imidazolepyruvic acid each producing a green colour. Salicyluric acid (following salicylate ingestion) gives a purple colour.

3. *Dinitrophenylhydrazine for α-oxo-acids*. Add equal volumes of urine and dinitrophenylhydrazine reagent (5 g 2,4-dinitrophenylhydrazine in 100 ml 2 mol/l hydrochloric acid, filtered) and stand for 10 min at room temperature. α-Oxo acids produce dinitrophenylhydrazones forming a yellow precipitate. A positive test can be given by phenylpyruvic acid, *p*-hydroxyphenylpyruvic acid and branched-chain oxo-acids. Acetoacetate and acetone (excreted in ketosis) will also give a positive reaction. Dinitrophenylhydrazones can be extracted with ethyl acetate and further identified by thin-layer chromatography (Dancis *et al.*, 1963).

6. Analysis of Organic Acids by Gas Chromatography

Many inherited disorders of amino acid metabolism are caused by an enzyme deficiency subsequent to removal of the amino group and cannot be identified with ninhydrin. These are often characterised by accumulation in blood and urine of a ninhydrin-negative compound, often an organic acid which can be detected by gas chromatography. For example, propionic acidaemia and methylmalonic acidaemia are both disorders of metabolism of propionate, which is derived from several precursors including odd-chain fatty acids, methionine, threonine and isoleucine. Isovaleric acidaemia and β-methylcrotonic aciduria are both disorders of leucine metabolism, whereas methyl acetoacetyl CoA thiolase deficiency is a disorder of isoleucine degradation. Organic acid disorders have been reviewed by Tanaka *et al.* (1980a). A useful application of this method is the quantitative determination of phenolic acids and other metabolites of phenylalanine and tyrosine. The methods most widely used employ extraction by organic solvent or ion-exchange (Thompson and Markey, 1975; Tanaka *et al.*, 1980b) with formation of methyl- or trimethyl silyl-esters to increase volatility. Packed or capillary columns with polar or non-polar silicone liquid phases are used with detection by flame ionisation or preferably with mass spectrometric analysis (Goodman and Markey, 1981).

ABNORMALITIES OF AMINO ACID METABOLISM AND TRANSPORT

These can be classified as those caused by primary abnormalities of amino acid metabolism or transport due to a genetic defect, and those secondary to exogenous or endogenous factors which can also be genetic.

Aminoaciduria

Aminoaciduria refers to excessive urinary excretion of one or several amino acids. There are broadly two groups, 'overflow' and 'renal'. *Overflow aminoaciduria* refers to increased excretion of amino acids consequent upon increased plasma concentrations, either generalised as in liver disease or specific in inherited disorders affecting a single or a few amino acids. In *renal aminoaciduria* increased amino acid excretion can either be due to specific primary defects of renal tubular reabsorption or to generalised tubular damage as in Fanconi syndrome. Mixed types also occur whereby excessive plasma concentration of an amino acid saturates its renal tubular reabsorption site thereby causing loss of another amino acid which shares the same site, e.g. increased excretion of glycine and hydroxyproline in hyperprolinaemia (Scriver and Rosenberg, 1973c). Importantly, this phenomenon can also result in the same pattern of amino acid excretion in different disorders. For example, cystine-basic aminoaciduria is found in hyperornithinaemia, hyperlysinaemia, and hyper-argininaemia as well as in cystinuria.

Aminoaciduria Secondary to Other Disorders

There are many examples of deranged amino acid metabolism or transport not due to abnormalities in processing of the amino acids themselves, but caused by other factors or diseases.

A *generalised aminoaciduria* can reflect renal damage caused by several toxic agents including heavy metals, nitrobenzene or salicylate. Reversible generalised aminoaciduria has been reported in malnutrition, e.g. kwashiorkor, scurvy and rickets and in pernicious anaemia (Scriver and Rosenberg, 1973d). Generalised aminoaciduria may also be a feature of conditions characterised by tissue breakdown, e.g. wasting disease, hyperthyroidism, trauma or muscle atrophy (Meister, 1965b). D-Isomers of amino acids (sometimes used in intravenous alimentation) are excreted largely unchanged due to specificity of metabolic and transport systems for the L-isomers. Generalised hyperaminoacidaemia and aminoaciduria has been observed in acute hepatic disorders (Munro, 1970) and in Reye's Syndrome (Romshe *et al.*, 1981). Increased excretion of cystine, taurine, β-aminoisobutyric acid, methylhistidine and ethanolamine was reported in patients with mild hepatic disease (Meister, 1965b). More specific increases of tyrosine and methionine may be observed in some forms of liver disease (Yu *et al.*, 1971; Thoene *et al.*, 1978). At the metabolic level, drug-inhibition of an enzyme may cause increased excretion of a specific amino acid, e.g. homocystinuria following 6-azauridine intake (Hyanek *et al.*, 1969).

In several conditions which result in cellular accumulation of toxic compounds there may be associated renal tubular damage causing generalised aminoaciduria. For example galactose-1-phosphate accumulates in galactosaemia, fructose-1-phosphate in hereditary fructose intolerance, copper in Wilson's disease, cystine in cystinosis and less well defined compounds in tyrosinaemia and the oculo-cerebro-renal syndrome (Lowe's) (Scriver and Rosenberg, 1973d).

More specifically, hyperglycinaemia and hyperglycinuria are found in a number of organic acid disorders, alanine may be increased secondary to disturbed pyruvate metabolism and increased glutamine may reflect ammonia accumulation in urea cycle disorders.

Inherited Disorders Producing Aminoaciduria

There are many inherited disorders of amino acid metabolism and transport, usually transmitted in an autosomal recessive manner. The more important conditions are described in the remainder of this chapter.

Phenylalanine Disorders

Phenylketonuria (see Scriver and Clow, 1980 for a review)

Classical phenylketonuria is caused by deficiency of the liver enzyme phenylalanine hydroxylase. This enzyme has been well characterised at the protein (Woo *et al.*, 1974) and DNA level (Robson *et al.*, 1984; Kwok *et al.*, 1985) and requires tetrahydrobiopterin as a cofactor. It catalyses the conversion of phenylalanine to tyrosine. Deficiency causes accumulation of phenylalanine in body fluids, plasma concentrations ranging widely from 300 to 5000 μmol/l (normal, less than 120 μmol/l). This reflects much genetic variation at the phenylalanine hydroxylase locus itself as well as other variant forms (see p. 389). Urinary excretion of phenylalanine can also be increased but often less markedly due to its high renal threshold. Metabolites resulting from alternative pathways of phenylalanine metabolism are also excreted, including phenylpyruvic acid, phenyllactic acid, phenylacetic acid, sometimes as its conjugate phenylacetylglutamine, and *o*-hydroxyphenylacetic acid. Their concentrations tend to be lower in neonates, reaching higher levels with increasing age.

Untreated, the condition exhibits marked clinical features including severe mental retardation, neurological abnormalities, blond hair and blue eyes. Furthermore, there is a severe teratogenic effect of phenylalanine *in utero*, babies born to mothers with phenylketonuria commonly exhibiting mental retardation, microcephaly and congenital abnormalities, e.g. heart disease (Lipson *et al.*, 1984).

Screening of newborn populations and dietary treatment of detected cases, introduced in many countries during the last two decades, has proved extremely effective in preventing the symptoms of the disorder.

Screening Methods. Capillary blood can be collected in drops on filter paper, e.g. Schliecher and Schuell 903, giving 10 to 12 mm wide spots allowing punching of discs of known diameter for analysis. Standard forms with filter paper are ideal for postal transport and long-term storage. Alternatively, blood for liquid plasma can be collected in heparinised glass tubes (75 × 1·3 mm) sealed with plasticine and transported in special carrier tubes or in corrugated paper. Plasma is then obtained by centrifugation of flame-sealed tubes in a haematocrit rotor. The latter method has the disadvantage of unsuitability for long-term storage.

The most commonly used laboratory methods are microbiological, chromato-graphic or fluorimetric, all proving very satisfactory for screening. Selection of a method depends on laboratory experience and availability of equipment but chromatographic methods have the advantage of detection of other disorders in addition to phenylketonuria.

1. *Guthrie microbiological inhibition assay* (Guthrie and Susi, 1963; Newman and Starr, 1971). Filter-paper discs of blood are placed on an agar plate seeded with a *Bacillus subtilis* strain (ATCC 6051) and containing the growth inhibitor thienylalanine. Phenylalanine counteracts this inhibition so that after overnight incubation at 37°C, growth zones around each sample disc are proportional to the blood phenylalanine concentration. Alternative inhibitors or mutant bacteria have been used to detect other disorders, albeit requiring a separate test for each amino acid (Guthrie 1967a; Guthrie 1967b).

2. *Chromatography.* On paper with liquid plasma (method described p. 371, Komrower *et al.*, 1979) or on thin-layer plates with plasma or eluates of filter paper blood (method described p. 375, Ireland and Read, 1972). These methods are simple and reliable for detection of hyperphenylalaninaemia as well as some other amino acid disorders in a single test. Furthermore, identification of the overall amino acid pattern aids interpretation dis-tinguishing specific hyperphenylalaninaemia from increases secondary to tyrosinaemia or generalised hyperaminoacidaemia.

   In the north west of England the paper chromatographic method has been used to screen 900 000 infants during the past 15 years. The following positive cases have been detected: 118 cases of phenylketonuria (incidence approximately 1:8000); 9 cases of homocystinuria (1:100 000); 73 cases of histidinaemia (1:12 000); 6 cases of tryptophanaemia (1:150 000); 5 cases of branched-chain aminoacidaemia (1:180 000); 30 cases of prolinaemia (1:30 000) (Sardharwalla and Fowler, unpublished observations).

3. *Spectrofluorimetric assay.* Using liquid plasma or dried blood on filter paper, the method referred to above (p. 382) for phenylalanine and tyrosine has been adapted for autoanalysis by Hill *et al.* (1965). See also Searle *et al.* (1967) and Holton and West (1970).

Screening is usually performed in the UK at 6 to 10 days of age (earlier in some other countries) and phenylalanine levels above 240 μmol/l should be followed-up by confirmation in fasting blood using quantitative analysis. This will allow distinction of those cases with hyperphenylalaninaemia secondary to hypertyrosinaemia.

Classification of Hyperphenylalaninaemia. This has been the subject of much study and debate. Essentially, when transient forms are excluded, blood levels of phenylalanine reflect the degree of residual activity of phenylalanine hydroxylase in the liver, reflecting different mutations. Trefz and coworkers (1985) classified patients based on phenylalanine levels after introduction of normal milk intake at 6 months of age, loading studies with deuterated phenylalanine and liver phenylalanine hydroxylase assay. They define three groups based on plasma phenylalanine levels after loading, and on phenylalanine hydroxylase activity in relation to control values as follows

1. *Classical phenylketonuria.* Post-load greater than 1200 μmol/l; no detectable activity.
2. *Mild phenylketonuria.* Post-load 600 to 1200 μmol/l; activity 1 to 3%.
3. *Hyperphenylalaninaemia.* Post-load below 600 μmol/l; activity more than 3%.

Monitoring of Treatment. Regardless of the classification of an individual with hyperphenylalaninaemia, it would seem prudent to treat empirically all patients with plasma phenylalanine concentrations above 600 μmol/l. However it is vital to determine the 'tolerance' of phenylalanine by titration of intake against plasma levels, monitored at weekly intervals in early age, less frequently later. One-dimensional thin-layer chromatography of plasma (1 μl) together with graded amounts of aqueous phenylalanine standard solutions added to control plasma followed by comparison of spot intensity provides a simple, reliable method for monitoring of phenylalanine levels during treatment (see Fig. 18.4). Such monitoring is essential for proper management and to ensure that over-restriction of phenylalanine does not occur but importantly it will identify patients with a transient abnormality. O'Flynn *et al.* (1980) emphasised the need to carry out a challenge with milk at 6 months of age. However, this should not be necessary since the tolerance of phenylalanine can also be used to distinguish classical phenylketonuria and hyperphenylalaninaemia (Guttler, 1980a). Other subjects with hyperphenylalaninaemia (below 600 μmol/l) should be monitored to distinguish transient from persistent forms. Both of these groups seem to develop normally without any dietary restriction.

The incidence of persistent hyperphenylalaninaemia requiring dietary treatment is about 1:10 000 on average in several countries. There is strong evidence that effective treatment (phenylalanine levels kept between approximately 120 to 300 μmol/l) introduced by 3 weeks of age will prevent the symptoms of the condition (Dobson *et al.*, 1977). However, there is increasing evidence that relaxation of dietary treatment, previously thought to be possible at 5 years of age, will cause significant decreases in IQ (Smith *et al.*, 1978; Koch *et al.*, 1982).

Genetic Aspects. The condition is transmitted in an autosomal recessive manner and distinction of heterozygotes has been possible, although with a small degree of ambiguity, e.g. using phenylalanine and tyrosine measurements in the fasting state with discriminant analysis (Gold *et al.*, 1974; Freehauf *et al.*, 1984), or after loading with phenylalanine (Guttler, 1980b).

Recent developments in the application of DNA technology have opened the way to reliable heterozygote detection and prenatal diagnosis. Woo *et al.* (1983) reported cloning of the phenylalanine hydroxylase gene and restriction fragment length polymorphism in the phenylalanine hydroxylase locus which was informative in 75% of families. This has been subsequently applied to prenatal diagnosis (Lidsky *et al.*, 1985). Furthermore, studies of gene transfer and expression of human phenylalanine hydroxylase in mouse cells underlines the potential for future gene replacement therapy (Ledley *et al.*, 1985).

Defects in Tetrahydrobiopterin Synthesis

Proper function of the phenylalanine hydroxylase system (as well as tyrosine and tryptophan hydroxylases) requires tetrahydrobiopterin. This co-factor is synthesised in humans by a series of enzyme reactions. Once formed it is maintained in its active tetrahydro form by the NADH-dependent dihydropteridine reductase (Kaufman, 1985). To date, three different enzyme deficiencies in the biopterin pathway have been described (Niederwieser *et al.*, 1985b): guanosine triphosphate cyclohydrase, the phosphate-eliminating component of the multi-enzyme dihydrobiopterin synthase system (Niederwieser *et al.*, 1985a), and dihydropteridine reductase. The net result of each is a deficiency of tetrahydro-biopterin causing a malfunction of the three aromatic amino acid hydroxylases.

Approximately 1 to 3 % of patients with hyperphenylalaninaemia are thought to have a biopterin synthesis defect. Therefore all cases of hyperphenyl-alaninaemia detected on screening should be tested for these variant forms by: (1) measurement of plasma biopterin which is deficient in each form, (2) analysis of biopterins in urine by high-performance liquid chromatography, (3) response of plasma phenylalanine to oral loading with tetrahydrobiopterin, when a marked fall is seen in these variants in contrast to unaltered levels in phenylalanine hydroxylase deficiency (Niederwieser *et al.*, 1985b).

Clinical features include severe neurological abnormalities, probably reflecting neurotransmitter deficiencies, which do not respond to dietary restriction of phenylalanine alone. Treatment is by administration of tetrahydrobiopterin or an analogue with or without neurotransmitters (Kaufman, 1985). Early results suggest a less satisfactory outcome compared with the common form of phenylketonuria, probably due to an insufficient correction of brain levels of biopterin and/or neurotransmitters.

Tyrosine Disorders

Conditions which exhibit hypertyrosinaemia have been classified in three main groups (see Goldsmith, 1983 for a review and details of normal and abnormal tyrosine metabolism).

Neonatal Transient Tyrosinaemia

This is the most common form (found in from 0·2 to a few per cent of different populations) often related to prematurity, immaturity or high protein intake. Plasma concentrations of tyrosine (up to 3300 μmol/l; normal less than 120 μmol/l) and phenylalanine and urinary excretion of phenolic acids, including p-hydroxyphenylpyruvic acid, p-hydroxyphenyllactic acid and p-hydroxyphenyl-acetic acid are all increased. This probably reflects immaturity of p-hydroxy-phenylpyruvate dioxygenase, a key enzyme in tyrosine catabolism which is low in fetal liver normally maturing around birth. The abnormality is usually corrected by one month of age (vitamin C supplementation may speed up correction but this is not proven) although exceptionally it may persist for up to six months. The condition is thought to be symptom-free but this has been questioned.

Hereditary Tyrosinaemia Type I—Tyrosinosis (Berger, 1985)

This form presents acutely in the neonatal period with severe liver and kidney disease. Symptoms include failure to thrive, vomiting, diarrhoea, hepatospleno-megaly and nephropathy with Fanconi syndrome. The platelet count can be high, the prothrombin time prolonged and plasma α-fetoprotein may be elevated. Death usually occurs in the first year of life. Thus it mimics other forms of liver disease, e.g. congenital infections, fructosaemia and galactosaemia in which accumulation of tyrosine and methionine may also occur. In the chronic form, symptoms may be milder with later onset, death occurring in the first or second decade with hepatoma reported in about 40% of these cases.

There are elevated plasma concentrations of tyrosine (300 to 600 μmol/l) and sometimes phenylalanine and/or methionine. Excretion of phenolic acids derived from tyrosine and, importantly, succinylacetone and succinylacetoacetate is increased. These latter two compounds reflect the probable basic defect, deficiency of fumarylacetoacetate hydrolase, demonstrated in liver and cultured fibroblasts. Metabolites which accumulate, e.g. succinylacetone or fumaryl-acetoacetate are thought to inhibit other enzymes explaining increased plasma concentration of methionine or urinary excretion of δ-aminolaevulinic acid as well as the generalised aminoaciduria which is found. Since the chemical and biochemical findings are both variable and non-specific, correct diagnosis of this form of tyrosinaemia must depend on enzyme assay and succinylacetone determination. Treatment with dietary restriction of tyrosine and phenylalanine or liver transplantation has been attempted without dramatically improving the outcome. The incidence of this condition is estimated to be less than 1:100 000 although many cases may not be diagnosed.

Tyrosinaemia Type II—(Richner–Hanhart Syndrome) (Buist *et al.*, 1985)

The very characteristic clinical features include eye lesions with keratitis or conjunctivitis, skin lesions with hyperkeratosis and, usually, mental retardation. Plasma concentrations of tyrosine are elevated (600 to 3300 μmol/l) with increased urinary excretion of phenolic acid derivatives of tyrosine due to deficiency of cytosolic tyrosine aminotransferase, demonstrated in the liver of some affected patients. Treatment by dietary restriction of tyrosine and phenylalanine has effectively corrected both the biochemical and clinical abnormalities. The condition is very rare but seems to be more prevalent in particular populations, e.g. in Italy.

Urea Cycle Disorders

The urea cycle plays a vital role by removing highly toxic ammonia produced by many catabolic processes. This cycle is a highly controlled sequence of six reactions closely inter-related with other pathways: (1) *N-acetylglutamate synthetase*—catalysed formation of *N*-acetylglutamate, an activator for (2) *carbamoylphosphate synthetase* which acts on ammonia, HCO_3^- and ATP to form carbamoyl phosphate, (3) *ornithine carbamoyl transferase* acts on ornithine and carbamoyl phosphate to form citrulline, (4) *argininosuccinate synthetase* condenses citrulline with aspartate, (5) argininosuccinate is hydrolysed to arginine and fumarate by a *lyase* and (6) arginine is hydrolysed by *arginase* to release urea and ornithine.

Deficiency of each of these enzymes is known. The major clinical signs are due to ammonia intoxication, i.e. lethargy, poor feeding, vomiting, hypotonia, convulsions, coma, then death, or can be less specific, e.g. neurological features or mental retardation. The degree of ammonia accumulation and threat to life are greatest with deficiency of early steps; least when the end of the cycle is involved. The ammonia levels approach 1000 μmol/l in carbamoyl phosphate synthetase deficiency with death in the first few days of life whereas in arginase deficiency ammonia may be normal or only slightly increased without life-threatening episodes.

In carbamoyl phosphate synthetase and ornithine carbamoyltransferase deficiencies there are no primary amino acid changes although plasma concentrations of alanine and glutamine may be high with low plasma levels of citrulline. Ornithine carbamoyltransferase deficiency is characterised by a marked increase of orotic acid excretion (detected by high voltage electrophoresis or high-performance liquid chromatography). Liver is required for enzyme assay. In contrast, deficiencies of the last three enzymes of the cycle are characterised by increased plasma and urine concentrations of citrulline, argininosuccinic acid and arginine respectively. In the last of these, urinary excretion of other basic amino acids and cystine may also be increased due to saturation of the group-specific renal tubular reabsorption site, a possible pitfall in its diagnosis.

It should be noted that ornithine carbamoyl transferase deficiency is inherited as an X-linked condition; hemizygous males are usually severely affected and carrier females may also exhibit less severe abnormalities (Walser, 1983).

Branched-chain Amino Acid Disorders

Maple Syrup Urine Disease. This is caused by deficiency of the three branched-chain oxo-acid decarboxylases resulting in accumulation in body fluids of leucine (usually predominating), isoleucine and valine and their oxo-acid analogues. The oxo-acids can be detected by the dinitrophenylhydrazine test on urine, thin-layer chromatography of the DNP-hydrazones or quantitative analysis can be done by gas chromatography after conversion to oximes. There are acute (life-threatening with severe acidosis in neonates if untreated), mild, intermittent and thiamine-responsive forms. Dietary restriction of branched-chain amino acids with frequent monitoring and symptomatic treatment during acute episodes of illness can improve the clinical outcome (Clow *et al.*, 1981).

Hypervalinaemia. This is due to defective transamination and has been described in a single patient.

Other Disorders. Other disorders of branched-chain amino acid metabolism are known in which the free amino acids themselves do not accumulate, e.g. isovaleric acidaemia, β-oxothiolase deficiency, β-methylcrotonylglycinuria and propionic acidaemia (Goodman and Markey, 1981).

Methionine Disorders

This essential amino acid is converted to cysteine by transsulphuration. First, methionine is converted to homocysteine via their *S*-adenosyl derivatives. Homocysteine can be remethylated to methionine or condensed with serine to form cystathionine. This thioether is hydrolysed to 2-oxobutyrate and cysteine which is catabolised eventually to inorganic sulphate. Deficiencies of many of the enzymes of this pathway are known (see Mudd and Levy, 1983).

Homocystinuria—Cystathionine β-Synthase Deficiency. This type of homocystinuria is one of the more common amino acid disorders. Characteristic symptoms include dislocated lenses, mental retardation, skeletal abnormalities and vascular disorders, the last often causing early death. Methionine and homocystine accumulate in body fluids with low levels of cystine. There are mild and severe forms probably reflecting the degree of residual cystathionine-β-synthase activity (Fowler, 1985). Some patients, often more mildly affected, respond to pyridoxine; others do not and require treatment by restriction of dietary methionine and/or betaine administration. Dietary treatment can prevent symptoms if introduced early in patients detected on newborn screening. Note that the pyridoxine-responsive form is probably missed on screening due to lower methionine levels in the neonatal period. Diagnosis can be made by detection of homocystine in urine (e.g. using high-voltage electrophoresis or one-dimensional paper chromatography with iodoplatinate staining) together with increased plasma concentration of methionine. Exceptionally, mild cases may require methionine-loading before abnormalities can be detected.

Homocystinuria—Other Forms. In less common forms, homocystinuria can be due to deficient remethylation of homocysteine to methionine caused by two defects. (1) *Methylenetetrahydrofolate reductase deficiency.* This enzyme is required to produce methyltetrahydrofolate, a substrate for the methyl-transferase. The clinical symptoms vary considerably, ranging from severe neurological abnormalities and death in the first year to mild psychiatric problems in adulthood. Some milder patients have responded to folate treatment. (2) *Deficiency of methyltetrahydrofolate:homocysteine methyltransferase* due to disorders resulting in low levels of methylcobalamin usually associated with methylmalonic acidaemia and responsive to hydroxocobalamin.

In contrast to cystathionine synthase deficiency, remethylation defects are associated with low or normal plasma methionine concentrations and sometimes a small degree of cystathioninuria.

Hypermethioninaemia. This is probably due to deficiency of *S-adenosyl-methionine synthase*, the first step in methionine metabolism, most cases being transient and detected on newborn screening. More rarely, persistent cases have been described which appear to have no consistent pattern of clinical symptoms. Plasma and urine levels of methionine are grossly elevated and α-oxomethylthiol-butyric acid can be detected in urine without increased excretion of homocystine.

Cystathioninuria. This is caused by deficiency of γ-*cystathionase* and is characterised by massive excretion of cystathionine, often responding to high doses of pyridoxine. There appear to be no clear clinical symptoms associated. Several non-genetic factors can result in excessive excretion of cystathionine, e.g. prematurity, vitamin B_6 deficiency and neural tumours.

Cystine Disorders

Cystinosis. This is characterised by widespread intra-lysosomal deposition of ·cystine crystals causing renal disease in the more severe forms. Plasma cystine concentrations are normal and excretion of cystine may be increased only as part of a generalised Fanconi type of aminoaciduria. Quantitative determination of cystine in white cells by column chromatography may aid diagnosis (Schneider and Schulman, 1983).

Cystinuria. This is a relatively common disorder of transport characterised by greatly increased excretion of cystine, lysine, arginine and ornithine which share common renal and intestinal transport sites. The low solubility of cystine results in calculi formation in the urinary tract. This has been treated by measures to keep the urinary cystine concentration below saturation, i.e. 1·25 mmol/l, either by high fluid intake to increase urine dilution, or by measures which increase the solubility of cystine, e.g. by maintaining a urine pH above 7·5 or by administration of penicillamine which combines with cysteine to form the more soluble penicillamine–cysteine mixed disulphide. Unfortunately, toxicity of penicillamine has been reported so that its use requires careful appraisal to detect any adverse reaction. Much genetic variation is known and three distinct types have been classified which can sometimes occur as genetic compounds. In *type I*, defective intestinal transport of cystine, lysine and arginine is found with normal excretion of dibasic amino acids in heterozygotes. In *type II*, intestinal transport of lysine is reduced but that of cystine is normal and there is cystine-basic aminoaciduria in heterozygotes although to a much lower degree than that seen in homozygotes. In *type III* there is active intestinal transport of cystine, lysine ‸ and arginine and cystine-basic aminoaciduria is present in heterozygotes but to a lesser degree than in type II heterozygotes (Scriver and Rosenberg, 1973e).

Tryptophan Disorders

This aromatic amino acid is metabolised by three main pathways in humans: the major degradative 'kynurenine' pathway, the 5-hydroxytryptamine (serotonin) pathway and the indole pathway.

There is considerable interest in this amino acid, due not only to inherited disorders, but also because of the implicated role of tryptophan or 5-hydroxytryptamine in many diseases. Further, excessive 5-hydroxyindole excretion has proved a useful marker for carcinoid tumours.

Hartnup Disease. This disorder of transport is characterised clinically by a 'pellagra-like' rash and variable neurological features. There is markedly increased excretion of neutral monoamino monocarboxylic acids namely, glutamine, asparagine, valine, isoleucine, leucine, phenylalanine, tyrosine, tryptophan, threonine, serine, alanine and histidine whereas that of dibasic and dicarboxylic amino acids, the imino acids and glycine is normal. This reflects defective intestinal and renal transport of this group of amino acids. Intestinal degradation of tryptophan leads to a characteristic excessive excretion of indolic compounds which are easily detected after chromatography using Ehrlich's stain.

Xanthurenic Aciduria. Excessive urinary excretion of several metabolites of the kynurenine pathway proximal to kynureninase has been found in patients thought to have a deficiency of this enzyme. Xanthurenic acid, hydroxy-kynurenine, kynurenine, kynurenic acid and some *N*-acetyl derivatives of these produce a dramatic characteristic pattern on chromatograms when viewed under ultraviolet light, in some patients only seen after tryptophan loading. In most cases, the abnormalities are corrected by treatment with pyridoxine (Komrower *et al.*, 1964).

Hypertryptophanaemia. Increased plasma concentration of tryptophan with increased urinary excretion of indoles and elevated whole blood levels of 5-hydroxytryptamine has been found in several adults and children who have no obvious clinical symptoms. Indirect evidence suggests a defect in the first or second step in the kynurenine pathway (Sardharwalla and Fowler, unpublished observations). Similar biochemical abnormalities have also been reported in two mentally subnormal patients (Snedden *et al.*, 1983).

Other Disorders

Many other amino acid disorders have been described (see Wellner and Meister, 1981, who include 122 different disorders in a survey). A few examples follow.

Histidinaemia. This is characterised by increased plasma concentrations of histidine, urinary excretion of imidazoles (detected after chromatography by

Pauly's reagent) and is caused by deficiency of histidine α-deaminase. Mental retardation and speech disorders were previously reported in many patients, but experience with patients detected on newborn screening who were untreated points to the condition being asymptomatic (Tada, 1982).

Hyperglycinaemia. Non-ketotic hyperglycinaemia is a primary disorder due to deficiency of the glycine-cleavage system. There are severe neurological features, often life-threatening in neonates, and glycine accumulates markedly in body fluids. However, hyperglycinaemia can also occur secondary to a number of organic acid disorders, e.g. propionic acidaemia. These two forms can be distinguished by the high level of glycine found in the cerebrospinal fluid only in the non-ketotic form.

Hyperprolinaemia. There are two forms both with increased excretion of hydroxyproline and glycine as well as proline, due to the shared renal transport system. *Type I* is due to deficiency of the first enzyme of proline degradation, proline oxidase, *type II*, the second step, pyrroline 5-carboxylic acid oxidase. The latter results in excretion of pyrroline-5 carboxylate which can be measured spectrophotometrically with *o*-aminobenzaldehyde to distinguish the two types.

Hyperornithinaemia. This is caused by deficiency of ornithine δ-aminotransferase and is associated with gyrate atrophy of the choroid and retina. Ornithine is elevated 5- to 20-fold in plasma. There is increased urinary excretion of cystine, lysine and arginine as well as ornithine due to the common renal transport system. Some patients respond to pyridoxine treatment.

Ornithine can also be increased in body fluids in the hyperornithinaemia—hyperammonaemia—hypercitrullinuria syndrome.

5-Hydroxyindoles

These substances are excreted in greatly increased quantities by patients with metastasising carcinoid tumours, often in association with the *carcinoid syndrome* which includes such features as diarrhoea, cardiac valvular damage and flushing attacks of various types. The syndrome is more marked when metastases are extensive. These tumours secrete 5-hydroxytryptamine (5HT) or, much less commonly, 5-hydroxytryptophan (5HTP). The most common metastasising tumours are of ileal origin and secrete 5HT but those of foregut origin, gastric and bronchial carcinoids, are rarer and usually secrete 5HTP. Some carcinoids also produce ACTH, MSH, insulin or histamine.

5HTP is formed from tryptophan by a hydroxylase. That derived from tumour tissue is specific and differs from phenylalanine hydroxylase which can also bring about the reaction. Both enzymes are inhibited by *p*-chlorophenylalanine, used to treat the carcinoid syndrome. 5HTP is converted to 5HT by a decarboxylase. Again, tumour decarboxylase is relatively specific for 5HTP and is inhibited by α-methyldopa, also used in treating these cases. Those tumours secreting 5HTP as such may have some conversion to 5HT in the rest of the body by a widespread decarboxylase, also active against dopa, phenylalanine, tyrosine, tryptophan and histidine. 5HT entering the circulation is normally converted by the widespread enzyme, monoamine oxidase, to 5-hydroxyindolyl acetic acid (5HIAA). This is the main excretory product in tumours secreting 5HT but in the rarer tumours producing 5HTP, the urine contains in addition, 5HTP excreted unchanged and 5HT, perhaps released by kidney decarboxylase. The diarrhoea and valvular lesions are caused by excessive quantities of 5HT but there is good evidence that the flushing attacks are caused by tumour release of other substances including histamine, prostaglandins and especially the enzyme kallikrein which releases bradykinin from a plasma precursor.

Simple colorimetric methods for the detection and determination of urinary total 5-hydroxyindoles (5HTP, 5HT + 5HIAA) or of 5HIAA and 5HT separately use their reaction with 1-nitroso-2-naphthol in the presence of nitrous acid to produce a purple colour.

Test for Increased Total 5-Hydroxyindole Excretion

After reacting with 1-nitroso-2-naphthol, excess yellow reagent is removed with ethyl acetate.

Reagents.
1. 1-Nitroso-2-naphthol, 1 g/l solution in ethanol.
2. Sodium nitrite solution, 25 g/l. Prepare freshly at frequent intervals.
3. Sulphuric acid, 1 mol/l.
4. Nitrous acid reagent. Immediately before use, mix 0·2 ml of the nitrite solution and 5 ml sulphuric acid.
5. Ethyl acetate.
6. Standard solution of 5HT. Dissolve 20·3 mg 5HT creatinine sulphate monohydrate in 10 ml hydrochloric acid, 100 mmol/l. Dilute 1 ml to 100 or 50 ml with water for use to give 5HT concentrations of 50 or 100 μmol/l.

Technique. To 1 ml fresh overnight specimen of urine add 1 ml water and 1 ml nitrosonaphthol solution. Mix and add 1 ml nitrous acid reagent. Stand for 10 min. Shake twice with 5 ml ethyl acetate, removing and discarding the ethyl acetate layers. Only a faint pinkish colour remains in the aqueous layer in normal urines. Urines from patients with metastasising carcinoid tumours show marked purple colours.

For an *approximate quantitative test* add 1 ml urine to 1 ml of each dilute standard and to 1 ml water and proceed as before. As a blank add 1 ml urine to 1 ml water and 1 ml sulphuric acid, mix, add the nitrosonaphthol and proceed as before. After 30 min read test and standards against the blank at 540 nm. The increment in the reading for 50 and 100 μmol/l is used to calculate the 5-hydroxyindole content of the urine. If a random rather than a 24 h specimen of urine is used, it is advisable to express the total 5-hydroxyindole excretion per unit of creatinine.

INTERPRETATION

This simple test has proved useful in screening suspected cases of carcinoid tumour. Normal urines contain less than 6·4 mmol/mol creatinine, whereas figures over ten times greater may be found in patients with metastasising carcinoid tumour. A normal result may occur with a localised tumour.

Determination of 5-Hydroxyindolyl-3-acetic Acid (Udenfriend *et al.*, 1955)

In this more specific method for 5HIAA, urine is first treated with dinitrophenyl-hydrazine to remove keto-acids which would interfere later. Any indolylacetic acid present is removed into chloroform. After saturating with sodium chloride, 5HIAA is extracted into ether and then returned to buffer pH 7·0 for colorimetry.

Reagents.
1. 2,4-Dinitrophenylhydrazine, 5 g/l in hydrochloric acid, 2 mol/l.
2. Chloroform.
3. Solid sodium chloride.

4. Ether, peroxide-free.
5. Phosphate buffer, 500 mmol/l, pH 7·0. Mix 61·1 ml of a solution of Na_2HPO_4, $2H_2O$ (89·07 g/l) and 38·9 ml of a solution of KH_2PO_4 (68·09 g/l).
6. Standard HIAA solution, 60 μmol/l. Dissolve 5·74 mg HIAA in 20 ml glacial acetic acid. Dilute 1 to 25 with water just before use.
7. Other reagents are reagents 1 to 5 for the total 5-hydroxyindole method.

Technique. In a 50 ml glass stoppered tube place 6 ml urine and 6 ml reagent (1). After 30 min add 25 ml chloroform, shake for a few minutes and centrifuge. Remove the chloroform layer and re-extract with 25 ml chloroform. After centrifuging, transfer 10 ml aqueous layer to a 50 ml glass stoppered centrifuge tube, add 4 g sodium chloride and 25 ml ether. Shake for 5 min. Transfer 20 ml ether extract to another 50 ml stoppered tube, add 3 ml buffer, shake for 5 min, centrifuge and remove the ether layer. Transfer 2 ml aqueous phase to a 15 ml glass stoppered centrifuge tube containing 1 ml nitrosonaphthol reagent, add 1 ml nitrous acid reagent, mix and keep at 37 °C for 5 min. Add 5 ml ethyl acetate, shake, allow the layers to separate and remove the ethyl acetate layer. Re-extract with 5 ml ethyl acetate. Transfer the final aqueous layer to a cuvette and read at 540 nm. Prepare a blank from 6 ml water and a standard using 6 ml dilute standard and carry both through the full procedure.

MacFarlane *et al.* (1956) omit the removal of keto-acids as they are only present infrequently.

Calculation.

$$\text{Urinary 5HIAA }(\mu\text{mol/l}) = \frac{\text{Reading of unknown}}{\text{Reading of standard}} \times 60.$$

Note. Collect 24 h urine specimens in a container bottle containing 25 ml glacial acetic acid, otherwise 5HIAA decomposes quickly on storage.

INTERPRETATION

Normal urines contain less than 50 μmol/24 h. In patients with metastasising carcinoid tumours the increase is often considerable, but occasionally only slight. The proportion of individual hydroxyindoles varies. In most cases. 5HIAA markedly predominates but occasionally considerable amounts of 5HTP and 5HT occur and are included in the greatly increased total 5-hydroxyindole excretion. For a review of the clinical chemistry of carcinoid tumours see Gowenlock and Platt (1963) and Grahame-Smith (1972).

Determination of 5-Hydroxytryptamine

5HT is separated by chromatography on Amberlite IRC50 and determined using the nitrosonaphthol reagent.

Reagents.
1. Amberlite IRC50 resin, prepared in bulk. Wash with water, stand and decant. Stir with 5 volumes of 6 mol/l hydrochloric acid for 30 min, remove excess acid and wash several times with water, decanting each time. Add 3 volumes of water followed by 2 volumes 10 mol/l sodium hydroxide added over 15 min with constant stirring. Wash again with water several times. Suspend the resin in an equal volume of water and add orthophosphoric acid (syrupy, 89%) until the pH reaches 6·5 and remains constant while stirring for 30 min continuously.
2. Sodium hydroxide solution, 1 mol/l.

3. Sulphuric acid, 500 mmol/l.
4. Other reagents as for total 5-hydroxyindoles.

Technique. Prepare a 5 × 1 cm column of the resin, drain and wash with 25 ml water. Adjust 10 ml urine to pH 6·5 with sodium hydroxide and run through the column at 2 to 3 ml/min. Wash with 50 ml water and then elute with reagent (3), discarding the first 5 ml and collecting the next 20 ml. To 2 ml eluate (≡ 1 ml urine) add 1 ml nitrosonaphthol reagent and complete the determination as for total 5-hydroxyindoles. For the standard, use the 50 μmol/l solution and carry 10 ml through the whole procedure. For a blank, treat 2 ml sulphuric acid in the same way as 2 ml eluate.

Calculation.

$$\text{Urinary 5HT } (\mu mol/l) = \frac{\text{Reading of unknown}}{\text{Reading of standard}} \times 50$$

Note. Normal urines contain 0·3 to 0·9 μmol/24 h. The method is intended for urines which show an increased excretion of 5-hydroxyindoles.

REFERENCES

Adams R. F. (1974). *J. Chromatogr*; **95**: 189.
Albanese A. A., Irby V. (1944). *J. Biol. Chem*; **153**: 583.
Archibald R. M. (1944). *J. Biol. Chem*; **156**: 121.
Bellon G., Malgras A., Randoux A., Borel J. P. (1983). *J. Chromatogr*; **278**: 167.
Berger R. (1985). In *Inherited Diseases of Amino Acid Metabolism*. (Bickel H., Wachtel U. eds) p. 192. Stuttgart, New York: Georg Thieme, Verlag.
Beutler H. (1985). In *Methods of Enzymatic Analysis*, 3rd ed., Vol. VIII. (Bergmeyer H. U., ed.) pp. 369–376. Weinheim, Fed. Rep. Germany: VCH Publishers.
Bidlingmeyer B. A., Cohen S. A., Tarvin T. L. (1984). *J. Chromatogr*; **336**: 93.
Brandt N. J., Christensen E. (1984). *Lancet*; **1**: 450.
Brodehl J., Gellissen K. (1968). *Pediatrics*; **42**: 395.
Buist N. R. M., Kennaway N. G., Fellman J. H. (1985). In *Inherited Diseases of Amino Acid Metabolism*. (Bickel H., Wachtel U., eds) p. 203, Stuttgart, New York: Georg Thieme, Verlag.
Ceriotti G., Spandrio L. (1957a). *Biochem. J*; **66**: 603.
Ceriotti G., Spandrio L. (1957b). *Biochem. J*; **66**: 607.
Chinard F. P. (1952). *J. Biol. Chem*; **199**: 91.
Clow C. L., Reade T. M., Scriver C. R. (1981). *Pediatrics*; **68**: 856.
Dancis J., Hutzler J., Levitz M. (1963). *Biochim. Biophys. Acta*; **78**: 85.
Dobson J. C., Williamson M. L., Azen C., Koch R. (1977). *Pediatrics*; **60**: 822.
Drescher M. J., Medina J. E., Drescher D. G. (1981). *Analyt. Biochem*; **116**: 280.
Dubin D. T. (1960). *J. Biol. Chem*; **235**: 783.
Duggan D. E., Udenfriend S. (1956). *J. Biol. Chem*; **223**: 313.
Faulkner W. R. (1965). In *Standard Methods of Clinical Chemistry*, Vol. 5. (Meites S. ed.) p. 199. New York, London: Academic Press.
Fernandez A. A., Henry R. J. (1965). *Analyt. Biochem*; **11**: 190.
Fowler B. (1985). *J. Inher. Metab. Dis*; **8**: Suppl. 1, 76.
Fowler B., Robins A. J. (1972). *J. Chromatogr*; **72**: 105.
Frame E. G., Russell J. A., Wilhelmi A. E. (1943). *J. Biol. Chem*; **149**: 255.
Freehauf C. L., Lezotte D., Goodman S. I., McCabe E. R. B. (1984). *Amer. J. Hum. Genet*; **36**: 1180.
Frisell W. R., Mackenzie C. G. (1958). In *Methods of Biochemical Analysis*, Vol. 6. (Glick D. ed.). London: Interscience Publishers Ltd.
Gade G. (1985). In *Methods of Enzymatic Analysis*, 3rd ed., Vol. VIII. (Bergmeyer H. U. ed.) pp. 425–431. Weinheim, Fed. Rep. Germany: VCH Publishers.

Gerritsen T., Vaughan J. G., Waisman H. A. (1963). *Arch. Biochem. Biophys*; **100**: 298.
Gold R. J. M., Maag U. R., Neal J. L., Scriver C. R. (1974). *Ann. Hum. Genet*; **37**: 315.
Goldsmith L. A. (1983). In *The Metabolic Basis of Inherited Disease*, 5th ed. (Stanbury J. B., *et al.* eds.) pp. 287–299. New York: McGraw-Hill Inc.
Goodman S. I., Markey S. P. (1981). *Laboratory and Research Methods in Biology and Medicine*, Vol. 6. Diagnosis of organic acidemias by gas-chromatography-mass spectrometry. New York: A. R. Liss Inc.
Goodwin J. F. (1968). *Clin. Chem*; **14**: 1080.
Goodwin J. F. (1970). In *Standard Methods of Clinical Chemistry*, Vol. 6. (MacDonald R. P. ed.) p 89. New York, London: Academic Press.
Gowenlock A. H., Platt D. S. (1963). *The Clinical Chemistry of the Monoamines.* (Varley H., Gowenlock A. H. eds) p. 140. Amsterdam: Elsevier.
Grahame-Smith D. G. (1972). *The Carcinoid Syndrome.* London: William Heinemann Medical Books.
Guthrie R. (1967a). *Screening of Inborn Errors of Metabolism in the Newborn Infant-A Multiple Test Programme.* Memorandum from the State University of New York at Buffalo.
Guthrie R. (1967b). *Proceedings of International Conference on Inborn Errors of Metabolism.* US Department of Health, Education and Welfare.
Guthrie R., Susi A. (1963). *Pediatrics*; **32**: 338.
Gutteridge J. M., Wright E. B. (1970). *Clin. Chim. Acta*; **27**: 289.
Guttler F. (1980). *Acta. Paediat. Scand*; Suppl. 280, (a) p. 29; (b) p. 56.
Hill J. B., Summer G. K., Pender M. W., Roszel N. O. (1965). *Clin. Chem*; **11**: 541.
Holton J. B., West P. M. (1970). *J. Clin. Path*; **23**: 440.
Hyanek J., Bremer H. J., Slavik M. (1969). *Clin. Chim. Acta*; **25**: 288.
Ireland J. T., Read R. A. (1972). *Ann. Clin. Biochem*; **9**: 129.
Kaufman S. (1985). *J. Inher. Metab. Dis*; **8**: Suppl. 1, 20.
Koch R., Azen C. G., Gross Friedman E., Williamson M. L. (1982). *J. Pediat*; **100**: 870.
Komrower G. M., Fowler B., Griffiths M. J., Lambert A. M. (1968). *Proc. Roy. Soc. Med*; **61**: 294.
Komrower G. M., Sardharwalla I. B., Fowler B., Bridge C. (1979). *Brit. Med. J*; **2**: 635.
Komrower G. M., Wilson V., Clamp J. R., Westall R. G. (1964). *Arch. Dis. Childh*; **39**: 250.
Kwok S. C. M. *et al.* (1985). *Biochemistry*; **24**: 556.
Ledley F. D. *et al.* (1985). *Science*; **228**: 77.
Lidsky A. S. *et al.* (1985). *Amer. J. Hum. Genet*; **37**: 619.
Lipson A. *et al.* (1984). *J. Pediat*; **104**: 216.
Lorentz K., Flatter B. (1974). *Clin. Chem*; **20**: 1553.
McCaman M. W., Robins E. (1962). *J. Lab. Clin. Med*; **59**: 885.
MacFarlane P. S. *et al.* (1956). *Scot. Med. J*; **1**: 48.
Matthews D. M. (1971). *Brit. Med. J*; **3**: 659.
Mecke D. (1985). In *Methods of Enzymatic Analysis*, 3rd ed., Vol. VIII. (Bergmeyer H. U. ed.) pp. 364–369. Weinheim, Fed. Rep. Germany: VCH
Meister A. (1965). *Biochemistry of the Amino Acids*, 2nd ed., Vols I and II. (a) pp. 1–199; (b) p. 1030. New York, London: Academic Press.
Mollering H. (1985). In *Methods of Enzymatic Analysis*, 3rd ed., Vol. VIII. (Bergmeyer H. U. ed.) pp. 350–357. Weinheim, Fed. Rep. Germany: VCH Publishers.
Mudd S. H., Levy H. L. (1983). In *The Metabolic Basis of Inherited Diseases*, 5th ed. (Stanbury J. B. *et al.* eds) pp. 522–559. New York: McGraw-Hill Inc.
Munro H. N. (1970). In *Mammalian Protein Metabolism*, Vol. IV. (Munro H. N., ed) pp. 299–387. New York, London: Academic Press.
Neidig B. A., Hess W. C. (1952). *Analyt. Chem*; **24**: 1627.
Newman R. L., Starr D. J. T. (1971). *J. Clin. Path*; **24**: 564.
Niederwieser A. *et al.* (1985a). *Eur. J. Pediat*; **144**: 13.
Niederwieser A., Ponzone A., Curtius H.-Ch. (1985b). *J. Inher. Metab. Dis*; **8**: Suppl. 1, 34.
O'Flynn M. E. *et al.* (1980). *Amer. J. Dis. Childh*; **134**: 769.
Parry T. E. (1957). *Clin. Chim. Acta*; **2**: 115.
Perry T. L., Hansen S. (1969). *Clin. Chim. Acta*; **25**: 53.

Potter J. L. (1974). *J. Paediat*; **84**: 250.

Rattenbury J. M., ed. (1981). *Amino Acid Analysis*. New York: Halstead Press.

Robson K. J. H. *et al.* (1984). *Biochemistry*; **23**: 5671.

Romette J. (1985). In *Methods of Enzymatic Analysis*; 3rd ed., Vol. VIII. (Bergmeyer H. U. ed.) pp. 393–399. Weinheim, Fed. Rep. Germany: VCH Publishers.

Romshe C. A. *et al.* (1981). *J. Pediat*; **98**: 788.

Rose W. C. (1938). *Physiol. Rev*; **18**: 109.

Rosenberg H., Ennor A. H., Morrison J. F. (1956). *Biochem J*; **63**: 153.

Russell J. A. (1944). *J. Biol. Chem*; **156**: 467.

Schneider J. A., Schulman J. D. (1983). In *The Metabolic Basis of Inherited Disease*, 5th ed. (Stanbury J. B., *et al.* eds) pp. 1844–1866. New York: McGraw-Hill Inc.

Schonberg A., Singer E. (1978). *Tetrahedron*; **34**: 1285.

Scriver C. R., Clow C. L. (1980). *New Engl. J. Med*; **303**: 1336 and 1394.

Scriver C. R., Davies E., Cullen A. M. (1964). *Lancet*; **2**: 230.

Scriver C. R., Rosenberg L. E. (1973). *Amino Acid Metabolism and its Disorders*; (a) pp. 1–94; (b) pp. 384–386; (c) pp. 178–186; (d) pp. 198–199; (e) pp. 155–177. Philadelphia: W. B. Saunders Co.

Searle B., Mijuskovic M. B., Widelock D., Davidow B. (1967). *Clin. Chem*; **13**: 621.

Shen R., Abell C. W. (1985). In *Methods of Enzymatic Analysis*; 3rd ed., Vol. VIII. (Bergmeyer H. U., ed) pp. 405–411. Weinheim, Fed. Rep. Germany: VCH Publishers.

Smith I. *et al.* (1978). *Brit. Med. J*; **2**: 723.

Smith I., Seakins J. W. T., eds. (1976). *Chromatographic and Electrophoretic Techniques*, 4th ed. (a) pp. 88–94; (b) pp. 145–146. London: William Heinemann Medical Books.

Snedden W., Mellor C. S., Martin J. R. (1983). *Clin. Chim. Acta*; **131**: 247.

Snyderman S. E. *et al.* (1963). *Pediatrics*; **31**: 786.

Sobel C., Henry R. H., Chiamori N., Segalove M. (1957). *Proc. Soc. Exp. Biol. Med*; **95**: 808.

Stanbury J. B. *et al.*, eds. (1983). *The Metabolic Basis of Inherited Disease*, 5th ed. New York: McGraw-Hill Inc.

Szekely M. (1980). *From DNA to Protein*, London: Macmillan Press Ltd.

Tada K. (1982). *J. Pediat*; **101**: 562.

Tanaka K., Hine D. G., West-Dull A., Lynn T. B. (1980a). *Clin. Chem*; **26**: 1839.

Tanaka K. *et al.* (1980b). *Clin. Chem*; **26**: 1847.

Thoene J. *et al.* (1978). *J. Pediat*; **92**: 108.

Thompson J. A., Markey S. P. (1975). *Analyt. Chem*; **47**: 1313.

Toennies G., Kolb J. J. (1951). *Analyt. Chem*; **23**: 823.

Trefz F. K. *et al.* (1985). In *Inherited Diseases of Amino Acid Metabolism*; (Bickel H., Wachtel U., eds) p. 86. Stuttgart, New York: Georg Thieme, Verlag.

Tudball N., Beaumont A. (1979). *Biochim. Biophys. Acta*; **588**: 285.

Turnell D. C., Cooper J. D. H. (1982). *Clin. Chem*; **28**: 527.

Udenfriend S. *Fluorescence Assay in Biology and Medicine*; Vol. 1 (1962), Vol. 11 (1969). New York, London: Academic Press.

Udenfriend S., Titus E., Weissbach H. (1955). *J. Biol. Chem*; **216**: 499.

Von Arx E., Neher R. (1963). *J. Chromatogr*; **12**: 329.

Wadman S. K., Fabery de Jonge H., De Bree P. K. (1969). *Clin. Chim, Acta*; **25**: 87.

Walser M. (1983). In *The Metabolic Basis of Inherited Disease*, 5th ed. (Stanbury J. B. *et al.*, eds) pp. 402–438. New York: McGraw-Hill Inc.

Wellner D., Meister A. (1981). *Ann. Rev. Biochem*; **50**: 911.

Wells M. G. (1969). *Clin. Chim. Acta*; **25**: 27.

Wong P. W. K., O'Flynn M. E., Inouye T. (1964). *Clin. Chem*; **10**: 1098.

Woo S. L. C., Gillam S. S., Woolf L. I. (1974). *Biochem J*; **139**: 741.

Woo S. L. C. *et al.* (1983). *Nature*; **306**: 5939.

Yu J. S., Walker-Smith J. A., Burnard E. D. (1971). *Arch. Dis. Childh*; **46**: 306.

19

PLASMA PROTEINS

The plasma proteins form an extraordinarily complex mixture of which our knowledge has increased considerably with the development of new techniques. Their very varied functions are summarised below.

1. *Nutrition.* The amino acids from the metabolism of protein enter the amino acid pool, part of which is used for the synthesis of new protein or other nitrogenous compounds while the remainder is deaminated to give substances which are either completely catabolised to carbon dioxide and water or used for the formation of glucose (gluconeogenesis). Both mechanisms provide part of the body's energy requirements.
2. *Control of body water distribution.* The colloid osmotic pressure (oncotic pressure) of the plasma proteins counteracts the hydrostatic blood pressure thus maintaining the required circulating blood volume. Albumin, because of its higher concentration and lower molecular weight than most of the other proteins, is the major contributor.
3. *Transport.* While albumin transports a wide range of substances, other proteins have a specific transport function, e.g. transferrin for iron. Important groups of substances transported by plasma proteins include hormones such as cortisol and thyroxine, lipids, fat-soluble vitamins, metals and drugs. In this way substances which are insoluble in water or would be excreted too rapidly are able to reach their target organs. Also some toxic substances are rendered harmless by binding to protein.
4. *Blood coagulation.* Many of the coagulation factors are proteins.
5. *Protection.* The immunoglobulins are antibodies which provide a defence against infection. The components of the complement system are also proteins.
6. *Buffers.* Proteins play a part in maintaining the plasma pH. They are negatively charged at body pH and therefore act as bases, accepting hydrogen ions.
7. *Enzymes.* The wide range of enzymes present in plasma are proteins.

Most plasma proteins are synthesised in the liver; immunoglobins are produced by the reticuloendothelial system, the lymph nodes and plasma cells; enzymes are released from various organs. Some proteins consist only of amino acids linked by peptide bonds, e.g. albumin, while others contain additional substances bound to the polypeptide portion. Thus proteoglycans contain carbohydrates, lipoproteins contain lipids, and metalloproteins contain iron, copper or zinc.

Proteoglycans are proteins containing a varying amount of carbohydrate such as hexosamines—galactosamine, glucosamine; hexoses—galactose, mannose; fucose and sialic acids, derivatives of *N*-acetyl neuraminic acid. The term glycoprotein is used when the carbohydrate content is less than 4% and mucoprotein when it is greater than this. Like the other proteins it is now more appropriate to measure individual proteoglycans rather than as a group, but details of the earlier techniques are available in the 5th edition of this book.

Lipoproteins are considered separately in Chapter 21.

FRACTIONATION OF PLASMA PROTEINS

The techniques used to separate the various groups of proteins from each other and to demonstrate the presence of particular proteins in them rely on certain properties of the proteins. These depend mainly on (1) the kind of electrically charged groups present in the protein molecule, which determines the type and strength of the net charge this carries, whether it is hydrophobic or hydrophilic, and (2) the weight and shape of the protein molecule. Groups which can become electrically charged include the terminal amino and carboxyl groups of the polypeptide sequences—all other such groups are linked in the peptide bonds. At the isoelectric point the terminal amino groups, being proton acceptors, are positively charged, NH_3^+, but lose a proton at higher pHs, while the carboxyl groups as proton donors are negatively charged, COO^-, but accept protons at a lower pH. Other groups which can be positively charged are the amino groups in the side-chains present in lysine and ornithine, the guanidino group in arginine, and the imidazole group of histidine, while groups which can be negatively charged include the carboxyl groups in the side-chains when glutamic and aspartic acids are present, in neuraminic acid in the proteoglycans and phosphoric acid in the lipoproteins. Another factor which can influence the total charge is the extent to which glutamic and aspartic acids are present as their amides, glutamine and asparagine. For each protein there is a pH, the isoelectric point (pI), at which the sums of the positive and negative charges are equal so that the net charge is zero. This is altered a little when small ions are present but the pI is mainly determined by the amino acids present in the molecule, the greater the proportion of groups which can become positively charged the higher the pI and vice versa. Examples of isoelectric points (Table 19.1) are: albumin 4·7, pre-albumin 4·7, α_1-acid glycoprotein 2·7, ceruloplasmin 4·4, transferrin 5·5, fibrinogen 5·5, immuno-globulins 5·8 to 7·3.

Because of the electric charge on the protein molecules these move in an electric field, towards the anode when the pH is above the pI, and to the cathode when it is below. The rate of movement is also influenced by the size and shape of the molecule. Molecular weights of proteins vary widely, but are usually above 5000; below this the substances are referred to as polypeptides. Molecular weights of the more common plasma proteins are given in Table 19.1.

Whether a protein is hydrophilic or hydrophobic depends largely on the number of polar groups in the surface of the molecule; fewer polar groups imply a more hydrophobic character. Therefore the more amino and carboxyl groups of the dibasic and diacidic acids and the hydroxyl groups of serine, threonine and tyrosine are present, the more hydrophilic the protein and the more soluble in water it will be.

Salt Fractionation

The separation of serum proteins into albumin and globulins by this means was one of the first to be made. Albumin is soluble in water whereas globulins are not but are soluble in weak salt solutions, going into solution at concentrations of

TABLE 19.1
Properties and Composition of Selected Plasma Proteins

Protein	Physical Properties					Composition					
	Mol. wt. $\times 10^{-3}$	$S^{\circ}_{20,w}$	EM^a	A^b	pI^c	Total peptide (%)	Tyrosine (%)	N (%)	BC^d	TCH^e (%)	Concentration in Adult Serum $(1^{-1})^h$
Prealbumin	55.0	3.9	7.6	3.2	4.7	99	5.51	14.9	96	0	0.1–0.4 g
Albumin	66.3	4.6	5.92	5.8	4.7	100	4.03	16.0	100	0	35–50 g
α_1-Acid glycoprotein	40.0	3.5	5.7	8.9	2.7	62	4.1	10.1	62	41.5	0.3–1.0 g
α_1-Antitrypsin	54.0	3.4	5.42	4.4	4.8	86	1.9	16.3	86	12.3	2.0–4.0 g
α_1-Fetoprotein	64.0	4.5	α_1	5.3						3.4	<10 µg
Transcortin	55.7		α_1			86					70 mg
Thyroxine-binding globulin	58.0	3.9	α_1	8.9	4.0	73	1.9		85	22.7	10–20 mg
α_1-Antichymotrypsin	68.0	6.4	α_1			91			90	9.1	0.3–0.6 g
Inter-α trypsin inhibitor	≈160	3.2	α_1-α_2	18	3.8	85	6.2	12.6		18.2	
Zn-α_2 glycoprotein	41.0	3.3	4.2	5.6	4.2	87	2.3	12.8	86	13.4	0.4–0.85 g
α_2-HS glycoprotein	49.0	4.1	4.2			85					0.17–0.3 g
α_2-Antithrombin	≈65		α_2								
Haptoglobin types											
1-1	100	4.4	4.5	12.0	4.1	81	5.55	11.2	81	19.3	1.0–2.2 g
1-2	≈200	4.3, 6.5			4.1						1.6–3.0 g
2-2	≈400	7.5									1.2–2.6 g
Ceruloplasmin	≈150	7.1	4.6	14.9	4.4	89	8.9	16.9	89	8.0	0.15–0.60 g
Cholinesterase	348	12	3.1		3.0	76					5–15 mg
α_2-Macroglobulin	725	19.6	4.2	8.1	5.4	92	4.84	16.7	92	8.4	1.5–4.2 g
Transferrin	76.5	5.3	3.1	11.2	5.5	95	4.6	15.4	95	5.87	1.4–3.6 g
Hemopexin	57	4.8	3.1	19.7		77	5.3		80	22.6	0.5–1.2 g
Plasminogen	87	4.2	3.7	17.0	5.6	91	3.74				0.1–0.4 g
Fibrinogen	341	7.9	2.1	15.5	5.5	97	4.95	16.7		2.5	2.0–4.5 g

TABLE 19.1 (*Continued*)

Protein	Physical Properties					Composition					
	Mol. wt. $\times 10^{-3}$	$S^{o}_{20,\,w}$	EM[a]	A[b]	pI[c]	Total peptide (%)	Tyrosine (%)	N (%)	BC[d]	TCH[e] (%)	Concentration in Adult Serum (l^{-1})[h]
Immunoglobulins:											
IgG	160	6·6	1·1	13·8	5·8–7·3	97	6·1	16·5	110	2·9	6–16 g
IgA	160[f]	7–15		13·4		92	5·0	17·4		7·5	1·0–4·5 g
IgM	950[g]	19, 26	2·1	13·3		88	4·9	16·7		11·8	0·5–2·0 g
IgD	170				13–15	89				11·3	< 150 mg
IgE	190	7·86				88				12·1	< 160 μg

a EM = electrophoretic mobility.
b A = absorbance at 280 nm at concentration of 10 g/l in 1 cm cell.
c pI = isoelectric point.
d BC = biuret colour at constant concentration in comparison to albumin (100).
e TCH = total carbohydrate content.
f mol. wt. for monomer, S for monomer and polymers.
g mol. wt. for pentamer, S for pentamer and greater polymers.
h author's reference data.
Data complied mainly from Putnam (1975), Schultze and Heremans (1966) and Table of Proteins of Human Plasma (Hoechst, Behringwerke).

electrolytes of about 0·1 mol/l. This phenomenon, called 'salting in', is due to electrostatic attraction between the salt ions and the charged groups of the protein molecule which decreases the attraction of the protein molecules for each other. As the salt concentration increases, however, the salt ions compete for the water molecules of the hydrated polar groups of the protein so that these become dehydrated and the protein less soluble—the phenomenon of 'salting out'.

The large but obsolete literature on this topic and its now out-moded application to clinical biochemical practical methods is discussed in the 5th edition of this book.

Electrophoresis

Tiselius first separated albumin from the other proteins, the globulins, which were themselves split into three fractions designated α, β and γ, in decreasing mobility. With a buffer of pH 8·6 the α-fraction separates into two parts, termed α_1 and α_2. Further division can be achieved by using buffers containing ions which interact with some proteins, e.g. splitting of the β band into β_1 and β_2 components by adding calcium ions or borate to the barbitone buffer.

At pH 8·6, all the proteins are negatively charged and tend to move towards the anode. At a higher pH there is increasing danger of denaturation of the proteins. Barbitone buffers of ionic strength between 50 and 140 mmol/l have been mostly used. At lower ionic strengths the buffering capacity is too low, at higher ones too much heat is developed so that the possibility of denaturation increases. Demarcation of the bands sharpens with increasing ionic strength.

The rate of movement is mainly dependent on the charge on the protein molecule, the greater the charge the more rapidly it moves, but it is also influenced by the mass and shape of the molecule, increase in mass exerting a retarding effect. Also opposing the movement of these proteins is the electroendosmotic flow from anode to cathode (see p. 73) as a result of which the slowest moving γ-fraction although negatively charged may remain at the origin or even move slightly toward the cathode.

A variety of support media has been used for protein separations, among which are cellulose acetate, agar gel, agarose, starch gel and acrylamide gel, the relative merits of which have been discussed in Chapter 4 (p. 70). The major difference is that in the last two the smaller pore size superimposes a molecular sieve effect. This enables molecules of the same charge but different size to be separated. Compared with starch, acrylamide has finer pore size and greater resolving power. In the form of disc electrophoresis (p. 78) it gives greater detail than other forms of electrophoresis, but may be rather difficult to interpret. Immunoelectrophoresis using specific antisera usually gives clearer information.

Staining of the strips is by acid dyes with sulphonic acid groups which react with basic groups in the protein molecule. Denaturation of the protein is necessary to ensure adequate staining. Appropriate stains for carbohydrate moieties, Schiff's reagent, and fat stains for lipoproteins can be used for the recognition of such fractions.

Isoelectric Focusing

The principles of isoelectric focusing are described in Chapter 4 (p. 81). This is an extremely powerful tool separating proteins by virtue of their pI value. Its main use is in analytical work but preparative isoelectric focusing can be achieved. Focusing over a narrow pI range allows separation of closely related proteins such as allotypes. The technique is used to identify the allotypes of α_1-antitrypsin with a pI range of 4 to 5.

Ultracentrifugation

In the ultracentrifuge, proteins in a buffered solution are centrifuged at speeds up to 60 000 rpm and forces up to 160 000 g. As centrifugation proceeds, a boundary of sedimenting protein moves outwards and can be observed by the Schlieren optical system as a peak due to a change in the refractive index. If several proteins are present, a series of peaks is observed as the movement proceeds, corresponding to the different sedimentation velocities of the components.

The sedimentation velocity depends on the gravitational field, and the ratio of the velocity to the field is the sedimentation constant. This has the dimension of time (second) but is usually more conveniently expressed in Svedberg units, S, of which one equals 10^{-13} seconds. The sedimentation constant depends on the molecular weight, density and surface properties of the protein and on the viscosity of the solvent, with molecular weight the main factor. The greater the molecular weight, the greater is the S value. The constant for a particular protein is corrected to standard conditions (water at 20°C), the effect of viscosity being eliminated by extrapolation to infinite dilution. The result is then given as $S_{20,w}$. Serum proteins fall into three main groups: 4–5 S, 6–8 S and 17–40 S, usually referred to as 4 S, 7 S, and 19 S (see Table 19.1). The fastest moving 19 S group contains α_2-macroglobulin and the IgM immunoglobulins, followed by the 7 S group comprising mostly immunoglobulins IgG and IgA, then the main peak with the 4 S proteins containing albumin and some globulins with molecular weights in the range 50 000 to 90 000. Small amounts of very large proteins and some with S values below 3·5 do not show in patterns given by normal sera.

In the above technique, the proteins have a higher density than the solvent. However, the ultracentrifuge has also been used to study the flotation of proteins with lower densities than the medium in which they are placed as in the classification of the lipoproteins (see Chapter 21, p. 454).

Gel Filtration

Different grades of Sephadex have been used to separate proteins according to the size of their molecules affording a technique which, unlike the ultracentrifuge, is readily applicable to use in the routine laboratory. In this case, since they are less able to enter the pores of the gel, the larger molecules pass through a Sephadex column more quickly and so are collected first to be followed in order of diminishing size by the other components. Equal volumes of eluate are collected and the absorbance is measured at 280 nm. Peaks corresponding to the various S groups are obtained; the amount in each peak can be calculated from the absorbances and the volumes of eluates, thus permitting quantitation of the various fractions.

DETERMINATION OF PLASMA PROTEINS

Determination of Total Protein

The most commonly used method for plasma or serum total protein employs the biuret reaction. Substances which contain two $-CO \cdot NH_2$ groups joined together directly or through a single carbon or nitrogen atom, and those which contain two or more peptide links, give a blue to purple coloured compound with alkaline copper solutions. The reaction takes its name from the fact that the simple substance, biuret ($NH_2 \cdot CO \cdot NH \cdot CO \cdot NH_2$), gives the same kind of colour with cupric ions. One copper atom complexes with four molecules of biuret, the linkages being to the central nitrogen atom. It is thus given by proteins, the shade of colour being different with different proteins. The amount of colour given by the biuret reaction also varies appreciably for different proteins. It is mainly differences in the amount of lipoproteins and to a lesser extent the proteins containing significant amounts of carbohydrate which are responsible for these variations. However, the method is reliable, reproducible and useful in the clinical field.

Other techniques used to determine total protein depend on light absorption in the ultraviolet and measurement of the refractive index. Details of the Kjeldahl–Nesslerisation method are given in earlier editions of this book.

Manual Biuret Method (Reinhold, 1953).

Reagents.
1. Stock biuret reagent. Dissolve 45 g sodium potassium tartrate in about 400 ml of 200 mmol/l sodium hydroxide and add 15 g copper sulphate (finely powdered $CuSO_4$, $5H_2O$), stirring continuously until solution is complete. Add 5 g potassium iodide and make to a litre with 200 mmol/l sodium hydroxide.
2. Working biuret reagent. Dilute 200 ml of stock reagent to 1 litre with 200 mmol/l sodium hydroxide containing 5 g potassium iodide/l.
3. Tartrate-iodide solution. Dissolve 9 g sodium potassium tartrate in 1 litre of 200 mmol/l sodium hydroxide containing 5 g potassium iodide/l.
4. Bovine or human albumin standard, 80 g/l.

Technique. Set up separate tubes as follows:

(a) *Test.* Add 0·1 ml serum to 5·0 ml working biuret solution.
(b) *Serum blank.* Add 0·1 ml serum to 5·0 ml tartrate-iodide solution.
(c) *Standard.* Add 0·1 ml standard to 5·0 ml working biuret solution.
(d) *Standard blank.* Add 0·1 ml standard to 5·0 ml tartrate-iodide solution.
(e) *Reagent blank.* Add 0·1 ml water to 5·0 ml working biuret solution.

Incubate all tubes at 37°C for 10 min. After cooling to room temperature measure the absorbances at 555 nm using the reagent blank to set the zero.

Calculation.
Serum total protein (g/l)
$$= \frac{\text{Reading of (a)} - \text{Reading of (b)}}{\text{Reading of (c)} - \text{Reading of (d)}} \times \text{Concentration of standard}$$

Notes.
1. The rate of colour development varies with time and temperature.

2. Only the peptide part of the protein molecule gives this reaction. The presence of lipid and carbohydrate components reduces the amount of colour given by proteins containing them. The biuret equivalent of several proteins compared with albumin, 100, is given by Schultze and Heremans (1966) as α_1-B glycoprotein, 89; G_c-globulin, 96; β_2-glycoprotein 1, 82. Further information appears in Table 19.1 (p. 403).

3. An average between-batch coefficient of variation for the method is 3·7% at normal levels of total protein.

Automated Methods

The biuret reaction is used in most automated techniques. As the details vary with the equipment, the reader is referred to those provided by individual instrument manufacturers.

Ultraviolet Absorption Techniques

Most proteins absorb light in the ultraviolet. In the region 260 to 280 nm, this arises from tyrosine and tryptophan in the molecule. As the proportion of tyrosine and tryptophan varies widely, there can be appreciable differences in the molar absorptivities of different proteins at this wavelength. Between 200 and 225 nm however, absorption is mainly due to the peptide links. As the absorbance is higher at these wavelengths, a higher dilution can be used to eliminate the effect of other substances which also absorb in this region. Most serum proteins have similar molar absorptivities at 210 nm. This method is useful for measuring protein fractions from chromatographic separations but is not recommended for measuring total protein in serum.

Refractive Index Techniques

The refractive index of water is increased by solutes proportionally to their mass concentration, at least in dilute solutions. As proteins form 85% of plasma solutes and the concentrations of others vary only moderately, it is possible to use the measurement of refractive index to show changes in the plasma protein concentration. Reiss used the refractometer in 1913 to determine total protein in a detailed study covering many disorders. Subsequently, several workers (e.g. Martinek, 1965; Lines and Raine, 1970) obtained good agreement with other methods. The latter authors determined the refractive index of urea, glucose, sodium chloride, albumin, lipid and γ-globulin over the range of concentration found in serum, obtaining a linear relationship in each case. Comparison of refractometric, biuret and Kjeldahl techniques using 102 normal and pathological sera showed refractometry to be as accurate and precise as the other two methods. The method is simple, requires only 50 μl of serum, and is useful for paediatric work.

Determination of Albumin Using Dye-binding

Many dyes bind to proteins and this is utilised in the staining procedures employed in electrophoresis described below. Such dyes have an affinity for most serum proteins. A more selective form of binding has been exploited for the determination of albumin.

At a pH lower than its pI, albumin is positively charged and has an affinity for anions. On combination several anionic dyes undergo changes in colour. However, if the dye is an indicator the anionic (I^-) and undissociated (HI) forms, which are of different colours, are normally in equilibrium,

$$HI \rightleftharpoons H^+ + I^-$$

and if I^- is bound, the equilibrium is disturbed. The colour change may then be even more marked. This effect of albumin on certain indicators, especially at a pH below 5, causes difficulty in measuring pH and is known as the 'protein error' of indicators. Most of the dye-binding methods rely on this affinity for the anionic form of indicators at a pH below 5, but with particular indicators some binding occurs at higher pHs, suggesting that binding affinities other than simple electrostatic ones are operative. Dye-binding techniques would be expected to be sensitive to the nature and pK of the indicator, the pH at which the reaction is carried out and the presence of other competing anions. Although the physical chemistry is complicated, the methods have been widely employed because of their practical simplicity.

Early methods using *methyl orange* at pH 3·5, its pK value, or 2-(4'-*hydroxyazobenzene)benzoic acid* (*HABA*) at pH 6·2 were unsuitable because of non-specificity and interferences.

Bromocresol green (*BCG*) is most commonly used. The pK value is 4·7 and like the related sulphonephthalein indicator, bromophenol blue, the colour change is from yellow to blue on adding alkali. The blue form is the divalent anion, the yellow has the phenol group undissociated.

Bromocresol green: R = CH$_3$
Bromophenol blue: R = H

The latter indicator forms a blue complex with albumin which is used to indicate its position during electrophoresis and the blue anion of BCG is similarly bound by albumin. At a pH near the pK value, BCG solutions show absorption peaks at 430 and 615 nm. The latter is due to the blue, divalent anion, the former to the yellow, monovalent anion; the relative amounts will depend on the pH. Binding of the blue anion to albumin alters the absorption peak to 627 nm and reduces the absorbance by about one-third.

Rodkey (1965) first used BCG (45 μmol/l) in a phosphate buffer at pH 7·0 to 7·1, when it is entirely present as the blue anion, and measured the reduction in absorbance at 615 nm resulting from the change in the absorption curve as binding occurred. Most other investigators use a pH less than the pK value of BCG. Only a minor part of the indicator is then in the blue form but binding upsets the equilibrium as outlined earlier. The net effect is to increase absorbance in the region of 630 nm in proportion to the amount of albumin present. The absorbance of other coloured substances present in the specimen is likely to be low at this wavelength. It is possible that inhibition of the binding of BCG anions to the albumin by other anions is also less at the lower pH. The method is prone to interference at low albumin concentrations when binding of BCG to other proteins such as transferrin and lipoproteins becomes important (Slater *et al.*, 1975; Webster, 1974). This results in over-estimation of albumin. Another important factor is the nature of the buffer anion as well as its concentration although increase in the latter displaces BCG from albumin (Spencer and Price, 1977). Succinate is the least likely of the usual buffer anions to compete for binding sites, thereby increasing the sensitivity of the method (Doumas *et al.*, 1971).

Bromocresol purple (BCP) was first used by Louderback *et al.* (1968) to measure serum albumin. Since then, manual (Carter, 1970) and automated (Pinnell and Northam, 1978) methods have been described. The reaction of BCP with albumin is immediate and appears to be specific. Several workers have found excellent agreement between the BCP method and immunochemical assays (Pinnell and Northam, 1978; Pascucci *et al.*, 1980; Hill and Wells, 1983). Perry and Doumas (1979) found a mean increase of 4·2 g/l in heparinised plasma samples when compared with serum, and Hill and Wells (1983) showed that this was due to turbidity appearing on addition of plasma to the BCP reagent as a result of the precipitation of fibrinogen. By increasing the ionic strength of the acetate buffer using sodium chloride (0·15 mol/l), the precipitation can be prevented. The reaction of BCP with bovine or equine albumin is much less than with human albumin by 26 to 41 % and therefore human albumin must be used for calibration and control material (Pinnell and Northam, 1978; Duggan and Duggan, 1982).

In many ways the choice between BCG and BCP is a matter of personal preference. The authors have again selected a BCG method for inclusion here. Bartholomew and Delaney (1966) found BCG to be the best of several sulphonephthaleins and used a 60 μmol/l solution in citrate buffer at pH 3·8, reading the absorbance at 637 nm. Their method was applicable to the AutoAnalyzer but Northam and Widdowson (1967) found that trouble arose from the deposition of BCG from the reagent on the wall of the tubing. This was subsequently removed by the first serum specimen resulting in a falsely high peak. Following a series of sera, the baseline fell below the initial level as BCG was re-taken up by the tubing until a new steady state was achieved. This effect was minimised by including Brij 35 in the buffered BCG reagent at a carefully selected concentration. Harding and Keyser (1968) also used Brij 35. By reading each test against the serum diluted with citrate buffer only, they found a good correlation with electrophoretic and immunoprecipitation methods. In a careful study of the effect of variations in the composition of buffered BCG reagents including Brij 35, Spencer and Price (1977) found the best sensitivity and linearity with citrate buffer occurred with 40 μmol/l of BCG in 25 mmol/l citrate buffer at pH 4·1 with a concentration of Brij 35 of 1 to 2 ml/l. They preferred to use succinate buffer because of the 70 % greater sensitivity and found the optimal conditions to be 80 μmol/l BCG in 50 mmol/l succinate buffer, pH 4·15 containing 2·5 ml/l of Brij 35. Careful checking of the reagent is necessary to maintain good performance, and details are given below.

The Determination of Serum Albumin using Bromocresol Green—Manual Method of Doumas *et al.* (1971), modified Spencer and Price (1977).

Reagents.
1. Stock succinate buffer, pH 4·10, 0·5 mol/l. Dissolve 10 g sodium hydroxide and 56 g succinic acid in 800 ml water. Adjust to pH 4·10 ± 0·05 at 20°C with 1 mol/l sodium hydroxide and make up to 1 l with water. Store at 4°C.

2. Stock BCG dye solution, 10 mmol/l. Dissolve 1·75 g BCG (Indicator grade) in 5 ml 1 mol/l sodium hydroxide and make up to 250 ml with water. When diluted 1/1000 with succinate buffer, pH 5·3, 0·2 mol/l, and read against water at 615 nm in a 1 cm cell this solution should have an absorbance of 0·315 ± 0·015.

3. Stock sodium azide. Dissolve 40 g sodium azide in 1 litre water.

4. Stock Brij 35, 250 g/l. Warm 25 g solid Brij 35 in water to dissolve and make up to 100 ml with water.

5. Working BCG dye solution, 80 μmol/l. To 2 l water in a 5 l volumetric flask add: (1) 500 ml stock succinate buffer, (2) 40 ml stock dye solution (volumetrically) removing all traces of the dye from the pipette walls by washing with water, (3) 12·5 ml stock sodium azide, (4) 12·5 ml stock Brij 35. Make up to volume with water, mix thoroughly and check that the reagent fulfils the following criteria: pH, 4·15 ± 0·05 at 20°C; absorbance, 1·347 ± 0·068 at 430 nm and 0·202 ± 0·023 at 615 nm in 1 cm cells.

6. Stock standard albumin solution, 100 g/l. Dissolve 10 g human serum albumin corrected for moisture content and 50 mg sodium azide in water and make up to 100 ml.

7. Working albumin standards, 20, 30, 40, 50 and 60 g/l prepared by diluting the stock standard with a 500 mg/l solution of sodium azide in water. Store the standard solutions at 4°C.

Technique. Add 20 μl serum to 4 ml working dye solution, mix, stand at 25°C for 10 min and read the absorbance at 632 nm against a blank of working dye solution. Prepare a serum blank for lipaemic or turbid sera by adding 20 μl serum to 4 ml buffer. If the standard curve is linear use 20 μl of the 40 g/l standard and 4 ml working dye solution for single point calibration.

Calculation.

$$\text{Serum albumin (g/l)} = \frac{\text{Reading of unknown}}{\text{Reading of standard}} \times 40$$

Notes.

1. The coloured solution from the 60 g/l albumin standard should give an absorbance of 0·811 ± 0·035 in a 1 cm cell.

2. An average between-batch coefficient of variation for the method at normal albumin levels is 4·5%.

Automated Methods

BCG is used much more frequently than BCP, usually with a succinate buffer. Although a single channel AutoAnalyzer method was given in the 5th edition of this book, this is now uncommon. Laboratories use either a continuous flow multi-channel system, a discrete analyser or a centrifugal analyser. The reader is therefore referred to the practical details provided by the manufacturers of specific equipment. The precision of automated methods is, in general, better than that of the manual technique.

Calibration of Albumin Methods

Commercial preparations of crystalline albumin contain aggregates which can introduce bias into albumin methods if they are used for calibration. Bovine albumin is often used for the calibration of BCG methods although Spencer and

Price (1977) showed that the BCG binding characteristics of human and bovine albumin differ. Human albumin must be used for BCP and immunochemical methods.

An IFCC Expert Panel prepared a human serum pool designated IFCC 74/1 (Hobbs *et al.*, 1979) and assigned an albumin value using a specially selected calibration material. IFCC 74/1 has been used as a reference preparation to calibrate working standards in laboratories throughout the world. More recently, Ward *et al.* (1984) prepared a serum pool (SPS–01) for use as a national working calibrant for specific protein assays in the UK. This seems to be satisfactory for BCG methods but is unsuitable for BCP methods due to altered dye-binding characteristics caused by the preservative, phenylmethylsulphonyl fluoride (Hill, 1985). The WHO has also produced a protein reference preparation calibrated in International units.

Electrophoresis of Serum Proteins

The general principles of this technique and the different media used are discussed in Chapter 4 (p. 68). Only cellulose acetate and agarose methods are described further here.

Cellulose Acetate Electrophoresis

Details of the application to serum proteins are as follows:

Buffers. A suitable buffer contains 1·84 g diethylbarbituric acid and 10·3 g of its sodium salt per litre, to which 5 ml of a solution of thymol in isopropanol (50 g/l) has been added. This has ionic strength 0·05 mol/l and pH 8·6.

Stains. A drop of bromophenol blue added to one of the specimens prior to electrophoresis provides a marker for the movement of albumin. Following separation, there are several stains suitable for revealing the separation such as Ponceau S, bromophenol blue, amidoschwarz and azocarmine, all at a concentration of 2 g/l for 10 min. Nigrosin is a much more sensitive stain for proteins.

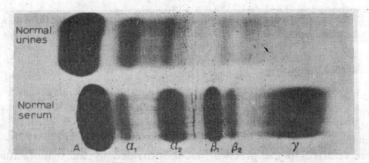

Fig. 19.1. Electrophoretic Separation of Serum and Urinary Proteins on Agarose. (Reproduced with permission from Schultze and Heremans, 1966; Fig. 328.)

Ponceau S, 2 g/l in trichloracetic acid (30 g/l in water) is allowed to act for 10 min after first soaking the strip by flotation. If the protein band is too intense, the dye may not bind properly resulting in imperfect staining. This may be overcome either by treating the strip with a few drops of methanol before restaining or by placing another strip in methanol for a short time before staining. Wash in acetic acid (50 ml/l in water) until the background is clear, changing the bath two or three times until the fluid stays colourless. This generally takes only a few minutes. Rinse in distilled water.

Nigrosin, 10 to 20 mg/l in acetic acid (20 ml/l in water) is more sensitive but requires a much longer staining time so that strips may be left in the stain overnight. Wash with water. With the 10 mg/l stain, a quick rinse in running tap water may be sufficient since the background stays white. After washing, blot between filter papers to remove excess moisture and allow to dry.

Equipment. A wide variety of equipment is available commercially. There are advantages in using a very small sample volume as in the microzone system. The essential elements are a fine wire applicator and cellulose polyacetate strips such as Sepraphore III. The pores are smaller than in other cellulose acetate strips giving better resolution with the very small sample volumes used (0·5 μl). Run using a barbiturate buffer at 120 V/cm (about 200 V). Stain with Ponceau S for 5 min and wash as described above.

Assessment of the separation. Visual inspection is usually sufficient, once the worker becomes familiar with the stain used, and is adequate for most clinical purposes. Abnormal bands such as are seen in myeloma and macroglobulinaemia are usually easily recognised while quantitative changes in the usual bands are readily assessed, particularly if several sera, including a known normal, are run together on a single strip by using a multi-applicator.

Densitometric scanning, if required, may use transmitted or reflected light. The strips can be made transparent by impregnating with oil, suitable ones being Whitmore Oil (Shell) and Ondina Oil 17 (Shell) which have the same refractive index as the strip. Float the strip on the surface of the oil until it becomes completely transparent before placing between glass plates for scanning. A variety of densitometers is available which can use either kind of optical path. The different proteins take up a different amount of dye per unit weight. Thus albumin stains more intensely than the globulins. With reflected light more accurate results are obtained with transparent strips, since otherwise the more intense bands are undervalued as only the surface layers reflect. Quantitation of the separated bands is only useful for paraproteins. Due to differences in dye uptake by different proteins, it is not recommended for determining protein fractions. Quantitation of individual proteins using immunochemical methods should be used.

Electrophoresis on Agar or Agarose Gel

Buffers. A barbitone buffer, pH 8·6, ionic strength 0·05 mol/l (1·84 g diethyl-barbituric acid and 10·3 g sodium diethylbarbiturate/l) is usually used. Barbitone-sodium acetate buffer (5 g sodium diethylbarbiturate, 34·2 ml 100 mmol/l hydrochloric acid and 3·25 g sodium acetate, CH_3COONa, $3H_2O$ per litre; ionic strength 0·05 mol/l) and barbiturate-calcium lactate buffer (12·76 g sodium diethylbarbiturate, 1·66 g diethylbarbituric acid and 0·384 g calcium lactate per litre) are less frequent alternatives.

Technique. For ordinary electrophoresis of proteins cut a 5 mm slot across the middle of the slide and insert 2 to 3 μl serum into this using a fine capillary Pasteur pipette. Invert the slide and lay across wicks of Whatman 3MM paper in the usual type of tank (p. 69). Using a constant current setting, apply the voltage, adjusting the current to 7 mA per slide if possible. Run for 60 min or until a bromophenol blue marker shows that the albumin band has moved 25 to 30 mm. Switch off the current, remove the slide and place in cold dilute acid ethanol (ethanol–water–acetic acid, 70/25/5 v/v) for 30 min. Then dehydrate by immersing in acetone–water, 90/10 v/v, for 4 h and finally dry at 37 °C.

Plastic-backed agarose films are available commercially making handling much simpler.

Stains. Two staining methods are particularly useful.

Amidoschwarz 10B. Dissolve 5 g in a litre of water containing 50 g mercuric chloride and 50 ml glacial acetic acid. Filter before use. Immerse the slide for 30 min, then wash by immersing three times in fresh portions of acetic acid (20 ml/l in water) for 5 min. Rinse for 10 min in water and dry at 37 °C.

Coomassie Brilliant Blue R250. Dissolve 5 g in 1 l of methanol–water–glacial acetic acid solution (9/9/2 v/v). Filter before use. Immerse the slide for 10 min, then wash in the same methanol–water–glacial acetic acid solution until the background is clear. Rinse in water and dry at 60 °C.

For scanning, the slide can be cleared by placing in xylene. Remove and mount in depex using a 64 × 22 mm cover glass.

This technique separates the β-globulins into β_1 and β_2 bands. The latter and the γ-globulins move towards the cathode since with agar electro-endosmotic flow is greater.

Immunoelectrophoresis

The principles of this technique appear in Chapter 5 (p. 96). The practical details are as follows:

Using a Pasteur pipette cut two sample wells 1 to 2 mm in diameter, half-way along an agar slide, 15 mm apart. Suck out the cores and fill each with a sample until the meniscus flattens. A 1 ml syringe with a fine needle is satisfactory. Invert the slide and run as above. Using two razor blades bound to a glass slide by adhesive tape, then cut a slot 1·5 mm wide and 65 mm long along the mid-line of the slide (Fig. 5.7, p. 99), stopping just short of each end. Alternative cutting devices are commercially available. Remove the agar strip using a 22 gauge needle and suction, and fill the resulting trough with 0·1 ml antiserum, tilting gently to ensure even spread along the trough. The antiserum will be rapidly taken up by the agar but no more should be applied. Place in a moist chamber on a level surface and leave undisturbed overnight.

Before staining, place a sheet of moist filter paper over the agar, followed by several layers of absorbent paper, and press with a heavy weight. Most of the soluble proteins pass into the paper and washing of the agar is unnecessary. The film of dry agar is very thin and adheres well to the slide so that any fluff from the paper adhering to the agar surface can easily be removed by a quick rinse in cold water.

Stain by placing the slide for 10 min in the amidoschwarz 10B solution above. Decolourise with two 10 min rinses in methanol–acetic acid (9/1 v/v). Alternatively, stain with Light (Lissamine) green (2 g/l in acetic acid 50 ml/l) for 10 min and decolourise with acetic acid (50 ml/l). The fine arcs of antigen–antibody precipitate stain well against a transparent background. The final slides are conveniently stored in a microscope slide box.

Electroimmunoassay

The principles of rocket electrophoresis appear in Chapter 5 (p. 104). The amount of protein present is measured by the peak height. For details of the equipment and methods see Weeke (1973) from which the following method for albumin is derived.

Reagents

1. Buffer A. Dissolve 4·19 g diethylbarbituric acid (barbitone) in about 200 ml of boiling water, add 26 g sodium barbitone, cool and make up to 1 litre.
2. Buffer B. Dissolve 112 g glycine and 90·4 g tris in 1 litre of water.
3. Working buffer, pH 8·8 ionic strength 0·08 mol/l. Mix equal volumes of A and B and dilute 1:1 with water. This buffer has a low ionic strength but high buffering capacity.
4. Agarose, 15 g/l. Add 15 g agarose to 1 l buffer and bring to the boil on a boiling water bath or on a heated magnetic stirrer to clarify the agarose. Dispense into suitable containers in portions of 20 to 25 ml.
5. Antiserum. Anti-human albumin.
6. Buffered agarose containing antiserum. Mix, at 56 °C, 15 ml buffer (3) 15 ml agarose (4) and 0·2 ml antiserum (5). This volume gives a 1.5 mm thick gel on a 200 × 100 mm plate. The amount of antiserum is variable depending on the source and the experimental conditions. It is determined by trial and error to obtain adequate sensitivity.
7. Human albumin standard, Hoechst purified dried human albumin. This standard is dissolved in water and calibrated by reading at 280 nm and using an absorptivity index of $0·58 \, l \, cm^{-1} \, g^{-1}$. The standard solution is then diluted to give solutions containing 10, 20, 30, 40 and 50 g/l.
8. Acid ethanol wash solution and dye solvent. Mix 450 ml ethanol (960 ml/l), 100 ml glacial acetic acid and 450 ml water.
9. Stain. To 1 l acid ethanol solution (8) add 5 g Coomassie Brilliant Blue R-250, mix well and leave to stand overnight. Filter and store in a sealed container.

Technique. Prepare a 1·5 mm gel by pouring the required amount of heated antibody-containing agarose on to a previously levelled plate of appropriate dimensions (see note 2, p. 416). Once the gel has set cut the number of holes appropriate for its size using a template and stainless steel punch to make 3 mm diameter wells set 5 mm between centres. These should be placed 10 mm from the cathodal edge of the plate and the outside wells should be located not less than 10 mm from the outside edge to avoid undue distortion. Dilute the standards and serum samples 1 to 300 with buffer. Locate the plate in a suitable electrophoresis tank, turn on the cooling water, connect up with 5 thicknesses of Whatman 3 MM paper wicks soaked in buffer and switch on the power supply to 70 to 100 V (corresponding to 2 V/cm gel). Apply samples with the power on to avoid forming diffusion rings round the wells. Pipette 5 μl of standards and samples into the wells, replace the cover and adjust the voltage to 280 to 300 V (8 to 10 V/cm gel) for 2 to 4 h. For particular equipment and conditions the meter voltage reading should be noted while measuring the actual voltage across the gel as this is the controlling factor in the separation. Alternatively the voltage can be left at 70 to 100 V for about 18 h. In either case continue the run until the sample with the highest concentration completes its migration. After switching off the current, remove the plate, cover successively with filter paper, folded blotting paper and either a sheet of plate glass or a book to give a pressure of about 10 g/cm². After 10 to 15 min remove the weight and blotting paper and carefully remove the filter paper from the pressed gel. Dry with warm air from a suitable dryer, place in a staining box with Coomassie Blue for 10 min then drain and destain. The destaining process using acid ethanol must be controlled by experience until a compromise of faint bluish tint of the background is balanced against any loss of dye from the rockets. Measure the distance from the top of the well to the tip of the rocket for standards and tests. Calculate the albumin concentration of the test samples from the calibration curve obtained.

Notes.

1. Most workers have used barbitone buffers of low ionic strength with agarose gels to enable electrophoresis to be carried out for periods up to 18 h without overheating. Such buffers have poor buffering capacity, allowing the pH to rise to more than 10 on the cathodic side of the plate. At this pH the precipitates redissolve. This is avoided in the method above by using the combined buffer with the higher buffering capacity.

2. To prepare 1·5 mm gels on different sized plates the following amounts of buffered agarose containing antisera (Reagent 6) are required:

    70×100 mm, 10 ml; 100×100 mm, 15 ml; 200×100 mm, 30 ml. The optimum number of wells for each size of plate is 10 to 12, 16 to 18, and 32 to 34, respectively.

Main Electrophoretic Components of the Plasma Proteins

The main components of the plasma proteins are listed in Table 19.1 (p. 403) and normal electrophoretic patterns using a barbitone buffer, pH 8·6 on cellulose acetate and barbiturate-calcium lactate buffer (p. 413) on agarose, are shown in Figs. 19.3 (p. 424) and 19.1.

The main components of the α_1 region are α_1-lipoproteins, α_1-antitrypsin and α_1-acid glycoprotein. Of these, α_1-antitrypsin contributes most to the intensity of the band since the last with its much greater carbohydrate content stains less strongly, and the α_1-lipoproteins are more heterogeneous and cover a wider range, extending into the region between the main α_1 band and albumin.

The main component of the α_2 band is α_2-macroglobulin, a 19 S protein forming up to 75 % of the α_2 globulins. Next are the haptoglobins which exist in three main types 1–1, 2–1 and 2–2 (see p. 423) of which the latter two are polymers of the first. Of these, 2–2 moves slowest and 1–1 fastest. In some diseases ceruloplasmin (p. 424) also makes a significant contribution. With the lactate-containing buffer two faint bands may be seen on the anodic side of the α_2 band, due to antichymotrypsin, an inhibitor of some proteases, inter-α-trypsin inhibitor, and small amounts of proteoglycans termed group specific components (G_c globulin).

A faint band which may be seen midway between the α_2 and β regions has been shown to be due to a cold-insoluble globulin.

The β band on cellulose acetate is mainly due to transferrin (see p. 425) and β_2-lipoproteins. With the above buffer the transferrin is responsible for most of the band as it stains more intensely than hemopexin, which has the same mobility but contains more carbohydrate (22·6 % compared with 5 % for transferrin). The β-lipoproteins are in the β_2 region in which there are also complement factors 3 and 4 giving a band sharp at the cathodic edge but less so at the anodic one.

If plasma is used fibrinogen forms an intense band between the β and γ regions. The greater part of the immunoglobulins are in the γ but contribute to some extent, though diminishingly towards the anode, to the background colour stretching as far as the α_2 region. CRP (p. 425) may be seen in the mid-γ region.

Gel Filtration of Serum Proteins

The serum proteins can be separated into the major fractions obtained by ultra-centrifugation using gel filtration on Sephadex 200. This may be in the form of a column or a thin layer.

Column Chromatography using Sephadex G200

Reagents.
1. Sephadex G200 (200 to 400 mesh), Pharmacia.
2. Eluting buffer, 100 mmol/l tris-hydrochloric acid, pH 8·0 in 200 mmol/l sodium chloride.
3. Sucrose solution, 200 g/l in water.
4. Blue dextran 2000, Pharmacia.

Technique. A column of Sephadex 45 cm long, internal diameter 1·75 cm and bed volume of 100 ml is used. A sintered glass disc at the bottom can support the gel but has the disadvantage that it adsorbs lipoproteins. A sheet of terylene, finer than 400 mesh, stretched over a plastic stopper (Fig. 19.2) fashioned out of perspex and sealed in with Araldite is suitable. Allow 6 g Sephadex to swell in eluting buffer for three days. Stopper the bottom of the columns and pour in 20 ml buffer. Fit a 25 cm extension tube to the top of the column and pour in the swollen gel slurry. When a layer of packed gel has formed, open the outlet and add more slurry. When the gel reaches 3 cm below the top of the column remove the extension tube and fit a constant head reservoir. Before doing so a thin layer of powdered Pyrex glass can be placed on the gel surface. This prevents its disturbance and allows a narrower band of material to be formed so that a more even passage down the column results. Wash the column with buffer overnight.

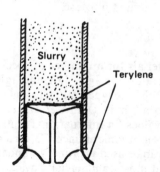

Fig. 19.2. Stopper for Sephadex G200 Column.

An estimate of the dead volume space can be obtained by applying the blue dextran. This has a larger molecular weight than the macroglobulins and appears several ml before them. This gives the time for which elution can be carried on before collection of specimens need begin. This can be included with the test specimen so that there is visible indication when to start collecting. Then layer 0·2 ml serum plus 0·2 ml sucrose solution on to the upper surface of the column. The sucrose increases the specific gravity so that the mixture can be layered more sharply. Elute by washing through with the buffer. Allow the dead volume to escape then collect 2 ml volumes. Read their absorbance at 280 nm and plot against the cumulative elution volume or sample number on the abscissa. Peaks corresponding to 19 S, 7 S and 4 S proteins are obtained. Normal sera show only a very slight rise for the first, a good peak for 7 S and a larger one for the 4 S (albumin). Haemoglobin, if present, appears very slightly after the albumin.

Standardise the technique for each column prepared. If a little chloroform is added to the eluting buffer, this enables the column to be used repeatedly for weeks provided it is kept moist.

Note. Sephadex separation can also be performed on thin layers. Its use has diminished but details are available in the 5th edition of this book.

Immunochemical Methods

With the availability of high quality specific antisera, many individual proteins can now be measured. Radial immunodiffusion plates are available from several companies but the technique suffers from imprecision in the reading of the precipitin rings. Diffusion takes up to 48 h which can be a disadvantage. Electroimmunoassay or rocket electrophoresis is faster with runs of 4 to 16 h. Both immunochemical methods are somewhat limited in the number of specimens which can be assayed in one day so that automated immunoprecipitation methods are more appropriate for large numbers of specimens. Methods using nephelometry or turbidimetry can be used on many of the currently available analysers such as centrifugal and discrete analysers (Chapter 8, p. 000). Dedicated protein analysers are also available. Such automated methods are faster, more precise and usually more economical in their use of antisera. The limit of sensitivity of immunoprecipitation methods is about 10 mg/l making them unsuitable for proteins such as α-fetoprotein and carcinoembryonic antigen which are present in lower concentrations. Radioimmunoassay is then usually needed to achieve the required level of sensitivity, although methods employing fluorescent labels are also coming into use.

Calibration Materials

Reference calibration materials for a number of specific proteins are available. There is an IFCC preparation for IgG, IgA and IgM which is calibrated in International units. SPS–01 has assigned values for IgG, IgA, IgM, C3, C4 and α_1-antitrypsin in addition to albumin (Ward *et al.*, 1984). The WHO reference preparation has assigned values (in International units) for IgG, IgA, IgM, IgD, IgE, α-fetoprotein, carcinoembryonic antigen, C3, ceruloplasmin, transferrin, and albumin. These materials can be used as primary standards to calibrate secondary standard preparations and most commercially available standards have values assigned in this way.

Choice of Techniques for the Study of Plasma Proteins

The biuret method is the method of choice for the determination of total protein but the situation with albumin is not as clear.

The dye binding methods lend themselves to automation and the most satisfactory dyes are BCG and BCP although they are not without problems. BCG provides a useful screening method giving reliable results in the normal range. The difficulty of standardisation has already been discussed as has the reaction of BCG with other protein fractions. Although Gustafsson (1976) has suggested that these react more slowly than albumin making the interactions less important if the reaction time is minimised, they can cause serious overestimation of albumin at low levels, particularly in the presence of increased amounts of α and β globulins. Immunochemical or BCP methods must be used for investigating specimens with low albumin levels.

The most specific determination of albumin is made by immunochemical techniques. Radial immunodiffusion plates are commercially available but the results are somewhat imprecise. Rocket electrophoresis requires additional apparatus and a means of preparing agarose plates if appreciably increased costs are to be avoided. Reading by rocket height improves precision compared with radial immunodiffusion. Automated immunoprecipitation techniques are simple to operate. Dedicated equipment is fairly costly as is the monospecific high affinity antiserum required but immunoturbidimetric and, sometimes, immunonephelometric methods can be adapted to general clinical laboratory instruments such as centrifugal analysers.

Apart from the determination of total protein and albumin just discussed, important clinical information can be gained from the specific quantitation of other proteins. In many cases, good quality specific antisera are available and immunochemical methods are then the technique of choice.

INTERPRETATION OF PLASMA PROTEIN RESULTS

Details of the various proteins present in plasma are given in Table 19.1 (p. 403). The total plasma protein concentration normally ranges from 60 to 80 g/l. Albumin ranges from 35 to 50 g/l and globulins from 20 to 35 g/l.

The measurement of total protein concentration is of limited value. It may be altered by changes in plasma volume, an increase is caused by dehydration and a decrease from overloading with water. Total protein concentration is higher when a person is standing than when recumbent, about 2 h being required in either position for the maximum change to take place. A short spell of vigorous exercise increases the total protein concentration by 5 to 10%, as does excessive stasis while taking the blood specimen. Some anticoagulants withdraw water from the red cells resulting in the plasma and serum protein concentrations being similar in spite of the fibrinogen in the former. Heparin in anticoagulant concentrations does not have this effect.

Otherwise, significant increases in total protein concentration in disease arise from an increase in total globulins, usually of the γ-globulins. A decrease in total protein concentration is usually the result of a fall in albumin, or sometimes γ-globulins. Changes are best discussed in terms of individual proteins or groups of similar proteins.

Albumin

The functions of albumin include regulation of the distribution of extracellular fluid by its effect on the plasma oncotic pressure, contribution to the amino acid pool, and transport of a wide range of naturally occurring substances and drugs. The former include bilirubin, fatty acids, urate, calcium and magnesium. Although some substances have a high affinity for specific plasma proteins, many also have a low affinity for albumin, e.g. thyroxine, T3, cortisol and iron. The drugs which bind to albumin include barbiturates, digoxin, histamine, PAS, radio-opaque contrast media, salicylate, sulphonamides and such antibiotics as chloramphenicol, penicillins, streptomycin, and tetracyclines.

Albumin is the main contributor to the plasma colloid osmotic pressure (the oncotic pressure), counteracting the effect of the capillary blood pressure which tends to force water into the tissue spaces. While no definite figure can be given owing to the operation of other factors, oedema is probable when the albumin concentration falls below 20 g/l.

An *increase* in albumin concentration is almost invariably a consequence of dehydration when it is part of a general increase in plasma protein concentration due to the reduced plasma water content. However, other factors causing the dehydration may counteract this increase. Thus chronic vomiting and diarrhoea may impair intestinal absorption of amino acids so reducing plasma albumin formation.

A *decrease* in plasma albumin concentration can be due to increased loss, reduced synthesis or increased catabolism. Excessive loss of albumin can occur (1) in the urine as in the nephrotic syndrome (p. 783); (2) into the intestine as in protein-losing enteropathy (p. 708); (3) from the skin in widespread burns; (4) in severe haemorrhage. Defective anabolism may be due to (1) reduced synthesis in liver disease (Chapter 28, p. 741); (2) impaired intake of proteins in malnutrition; (3) defective digestion or malabsorption (Chapter 27, p. 698). Increased catabolism of protein occurs in fevers and after injury. A small decrease in albumin is not easily recognised on electrophoresis as the intensity of the albumin band must be about 30% weaker for a change to be clearly seen.

The amount of albumin lost in the urine in the nephrotic syndrome can be considerable with 10 to 20 g/24 h not being unusual. Since synthesis of albumin cannot match the rate of loss, the plasma albumin level falls, particularly in older people.

Plasma albumin concentration is appreciably reduced shortly after severe haemorrhage. The plasma volume is restored more quickly than the plasma proteins, the concentration of which may take some time to return to normal. A similar effect is observed in the early stages of shock, whether post-operative, following extensive burns or after trauma. In all these conditions there is, in addition to any direct loss, the metabolic response to injury which includes a negative nitrogen balance due to increased protein catabolism, often causing an increase in the serum urea. The patient loses considerable amounts of nitrogen in the urine, commonly about 20 g/day and occasionally over 30 g. A similar increased catabolism of protein occurs in the febrile stages of acute infections, in untreated diabetes mellitus and in hyperthyroidism.

The impaired synthesis of albumin found in severe liver disease contributes to the development of oedema and, with portal venous hypertension, to the development of ascites. The ascitic fluid contains a high concentration of protein, particularly albumin, and if this is repeatedly aspirated there is significant loss of protein. Although the concentration of serum albumin is reduced in severe liver disease, that of the globulins is usually increased so that the total protein concentration is rarely low and is often high (p. 429).

A low plasma albumin concentration can be due to insufficient protein intake, e.g. in kwashiorkor, or due to impaired absorption as in carcinoma of the stomach or pancreas, peptic ulcer, enteritis and steatorrhoea. Loss of protein into the alimentary tract, protein-losing enteropathy, is a feature of several diseases of the stomach and intestine and may also be a primary condition.

The plasma albumin of hospital in-patients is often in the range 30 to 40 g/l, lower than in hospital out-patients and in the normal population. In chronic disease, one or more of the above causes of a low albumin may contribute and recumbency also lowers the level. In pregnancy, there is a fall of as much as 10 g/l, especially in the last trimester, due partly to increased requirements and partly to an increased plasma volume. There is a rapid return to normal levels after delivery.

Rare congenital disorders affecting albumin include:

Analbuminaemia, in which plasma albumin in homozygotes is almost completely absent because of impaired synthesis, though small amounts can be detected by sensitive immunological techniques. There is some increase in globulins but oedema is slight as are any other symptoms. Heterozygotes have normal values for plasma albumin.

Bisalbuminaemia, in which the albumin appears as two roughly similar peaks each about half as intense as the normal band. Immunologically they react similarly but structural analysis has shown that one band is normal albumin and the other is a genetic variant usually with a single amino acid changed. Depending on the nature of the change the abnormal albumin has a greater or lesser mobility than normal. Other amino acid alterations which do not alter the molecular charge would not be easily detected. The condition represents the heterozygous state of this genetic abnormality and usually has little clinical significance (but see p. 801). In another form, acrylamide and starch gel electrophoresis have shown an albumin dimer of lower mobility and much weaker than the normal band but identical immunologically (Bearn and Cleve, 1972a; Fraser *et al.,* 1959; Laurell and Nikkilin, 1966).

Prealbumin

This minor band can be seen running ahead of albumin when resolution is good and the background is unstained. Its major component is thyroxine-binding prealbumin (TBPA, mol. wt. 55 000) which is a minor transport protein for this hormone. It also binds retinol-binding protein (RBP, mol. wt. 21 000) present in a concentration of 20 to 80 mg/l. RBP, which transports vitamin A (retinol), forms a 1:1 complex with TBPA.

Prealbumin is synthesised in the liver and its production is decreased during synthesis of acute phase proteins (p. 425). There is a fall in plasma level one to two days after the onset of an acute inflammatory state or following injury, with later rise during clinical recovery. In progressive chronic inflammatory states the fall persists. Impaired liver synthesis with low levels of prealbumin occurs in hepatitis and in early cirrhosis. Low levels are also a feature of thyrotoxicosis, pregnancy or oestrogen administration, and in selective proteinuria. The concentration increases in acromegaly, in alcoholism and during corticosteroid therapy.

Zinc is required for RBP synthesis and both RBP and vitamin A concentrations are low in zinc deficiency. Urinary levels of RBP (and other small globulins) increase in tubular proteinuria. The half-lives of RBP (10 h) and prealbumin (2 days) are much shorter than for albumin and both these proteins provide a more sensitive indicator of malnutrition than does albumin.

Proteins in the Albumin-α_1 Interzone

These include high density lipoprotein (Chapter 21, p. 456), fast genetic variants of α_1-antitrypsin (see below) and α-fetoprotein.

α-**Fetoprotein.** This glycoprotein is present in fetal and maternal blood and in amniotic fluid, being formed chiefly in the fetal liver. Its concentration in infant serum diminishes steadily over two years reaching levels of less than 10 μg/l which remain throughout adult life, but may increase a little in old age.

Increased amounts are present in maternal plasma and amniotic fluid in pregnancies in which the fetus has a neural tube defect or a 45/XO chromosomal constitution and in the plasma of pregnant women with a multiple pregnancy, with diabetes or Rh immunisation (Chapter 33, p. 868). In the non-pregnant state increases above 10 μg/l are found in the serum of patients with a variety of tumours, especially primary hepatomas of which about 90% produce α-fetoprotein, and in teratoblastomas (about 80%). Increases also occur in ulcerative colitis and Crohn's disease and in such liver diseases as viral hepatitis, alcoholic cirrhosis and chronic active hepatitis but not in extrahepatic obstruction. Its mol. wt. is low enough for it to be excreted in the urine.

Proteins in the α_1 Zone

In addition to the specific proteins considered below, this zone includes several other glycoproteins, α_1-microglobulin, transcobalamin I (binding vitamin B_{12}) and α-antichymotrypsin.

α_1-**Antitrypsin.** This protein (2·0 to 4·0 g/l) forms about 75% of the α_1-globulins and is responsible for most of the observable changes in the intensity of this electrophoretic band. It is the major natural inhibitor of plasma proteases including plasmin, elastase, collagenase, renin, thrombin and kallikrein. This mucoprotein is an acute phase protein, plasma levels increasing two to three-fold within days after trauma, acute infection or inflammation. It is persistently elevated in many malignant and chronic conditions and in pregnancy or after oestrogen administration.

Most clinical interest is related to the lowered plasma levels of α_1-antitrypsin associated with genetic variations. Severe deficiency (less than 0·6 g/l) is associated with progressive lower lobe panlobular emphysema and, occasionally, micronodular cirrhosis in adults. Children can present with neonatal cholestasis or progressive juvenile cirrhosis. The genetic system describing the polymorphism is the Pi (protease inhibitor) system and 31 alleles or sub-alleles are officially recognised. The commonest allele in all populations is designated PiM, and an alphabetic nomenclature for the other alleles is based on their isoelectric points relative to PiM. The full Pi system is of interest in anthropogenetics but only the deficiency ones are of clinical interest. These are S, Z and null(⁻), with 3 others under consideration (Mlike, Mduarte, Mmalton). Pi null (Pi⁻) is the complete deficiency allele. Homozygotes for any of these alleles or heterozygotes for two will have severe deficiency of α_1-antitrypsin. Combination of one of the deficiency alleles with any other allele results in intermediate plasma α_1-antitrypsin levels.

The different alleles can be identified by acid starch gel electrophoresis or isoelectric focusing. Complete identification requires agarose gel electrophoresis and immunochemical quantitation. Family studies should be performed whenever a homozygote or heterozygote with α_1-antitrypsin deficiency is identified.

Low levels are also seen in premature infants with the respiratory distress syndrome.

α_1-**Acid Glycoprotein.** The exact function of this protein (0·3 to 1·0 g/l), formerly called orosomucoid, is uncertain but it is an acute phase protein and also rises in late pregnancy. Reduced plasma levels are found in hepatitis and cirrhosis due to reduced hepatic synthesis and in the nephrotic syndrome due to protein loss. α_1-Acid glycoprotein is usually high in patients with cancer, particularly of the lung, but its general usefulness as a tumour marker has not yet been established.

Proteins in the α_1-α_2 Interzone

This poorly staining zone contains glycoproteins, including a pregnancy-associated one, enzyme inhibitors such as inter-α trypsin inhibitor (Table 19.1, p. 403) and antithrombin III, and transport proteins, namely transcortin (70 mg/l) or corticosteroid-binding globulin (Chapter 31, p. 812), and thyroxine-binding globulin (10 to 20 mg/l) important in transport of thyroid hormones (Chapter 30, p. 790). The faster genetic variants of haptoglobin may extend into this region.

Proteins in the α_2 Zone

The main components are α_2-macroglobulin and haptoglobin with smaller amounts of ceruloplasmin (see below), various glycoproteins including Zn-α_2 glycoprotein and α_2-HS glycoprotein (Table 19.1, p. 403), and α_2-antiplasmin. The group specific component Gc globulin (0·2 to 0·6 g/l) occurs in genetic variant forms, acts as a transport protein for vitamin D_3, and shows acute phase properties.

α_2-**Macroglobulin.** Present in concentration 1·5 to 4·2 g/l, this protein is a polymer containing five 7 S sub-units. Although its function is uncertain it binds proteases including trypsin, chymotrypsin, plasmin, thrombin and, possibly, insulin. Its concentration varies with age falling from a maximum between 1 and 3 years over the next 20 years. It behaves as an acute phase protein but increases are also seen in pregnancy and oestrogen therapy, cirrhosis, malignancy, diabetes and, most markedly, in the nephrotic syndrome in which it is responsible for the much increased α_2 band (Fig. 19.3). Low levels have been reported in myeloma, peptic ulcer, disseminated intravascular coagulation, pre-eclampsia and shortly before death.

Haptoglobin. The amount present (1·0 to 3·0 g/l) comprises about 25 % of the α_2-globulin band.

Genetic polymorphism results in three phenotypes of haptoglobin: Hp 1–1, Hp 2–1 and Hp 2–2, with Hp 2–1 and Hp 1–1 occurring in 35 and 15 % of Caucasians respectively. Each haptoglobin molecule consists of two types of polypeptide chain, α and β. The β chain is invariant with a mol. wt. of 65 000 and has two binding sites for the α chains. These occur as three variants, α^{1F}, α^{1S} and α^2. The α^2 chain appears to be formed by combination of an α^{1F} with an α^{1S} chain with loss of some amino acids. The α^1 chains, mol. wt. about 9000, have a single binding site for attachment to a β chain. The Hp 1–1 phenotype comprises three subgroups each with a monomeric haptoglobin: α^{1F}–β–α^{1F}, α^{1F}–β–α^{1S} and α^{1S}–β–α^{1S}. The α^2 chain, mol. wt. about 18 000, has two binding sites permitting binding of two β chains. Polymeric products exist with molecules containing α^2 chains. In Hp 2–2 only α^2 and β chains exist in a series of molecules of general form $(\alpha^2\beta)_n$. In Hp 2–1, β chains are found with α^2 and either α^{1F} or α^{1S} chains. Haptoglobins containing the α^2 chain are unique to man and may confer the advantage of ensuring that the complex with haemoglobin is unlikely to pass the glomerulus even if this is abnormally permeable.

Haptoglobins of all three phenotypes bind haemoglobin similarly if this enters the plasma. The complex is rapidly removed by the reticuloendothelial cells. Its configuration is such that the haem residues are more readily exposed to the

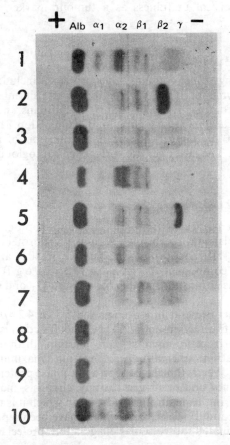

Fig. 19.3. Electrophoretic Separation of Serum Proteins on Cellulose Acetate.
Five patterns are normal but 2, 4, 5, 7, 10 show abnormalities:
4: reduced albumin and γ-globulins with raised α_2-globulin in the nephrotic syndrome,
2 and 5: paraproteinaemia in multiple myeloma,
7 and 10: polyclonal increases in γ-globulins, with increased α_2-globulin in 10, in rheumatoid arthritis.

enzyme α-methenyl oxygenase than in haemoglobin, thus facilitating the breakdown to biliverdin. The rate of removal of circulating complex greatly exceeds the rate of hepatic synthesis of new haptoglobin.

Earlier colorimetric methods for the determination of haptoglobin have been replaced by immunochemical methods which are now the techniques of choice.

Haptoglobin behaves as an acute phase protein and high levels are also seen in steroid therapy, pregnancy and biliary obstruction. Low levels occur in haemolytic states, congenital or acquired, and in some cases of vitamin B_{12} and folate deficiency.

Ceruloplasmin. This copper-binding protein (0·15 to 0·60 g/l) is present in low concentration in the neonate, slowly increasing to adult levels by about the age of 12. It is increased in pregnancy and is an acute phase protein. The chief clinical interest is in differentiating Wilson's disease, in which its concentration is low, from chronic active liver disease in which it is somewhat increased.

Proteins in the α_2-β Zone

This region contains small quantities of glycoproteins, fibronectin, and cholinesterase (p. 504). Any free haemoglobin in the sample appears here.

Proteins in the β Zone

In addition to the major compounds discussed below, this region contains several glycoproteins, including one pregnancy-associated protein, β_2-microglobulin, transport proteins such as LDL (Chapter 21, p. 456), sex hormone binding globulin and transcobalamin II as well as plasminogen (Table 19.1, p. 403).

Transferrin. Present as a well-defined band at the anodal end of the zone, this protein of hepatic origin (1·4 to 3·6 g/l) transports iron (Chapter 25, p. 627). A large number of genetic variants exists. Increased serum levels are seen particularly in iron deficiency anaemia and in pregnancy. Low transferrin levels occur in conjunction with an increase in acute phase proteins, in chronic infections and in malnutrition. Impaired liver function as in cirrhosis and selective protein loss also cause low levels.

Hemopexin. This protein (0·5 to 1·2 g/l) binds haem but not haemoglobin. Increased levels have been reported in haematological malignancies, diabetes and in pregnancy, while low levels occur in haemolytic states and when liver synthesis is impaired.

Fibrinogen. Although synthesised in the liver, the plasma level of this important coagulation protein only falls below the usual range (2·0 to 4·5 g/l) when liver damage is severe as in acute liver necrosis or advanced chronic liver disease. Congenital deficiency of fibrinogen has been described (Ratnoff, 1972). In typhoid fever, unlike other acute infections, plasma fibrinogen is low.

Another cause of reduced fibrinogen concentration is increased catabolism. This may be due to increased conversion to fibrin as in the disseminated intravascular coagulation syndrome. Alternatively, destruction of fibrinogen or fibrin by plasmin occurs with the formation of fibrin(ogen) degradation products (FDP) in a variety of disorders. FDP show marked anticoagulant activity leading to bleeding complications. For such reasons an abrupt fall in fibrinogen to below 1·0 g/l sometimes occurs in antepartum haemorrhage, or eclampsia and a slow fall may follow fetal death *in utero* and reach similarly dangerously low levels in five to six weeks. Usually, there is a quick return to normal after delivery. A rapid test to show the presence of a low plasma fibrinogen may be valuable. Alternatively, FDP may be measured in serum.

Fibrinogen is another acute phase protein so that increased concentrations are found in most acute inflammatory states particularly in pneumonia, in active rheumatic disease and in tuberculosis. Fibrinogen is the plasma component with the greatest effect on the red cell sedimentation rate. This is much increased in conditions with raised plasma fibrinogen, hence its use in rheumatic disease in assessing the severity and course of the condition. Increase in fibrinogen has been observed in the nephrotic syndrome and there is often a slight increase in pregnancy.

Acute Phase Proteins

Several members of this group of proteins have already been mentioned but an important member of the group has γ-mobility and is called C-reactive protein.

C-Reactive Protein (CRP). This protein (less than 10 mg/l) was so named because of its ability to bind the C-polysaccharide of the cell wall of *Streptococcus pneumoniae*. CRP is the most responsive of the acute phase proteins, with increased levels usually appearing 6 to 10 h after injury or infection. Increases in CRP can be much greater than the other proteins, levels over 100 mg/l frequently being found. Thus CRP is a sensitive marker of inflammation and is a useful indicator of the extent of activity in such disorders as rheumatoid arthritis and systemic lupus erythematosus. It is also useful in differentiating bacterial from viral infections being raised only in the former. Unlike many other proteins, the CRP response occurs in the neonate.

General features of acute phase proteins. The physiological response stimulated by trauma, surgery, infection and other inflammatory states is complex but results in a fairly consistent pattern of changes in the plasma proteins. The acute phase proteins are all rich in carbohydrate (proteoglycans) and are nearly all synthesised in the parenchymal cells of the liver. They include the protease inhibitors to phagocytic enzymes and are all increased to a greater or lesser degree when phagocytes are activated. The plasma concentration of a protein is dependent on synthesis, degradation and loss, therefore the change in individual proteins will be different. Protein synthesis is switched to the protective proteins at the expense of transport proteins therefore there is a concomitant fall in prealbumin, albumin and transferrin. The typical plasma protein response to trauma is shown in Fig. 19.4. The changes in the acute phase proteins being a general response to inflammation therefore do not aid in the differential diagnosis. However, measurement of those which show a large and early rise, e.g. CRP, is useful in monitoring high risk groups and the response to treatment. For a review of the acute phase proteins see Laurell (1985).

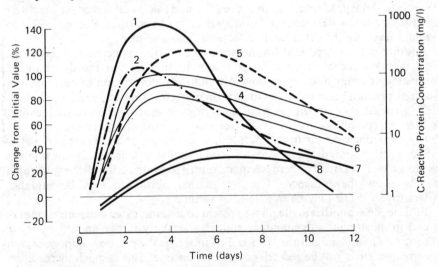

Fig. 19.4. Time Course of the Acute Phase Plasma Protein Response to Trauma. 1. C-Reactive protein (CRP) on logarithmic ordinate. 2. Antichymotrypsin. 3. α_1-Acid glycoprotein (orosomucoid). 4. Fibrinogen, 5. Haptoglobin. 6. α_1-Antitrypsin. 7. Ceruloplasmin. 8. Third complement factor. (Adapted from Laurell (1985), with permission.)

The Complement System

At least 20 components make up the complement system and interact with antigen–antibody complexes and with each other in a complex cascade to destroy bacteria and viruses. The components of complement are normally functionally inactive until activated by antigen–antibody complexes (IgG or IgM) or by C-reactive protein. Complement activation follows two distinct sequences, the 'classical' and the 'alternative' pathways, each having its own activators and inhibitors. For details of the pathways and the pathophysiology of complement the reader should refer to a text book of immunology.

The Immunoglobulins

These are proteins which function as antibodies or are chemically related to antibodies. On electrophoresis although they mainly have mid γ mobility, small amounts are also found in the extreme slow γ region and on the other hand, stretching across the β to the α_2 zone.

Structure. Monomeric immunoglobulin (Ig) molecules are composed of two identical short polypeptide chains of mol. wt. about 23 000 and two identical longer chains of mol. wt. about 55 000, the chains being linked by disulphide bonds as shown in Fig. 19.5. Because of their relative behaviour in the ultracentrifuge the shorter chains are termed light chains, and the longer, heavy chains. The C terminal half of the light chains of different Ig molecules occurs in two distinct types recognisable by their antigenic properties and designated

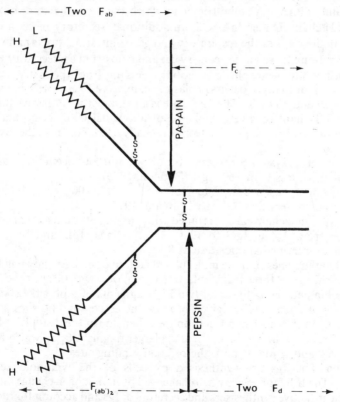

Fig. 19.5. Schematic Diagram Showing Part of the Structure of IgG.
  The N-terminal ends of the chains are to the left. L = light chain (κ or λ), H = heavy chain (γ in this case), S–S = disulphide link. The highly variable antibody-combining sites are the parts of the chain as shown ∿∿∿ . Papain cleaves the molecule to the left of the disulphide bond linking the heavy chains while pepsin acts on the area to the right of this bond.

kappa, κ, and lambda, λ. In the usual mixture of Igs about 70% of the light chains are type κ and only 30% λ. The N terminal half of the chain is highly variable and its composition is unique to each individual antibody. Similarly the heavy chains contain a highly variable N terminal portion but the C terminal part is of much more constant composition and allows broad classification into five antigenically distinguishable forms: gamma, γ; alpha, α; mu, μ; delta, δ; epsilon, ε. Within a single type, sub-classes may occur as a result of variation in a small part of this group-characteristic amino acid sequence. Each Ig molecule has two light chains (κ or λ) and two heavy chains of a single type. The type of heavy chain present divides the Igs into five main groups: IgG, IgA, IgM, IgD and IgE. The first three are present in much greater concentration than IgD and IgE. In these group names, the English capital letter corresponds to the Greek letter designating the antigenic type of heavy chain.

IgG, $\gamma_2\kappa_2$ or $\gamma_2\lambda_2$, is a 7 S protein, mol. wt. about 160 000, and the normal concentration in adult serum is 6 to 16 g/l. It occurs in four subgroups and although mainly found in the mid γ region it spreads from the slow γ almost to the α_2 area.

IgA, $(\alpha_2\kappa_2)_n$ or $(\alpha_2\lambda_2)_n$ exists in plasma mainly as a 7 S protein, mol. wt. 160 000, in normal concentrations of 1·0 to 4·5 g/l. It also exists in polymeric forms, mainly dimer but some trimer in which the monomers are linked by a junction (J) chain. Dimer IgA with an additional 'secretory piece' attached is produced in the walls of the respiratory and gastrointestinal tracts and is present in their secretions as well as in tears, sweat and colostrum as 'secretory IgA'. The IgA in plasma has electrophoretic mobility varying from the fast γ to the α_2.

IgM, $(\mu_2\kappa_2)_n$ or $(\mu_2\lambda_2)_n$, occurs in plasma mainly as a 19 S protein but some has S values of 29 and 35 to 40. The 19 S type is a pentamer with the five monomers linked by a J chain to give a mol. wt. of about 950 000. Its normal plasma concentration is 0·5 to 2·0 g/l. Electrophoretically it extends from the fast γ to the slow β region.

IgD, $\delta_2\kappa_2$ or $\delta_2\lambda_2$, a 7 S protein of mol. wt. 170 000, occurs in plasma at a concentration of less than 150 mg/l (Putnam, 1975).

IgE, $\varepsilon_2\kappa_2$ or $\varepsilon_2\lambda_2$, an 8 S protein of mol. wt. 190 000 occurs in plasma in concentrations of less than 60 μg/l (Putnam, 1975).

The polypeptide chains are combined with varying amounts of carbohydrate. This varies from 3% in IgG to 12 to 13% in IgM, IgD and IgE with IgA occupying an intermediate position at 8%.

Proteolytic enzymes split the molecules at certain points. As shown in Fig. 19.5, (p. 427), papain gives three fragments, one F_c of mol. wt. 48 000 so called because it can be obtained crystalline, and two F_{ab} fragments of mol. wt. 42 000, the ab standing for antigen-binding, given because the active binding sites are in this part. Pepsin, on the other hand, acts on the other side of the disulphide bridge to give two portions of heavy chain, F_d, and a larger fragment $F_{(ab')2}$ which has a mol. wt. of 91 000 and contains both the original binding sites.

Function. The Igs are synthesised by cells of the lymphoid series (see Chapter 5). The B-lymphocytes when challenged by immunogen change into plasma cells which are active synthesisers and secretors of Igs and account for most of the production. The B-lymphocytes themselves may produce a little Ig which is present on their surface . Most of these bear IgM in monomer form but others carry other Ig groups. The heavy and light chains are produced on separate ribosomes and are assembled into the final product in the Golgi apparatus in the plasma cell before extrusion. A particular plasma cell and its progeny, referred to as a clone, produces only one class of Ig with a unique structure in the variable part of the light and heavy chains. The antibody specificity is determined by these variable parts.

The invariant portion defines the type of light chain and the class of Ig by the type of heavy chain. Various parts of the constant part of the heavy chain called 'domains' are produced by intra-chain disulphide bonds and confer particular biological properties on the Ig. Other properties are determined by the size of the molecule, the number of antibody binding sites per molecule and resistance to proteolytic attack (Hobbs, 1970, 1971). Thus IgG is mainly effective against soluble antigens, particularly in interstitial fluid. It fixes complement and assists in the binding of foreign organisms to macrophages while its smaller molecular weight allows it to cross the placenta so that neonatal Ig reflects the maternal IgG. IgA is mainly important in protecting body surfaces by its presence in seromucous secretions. It binds micro-organisms and prevents their adherence to mucosal cells while it is itself protected from proteolytic enzymes by the secretory piece. IgM having 5 to 10 binding sites per molecule is an effective agglutinator of bacteria thereby preparing them for removal from the blood within which IgM is largely confined in view of its high mol. wt. It also actively fixes complement, and is the first Ig to increase following challenge with an immunogen. The role of IgD is currently uncertain but IgE binds firmly to mast cells. Contact with the antigen stimulates release of vasoactive amines from the mast cell producing the symptoms of atopic allergy, thus IgE is the reaginic antibody.

Changes in Disease States. Increases in Igs can produce two different types of electrophoretic picture, either a general increase in staining of the whole normal γ region or a more intense but narrow band. These patterns are termed respectively polyclonal and monoclonal. In the former there is a generalised increase in the activity of a large number of clones of plasma cells whereas in the latter a single clone proliferates in an uncontrolled fashion to produce a greatly increased amount of a single Ig, hence its electrophoretic uniformity. Such proliferation is often accompanied by interference with the function of other, normal, plasma cells demonstrated by reduced synthesis of other immunoglobulins producing a relative hypogammaglobulinaemia (see p. 434).

A **generalised polyclonal increase** is seen characteristically in response to infections of any kind. Often this is a small to moderate one but in certain tropical diseases, a considerable increase may be found taking the total globulins to over 100 g/l. In chronic liver disease a similar diffuse band is often seen (Fig. 19.3, p. 424) with total globulins between 35 and 70 g/l, mainly γ-globulins. In acute infective hepatitis any increase in γ-globulins is smaller and temporary. Diseases of connective tissue show small polyclonal increases giving total γ-globulins not usually exceeding 50 g/l; this is often accompanied by some increase in intensity of the α_2 band (Fig. 19.3, p. 424) attributable to an increase in glycoproteins.

In most generalised infections there is a roughly similar percentage increase in IgG, IgA and IgM but in those affecting the mucous surfaces the predominant increase is in IgA while in those in which the blood stream is involved, e.g. malaria, IgM is increased with the others staying within normal limits.

Determination of Igs is useful in diagnosing perinatal infections whether acquired *in utero* or during the first 6 weeks of life when clinical diagnosis is difficult. IgA and IgM are normally low at birth but intra-uterine infection is suggested by an increased IgM. Infections developing in the early post-natal period are revealed by rising IgM levels starting from a normal baseline. After 18 weeks the infant responds to antigens in the environment by increases in IgM and later by increases in IgG and IgA. The maturation of serum Ig levels is illustrated in Fig. 19.6.

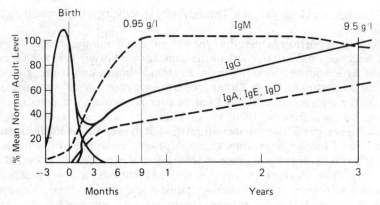

Fig. 19.6. Maturation of Serum Immunoglobulin Levels.
Normal adult levels are reached for IgG by 3 years and for IgA, IgD and IgE by puberty. Salivary IgA (not shown) matures by about 6 weeks. (Reproduced with permission from Hobbs, 1969 as modified by Keyser, 1979.)

A variety of changes is found in liver disease. Hobbs (1970, 1971) described four distinctive patterns. In acute viral hepatitis there is an initial increase in IgM followed by a fall to normal within about two months. IgG and IgA are not more than slightly increased, often remaining normal in patients who recover uneventfully. An increase in IgG as IgM falls is a sign of possible development of chronic hepatitis. In hepatitis B antigen-negative cases, IgM levels are higher following the onset of jaundice but remain normal in antigen-positive cases (Iwarson and Holmgren, 1972). In chronic aggressive hepatitis (juvenile, macronodular cirrhosis) the major increase is in IgG with the mean value of IgM lying in the upper normal range, and the mean IgA little altered. This response is also seen in systemic lupus erythematosis.

In the micronodular Laennec type of cirrhosis seen in haemochromatosis, Wilson's disease, or as a result of alcohol, the main increase is in IgA with a lesser one in IgG and little change in IgM. In primary biliary cirrhosis a more marked increase in IgM is found than in acute hepatitis with values ranging from 3 to 15 times the mean average normal in the former compared with 1·75 to 5 times in the latter. There is little change in IgG and IgA.

A monoclonal increase occurs in several conditions. The term 'paraprotein' describes these single types of Ig, intact molecules or portions thereof, which give an intense band on electrophoresis. Table 19.2 shows the primary diagnosis in 691 cases with such an increase (Hobbs, 1971).

The most common cause is *myeloma*, the proliferation of a single clone of malignant plasma cells. The increase in total protein found in at least half of the cases is due entirely to the paraprotein. Most of these have a total protein between 80 and 120 g/l but values up to 160 g/l occur. The albumin is usually slightly reduced and the paraprotein band seen on electrophoresis is most often in the γ region, then in diminishing frequency between the γ and the β, in the β, and beyond the β towards the α_2. Often the staining of the rest of the γ-globulin region is diminished due to reduced synthesis of other Igs (immuneparesis).

According to Hobbs (1971), 53% of the paraproteins in myeloma are of type IgG, 22% IgA, 1·5% IgD, 0·5% IgM and 0·1% IgE. In about 20% only light chains are produced; these are rapidly cleared from the plasma and are recognised in the urine as Bence–Jones protein. In a few cases more than one monoclonal

TABLE 19.2
Diagnoses in 691 Patients with Paraproteins

A. Malignant immunocytomata (74%)	
Myeloma (including 5 plasma cell leukaemia)	420
Waldenström's macroglobulinaemia	32
Lymphosarcoma	26
Soft-tissue plasmacytoma	20
Reticulosarcoma (including 5 atypical Hodgkin's)	6
Chronic lymphatic leukaemia	5
Arabian lymphoma of gut (α-chain disease)	3
Atypical myelosclerosis	2
Giant follicular lymphoma	1
B. Benign immunocytoma (23%)	
(i) Followed up for at least 5 years	112
(ii) Monoclonal antibody	
Primary cold agglutinins (8 others had lymphoma)	37
Lichen myxoedematosis	4
Transient paraproteins	5
C. Uncertain (3%)	18

protein is present, and in about 1% no paraprotein is detectable. The malignant plasma cell may show a much greater rate of production of light chains than heavy chains and then the excess light chains which enter the plasma are excreted in the urine, usually in dimer form as Bence–Jones protein. Some malignant plasmacytomas (20%) fail to synthesise any heavy chains and are the Bence–Jones myelomas referred to above. Much more rarely the production of light chains is halted and only heavy chains, usually in incomplete form, are released; these are discussed below under 'heavy chain disease' (p. 433). Other than this type, the soft-tissue plasmacytomas and the usual myelomas, those malignant immunocytomas in which a paraprotein is present are almost always associated with the IgM type. Again Bence–Jones proteinuria may occur.

Immunochemical methods (Chapter 5) are invaluable in the investigation of patients with paraproteinaemia. The Ig class of the paraprotein can be determined and the amounts of Ig in the other classes may be subnormal. The apparent amount of paraprotein determined by immunochemical methods depends on the avidity of the particular antiserum for that paraprotein. For serial studies the same antiserum should be used throughout. A less biased result is obtained by scanning the electrophoretic strip after staining and recording the paraprotein peak area. Difficulties arise with small amounts of paraprotein as in the benign immunocytomas or during remission following cytotoxic therapy. Normal Ig of the same class as the paraprotein may then be present and immunochemical measurement of that class as a group will overestimate the paraprotein. In scanning, the presence of polyclonal Igs up to normal amounts may make recognition and quantitation of the paraprotein peak difficult. Immunoelectrophoresis or immunofixation is essential in the detection and typing of paraproteins. The class can be recognised from the distortion of the arc produced (immunoelectrophoresis) or from the single band stained (immuno-fixation) with antisera specific for the heavy chain. Anti-κ and anti-λ sera should be used to type the light chain as the paraprotein will be entirely of one light chain type. If light chain production is disproportionate or the sole feature of the malignant plasmacytoma, it is often possible to demonstrate its presence in serum by the distorted anti-κ or anti-λ arc at a position different from that occupied by any complete paraprotein molecules. Alternatively, immunofixation will demonstrate a band not seen with antisera directed against heavy chains. The light chains are, however, best detected in the urine. Simple tests (p. 438) may be positive, but definitive detection requires concentration of the urine followed by electrophoresis and the use of anti-κ and anti-λ sera either by immunoelectrophoresis (Fig. 5.8C and D, p. 102) or immunofixation. The presence of a discrete band on electrophoresis which reacts with only one of the antisera indicates monoclonal light chains or Bence–Jones proteinuria. Normal urine if concentrated sufficiently may show the presence of minor bands on electrophoresis and these include normal light chains (Chapter 20, p. 436). The latter will, however, react with both anti-κ and anti-λ sera. Paraproteinaemia may be associated with abnormal renal function including the nephrotic syndrome. Then the paraprotein itself, if present as monomer, may pass through the glomerulus and can be demonstrated in the urine as well as in the serum. Such bands have the same mobility in serum and urine and give abnormal arcs on electrophoresis with the appropriate anti-heavy chain serum (Fig. 5.8D, p. 102). The Bence–Jones protein in the urine may have a different mobility from that of the intact paraprotein in the serum. Finally, confusion with Bence–Jones protein may arise from discrete bands in the β region due to the presence of transferrin or haemoglobin. They do not react with the anti-light chain sera and are often accompanied by some albumin.

The differentiation of benign and malignant immunocytomas is not always easy but in the latter, demonstrable Bence–Jones proteinuria, and increase in paraprotein concentration with time in the absence of therapy are common while being very rare in the benign type. Radiographic examination of the skeleton and histological assessment of the bone marrow are essential investigations in looking for evidence of dissemination or cytological features of malignancy. Suppression of other Igs and a paraprotein concentration greater than 10 g/l are much more common in the malignant type. The prognosis in myeloma is generally poor but particularly so in patients in whom anaemia, uraemia, hypoalbuminaemia or Bence–Jones proteinuria above 2 g/l are present when the diagnosis is made.

In *Waldenström's macroglobulinaemia* the excessive production of IgM is due to the malignant proliferation of lymphocytoid cells. The serum IgM lies between 7 and 100 g/l. Since it is often present in aggregates, the IgM may not enter the gel during electrophoresis and the serum should be preincubated with mercaptoethanol. Ultracentrifugal studies show the presence of a protein with high S value, mainly around 19 but with some higher.

The *Sia test* is often positive. For this test let a drop of serum fall into about 100 ml deionised water in a measuring cylinder. A white precipitate forming at once constitutes a positive test, but false negative and false positive results can occur. The *viscosity of the serum* is increased and many of the clinical features of this condition result from this change. Measurement of the serum viscosity can be used to detect macroglobulinaemia.

Cryoglobulins. These are globulins which come slowly out of solution when the serum or plasma is cooled below 37 °C, usually as white flakes or an amorphous precipitate but sometimes as a gel. The process is reversible, the precipitate redissolving on warming to 37 °C. To show the presence of cryoglobulins collect the blood in a warmed syringe and place into a tube in a water bath at 37°C while clotting occurs. Then centrifuge warm, separate the serum and cool half to 4°C for a few hours keeping the other warm. If present, cryoglobulins will precipitate. Measure the supernatant cold serum and the warm serum Ig content. The difference corresponds to the cryoglobulin concentration.

Cryoglobulins are most often found in multiple myeloma, though only in a minority of cases, but occur occasionally in a variety of conditions in which an IgM paraprotein is present, e.g. chronic lymphatic leukaemia, lymphosarcoma, and Waldenström's macroglobulinaemia. Their presence may be suspected when it is difficult to separate the serum at room temperature.

Cryofibrinogens have also been reported. Collect heparinised or oxalated plasma at 37 °C and cool at 4 °C for several hours. A precipitate in the plasma but not in similarly collected serum indicates the presence of cryofibrinogen. This also redissolves on warming.

Pyroglobulins. This term is given to globulins coagulable on heating to 56 °C, the existence of such proteins having been noted by several workers when serum complement was being inactivated by heating for 30 min at 56 °C. Pyroglobulins are found most often in myeloma but occur in other cases of hyperglobulinaemia and chronic infections. They bear no constant relationship to the degree of hyperglobulinaemia or to the presence of Bence–Jones protein.

Heavy Chain Disease. Some patients with neoplasms of lymphocytes or plasma cells produce a homogeneous population of fragments of heavy chains, normal or abnormal, without light chains. These form the group of heavy chain diseases. Those derived from α-chains are the most common with those from γ-chains a little less common and from μ-chains much less frequently seen. For a review of γ and μ-chain diseases see Franklin (1975) and of α-chain disease, Seligman (1975).

In alpha-chain disease, the protein has a mol. wt. of 29 000 to 34 000, about two-thirds that of a single normal α chain. This is a consequence of the deletion of the variable part and the first section of the constant part of the usual α chain. The part found in dimer form as the F_c component of IgA is intact. Cellulose acetate electrophoresis may reveal an abnormal, diffuse band in the α_2-β region but the characteristic monoclonal band is absent probably as a result of varying degradation of the monoclonal protein after synthesis. Immunoelectrophoresis (Chapter 5, p. 96) is more helpful. The clinical presentation is usually as severe intestinal malabsorption.

Gamma heavy chain disease behaves rather like a malignant lymphoma. Varying deletions from the normal γ chain have been noted and result in fragments of mol. wt. varying from 45 000 up to 80 000 when present as the dimer. Cellulose acetate electrophoresis usually shows a rather broad band in the β or fast γ region and the protein may be detected in the urine. Immunoelectrophoresis is needed for further characterisation.

The rare μ heavy chain disease has usually been associated with chronic lymphatic leukaemia and unlike the other two types, Bence–Jones proteinuria may occur. The nature of the chemical change is uncertain but the protein appears to be an 11·5 S pentamer of mol. wt. 180 000 to 300 000. This is absent from the urine and often is not detectable on cellulose acetate electrophoresis although other Igs may be present in reduced amounts.

Benign Paraproteinaemias. A benign form of monoclonal increase is found when any large number of sera, particularly from the elderly, are screened. The increase is most often of IgG but may be one of the others. Differentiation from myeloma can be difficult though in general the quantity of paraprotein is below 10 g/l and there is little tendency for it to increase. Bence–Jones proteinuria is absent and other Igs are not suppressed. The diagnosis can only be made with confidence if its lack of progress can be demonstrated over many years.

Immune Deficiency Diseases. Hypogammaglobulinaemia. These diseases are characterised by recurrent infections and a much reduced concentration of plasma immunoglobulins. The normal infant at birth has a plasma IgG of 8 to 10 g/l which is of maternal origin. The level falls to about 35% during the first 6 months until synthesis of IgG which begins at 2 to 3 months exceeds catabolism. The concentration rises to about 60% of the normal adult value by one year and then more slowly reaching its final level about the third year. IgM, absent at birth, increases more rapidly reaching 70% of the adult level at about 1 year and 100% by puberty. IgA, also absent at birth, rises more slowly only reaching 20% of the adult value at 1 year and being below this until the later teens. Occasionally this development is delayed. Other cases of hypogammaglobulinaemia may be congenital or acquired. Congenital forms may be general, involving all classes of immunoglobulins, or selective. There are several varieties of the latter. Type I has decreased IgA and IgM with normal IgG; Type II, decreased IgG and IgA but increase in IgM and IgD; Type III, practically no IgA but normal IgG and IgM; Type IV, deficiency only of IgA; Type V, deficiency only of IgM; Type VI, deficiency of quality; Type VII, deficiency of IgG and IgM (Hobbs, 1971). In Bruton's disease (a sex-linked form) all types of immunoglobulin are very low.

A secondary or acquired hypogammaglobulinaemia can develop in a number of diseases. Thus in monoclonal gammopathies, synthesis of the normal immunoglobulins is often severely reduced as it is in conditions in which there is severe loss of protein, as in nephrosis and protein-losing enteropathies.

The Effect of Steroids on Plasma Proteins

The rate of synthesis and volume of distribution of many plasma proteins are altered by steroids, either endogenous or exogenous. Pregnancy and the contraceptive pill are probably the most frequently encountered but corticosteroid therapy and androgen excess should also be considered when interpreting plasma protein results. The effects on individual proteins are shown in Table 19.3, which is adapted from Whicher (1983).

TABLE 19.3

The Effect of Various Steroids on Plasma Protein Concentration

Protein	Pregnancy	Contraceptive pill	Androgens	Corticosteroids
Prealbumin	−	N	+	−
Albumin	−	−	N	−
α-Lipoprotein	+	+	−	N
α_1-Acid glycoprotein	−	−	+	+
α_1-Antitrypsin	+ +	+	+	N
Haptoglobin	N	−	+ +	+
Ceruloplasmin	+ + +	+ + +	N	N
Transferrin	+	+	+	N
β-Lipoprotein	N	N	+	+ +
IgG	N	N	N	−

+ = increased concentration
N = no change
− = decreased concentration

REFERENCES

Bartholomew R. J., Delaney A. M. (1966). *Proc. Austral. Assn. Clin. Biochem*; 1: 214 (see also p. 64).

Bearn A. G., Cleve H. (1972). In *The Metabolic Basis of Inherited Disease*, 3rd ed. (Stanbury J. B., Wyngaarden J. B., Frederickson D. S. eds) (a) p. 1629; (b) p. 1637. New York: McGraw Hill.

Carter P. (1970). *Microchem. J*; 15: 531.

Doumas B. T., Watson W. A., Biggs H. G. (1971). *Clin Chim. Acta*; 31: 87.

Duggan J., Duggan P. (1982). *Clin. Chem*; 28; 1407.

Franklin E. C. (1975). In Disorders of Protein Metabolism. (McGowan G. K., Walters G. eds) p. 65. *J. Clin. Pathol*; 28: suppl. (*Ass. Clin. Path.*); 6.

Fraser G. R., Harris H., Robson E. B. (1959). *Lancet*; 1: 1023.

Gustafsson J. E. C. (1976). *Clin. Chem*; 22: 616.

Harding J. R., Keyser J. W. (1968). *Proc. Ass. Clin. Biochem*; 8: 51.

Hill P. G. (1985). *Ann. Clin. Biochem*; 22: 565.

Hill P. G., Wells T. N. C. (1983). *Ann. Clin. Biochem*; 20: 264.

Hobbs J. R. (1969). In *Developmental Biology*. (Adinolfi A. ed) p. 114. London: Spastics International Press.

Hobbs J. R. (1970). *Brit. J. Hosp. Med*; 3: 669.

Hobbs J. R. (1971). In *Advances in Clinical Chemistry*. (Bodansky O., Latner A. L. eds) 14: 219. New York and London: Academic Press.

Hobbs J. R., Harboe N., Alper C., Johansson B. G. (1979). *Clin. Chim. Acta*; 98: 179.

Iwarson S., Holmgren J. (1972). *J. Infect. Dis*; 125: 178.

Keyser J. W. (1979). *Human Plasma Proteins*, p. 2. Chichester, New York: John Wiley and Sons.

Laurell C.-B. (1985). In *Recent Advances in Clinical Biochemistry*, Vol. 3. (Price C. P., Alberti K. G. M. M. eds) p. 103. Edinburgh: Churchill Livingstone.

Laurell C.-B., Nikkilin J. E. (1966). *J. Clin. Invest*; 45: 1935.

Lines J. G., Raines D. N. (1970). *Ann. Clin. Biochem*; 7: 6.

Louderback A., Mealey E. H., Taylor N. A. (1968). *Clin. Chem*; 14: 793.

Martinek R. G. (1965). *Proc. Ass. Clin. Biochem*; 3: 264.

Northam B. E., Widdowson G. M. (1967). Technical Bulletin, No. 11. Association of Clinical Biochemists. Professional and Scientific Publications, BMA House, Tavistock Square, London WC1H 9JR.

Pascucci M. W., Grisley D. W., Rand R. N. (1980). *Clin. Chem*; 26: 1058.

Perry B. W., Doumas B. T. (1979). *Clin. Chem*; 25; 1520.

Pinnell A. E., Northam B. E. (1978). *Clin. Chem*; 24: 80.

Putnam F. W. ed. (1975). *The Plasma Proteins. Structure, Function and Genetic Control*, 2nd ed., Vol. 1, p. 83. New York and London: Academic Press.

Ratnoff O. D. (1972). In *The Metabolic Basis of Inherited Diseases*, 3rd ed. (Stanbury J. B., Wyngaarden J. B., Frederickson D. S. eds) p. 1690. New York: McGraw Hill.

Reinhold J. G. (1953). In *Standard Methods of Clinical Chemistry*. (Reiner M. ed) 1: p. 88. New York and London: Academic Press.

Rodkey F. L. (1965). *Clin. Chem*; 11: 478.

Schultze H. E., Heremans J. F. (1966). *Molecular Biology of Human Proteins*, Vol. 1. Amsterdam: Elsevier.

Seligman M. (1975). In Disorders of Protein Metabolism. (McGowan G. K., Walters G. eds) p. 72. *J. Clin. Pathol*; 28, suppl. (*Ass. Clin. Path.*); 6.

Slater L., Carter P. M., Hobbs J. R. (1975). *Ann. Clin. Biochem*; 12: 33.

Spencer K., Price C. P. (1977). *Ann. Clin. Biochem*; 14: 105.

Ward A. M. *et al.* (1984). *Ann. Clin. Biochem*; 21: 254.

Webster D. (1974). *Clin. Chim. Acta*; 55: 109.

Weeke B. (1973). *Scand. J. Immunol*; 2, suppl. 1, pp. 15, 36.

Whicher J. T. (1983). In *Biochemistry in Clinical Practice*. (Williams D. R., Marks V. eds) p. 223. London: William Heinemann Medical Books.

20

PROTEINS IN URINE, CEREBROSPINAL FLUID AND OTHER FLUIDS

URINE

Proteins in Normal Urine

Normally only a small amount of protein is excreted in the urine (up to about 150 mg/day) and three factors contribute to this:

1. Small amounts of some plasma proteins pass into the glomerular filtrate.
2. Some of the protein in the glomerular filtrate is reabsorbed in the proximal tubules.
3. Some proteins are secreted by the tubules and the rest of the renal tract.

Glomerular Filtration. The glomerular membrane acts as an ultrafilter for plasma proteins and is almost impermeable to proteins with a molecular size of albumin (66 000) or greater. However, a small but significant amount of albumin is passed into the glomerular filtrate due to its high plasma concentration, as is some transferrin due to its similar mol. wt. (76 500). Smaller amounts of haptoglobin, α_2-lipoprotein, hemopexin, IgG and IgA are also present in the filtrate. Very few proteins of mol. wt. above 200 000 are present.

Proteins smaller than albumin pass through the glomeruli in amounts inversely proportional to their molecular weight but are present in the filtrate in lesser amounts due to their lower plasma concentrations. Immunoglobulin fragments with antigenic properties similar to F_{ab} fragments and to kappa and lambda light chains can also be detected.

Tubular Reabsorption. The low molecular weight proteins are actively reabsorbed from the glomerular filtrate and catabolised by the proximal tubules. Albumin is incompletely reabsorbed and therefore makes up the majority of the protein in normal urine.

Renal Tract Secretion. The major protein secreted by the renal tract, probably by the distal tubule, is Tamm–Horsfall protein (uromucoid) which is the main constituent of urinary casts. In men, secretions from the prostate and seminal vesicles also contribute to some extent to the protein excreted.

Urine Proteins in Disease

Increased amounts of protein in the urine (proteinuria) can be caused by increased glomerular permeability, reduced tubular reabsorption, increased secretion of protein from the renal tract or increased concentration of low molecular weight proteins in the plasma.

Glomerular Proteinuria. This is the most common type of proteinuria and because most of the protein is albumin it is often referred to as albuminuria. Various disease processes increase the permeability of the glomerular 'membrane'. In glomerulonephritis, immune complexes and complement are deposited in the glomerular membrane. Diabetic nephropathy and immune-complex diseases are often associated with glomerular damage. The permeability of the glomeruli often increases progressively so that while albumin is lost in increased amounts in the early stages, the larger molecular weight proteins appear with increasing damage. When the glomeruli can retain larger proteins the proteinuria is termed *selective* but when selectivity is lost and large molecular weight proteins are excreted there is *non-selective* proteinuria. Loss of large amounts of plasma albumin results in oedema in the nephrotic syndrome.

If the glomeruli are severely damaged, e.g. in acute glomerulonephritis, blood may pass directly into the glomerular filtrate and the urine. Lesions of the ureters or the bladder may also result in blood passing into the urine causing *haematuria*. This is often visible but small amounts of blood may only be detected microscopically. Once the binding capacity of haptoglobin is exceeded in intravascular haemolysis, haemoglobin will be filtered by the glomeruli and appear in the urine without red blood cells (*haemoglobinuria*). In haematuria, haemoglobin may be liberated after the blood has been mixed with the urine and will increase on standing. Haemoglobin may be oxidised to methaemoglobin in the cells (see p. 659). If these are haemolysed, methaemoglobin will be liberated and be excreted in the urine. The same change may occur to haemoglobin in urine which is allowed to stand.

Myoglobin (see p. 660) is also sometimes found in urine, being liberated into the plasma following severe muscle cell breakdown. It is much more readily filtered at the glomeruli than haemoglobin since its molecular weight is only a quarter of that of haemoglobin and it does not bind to haptoglobin. In some states myoglobin may be oxidised before or after excretion giving metmyoglobinuria.

Proteinuria due to renal disease is usually continuously present from day to day and should be distinguished from less serious, intermittent proteinurias. Postural or orthostatic proteinuria is a benign form of glomerular proteinuria which occurs when the subject is standing or ambulant but is absent when recumbent. Protein loss is generally small but may be as much as 5 g/l. It is most common in adolescents, especially those with lumbar lordosis, and in most cases disappears in early adulthood. The condition has been attributed to inferior vena caval compression between the liver and the vertebral column in a lordotic posture. There are no other symptoms or signs of renal disease, serum urea and blood pressure being normal. Haematuria is absent but hyaline and granular casts are often present. The degree of proteinuria may vary from day to day but characteristically vanishes at night. The proteinuria of reversible renal glomerular disease may also pass through an orthostatic stage on the way to full recovery. Also, some patients with continuous proteinuria show more marked loss during the day, when ambulant, but nocturnal loss continues. Stress proteinuria is also intermittent and follows severe exercise, exposure to cold or pyrexia.

In normal pregnancy, urine protein excretion may increase slightly to about 300 mg/day. However, more severe proteinuria of several grams per day occurs in pre-eclamptic toxaemia.

Tubular Proteinuria. This type of proteinuria can occur alone but is usually associated with glomerular proteinuria. The proteins excreted are of low molecular weight such as β_2-microglobulin (mol. wt. 11 800), retinol-binding protein (mol. wt. 21 000), lysozyme (mol. wt. 14 500), α_1-microglobin (mol. wt. 27 000) and α_1-acid glycoprotein (mol. wt. 40 000).

Post-renal Proteinuria. This is usually caused by inflammatory conditions or malignancy. Lesions of the renal pelvis, bladder, prostate and urethra can cause such proteinuria. Microscopic examination of urinary sediment for pus or malignant cells can often indicate the cause. Drainage of lymph into the renal tract can cause chyluria.

Methods for Detecting and Measuring Urine Proteins

1. Stick Tests

Albumin. Albustix (Ames) is a plastic strip bearing at one end an absorbent cellulose area impregnated with the indicator, bromophenol blue, and a citrate buffer, pH 3·5. A similar area is present on several multi-test strips produced by the same company. At pH 3·5, the indicator is yellow but changes to blue through various intermediate shades of green in the presence of increasing amounts of protein. This is the result of the *divalent anionic (blue)* form of the indicator combining with protein producing further dissociation of the yellow monovalent anion into the blue divalent anion; the 'protein error' of an indicator. A related indicator with similar properties is incorporated into the Albym-test (Boehringer) strip for protein detection and as an area in several multi-test strips.

To perform the test, dip the strip in the urine for about a second and remove excess urine by tapping the edge against the container. Compare the colour with the test chart within 60 s. The colour intensity changes with protein concentration but is most sensitive to albumin while Bence–Jones proteins, globulins and glycoproteins are much less readily detected. A result designated as positive corresponds to an albumin concentration of 0·3 g/l. Difficulties arise in the interpretation of 'trace' results. An albumin concentration of 0·1 to 0·2 g/l may be detected under ideal conditions but a slightly greenish colour change is apparent in concentrated urines containing only physiological concentrations of protein.

False negative results are likely if the urine is acidified or if the protein is not albumin. False positive results are given by very alkaline, infected urines (pH 9 or higher). Other agents giving a false positive result are polyvinylpyrrolidone and quaternary ammonium compounds including a few drugs and Cetavlon (ICI Limited), which is sometimes used to clean and sterilise urine containers. Such compounds bind the indicator in the same way as albumin.

Haemoglobin. Tests include microscopic examination of uncentrifuged, well-mixed urine for red blood cells (see p. 754), spectroscopic examination for blood pigments (see p. 661) and chemical tests (see p. 663). The most sensitive test if red cells are present is microscopic examination; red cells may still be seen when both other tests are negative.

Ames produce the Hemastix strip test for blood in urine and a corresponding area is also incorporated in some of their multi-test strips. The test area of cellulose on a plastic strip is impregnated with a buffered mixture of organic peroxide and *o*-tolidine. Haemoglobin and myoglobin have peroxidase-like activity and catalyse the oxidation of *o*-tolidine to a blue compound. Boehringer produce a similar plastic strip incorporated in the BM multi-test strips. This employs a different chromogen but the principle is the same. Both tests are more sensitive to free haemoglobin than to intact red cells. A positive test is given by a haemoglobin concentration in solution of 0·2 mg/l which would result from haemolysis of about 50 erythrocytes/μl urine. This number of intact cells gives a speckled appearance to the test area and a generally fainter test. In good conditions it may be possible to detect 5 to 10 erythrocytes/μl urine, a sensitivity approaching that of the microscopic examination.

To perform the test, dip the stick in fresh, well-mixed, uncentrifuged urine for a second, tap the edge of the strip against the container to remove excess urine and compare with the colour chart at exactly 30 s (Ames) or between 30 and 60 s (Boehringer). If urine is not tested on receipt, store at 4° C but return to room temperature before testing. False negative results may be obtained if the urine contains excess ascorbate or nitrite, the latter in association with urinary tract infection. False positive results are obtained if the urine container is contaminated with oxidising cleansing agents, particularly hydrogen peroxide.

2. Spectroscopy

Myoglobin. This can be detected by spectroscopic examination and the stick tests for haemoglobin. The slight differences in the spectra of this and its met- and carboxy-derivatives from those of the corresponding haemoglobin derivatives are shown on p. 661. Oxyhaemoglobin and myoglobin have different solubilities in ammonium sulphate. Whereas haemoglobin and methaemoglobin are completely precipitated at 80% saturation with ammonium sulphate, only minor amounts of myoglobin or metmyoglobin are precipitated. To 5 ml urine add 2·8 g ammonium sulphate and shake to dissolve. Filter or centrifuge. If the abnormal colour and spectra are still present in the filtrate, myoglobin or metmyoglobin is probably present. It is necessary to show that the abnormal haem pigment is combined with protein by precipitating it with sulphosalicylic acid. Urine should be tested fresh or preserved by adjusting to pH 7·0 to 7·5 with dilute sodium hydroxide and stored at 4 °C. However, these methods are not very reliable especially if both haemoglobin and myoglobin are present. Myoglobin can also be distinguished from haemoglobin by electrophoresis (p. 443), by gel filtration through a column of Sephadex, by thin-layer chromatography on Sephadex, by HPLC separation or by reaction with antiserum raised against myoglobin.

3. Electrophoresis and Immunoelectrophoresis

The type of proteinuria can often be determined by electrophoresis, since excretion of albumin alone or along with other proteins in a pattern similar to that of the plasma proteins is indicative of glomerular proteinuria. Urine usually needs to be concentrated by 50 to 100 times to study excretion by electrophoresis. If the presence of monoclonal light chains (Bence–Jones proteins) is suspected, electrophoresis and immunoelectrophoresis or immunofixation should be performed. Tests based on heating or precipitation are not recommended because they have high rates of false positives and false negatives.

4. Immunoassay

If the quantitation of specific proteins is of interest, immunoassay methods can be used. Because of the small quantities of some of the proteins present in urine, the sensitivity of radioimmunoassay or enzymeimmunoassay is usually required, e.g. for β_2-microglobulin. Nephelometry, radial immunodiffusion and electroimmunoassay are sufficiently sensitive for albumin, transferrin and IgG.

Total Protein

The quantitation of urine total protein is difficult as urine contains a complex and variable mixture of proteins. Different proteins may give different responses in a particular method and other substances such as urinary pigments may interfere. Calibrant materials can also affect results due to differences in reactivity between individual proteins or between species. External quality assessment surveys for urine proteins in the USA, Australia and the UK have shown poor agreement between laboratories and poor intralaboratory precision (Glenn and Hathaway, 1977; Glenn, 1978, 1979, 1980; Shephard et al., 1981, 1982; Whicher, 1985).

Many methods have been used including turbidimetry, protein precipitation and dye binding methods. Turbidimetry using sulphosalicylic acid has very poor precision and poor sensitivity. Precision is slightly improved by the addition of sodium sulphate and variation of reaction between different proteins is reported to be reduced. This method shows a marked difference between human and bovine serum albumins, making bovine serum albumin unsuitable as a calibration material (Dilena et al., 1983). In a comparison of turbidimetric methods using sulphosalicylic acid/sodium sulphate, trichloracetic acid and alkaline benzethonium chloride, Nishi and Elin (1985) showed that the benzethonium chloride method of Iwata and Nishikaze (1979) had the best sensitivity and most consistent bias with different globulin fractions. McElderry et al. (1982) obtained a coefficient of variation of 4·4% at a protein concentration of 0·81 g/l using benzethonium chloride.

Precipitation of urine proteins by trichloracetic or sulphosalicylic acid followed by the biuret reaction has the advantages of less variation between different proteins and species and improved linearity up to about 5 g/l (McElderry et al., 1982; Dilena et al., 1983). However, the methods are relatively insensitive at normal levels of urine protein. Blanks are required for all standards, tests and control materials. The biuret reaction applied directly to urine without prior precipitation is not appropriate due to the presence of interfering substances (Doetsch and Gadsden, 1973). Although precipitation methods have certain advantages over turbidimetric methods they are more time consuming and are not readily adaptable to automation.

Dye binding methods are simple and readily applied to large batches. Ponceau S (Pesce and Strande, 1973) and Coomassie Brilliant Blue (Bradford, 1976) have been most used and commercial kits are available. However, they suffer from the same problems as turbidimetric methods of variable response to different proteins (McElderry et al., 1982) and in some forms the Coomassie Brilliant Blue method has limited linearity or is non-linear (Dilena et al., 1983; McElderry et al., 1982).

Protein Precipitation Followed by Biuret Reaction (Bell and Baron, 1968).

Reagents.
1. Trichloracetic acid (TCA), 200 g/l.
2. Sodium hydroxide, 1 mol/l. Dissolve 40 g in 1 litre distilled water.
3. Sodium hydroxide, 0·2 mol/l. Dissolve 8 g in 1 litre distilled water.
4. Stock biuret reagent. Dissolve 45 g potassium sodium tartate, 5 g potassium iodide, 15 g copper sulphate and 8 g sodium hydroxide in 1 l distilled water.
5. Potassium iodide solution. Dissolve 5 g potassium iodide and 80 g sodium hydroxide in 1 litre distilled water.

6. Working biuret reagent. Add 80 ml potassium iodide solution to 200 ml stock biuret reagent and make up to 1 litre with distilled water.

7. Standard albumin solution. Prepare a bovine albumin solution of 3·0 g/l.

Technique. Test each sample of urine with Albustix. The volume of urine to be used depends on the Albustix result

Result	+ + + +	+ + +	+ +	+ or trace
Volume (ml)	1	2	3	6

Add the appropriate volume of urine to a graduated centrifuge tube. Add an equal volume of trichloracetic acid to the urine and mix. For the standard, add 3 ml of this acid to 3 ml standard in a graduated centrifuge tube and mix. Cover the tops of the centrifuge tubes and allow to stand overnight at 4 °C.

Centrifuge the tubes for a minimum of 5 min to ensure that the protein precipitate is secured at the base of the tube. Discard the supernatant and allow to drain by inverting the tube. Dissolve the protein precipitate in approximately 1 ml reagent (2). Mix by sucking the liquid up and down a Pasteur pipette. Make up to exactly 2 ml with reagent (2) and mix. Accurately transfer 1 ml to another tube. This is portion A. The remaining 1 ml in the centrifuge tube is portion B. Add 5 ml working biuret reagent to all A tubes and mix. Add 5 ml reagent (3) to all B tubes and mix.

Set up two blanks

Blank A: 1 ml reagent (2) + 5 ml working biuret reagent.

Blank B: 1 ml reagent (2) + 5 ml reagent (3).

Allow all tubes to stand for 30 min. Read absorbances (Abs) at 540 nm, reading the A tubes against blank A and the B tubes against blank B.

Calculation.

Urinary total protein (g/l) =

$$\frac{(Abs_A - Abs_B) \text{ unknown}}{(Abs_A - Abs_B) \text{ standard}} \times 3\cdot0 \times \frac{3}{\text{Urine volume (ml)}}$$

Albumin

Although the measurement of urine total protein is satisfactory in most clinical situations there is considerable evidence that even small increases in the loss of albumin in insulin-dependent diabetics can be pathological and predictive of later development of diabetic nephropathy (Viberti *et al.*, 1982; Mogensen and Christensen, 1984). This is sometimes, misleadingly, termed microalbuminuria. The normal excretion of albumin is less than about 20 mg/l which is below the sensitivity limits of urine total protein methods and dipstick techniques. To achieve the degree of sensitivity required for detecting small increases in urine albumin, immunochemical methods are required. Enzyme immunoassay (Fielding *et al.*, 1983; Townsend, 1986), radioimmunoassay (Keen and Chlouverakis, 1963; Miles *et al.*, 1970; Nargessi *et al.*, 1978; Berglund *et al.*, 1984; Christiansen and Ørskov, 1984) and immunoturbidimetric (Teppo, 1982; Bell *et al.*, 1986; Sathianathan *et al.*, 1986) techniques have been used.

Tubular Proteins

β_2-Microglobulin is a low mol. wt. protein (11 800) present on cell surfaces. It is the light chain of human leucocyte antigen (HLA) and because of its low mol. wt. it passes through the glomerulus. However, normally more than 99% is reabsorbed and catabolised by the renal proximal tubules. Urinary excretion of β_2-microglobulin can be used as an indicator of renal tubular damage and it has been used in evaluating damage by nephrotoxic drugs and heavy metals. Recent evidence suggests β_2-microglobulin is unstable in acid urines (Bernard *et al.*, 1982) and that retinol-binding protein is more suitable for investigating tubular function. Radioimmunoassay or techniques with similar sensitivity are required for measuring both proteins in urine.

Glomerular Selectivity

In children with nephrotic syndrome, assessment of the degree of glomerular selectivity for proteins can be helpful in diagnosis and in predicting prognosis. The less damage to the glomerulus, the greater the selectivity; therefore protein excretion is limited to proteins with mol. wt. below 100 000. Selectivity is usually measured by comparing the clearances of two proteins of different molecular size. Albumin or transferrin is usually used being of a size which is normally just retained by the glomerulus and the larger IgG which is well retained. A random urine sample and a serum sample are collected at the same time and both proteins measured in each specimen. Nephelometry, radial immunodiffusion and rocket immunoelectrophoresis are sufficiently sensitive.

The selectivity ratio is calculated as:

$$\frac{\text{Clearance of IgG}}{\text{Clearance of albumin}} = \frac{\dfrac{UV}{S}\,(\text{IgG})}{\dfrac{UV}{S}\,(\text{Albumin})}$$

where U = urine concentration, S = serum concentration and V = volume of urine per minute. Thus

$$\text{Selectivity ratio} = \frac{(\text{Urine IgG}) \times (\text{serum albumin})}{(\text{Serum IgG}) \times (\text{urine albumin})}$$

Thus a high selectivity ratio reflects an increased loss of IgG whereas a low ratio reflects a selective proteinuria. A ratio of less than 0·2 is usually considered selective and associated with steroid-responsive minimal change glomerulonephritis.

Separation Procedures for Urine Proteins

Various forms of electrophoresis on cellulose acetate, agar gel and starch gel, and both column and thin-layer gel filtration have been used in studying the various protein fractions present in urine. Concentration of the urine is necessary before applying these procedures.

Concentration of Urine Specimens

When only a small volume needs to be concentrated, dialysis against dextran, polyvinylpyrrolidone or carboxymethylcellulose can be used. Place an appropriate volume of urine, 20 to 40 ml depending on the concentration of protein, into Visking tubing, 19 mm diameter, and concentrate to between 0·2 and 2·0 ml to obtain a protein concentration of about 5 g/l, by extracting into a 150 g/l solution of carboxymethylcellulose, or a 250 g/l solution of polyvinylpyrrolidone. Perform the dialysis at 4 °C.

Alternatively Lyphogel (Gelman Limited) avoids the use of Visking tubing. This dried polyacrylamide gel is added to a measured volume of urine as weighed granules. Water and small molecules are attracted into the gel by osmosis but those of mol. wt. greater than 20 000 are excluded by the pore size. As 1 g of gel absorbs 5 ml water, the required concentration can be planned and is achieved in about 5 h. The concentrated urine lies between the swollen gel pellets which may be removed either by forceps or by decantation through a mesh. Small volumes of urine can also be removed directly into a capillary tube passed between the pellets.

Ultrafiltration membranes with varying cut-off characteristics for molecular size can also be used. In its simplest form, the Minicon-B Clinical Sample Concentrator (Amicon Limited) has an ultrafiltration membrane separating a cell holding up to 5 ml urine from an absorbent pad. The cut-off point is about mol. wt. 15 000 and concentration is up to a maximum of 100-fold in 2 to 4 h.

Electrophoresis of Urine Proteins

Any of the techniques for serum proteins can be used with concentrated urine specimens; their relative merits are the same. Separation of the globulin fractions is, however, less satisfactory than with serum. The proportion of prealbumin is less than with serum; the two α bands are well marked with the α_1 particularly prominent, while the β band is only faint as is the γ band. Separation on cellulose acetate is shown in Fig. 20.1. As with serum, starch and polyacrylamide gels give more effective separation but the pattern may be so detailed as to make recognition of the components difficult.

Electrophoresis is useful: (1) to distinguish glomerular and tubular proteinuria when present in renal disease and in conditions affecting renal function; (2) to show the presence of Bence–Jones protein and other immunoglobulin fragments; (3) to distinguish haemoglobin and myoglobin and (4) to study lipoproteins and protein–carbohydrate complexes. In most cases, it is useful to put up serum from the patient at the same time so that a direct comparison of the two can be made.

CEREBROSPINAL FLUID

Production of Cerebrospinal Fluid

The surface of the central nervous system is covered by the meninges, three layers referred to as the pia mater, arachnoid mater and dura mater. The last is the outermost and the cerebrospinal fluid (CSF) is found between the pia and the arachnoid mater. It is formed by active secretion from the cells of the choroid plexus, vascular structures lying within the ventricles of the brain. Fluid from the lateral ventricles passes via the third ventricle to join fluid secreted in the fourth ventricle from which it emerges into the subarachnoid space through three

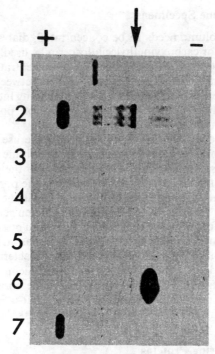

Fig. 20.1. Cellulose Acetate Electrophoresis of Urine Concentrates after Staining with Nigrosin.

The lines of application lie vertically below the arrow.

1. Albumin, transferrin and monoclonal free light chains of mid to fast γ-mobility.
2. Heavy proteinuria (non-selective) showing a similar pattern to serum.
3,4. Normal urines showing a faint albumin band only.
5,6. Monoclonal free light chains in amounts in excess of albumin.
7. Selective proteinuria showing mainly albumin.

apertures. This space is deep near the base of the brain and the spaces created are known as cisterns. The largest, the cisterna magna, lies beneath the cerebellum and can be sampled by inserting a needle into the back of the neck and passing it through the foramen magnum.

Some of the fluid passes upwards over the brain in the subarachnoid space. In so doing it is in communication with the perivascular spaces around all blood vessels entering and leaving the brain. Cells and protein are believed to pass from the brain substance into these spaces and hence into the CSF, a process which is more marked in inflammation of the meninges (meningitis). When the fluid reaches the top of the brain it is reabsorbed through the arachnoid granulations which project into the venous sinuses at this site.

Part of the CSF passes downwards in the subarachnoid space around the spinal cord and is eventually reabsorbed into the venous plexuses surrounding the dura in the spinal canal. The spinal cord ends near the 1st lumbar vertebra and the accumulation of fluid below this, the lumbar fluid, is the portion of the CSF most often examined. It is obtained by passing a needle between the 3rd and 4th lumbar vertebrae into the subarachnoid space.

The composition of lumbar, cisternal and ventricular fluids varies, probably from contributions from the perivascular spaces and absorption of water. Thus the protein content of ventricular fluid is 0·10 to 0·20 g/l increasing to 0·15 to 0·25 g/l in cisternal fluid and to 0·15 to 0·45 g/l in lumbar fluid. The total volume of CSF is about 130 ml of which on average 25 ml is ventricular. Evidence suggests that the daily secretion is about 750 ml implying a fairly rapid turnover. The secretory process is selective and a 'blood–CSF barrier' exists for many substances including drugs so that their concentration in CSF is lower than in plasma. Other substances, e.g. chloride and folate, are present in increased concentration. These differences may be less marked if the blood–CSF barrier is impaired as in inflammatory states. Even though there are differences between plasma and CSF values, substances such as chloride and glucose change in a similar fashion to any change in plasma concentration.

Pathological Conditions Involving Cerebrospinal Fluid Examination

A wide range of disorders can produce changes in CSF composition and the type and extent of change is often not specific for a single pathological condition. However, it is useful to review the types of disorder for which the examination is often helpful. Most can be classified as infections, other inflammatory states, degenerative disorders, tumours, vascular disorders and trauma.

Infections. Many different infective agents are involved. They may attack the meninges or the central nervous system (brain or spinal cord) itself. In the former case, meningitis, the changes in the CSF are more marked as the meninges are in close proximity to the CSF. Infections of the central nervous system are divided into those affecting the brain, encephalitis, and those affecting the cord, myelitis. All these infections may be acute, subacute or chronic, the more florid changes in CSF composition occurring in the acute types. (For fuller details, see the 5th edition of this book.)

Other Inflammatory States. An acute or chronic inflammatory response, usually of mild degree, is seen if the meninges are irritated by the presence of a tumour, by a prolapsed intervertebral disc or by trauma. An inflammatory state of doubtful aetiology, but probably a hypersensitivity reaction, is acute post-infective polyneuritis (Guillain–Barré syndrome), one of the most common forms of polyneuritis. Acute lead toxicity, especially in children, produces an acute inflammatory reaction.

Degenerative Disorders. The most important condition in which CSF examination is helpful is multiple sclerosis characterised by patches of demyelination occurring throughout the central nervous system. Schilder's disease in children may be an acute form of multiple sclerosis. Other degenerative disorders include syringomyelia and cerebral infarction.

Tumours. Primary neoplasms of the nervous system include the benign meningioma and the malignant glioma. Secondary deposits arising from carcinoma elsewhere in the body may involve the brain or spinal cord direct or may infiltrate the meninges. Other space-occupying lesions may occur within the brain, e.g. the tuberculoma, a localised tuberculous abscess, which may calcify.

Vascular Disorders. These involve either rupture of a vessel or its obstruction by thrombosis. Subarachnoid haemorrhage with bleeding directly into the CSF occurs following rupture of one of the arteries forming the circle of Willis at the base of the brain. Such bleeding may also occur into the brain substance and this form of cerebral haemorrhage from other arteries is also associated with hypertension. Then the blood may often break through into the lateral ventricle and hence into the CSF. Atheroma of cerebral, internal carotid or vertebral arteries predisposes to sudden, thrombotic occlusion of an artery with the development of a cerebral infarct of size depending on the calibre and site of the obstructed vessel.

Trauma. Head injury may result in bleeding directly into the CSF or in the development of a subdural haematoma between the dura and the arachnoid. Some bleeding into the CSF occurs during neurosurgical operations. To a minor degree this may happen if a vein is damaged during lumbar puncture. Trauma may also damage the intervertebral discs with prolapse of the central softer material.

Changes in Cerebrospinal Fluid in Disease

Appearance

Normal cerebrospinal fluid is clear and colourless and gives no coagulum or sediment on standing, if kept sterile. Abnormalities in appearance may arise in regard to colour, turbidity and the presence of a coagulum.

Colour. The presence of blood is the main cause of an abnormal colour. Normally no red blood cells should be present. Some may be introduced as a result of trauma while obtaining the fluid. In such cases, the first few drops are most contaminated so that if the first millilitre or two is collected separately, the subsequent fluid should be almost, if not completely, clear. Centrifugation reveals small numbers of cells not easily visible to naked eye inspection. They are, of course, seen on microscopic examination.

Pathologically, blood may be present in subarachnoid haemorrhage, in haemorrhage into the ventricles and following neurosurgical operations. Such blood is more homogeneously mixed with the fluid than is that introduced during collection so that there is not the same disappearance of red cells after the first millilitre or two of fluid has been withdrawn. Furthermore, haemolysis often occurs and the haemoglobin liberated is converted into bilirubin, so that within a day after such a haemorrhage, the supernatant fluid obtained on centrifugation becomes yellow coloured (xanthochromic) to a depth out of proportion to the diminishing number of red cells present. These eventually disappear completely. Xanthochromic fluids are also obtained from the lumbar region when there is a complete block due to spinal tumour.

Cell content. In normal CSF this is only 0 to 4×10^6 /l, present as mononuclears or lymphocytes. In disease states, the number may increase and other normal blood cells may be present, sometimes accompanied by bacterial cells.

In addition to the entry of red cells just discussed, an increase in leucocytes occurs in meningeal irritation, most markedly in acute meningitis. In bacterial meningitis, the cell response is predominantly of polymorphs but in viral meningitis and in tuberculous meningitis the response is mainly lymphocytic and of varying degree. Acute encephalitis produces only small increases in cells, usually mononuclears or lymphocytes, but this non-specific response occurs also in non-infective inflammatory states, and in multiple sclerosis, tumours and following injury of the meninges.

Turbidity. Turbidity is seen when there is marked increase in the number of polymorphs present and so is found in meningitis, more especially in the coccal forms. Fluids from patients with viral or tuberculous meningitis in which the cell response is lymphocytic are not as a rule turbid. At least 400 to 500 polymorphs $\times 10^6$/l are needed to give visible turbidity. Highly purulent fluids may be obtained, e.g. in streptococcal meningitis before antibiotic treatment is started. Small numbers of red cells also give fluids an opalescent appearance. If traces of substances such as alcohol are mixed with the fluid during its collection some opalescence may result.

Coagula. On standing, fibrin clots may form in pathological fluids containing fibrinogen, which is usually only found when there is a considerable increase in protein. The fluids with a very high protein content obtained in patients with spinal tumours may set solid on standing. In tuberculous meningitis a fine web-like coagulum sometimes forms if the fluid is allowed to stand overnight. Such a web may entangle tubercle bacilli, making them more easily seen microscopically than by direct examination of the fluid itself. Hence it may be useful to leave part of the specimen to stand overnight while examining the rest immediately.

Total Protein

Determination of Total Protein

Turbidimetric methods are mainly used. Meulemans (1960) compared several turbidimetric techniques and concluded that trichloracetic acid 30 g/l, was preferable to the earlier reagent, sulphosalicylic acid, also 30 g/l, since different proteins, in this case albumin and globulins, gave a similar degree of turbidity with the former but not the latter unless sodium sulphate was added to a concentration of 70 g/l. However Gerbaut and Macart (1986) have reported differences between human serum albumin, bovine serum albumin and human serum using sulphosalicylic acid/sodium sulphate.

Colorimetric methods include the biuret and Lowry methods. The former are less sensitive and often employ preliminary protein precipitation. The Lowry methods use the Folin-Ciocalteu reagent after alkaline copper treatment and are much more sensitive. Interference from drugs may require a blank prepared from the deproteinised CSF. Dye binding methods include Coomassie Brilliant Blue and Ponceau S. Macart and Gerbaut (1982) reported that addition of sodium dodecyl sulphate to Coomassie Brilliant Blue reduced protein variability. The most sensitive methods utilise the absorption of the peptide bond at 220 nm. Interference from non-protein substances requires either a deproteinised CSF as the blank or preliminary separation of CSF proteins on Sephadex G-50.

Reagents.
1. Sulphosalicylic acid–sodium sulphate solution. Dissolve 30 g sulphosalicylic acid and 70 g anhydrous sodium sulphate in water and make up to 1 l. Filter and store in a dark bottle. Discard if any colour or turbidity develops.
2. Sodium chloride solution, 8·8 g/l.
3. Standards. Dilute serum of known protein content with sodium chloride to obtain solutions containing 1 and 2 g/l.

Technique. Add 0·5 ml centrifuged CSF to 3·5 ml sulphosalicylic acid reagent. Mix immediately and read after 10 min against a reagent blank in a spectrophotometer at 660 nm.

Notes.
1. Although turbidimetric methods are simple and quick they are affected by several factors which modify the particle size produced. Temperature affects the turbidity so that samples and standards should be measured at the same temperature. The turbidity may alter with time and this should be standardised.

2. Standardisation with purified albumin may give different results as it may be partly denatured during preparation. The use of diluted serum is preferred.
3. Interference occurs from the presence of red cells and bacteria.
4. Contamination of CSF with blood invalidates protein results due to the presence of plasma proteins.

INTERPRETATION

Normal lumbar CSF has a protein content of 0·15 to 0·45 g/l, although most are in the range 0·25 to 0·30 g/l. The average figures for cisternal and ventricular fluids are 0·20 and 0·10 g/l respectively. Rather more than half the protein is albumin.

An increase in total protein is the most common abnormality in CSF and results from a breakdown of the blood–CSF and brain–CSF barriers, usually as a consequence of an inflammatory reaction but occasionally if the flow of CSF is obstructed. Albumin is still the predominant protein but depending on the abnormality, globulins appear in varying amount. If the permeability of the barriers is markedly increased, fibrinogen is present and is the precursor of the clot or coagulum found after such an abnormal CSF is allowed to stand. In many conditions the concentration does not exceed 1 g/l though increases of up to 4 g/l are not infrequent in acute meningitis, in polyneuritis, and in the presence of such tumours as acoustic neuroma and meningioma. Values higher than this are rare though occasionally with tumours compressing the spinal cord, the lumbar fluid below the block may have a protein content between 10 g/l and that of plasma, following the passage of proteins through the walls of capillaries drained by obstructed venous plexuses associated with the dura. Such a high protein content accompanied by xanthochromia is referred to as Froin's syndrome.

The increase in CSF protein content is not always accompanied by an increase in cells. Both increase in many infections. Small increases in cells and protein may occur in multiple sclerosis. A disproportionate increase in protein compared with cells is found most commonly in tumours, particularly spinal ones, following cerebral infarction, and in acute post-infective polyneuritis (Guillain–Barré syndrome).

Immunoglobulins

Electrophoresis of CSF shows the presence of many different globulins. Normal CSF consists of approximately 60% albumin, 8% immunoglobulins and 32% other proteins. With careful electrophoresis on agar or agarose gels the immunoglobulins can be further resolved and shown to be of mid- to fast-γ mobility and one or sometimes two faint bands may be visible. Some diseases are associated with a selective increase in γ-globulins with the appearance of slow-γ components and often the presence of extra bands, the so-called 'oligoclonal' pattern. The predominant immunoglobulin is IgG in a concentration of about 30 mg/l with smaller amounts of IgA, about 4 mg/l.

Changes in CSF immunoglobulins are of particular interest in multiple sclerosis. The predominant changes are in IgG. Two main conditions need to be differentiated. There may be an increase in IgG in proportion to the increase in other proteins if the blood–CSF barrier is impaired as occurs in many inflammatory states; alternatively, the barrier may be intact but proteins reach the CSF directly from nervous tissue via the perivascular spaces. Such proteins are usually IgG antibodies accumulating in nervous tissue in association with the disease process. In multiple sclerosis they may be anti-myelin antibodies which accumulate in the plaques of demyelination (McAlpine *et al.*, 1972). The result is a disproportionate increase in CSF IgG. A third factor is the effect of changes in a particular CSF protein concentration as a result of a change in its serum concentration.

It is useful therefore to measure CSF IgG in relation to either the total protein content or the albumin concentration. Rocket immunoelectrophoresis (p. 104) or radial immunodiffusion (p. 93) are usually used for IgG and albumin using appropriately sensitive methodology and standards for the lower levels in CSF than in serum.

INTERPRETATION

The difficulty is to define an index which gives good discrimination between multiple sclerosis and neurosyphilis and other neurological conditions. Fischer-Williams and Roberts (1971) measured the ratio of IgG to total protein and took 14% as the upper limit. A higher result was found in 75% of patients with multiple sclerosis but also in 23% with other conditions. Riddoch and Thompson (1970) took 13% of the total protein content as the dividing line. They obtained higher figures in 62% of patients with multiple sclerosis and in 14% of other neurological disorders and noted the high level of CSF IgG in two cases of IgG myeloma.

Better discrimination is found if serum protein concentrations are also measured. Ganrot and Laurell (1974) plotted the CSF/plasma ratio of IgG against that of albumin and clearly separated the results from patients with multiple sclerosis from those with no detectable neurological disease. This has been taken further, to define an IgG index as:

$$\frac{\text{CSF IgG} \times \text{serum albumin}}{\text{serum IgG} \times \text{CSF albumin}}$$

Tibbling *et al.* (1977) found this to be independent of age and to be the least variable measurement in a reference population with a mean of 0·46 and an SD of 0·06. If there is impairment of the blood–CSF barrier, as in many inflammatory conditions, the IgG index usually remains normal although the CSF/serum ratios for both albumin and IgG increase (Link and Tibbling, 1977a). Synthesis of IgG within the nervous system as in multiple sclerosis is associated with an increase in the IgG index (Link and Tibbling, 1977b). This is the most sensitive of the various indices detecting 86% of patients. The index was slightly increased in 20% of other conditions but rarely more than 3 SD from the mean.

Further information can be obtained using agarose gel or polyacrylamide gel electrophoresis of concentrated CSF followed by conventional staining techniques, or by silver staining (Mehta *et al.*, 1984), immunofixation or immunoblotting of unconcentrated samples. About 90% of multiple sclerosis patients show an oligoclonal pattern of bands in the γ-globulin region of the CSF (Thompson *et al.*, 1979). This picture is not unique to multiple sclerosis and may occur in infections of the nervous system and in combination with a high IgG index in systemic lupus erythematosus (Link and Tibbling, 1977b). The oligoclonal bands in multiple sclerosis are much more likely to have an abnormal kappa/lambda proportion in their light chains than in infections (Link and Muller, 1971) but such an altered ratio is found less often than the increase in IgG index.

Myelin basic protein (MBP) is a component of the myelin sheath and its use in following fluctuations in the activity of multiple sclerosis has been described (Cohen *et al.*, 1976, 1980; Whitaker *et al.*, 1980). However radioimmunoassay of this protein is complicated by *in vivo* fragmentation of MBP and difficulties of raising antisera specific to MBP.

EFFUSIONS

In health, there is little protein in the small amount of fluid in the body cavities and tissue spaces, but in inflammatory disease this can increase up to that found in plasma as a consequence of the passage of protein through the capillary walls into the fluid collection. It is customary to take an arbitrary dividing line for protein content of 20 g/l below which effusions are described as *transudates* and above which they are called *exudates*. There is, in fact, a continuous spectrum of protein content and a varying degree of vascular permeability. If fibrinogen can enter the fluid, it clots on removal and is referred to as a fibrinous exudate. Cells may also enter; if these are polymorphs, the exudate is purulent and if they are red cells, it is referred to as a haemorrhagic exudate. In hypoproteinaemia, e.g. in the nephrotic syndrome, the protein content of the transudate is low, often below 1 g/l, and resembles an ultrafiltrate of plasma. The protein content can be measured by diluting the fluid and applying the turbidimetric method given for CSF (p. 447) or by the biuret reaction (p. 407).

Many substances are present in similar concentrations to those in plasma, except that the chloride content may be somewhat higher in transudates as a consequence of the Donnan equilibrium. The glucose content of infected exudates is often low. Most exudates do not contain fat. Those that do are of various types. True chylous fluids result from admixture with triglyceride-rich chyle from the thoracic duct. Some fat may be present as a result of cell degeneration producing a chyliform fluid. Opalescence may be due to the presence of lecithin or cholesterol, and such fluids are termed pseudochylous. The presence of fat may be suspected by the clarification achieved following shaking with ether and centrifugation.

REFERENCES

Bell J. L., Baron D. N. (1968). *Proc Assoc. Clin. Biochem*; **5**: 63.
Bell J. L., McNeill D. P. O., Dandona P., Wojdyla J. W. (1986). *Clin. Chem*; **32**: 1412.
Berglund A. B., Carlsson L. A., Dahlquist G. G. (1984). *Diabetic Nephropathy*; **3**: 89.
Bernard A. M., Moreau D., Lauwerys R. (1982). *Clin. Chim. Acta*; **126**: 1.
Bradford M. M. (1976). *Anal. Biochem*; **72**: 248.
Christiansen C. K., Ørskov C. (1984). *Diabetic Nephropathy*; **3**: 92.
Cohen S. R., Herndon R. M., McKahnn G. M. (1976). *New Engl. J. Med*; **295**: 1455.
Cohen S. R., Brooks B. R., Herndon R. M., McKahnn G. M. (1980). *Ann. Neurol*; **8**: 25.
Dilena B. A., Penberthy L. A., Fraser C. G. (1983). *Clin. Chem*; **29**: 553.
Doetsch K., Gadsden R. H. (1973). *Clin. Chem*; **19**: 1170.
Fielding B. A., Price D. A., Houlton C. A. (1983). *Clin. Chem*; **29**: 355.
Fischer-Williams M., Roberts R. C. (1971). *Archs Neurol. Chicago*; **25**: 526.
Ganrot K., Laurell C.-B. (1974). *Clin. Chem*; **20**: 571.
Gerbaut L., Macart M. (1986). *Clin. Chem*; **32**: 353.
Glenn G. C. (1978). *Amer. J. Clin. Pathol*; **70**: 513.
Glenn G. C. (1979). *Amer. J. Clin. Pathol*; **72**: 299.
Glenn G. C. (1980). *Amer. J. Clin. Pathol*; **74**: 531.
Glenn G. C., Hathaway T. K. (1977). *Amer. J. Clin. Pathol*; **68**: 153.
Iwata J., Nishikaze O. (1979). *Clin. Chem*; **25**: 1317.

Keen H., Chlouverakis C. (1963). *Lancet*; **2**: 913.

Link H., Muller R. (1971). *Archs Neurol. Chicago*; **25**: 326.

Link H., Tibbling G. (1977). *Scand. J. Clin. Lab. Invest*; **37**: 391(a), 397(b).

Macart M., Gerbaut L. (1982). *Clin. Chim. Acta*; **122**: 93.

McAlpine D., Lumsden C. E., Acheson E. D. (1972). *Multiple Sclerosis. A Reappraisal*, 2nd ed. Chapters 13 to 16. Edinburgh and London: Churchill Livingstone.

McElderry L. A., Tarbit I. F., Cassells-Smith A. J. (1982). *Clin. Chem*; **28**: 356.

Mehta P. D., Mehta S. P., Patrick B. A. (1984). *Clin. Chem*; **30**: 735.

Meulemans O. (1960). *Clin. Chim. Acta*; **5**: 757.

Miles D. W., Mogensen C. E., Gundersen H. J. G. (1970). *Scand. J. Clin. Lab. Invest*; **26**: 5.

Mogensen C. E., Christensen C. K. (1984). *New Engl. J. Med*; **311**; 89.

Nargessi R. D., Landon J., Pourfarzaneh M., Smith D. S. (1978). *Clin. Chim. Acta*; **89**: 455.

Nishi H. H., Elin R. J. (1985). *Clin. Chem*; **31**: 1377.

Pesce M. A., Strande C. S. (1973). *Clin. Chem*; **19**: 1265.

Riddoch D., Thompson R. A. (1970). *Brit. Med. J*; **1**: 396.

Sathianathan P., Rege V. P., Barron J. L. (1986). *Clin. Chem*; **32**: 202.

Shephard M. D. S., Penberthy L. A., Fraser C. G. (1981). *Pathology*; **13**: 543.

Shephard M. D. S., Penberthy L. A., Fraser C. G. (1982). *Pathology*; **14**: 327.

Teppo A. M. (1982). *Clin. Chem*; **28**: 1359.

Thompson E. J. *et al.* (1979). *Brit. Med. J*; **1**: 16.

Tibbling G., Link H., Ohman S. (1977). *Scand. J. Clin. Lab. Invest*; **37**: 385.

Townsend J. C. (1986). *Clin. Chem*; **32**: 1372.

Viberti G. C. *et al.* (1982). *Lancet*; **1**: 1430.

Whicher J. T. (1985) *United Kingdom External Quality Assessment Scheme (UKEQAS) Report* (unpublished).

Whitaker J. N., Lisch R. P., Bashir R. M. (1980). *Ann. Neurol*; **7**: 58.

21

LIPIDS AND LIPOPROTEINS

The plasma lipids are present as complexes with protein molecules, the lipoproteins, the means by which these mostly insoluble substances are kept in solution. These complexes form large to very large molecules with molecular weights up to 400×10^6. Since changes in plasma lipid concentration in disease reflect alterations in the concentration of the various types of lipoproteins present, it is most satisfactory to consider lipids and lipoproteins together.

LIPIDS

The lipids form a heterogeneous group of substances which, while mostly insoluble in water, are soluble in a group of solvents, the 'fat solvents', among which are chloroform, ether, benzene, light petroleum and hexane. The lipids include fatty acids and some of their esters and some substances which can form such esters. The main groups are:

Non-esterified Fatty Acids (NEFA) or Free Fatty Acids (FFA)

These are straight-chain fatty acids with the formula $C_nH_{2n+1}COOH$ for the saturated fatty acids and $C_nH_{2n-x}COOH$ for the unsaturated in which n is always an odd number, and $x = 1, 3, 5$, or 7 depending on whether there are 1, 2, 3, or 4 double bonds. Fatty acids with two or more double bonds are known as polyunsaturated fatty acids. Examples of fatty acids present in fats are given in Table 21.1. Numbering of fatty acids is from the carboxyl group, the carbon of which is C–1.

The Triglycerides (TG)—Neutral Fat

As their name indicates, these are esters of glycerol with the group formula shown, where R_1, R_2, R_3, are fatty acid radicles. The three fatty acids may be the same or different. The melting point of fat depends on the fatty acids present, the greater the proportion of unsaturated fatty acids the lower the melting point. The melting point also depends, to a lesser extent, on the length of the hydrocarbon chain, the longer this is the higher the melting point. Thus tristearin with three stearic acids melts at 71°C, tripalmitin with three palmitic acids at 60°C, whereas triolein with three oleic acids is liquid at ordinary temperatures.

Oleic acid is the fatty acid found most abundantly in fats with palmitic acid the second most abundant. Both are present in most fats. Of the saturated fatty acids, stearic acid is commonly present in animal fats but only found in small amounts in vegetable fats. The polyunsaturated fatty acids are relatively abundant in fish and vegetable oils but hardly present at all in mammalian fats. Polyunsaturated

TABLE 21.1

Fatty Acids Present in Lipids

I. *Saturated Fatty Acids*, C_nH_{2n+1}. COOH

		n		M. Pt. (°C)
Acetic	*n*-duanoic	1	CH_3.COOH	16·6
Butyric	*n*-tetranoic	3	C_3H_7.COOH	−4·7
Caproic	*n*-hexanoic	5	C_5H_{11}.COOH	−1·5
Caprylic	*n*-octanoic	7	C_7H_{15}.COOH	16·5
Capric	*n*-decanoic	9	C_9H_{19}.COOH	31·5
Lauric	*n*-dodecanoic	11	$C_{11}H_{23}$.COOH	43·6
Myristic	*n*-tetradecanoic	13	$C_{13}H_{27}$.COOH	58·0
Palmitic	*n*-hexadecanoic	15	$C_{15}H_{31}$.COOH	62·9
Stearic	*n*-octadecanoic	17	$C_{17}H_{35}$.COOH	69·9
Arachidic	*n*-eicosanoic	19	$C_{19}H_{39}$.COOH	75·2

II· *Unsaturated Fatty Acids*, C_nH_{2n-x}. COOH

		n	x	
Palmitoleic	Δ^9-hexadecenoic	15	1	$C_{15}H_{29}$.COOH
Oleic	Δ^9-octadecenoic	17	1	$C_{17}H_{33}$.COOH
Linoleic	$\Delta^{9,12}$-octadecadienoic	17	3	$C_{17}H_{31}$.COOH
Linolenic	$\Delta^{9,12,15}$-octadecatrienoic	17	5	$C_{17}H_{29}$.COOH
Arachidonic	$\Delta^{5,8,11,14}$-eicostetraenoic	19	7	$C_{19}H_{31}$.COOH

fatty acids have an important physiological role as precursors of the prostaglandins and, since the human body is unable to synthesise them, they are essential dietary constituents.

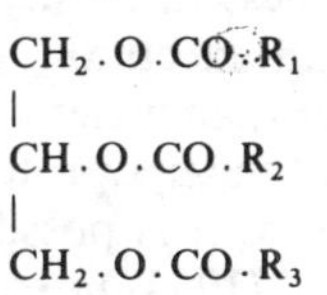

$$CH_2.O.CO.R_1$$
$$|$$
$$CH.O.CO.R_2$$
$$|$$
$$CH_2.O.CO.R_3$$

A triglyceride

$$CH_2.O.CO.R_1$$
$$|$$
$$CH.O.CO.R_2$$
$$|\quad\quad O$$
$$\quad\quad\quad \|$$
$$CH_2-O-P-O-\text{Nitrogen base}$$
$$|$$
$$OH$$

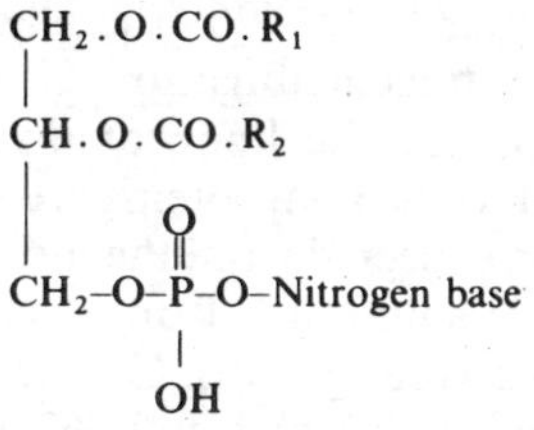

A phospholipid

Phospholipids

Two important groups among the lipids that contain phosphorus are the phosphoglycerides and the sphingomyelins.

The *phosphoglycerides* are esters of glycerol containing two fatty acids and one phosphoric acid to which is linked a nitrogenous base. The latter is choline in the lecithins, the most common of these compounds, and ethanolamine or serine in the cephalins.

The *sphingomyelins* do not contain glycerol; instead they possess a long chain aliphatic aminoalcohol, sphingosine. In the sphingomyelins a fatty acid forms an amide with the amine group, phosphate forms an ester link with the hydroxyl group and choline is attached to the phosphate.

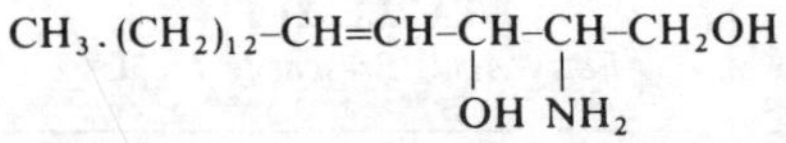

$$CH_3 . (CH_2)_{12}-CH=CH-CH-CH-CH_2OH$$

$$OH \quad NH_2$$

Sphingosine

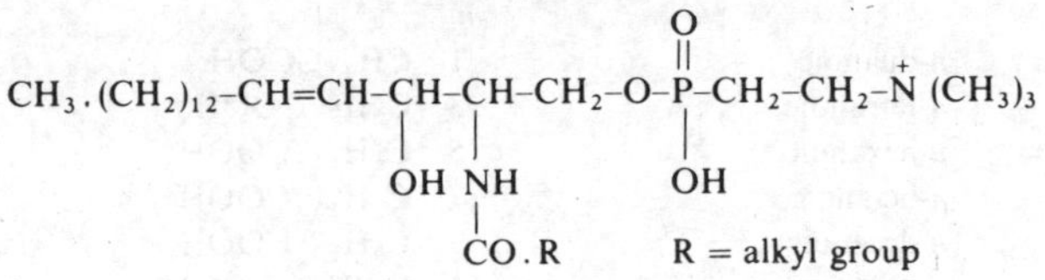

$$O$$
$$\|$$
$$CH_3 . (CH_2)_{12}-CH=CH-CH-CH-CH_2-O-P-CH_2-CH_2-\overset{+}{N}(CH_3)_3$$

$$OH \quad NH \qquad\qquad OH$$

$$CO . R \qquad R = alkyl\ group$$

Sphingomyelins

Cholesterol and Cholesterol Esters

Steroids, of which cholesterol is one, are soluble in fat solvents. As an alcohol it forms esters, those present in the body being with oleic, linoleic and palmitic acids in the main, although small amounts of other fatty acids are also present.

Other Lipids

Several other compounds may be found in tissue extracts using fat solvents. These include other sterols, other sphingolipids, fat-soluble vitamins, carotenes, prostaglandins and bilirubin.

PLASMA LIPOPROTEINS

As shown in Chapter 19 (p. 406), the plasma proteins have been separated into several groups by ultracentrifugation. Usually the S value increases with the mol. wt. of the protein but the lipoproteins are an exception. In these, the lipid fractions attached to the apoproteins are lighter than water so that the S value is less than would be expected from the mol. wt. of the lipoprotein. By centrifuging in sodium chloride solutions of different density, it is possible to separate the lipoproteins into several groups. Gofman *et al.* (1954) introduced the use of a solution the density of which was 1·063 g/ml. This divides the lipoproteins into two main groups, those which float (lower density), and those which sediment. The lighter fraction is further separated in terms of the $S_f(d = 1·063)$, the Svedberg flotation index in the fluid. This index is higher the lower the density of the particles and allows division into chylomicrons, very low density lipoproteins (VLDL), intermediate density lipoproteins (IDL) and low density lipoproteins (LDL). By using a solution of density 1·21 g/ml, the higher density fraction is further separated in terms of the d = 1·21 values. The resulting subdivisions are shown in Tables 21.2 and 21.3.

Chylomicrons

These exogenous fat particles are formed in the intestinal mucosa following re-synthesis of triglycerides from the products of fat digestion in the small intestine. With a diameter of up to one micrometre, they are kept in emulsion form by a hydrophilic surface layer of protein. Chylomicrons pass into the lacteals of the

TABLE 21.2

Physical Characteristics of Lipoproteins

	Density (g/ml)	S_f (d = 1·063)	Electrophoretic mobility	Mol. Wt.	Diameter (nm)
Chylomicrons	0·95	400	Origin	4×10^8	75–1000
VLDL	0·95–1·006	20–400	Pre-β	5–10×10^6	25–70
IDL	1·006–1·019	12–20	β	$3·9$–$4·8 \times 10^6$	22–24
LDL	1·019–1·063	0–12	β	$2·75 \times 10^6$	20–22
HDL	1·063–1·21		α_1		
HDL$_2$	1·063–1·125	4–20*		$3·6 \times 10^5$	7·5–10
HDL$_3$	1·125–1·21	0–4*		$1·75 \times 10^5$	4–7

* Values determined at d = 1·21.

TABLE 21.3

Chemical Composition of Lipoproteins
(Figures are per cent of total)

	Protein	Triglyceride	Phospholipid	Cholesterol Free	Ester	NEFA
Chylomicrons	2	87	7	1	3	—
VLDL	8	54	18	7	12	1
IDL	11	26	24	10	28	1
LDL	21	10	23	8	37	1
HDL	50	6	24	2	18	—
HDL$_2$	33	11	27	6	21	1
HDL$_3$	56	6	22	4	10	2

intestinal villi to enter the thoracic duct which drains into the great veins at the root of the neck. They are responsible for the visible opalescence of plasma following a meal rich in fat. As they circulate in the blood, triglycerides are stripped off by the action of lipoprotein lipase present on the endothelium of extrahepatic tissues leaving remnant particles that are, for the most part, metabolised in the liver.

Very Low Density Lipoproteins

These endogenous fat particles cover a wide range of size, density and S_f values, merging at one end of their range with the chylomicrons and at the other end with IDL. They appear to be mostly synthesised in the liver and are rich in triglycerides formed from fatty acids reaching that organ by the circulation or formed in the liver from carbohydrate present in excess of the body's immediate requirements. They therefore act as transporting agents for endogenously formed triglycerides.

Intermediate Density Lipoproteins

These are lower in their triglyceride content and richer in cholesterol than VLDL from which they are produced by the action of lipoprotein lipase. They are virtually absent in plasma from normal fasting subjects, but are present at high concentration in patients with type III hyperlipoproteinaemia (p. 470).

Low Density Lipoproteins

These are produced by the further removal of triglyceride from IDL, probably by the action of hepatic triglyceride lipase. In addition to the removal of triglycerides, the conversion of VLDL to LDL is accompanied by other changes affecting the lipid and apoprotein composition of the particle (Fig. 21.1). LDL are particularly rich in cholesterol which on average forms 40–50 % of their weight, with ester cholesterol about three-quarters of this. They are also rich in phospholipids. ,

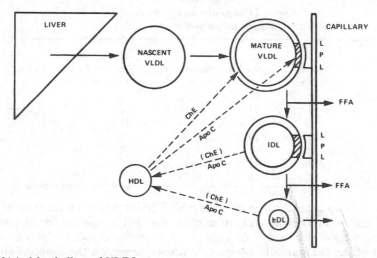

Fig. 21.1. Metabolism of VLDL.
Maturation of nascent VLDL follows transfer of cholesterol ester (ChE) and apoprotein C (Apo C) from HDL. Apo C activates lipoprotein lipase (LPL) in the capillary wall allowing free fatty acids (FFA) to enter tissues. The end product is LDL but during the degradation some ChE and Apo C is transferred back to HDL from intermediate density lipoprotein (IDL) and LDL.

High Density Lipoproteins

These contain the highest protein concentration. The division into three sub-fractions is based on ultracentrifugal behaviour. HDL$_1$, the least dense, is only a very minor component. HDL$_3$ is the form in which HDL are released from the liver where they are formed. Conversion into HDL$_2$ is accompanied by an increase in cholesterol ester content. This results from the activity of the plasma enzyme, lecithin-cholesterol acyl transferase (LCAT), which transfers a fatty acid (mainly linoleic acid) from lecithin to free cholesterol.

$$
\text{Cholesterol} + \begin{array}{l} CH_2.O.COR_1 \\ | \\ CH.O..COR_2 \\ | \\ CH_2.O.\textcircled{P}.\text{choline} \end{array} \xrightarrow{\text{LCAT}} \text{Cholesterol ester} + \begin{array}{l} CH_2.O.COR_1 \\ | \\ CHOH \\ | \\ CH_2.O.\textcircled{P}.\text{choline} \end{array}
$$

Lecithin   ($R_2.CO-$ form)   Lysolecithin

The free cholesterol is partly derived from HDL_3 and, in part, from other plasma sources which are in equilibrium with the tissue pools of cholesterol. HDL are thus concerned with the mobilisation of tissue cholesterol and its transfer to the liver where HDL_2 are degraded (Fig. 21.2). The released cholesterol is partly converted to bile acids and salts and appears in the bile with them. Another important function of HDL is to act as a source of cholesterol esters and apolipoprotein C for transfer to newly formed VLDL.

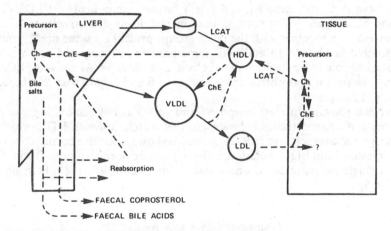

Fig. 21.2. Mobilisation of Cholesterol from Tissue Pools.
LDL is degraded in tissues releasing cholesterol into the tissue pool which is in equilibrium with the free cholesterol of plasma. Removal of this involves its uptake and esterification by HDL and LCAT and final degradation of the HDL in the liver releasing cholesterol into the liver pool. Cholesterol is partly converted to bile salts and these are excreted into the bile with unchanged cholesterol. Some intestinal reabsorption occurs and the remainder is degraded and excreted in the faeces.

Lp(a) Lipoprotein

This protein is also known as 'sinking pre-β' because it has pre-β mobility on electrophoresis, but unlike VLDL, which share its position on electrophoresis, it sediments on ultracentrifugation in a medium of density 1·006. Its lipid content is similar to LDL but its protein composition differs: 65 % is apo-B, 15 % is albumin and 20 % is a specific apoprotein (Albers and Hazzard, 1974). Serum levels of Lp(a) show a skewed distribution and are reported to be subject to genetic regulation. A number of reports suggests an increased risk of coronary heart disease in patients with high levels. The physiological significance of Lp(a) is poorly understood. There is evidence of a relationship between Lp(a) and serum insulin and glucose levels (Dahlen and Berg, 1979).

Lipoprotein-X

This lipoprotein is not detectable in serum from normal subjects but is present in the majority of patients with obstructive jaundice and those with LCAT deficiency. The molecule consists of 66 % phospholipid, 22 % free cholesterol, 3 % cholesterol ester, 6 % protein, 3 % triglyceride and 2–3 % bile acid. The protein is 40 % albumin and 60 % apolipoprotein C (Seidel *et al.*, 1973).

Apolipoproteins

Currently, some ten peptides have been identified as comprising the apolipo-protein population. Those that have been most studied are AI, AII, B, CI, CII, CIII and E. HDL have AI and AII as major components, with C and E as minor components. Apo-B forms most or all of the protein in LDL. Chylomicrons and VLDL have B, C and some AI, and E is a further component of VLDL. The apolipoproteins play an important part in stabilising the structures of the lipoproteins and, together with the polar groups present on some lipids, render them soluble in plasma. In addition, some have been recognised as having a physiological role in lipoprotein metabolism. For example: AI activates LCAT, CII is a cofactor for lipoprotein lipase, and both B and E have sites that bind to specific cell receptors.

There is a growing interest in apo-A1 and apo-B as risk factors in coronary thrombosis. A1 concentrations show a positive correlation with HDL, which is well recognised as a negative risk factor, and B shows a positive correlation with total cholesterol and LDL cholesterol. There is some evidence the apo-B might be the best single indicator of coronary risk (Sniderman *et al.*, 1980; Durrington *et al.*, 1986).

Non-esterified Fatty Acids

Non-esterified fatty acids (NEFA) are bound to albumin and, because of their rapid turnover, are present in plasma in very small amounts (less than 1 mmol/l). Nevertheless, they form a readily available source of energy to muscle and other tissues when the supply of glucose is reduced and they are an important means by which a source of energy is transported from adipose tissue to other organs.

DIAGNOSTIC TESTS IN DISORDERS OF LIPID METABOLISM

For many years, clinical investigation was limited to the measurement of the lipids. More recently, however, attention has focused on the lipoproteins as the classification of disorders has been increasingly based on changes in the concentrations of one or other of the various fractions.

In research laboratories, the preferred method for measuring lipoproteins is ultracentrifugation but this procedure is not suitable for routine analysis in hospital laboratories. An alternative and more convenient method is lipoprotein electrophoresis; but this technique is not quantitative, and attempts to make it so (e.g. by densitometry) have generally not been very successful. A third approach, described in detail in the 5th edition of this book, was introduced by Stone and Thorp (1966). Medium and large particles, corresponding to VLDL and chylomicrons, are measured nephelometrically after separation by membrane filtration. Small particles corresponding to LDL are estimated from the total cholesterol concentration after making an allowance for the cholesterol contained in the VLDL. The technique is simple to perform and in practice has proved to be a useful diagnostic procedure. The main disadvantages are that it is somewhat time consuming, and it does not provide a measure of HDL.

At the present time, the approach which appears to be gaining widest favour is to measure total cholesterol, total triglycerides and, after chemical precipitation of lipoproteins of lower density, HDL-cholesterol. From these results, LDL-cholesterol can be calculated, provided that severe hypertriglyceridaemia is not present. This analysis enables the lipoprotein composition of most specimens sent for routine analysis to be assessed with reasonable confidence. The exceptions are specimens that show severe mixed hyperlipidaemia, and for these electrophoresis may be used to provide further information.

Determination of Serum Cholesterol

Until recent years, methods were for the most part based on the ability of cholesterol to be converted to highly coloured substances in strong acid solvents that possess dehydrating, oxidising and sulphonating properties. The Liebermann–Burchard reaction, which gives a green colour, and the Salkowski reaction, which gives a red colour, have long been known as qualitative tests and have been the basis of many quantitative methods. The solvent system includes acetic acid, acetic anhydride and sulphuric acid to which, in some cases, is added another acid, usually an aromatic sulphonic acid. The reaction involves the '3-hydroxy-5-ene' part of the cholesterol molecule which is first dehydrated to form cholesta-3,5-diene and then oxidised by the sulphuric acid to link two molecules together as bis-cholesta-3,5-diene. This material can be sulphonated by the

Cholesterol

sulphuric acid or added sulphonic acid to produce mono- and di-sulphonic acids which are highly coloured. The former are green (Liebermann–Burchard reaction) but in the presence of more sulphuric acid and by the catalytic action of added metal ions, particularly Fe^{3+}, the disulphonic acids are preferentially formed and are red (Salkowski reaction). The red product has the higher molar absorption coefficient but in each reaction the products are probably not single substances because side-reactions, often difficult to control, also occur. The reaction conditions therefore need to be carefully adhered to and this may be easier to achieve by automated procedures.

Other difficulties arise when assaying serum specimens. Lipoprotein cholesterol exists in esterified and 'free' (non-esterified) forms that may react differently; other sterols present in small quantities may also react, and the presence of coloured substances such as bilirubin or haemoglobin may cause interference. Preliminary extraction of lipids and hydrolysis of the ester cholesterol to the 'free' form are among the steps that have been taken to improve specificity, but such improvements are often at the expense of time. Furthermore, increased complexity of method can result in poor precision in inexperienced hands. Over recent years, enzymatic methods have been introduced and these, as a result of their ease of use, precision and relative specificity, have largely replaced the older methods in clinical laboratories. For those who require further information about the non-enzymatic methods, the 5th edition of this book provides details. The remainder of this section will be concerned with enzymatic methods.

Enzymatic Methods

Assays have been developed by Richmond (1972) and Flegg (1973) in which cholesterol oxidase (EC 1.1.3.6) obtained from the bacterium *Nocardia erythropolis* is used to convert cholesterol into cholest-4-en-3-one with formation of hydrogen peroxide. The cholest-4-en-3-one formed has been measured by reading at 240 nm after extracting into isopropanol (Flegg, 1973). Alternatively, the hydrogen peroxide has been quantified by formation of a chelate complex with quadrivalent titanium and xylenol orange (Richmond, 1973); by the reaction with peroxidase in the presence of *o*-dianisidine (Tarbutton and Gunter, 1974); by its reaction with methanol in the presence of catalase to give formaldehyde, which is estimated by the Hantzsch reaction; and finally, as used by Allain *et al.* (1974), by determining the hydrogen peroxide with Trinder's reagents: 4-aminophenazone, phenol, and peroxidase. The latter seems to be the best technique for the final stage in the enzymatic method and is now used in the kits available from several manufacturers.

The enzyme reacts only with free cholesterol so, for the determination of total cholesterol, the ester cholesterol has to be hydrolysed. This can be done chemically using ethanolic potassium hydroxide, or by using cholesterol ester hydrolase (EC 3.1.1.13). This enzyme was isolated from pig pancreas and rat pancreatic juice by Hernandez and Chaikoff (1957) and applied to the hydrolysis of these esters by Allain *et al.* (1974). The kits referred to above are fully enzymatic with a colorimetric end-point.

Manual Method for Cholesterol (Allain *et al.*, 1974)

Reagent. The composition of the single reagent solution is: sodium cholate 3 mmol/l, 4-aminophenazone 0·82 mmol/l, phenol 14 mmol/l, Na_2HPO_4 50 mmol/l, NaH_2PO_4 50 mmol/l, Carbowax-6000 0·17 mmol/l, cholesterol ester hydrolase 33U/l, cholesterol oxidase 117 U/l, peroxidase 67 000 U/l; pH 6·7. The reagent blank solution is similar but the cholesterol esterase and oxidase are omitted.

Technique. Add 30 μl serum to 3 ml reagent solution and 3 ml reagent blank solution. Incubate for 10 min at 37°C. Measure the absorbance at 500 nm of the test against the reagent blank.

Notes.
1. Several manufacturers supply the reagents for this procedure (sometimes with modifications) ready made up as kits and most laboratories prefer to use the commercial products.
2. In the original method, Allain *et al.* (1974) employed a standard curve using cholesterol diluted in isopropanol in place of the test sample. However, single-point calibration may be used over the linear part of the curve and

this extends from 0 to nearly 20 mmol/l with some commercial kits. Some manufacturers recommend that the result be calculated from the absorbance change using the absorption coefficient.

3. In the original paper, reagent stability was given as 6 h at room temperature or 24 h at 4°C. Commercial kits are stable for some weeks.

4. *Specificity.* Cholesterol oxidase is specific for 3β sterols and requires a double bond at Δ^4 or Δ^5. Consequently, a number of other sterols will be measured with cholesterol but these are present in comparatively low concentration in normal serum.

Automated Methods

The enzymatic procedure has been adopted for automation on a wide range of instruments including continuous flow and discrete analysers. Most manufacturers of commercial kits provide details of modifications to their methods appropriate to at least some individual machines. Generally, automated methods produce results of better quality than manual methods, particularly when the machine employed offers facilities for reagent and, ideally, sample blanking. In this respect, certain centrifugal analysers are particularly suitable. The average between-batch precision for automated methods is 0·10 mmol/l compared with 0·18 mmol/l for manual techniques. Continuous flow methods give results on average about 0·1 mmol/l higher than those using discrete analysers or manual techniques.

Another advantage provided by many modern analytical machines is low reagent consumption, which provides cost benefits. To some extent, the choice of method for individual laboratories will be a matter of selecting commercial reagents that enable the method most suited to the analysers they possess to be used. Most of the methods in use are based on the cholesterol esterase/cholesterol oxidase procedure described above.

Determination of HDL Cholesterol.

LDL, VLDL, and chlyomicrons are precipitated by polyanions in the presence of metal ions to leave HDL in solution. The cholesterol content of the supernatant fluid is then determined by the enzymatic method. The two most commonly used precipitants are phosphotungstate/magnesium (see Burstein *et al.*, 1970) and heparin/manganese (see also Warnick and Albers, 1978). They are discussed in the News Sheet, Association of Clinical Biochemists, London: No. 190 (1979).

1. Phosphotungstate/Magnesium Method

Reagents.
1. Phosphotungstate reagent. Dissolve 22·5 g phosphotungstic acid AR grade in 200 ml water, add 80 ml 1 mol/l sodium hydroxide and make to 500 ml with water.
2. Magnesium chloride solution, 2 mol/l. Dissolve 101·7 g $MgCl_2$, $6H_2O$ in water and make to 250 ml.
3. Tris buffer, 10 mmol/l, pH 7·6. Dissolve 1·21 g tris in 900 ml water, adjust to pH 7·6 with 1 mol/l hydrochloric acid and dilute to 1 litre.

Technique. Place 1 ml serum in a centrifuge tube, add 0·1 ml reagent (1) and mix on a vortex mixer for 10 s. Add 50 μl reagent (2) and re-mix similarly.

Centrifuge at ambient temperature for 30 min at 1500 g ensuring that the temperature does not increase appreciably. Carefully remove the clear supernatant for analysis, avoiding any surface deposit. If the supernatant is not clear, recentrifuge at a higher speed and, if still slightly turbid, repeat the analysis on serum diluted with an equal volume of the tris buffer. Analyse for cholesterol by an enzymatic method bearing in mind the dilution factor of 1·125 (or 2·25 if diluted serum is used).

2. Heparin/Manganese Method

Reagents.
1. Heparin solution. Dilute one vial of sodium heparin (Grade 1, Sigma London Chemical Co., cat no. H3125) with sodium chloride solution 9 g/l, to give a final concentration of 7500 USP units in each ml.
2. Manganous chloride solution, 2·02 mol/l. Dissolve 40·1 g $MnCl_2$, $4H_2O$ in water and make to 100 ml.

Technique. To 1 ml serum in a centrifuge tube add 0·1 ml reagent (1) and vortex mix for 10 s. Add 50 μl reagent (2) and re-mix similarly. Place in an ice bath for 30 min and then centrifuge at 4°C for 30 min at 1500 g. Carefully remove the clear supernatant for analysis, avoiding any surface deposit. If the supernatant is not clear, re-centrifuge at a higher speed and, if still slightly turbid, repeat the analysis on serum diluted with an equal volume of sodium chloride solution, 9 g/l. Analyse for cholesterol by an enzymatic method bearing in mind the dilution factor of 1·10 (or 2·20 if diluted serum is used).

Calculation. HDL cholesterol (mmol/l) = cholesterol result (mmol/l) × the dilution factor. This is valid for both methods.

Notes.
1. Serum is preferable to plasma and should be stored at 4°C prior to analysis, which should be carried out within 7 days.
2. The patient should preferably be fasting overnight and have been sitting for at least 3 min before venepuncture, rather than lying or standing, in order to reduce the non-analytical variables.
3. Some HDL may be precipitated by the phosphotungstate/Mg^{2+} method and some other lipoproteins present in high concentration are not always fully precipitated by heparin/Mn^{2+} but over a range of samples, the accuracy of the two methods is similar.

Calculation of LDL-Cholesterol Concentration

In specimens in which the triglyceride level does not exceed 4·5 mmol/l, the LDL-cholesterol can be calculated from the following formula (Friedewald *et al.*, 1972):

LDL-Cholesterol = total cholesterol − HDL-cholesterol − 0·46 × triglyceride (all values are in mmol/l).

INTERPRETATION

Total Cholesterol. If conventional criteria for assessing 'normal' values are applied, the range for young adults is around 3·8 to 6·2 mmol/l, being a little higher in men than in women. Values increase with age and the rise is greater in men than in women during the reproductive years; thereafter, levels in women increase to those in men. Levels are highest in the 6 to 7th decades when the upper limits exceed 7·8 mmol/l. However, conventional methods of ascribing reference values may be inappropriate for cholesterol because there is growing evidence to support the view that the nature of the diet in the countries of the affluent West leads to serum cholesterol levels that exacerbate the development of atherosclerosis. Consequently, many authorities have proposed that reference ranges should be based on values that have been shown in epidemiological studies not to be associated with an increased risk of premature atherosclerosis. Upper limits put forward by the NIH Consensus Development Conference (1984) range from 5·17 mmol/l for age 20 to 29 to 6·72 mmol/l at age 40 and over. The issue is too complex for discussion in the space available here, but it should be recognised that if the proposed levels are accepted, there will be a large number of individuals who will, by definition, have hypercholesterolaemia and to provide treatment aimed at lowering serum cholesterol in those individuals would make heavy demands on resources. In the absence of a nationally agreed policy for intervention in hypercholesterolaemia, it would be advisable for laboratories to be cautious in quoting reference values.

Hypercholesterolaemia. Increases are found most characteristically in the primary hyperlipoproteinaemias described on p. 469 and in the nephrotic syndrome, myxoedema, obstructive jaundice and diabetes mellitus, but less consistently and markedly in some other conditions. In the nephrotic syndrome when oedema is present values up to 15 to 18 mmol/l are common and may occasionally reach and exceed 25 mmol/l. Otherwise in chronic glomerulonephritis the cholesterol is within normal limits or slightly increased. This is also the case in most patients with acute glomerulonephritis, at least in the acute phase, but should the disease pass into the subacute stage marked increases can be seen. In diabetes mellitus, levels are by no means invariably increased although values in excess of 10 mmol/l may be seen on occasions. In jaundice, increases occur most commonly when there is obstruction of the large bile ducts. The increase roughly parallels the rise in serum bilirubin. In parenchymatous liver disease findings are more variable. While serum cholesterol may be normal, in many cases increases are seen of appreciable proportion particularly during recovery. Very high values are found in primary (xanthomatous) biliary cirrhosis rising to 26 to 52 mmol/l and somewhat smaller rises are associated with drug-induced cholestasis. Values up to 13 mmol/l occur in myxoedema, the rise roughly paralleling the severity. Smaller increases may be found in hypopituitarism, usually in the range 6·5 to 9·0 mmol/l.

Xanthomatosis is frequently associated with an increase (see Zollner and Wolfram, 1970). Primary xanthomatosis is divided into two groups, in one of which there is raised serum cholesterol, whereas in the other it is within normal limits. In secondary xanthomatosis, the condition accompanies hypercholesterolaemia, arising from one of the conditions mentioned above.

Hypocholesterolaemia. Decreases are not so well defined. Because of the rather wide normal range an appreciable fall may occur in some individuals before the concentration goes below the lower limit of normal. Thus the effect of hyperthyroidism is to reduce the serum cholesterol so that values below 2·6 mmol/l may be found in the severest cases. Most results remain within the normal range and the determination is of limited value in this condition. Low values are not infrequently obtained in pernicious anaemia and other anaemias, in haemolytic jaundice, in the malabsorption syndrome, severe malnutrition, acute infections and in terminal states. Figures falling below 2·6 mmol/l are seen in some cases.

Very low figures occur in abetalipoproteinaemia and, to a lesser degree, in familial hypobetalipoproteinaemias. Therapeutic reduction of serum cholesterol is seen during administration of clofibrate, cholestyramine, nicotinic acid and D-thyroxine and sometimes accompanies chlorpropamide or phenformin therapy.

HDL Cholesterol. Interest in HDL cholesterol has largely arisen from the finding that the serum concentration is a negative risk factor for coronary heart disease (Miller *et al.,* 1977; Gordon *et al.,* 1977). A number of studies indicate that the mean serum level for men lies between 1·1 and 1·2 mmol/l, with mean values for women 20 to 30 % higher. Gordon *et al.* (1977) showed that the incidence of coronary heart disease increased as values fell progressively below 1·17 mmol/l, and diminished as levels increased above this figure. The risk for subjects with values of 0·91 mmol/l or less was more than eight times that for subjects with levels of 1·68 mmol/l or greater.

Determination of Triglycerides

Earlier methods for triglycerides were indirect. Saponification liberated glycerol from triglycerides and phospholipids and converted the fatty acids from them, and from cholesterol esters, to soaps. Subsequent acidification freed the fatty acids so that total fatty acids could be titrated. Alternatively, total esterified fatty acids were determined by the hydroxamic acid method of Stern and Shapiro (1953). In each case, phospholipids and cholesterol esters had to be determined and the fatty acids present in them calculated and subtracted using factors derived from the average mol. wt. of the fatty acids present. As several estimations thus had to be made, precision was poor, particularly at low values, although in hypertriglyceridaemia useful results could be obtained.

Later, such methods were largely superseded by techniques in which the glycerol liberated by saponification was measured chemically. Phospholipids were first removed by absorption onto zeolite, which was sometimes mixed with other absorbents such as Lloyd's reagent (hydrated aluminium silicate). The triglycerides were then saponified, usually by alcoholic potassium hydroxide. Fatty acids and cholesterol were removed by a dilute acid/organic solvent partition procedure in which the contaminants passed into the organic phase leaving glycerol in the aqueous phase. Finally, glycerol was oxidised by metaperiodate to formaldehyde, which was measured colorimetrically following its reaction with chromotropic acid or, alternatively, either colorimetrically or fluorimetrically after treatment with acetyl acetone and ammonia (the Hantzsch reaction).

Enzymatic methods. The chemical methods outlined above have now been replaced by enzymatic assays in the majority of clinical laboratories. These methods employ lipase for the hydrolysis of the triglycerides coupled with enzymatic procedures for measuring the glycerol released.

In one of the earliest enzymatic methods it was reported that none of the lipases investigated (from *A. niger, G. candidum,* hog pancreas and *R. delemar*) would produce complete hydrolysis of the triglycerides but it was demonstrated that the enzyme from *R. delemar* would do so in the presence of alpha chymotrypsin (Bucolo and David, 1973). Subsequently, other authors have used lipases that were found to produce complete hydrolysis without requiring a proteolytic enzyme: Megraw *et al.* (1979) used the enzyme from *R. arrhizus;* Fossati and Prencipe (1982) used *C. viscosum* lipase. Currently, triglyceride methods fall into two groups depending on whether glycerol measurement is based on glycerol dehydrogenase (EC 1.1.1.6) or glycerol kinase (EC 2.7.1.30).

Glycerol dehydrogenase acts on glycerol in the presence of NAD^+ to produce dihydroxyacetone and NADH. The reaction is measured by the change in absorbance at 340 nm (Grossman *et al.*, 1976). The method has been criticised because of unfavourable equilibrium due to product inhibition, sensitivity to pH and lack of linearity.

Glycerol kinase, which is used much more frequently, acts on glycerol in the presence of ATP to produce glycerol-3-phosphate and ADP. Either of these products may be measured by further enzymatic reactions. ADP was measured in the method described by Bucolo and David. In the presence of phosphoenol pyruvate and pyruvate kinase (EC 2.7.1.40), ADP is converted to ATP and pyruvate is generated. Pyruvate is then converted to lactate by the action of lactate dehydrogenase (EC 1.1.1.27) with the equimolar conversion of NADH to NAD^+. The reaction is monitored by the change in absorbance at 340 nm. A disadvantage of this method is that serum components cause NADH consumption additional to that due to glycerol: ideally, a specimen blank should be run with lipase omitted from the reagent mixture.

Methods which measure the glycerol-3-phosphate produced by glycerol kinase are divided into those that use glycerol phosphate dehydrogenase (EC 1.1.1.8; GPDH) and those that use glycerol-3-phosphate oxidase (EC 2.7.1.30; GPO) for the next step.

Glycerol-3-phosphate is converted by GPDH to dihydroxyacetone phosphate with the equimolar reduction of NAD^+, which can be measured by the change in absorbance at 340 nm. A modification of this procedure was introduced by Megraw *et al.* (1979), who added diaphorase (EC 1.6.4.3) and INT (2-(*p*-iodophenyl)-3-(*p*-nitrophenyl)-5-phenyltetrazolium) to the reaction mixture. In the presence of diaphorase, the NADH generated by the earlier reactions reduces the INT to formazan, which is measured colorimetrically at 500 to 550 nm. An evaluation of five commercial kits based on this method was reported by Walker *et al.* (1982). The results showed a close correlation with those obtained by a fluorimetric method and three gave coefficients of variation better than 5%. Sample blanks were not included in any of the methods used in the study.

In GPO methods, glycerol-3-phosphate is converted in the presence of oxygen to dihydroxyacetone and hydrogen peroxide. In turn, the hydrogen peroxide is acted on by peroxidase in the presence of a suitable chromogen which is oxidised to a coloured product. Fossati and Prencipe (1982) used 4-aminophenazone, 3,5-dichloro-2-hydroxy-benzene sulphonic acid and potassium ferrocyanide as the chromogenic mixture from which the coloured product is quinone monoimine, which gives maximum absorbance at 510 nm. They investigated a number of substances for possible interference with the assay and concluded that ascorbic acid was the only material that might interfere at 'clinically realistic' concentrations but even at an ascorbate concentration of 380 μmol/l they recovered an average of 90% of triglyceride. Bilirubin and haemoglobin gave no interference at levels up to 170 μmol/l and 10 g/l respectively. The method has become known as the GPO–PAP method.

A problem that relates to all of the methods described above is that free glycerol present in the specimens will be measured as triglyceride unless modifications to the methods are introduced. In normal subjects the concentration of free glycerol in serum is low and it is common practice to reduce the triglyceride result by 0·11 mmol/l to allow for it. However, recent reports (Elin *et al.*, 1983; ter Welle *et al.*, 1984) indicate that patients with lipid disorders may have significantly higher levels. Free glycerol may be determined in a separate assay using the reagents employed in the triglyceride assay but omitting the lipase. Sulivan *et al.* (1985) introduced a modification to the GPO-PAP method in which the specimen is pre-incubated with GPO and peroxidase to destroy the free glycerol. Lipase and the chromogenic substrate are then added to measure triglyceride.

At the present time it is difficult to recommend a method for triglyceride measurement. A number of improvements in methodology have appeared only recently and consequently there are no up-to-date reports of comparisons that include the latest methods. Most of the methods described above, sometimes with modifications, appear among the kits of commercial manufacturers, and some manufacturers include more than one method in their catalogue, emphasising perhaps that no method has yet become established as the best.

If an automated method is to be used, the choice of method must obviously be related to the machine on which the analysis is to be performed. Methods exist for all analysers in common use, and most reagent manufacturers will provide method sheets that enable their reagents to be used on at least some of these machines. The suitability of any machine for any particular method may depend on such factors as its capability to handle sample and reagent blanking, its ability to carry out multiple reagent additions, and whether it will perform kinetic analysis or end-point determinations only. The range of possible combinations of methods and machines is too wide to discuss here: a study of reports from interlaboratory QC schemes will give some guide to successful combinations.

In general, automated methods using any of the enzyme systems described above have an average between-batch precision of 0·06 mmol/l with the exception of glycerol kinase kinetic methods (0·09 mmol/l). Manual enzymic methods, as expected, show somewhat worse precision, an average figure being 0·11 mmol/l for both kinetic and end-point methods.

INTERPRETATION

Serum or plasma should be obtained from fasting patients as otherwise physiological chylomicronaemia may be difficult to distinguish from an increase in VLDL. The normal range for triglycerides may be taken as 0·11 to 1·60 mmol/l up to the age of 30, with an increase at the upper end with increasing age to 1·83 mmol/l at 50, and 2·17 mmol/l at 60. The normal range for endogenous glycerol is 0·05 to 0·18 mmol/l.

Moderate increases are seen in obesity and these will often return to normal following weight reduction. Other increases may be primary (discussed below, p. 469) or secondary. The most common secondary hypertriglyceridaemia accompanies diabetes mellitus and is greater the less satisfactory the treatment. A similar increase is seen in Von Gierke's disease (Type 1 glycogen storage disease), alcoholism and in hypothyroidism. Increases up to 3·4 to 4·6 mmol/l occur in the nephrotic syndrome, in general paralleling the degree of hypoalbuminaemia. There is a well recognised association between hyperuricaemia and hypertriglyceridaemia.

Serum triglyceride values are decreased following large doses of ascorbic acid and during the administration of halofenate, heparin, oral hypoglycaemic drugs such as metformin and phenformin, and oxandrolene or oxymethalone. Therapeutic agents which are intended to reduce high levels of triglyceride include clofibrate and bezafibrate. Increases in serum triglycerides occur during oestrogen administration, including oral contraceptive preparations, and following ethanol ingestion. Other drugs which may cause hypertriglyceridaemia include the beta-blockers, thiazides and synthetic retinoids.

Determination of Phospholipids

The technique most used for phospholipids has been to extract them into a suitable solvent, e.g. ethanol–ether, and then to digest an aliquot of the extract with sulphuric acid and hydrogen peroxide to oxidise the phosphorus to inorganic phosphate, which can be measured by a variety of methods. Youngberg and Youngberg (1930) used the Fiske and Subbarow technique (1925); others have applied Gomori's method (1942) using metol, e.g. Varley (1967), while Henry (1964) used N-phenyl-p-phenylene diamine (semidine) a reagent introduced by Dryer *et al.* (1957). A different approach is that of Zilversmit and Davis (1950) who precipitated proteins with trichloracetic acid and digested the precipitate, which contains the phospholipids, with a sulphuric-perchloric acid mixture. Again, the inorganic phosphate formed is determined by one of the techniques used to determine serum inorganic phosphate.

Currently, enzymatic methods are being introduced. For example, in the phospholipids B-test marketed by Wako Pure Chemical Industries Limited, phospholipase D reacts with phospholipids to release choline which in turn reacts with choline oxidase to yield betaine and hydrogen peroxide. The latter product is then measured colorimetrically by its reaction with phenol and aminophenazone in the presence of peroxidase. An alternative approach was described by Blaton *et al.* (1983) who used phospholipase C and sphingomyelinase to release choline phosphate, which was hydrolysed by alkaline phosphatase to choline and phosphate. Phosphate could then be measured colorimetrically by ammonium vanadate, or choline measured by the choline oxidase method as described above.

INTERPRETATION

Normal values for serum lipid phosphorus in the post-absorptive state are 1·9 to 3·6 mmol/l. There is rather more in whole blood since the cells contain about twice as much as the plasma. The serum phospholipid bears a close relationship to the serum cholesterol and increases in those conditions in which the cholesterol is increased, although to a lesser degree. This applies to liver and biliary tract disease, diabetes mellitus and myxoedema.

Investigation of Lipoproteins

Visual Inspection of Plasma or Serum

Valuable information can be gained simply by looking at the specimens to be analysed. Because of their large molecular size, the exogenous and endogenous particles (chylomicrons and VLDL) scatter light and are responsible for the turbidity of serum. In fasting specimens from normolipaemic subjects, chylomicrons are absent and the concentration of VLDL is sufficient to confer at most only slight turbidity. The presence of increased turbidity is indicative therefore of an increase in either or both of these lipoproteins. If the specimen is left to stand overnight in the refrigerator, chylomicrons will float to the surface to form a creamy layer whereas VLDL will remain dispersed throughout the specimen. In a small minority of specimens, increased turbidity is the result of elevated levels of IDL—the significance of this finding will be discussed below (p. 470).

Electrophoresis

Paper electrophoresis was used as early as 1952 by Fasoli, who used the stain Sudan III; Swahn, who used Sudan Black and Durrum *et al.* who used Oil Red O. The run was carried out on fairly wide strips, which were then cut lengthwise in two, one half being stained for proteins and the other for lipoproteins so that, on realigning the strips, the protein fraction to which the lipoproteins belonged could be seen. Later, Hatch and Lees (1968) added albumin to the buffer, a modification found by several workers to improve resolution. Oil Red O was the stain, used.

Electrophoresis on *cellulose acetate* was found to have several advantages including a shorter running time, a smaller sample, better resolution, and less trouble from adsorption of the lipoproteins on to the medium. There are, however, problems in staining the strips. Because of the lipophilic nature of cellulose acetate, it resists destaining when fat stains have been used. Kohn and Feinberg (1965) resolved the difficulty by staining with Schiff's reagent after first oxidizing the lipids with ozone liberated from barium peroxide by concentrated sulphuric acid. However, the technique is rather unsatisfactory as the reagents are unpleasant and hazardous to use and, in addition, it is difficult to achieve uniform staining of the bands. A more acceptable procedure makes use of the finding that alkali treatment of cellulose acetate enables destaining to be carried out when fat stains, such as Fat Red B, are used (Golfs and Verheyden, 1967). The disadvantage of this approach is that the cellulose acetate strip becomes very limp but plastic sheets can be used to provide support. Reagents for this method, including cellulose acetate strips ready prepared with plastic backing, may be purchased from Gelman Sciences and Helena Laboratories.

Agar gel was soon applied to the separation of lipoproteins (Giri, 1956; Cawley and Eberhardt, 1962; Noble, 1968). With the removal of anionic groups (mainly sulphate) from agar to give agarose, the rate of electroendosmosis and the interaction between the medium and the lipoproteins were lessened. *Agarose* has been used by several workers including Rapp and Kahlke (1968), Noble (1968), McGlashan and Pilkington (1968) and Papadopoulos and Kintzios (1969). Rapp (1967) included bromophenol blue-stained albumin and vitamin B_{12} as markers in each run. The albumin showed the limit of protein migration to the anode while the coloured vitamin B_{12} showed the effect of electroendosmosis.

Agarose Gel Electrophoresis

Reagents.
1. Tris-barbitone buffer, pH 8·8. Dissolve 57·8 g tris(hydroxymethyl)methyl-amine and 97·6 g sodium barbitone in distilled water and make up to 10 l.
2. Agarose in tris-barbitone buffer, 1%. Dissolve 5 g agarose in 500 ml buffer by heating in a boiling water bath. Store in 10 ml aliquots at 4°C.
3. Stain. Fat Red 7B, 0·225 g/l in methanol. Dilute 30 ml with 6 ml distilled water immediately prior to use.
4. Rinse solution, 50% methanol in water.
5. Equipment (e.g. Shandon). Electrophoresis tank, levelling table, micro-applicators, power pack.

Technique. Melt a tube of agar and pour onto a glass slide (9 cm × 9 cm) on a level surface. Allow to set and place in a refrigerator for 15 min to harden. Lay the plate on a sheet of graph paper and apply the specimens in a row 3 cm from the end of the plate using a microapplicator. One of the specimens should be from a normolipaemic subject to act as a control. A small crystal of bromophenol blue added to this specimen prior to application will stain the albumin blue and act as a marker. Carry out electrophoresis at 200 V until the stained albumin in the marker specimen has migrated 3·5 to 4 cm. Remove the plate and dry under a warm air blower. Place the plate in the staining solution for 3 to 5 min, then wash in the rinse solution until the background is clear. Finally, dry in air.

Notes.

1. An alternative approach is to apply the samples to slots in the gel. These are formed by placing a broad-toothed 'comb' across the breadth of the gel before it has set (Mills *et al.*, 1984; this reference provides a detailed discussion of electrophoresis and other lipoprotein techniques).
2. Instead of glass plates, Gel-bond film may be used to support the gel. This is a less bulky material and is therefore more convenient for storage.
3. Commercially prepared plates may be obtained from Corning (Universal electrophoretic film, agarose). These may be used with a variety of electrophoretic tanks but the model that was designed specifically for them is particularly convenient. The gels are supplied moulded to templates that form slots for the specimens.

INTERPRETATION

In fasting serum from normal individuals, three bands are seen. These represent, in order of increasing mobility, the β, pre-β and alpha lipoproteins, corresponding to LDL, VLDL and HDL respectively. The β lipoprotein band is more intense than the other two and the pre-β band may be very faint. In non-fasting specimens, and certain pathological sera, a fourth band may be present at the origin due to the presence of chylomicrons.

Variations in concentrations of the lipoproteins will produce variations in the intensity of staining of the various bands, but it is not easy to gauge minor changes precisely. Caution must be exercised in interpreting an increased intensity of the pre-β band because, in a minority of the population, this increase may be due not to an increase in VLDL, but to the presence of high levels of Lp(a). In such cases the serum triglyceride level is usually less elevated than would be expected were the VLDL increased. In some cases with pronounced hyper-triglyceridaemia, atypical patterns may be seen. These will be discussed below.

CLASSIFICATION OF HYPERLIPOPROTEINAEMIA

The association between certain types of hyperlipidaemia and the accelerated development of atherosclerosis has been recognised for many years. In order to identify more precisely the disorders that carry an increased risk of arterial disease, Fredrickson and Lees (1965) introduced the following classification of hyperlipoproteinaemia based on the appearance of the lipoprotein patterns seen on electrophoresis. Paper electrophoresis was used originally, but similar patterns are obtained with agarose gel or cellulose acetate. Specimens may also be classified by ultracentrifugation (Fredrickson and Levy, 1972). 469

Type I is a rare condition characterised by a pronounced increase in chylomicrons. It results from an inherited defect in chylomicron metabolism, due to lipoprotein lipase deficiency or to apolipoprotein CII deficiency. Clinically, the condition is usually seen in childhood and the patient may suffer from eruptive xanthomata and recurrent bouts of abdominal pain due to pancreatitis.

Type II is characterised by an elevation of β lipoprotein (LDL). In some cases, pre-β lipoprotein (VLDL) is also increased. Consequently, Type II has been subdivided into IIa (VLDL not increased) and IIb (VLDL increased). A common condition giving rise to a Type II pattern is familial combined hyperlipoproteinaemia, in which there is polygenic inheritance. Less common, but usually severe, is monogenic familial hypercholesterolaemia (FH). This condition is due to a cellular deficiency of the apolipoprotein B receptor. Inheritance is by an autosomal codominant gene which is present in about 1 in 500 of the population. The homozygous genotype is rare. Patients with FH frequently develop tendon xanthomata and corneal arci.

Type III is an uncommon condition in which an abnormal electrophoretic pattern is observed, with a single broad-β band overlapping the β and pre-β regions. This appearance is due to elevated levels of IDL and is the result of impaired hepatic clearance of these particles. The abnormality is often referred to as dys-β-lipoproteinaemia. Patients often have palmar and tubero-eruptive xanthomata.

Type IV is a common abnormality in which there is an elevation of pre-β lipoprotein (VLDL). The underlying disorder is unknown, but there appears to be over-production of VLDL. Many of the milder cases are probably nutritional in origin.

Type V is due to an increase in both pre-β lipoprotein and chylomicrons. In addition to showing a chylomicron band at the origin, the electrophoretic strip shows an atypical smear of stained lipoprotein extending from the origin to the pre-β region. The condition is fairly uncommon. In a minority of cases, the abnormality may be a manifestation in the adult of the Type I hyperlipoproteinaemia of childhood. As in that disorder, patients may suffer eruptive xanthomata and recurrent pancreatitis.

Typing Patient Specimens

Although the classification described above was based on electrophoresis, the majority of specimens from untreated patients can be classified with reasonable accuracy from a knowledge of the lipid results. Most patients who have raised cholesterol with normal triglyceride values will have a Type IIa hyperlipoproteinaemia. Patients with triglyceride levels between 2·0 and 4·5 mmol/l, generally, but not inevitably, have either a Type IIb or a Type IV pattern. In such cases, a calculated LDL-cholesterol value is helpful. In Type IV, LDL-cholesterol is usually less than 4·5 mmol/l and in Type IIb it is generally greater than 4·5 mmol/l. Electrophoresis will usually serve only to confirm the patterns anticipated from the lipid results but may have some value in cases showing mild hypertriglyceridaemia, because the presence of chylomicrons will act as a warning that the patient may not have been fasting when the specimen was taken and other types may occasionally be detected.

Patients who have triglyceride levels greater than 4·5 mmol/l are a minority, but typing them can be more of a problem. Visual inspection of the specimen that has stood overnight at 4°C will reveal a pronounced supernatant layer of cream in Types I and V, reflecting the marked increase in chylomicrons. Electrophoresis is helpful in the investigation of patients with marked hypertriglyceridaemia, but it should be recognised that the broad β band referred to above is not a totally reliable parameter for Type III as both false positive and false negative results can be obtained.

Further tests that may be of value in this group of patients include lipoprotein lipase measurement after heparin administration (Mount *et al.*, 1982) and isoelectric focusing of apolipoproteins . Lipoprotein lipase deficiency is the usual cause of Type I hyperlipoproteinaemia and an unusual cause of Type V. Isoelectric focusing is used to identify apo-CII deficiency or apo-E abnormality. The former is sometimes present in Type I hyperlipoproteinaemia (Breckenridge *et al.*, 1978), the latter usually present in Type III (see Havel, 1982).

OTHER LIPID AND LIPOPROTEIN METHODS

Determination of Apolipoproteins A1 and B

Apolipoprotein A1

Several immunochemical methods have been used to measure apo-A1, including radial immunodiffusion, electroimmunoassay, radioimmunoassay, immuno-turbidimetry and nephelometry (see Steinberg *et al.*, 1983). One of the major problems encountered is that not all of the antigenic sites present on the pure peptide are exposed when the molecule is a component of HDL. Consequently, the apo-A1 in patients' specimens will react with antiserum differently to the purified apo-A1 used as a primary standard. The difficulty is compounded by variations in specificity shown by different antisera. To overcome this problem, a number of procedures have been used to increase exposure of the antigenic sites. These include delipidation, heating, and treatment with high concentrations of urea or guanidine HCl. Fesmire *et al.* (1984) report that the use of reference sera as secondary standards in the electroimmunoassay method resolves many of the problems associated with primary standardisation.

Electroimmunoassay of Apolipoprotein A1 (based on Miller *et al.*, 1980).

Reagents.
1. Agarose gel and tris-barbitone buffer as for lipoprotein electrophoresis (see p. 468).
2. Sheep antihuman apolipoprotein A1 (Seward).
3. Urea solution (9 mol/l). Dissolve 54·05 g urea (Aristar, BDH Chemicals Limited) in 500 ml buffer.
4. Secondary standard supplied by Immuno AG. Value depends on batch, about 1 g/l.
5. Stain. Amidoblack 10B, 2 g/l in reagent (6).
6. Acetic acid, 50 g/l in water.
7. Sodium chloride solution, 150 mmol/l.

Technique. *Preparation of specimens and standards.* Specimens are diluted 1:30 in urea solution. The secondary standard is diluted 1:30, 1:25 and 1:20 in urea solution to provide standards 3, 4 and 5. Standard 2 is prepared by diluting a portion of standard 3 with an equal volume of urea solution, and standard 1 similarly prepared from standard 2.

Melt 10 ml agarose gel in a beaker of boiling water, then cool in a water bath at 56 °C. Add the antiserum and mix thoroughly by pouring the mixture into a warmed test tube and back again three times, then pour onto a glass plate resting on a level surface and spread completely over the surface. Cool and place at 4 °C for 15 min to harden the gel. Punch a row of holes across the plate 3 cm from the end with a 1·5 mm punch (maximum of 11 holes evenly spaced). Remove the agar from the wells by suction applied via a fine tipped Pasteur pipette. Fill the wells with pretreated standards and specimens, 3 µl per well. Perform electrophoresis at 130 V for 6 h or at 90 V overnight. Remove the plate, lay moist filter paper on the surface of the gel and dry with a warm air blower. Wash the plate in saline for 1 h, then stain for 5 min. Allow the plate to dry in air, then wash in acetic acid until the background is clear. Dry in air and measure the height of the rockets. Plot a standard curve and read the concentrations of apo-A1 in the samples from the rocket heights.

Notes.
1. Further details of the 'rocket' electroimmunoassay technique can be found in Chapter 5 (p. 104).
2. The volume of antiserum to be added to the gel is determined by trial and error to give a satisfactory standard curve with a height for the top standard of about 20 mm or more. The volume required is likely to be about 300 µl.

Apolipoprotein B

As with apo-A1, a variety of immunochemical techniques has been used to measure apo-B, including radioimmunoassay, electroimmunoassay, radial immunodiffusion, immunonephelometry and enzyme-labelled immunosorbent assay.

The insolubility of apo-B in aqueous media presents a problem in standardisation, and LDL prepared by ultracentrifugation within a narrow density range (1·030 to 1·050) are generally used as a primary standard. However, purified LDL are stable for only a relatively short period and in practice, secondary serum standards are generally used. A further problem relates to the question of whether apo-B present in VLDL and chylomicrons is as accessible to antibodies as that present in LDL. For electroimmunoassay and radial immunodiffusion, the issue is further complicated by reports that the different lipoproteins penetrate agarose gel to varying extents depending on the agarose content of the gel. It is difficult to assess the degree of inaccuracy that results from these effects because reviews on the subject are not entirely in agreement. Some authors have pretreated specimens with lipase or detergents in an attempt to reduce the size of VLDL to that of LDL. For a more detailed discussion, see Rosseneu *et al.* (1983).

Electroimmunoassay of Apolipoprotein B

The reagents and procedure are the same as in the method for apo-A1 described on p. 471 but with the following differences:

1. Antiserum to apo-B replaces antiserum to apo-A1. The amount of antiserum to be added to the gel will be less because apo-B is a stronger immunogen and antisera have higher titres.
2. Samples are not pretreated with urea. They are applied undiluted to the wells, unless they have an apo-B concentration greater than the top standard, in which case they are diluted with an equal volume of saline.
3. Standardised serum supplied by Immuno AG may be used to provide a standard curve. However, the apo-B level is not very high (about 1 g/l) and it is more satisfactory to use it to calibrate a pool of serum with high apo-B concentration for use as a tertiary standard. Serum from subjects with pronounced hypercholesterolaemia will be found suitable.

INTERPRETATION

Reported values for mean levels of apo-A1 in men range from around 1·15 g/l to about 1·35 g/l; values for women are about 0·2 g/l higher. There is a slight increase with age (see Steinberg *et al.*, 1983). For apo-B, reported mean adult levels tend to be between 0·85 g/l and 1 g/l, although higher values have been reported with immunonephelometry (see Rosseneu *et al.*). Apo-B levels show a positive correlation with total cholesterol and with LDL cholesterol. The growing interest in these apolipoproteins as risk factors in atherosclerotic diseases has already been mentioned. Disorders producing marked changes in serum concentrations of apo-B include familial hypercholesterolaemia, in which levels may sometimes exceed 3 g/l; homozygous hypobetalipoproteinaemia and familial abetalipo-proteinaemia, in both of which levels are very low. Low concentrations of apo-A1 are seen in Tangier disease, in which an abnormal A1 is present, and familial hypoalphalipoproteinaemia (see Schaefer and Levy, 1985).

Non-esterified Fatty Acids (NEFA)

NEFA are present in serum at about 500 μmol/l so sensitive methods are needed if the use of large specimens is to be avoided. It is also necessary to avoid interference from other lipids and to prevent lipolysis of the more abundant esterified fatty acids present. Specimens should be separated and analysed shortly after collection or, alternatively, stored as plasma at $-20\,°C$.

Titrimetric and colorimetric methods are described in the 5th edition of this book. More recently, an enzymatic method has been developed and is produced commercially as the NEFA C-Test by Wako Pure Chemical Industries Limited (available in the UK from Alpha Laboratories). In this method, fatty acid is converted to acyl CoA by acyl CoA synthetase in the presence of CoA and ATP. Acyl CoA is then acted on by acyl CoA oxidase to produce 2,3-transenoyl-CoA and hydrogen peroxide, which is measured colorimetrically by a peroxidase technique. The method is sensitive, simple to perform and can be readily automated.

INTERPRETATION

In adults, the normal range is 400 to 900 μmol/l. In children, it is a little higher. In untreated diabetics, it may rise to 1·5 mmol/l. Raised values are also found during starvation, during exercise, and in states of emotional stress. They are also increased in hyperthyroidism and following injection of adrenaline or isoproterenol, after giving growth hormone and about 3 h after glucose ingestion. Increases are seen also following administration of amphetamines, caffeine, carbutamide, diazoxide, ethanol, heparin, nicotine or tolbutamide. High values often occur during oral contraception after the first three months have elapsed.

Decreases in NEFA follow shortly after giving insulin or glucose. Aspirin lowers values by increasing fatty acid oxidation and diminishing lipogenesis, while clofibrate lowers them by displacing NEFA from albumin. Other drugs causing reduced levels are nicotinic acid and propranolol.

Determination of Free and Ester Cholesterol

Originally, methods were based on digitonin precipitation of free cholesterol or adsorption of ester cholesterol on alumina columns (see the 5th edition of this book). Free cholesterol can now be measured more conveniently by using a modification of the enzymatic method for total cholesterol, in which cholesterol esterase is omitted from the reagent mixture.

Free cholesterol forms 20 to 40% of the total in normal specimens. The proportion is increased in liver disease and LCAT deficiency.

Lp(a) Lipoprotein

Lp(a) has been measured by radioimmunoassay (Albers *et al.*, 1977), counter-immunoelectrophoresis (Molinari *et al.*, 1983), and electroimmunoassay (Walton *et al.*, 1974). Antisera have generally been raised against purified Lp(a) and subsequently absorbed with Lp(a)-negative sera to remove reactivity against apo-B and other proteins.

Lipoprotein-X

Qualitatively, Lp-X may be identified as a cathodally migrating protein on agar gel electrophoresis. Following the electrophoretic run, a solution containing 0·54 mol/l of magnesium chloride and 40 g/l of phosphotungstic acid is layered on the gel and if Lp-X is present, a characteristic arc of precipitation may be seen (Hashiguchi *et al.*, 1982). Materials for performing this test can be obtained from Immuno AG. An alternative procedure is immunoelectrophoresis against antiserum to Lp-X, which can be purchased from Behringwerke AG. The presence of Lp-X is shown by an arc of immunoprecipitation in the cathodal region. For quantitative assessment, Hashiguchi *et al.* described a method based on differential precipitation. Another technique, published by Talafant and Tovarek (1978), was based on the observation that the phospholipids of Lp-X can be extracted from serum with ether in the presence of cetyltrimethylammonium bromide.

Fat in Urine

Fat has been said to occur in urine (lipuria) after large amounts of fat have been taken; in conditions such as the nephrotic syndrome and diabetes mellitus in which there is an increase in triglycerides; and following injuries in which there has been considerable crushing of subcutaneous fat. Lipuria if it occurs, is certainly a rare condition. There are many ways in which urine may appear to be contaminated with extraneous fat, e.g. from liquid paraffin used as laxative, lubricants used in passing catheters, and even from deliberate addition of fat.

A particular example of lipuria is chyluria, the term given to milky urines resulting from admixture with chyle from ruptured lymphatics in the kidneys or bladder. In chyluria, there are also red blood cells present, and in some cases there may be enough fibrinogen to form clots. The amount of fat present may reach a few per cent, but varies considerably with changes in fat absorption. The fat is said to be more finely dispersed in chyluria than in other cases of lipuria. For recognising this condition, Sudan III has been given with fat in the food. Thus, Harrison (1947) gave 100 mg with 10 g butter. The Sudan III is excreted with the fat in the urine and can be extracted into ether.

REFERENCES

Albers J. J., Adolphson J. L., Hazzard W. R. (1977). *J. Lipid Res*; **18**: 331.
Albers J. J., Hazzard W. R. (1974). *Lipids*; **9**: 15.
Allain C. C., *et al.* (1974). *Clin. Chem*; **20**: 470.
Blaton V., De Buyzere M., Spincemaille J., Declerq B. (1983). *Clin. Chem*; **29**: 806.
Breckenridge W. C., *et al.* (1978). *New Engl. J. Med*; **298**: 1265.
Bucolo D., David H. (1973). *Clin. Chem*; **19**: 476.
Burstein M., Scholnick H. R., Morfin R. (1970). *J. Lipid Res*; **11**: 583.
Cawley L. P., Eberhardt L. (1962). *Amer. J. Clin. Path*; **38**: 539.
Dahlen G., Berg K. (1979). *Clin. Genet*; **16**: 418.
Dryer R. L., Tammes A. R., Routh J. I. (1957). *J. Biol. Chem*; **225**: 177.
Durrington P. N., *et al.* (1986). *Br. Heart J*; **56**: 206.
Durrum E. L., Paul M. H., Smith E. R. B. (1952). *Science*; **116**: 428.
Elin R. J., Ruddel M., McLean S. (1983). *Clin. Chem*; **29**: 1174.
Fasoli A. (1952). *Lancet*; **1**: 106.
Fesmire J. D., McConathy W. J., Alaupovic P. (1984). *Clin. Chem*; **30**: 712.
Fiske C. H., Subbarow Y. (1925). *J. Biol. Chem*; **66**: 375.
Flegg H. M. (1973). *Ann. Clin. Biochem*; **10**: 79.
Fossati P., Prencipe L. (1982). *Clin. Chem*; **28**: 2077.
Fredrickson D. S., Lees R. S. (1965). *Circulation*; **31**: 321.
Fredrickson D. S., Levy R. I. (1972). Familial hyperlipoproteinaemia. In *The Metabolic Basis of Inherited Disease*, 3rd ed. (Stanbury J. B., Wyngaarden J. B., Fredrickson D. S. eds) New York: McGraw-Hill.
Friedewald W. T., Levy R. I., Fredrickson D. S. (1972). *Clin. Chem*; **18**: 499.
Giri K. V. (1956). *J. Lab. Clin. Med*; **48**: 775.
Gofman J. W., *et al.* (1954). *Plasma*; **2**: 413.
Golfs B., Verheyden J. (1967). *Clin. Chim. Acta*; **18**: 325.
Gomori G. (1942). *J. Lab. Clin. Med*; **27**: 955.
Gordon T., *et al.* (1977). *Amer. J. Med*; **62**: 707.
Grossman S. H., Mollo E., Ertingshausen G. (1976). *Clin. Chem*; **22**: 1310.
Harrison G. A. (1947). *Chemical Methods in Clinical Medicine*, 3rd ed., p. 278. London: Churchill Livingstone.
Hashiguchi Y., *et al.* (1982). *Clin. Chem*; **28**: 606.
Hatch F. T., Lees R. S. (1968). In *Advances in Lipid Research*, Vol. 6, (Paoletti R., Kritchevsky D., eds) p. 30. New York, London: Academic Press.
Havel R. J. (1982). *Med. Clinics. N. Amer*; **66**: 441.
Henry R. J., ed. (1964). In *Clinical Chemistry, Principles and Technics*, p. 841. New York, London: Harper Row.
Hernandez H. H., Chaikoff I. L. (1957). *J. Biol. Chem*; **228**: 447.
Kohn J., Feinberg J. G. (1965). *Electrophoresis on Cellulose Acetate*. Shandon Instrument Application, No. 11. Shandon Scientific Co., London.
McGlashan D. A. K., Pilkington T. R. E. (1968). *Clin. Chim. Acta*; **22**: 646.
Megraw R. E., Dunn D. E., Biggs H. G. (1979). *Clin. Chem*; **25**: 273.
Miller N. E., Forde O. H., Thelle D. S., Mjos O. D. (1977). *Lancet*; **1**: 965.
Miller J. P., Mao S. J. T., Patsch J. R., Gotto A. M. (1980). *J. Lipid Res*; **21**: 775.
Mills G. L., Lane P. A., Weech P. K. (1984). [*A Guidebook to Lipoprotein Technique*] *Laboratory Techniques in Biochemistry and Molecular Biology*, Vol. 14, Amsterdam: Elsevier.
Molinari E., Pichler P., Krempler F., Kostner G. (1983). *Clin. Chim. Acta*; **128**: 373.
Mount J., *et al.* (1982). *Laboratory Investigation of Lipid Disorders*. Broadsheet 101, Association of Clinical Pathologists, London.
NIH Consensus Development Conference Statement (1984), Vol. 5, No. 7.
Noble R. R. (1968). *J. Lipid Res*; **9**: 693.
Papadopoulos N. M., Kintzios J. A. (1969). *Anal. Biochem*; **30**: 421.
Rapp W. (1967). *Clin. Chim. Acta*; **15**: 177.
Rapp W., Kahlke W. (1968). *Clin. Chim. Acta*; **19**: 493.

Richmond W. (1972). *Scand. J. Clin. Lab. Invest*; **29**: Suppl. **126**, *Abstract* **3**: 25.
Richmond W. (1973). *Clin. Chem*; **19**: 1350.
Rosseneu M., Vercaemst R., Steinberg K. K., Cooper G. R. (1983). *Clin. Chem*; **29**: 427.
Schaefer E. J., Levy R. I. (1985). *New Engl. J. Med*; **312**: 1300.
Seidel D., Gretz H., Ruppert C. (1973). *Clin. Chem*; **19**: 86.
Sniderman A., *et al.* (1980). *Proc. Natl. Acad. Sci. USA*; **77**: 604.
Steinberg K. K., Cooper G. R., Graiser S. R., Rosseneu M. (1983). *Clin. Chem*; **29**: 415.
Stern I. S., Shapiro B. (1953). *J. Clin. Path*; **6**: 158.
Stone M. C., Thorp J. M. (1966). *Clin. Chim. Acta*; **14**: 812.
Sulivan D. R., *et al.* (1985). *Clin. Chem*; **31**: 1227.
Swahn B. (1952). *Scand. J. Clin. Lab. Invest*; **4**: 98.
Talafant E., Tovarek J. (1978). *Clin. Chim. Acta*; **88**: 215.
Tarbutton P. H., Gunter C. R. (1974). *Clin. Chem*; **20**: 725.
ter Welle H. F., Baartscheer T., Fiolet J. W. T. (1984). *Clin. Chem*; **30**: 1102.
Varley H. (1967). *Practical Clinical Biochemistry*, 4th ed. London: William Heinemann Medical Books.
Walker R. E., Bachorik P. S., Kwiterovich P. O. (1982). *Clin. Chem*; **28**: 2299.
Walton K. W., Hitchens J., Magnani H. N., Khan M. (1974). *Atherosclerosis*; **20**: 323.
Warnick G. R., Albers J. J. (1978). *J. Lipid Res*; **19**: 65.
Youngberg G. E., Youngberg M. V. (1930). *J. Lab. Clin. Med*; **16**: 158.
Zilversmit D. B., Davies A. K. (1950). *J. Lab. Clin. Med*; **35**: 155.
Zollner N., Wolfram G. (1970). In *Biochemical Disorders in Human Disease*, 3rd ed. (Thompson R. H. S., Wootton I. D. P. eds) p. 609. London: Churchill Livingstone.

22

ENZYMES

The first enzymes to be determined for diagnostic purposes appear to have been the digestive enzymes amylase and lipase, some techniques for which go back to the last century. In the 1930s the phosphatases began to be widely determined but it was with the introduction of techniques for determining aminotransferase and lactate dehydrogenase activities in the 1950s that a considerable increase in the use of enzyme assays began. This involved intracellular enzymes of which in health only small amounts are present in the blood plasma. When an organ is diseased, however, a greater amount of its enzymes may escape so that there is an increase, often marked, in their activity in the plasma. Since some of these catalyse steps in the metabolism of carbohydrate and protein they are present in most tissues, though the amount in different organs can vary widely. As a result an increased activity of such enzymes is found in a number of diseases. However, the pattern of the increase may be sufficiently typical for information of diagnostic value to be obtained, or taken in conjunction with clinical findings clearly to indicate the organ involved. Occasionally an enzyme may have a much more restricted occurrence and even be mainly found in a single organ. Examples of such organ-specific enzymes are sorbitol dehydrogenase, glucose-6-phosphatase, and enzymes of the urea cycle, all in the liver. Also an enzyme may occur in different forms, isoenzymes, according to the tissue from which it is derived.

The rise in serum activity does not only depend on the concentration of the enzyme in the tissue and on the severity of the disease process. The great difference in the mass of different organs has to be borne in mind and the rate at which an enzyme escapes from diseased tissues is affected by its intracellular location and by changes in the permeability of the cell membrane. Other factors which influence the extent and duration of an increase include the rate at which an enzyme is removed from the plasma either by metabolism or by renal excretion. Increased synthesis of enzyme is responsible for the increase in serum alkaline phosphatase in biliary tract obstruction and for an increase in gamma-glutamyl transferase after taking phenobarbitone or alcohol regularly. On the other hand, there are enzymes which are normally released into the blood, e.g. cholinesterase, and enzymes involved in blood coagulation, e.g. plasminogen, for which there is reduced plasma activity when the organ concerned, in these cases the liver, is diseased.

For works on enzymes and enzyme-catalysed reactions see Dixon and Webb (1964), Plowman (1972) and Wong (1975) and for clinical applications see Wilkinson (1976).

CLASSIFICATION AND NOMENCLATURE

The Recommendations (1972) of the Commission on Biochemical Nomenclature and Classification of Enzymes together with their Units and the Symbols of Enzyme Kinetics (see Florkin and Stotz, 1973), a revision of the

Recommendations of the International Union of Biochemistry (IUB, 1964), have been generally accepted. The basic classification of enzymes is into six groups:

1. Oxidoreductases

The general reaction can be stated:

$$AH_2 + B \rightleftharpoons A + BH_2$$

in which A is the hydrogen donor and B the hydrogen acceptor. The latter may be molecular oxygen but more often in the body is a coenzyme of which nicotinamide adenine dinucleotide (NAD$^+$) and nicotinamide adenine dinucleotide phosphate (NADP$^+$) are the most common. There are three types of oxidoreductase:

(a) **Aerobic Oxidases.** These can only use molecular oxygen as a hydrogen acceptor, water being formed. Examples are tyrosinase which oxidises tyrosine to dihydroxyphenylalanine quinone,

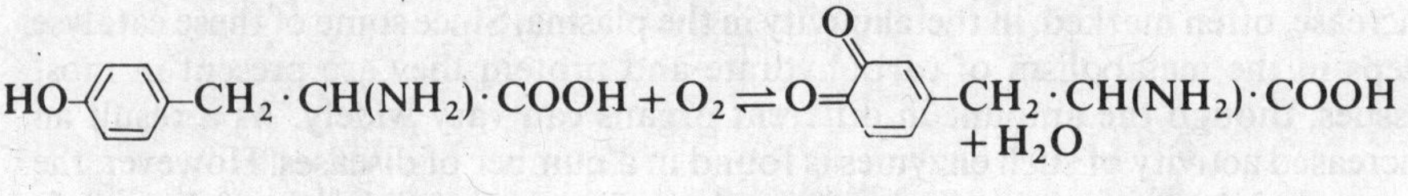

$$HO\text{–}\langle\bigcirc\rangle\text{–}CH_2\cdot CH(NH_2)\cdot COOH + O_2 \rightleftharpoons O=\langle\bigcirc\rangle\text{–}CH_2\cdot CH(NH_2)\cdot COOH + H_2O$$

a stage in the formation of melanin from tyrosine; ascorbate oxidase which oxidises ascorbic acid to dehydroascorbic acid; and homogentisate oxidase.

(b) **Aerobic Dehydrogenases.** Molecular oxygen again acts as hydrogen acceptor but forms hydrogen peroxide, which is then removed by other enzymes such as peroxidase and catalase. Examples are glucose oxidase and xanthine oxidase. Unlike the aerobic oxidases these can use methylene blue as hydrogen acceptor for experimental purposes.

(c) **Anaerobic Dehydrogenases.** These cannot use molecular oxygen and so require the presence of a suitable coenzyme as hydrogen acceptor. Examples are lactate dehydrogenase and malate dehydrogenase which require NAD$^+$, and glucose-6-phosphate dehydrogenase which requires NADP$^+$ or NAD$^+$ depending on the source of the enzyme.

2. Transferases

These transfer a group from one type of organic compound to another:

$$AX + B \rightleftharpoons A + BX$$

Important groups thus transferred include methyl, amino, phosphate and glycosidyl. Examples are the aminotransferases; the phosphotransferases, often referred to as kinases, e.g. creatine kinase and pyruvate kinase; hexose-1-phosphate uridylyl transferase; and transketolase.

3. Hydrolases

These hydrolyse their substrates:

$$AB + H_2O \rightleftharpoons AH + BOH$$

They include enzymes acting on ester bonds, e.g. lipase and the cholinesterases; those acting on glycoside links, e.g. α-amylase and the disaccharidases; those acting on peptide bonds, e.g. pepsin, trypsin and thrombin; and those acting on C–N bonds other than peptides, e.g. urease.

4. Lyases

These remove groups without hydrolysis, leaving a double bond. Examples are decarboxylases such as pyruvate decarboxylase:

$$CH_3.CO.COOH \rightleftharpoons CH_3.CHO + CO_2$$

5. Isomerases

These convert one of a pair of isomers into the other. They include racemases and epimerases; cis-trans isomerases; intramolecular oxidoreductases interconverting aldoses and ketoses to which belong the isomerases – triosephosphate isomerase interconverting D-glyceraldehyde-3-phosphate and dihydroxyacetone phosphate, and glucose phosphate isomerase interconverting D-glucose-6-phosphate and D-fructose-6-phosphate. Other isomerases include intramolecular transferases and enzymes interconverting keto and enol groups and transposing C=C bonds.

6. Ligases

Also known as synthetases, these catalyse the linking together of two molecules, a reaction coupled with the breakdown of a phosphate bond in substances such as ATP. Examples are acetyl CoA synthetase which catalyses the reaction:

$$Acetate + CoA + ATP \rightleftharpoons Acetyl\text{-}CoA + AMP + Pyrophosphate$$

succinyl-CoA synthetase (ADP-forming) which catalyses the reaction:

$$Succinate + CoA + ATP \rightleftharpoons Succinyl\text{-}CoA + ADP + Orthophosphate$$

and succinyl-CoA synthetase (GDP-forming), which catalyses the reaction:

$$Succinate + CoA + GTP \rightleftharpoons Succinyl\text{-}CoA + GDP + Orthophosphate$$

NUMBERING SYSTEM

The Commission adopted a numbering system in which each enzyme is given four numbers separated by dots. The first number is one of the above six major groups; the second indicates the kind of group acted on, e.g. the dehydrogenases 1.1 act on the CHOH group of donors, 1.2 on the aldehyde or keto group, 1.3 on the =CH–CH= group, 1.4 on the =CH–NH$_2$ and so on; the third number breaks these down a stage further, e.g. in the dehydrogenases to show the type of acceptor, 1.1.1 with NAD$^+$ or NADP$^+$, 1.1.2 with a cytochrome, 1.1.3 with oxygen; finally the fourth is for individual enzymes. (See the 5th edition of this book for a table giving the Enzyme Commission number, the systematic name and the recommended name of a number of enzymes relevant to clinical biochemistry.)

NOMENCLATURE OF THE NICOTINAMIDE NUCLEOTIDE COENZYMES

Suggestions were also made in the Report for the names to be used for other substances important in enzyme chemistry. Two common coenzymes were renamed nicotinamide adenine dinucleotide (NAD^+) and nicotinamide adenine dinucleotide phosphate ($NADP^+$). The structural formulae of these are shown in Fig. 22.1, together with the changes to produce the reduced form of these coenzymes. For example the reactions are written as follows:

$$\text{L-Lactate} + NAD^+ \rightleftharpoons \text{Pyruvate} + NADH + H^+$$

$$\text{Isocitrate} + NADP^+ \rightleftharpoons \text{Oxalosuccinate} + NADPH + H^+$$

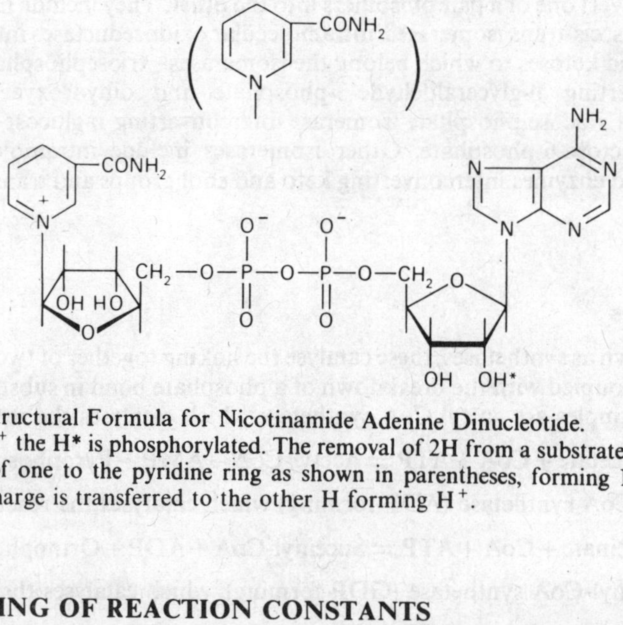

Fig. 22.1. Structural Formula for Nicotinamide Adenine Dinucleotide.
In $NADP^+$ the H* is phosphorylated. The removal of 2H from a substrate involves the addition of one to the pyridine ring as shown in parentheses, forming NADH. The positive charge is transferred to the other H forming H^+.

NUMBERING OF REACTION CONSTANTS

The Commission also recommended that reaction constants for enzyme reactions should be labelled k_{+1}, k_{+2}, k_{+3}, etc., for the forward direction of a sequence of reactions, and k_{-1}, k_{-2}, k_{-3}, etc., for the reverse reactions as being less likely to be misleading than k_1 and k_2, k_3 and k_4, k_5 and k_6, and so on for successive reactions.

FACTORS AFFECTING THE DETERMINATION OF ENZYME ACTIVITIES

Since enzymes are usually determined indirectly by measuring some result of their activity, several factors must be carefully controlled.

1. Substrate Concentration

Initially, there is a combination between the enzyme (E) and the substrate (S). When the enzyme acts on only one substrate this can be written:

$$E + S \underset{k_{-1}}{\overset{k_{+1}}{\rightleftharpoons}} ES \tag{1}$$

If e is the initial, i.e. the total, concentration of enzyme, s the concentration of free substrate, and c the concentration of the complex ES, the velocity of the forward reaction will be given by $k_{+1}s(e-c)$, that of the reverse reaction by $k_{-1}c$ and the overall rate by $k_{+1}s(e-c) - k_{-1}c$.

The complex is unstable so that it breaks down:

$$ES \overset{k_{+2}}{\rightarrow} E + P \tag{2}$$

where P represents the products of the action. The velocity of this reaction is given by:

$$v = k_{+2}c \tag{3}$$

It is assumed in the Michaelis–Menten theory of enzyme action that when k_{+2} is small enough for it not to affect the equilibrium of reaction (1) a steady state will be maintained, c will remain constant, and $k_{+2}c$ will equal $k_{+1}s(e-c) - k_{-1}c$ which rearranges to:

$$\frac{s(e-c)}{c} = \frac{k_{-1} + k_{+2}}{k_{+1}} = K_s \tag{4}$$

where K_s is the dissociation constant of the enzyme–substrate complex. Rearranging again we get:

$$es = cK_s + cs \tag{5}$$

Now let us consider what happens as the concentration of substrate increases. At low concentrations few of the active enzyme sites will be combined with substrate molecules and newly added molecules will easily find sites with which to complex. Concentration of ES at first will increase linearly but as sites become increasingly occupied the rate of increase will taper off and finally cease. The active sites will become saturated with substrate, c, the concentration of ES, becomes equal to the concentration, e, and the velocity v reaches a maximum. If we let this maximum velocity be V_{max} we have as a special example of equation (3):

$$V_{max} = k_{+2}e \tag{6}$$

Combining this with (3) we have:

$$\frac{v}{V_{max}} = \frac{c}{e}$$

Rearranging equation (5) we get:

$$s = \frac{c}{e}(K_s + s)$$

Inserting v/V_{max} for c/e gives us:

$$s = \frac{v}{V_{max}}(K_s + s)$$

so that:

$$v = \frac{sV_{max}}{K_s + s} \quad \text{or} = \frac{V_{max}}{1 + K_s/s} \tag{7}$$

These are forms of the Michaelis–Menten (1913) or Briggs–Haldane (1925) equation. From them we see that when s is equal to K_s, v equals $V_{max}/2$. This substrate concentration at which the rate of reaction is half the maximum is termed the Michaelis constant, K_m. It should be noted that K_m and K_s are not necessarily the same. This is only so when the conditions are as before, when the breakdown of ES is slow enough for a true equilibrium of reaction (1) to build up. The equation (7) can then be written:

$$v = \frac{sV_{max}}{s + K_m} \tag{8}$$

When this equation is plotted as in Fig. 22.2 with concentration of substrate as abscissa and velocity of the reaction as ordinate we get a rectangular hyperbola, a special kind of hyperbola in which the two asymptotes are at right angles to one another. At high substrate concentrations the curve becomes asymptotic to a line parallel to the abscissa at height V_{max} and at low concentrations it approaches the origin. The mathematical curve then becomes asymptotic to a line parallel to the ordinate and passing through the abscissa at $-K_m$. V_{max} and K_m are constants which determine the shape of the curve and are termed the kinetic constants. From this we see that the velocity of the reaction at high values of s becomes independent of the substrate concentration and is the maximum possible for the conditions of the assay. The reaction is then said to show zero order kinetics or to be zero order with respect to substrate concentration (i.e. v is proportional to s^0, the zero power of the substrate concentration). The deviation from zero order

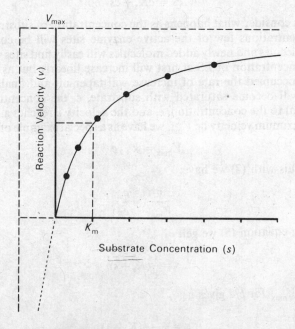

Fig 22.2. **The Relationship Between Reaction Velocity (v) and Substrate Concentration (s).**
  The curve, defined by the equation $v = s\,V_{max}/(s + K_m)$, is a rectangular hyperbola related to the axes shown by the broken lines; the horizontal one lies V_{max} above the abscissa and the vertical one lies $-K_m$ from the ordinate. The markings on the abscissa are in multiples of K_m, the value of which corresponds to a reaction velocity of $V_{max}/2$.

kinetics is just under 1 % when $s = 100\ K_m$ and below 9 % when $s = 10\ K_m$. At the other extreme when s is small compared to K_m the equation reduces to:

$$v = \frac{s \cdot V_{\max}}{K_m}$$

Then v is proportional to s, i.e. to the first power of s, and the reaction is said to be a first order one or to show first order kinetics. The deviation from this is less than 1 % when s is below $0.01\ K_m$ and below 9 % when $s = 0.1\ K_m$. Between the two extremes of zero and first order the reaction order is indeterminate.

The curve shown opposite (Fig. 22.2) agrees well with that found by measuring the initial reaction rates at different substrate concentrations. By inspection it is clear that it is only when zero order kinetics apply that constant activity will be demonstrable during the period of incubation. We have seen that to approximate to zero order kinetics substrate concentrations in the upper part of the range 10 to 100 times the K_m are needed. Between 25 and 100 times the K_m the deviation from zero order is between 4 and 1 %, so, if possible, a concentration of substrate in this range should be used. If, as may be the case, the solubility of the substrate does not allow this concentration to be reached or at such a concentration, inhibition of the reaction by the substrate occurs, as is illustrated in Fig. 22.3 it will be necessary to use a concentration less than the optimum.

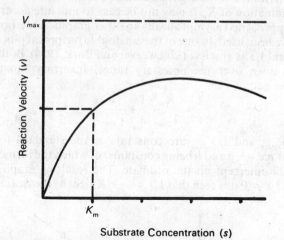

Substrate Concentration (s)

Fig. 22.3. The Relationship Between Reaction Velocity (v) and Substrate Concentration (s) When Inhibition Occurs at Higher Substrate Concentrations.
The early part of the curve is as in Fig. 22.2 opposite but the reaction velocity lies substantially below $V_{\max}$, even at its peak.

Whether or not zero order kinetics are being followed can be checked by studying the time course of the reaction (Fig. 22.4) by plotting the amount of product formed against the time of incubation. A linear response corresponds to the period of zero order. Should there be an initial lag period as occurs with some enzyme actions, there will be a relatively short early period when the reaction rate is less than the zero order rate. Examination of the time course of a reaction allows the analyst to calculate the amount of product which can be formed before the rate of reaction decreases. The incubation time can then be decided from a

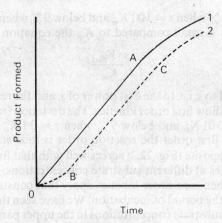

Fig. 22.4. Formation of Reaction Product with Time.
Curve 1 shows zero order reaction between 0 and A but in Curve 2 there is an initial lag period so that zero order kinetics are only obeyed between B and C.

consideration of the enzyme activities likely to be encountered in practice. The presence of a lag period can be seen and the time at which the linear response starts can be determined for use with automatic analysers.

For the determination of K_m it may not be easy to measure accurately a value which is being approached asymptotically so other graphical methods of finding K_m and V_{max} have been used. In one of these a double reciprocal plot is made with $1/v$ as ordinate and $1/s$ as abscissa (Lineweaver and Burk, 1934). Both of these can be accurately known over the necessary range. Inverting equation (8) and rearranging it we get:

$$\frac{1}{v} = \frac{K_m}{V_{max}} \cdot \frac{1}{s} + \frac{1}{V_{max}}$$

which, as K_m/V_{max} and $1/V_{max}$ are constants, is the standard formula for a straight line ($y = ax + b$, a and b being constants) of which the former is the slope and the latter the intercept on the ordinate. The resulting graph is shown in Fig. 22.5. When $1/v = 0$ it is seen that $1/s = -1/K_m$. So by measuring v at several

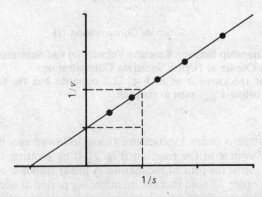

Fig. 22.5. Lineweaver–Burk Plot for Determination of K_m.
The markings on the abscissa are in multiples of $1/K_m$ and on the ordinate in multiples of $1/V_{max}$. From the equation (see text), when $1/s$ equals $1/K_m$ then $1/v$ equals $2/V_{max}$ as indicated by the broken lines.

substrate concentrations as shown on the graph we can find K_m. This appears to have been the type of graph most used. Others are described in Dixon and Webb (1964), Plowman (1972) and Wong (1975).

K_m is important as an indicator of enzyme–substrate affinity. If an enzyme acts on two different substrates (1) and (2) and the K_m for (1) is greater than for (2) then to get the same rate of reaction, (1) must be taken to a higher concentration of substrate than (2) as shown in Fig. 22.6. So a higher K_m indicates a lower enzyme–substrate affinity and *vice versa*. In the case of a metabolic process involving a sequence of enzyme actions the rate-limiting reaction is that with the highest K_m.

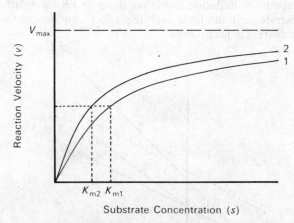

Fig. 22.6. The Effect of Substrate Composition on Reaction Velocity.
In this instance V_{max} is taken as the same for the substrates 1 and 2. Substrate 1 has a greater K_m than substrate 2. At sub-optimal concentrations, a higher concentration of substrate 1 than substrate 2 is needed to achieve the same reaction velocity.

The theory discussed in this section deals only with the case of an enzyme with one substrate and cannot generally be applied to enzymes which catalyse reactions in which more than one substrate is involved. The nomenclature and rate equations for the kinetics of enzyme-catalysed reactions with two or more substrates are discussed by Cleland (1963).

By combining equations (6) and (8) it can be seen that under the usual *in vitro* assay conditions the rate of reaction will be directly proportional to the amount of enzyme present and this fact can be used to assay enzyme activity in serum. It should be stressed that the relationship between the rate of reaction and the amount of enzyme is linear only if the initial velocity is used, since this is implicit in the derivation of the Michaelis–Menten equation. Since the instantaneous initial velocity is difficult to measure it is considered acceptable to use the rate during that part of the progress curve when zero order applies.

2. Concentration of Product

As the concentration of the product of the enzyme action increases and substrate is used up the rate of the reverse reaction:

$$E + P \underset{k_{-2}}{\overset{k_{+2}}{\rightleftharpoons}} EP$$

increases and is proportional to $k_{+2} \cdot p$ where p is the concentration of product. We now have a phenomenon which has been termed 'product inhibition'. The formulae applicable to this state are given for example by Dixon and Webb (1964) and by Plowman (1972) which can be consulted by those who wish to see how they are derived. The phenomenon belongs to the type of inhibition described as competitive inhibition on p. 488, so that as the Lineweaver and Burk reciprocal plot shows in Fig. 22.7 the velocity is not altered but the apparent K_m is greater. Increase in the product concentration can be analysed like substrate concentration to derive K_p analogous to K_m. According to Plowman, measurable inhibition is only found when p is greater than approximately $0.1\ K_p$. As we see on p. 488 with competitive inhibition the effect depends on the relative concentrations of substrate and inhibitor and the effect can be counteracted by increasing the substrate concentration.

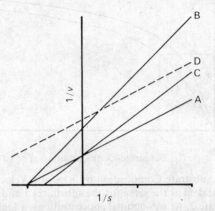

Fig. 22.7. **Lineweaver–Burk Plot Showing Different Types of Inhibition.**
The axes are marked as in Fig. 22.5. Line A shows the uninhibited reaction and crosses the abscissa at $-1/K_m$. Line B shows the effect of a non-competitive inhibitor, K_m remaining unchanged. Line C shows competitive inhibition with an increase in K_m but V_{max} is unaltered. Line D shows the situation with an uncompetitive inhibitor with proportional changes in V_{max} and K_m so that the slope of the line (K_m/V_{max}) is unaltered.

3. Concentration of Enzyme

So long as the other factors which influence the enzyme action remain the same, the initial rate of reaction is proportional to the concentration of the enzyme.

4. pH

Enzymes are only active over a limited pH range in which activity reaches a maximum at the optimum pH and on each side of which it falls away. The optimum pH for an enzyme may vary with different substrates and with different ionic strengths. Thus for alkaline phosphatase it is 8·1 using ethyl phosphate, 8·6 with sodium β-glycerophosphate and 9·8 for sodium phenyl phosphate. In fact the optimum pH and the rate of reaction rises as the pK of the ester falls. Furthermore, the optimum pH is not always the same for both directions of an enzyme action. In addition to being the pH with greatest activity, the optimum pH has the advantage that small errors in reagent preparation result in the smallest variation in activity.

5. Temperature

The velocity of enzyme-catalysed reactions at first increases as the temperature rises above ordinary room temperature. It is found that between 20 and 45 °C the temperature coefficient, Q_{10}, for a rise of 10 °C is between 1·5 and 3·0, but may not be the same for different ranges, e.g. for the range 25–35 °C as for 35–45 °C. However, as the temperature rises, denaturation of the protein and hence inactivation of the enzyme also increases. The result is that for a given set of experimental conditions there is a temperature for which the rate of reaction is greatest. This varies with the time of incubation. Some denaturation may take place over longer periods even at 37 °C and lower, and in general the longer the period of incubation the greater the effect of denaturation and the lower the optimum temperature.

There has been considerable discussion about the temperature to be recommended for general adoption in the determination of enzyme activities (e.g. see Bowers, 1972; Bergmeyer, 1973; Duggan, 1979; Haeckel *et al.*, 1982). The IUB (1961) in agreement with the International Federation of Clinical Chemistry (IFCC) recommended 25 °C, then replaced this by 30 °C in 1965. The latter temperature was also recommended by the IFCC Expert Panel on Enzymes in 1978 for the performance of IFCC-optimised methods. This was not supported by the IFCC Expert Panel on Instrumentation which for operational and economic reasons endorsed 37 °C as the preferred temperature. Haeckel *et al.* (1982) after a survey of current practice suggested that for most enzymes the temperature for reference methods should be 30 °C, but that routine determination of enzyme activity could be performed at 37 °C. The higher temperature has the advantage of giving higher activity and shorter lag periods making for more rapid processing and potentially better precision. It is also the only temperature at which a valid identification of cholinesterase variants is obtained (Silk *et al.*, 1979). A disadvantage is the effect on the clinical value of the Wilkinson quotient for 2-hydroxybutyrate–lactate dehydrogenase (see p. 526) which is less commonly used than formerly. Thus it may not be desirable to use the same temperature in all cases even for routine analysis. The authors aim to use either 25°C or 37°C for most assays. The use of temperature correction factors published by other workers is not recommended.

6. Activators, Coenzymes, Prosthetic Groups

In many enzyme-catalysed reactions other co-factors besides the enzyme and its substrate are required. These form three groups:

(a) **Activators**. These are simple substances, often inorganic and mostly metal ions. Some enzymes are active whether salts are present or not, others remain inactive unless a particular ion or one of a group of ions is present and its removal by dialysis inactivates the enzyme. The cationic activators, Mg^{2+}, Mn^{2+}, Zn^{2+}, K^+, Co^{2+}, Ca^{2+}, Fe^{2+}, and Ni^{2+} are most common in roughly that order of frequency. Mg^{2+} activates creatine kinase and other kinases, K^+ pyruvate kinase, alkaline phosphatase and 5′-nucleotidase, and Mn^{2+} the decarboxylation stage in the action of isocitrate dehydrogenase. Anions may also activate. Thus Cl^-, Br^- and NO_3^- activate amylase. Often there is an optimum concentration above which inhibition can occur, and while some ions may activate, others can inhibit.

(b) **Coenzymes**. In addition, organic substances may be activators. These play a part in the reaction and in the body may need to be reconverted to the original form. They are usually carriers of a particular group such as hydrogen, amino or phosphate. Many are nucleotides, the most common being the hydrogen-carrying nucleotides NAD^+ and $NADP^+$, and adenosine diphosphate which transfers a phosphate group by taking up a further phosphate to form adenosine triphosphate. Others include the flavin nucleotides, FMN and FAD, thiamine pyrophosphate, and pyridoxal phosphate. For a full description see Dixon and Webb (1964).

(c) **Prosthetic Groups.** In some enzymes, a group acting as a coenzyme is firmly attached to the protein part of the molecule. Such groups have been termed prosthetic groups. Examples are thiamine pyrophosphate in carboxylase; flavin adenine dinucleotide in glucose oxidase and xanthine oxidase; pyridoxal phosphate in the aminotransferases; and haem in peroxidase. Although in the above examples the group is firmly bound, the dissociation constant of the prosthetic group varies so there is no sharp dividing line between prosthetic groups and coenzymes.

Concentration of coenzymes and other activators can be treated in the same way as substrate concentration (p. 480) to define K_m values and arrive at optimal concentrations to use in assays.

7. Inhibitors

In contrast, some substances inhibit the enzyme action. These can be competitive, uncompetitive or non-competitive, reversible (i.e. removed by dialysis or chelation) or irreversible, and they can act on the enzyme itself or on the substrate, activator, or coenzyme.

Competitive inhibitors bind to the same site in the enzyme as the substrate thus blocking it. The extent of the inhibition depends on the relative concentrations of inhibitor and substrate so that by increasing the concentration of the latter the amount of inhibition can be reduced. The inhibitor in these cases may be similar in structure to the substrate. Thus the action of succinate dehydrogenase on succinate ($^-OOC.CH_2.CH_2.COO^-$) is inhibited by malonate ($^-OOC.CH_2.COO^-$).

In non-competitive inhibition, substrate and inhibitor bind reversibly, randomly and independently at different sites. Binding of the inhibitor to either the free enzyme or to the enzyme–substrate complex produces an inactive enzyme molecule. The effect is to decrease the apparent amount of enzyme present. In uncompetitive inhibition the inhibitor cannot bind to the free enzyme but binds reversibly to the enzyme–substrate complex yielding an inactive complex. This form of inhibition is rare in single substrate reactions but was found by Elliot and Wilkinson (1961) when studying the properties of 2-oxobutyrate as a substrate for the isoenzymes of lactate dehydrogenase.

The reciprocal plot described above (p. 484) can be used to differentiate between these different types of inhibition as will be seen from Fig. 22.7 (p. 486). The K_m is unaltered but the maximum velocity is reduced in the presence of a non-competitive inhibitor; in the competitive type, K_m as measured (the apparent K_m) is the sum of the dissociation constants of the enzyme–substrate complex and the enzyme–inhibitor complex and is increased but does not alter the maximum velocity; in the uncompetitive type a line parallel to and to the left of that for the uninhibited reaction is obtained so that both K_m and the maximum velocity are reduced. A substance which binds irreversibly with an enzyme may resemble a non-competitive inhibitor because V_{max} is decreased but K_m remains the same.

Metal ions form an important group of inhibitors. Some act by binding at a site which would otherwise be occupied by an activating ion. Thus Ca^{2+} may inactivate an enzyme activated by Mg^{2+}. Some ions are very selective. Thus Zn^{2+} inhibits creatine kinase, Ni^{2+} 5'-nucleotidase. These can therefore be used when it is necessary to inhibit an enzyme to prevent it from interfering in the assay of another enzyme. Another point to note is that metal ions may be removed by dialysis or by a chelating agent.

The dramatic effect of cyanide is due to its inhibition of metalloenzymes containing iron, copper, and zinc. Among these is cytochrome oxidase, so that aerobic oxidation in the body is stopped causing death within a few minutes. Sodium azide also acts by inhibiting metalloenzymes.

Many enzymes require the presence of –SH groups so that substances such as iodoacetate and *p*-chloromercuribenzoate which react with these inhibit their activity. Also some anticoagulants are enzyme inhibitors, particularly oxalate and fluoride, while EDTA acts by chelating Ca^{2+}

Finally, drugs which can act as inhibitors may be taken by a patient and be present in the specimen being tested; impurities in reagents used in the assay may also inhibit; and as we have seen, excess substrate may inhibit an enzyme reaction.

8. Specificity

A characteristic property of enzymes is their specificity. A particular enzyme catalyses only a limited number of reactions, in some cases one only. If we take a group of compounds with the general formula A–B which are acted on, there are three types of specificity:

(1) that involving only one kind of bond: bond specificity,
(2) that involving the bond and one of the groups A or B: group specificity,
(3) that involving the bond and both groups A and B: absolute specificity.

Thus esterases act on many esters of aliphatic alcohols and fatty acids, glucosidases act only on esters of glucose, while the highly specific enzyme urease acts only on urea and not on substituted ureas such as $RNH.CO.NH_2$.

Some enzymes show stereochemical specificity. Thus lactate dehydrogenase only acts on $L(+)$ lactate not on the $D(-)$ form or it converts optically inactive pyruvate only to $L(+)$ lactate. Furthermore, if a substance exists in *cis* and *trans* forms only one will be acted on. Thus fumarate hydratase acts on fumarate (the *trans* form) but not on maleate (the *cis* form), and succinate dehydrogenase converts succinate to fumarate, not to maleate. For a discussion of specificity see Dixon and Webb (1964).

UNITS

Units of enzyme activity have been expressed in many ways. Units were often given the name of the author of the method so that there have been several such units for a particular enzyme using different substrates and buffers. Each unit has its own reference range. The Recommendations (1966) of the Commission on Clinical Chemistry of the International Union of Pure and Applied Chemistry and of the IFCC (see Dybkaer and Jørgensen, 1967) were that all activities should be expressed in terms of International Units (U) one such unit being the activity which transforms one micromole of substrate per minute under defined conditions. The enzyme concentration was conveniently expressed as units per ml (U/ml). However, as is often the case, milli-International units (mU) can be used if these give a more convenient figure. One mU corresponds to the transformation of 1 nmol/min and enzyme concentration can be reported as mU/ml or, as in this book, U/l. In the case of some enzymes, the mol. wt. of the substrate may not be known and results are then expressed in micromoles of product. Units thus defined are still imperfect in several ways, the minute is not a basic SI unit, and standard conditions cannot be unambiguously defined.

The Commission recommended that the concept of 'enzyme unit' as a physically undefined 'amount of enzyme' should be abandoned and that 'enzyme activity' should be defined as the rate of reaction of substrate which may be attributed to catalysis by an enzyme. It is only with the enzymes which have been isolated, weighed, and chemically characterised, that we can go further. Then the specific and molar activities can be defined as the phenomenological coefficients which relate the activity under specified conditions respectively to the mass and to the amount of enzyme substance (usually expressed in moles).

The Katal. The Commission also proposed a new coherent SI unit of enzyme activity, the katal (symbol kat). One kat is defined as the catalytic amount of a system which has the amount of activity which produces a change of concentration of substrate or product of 1 mole per second. There is a fixed conversion for the International Unit and katal since the definitions imply rate measured in μmol/min and mol/s respectively. Thus one U corresponds to $1/60$ μmol/s or $1/60$ μkat or 16·67 nkat. So 1 U/l = 16·67 nkat/l and 1 katal = 6×10^7 U. This proposal has not been generally accepted yet.

The most commonly used units are U/ml and U/l. This definition of a unit has gone part way to allowing the comparison of results of different methods for measuring the same enzyme. However, the amount of enzyme which represents one unit varies with the conditions of the reaction, such as the type of substrate and its concentration, the type of buffer, pH, temperature and the presence or absence of activators. For this reason an enzyme for which many of these factors differ between methods may have a number of reference ranges quoted (see alkaline phosphatase, p. 534).

ISOENZYMES

Many enzymes exist in multiple forms. It has been recommended by the IUPAC-IUB Commission on Biochemical Nomenclature (CBN) (1976) that the term 'multiple forms of the enzyme' should be used as a general term covering all proteins catalysing the same reaction and occurring naturally in the same species. The term 'isoenzyme' (or less commonly, isozyme) should be applied only to those multiple forms of enzymes arising from genetically determined differences in the primary structure and not to those derived by modification of the same primary sequence. The multiple forms of the enzyme can differ in various ways. They can be genetically independent proteins such as cytosolic and mitochondrial aspartate aminotransferase. The enzyme can be a hybrid of two or more polypeptide chains non-covalently bound. Although the number of these units remains the same, the number of each type may vary as in lactate dehydrogenase and creatine kinase. Alternatively, genetic variants (allelo-enzymes) exist as with glucose-6-phosphate dehydrogenase. All the variations mentioned could be categorised as isoenzymes. Strictly speaking, the multiple forms of alkaline phosphatase are not all isoenzymes because the difference between some of them is due to different degrees of sialylation of the same gene product. The multiple forms of alkaline phosphatase will be described as isoenzymes in this chapter.

Isoenzymes can be measured and distinguished by their electrophoretic mobility, their behaviour towards different substrates, activators and inhibitors and by their heat stability. Recently, immunoinhibition has been used in the assay of isoenzymes by using antisera to inhibit the activity of one isoenzyme or subunit type. As the relative amounts of isoenzymes of a particular enzyme vary in different organs, the distribution of plasma isoenzymes found in disease tends to be similar to that in the organ from which they were released. This helps to identify the affected organ.

Electrophoretic mobility is also the basis for naming isoenzymes. The form having the greatest mobility towards the anode should be called number 1. This means that the fast-moving lactate dehydrogenase isoenzyme from heart muscle is lactate dehydrogenase 1 (or LD1) and the slow-moving liver isoenzyme is lactate dehydrogenase 5 (LD5). CBN recommends that isoenzymes should not be labelled on the basis of their tissue of origin since homologous forms may occur in different tissues in other species. This is not a problem in clinical chemistry and the forms of alkaline phosphatase are universally labelled by the tissue of origin.

Several electrophoretic techniques have been used to separate isoenzymes. Starch gel gives a clear separation and has been used with a variety of buffers (Latner and Skillen, 1968), as has cellulose acetate and agar gel. The presence of substances in the buffers which might inhibit one or other of the isoenzymes must be avoided, and since some isoenzymes are heat-labile the tank may need to be cooled. DEAE cellulose for column chromatography was applied to separate the isoenzymes of lactate dehydrogenase by Hess and Walter (1960, 1961) and DEAE Sephadex by Richterich *et al.* (1963). Gel filtration with various sizes of Sephadex G75-200 has also been used, as has isoelectric focusing (Dale and Latner, 1968).

For quantitation of isoenzymes, elution has been followed by estimation of each component by one of the techniques in use for the enzyme concerned. Alternatively, techniques have been developed for showing the isoenzyme bands *in situ* usually by staining. For lactate and other dehydrogenases tetrazolium salts have been used. These are easily reduced to poorly soluble formazans. The most sensitive are MTT, 2,5-diphenyl-3-(4',5'-dimethylthiazol-2-yl)-tetrazolium bromide, and the more sensitive INT, 2-(*p*-iodophenyl)-3-(*p*-nitrophenyl)-5-phenyltetrazolium chloride, and Nitro Blue Tetrazolium, NBT, 2,2'-di-*p*-nitrophenyl-5,5'-diphenyl-3,3'-(3,3'-dimethoxy-4,4'-diphenylene)ditetrazolium chloride, the structures of which are shown in Fig. 22.8. However, for dehydrogenases an intermediate is required since tetrazolium salts do not themselves react directly with NADH. A particularly useful hydrogen transport agent is *N*-methyl phenazonium methosulphate (phenazine methosulphate, PMS) (Latner and Skillen, 1961; Van der Helm, 1961). A suitable staining mixture for dehydrogenase enzymes contains the appropriate substrate; NAD^+ or $NADP^+$; MTT, INT or NBT; PMS; with hydrazine or cyanide as a carbonyl trapping agent. For lactate dehydrogenase the series of reactions is:

$$\text{Lactate} + NAD^+ \rightarrow \text{Pyruvate} + NADH + H^+$$

$$N\text{-Methylphenazonium methosulphate} + NADH + H^+ \rightarrow$$
$$N\text{-Methyldihydrophenazonium methosulphate} + NAD^+$$

$$N\text{-Methyldihydrophenazonium methosulphate} + \text{Tetrazolium salt} \rightarrow$$
$$N\text{-Methylphenazonium methosulphate} + \text{Formazan}$$

as shown in Fig. 22.9.

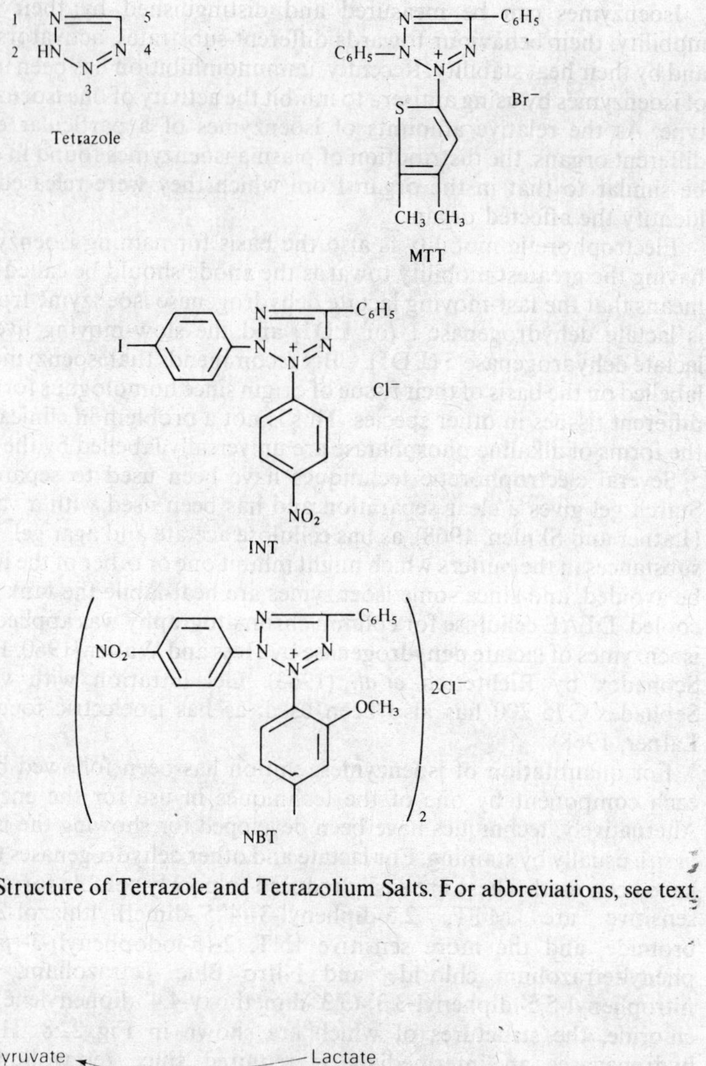

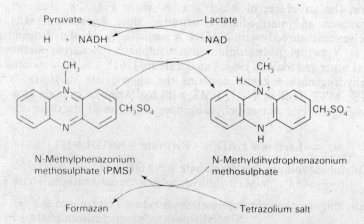

Fig. 22.8. The Structure of Tetrazole and Tetrazolium Salts. For abbreviations, see text.

Fig. 22.9. The Role of PMS as a Hydrogen Transport Agent.

A disadvantage of PMS is its sensitivity to light which has led to the use of Meldola Blue (Fast New Blue 3R, 8-dimethylamino-2,3-benzophenoxazine) which is unaffected by light (Fig. 22.10).

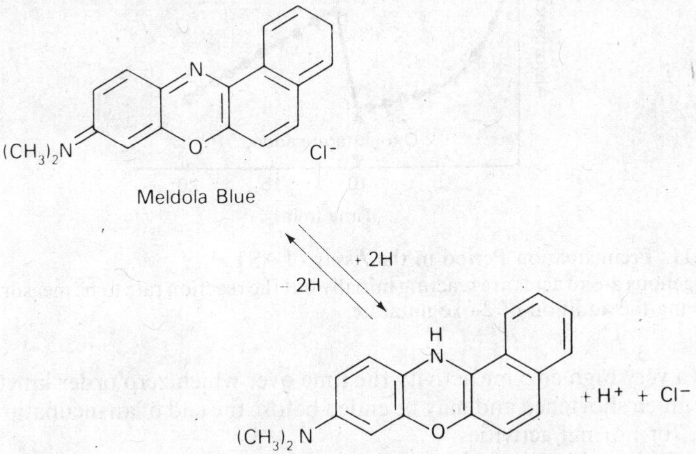

Fig. 22.10. Meldola Blue and its Reduction Product.
This dye can replace PMS in the reactions shown in Fig. 22.9.

Another staining technique widely applicable for esterases including phosphatases and cholinesterase, is to use a naphthyl ester as substrate and to couple the liberated naphthol with diazotised dianisidine. A strongly-coloured product is formed. Most commonly used techniques for quantitation of isoenzymes now involve immunoinhibition. See the sections on specific enzymes for details.

For full accounts of isoenzymes see the books by Latner and Skillen (1968), Moss (1982a) and Wilkinson (1970). Review articles are given for individual enzymes in the appropriate section.

TECHNIQUES FOR ENZYME ASSAY

Techniques for determining enzyme activity are of two types. In one, often termed 'two-point assays', the sample is incubated with the buffered substrate for a fixed period of time at the end of which the reaction is stopped and the amount of product formed or substrate used is measured. In the other, continuous monitoring or 'rate of reaction' assays, such changes are either measured at short intervals or are continuously monitored. In two-point assays it is necessary to know the range over which zero order kinetics are followed or serious errors may result. In rate reaction assays, any deviation from zero order kinetics can be seen by the appearance of non-linear rates of reaction. Therefore rate reaction methods are potentially more accurate and should, if possible, be used to check and standardise two-point assays. Two of the possible sources of error with enzyme assays should be considered in the development of an enzyme method. Firstly, one should allow a preincubation period (e.g. see Fig. 22.11) during which any side reaction will be allowed to go to completion before the substrate is added. Secondly, there may be a lag period before the full rate of reaction is reached (see p. 483). Care must be taken to ensure that the period of measurement does not begin until both processes are complete. Furthermore, in cases in which

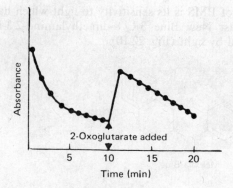

Fig. 22.11. Preincubation Period in the Assay of AST.
Endogenous α-oxo acids are reacting initially but the reaction rate to be measured is that following the addition of 2-oxoglutarate.

there is a very high enzyme activity the time over which zero order kinetics hold may be much shortened and may be ended before the end of an incubation period suitable for normal activities.

For samples with very high activity it may be desirable to shorten the time of incubation provided accurate timing is still possible. It may also be necessary to dilute the specimen although this should be avoided because dilution changes the concentration of activators and inhibitors in the specimen and may lead to a non-linear relationship between activity and dilution. By a combination of shorter incubation and dilution it is usually possible to obtain valid results even with the highest activities.

Reaction rate assays are generally superior to two-point assays and many instruments are now available which can continuously monitor reaction rates. However, as Moss (1972) noted in a review of the relative merits of the two types of assay, provided the limitations of the two-point assays are fully realised and methods are chosen to minimise the known sources of error, it is unlikely that clinically significant errors will result. If such methods are used, quality control procedures which include frequent comparison with a reaction rate method are advisable, and it may also be desirable to check very high results with a rate method so as to avoid as far as possible the need to dilute the specimen. Reaction rate assays depend on the ability to follow the reaction by using a convenient indicator reaction. This is not always possible and leads to the continued use of some two-point assays.

For a discussion of some general considerations concerning the determination of enzymes in serum see IFCC (1978).

General Techniques

The difference in the properties of the oxidised and reduced forms of NAD^+ and $NADP^+$ provides a convenient means of monitoring the activity of any enzyme using these coenzymes. Since the reduced form has an absorption peak at 340 nm and the oxidised form has little absorption at this wavelength (see Fig. 22.12), changes indicate the change in concentration of the reduced form due to the enzyme activity. The activity is calculated from the number of μmol coenzyme formed or removed per minute.

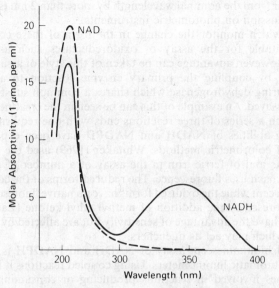

Fig. 22.12. Absorption Curves of NAD⁺ and NADH.

The molar absorptivity of NADH (and NADPH) is influenced by a rise in temperature which shifts the peak wavelength and reduces the molar absorptivity as does ionic strength and pH. This can lead to errors under some assay conditions. A number of revised values have been suggested and those currently recommended are given:

Wavelength	Value $\times 10^3$ l mol^{-1} cm^{-1}	
	NADH	NADPH
334 nm	6·18	6·18
(334·15 nm)		
340 nm	6·30	6·30
(339 nm)		
366 nm	3·40	3·50
(365·3 nm)		

Measurement of the change in absorbance over a few minutes has been widely used in rate of reaction assays. To convert such readings into U/l the following is used for a light path of 1 cm:

$$\text{Enzyme activity (U/l)} = \Delta A_{340}/\text{min} \times \frac{1000}{\text{Volume of serum used (ml)}}$$
$$\times \frac{\text{Total volume in the cuvette (ml)}}{6\cdot 3}$$

If readings cannot be made at 340 nm it is possible to read at 365 nm with some instruments. At this wavelength NADH has an absorbance a little over half that at 340 nm. Then 3·4 should be substituted for 6·3 in the above calculation.

Correct standardisation of enzyme assays using the molar absorption coefficient of a substrate, product or coenzyme relies entirely on the accuracy of the absorbance measurements. For greatest accuracy it is essential to use an instrument with a spectral bandwidth of not greater than 8 nm. The wavelength should not differ from the nominal wavelength by more than 2 nm (see Chapter 7 for further discussion on photometric instruments).

Techniques which monitor the change in the form of these coenzymes are particularly suitable for the assay of oxidoreductases such as lactate dehydrogenase. However, advantage can be taken of this style of assay to measure other enzymes by coupling the primary enzyme reaction to a NAD^+- or $NADP^+$- requiring dehydrogenase which shares a common substrate with the enzyme to be assayed. An example of this can be seen in the creatine kinase assay (p. 510) in which a series of three reactions ends with one requiring $NADP^+$.

The reducing abilities of NADH and NADPH have been exploited in the development of colorimetric methods. Whitaker (1969) used the reduction of tetrazolium salts and of ferric iron in the assay of a number of enzymes. An alternative approach uses fluorescence. The reduced forms of the coenzymes are naturally fluorescent while the oxidised forms have no native fluorescence but can be made to fluoresce by the addition of methyl ethyl ketone (Laursen, 1959). These methods have the advantage of sensitivity but are affected by the presence of substances which may act as quenchers.

The bacterial bioluminescent assay of NADH and NADPH is now readily performed on automatic luminometers. Using coupled reactions it is possible to measure enzymes involved in reactions producing or consuming NADH or NADPH. Similarly, enzymic reactions in which ATP is involved can be followed using firefly luciferase. This has been used for the assay of creatine kinase and its isoenzymes (e.g. see Tarkkanen *et al.*, 1979). Bioluminescent assays have the advantage of a 1000-fold increase in sensitivity over spectrophotometric assays but have not been adopted by clinical biochemistry laboratories. This is probably because the increased sensitivity is not required for this purpose and there is no incentive to change methodology or to buy dedicated equipment. For reviews on bio- and chemiluminescence see Gorus and Schram (1979), Whitehead *et al.* (1979) and Campbell *et al.* (1985).

Derivatives of 4-nitrophenol are often used as direct chromogenic substrates because above pH 7·2 the released phenolate ion absorbs strongly at 404 nm and the substrate has little absorbance at this wavelength. 4-Nitrophenyl phosphate is the preferred substrate for alkaline phosphatase and it can also be used for acid phosphatase. In the latter assay, the addition of a reagent to terminate the enzyme reaction also increases the pH to above 9·0 to produce the phenolate ion.

The absorbance or fluorescence of 4-methylumbelliferone has been used in the assay of esterases, lipases, phosphatases and a number of glycosidases. The anion of 4-methylumbelliferone absorbs maximally at 365 nm where the absorbance of the substrate is low. The anion also fluoresces with maximum emission at 448 nm. A cut-off filter is necessary to remove radiation below 405 nm since the substrate also fluoresces with maximum emission at 380 nm. The most common use for this technique in clinical biochemistry is probably the assay of β-N-acetyl-D-glucosaminidase.

Radioimmunoassay techniques have been applied for the determination of enzyme proteins (for reviews see Felber, 1973, and Landon *et al.*, 1977). It is important to realise the fundamental difference between such techniques which determine the actual concentration of the enzyme protein and other techniques which measure enzyme activity. Radioimmunoassay has the advantage of being more specific and more sensitive and avoids many of the problems concerning the conditions of the reactions such as the choice of substrate, buffer, coenzymes and temperature. Radioimmunoassay techniques are also less affected by haemolysed or lipaemic serum, the presence of inhibitors and the many drugs now in use.

However, the supply of purified enzymes required for antibody production is limited and the technique is costly.

Stability of Enzymes

Generally speaking it is best to do enzyme assays on the same day as the blood is taken. Of the enzymes dealt with in this chapter only acid phosphatase may not keep satisfactorily at room temperature for a few hours (see p. 542), though all the others can be stored overnight at 0–4 °C. Alanine aminotransferase is unstable forzen at − 25 °C but retains its activity satisfactorily at 4 °C. Creatine kinase should be stored at 4 °C and kept in the dark. The stability can be improved by reactivation with reagents containing a thiol group (see p. 510). Glucose-6-phosphate dehydrogenase is unstable at room temperature in red cell haemolysates, but is more stable in the intact red cell, so haemolysates should be prepared shortly before the assay is to be done and kept at 4 °C. Cholinesterase appears to be a robust enzyme since it is not only stable for 12 months at − 20 °C but is also unaffected by freezing and thawing (Turner *et al.*, 1984).

It should be borne in mind that isoenzymes may vary considerably in their heat lability and that the freezing of heteropolymers such as lactate dehydrogenase can change the distribution among the isoenzymes after thawing.

Current editions of the BCL catalogue include a table showing the average loss of activity of a number of enzymes stored at 4 °C and 25 °C.

Effect of Anticoagulants

Anticoagulants inhibit some enzymes and serum is generally considered preferable to plasma. Oxalate and fluoride inhibit a number of enzymes. Citrate inhibits amylase and EDTA inhibits some, e.g. alkaline phosphatase, but activates others according to whether it removes activating or inhibiting ions by its chelating action.

Some workers advocate the use of plasma since this overcomes the release of enzyme activity from platelets during the clotting process. If plasma is to be used, heparin is the recommended anticoagulant although it has been shown to inhibit enzymes such as creatine kinase and lactate dehydrogenase.

Effect of Haemolysis

As erythrocytes are much richer in some enzymes than plasma is, it is necessary to avoid haemolysis. This is particularly important for the assay of lactate dehydrogenase and the aminotransferases. Glutathione-activated creatine kinase methods are also affected by haemolysis. On storage some leakage of enzymes from red cells, platelets and leucocytes may occur. Generally, early separation of serum is recommended.

Instrumentation

Instruments suitable for enzyme assays are discussed in Chapter 7 (p. 199).

Quality Control

The quality control of enzyme assays has special problems. Since activity and not mass is usually measured the results are very dependent on reaction conditions and accuracy in the strict sense is unattainable. Reference serum with consensus values achieved using standardised methodology is substituted for primary or secondary standards. Various national and international bodies have published recommended methods for enzymes such as AST, ALT, ALP, LD, CK and GGT. The use of standardised optimised methodologies has been shown to decrease the interlaboratory imprecision for four enzymes (Strömme *et al.*, 1976). Reference and quality control materials may differ from human material with respect to stability, behaviour in enzyme assays and isoenzyme distribution. This may mean that slight changes in analytical conditions may affect the calibrant and control material in a different way from the effect on the patients' specimens. Lyophilised material has variable stability after reconstitution and rigid guidelines should be followed if the assigned values are to be achieved. Commercial liquid controls are now available. These are preserved in glycerol at sub-zero temperatures so the enzyme is not subjected to lyophilisation nor to the possible decrease in activity due to freezing and thawing.

External quality assessment schemes for enzymes are complicated by the method differences between laboratories. This can be overcome to some extent by expressing the activity obtained with one reference as a ratio or percentage of another. Alternatively a number of linearly related quality control sera can be used since, although the absolute figures will be different, the results should fall on a straight line. For a further discussion of this topic see Rosalki (1980) and Grannis (1976, 1977).

The quality of reagents is particularly pertinent in enzyme assays. Buffers and coenzymes have been shown to contain inhibitors (see p. 524). Substrates may contain the product of the reaction (pp. 485, 534). To avoid problems it is advisable to purchase high quality reagents and to store them according to the manufacturers' recommendations. If necessary, the quality of the reagent can be checked before use (pp. 501, 512, 519, 523, 534, 544).

REFERENCE RANGES FOR ENZYMES

While it is desirable for each laboratory to check carefully the normal range of results for any serum constituent, this is even more necessary for methods determining enzyme activity. Minor variations in technique can alter the accuracy of a method while the precision, which is rather poor for some methods, varies from one laboratory to another. Both factors influence the results and the range of values found in apparently healthy people. The 'normal ranges' quoted in this chapter should therefore be regarded as general guidelines rather than definitive reference ranges.

Results of enzyme assays can only be interpreted if a reference range is quoted and it is now usual to issue results on pre-printed stationery which displays reference ranges. To overcome the difficulty in interpretation, abnormal results will be given in multiples of the 'upper reference limit', URL, where appropriate.

Optimised Techniques

The early methods for measuring serum enzyme activity were sub-optimal in that the concentrations of the substrate, co-enzymes and activators were not adequate to achieve the maximum activity of the enzyme. Quality control studies showed a highly unsatisfactory performance of routine enzyme assays in several countries and steps were taken to establish a higher degree of precision and comparability in enzyme methods in use in clinical laboratories. The approach taken was to develop strictly defined methods for use as routine assays. These assays were optimised in that they would produce enzyme activities as close to V_{max} as was possible within the limits of reproducibility, practicability and clinical application. Practical aspects such as the solubility, absorbance and cost of the reagents are limiting factors. The introduction of such optimised methods has improved performance in national quality assessment schemes (Strömme *et al.*, 1976).

The methods used for optimising assays deserve some comment. Early attempts at optimisation used univariate methods in which the concentration of one component of the reaction was changed while the others were kept constant. This is an unsatisfactory approach since many of the conditions are interdependent. A more satisfactory method uses steady-state kinetic parameters which allow the prediction of measured catalytic activity at any substrate concentration but can only be applied to enzymes for which a detailed steady-state kinetic mechanism is known. If pure isoenzymes can be obtained it is possible to determine the optimal conditions for each. Then the conditions for total enzyme activity can be a compromise between those determined for the isoenzymes based on the clinical importance of each. Alternatively, differences in optimal conditions between isoenzymes can be used to design a differential assay. This method of optimisation requires much preliminary work in determining the Michaelis constants using pure enzyme, which may not reflect the enzymes in serum, and small errors in K_m or other parameters may lead to the recommendation of inappropriate conditions. This method has been used for AST (London *et al.*, 1975; Bergmeyer *et al.*, 1978).

An alternative approach to the selection of optimised conditions is the application of response-surface simultaneous optimisation, a multivariate method. With all enzymes it is found that any given activity can be achieved with many different combinations of two interdependent variables. For example, with AST, the stimulation by pyridoxal-5'-phosphate is pH-dependent and the same activity can be achieved with concentrations of pyridoxal phosphate ranging from 0·08 to 0·18 mmol/l as long as the pH is changed appropriately over the range pH 7·0 to 8·5 as the pyridoxal phosphate concentration increases. Thus, experiments are performed varying more than one concentration or condition at a time. A computer-generated contour plot can then be produced. This shows lines of 'iso-activity' from which optimal conditions can be chosen. This method is particularly useful for co-optimising variables which are difficult to predict from steady-state rate equations and has the advantage that rigorously determined Michaelis constants are not required. Rautela *et al.* (1979) applied this technique to the optimisation of a number of enzymes in human serum.

AMINOTRANSFERASES (TRANSAMINASES)
Aspartate Aminotransferase (2.6.1.1); Alanine Aminotransferase (2.6.1.2)

Transamination is the term given to the process in which an amino group is transferred from an α-amino acid to an α-oxo acid. As a result a different α-amino acid and a different α-oxo acid are formed. All naturally occurring α-amino acids can take part in such reactions, different enzymes being involved. Two clinically important examples are L-aspartate: 2-oxoglutarate aminotransferase (aspartate aminotransferase, AST) and L-alanine: 2-oxoglutarate aminotransferase (alanine aminotransferase, ALT). The former catalyses the reaction:

$$
\begin{array}{cccc}
\text{COO}^- & \text{COO}^- & \text{COO}^- & \text{COO}^- \\
| & | & | & | \\
\text{CO} & \text{CHNH}_2 & \text{CHNH}_2 & \text{CO} \\
| & | & | & | \\
\text{CH}_2 \; + & \text{CH}_2 \;\; \rightleftharpoons & \text{CH}_2 \; + & \text{CH}_2 \\
| & | & | & | \\
\text{CH}_2 & \text{COO}^- & \text{CH}_2 & \text{COO}^- \\
| & & | & \\
\text{COO}^- & & \text{COO}^- &
\end{array}
$$

2-Oxoglutarate   L-Aspartate   L-Glutamate   Oxaloacetate

and the latter the reaction:

$$
\begin{array}{cccc}
\text{COO}^- & \text{COO}^- & \text{COO}^- & \text{COO}^- \\
| & | & | & | \\
\text{CO} \; + & \text{CHNH}_2 \;\; \rightleftharpoons & \text{CHNH}_2 \; + & \text{CO} \\
| & | & | & | \\
\text{CH}_2 & \text{CH}_3 & \text{CH}_2 & \text{CH}_3 \\
| & & | & \\
\text{CH}_2 & & \text{CH}_2 & \\
| & & | & \\
\text{COO}^- & & \text{COO}^- &
\end{array}
$$

2-Oxoglutarate   L-Alanine   L-Glutamate   Pyruvate

Aminotransferases require pyridoxal-5′-phosphate as a co-factor. In most normal sera this is present in adequate amounts but it may be deficient in some pathological states leading to a reduced enzyme activity under the conditions used for its measurement. The recommended methods of the IFCC (1975, 1979) include pyridoxal phosphate to allow the measurement of the maximum potential activity of the sample. In Tris buffer, saturation of AST and ALT with pyridoxal phosphate produces average fractional increases of 1·4-fold and 1·2-fold respectively with considerable variation between individuals. The degree of stimulation of AST appears to be greatest in cases of heart disease and some workers feel this is sufficient to improve diagnostic discrimination.

Determination of Aminotransferases

Earlier colorimetric methods have been superseded by coupled-enzyme assays. The coupled enzymes used in these assays are malate dehydrogenase in the case of AST:

$$
\begin{array}{cc}
\text{COO}^- & \text{COO}^- \\
| & | \\
\text{CO} & \text{CHOH} \\
| & | \\
\text{CH}_2 \; + \text{NADH} + \text{H}^+ \;\; \rightleftharpoons & \text{CH}_2 \; + \text{NAD}^+ \\
| & | \\
\text{COO}^- & \text{COO}^-
\end{array}
$$

Oxaloacetate   Malate

and lactate dehydrogenase (LD) in the case of ALT:

$$\text{Pyruvate} + \text{NADH} + \text{H}^+ \rightleftharpoons \text{Lactate} + \text{NAD}^+$$

These allow the aminotransferase reactions to be followed by measuring the decrease in absorbance at 340 nm.

On incubating the mixture of serum, aspartate or alanine, NADH and the relevant dehydrogenase, there is an initial fall in the absorbance at 340 nm due to the NADH used up in the reduction of oxo acids in the serum. These side-reactions should be completed before the addition of 2-oxoglutarate and this is assisted by the inclusion of LD in the AST method to remove excess pyruvate present in the sample. In some cases the amount of NADH used in these side-reactions may be substantial and the remaining NADH may be insufficient to support maximum activity of the enzyme in the sample. To prevent this the analyst must determine the minimum initial absorbance below which the assay should not be continued. More NADH may need to be added before initiating the reaction by the addition of 2-oxoglutarate. Although the coupled enzyme assay is generally specific for aminotransferases, the presence of glutamate dehydrogenase (GLD) and ammonium ion can cause oxidation of NADH and therefore apparent aminotransferase activity. The reaction is:

$$\text{2-Oxoglutarate} + \text{NADH} + \text{NH}_4^+ \rightleftharpoons \text{L-Glutamate} + \text{NAD}^+$$

Since high levels of glutamate dehydrogenase can be present in serum in extrahepatic obstructive disorders and ammonium ion can be introduced by the use of ammonium sulphate preparations of malate and lactate dehydrogenases, glycerol solutions of the coupling enzymes are recommended.

The technique introduced by Karmen (1955) has been widely used and much studied and modified. Recommendations have been published by several authorities (e.g. see the following Recommended Method; IFCC, 1975 and 1979).

Recommended Method of the Committee on Enzymes of the Scandinavian Society for Clinical Chemistry and Physiology (1974)

Reagents.
1. Buffer substrate. *For AST*, Tris, 25 mmol (3·0 g); EDTA, disodium salt dihydrate, 6·25 mmol (2·3 g); L-aspartate, 250 mmol (33·3 g) L-aspartic acid/l. Dissolve these in 500 ml water, adjust the pH to 7·7 at 37 °C with 1 mol/l sodium hydroxide and make to a litre with water. *For ALT* use 500 mmol (44·6 g) L-alanine instead of the aspartic acid, otherwise proceed as above but adjust to pH 7·4 at 37 °C with 1 mol/l hydrochloric acid. Stored at 4 °C these keep for at least 6 weeks.
2. Working solutions. (a). *For AST* to 100 ml buffer substrate add 14 mg NADH disodium salt trihydrate, 75 units malate dehydrogenase (from pig heart 1100 U/mg) and 25 U lactate dehydrogenase (from pig muscle, 500 U/mg). Both the MD and LD supplied in glycerol should be free from AST, apoAST, and GLD. In the final mixture, the concentrations are L-aspartate, 250 mmol/l; NADH, 0·19 mmol/l; MD, 750 U/l; LD, 250 U/l.

   (b). *For ALT* to 100 ml buffer substrate add 14 mg NADH and 250 units lactate dehydrogenase (from pig muscle 500 U/mg free from ALT, apoALT, and GLD, supplied in glycerol). In the final mixture, the concentrations are L-alanine, 500 mmol/l; NADH, 0·19 mmol/l; LD, 2500 U/l.

   Stored at 4 °C well-stoppered these working solutions keep at least 3 days.
3. 2-Oxoglutarate solution 150 mmol/l. Dissolve 2·19 g 2-oxoglutaric acid in about 80 ml water and adjust at 37 °C to pH 7·7 for AST and 7·4 for ALT with 1 mol/l sodium hydroxide and make to 100 ml with water.

Technique. For both enzymes add 150 μl serum to 1 ml working solution, mix, and incubate for 5–15 min at 37°C. Then add 100 μl oxoglutarate, mix, transfer to a 1 cm cuvette and read the ΔA/min at 340 nm at 37 °C.

Calculation. Serum AST or ALT activity (U/l)

$$= \frac{\Delta A_{340}/\text{min}}{6 \cdot 3} \times \frac{\text{Total volume in the cuvette (ml)}}{\text{Volume of serum used (ml)}} \times 10^3$$

$$= \Delta A_{340}/\text{min} \times 1323$$

The molar absorption coefficient of NADH is $6 \cdot 3 \times 10^3$ l $\text{mol}^{-1}\text{cm}^{-1}$.

Notes.

1. The Scandinavian Committee on Enzymes, SCE (1981) used supplementation with pyridoxal phosphate at the preincubation stage. To Reagent 1 in the method given above add 50 ml pyridoxal phosphate, $2 \cdot 5$ mmol/l in Tris buffer, pH $7 \cdot 5$ (37 °C) before making to 1 litre. This reagent is stable at 4 °C for 2 weeks. Supplementation with pyridoxal phosphate is now recommended by the IFCC Expert Panel on Enzymes (e.g. IFCC, 1975). Earlier reports that addition of the coenzyme had no effect on aminotransferase activity can probably be explained by the use of phosphate buffer which inhibits the association of pyridoxal phosphate with the apoenzyme. Supplementation may give incorrect results with quality control materials which have been assigned values using a method which does not include pyridoxal phosphate.
2. There is general agreement that serum or EDTA, heparin, oxalate and citrated plasma are suitable for AST assay. However, heparin plasma has been reported to cause turbidity in the ALT method occasionally. The SCE could not confirm this but the IFCC recommendations prefer to avoid plasma (IFCC, 1979).
3. High activity specimens can be diluted up to 1 in 10 in 150 mmol/l sodium chloride solution. An activation of up to 10% may occur.
4. AST has been very closely studied with respect to the optimal conditions for assay. The application of steady-state kinetic models to the selection of optimal conditions for assay is given in a paper by Bergmeyer et al. (1978).

INTERPRETATION

The upper reference limit values quoted (Scandinavian Committee on Enzymes, 1981) for this method are:

	AST U/l	ALT U/l
Cord blood	50	25
Males (20–60 years)	40	40
Males (over 60 years)	35	35
Females	35	35
Pregnancy (third trimester)	40	45

Both these enzymes are found in most tissues but the relative values in U per 10^{-4} g wet tissue homogenates were given by Wroblewski (1958) for those tissues richest in these enzymes as follows:

	Heart	Liver	Skeletal muscle	Kidney	Pancreas	Spleen	Lung
AST	151	137	96	88	27	14	10
ALT	7	43	4·7	19	2	1·2	0·7

It can be seen that while the liver is by far the richest in ALT, several tissues are rich in AST, particularly heart.

Heart Disease. As would be expected the determination of serum AST activity is particularly useful in myocardial infarction. The increase begins 3–8 h after the onset of the attack and returns to normal in 3–6 days. The highest values are found on average some 24 h after the onset, the duration and extent of the increase being related to the size of the infarct. Values are most commonly from 1 to 5 times the upper reference limit (URL) but activities up to 15 times this value are reported. Enzyme determinations in the diagnosis of myocardial infarction are particularly useful when the ECG findings are equivocal. AST has had a central role in this area but is being replaced to some extent by the assay of total creatine kinase and CK–MB activity. Normal values are usual in heart conditions such as angina and pericarditis and in patients with pulmonary embolism and acute abdominal conditions.

In contrast, increase in ALT is found in only a minority of patients in the period immediately following a myocardial infarction and is mostly small. However, in some severer cases, damage to the liver due to hypoxia may cause an increase within a few days of the onset, and later congestive heart failure may also do so.

Liver Disease. Serum AST and ALT activities are sensitive indicators of parenchymal liver damage. Increases in both are commonly found in liver disease, with the increase in ALT being greater than that of AST, particularly in infective hepatitis. Levels from 10 to 100 times URL are reported with most being between 20 and 50 times this value. The increase begins in the prodromal period when the determination can be of great value in testing suspected cases in an outbreak of infective hepatitis in which a value in the normal range excludes the condition. It is maximal in the early stages of the jaundice, then falling if and when recovery takes place. So the determinations can be useful in showing the severity of the disease and in following its progress. Generally the enzyme activities do not return to normal until some time after the disappearance of the jaundice. Very high levels can also be found in hepatic ischaemia. Moderate increases, of 5 to 10 times URL are typical of infectious mononucleosis and hepatocellular damage secondary to cholestasis. The ALT level is usually slightly higher than the AST. In cirrhosis any elevation is less marked with activities of both enzymes being up to 5 times URL in alcoholic and cryptogenic cirrhosis and slightly higher in primary or secondary biliary cirrhosis. The ALT level is usually higher than the AST. In all forms of cirrhosis the serum AST and ALT activities may be normal.

Primary or secondary hepatic tumours cause an elevation of both enzymes with AST higher than ALT and usually less than 5 times URL. This rise occurs in only 50 % of anicteric patients with hepatic tumours but is almost invariable if the patient is jaundiced.

Both AST and ALT are excellent markers of liver damage caused by exposure to toxic substances. Several drugs and therapeutic substances affect serum aminotransferase activities in this way including opiates, salicylates, tetracyclines, heparin, chenodeoxycholic acid, penicillin, chloramphenicol, aminoglycosides and cephalosporins. Values comparable with those in infective hepatitis are seen in carbon tetrachloride poisoning but with similar increases in AST and ALT. A considerable increase is also found in paracetamol overdose. Chlorpromazine is an example of a drug which gives rise to intrahepatic cholestasis. Increase in AST and ALT is relatively small resembling that in post-hepatic jaundice. 17α-Alkylated steroids such as methyl testosterone also act in this way as do some of the steroids in the contraceptive pill (Hargreaves, 1970). Sometimes some degree of liver cell damage accompanies the cholestasis. For a comprehensive account of drug action with a list of those with some action on the liver see Hargreaves (1968).

De Ritis *et al.* (1958, 1972) used the ratio of AST to ALT activity as an aid to diagnosis in liver disease. There are several recent reports of the use of the De Ritis ratio (Ammann *et al.*, 1982; Gitlin, 1982; Matloff *et al.*, 1980).

Other Conditions. Diseases of skeletal muscle including muscular dystrophy and polymyositis may lead to increases in serum AST activity with normal ALT. A similar pattern is seen in muscle trauma, including surgery, and after severe exercise.

Low values of serum and erythrocyte AST activities have been associated with vitamin B_6 deficiency. However, stimulation of AST activity by added pyridoxal phosphate correlates better with vitamin status than does the absolute activity level (see Chapter 35, p. 913).

Isoenzymes of Aspartate Aminotransferase

Mammalian AST exists in two forms, one mitochondrial (m-AST) and the other of soluble or cytosolic origin (s-AST). These proteins are genetically distinct, true isoenzymes which differ in their amino acid composition and immunochemical properties and with considerable difference in their isoelectric points (pH 5·3 for s-AST and 9·3 for m-AST). Both isoenzymes are dimers composed of identical subunits and have been detected in nearly all mammalian tissues. In serum, m-AST contributes less than 12 % of the total AST activity but is the major fraction in human liver, heart, kidney, spleen and muscle.

AST isoenzymes have been separated and quantified using electrophoresis, chromatography, differential kinetics and immunochemical methods. Because of the large difference in their isoelectric points, semi-quantitative separation by electrophoresis and ion-exchange chromatography is readily achieved. In contrast to s-AST, m-AST has a lower pH optimum, a greater affinity for L-aspartate and a lesser affinity for 2-oxoglutarate. All have been exploited in differential kinetic methods. Martinez-Carrion *et al*. (1977) described a differential pH assay which includes adipate which, at low pH and ionic strength, inhibits s-AST but not m-AST. This procedure has been adapted for the Dupont aca analyser. Several immunochemical methods involve activity measurements after immuno-inhibition or immunoprecipitation of one of the isoenzymes (Rej, 1980). A comparison of six procedures for AST isoenzymes showed good correlation between immunoprecipation methods and the differential pH kinetic assay with adipate inhibition (Rej *et al*., 1981). An electrophoretic method was least accurate for measuring samples, the isoenzyme composition of which was known, and the chromatographic methods showed considerable positive bias for m-AST in human serum.

Studies in man suggest that serum m-AST more precisely reflects the extent and type of damage in liver disease, particularly alcoholic liver disease where it may be elevated while the total AST activity remains within the reference range (Ishii *et al*., 1978). Measurement of m-AST may have a role in the diagnosis of myocardial infarction especially since m-AST activity in human serum correlates with the extent of infarction more significantly than does CK-MB.

Nevertheless, m-AST assays are not yet generally used routinely because of the considerable shortcomings of their analysis.

CHOLINESTERASES (3.1.1.7 and 3.1.1.8)

Cholinesterases hydrolyse certain esters of choline, e.g. acetylcholine:

$$(CH_3)_3N^+ . (CH_2)_2 . O . CO . CH_3 + H_2O \rightarrow (CH_3)_3N^+ . (CH_2)_2 . OH$$
$$+ CH_3COOH$$

The two enzymes are *acetylcholinesterase* (3.1.1.7, acetylcholine hydrolase, 'true cholinesterase') present in nerve tissue and the red blood cells, and responsible for the hydrolysis of acetylcholine to choline at synapses and the neuromuscular junction, and *cholinesterase* (3.1.1.8, acylcholine acyl-hydrolase, 'pseudo-cholinesterase') present in liver and other non-nervous tissues and in the plasma.

Both enzymes act on several esters of choline and of other alcohols found in the human body but show wide differences in their affinity for different substrates. Thus acetylcholinesterase is most active with acetylcholine, or choline esters with acyl groups, whereas cholinesterase has greatest activity with butyrylcholine and also acts on benzoylcholine, with both of which acetylcholinesterase shows little activity. The reverse is the case with acetyl-2-methylcholine. Another difference is that acetylcholinesterase is inhibited by increasing concentrations of acetylcholine unlike cholinesterase which hydrolyses this substance at half the rate. Both enzymes, however, are specifically inhibited by physostigmine (eserine).

Several techniques have been used to determine serum cholinesterase activity (Silk *et al.*, 1979). The earlier ones measured the acid produced in the reaction by the change in pH, the colour change of indicators, or the volume of carbon dioxide released from bicarbonate. The choline ester remaining after enzyme action has been determined by the reaction of hydroxylamine with fatty acid esters in the presence of Fe^{3+} to produce the red to violet-coloured Fe^{3+} salts of hydroxamic acid. The amount of phenol liberated from a phenyl benzoate substrate has been estimated. Kalow and colleagues (Kalow and Lindsay, 1955; Kalow and Genest, 1957; Kalow and Davies, 1958; Davies *et al.*, 1960) introduced a reaction rate assay using benzoylcholine which has an absorption peak at 235 nm. Since diluted serum shows some absorption at this wavelength, measurements are usually made at 240 nm. These workers investigated various substrates and inhibitors, the latter being important in the recognition of genetic variants of cholinesterase. Dibucaine and fluoride have long been used, and the percentage inhibition by these substances is referred to as the dibucaine number (DN) and fluoride number (FN) respectively.

Dietz *et al.* (1973) preferred propionylthiocholine as substrate. The thiocholine produced reacts with 5,5'-dithiobis(2-nitrobenzoic acid) (DTNB) to give the 5-thio-2-nitrobenzoate anion, monitored by its absorbance at 410 nm. Others have been unable to achieve the precision cited in the original paper (Brown and Price, 1975; Price and Brown, 1975). The method of Kalow and colleagues is given since a large amount of experience has been gained with this method.

If it is desired to determine the red cell acetylcholinesterase, as in organophosphorus poisoning, acetylcholine or acetylthiocholine have been used as substrates with red cells or haemolysates (Dacie and Lewis, 1975; Demetriou *et al.*, 1974).

Determination of Serum Cholinesterase

Rate of Reaction Assay for Total Serum Cholinesterase and Dibucaine and Fluoride Numbers

Reagents.
1. Phosphate buffer, pH 7·4, 133 mmol/l, 19·19 g Na_2HPO_4, $2H_2O$ and 3·48 g KH_2PO_4/l.

2. Benzoylcholine chloride, 200 μmol/l, 48·8 mg/l in water. Keep the salt *in vacuo* over sulphuric acid. Prepare freshly for use.
3. Dibucaine hydrochloride, 40 μmol/l, 15·2 mg/l in water.
4. Fluoride solution, 200 μmol/l, 8·4 mg sodium fluoride/l in water.

Technique. Dilute the serum 1 to 100 with the phosphate buffer.

(a). *Determination of enzyme activity*. For the test add 1 ml water and 2 ml diluted serum (= 20 μl) to 1 ml benzoylcholine chloride solution (= 200 mmol). For the blank take equal volumes of water and diluted serum. Read the test at 240 nm at 25 °C in a 1 cm cuvette against the blank either by continuous recording or at least at minute intervals for 10 min to define the linear part of the slope of the curve.

Calculation. The hydrolysis of 200 nmol benzoylcholine gives a ΔA of 0·33 in a total volume of 4 ml. So

$$\text{Serum cholinesterase (kU/l)} = \frac{\Delta A/\min}{0\cdot33} \times \frac{200}{1000} \times \frac{1000}{20}$$

$$= \Delta A/\min \times 30\cdot3$$

Normal Ranges. At 25 °C the range is 0·6–1·4 kU/l and at 37 °C 1·08–2·4 kU/l.

(b). *Determination of dibucaine and fluoride numbers*. For these use 1 ml dibucaine or fluoride solution in place of 1 ml water.

Calculation.

$$\text{DN or FN} = \left(1 - \frac{\Delta A/\min \text{ with inhibitor}}{\Delta A/\min \text{ without inhibitor}}\right) \times 100$$

Determination of Red Cell Acetylcholinesterase
(Weber, 1966; Dacie and Lewis, 1975)

The rate of hydrolysis of acetylthiocholine by a red cell suspension at pH 7·2 is measured at 412 nm by the reaction of thiocholine with DTNB to give the yellow 5-thio-2-nitrobenzoate anion (molar absorptivity, $13\cdot6 \times 10^6$ l mol^{-1} cm^{-1}). The activity is expressed per litre of packed red cells.

Reagents.
1. Phosphate buffer, 50 mmol/l in 9 g/l sodium chloride; pH 7·20.
2. Substrate solution, acetylthiocholine iodide, 31 mmol/l. The stock reagent is available (Boehringer Corporation) at a concentration of 156 mmol/l. Dilute with water, 1 in 5, for use.
3. Colour reagent, DTNB, 250 μmol/l, in phosphate buffer, 50 mmol/l, pH 7·2. This is also available from Boehringer Corporation.
4. Sodium chloride solution, 9 g/l.

Technique. Determine the fractional packed cell volume (PCV) of the anticoagulated blood sample. Place 100 μl blood in a glass tube, 100 × 12 mm, and wash three times with saline, centrifuging between washes. Remove the last supernatant as completely as possible and resuspend the cells in 10 ml buffer, mixing well. To 1 ml suspension add 4 ml buffer and remix.

Into two silica cuvettes (1 cm optical path) pipette 2·0 ml (for test) or 2·1 ml (for blank) of the colour reagent and add 1·0 ml cell suspension to each, having ensured that it is homogeneous. Place the cuvettes in the thermostatted (30 °C) cuvette holder of a spectrophotometer set to 412 nm. After 3 min add 100 μl substrate to the test. Mix the contents of both cuvettes and determine the absorbance of the test against the blank. Repeat the readings every minute for at least 6 min, remixing the cuvette contents before each reading. Calculate the mean change of absorbance per min (ΔA_{412}/min).

Calculation. Red cell acetylcholinesterase (kU/l red cells)

$$= \frac{\Delta A_{412}/\text{min} \times 500 \times 10^3 \times 10^3 \times 3 \cdot 1}{\text{PCV} \times 13 \cdot 6 \times 10^6 \times 1}$$

$$= \frac{\Delta A_{412}/\text{min}}{\text{PCV}} \times 114$$

Normal Range. 8 to 13 kU/l.

Notes.

1. Blood may be anticoagulated by defibrination, heparin, EDTA or acid-citrate-dextrose (ACD) and may be kept at 20 °C for at least 3 days without loss of enzyme activity.
2. There is a slow non-enzymatic hydrolysis of substrate. If necessary, this is allowed for by setting up a further cuvette using 1 ml phosphate buffer instead of 1 ml cell suspension in the 'test' cuvette.

INTERPRETATION

Findings in disease are summarised by Brown *et al.* (1981). Low values have been found in uraemia and shock, in anaemia, tuberculosis and cancer, in malnutrition and cachexia, and also in pregnancy. Cholinesterase is formed in the liver and serum activity is reduced in liver damage. Normal values occur in obstructive jaundice unless there is also damage to the hepatocytes. A fall in plasma cholinesterase activity after burns is related to the severity of the injury. The sharp fall in the first 24 h suggests loss of enzyme from the capillaries and, perhaps, dilution due to intensive fluid therapy. It should be remembered that genetic variants of cholinesterase may also reduce its activity.

Serum cholinesterase activity is also reduced in poisoning by organo-phosphorus compounds used as insecticides. The determination should be carried out at intervals on workers making or using these substances to see if a significant fall has occurred. For this purpose a pre-exposure result can be useful in showing if a fall has taken place even if the later result is within the normal range. These organophosphorus compounds also inhibit acetylcholinesterase so that its determination in red cells is useful.

Increased levels of cholinesterase activity have been reported in obesity, thyrotoxicosis, essential hypertension, nephrosis and alcoholism (Silk *et al.*, 1979).

Currently, the main use of cholinesterase determinations relates to the use of the muscle relaxant suxamethonium (succinyl dicholine, scoline). This is rapidly hydrolysed and inactivated by cholinesterase but its brief action, 2 to 4 min in normal persons, allows easy endotracheal intubation in anaesthesia. In individuals with low serum cholinesterase activity arising from one of the conditions mentioned above, hydrolysis is retarded and apnoea may be appreciably prolonged.

A much longer period of apnoea, lasting over 3 h in some cases, occurs in a small number of patients not having one of these conditions. Often this is due to the presence of a genetic variant inherited as an autosomal recessive (Bourne *et al.*, 1952; Evans *et al.*, 1952). Two loci are responsible for the production of cholinesterase. Using the symbols E for esterase and E_1 and E_2 for the two loci, the gene at locus 1 is denoted E_1^u in the normal person, *u* standing for usual, while in the first genetic variant recognised, it is E_1^a, *a* standing for atypical. Thus the genotypes, $E_1^u E_1^u$, $E_1^u E_1^a$, $E_1^a E_1^a$, exist. The first (phenotype U) is found in most members of the population and the last (phenotype A) occurs in patients with prolonged apnoea. While in some individuals of phenotype A the cholinesterase activity is markedly reduced, it is not possible confidently to distinguish between these three genotypes on the basis of activity measurements alone. A sharper separation is obtained using inhibitors and Kalow and Genest (1957) found the $E_1^a E_1^a$ enzyme to be more resistant to dibucaine (lower DN) than the normal $E_1^u E_1^u$, with $E_1^u E_1^a$ (phenotype UA) lying in between (see also Table 22.1). This property of the enzymes is independent of their concentration; in the acquired conditions discussed earlier, serum activity is reduced but the DN is unaltered. Harris and Whittaker (1961) found the FN to behave similarly with regard to the 'atypical' variant but were able to identify another variant, the 'fluoride-resistant' form, by its different relationship between DN and FN. This allele, E_1^f, may occur in combination with itself, E_1^u, or E_1^a. The different sensitivities to dibucaine and fluoride of the various pairings are listed in Table 22.1.

TABLE 22.1

Percentage Inhibition of Cholinesterase Variants by Various Substances

Phenotype	Genotype	Dibucaine[1]	Fluoride[1]	Ro02–0683[1]	Scoline[2]
U	$E_1^u E_1^u$	80–83·5	57–63·5	93·5–97·5	85–95
UA	$E_1^u E_1^a$	58–68	45·5–53	66·5–80	54–79
A	$E_1^a E_1^a$	13·5–27	17–31·5	5–22·5	0–31
UF	$E_1^u E_1^f$	72–81	41·5–56·5	91–100	81–91
F	$E_1^f E_1^f$	64–67*	34–35*	75–86*	82–91
AF	$E_1^a E_1^f$	43–52	27–36·5	58–69	33–63
US	$E_1^u E_1^s$	77–84	51–67·5	94·5–99	–
FS	$E_1^f E_1^s$	61·5–70	30–43	92·5–100	–
AS	$E_1^a E_1^s$	14·5–26	21–32·5	4·5–28·5	–
AK	$E_1^a E_1^k$	47·5–58	33–48	49–66·5	52–66
AJ	$E_1^a E_1^j$	40–46·5	35·5–39	40–48·5	38–49
UK	$E_1^u E_1^k$	77·5–82	59–63	94·5–97	–
S	$E_1^s E_1^s$	no detectable enzyme activity			

Figures are from various sources:
1—Evans and Wardell (1984)
2—Owen (1986), unpublished data, Manchester Royal Infirmary
*—Lehmann and Liddell (1969)

A fourth allele, E_1^s, was later identified as the 'silent' gene since the rare homozygotes, $E_1^s E_1^s$, show extremely low or undetectable cholinesterase activity. This allele, which apparently exists in two forms, appears to act by suppressing the number of E_1^u molecules in the circulation by 95 to 100% (Rubinstein *et al.*, 1970). Thus in the phenotype US the enzyme activity is half the normal, and inhibitor studies are characteristic of the E_1^u allele. The change is a quantitative one rather than qualitative as with E_1^a and E_1^f. A second 'quantitative' variant, E_1^j (Garry *et al.*, 1976; Rubinstein *et al.*, 1976) was identified from family studies in which the E_1^u, E_1^a and E_1^f variants were also present. It causes a 65 to 70%

reduction in circulating E_1^u molecules but individuals of phenotype UJ cannot be differentiated from those of phenotype U who have developed acquired disorders reducing cholinesterase production. A third 'quantitative' variant named after Kalow, E_1^k (Rubinstein *et al.*, 1978), discovered in a similar fashion, suppresses circulating E_1^u molecules by about 33%. Other quantitative variants may be discovered later. They are usually recognisable only when present in combination with another variant allele. For a review of genetic variants see Brown *et al.* (1981).

The six alleles recognised can be combined in 21 different ways; some of the phenotypes appear in Table 22.1 opposite but others await investigation. Their discrimination is aided by two other inhibitors which are used in the assay system in the same way as dibucaine and fluoride. They are the dimethylthiocarbamate of (2-hydroxy-5-phenyl) trimethylammonium bromide (Hoffman La Roche, Ro 02–0683) in a concentration of 10 nmol/l (Liddell *et al.*, 1963), and scoline in a concentration of 4 mmol/l (King and Griffin, 1973). An earlier suggestion (Whittaker, 1968) to use also chloride (2 mol/l) has been mainly discarded.

The most common variant allele is E_1^a, with E_1^k probably the next most frequent, leaving E_1^f, E_1^j and E_1^s as the least common. In determining the genetic composition of a particular patient, the cholinesterase activity and its responses to inhibitors, preferably all four inhibitors listed in Table 22.1 opposite should be measured. Additional assistance is obtained by carrying out the same studies on close relatives, particularly if doubt exists as to classification. The use of DN and FN alone may cause errors, which are less likely when the effects of Ro 02–0683 and scoline are considered. They aid in the distinction between the pairs of phenotypes AJ/AF and UA/AK. Typing is probably best done in a specialised laboratory whose techniques are well established. It is also important that the incubation temperature is strictly controlled as the various enzymes have different responses to temperature increases (Dinwoodie, 1964; King and Morgan, 1970, 1971). For further details of phenotyping see Silk *et al.* (1979), Evans and Wardell (1984) and Turner *et al.* (1985).

Patients shown to belong to phenotypes A, F, S, AF, AJ, AK, and AS are very likely to show clinical sensitivity to suxamethonium and should be warned, preferably by the issue of a card which they can show to a responsible person should an anaesthetic be necessary at any time. The phenotype UA occurs in about 1 in 30 of the general population and may be associated with post-suxamethonium apnoea lasting up to about 8 min, although this may be a little longer in pregnancy with the fall in cholinesterase activity seen in that condition. Such cases and phenotype UF are not usually regarded as clinically sensitive. In the case of US, FS and remaining variants, clinical sensitivity may be variable and dependent on other factors affecting cholinesterase activity. Where there is a well-documented history of suxamethonium sensitivity in these cases, or even in other phenotypes not normally associated with sensitivity, it is sensible to advise future avoidance of this drug. It is possible that some cases of unexpected sensitivity represent other alleles as yet uncharacterised.

Another, unrelated cholinesterase genetic variant due to a gene at locus E_2 can be demonstrated in some people by electrophoresis (Harris *et al.*, 1962). It has been termed C_5, being the slowest moving component of five bands visible after starch gel separation. The usual situation is that C_4 contains most of the enzyme activity with C_1, C_2 and C_3 only minor components. C_5 is found in about 10% of individuals and has increased enzyme activity so that the total cholinesterase activity may be increased by up to 30%. Gel filtration (Harris and Robson, 1963) shows that C_4 and C_5 have the greatest mol. wt. with C_3, C_2 and C_1 in decreasing order. This genetic variant does not appear to have any special clinical importance.

ADENOSINE TRIPHOSPHATE: CREATINE N-PHOSPHOTRANSFERASE.
CREATINE KINASE, CREATINE PHOSPHOTRANSFERASE (2.7.3.2)

Creatine kinase (CK) catalyses the reaction:

Adenosine triphosphate (ATP) + creatine ⇌
$$\text{Adenosine diphosphate (ADP)} + \text{creatine phosphate}$$

The pH maximum of the forward reaction is 9·0, that of the reverse, which the equilibrium favours, is at 7·0. The enzyme is activated by Mg^{2+}

Determination of Serum Creatine Kinase

Several colorimetric methods were devised to determine the activity of CK in serum but these have been superseded by coupled enzyme assays using both forward and reverse reactions. These methods measure the rate of formation of ATP using the increase in absorbance at 340 nm of NADPH formed by the reactions:

$$\text{Creatine phosphate} + \text{ADP} \xrightarrow{\text{CK}} \text{ATP} + \text{creatine}$$

$$\text{ATP} + \text{glucose} \xrightarrow{\text{hexokinase}} \text{ADP} + \text{glucose-6-phosphate}$$

$$\text{G-6-P} + \text{NADP}^+ \xrightarrow{\text{G6PD}} \text{6-Phosphogluconate} + \text{NADPH} + \text{H}^+$$

or assay the rate of formation of ADP using the reaction sequence:

$$\text{Creatine} + \text{ATP} \xrightarrow{\text{CK}} \text{creatine phosphate} + \text{ADP}$$

$$\text{ADP} + \text{phosphoenol pyruvate} \xrightarrow[\text{kinase}]{\text{pyruvate}} \text{ATP} + \text{pyruvate}$$

$$\text{Pyruvate} + \text{NADH} + \text{H}^+ \xrightarrow{\text{LD}} \text{lactate} + \text{NAD}^+$$

The thermodynamically favourable reverse reaction has now been almost universally adopted. A dry chemistry method using this principle is available for the Ames Seralyser. A peroxidase/Trinder coupled method has recently been described (Wimmer *et al.*, 1985).

Interest in CK assays has focused on the most appropriate sulphydryl reagent to use as an activator, how to inhibit interference by adenylate kinase and whether EDTA should be present in the reaction mixture as a chelator. During storage, CK is rapidly inactivated by the oxidation of the sulphydryl groups at the active site of the enzyme. The need to reactivate the enzyme has been demonstrated and various sulphydryl reagents including cysteine, dithiothreitol, glutathione, 2-mercaptoethanol and *N*-acetylcysteine have been used. Cysteine was found to deteriorate rapidly in solution, dithiothreitol causes turbidity by precipitation of albumin and glutathione is unsuitable since it allows interference by glutathione reductase released from red cells in haemolysed specimens. 2-Mercaptoethanol causes turbidity and its decomposition products inhibit CK. *N*-Acetylcysteine suffers none of these shortcomings and is generally accepted to be the best thiol reagent for the maintenance and reactivation of CK activity in serum.

Adenylate kinase is present in many tissues and cells including skeletal and cardiac muscle, liver, brain and erythrocytes. The enzyme is also present in normal serum and may be markedly raised in haemolysed specimens. Adenylate kinase catalyses the reaction:

$$2ADP \rightleftharpoons AMP + ATP$$

and this could lead to an apparent increase in CK activity in the reaction schemes shown above. The method described below contains diadenosine pentaphosphate to inhibit red cell and muscle adenylate kinase and AMP to inhibit the liver enzyme. These inhibitors usually keep the serum blank reaction to less than 4 U/l at 37 °C although higher levels may occasionally be observed.

CK is readily inhibited by polyvalent cations such as Ca^{2+} and this can be prevented by the addition of EDTA which has the additional effect of protecting thiol reagents susceptible to oxidation by metal ions. The temperature during transport and storage is an important factor in maintaining CK activity in serum. Some workers have recommended that blood should be transported to the laboratory in ice/water mixtures and the serum frozen at $-20°C$, since the stability of CK in serum is better when stored at $-20°C$ than at either 20 °C or 4° C (Cho and Meltzer, 1979; Morin, 1977; Szasz *et al.*, 1978). Stability is improved by the addition of a thiol reagent before storage. It has been shown that pH, thiol and chelating agents have differential effects on storage and inactivation of the three isoenzymes of CK (Nealon *et al.*, 1981).

The determination of very high levels of CK activity is unsatisfactory because dilution causes a progressive increase in activity per unit volume. Dobosz (1974) showed that dilution of serum 1 : 5 with saline could give results which were up to 3.9 times the original activity. The method given below has a working range up to at least 3000 U/l, more than ten times the upper reference limit value for healthy males so dilution is rarely necessary.

Continuous Monitoring Method for Creatine Kinase (Scandinavian Committee on Enzymes, 1979)

Reagents.
1. Stock solution of imidazole-acetate buffer. Dissolve 8·72 g imidazole, 0·95 g EDTA (disodium salt, $C_{10}H_{14}O_8N_2Na_2$, $2H_2O$, mol. wt. 372·2) and 2·75 g magnesium acetate tetrahydrate in approximately 950 ml distilled water. Correct the pH to 8·0 at 25 °C with molar acetic acid and bring the volume to 1 l with distilled water. Mix and store at 4 °C or -20 °C when the stability will be 2 months and 6 months respectively.
2. Diadenosine pentaphosphate solution. Dissolve 11 mg of P^1,P^5-di(adenosine-5′) pentaphosphate (lithium salt, $C_{20}H_{26}N_{10}O_{22}P_5Li_3$, mol. wt. 934·2) in 10 ml of reagent (1) and store at -20 °C until used. Stable for 3 months.
3. Reagent mixture containing imidazole acetate (115 mmol/l), EDTA (2·3 mmol/l), magnesium acetate (11·5 mmol/l), N-acetylcysteine (23 mmol/l), ADP (2·3 mmol/l), AMP (5·8 mmol/l), diadenosine penta-phosphate (11·5 μmol/l), D-glucose (23 mmol/l), $NADP^+$ (2·3 mmol/l) at pH 6·5 (37 °C). For this, dissolve 98 mg adenosine-5′-diphosphoric acid, 211 mg adenosine-5′-monophosphoric acid monohydrate, 414 mg D-glucose, 181 mg nicotinamide-adenine dinucleotide phosphate (disodium salt, mol.

wt. 787·4) in 90 ml reagent (1). Add 1·0 ml reagent (2) and mix. Adjust the pH to 6·7 with molar acetic acid at room temperature. This reagent is stable at − 20 °C for one month.

4. Working reagent A. To the whole volume of reagent mixture (3) add 375 mg N-acetylcysteine and adjust the pH to 6·7 at 25 °C with molar acetic acid. Add 300 units of yeast hexokinase and 200 units of yeast D-glucose-6-phosphate dehydrogenase (D-glucose-6-phosphate: NADP 1-oxidoreductase) prepared from lyophilised material dissolved in aqueous glycerol, 500 ml/l. Make up to 100 ml with distilled water and mix gently. This reagent is stable for 30 h at room temperature and 5 days at 4 °C.

5. Working reagent B. Creatine phosphate (345 mmol/l). Dissolve 1·13 g creatine phosphate (disodium salt, $C_4H_8N_3O_5PNa_2$, $4H_2O$, mol. wt. 327·2) in 10 ml distilled water. The absorbance of the solution should be less than 0·150 at 340 nm. The reagent is stable for 3 months at 4 °C and at least one ·year at − 20 °C.

Technique. Add 0·05 ml serum to 1·0 ml reagent (4), mix and transfer to a cuvette with a 10 mm light path in a spectrophotometer with a temperature-controlled compartment set at 37 °C. Allow the cuvette contents to reach 37 °C and then add 0·1 ml reagent (5). Following the initial lag phase measure the absorbance at 1 min intervals for the next 5 min or record the change in absorbance continuously on a chart recorder. The reagent blank should be measured for each batch of reagents by repeating the above process but substituting water for serum. It is not usually necessary to check the serum blank but this can be done by replacing reagent (5) with water.

Calculation. Serum creatine kinase activity (U/l)

$$= \frac{\Delta A_{340}/\text{min}}{6\cdot3} \times \frac{\text{Total volume in the cuvette (ml)}}{\text{Volume of serum taken (ml)}} \times 10^3$$

For the above quantities:

$$\text{Serum creatine kinase (U/l)} = \Delta A_{340}/\text{min} \times 3651$$

Notes.
1. The Association of Clinical Biochemists (1980) recommended that blood should be collected into plain plastic tubes and kept at an ambient temperature below 30 °C. Separate the serum within 2 h, add 50 μmol acetylcysteine per ml of serum and store the specimen at 4 °C or − 18 °C. At 4 °C the enzyme is stable for 2 days and at − 18 °C for 1 month. Thaw frozen samples quickly in the 37 °C water bath in the dark, and do not use for further analysis if frozen and thawed a second time.

2. In lyophilised quality control materials the reactivation of CK may depend on the time of preincubation with thiol and the activity of CK after reconstitution is dependent on light and temperature. Liquid quality control materials containing CK in 50 % ethylene glycol need no reactivation and are stable for 6 months at − 20 °C (Lum, 1979).

3. A number of manufacturers make kits to this specification and these have been evaluated (DHSS, 1982).

Creatine Kinase Isoenzymes

CK is a dimeric molecule composed of two types of subunit, M and B. It is generally agreed that there are three isoenzymes in human tissue namely

CK–MM, CK–MB and CK–BB. These are also known as CK–3, CK–2 and CK–1 respectively under the convention that the most anodal isoenzyme is called isoenzyme-1 and the number increases with decreasing mobility. The M and B nomenclature will be used.

Significant amounts of CK–MM are found in heart muscle, the diaphragm and especially skeletal muscle (96% of total CK activity). CK–MB is predominantly found in cardiac muscle (20% of total CK activity) but is also present in small amounts in other tissues such as skeletal muscle and the diaphragm. CK–BB is the only isoenzyme found in brain tissue and is also present in the prostate, bladder and intestine (Jockers-Wretou and Pfleiderer, 1975; Tsung, 1976). CK–MM is the major isoenzyme in the sera of healthy persons and most studies agree that CK–MB and CK–BB are present in only very small amounts detectable using radioimmunoassay.

The methods used to separate and quantify CK isoenzymes include electrophoresis, ion-exchange chromatography, radioimmunoassay and immunoinhibition. Electrophoretic separation is readily achieved on cellulose acetate, agarose, agar and starch gel but is inconvenient for large numbers of assays and insufficiently precise in inexperienced hands. The separation of the isoenzymes, however, reveals the presence of atypical CK bands and macro-CK. The latter is a complex of CK–BB and IgG running between CK–MM and CK–MB and is detected in approximately 1·5% of all patients screened in some series (Wu and Bowers, 1982). No specific disorder is associated with the presence of macro-CK and its significance lies in the contribution it can make to B-unit activity in CK–MB assays (see below).

Ion-exchange chromatography methods using DEAE-Sephadex or DEAE-cellulose are based on selective elution by solutions of increasing ionic strength. CK–BB elutes with CK–MB, separately from CK–MM and interferes in the subsequent assay of CK–MB activity. Mercer (1976) has pointed out that the conditions of the separation must be very carefully controlled to prevent carry-over between fractions. The disadvantages of these methods include the relatively large sample size and the further dilution of the already low activity of the CK–MB fraction. Convenient column-chromatographic methods are commercially available.

Several immunological assays have been developed. Radioimmunoassay can be used but is inconvenient, time consuming and expensive. The mass of CK–MB has also been measured by enzyme immunoassay. CK–MB and CK–BB in the sample are bound by anti-CK–B antibodies coated on the inner surface of a test tube. Peroxidase-conjugated anti-CK–M is then added and this reacts with retained CK–MB but not with the retained CK–BB. Thus only molecules consisting of a combination of M and B subunits will have peroxidase bound to them. Unbound conjugate is removed by washing and a chromogenic substrate added to develop a colour proportional to the CK–MB concentration. Excellent diagnostic specificity and sensitivity are claimed for this method (Fenton *et al.*, 1984).

Immunoinhibition and immunoprecipitation methods measure the residual activity after subunit-specific antibodies have been allowed to bind to the enzyme. Immunoinhibition methods measure the B-subunit activity after the M-subunit is inhibited by anti-CK–MM antibodies. The non-inhibited activity is assumed to be solely that from the B-subunit of CK–MB, and the CK–MB result is obtained by multiplying the activity by two. However, about 2% of sera contain free CK–BB and other forms of CK which are not inhibited and contribute activity which will erroneously be assumed to derive from CK–MB.

Immunoprecipitation methods attempt to overcome the non-specificity of the immunoinhibition methods by using a second precipitation step. The first step is identical to that in immunoinhibition assays and this is followed by the addition of an antibody to remove all isoenzymes containing the M-subunit. After centrifugation the remaining activity in the supernatant is measured. By subtracting the result after precipitation from that after inhibition alone, the activity of the B-subunit of CK–MB is obtained. This is multiplied by two to give the CK–MB result.

In an evaluation and comparison of these two forms of CK–MB assay, Wu and Bowers (1982) concluded that immunoprecipitation is more specific, not readily automated, relatively time-consuming and more expensive. The immuno-inhibition method is cheaper, quicker, easily automated and equally good at detecting raised CK–MB levels. The major shortcoming is specificity but, since CK–B activity other than that from CK–MB occurs in less than 2% of all patients and exceedingly rarely in patients with myocardial infarction, the immuno-inhibition method is an acceptable assay of CK–MB.

See Lang and Würzburg (1982) for a review of the various forms of creatine kinase.

INTERPRETATION

Reference Ranges. Those for CK activity depend on age, sex and race. In neonates and infants the activity is considerably elevated, especially during the first 24 h post-partum and remains slightly elevated during the first year. The activity is constant between the ages of 5 and 12 years then rises with the increase in muscle mass during adolescence to reach levels greater than adult levels. From 20 to 60 years old reference values are unchanged. The reference range for women at all ages is lower than for men, presumably due to the smaller muscle mass. CK activity may be lower in early pregnancy and higher in the third trimester. Somewhat higher values are found in Negroes than in Caucasians.

The upper reference limit values (U/l) for different groups of healthy individuals using the Scandinavian Committee on Enzymes (1981) method are:

	Males (U/l)	Females (U/l)
Cord blood	570	570
12–14 years	370	250
20–60 years	270	150
Pregnant (third trimester)		265

There are several non-pathological reasons for raised CK-levels in serum. Normal persons after severe exercise can produce values considerably above the usually accepted URL. Maximum activity is attained up to 24 h after exercise and may remain elevated for up to 72 h. The activity of CK in serum can rise to 12 times the URL after the intramuscular injection of certain drugs. The enzyme comes from the muscle and the rise may be transient or last up to 8 days. Surgery leads to an increase in serum CK activity and many studies show such increases with maximum activities occurring between 24 and 48 h and returning to pre-operative levels after 5–6 days. The degree of elevation is very variable and shows no correlation with the degree of trauma.

Total CK activity shows an increase following myocardial infarction in which it is increased earlier than other enzymes (see table on p. 527) beginning within 6 h and peaking on average at 24 h and returning to normal within 2–3 days. The area under the peak and the slope of the initial rise are proportional to the size of the infarct. False negatives are rare and are usually due to technical factors such as errors in timing of blood collection. However, since CK, AST and LD are not peculiar to myocardial tissue, false positives are common and it is in the diagnosis of myocardial infarction that raised CK–MB levels are most useful. If the total CK activity is raised and CK–MB contributes more than 6 % of the activity then myocardial infarction is considered highly probable.

In progressive muscular dystrophy of the Duchenne type, which being sex-linked and recessive occurs mostly in males, increases in total CK activity up to 100-fold can be seen before the onset of clinical signs; several normal values almost certainly exclude the disease; Wilkinson (1976) recommends three determinations at weekly intervals. Increased values are found in about 75 % of female carriers (see Wilkinson, 1976). Smaller increases are seen in polymyositis and in other muscular dystrophies but values are mostly normal in muscle abnormalities secondary to nerve lesions.

Serum CK activity has been reported by several authors to be increased in hypothyroidism, but to be low in hyperthyroidism in which there is muscle wasting (Doran and Wilkinson, 1971). Increases have been reported in a wide variety of diseases, e.g. of the CNS, in motor neurone disease, hypothermia and hypoxia.

Increases, often considerable, occur in the rare condition of malignant hyperpyrexia particularly if halothane and suxamethonium are given as anaesthetic agents (Innes and Strömme, 1973).

For an extensive review of this enzyme see Bais and Edwards (1982). Griffiths (1986) has critically discussed the clinical utility of CK–MB assays.

GLUCOSE-6-PHOSPHATE DEHYDROGENASE (1.1.1.49)

Glucose-6-phosphate dehydrogenase (G6PD) catalyses the reaction:

Glucose-6-phosphate $+ NADP^+ \rightleftharpoons$
6-Phosphogluconolactone $+ NADPH + H^+$

The enzyme lactonase then adds water to convert the 6-phosphogluconolactone to 6-phosphogluconate. In the first stages in the pentose phosphate shunt this can then be acted on by 6-phosphogluconate dehydrogenase (1.1.1.44), which also requires $NADP^+$, and is converted to ribulose-5-phosphate, a process involving oxidation followed by decarboxylation. The whole sequence is as follows:

D-Glucose-6-phosphate · · · 6-Phosphoglucono-lactone · · · 6-Phosphogluconate · · · Ribulose-6-phosphate

Determination of Glucose-6-phosphate Dehydrogenase

Methods for the determination of G6PD use the rate of change of absorbance at 340 nm. A major difficulty is that the reaction product, 6-phosphogluconate, serves as a substrate for 6-phosphogluconate dehydrogenase which is also present, particularly in haemolysates. Both enzymes reduce $NADP^+$ so the NADPH produced must include a portion contributed by the second enzyme. However, conditions may be arranged for this effect to be minimised; pH 7·6 is lower than the optimum for 6-phosphogluconate dehydrogenase and cysteine, an activator for that enzyme and used in its assay, is omitted in the G6PD assay. Furthermore, in methods with short incubation times there is insufficient production of 6-phosphogluconate to allow significant activity of its dehydrogenase.

Several workers have used screening tests for the detection of G6PD deficiency. These include tests based on the decolorisation of dyes such as cresyl blue and 2,6-dichlorophenolindophenol or on the detection of the fluorescence of NADPH. These methods are efficient at detecting male hemizygotes and female homozygotes but are less reliable for the detection of heterozygotes and may fail to do so. The International Committee for Standardisation in Haematology (1979) recommended the fluorescent spot test of Beutler and Mitchell (1968). The dye decolorisation methods suffer from variation in batches of dye used.

Rate of Reaction Method (Kornberg and Horecker, 1955)

Reagents.
1. Triethanolamine buffer, pH 7·6, 50 mmol/l (7·45g/l) and containing EDTA, 5 mmol/l (1·861 g/l disodium salt dihydrate, mol. wt. 372·24).
2. $NADP^+$, 10 mmol/l (8·33 mg/ml) in water.
3. Glucose-6-phosphate (G6P), 31 mmol/l (9·42 mg of the disodium salt/ml) in water.
4. Digitonin solution: a saturated solution containing approximately 200 mg/l.
5. Sodium chloride solution, 150 mmol/l (9 g/l).

Technique. (a) *For serum.* Into a suitable test tube measure 2 ml buffer, 0·1 ml $NADP^+$ and 1 ml serum. Mix, stand for 5 min at 25 °C, add 50 μl G6P and after about 2 min begin to read the absorbance at 340 nm in a 1 cm cuvette every minute for 5 min or monitor continuously. Use as blank, serum plus buffer but without $NADP^+$ and G6P.

Calculation.

$$\text{Serum G6PD}(U/l) = \frac{\Delta A_{340}/\text{min}}{6·3} \times \frac{1000}{1} \times 3·15$$
$$= \Delta A_{340}/\text{min} \times 500$$

(b) *Red cell haemolysates.* Wash 0·2 ml finger blood three times with 2 ml sodium chloride solution, centrifuging at 3000 rpm. Suspend the washed cells in 0·5 ml digitonin solution and place in a refrigerator for 15 min to haemolyse them and again centrifuge for 10 min at 3000 rpm. Measure 3 ml buffer, 0·1 ml $NADP^+$ and 0·1 ml haemolysate into a suitable tube, mix, and proceed as above for serum using as blank, haemolysate plus buffer but without $NADP^+$ and G6P. Determine the red cell count separately.

Calculation. If the red cell count is $4·5 \times 10^{12}/l$, 0·2 ml blood contains 9×10^8 cells. These occupy approximately 0·1 ml so there will be about 0·6 ml haemolysate of which 0·1 ml is taken for the test. The number of red cells taken is thus $1·5 \times 10^8$, equal to 33 μl blood, and

Red cell G6PD activity (U/l whole blood or U/$4·5 \times 10^{12}$ cells)

$$= \frac{\Delta A_{340}/\text{min} \times 1000 \times 3·25}{6·3 \times 0·033} = \Delta A_{340}/\text{min} \times 15\,632$$

INTERPRETATION

Normal sera show barely detectable G6PD activity. An increase is observed in myocardial infarction which is less marked than that of aspartate aminotransferase or lactate dehydrogenase but may occur rather later.

Red cells contain 120 to 240 U/10^{12} cells. The main use of the determination is to recognise an inherited deficiency of the enzyme in the red cells which causes haemolytic anaemia following administration of some drugs. These include antimalarials such as primaquine, sulphonamides, and several other aromatic compounds. It is also found in favism in which anaemia follows eating fava beans. For an account of G6PD deficiency see Beutler (1983).

Over 200 G6PD variants have been recognised. Some of these have almost complete loss of enzyme activity, some varying degrees of diminished activity, and others have increased activity. Electrophoretically they may move more quickly, at the same speed, or more slowly than the normal enzyme. For a short account see Wilkinson (1976).

Screening Tests for Deficiency

Using Bromcresyl Blue (Bernstein, 1963)

Reagents.
1. Tris-hydrochloric acid buffer, pH 8·5, 200 mmol/l. Dissolve 2·42 g Tris in 54 ml 100 mmol/l hydrochloric acid and make to 100 ml. Check the pH.
2. Bromcresyl blue, 500 μmol/l (160 mg/l) in Tris buffer.
3. NADP$^+$, 2 mmol/l (1·67 mg/ml).
4. G6P, 50 mmol/l (152 mg anhydrous disodium salt, mol. wt. 304·1, or 179 mg trihydrate in 10 ml). Divide into small portions and keep with the NADP$^+$ in the deep freeze.
5. Dye reagent. Prepare immediately before use by mixing 8 volumes of the dye, 1 volume of the NADP$^+$ and 1 volume of G6P.

Technique. Haemolyse 20 μl fresh blood or 10 μl packed cells in the case of patients with anaemia, with 1 ml water and add 0·5 ml dye reagent. Mix, cover with liquid paraffin, incubate at 37 °C and note the time required for decolorisation to the sharp red-purple of reduced haemoglobin.

Dye from different sources was found to give different times for normal bloods. That from Sigma usually required to 30 to 50 min, occasionally up to 75 min, whereas some other sources took 2 to 3 h. Enzyme-deficient red cells needed more than 2 h with the former or over 5 h with the latter. No specimen decolorising in under 75 min was found to be enzyme-deficient but some in the range 75 to 120 min were. Bernstein checked these by determining the activity by one of the quantitative methods.

Using Fluorescent Screening (Beutler and Mitchell, 1968)

This uses the fluorescence of the NADPH formed by the action of G6PD on G6P.

Reagents.
1. G6P, 10 mmol/l (30·4 g anhydrous disodium salt/l).
2. NADP$^+$, 7·5 mmol/l (6·24 g/l).
3. Saponin, 10 g/l.
4. Tris-hydrochloric acid, 750 mmol/l, pH 7·8. Dissolve 90·85 g Tris in about 850 ml water, adjust to pH 8·5 with 6 mol/l hydrochloric acid and make to 1 litre.
5. Oxidised glutathione, 8 mmol/l (4·90 g/l).
6. Reagent for use. Mix freshly 1 volume of (1), 1 volume of (2), 2 volumes of (3), 3 volumes of (4), 1 volume of (5) and 2 volumes of water.

Technique. Incubate 10 μl blood with 0·1 ml reagent at room temperature. Take spots on Whatman paper No. 1 before and at 5, 10, and 30 min after beginning to incubate. Examine the spots under ultraviolet light at 365 nm. Specimens with G6PD activity less than 20 % of normal do not fluoresce as the small amount of NADPH formed is reoxidised by the glutathione under the action of glutathione reductase present in the blood.

γ-GLUTAMYL PEPTIDE: AMINO ACID
γ-GLUTAMYL TRANSFERASE
(γ-Glutamyl Transpeptidase, Glutamyl Transferase) (2.3.2.2)

γ-Glutamyl transpeptidase (GGT) catalyses the transfer of the γ-glutamyl group from γ-glutamyl peptides to another peptide or to L-amino acids or to water. The kidneys are richest in this enzyme with appreciable amounts in the liver, pancreas and prostate but with little in other tissues.

Determination in Serum

The determination of GGT was considerably simplified by the introduction of the directly chromogenic substrate L-γ-glutamyl-4-nitroanilide (glu-4-NA) by Orlowski and Meister (1965), and most methods now use this material or its carboxyl derivative, L-γ-glutamyl-3-carboxy-4-nitroanilide (glu-3-CA-4-NA). The most commonly used acceptor molecule is glycylglycine. The reaction is:

$$\text{HOOC.CH.CH}_2\text{.CH}_2\text{.CO.NH} \langle \bigcirc \rangle \text{NO}_2 + \text{CH}_2\text{.CO.NH.CH}_2\text{.COOH} \longrightarrow$$
$$\quad | \qquad\qquad\qquad\qquad\qquad\qquad | $$
$$\quad \text{NH}_2 \qquad\qquad\qquad\qquad\qquad\quad \text{NH}_2$$

L-γ-Glutamyl-4-nitroanilide   Glycylglycine

$$\text{NH}_2\langle \bigcirc \rangle \text{NO}_2 + \text{HOOC.CH.CH}_2\text{.CH}_2\text{.CO.NH.CH}_2\text{.CO.NH.CH}_2\text{.COOH}$$
$$\qquad\qquad\qquad\qquad\qquad | \qquad\quad \text{γ-Glutamyl glycylglycine}$$
$$\qquad\qquad\qquad\qquad\quad \text{NH}_2$$

4-Nitroaniline

Glu-4-NA is relatively insoluble at pH 7·6 to 7·9, the optimum pH range of the enzyme, but is more soluble in hydrochloric acid. Although the spontaneous hydrolysis of the substrate is markedly increased in acid solutions, some methods take advantage of the higher solubility to achieve the high concentrations necessary for use as a start reagent. While glu-3-CA-4-NA is highly soluble and can be used as a start reagent in aqueous solution, its higher absorbance at the wavelength used to monitor the reaction means unacceptably high absorbances can be reached in attempting to optimise the assay. Of the national and international bodies recommending GGT assays, all except IFCC have used glu-4-NA. Whichever is used, the preparation must be pure because the D-isomer of either substrate acts as a competitive inhibitor of the enzyme. Similarly, glycylglycine must not contain free glycine.

The wavelength must be chosen to minimise photometric interference by bilirubin and to ensure differentiation of the liberated product, 4-nitroaniline or 5-amino-2-nitrobenzoate, from unhydrolysed substrate. The range 405 to 410 nm is suitable since the absorbance of the substrate is minimal in this range whereas it is high at the absorbance maximum of the product, approximately 380 nm.

The cations Mg^{2+}, Ca^{2+}, Mn^{2+} and Zn^{2+} inhibit GGT slightly. Despite this, some assays include magnesium chloride in the reaction mixture (see p. 520). GGT activity in heparinised plasma is sometimes lower than in the corresponding serum (IFCC, 1983a). The reduction differs from specimen to specimen and from run to run and is greatest when the pre-incubation time is short. However, several published reports claim that heparinised plasma can be used for the assay of GGT activity (Rosalki, 1975; Schiele *et al.*, 1981; Association of Clinical Biochemists, 1980). The enzyme is stable and serum may be stored at 4 °C for seven days without loss of activity.

Method of the Committee on Enzymes of the Scandinavian Society for Clinical Chemistry and Clinical Physiology (1976)

Reagents.
1. Buffer, Tris 120 mmol/l, magnesium chloride 12 mmol/l and glycylglycine 90 mmol/l at pH 7·8 (37 °C). Dissolve 14·54 g Tris, 2·44 g $MgCl_2$, $6H_2O$ and 11·89 g glycylglycine in about 800 ml distilled water. Adjust the pH to 7·8 at 37°C and make to 1 litre with distilled water. It is stable for 24 h at room temperature and for at least 8 weeks at 4 °C.
2. Substrate. Dissolve 1·28 g L-γ-glutamyl-4-nitroanilide (anhydrous) in 0·15 mol/l hydrochloric acid and make to 100 ml with the acid. Considerable stirring may be required to dissolve the substrate. Divide into volumes suitable for one day's work and store at − 20 °C when it is stable for several weeks. The reagent is stable for only a few hours at room temperature.

Technique. Warm 100 μl serum and 1·0 ml buffer to 37 °C. Start the reaction by adding 0·1 ml substrate, mix and monitor the reaction continuously at 405 nm in a 1 cm cuvette so as to obtain the change in absorbance per minute.

Calculation. The molar absorption coefficient of 4-nitroaniline at 405 nm is 9900 l mol^{-1} cm^{-1}, so:

$$\text{Serum GGT (U/l)} = \Delta A_{405}/\text{min} \times \frac{1000}{0·1} \times \frac{1·2}{9·9} = \Delta A_{405}/\text{min} \times 1212$$

where 1·2 is the final volume in the cuvette (ml) and 0·1 the volume of serum.

Notes.
1. The Scandinavian Committee on Enzymes recommends that the value of the molar absorption coefficient be checked on the instrument used for the assay since the measurements are made on a steep part of the spectral curve. This can be done by dissolving 562·5 mg 4-nitroaniline in 10 ml concentrated hydrochloric acid and diluting to 1 litre with distilled water. A further 1 : 100 dilution is prepared in Tris buffer, pH 7·6 (37°C) to give a final

4-nitroaniline concentration of 0·04 mmol/l. The absorbance of this solution is measured in the spectrophotometer at 405 nm and the molar absorption coefficient calculated.

2. The rate of spontaneous hydrolysis of glu-4-NA is moderate in the recommended reagent 0·15 mol/l hydrochloric acid, and much less than in the reagent 0·5 mol/l hydrochloric acid, proposed by Rosalki and Tarlow (1974). The final pH of the reaction mixture should be 7·6.

3. GGT activity shows a pH optimum in the range 7·6 to 7·9. The lower end of this range is chosen so as to improve the solubility of glu-4-NA. The magnesium is added since it seems to prevent the precipitation of the supersaturated · solution of glu-4-NA, although concentrations of magnesium higher than 10 mmol/l may have a slight inhibitory effect on the enzyme.

INTERPRETATION

The activity of GGT in serum has been reported to be affected by age, sex, body weight, alcohol and drugs. The reference range for men is higher than that for women and increases with age and body weight. Alcohol and drugs such as warfarin and phenobarbitone cause hepatic enzyme induction. These facts should be considered in the determination of reference ranges for GGT and in the interpretation of results. Fasting does not appear to affect GGT levels.

Serum GGT is a sensitive but non-specific indicator of liver disease. Since elevated results are found in virtually all types of liver disease the test is of little value in the differential diagnosis of hepatobiliary disorders. The highest activities are seen in obstructive disorders with the increase generally being greater in intrahepatic cholestasis than in extrahepatic cholestasis. While the enzyme is less sensitive than the aminotransferases for the detection of hepatocellular disease, GGT may be the only biochemical abnormality in cirrhosis. When hepatic metastases are present, the rise in GGT is more pronounced than that of other liver enzymes so that if the GGT result is normal in a patient with established cancer, liver metastases are less likely to be present. GGT can be useful in helping to determine the tissue of origin of a raised alkaline phosphatase. This is particularly so when there are physiological reasons for a raised alkaline phosphatase as in childhood and pregnancy.

GGT determinations have been found to be appreciably more sensitive than other enzymes to the liver damage and enzyme induction caused by alcohol ingestion. In alcoholism 74 % showed an increased GGT activity compared with 29·5 % for AST, 20·5 % for ALT and 7·1 % for alkaline phosphatase. Very high levels reaching 20 to 30 times the URL have been found in alcoholics after recent drinking bouts. Moderate social drinking may slightly increase the serum GGT level but not usually to abnormal levels. Some workers have felt that GGT determination is useful for diagnostic confirmation in patients in whom excessive drinking is suspected but denied. Apparently healthy people, however, may have raised GGT levels even though their alcohol intake would not be considered excessive. Thus a patient should not be classed as an excessive drinker solely on the basis of a high serum GGT.

GGT activity in serum can be elevated in some non-hepatic disorders such as acute pancreatitis, carcinoma of the head of the pancreas, congestive cardiac failure, myocardial infarction and diabetes mellitus. Determination of GGT in these patients is of no clinical value. The mechanism of these increases in GGT is not understood but it is evident that in the case of acute pancreatitis the raised GGT activity may reflect concomitant hepatic damage in alcohol-associated pancreatitis or pancreatitis following biliary obstruction and so may not be specific to the pancreas. Similarly, in myocardial infarction, hypoxic damage to the liver could explain the raised GGT.

Although renal tissue contains the highest content of GGT, renal disorders do not cause elevated levels of GGT in serum. Increased urinary GGT activity has been reported in acute renal failure, pyelonephritis, Alport's syndrome, Wilm's tumour and glomerulopathies (Salgó and Szabó, 1982).

For a short summary of the clinical value of GGT assays see Penn and Worthington (1983) and for a more extensive review of this enzyme see Rosalki (1975).

γ-Glutamyl Transpeptidase Isoenzymes

Since GGT is believed to arise from a single gene locus the well-documented electrophoretic separation of variant forms is presumably due to post-transcriptional changes, probably differences in sialylation, glycosylation and the formation of complexes with lipids and small peptides. Thus, strictly speaking, the variants are not isoenzymes but this term will be used.

In healthy persons, two or three bands are found in the α_1- and α_2-globulin regions using agarose or cellulose acetate electrophoresis with γ-glutamyl-7-amino-4-methylcoumarin as substrate to obtain the greatest analytical sensitivity. Other GGT isoenzymes seen in disease have been studied in an attempt to improve the discriminatory power of the enzyme in liver disease. Unlike CK and lactate dehydrogenase the isoenzymes of GGT demonstrate no tissue-specific characteristics, but most of the serum GGT comés from the liver. There is still disagreement as to the clinical significance of various GGT isoenzyme patterns, due partly to the fact that the number and position of the bands can be altered by small changes in the method. No uniform numbering system for electrophoretic mobilities exists, they are either described relative to the main plasma protein bands or as a fraction of the mobility of albumin. Neither method has succeeded in unequivocally identifying the bands. Rosalki *et al.* (1981) described five bands using cellulose acetate electrophoresis; mobilities decreased from GGT-1 in the α_1/albumin zone through GGT-2 in the α_1 region, GGT-3 in the α_1-α_2 region, GGT-4 in the α_2 region to GGT-5 in the β region.

GGT-2 and GGT-4 are found in healthy individuals with GGT-3 also sometimes present as a faint band. GGT-2 may be increased in alcoholic liver disease but also in cholestatic disorders unrelated to alcohol ingestion. The GGT isoenzyme pattern varies in cholestatic disease. Several reports suggest that GGT-5 is a sensitive test for cholestasis, others claim an increase in GGT-2 is specific. The finding by Degenaar *et al.* (1976) that serum GGT-2 is higher in extrahepatic than intrahepatic obstruction was not confirmed by Park *et al.* (1984). Using polyacrylamide gel electrophoresis Wenham *et al.* (1985) identified a high molecular weight GGT, GGT–IIB, with mobility 0·45 to 0·55 relative to albumin. They claim that GGT–IIB is higher in obstructive than non-obstructive lesions and higher in extrahepatic than in intrahepatic obstruction. If confirmed this would be a valuable contribution to the differential diagnosis of liver disease.

Most reports of GGT isoenzyme studies in cases of liver malignancy show the presence of the slow-moving GGT-5 and in primary liver tumours GGT-1 is often observed. Unfortunately neither GGT-1 nor GGT-5 is sensitive or specific for liver malignancies; both have been observed in patients with non-malignant liver disease.

With current techniques a GGT isoenzyme assay would appear to have limited value because there is no clear relationship between GGT isoenzyme patterns and the various forms of liver disease. For a short review of this subject see Nemesánszky and Lott (1985).

LACTATE DEHYDROGENASE (1.1.1.27)

Lactate dehydrogenase (LD) catalyses the reaction:

$$CH_3.CHOH.COO^- + NAD^+ \rightleftharpoons CH_3.CO.COO^- + NADH + H^+$$
$$\text{Lactate} \qquad\qquad\qquad\qquad \text{Pyruvate}$$

The classical colorimetric methods are now obsolete and the enzyme activity is now almost invariably measured by monitoring the appearance or disappearance of NADH. The equilibrium is such that the pyruvate to lactate (P → L) reaction is more than twice as fast as the lactate to pyruvate (L → P) reaction and more workers use pyruvate as a substrate despite some disadvantages. Pyruvate in excess inhibits the reaction and this places a limit on the concentration that can be used. The consequent sub-optimal concentrations of pyruvate can lead to a non-linear rate of reaction. The formation of inhibitors in NADH solutions (or with damp solid NADH) can lead to falsely low reaction rates. To prevent this, NADH should be stored with a desiccant preferably under nitrogen. Inhibitors found in NAD$^+$ solutions can also interfere with the L → P reaction. A significant advantage of the P → L assays is the greater change in absorbance which allows better precision at low activities. The optimum pH with pyruvate as a substrate is 6·8 to 7·5 but with lactate is higher at 9·0 to 10·0. Reagents are less stable at the higher pH. Although NADH is more expensive than NAD$^+$ the cost of the P → L assay is less than that of the L → P assay since the concentration of the reagents is lower. All of the published recommended methods use pyruvate as substrate.

While phosphate buffer has been mostly used, others have been employed. The Scandinavian method below employs a Tris-EDTA buffer, and Amador and Wacker (1965), and Demetriou *et al.* (1974) used 2-amino-2-methyl-l-propanol. Martinek (1972) tested several buffers including these and those of Good *et al.* (1966) and found that a mixture of 2-amino-2-methyl-l-propanol and ortho-phosphate gave the highest value in the assay and assured better buffering, gave the same pH optimum, 6·8, for all the sera tested, and sharper pH optima with sera from patients with myocardial infarction.

Gerhardt *et al.* (1974) studied the formation of inhibitors and other contaminants under controlled conditions and the stability of NADH in several buffers at 37, 25, 4, and −20 °C. Tris-EDTA buffer was found preferable to phosphate.

For a discussion of earlier methods see the 5th edition of this book.

Determination of Serum Lactate Dehydrogenase Activity

Recommended Method (Optimised at 37 °C) cf the Committee on Enzymes of the Scandinavian Society for Clinical Chemistry and Clinical Physiology (1974).

Reagents
1. Tris (56 mmol/l)–EDTA (5·6 mmol/l) buffer, pH 7·4. Dissolve 6·8 g of Tris(hydroxymethyl)-aminomethane and 2·1 g EDTA, disodium salt dihydrate, in approximately 500 ml distilled water. Adjust to pH 7·4 at 37°C with

1·0 mmol/l hydrochloric acid and make up to 1 litre with distilled water. Stored at 4 °C in a tightly-capped dark bottle, it is stable for a minimum of 6 weeks.

2. Reduced nicotinamide adenine dinucleotide, 0·17 mmol/l. Dissolve 13 mg of NADH-disodium salt trihydrate, in 90 ml of reagent (1) and mix well. Calculate the concentration of NADH using the absorbance at 340 nm and the molar absorption coefficient, $6·3 \times 10^3 \; 1 \; mol^{-1} \; cm^{-1}$. Dilute the solution to give a concentration of 0·17 mmol/l. Stored at 4 °C in a tightly-capped dark bottle, it is stable for a minimum of 3 days (see note (2)).

3. Sodium pyruvate, 13·5 mmol/l. Dissolve 149 mg sodium pyruvate in 100 ml of distilled water. Stored at 4 °C in a tightly-capped bottle, it is stable for a minimum of 20 days or a few weeks if frozen at −20 °C.

Technique. Measure 2.0 ml of reagent (2) into a 1 cm path length spectrophotometric cuvette. Add 50 μl serum, mix and incubate at 37 °C for 5 to 15 min to remove endogenous oxo-acids. Add 0.2 ml sodium pyruvate solution prewarmed to 37 °C, mix and monitor the rate of change of absorbance at 340 nm.

Calculation. Serum lactate dehydrogenase activity (U/l)

$$= \Delta A_{340}/min \times \frac{1000}{\text{Volume serum used (ml)}} \times \frac{\text{Volume in the cuvette (ml)}}{6·3}$$

$$= \Delta A_{340}/min \times \frac{1000 \times 2·25}{0·05 \times 6·3} = \Delta A_{340}/min \times 7\,143$$

Since a decrease in rate may occur in the first minute of the reaction the Committee advised that the calculation should be based on the linear portion recorded from 15 to 30 s after initiating the reaction.

Notes.

1. For an explanation of the calculation see p. 495.

2. The dinucleotide salt suggested in reagent (2) is that recommended by the original workers. The anhydrous salt may be used. The quality of NADH can be checked using the control measurements recommended by the Scandinavian Society for Clinical Chemistry and Clinical Physiology (1974), *viz.*

(a) Reading the absorbance at 340 nm. The total A_{340} includes β-NADH, α-NADH plus any other substances absorbing at 340 nm. If the reading is made on the reaction mixture when the reaction is initiated with pyruvate as substrate and then again after complete oxidation of the NADH, thus giving the constant residual absorbance, the difference in readings is due to β-NADH, the amount of which can be calculated using the molar absorption coefficient. The above workers used 6·22 $\times 10^3 \, 1 \, mol^{-1} \, cm^{-1}$ (but see p. 495).

(b) Reading the absorbance at 260 nm (band width 0·5 nm) and 340 nm (band width 1·3 nm) with slit width 1·2 mm. The ratio A_{260}/A_{340} should be near to 2·30. Specimens with a value less than 2·30 have a high purity of NADH but could contain traces of inhibitors, while those with a value above 2·30 can contain impurities such as NAD^+ and other adenine nucleotides and inhibitors which absorb at 260 nm.

(c) Measuring the initial reaction rate with human LD–1 using the recommended LD method of the Society with the NADH being tested and with a certified NADH preparation. The former should be within 5% of the latter (Gerhardt *et al.*, 1974).

(d) Measuring the initial and residual fluorescence (see Gerhardt *et al.*, 1974).

On exposure to moist air, NADH forms inhibitors of LD and the salt acquires a yellow colour. Such changes must be avoided and Gerhardt *et al.* (1974) recommended that solid samples of NADH should be supplied in evacuated ampoules or in airtight containers filled with nitrogen and with a desiccant in the container. NADH of high purity bottled under nitrogen and specially suited for the assay of LD is now commercially available and should be used.

3. It is important to use serum free from haemolysed red cells since they may contain 100 to 150 times as much LD as the serum. It is therefore best to separate the serum as soon as possible. In the absence of haemolysis King (1959) did not find any increase in activity in serum which had remained in contact with the clot for 6 h. Serum has been said to keep up to 48 h at room temperature and up to 3 or 4 weeks at 0–4 °C but other workers have recommended measuring LD (and HBD, see p. 526) activities on the day the blood is taken and report a variable fall in activity if kept in the refrigerator for 3 to 4 days. If plasma must be used the sample must be centrifuged sufficiently to provide platelet-free plasma.

4. All determinations of total LD activity are necessarily a compromise because the isoenzymes differ with respect to optimum pH, optimum substrate concentration and thermal lability.

INTERPRETATION

LD, as expected from its involvement in glucose metabolism, occurs in all organ cells in man, but is especially plentiful in cardiac and skeletal muscle, liver, kidney, and red blood cells.

An increase in LD activity is found in myocardial infarction, beginning within 6 to 12 h and reaching a maximum at about 48 h. The extent of the increase is roughly similar to that of AST but it takes a longer time before normal values for LD are reached again. Thus King and Waind (1961) in a group of patients found AST activity raised from 3 to 9 days (average 5), LD from 6 to 14 (average 11). The increase is mostly in isoenzymes LD-1 and LD-2 and an increase in these may be seen when the total LD activity is within normal limits. An increase can be observed in progressive muscular dystrophy and in cases with gross rhabdomyolysis.

Increased activities are found in some forms of liver disease such as infective hepatitis, but these are not as great nor as predictable as the rise in aminotransferase activity. High values may occur in primary or secondary tumours of the liver and very high levels are seen in severe liver necrosis following exposure to carbon tetrachloride or overdose with paracetamol. Normal values, however, are often seen in cirrhosis or post-hepatic jaundice.

Increased activities are also seen in leukaemia, in pernicious anaemia and other megaloblastic and haemolytic anaemias, in renal disease, and in malignancy, particularly when metastases are present.

An increase in cerebrospinal fluid LD activity has been reported in the presence of tumours of the central nervous system.

Isoenzymes of Lactate Dehydrogenase

Five isoenzymes of LD, referred to as LD–1 to LD–5, exist in most tissues. They have different electrophoretic mobilities, LD–1 moving fastest towards the anode. As the LD molecule consists of four subunits of two different kinds, designated H (heart) and M (muscle), five different combinations of these exist: H_4, H_3M, H_2M_2, HM_3 and M_4, corresponding to LD–1 to LD–5 respectively. Cardiac muscle is richest in LD–1 and LD–2 with the former present in the largest amount and with only small diminishing proportions in the order LD–3 to LD–5. In liver the exact reverse is the case, LD–5 being the most plentiful. Red cells are similar in isoenzyme pattern to heart muscle; skeletal muscle to liver. Spleen, lung, pancreas, lymph nodes, adrenals, leucocytes and thyroid are richest in LD–3 and kidney in LD–2. The isoenzymes have different roles: LD–1 is associated with oxidative metabolism and LD–5 with anaerobic glycolysis.

In normal serum LD–2 is present in the greatest amount with others in diminishing quantities in the order – LD–2, 1, 3, 4, 5.

Isoenzyme Separation

Although the primary classification of LD isoenzymes was based on electrophoretic behaviour, other techniques have been investigated in the hope of providing simpler procedures for routine use.

Electrophoretic Separation of LD Isoenzymes. Latner and Skillen (1961) used starch gel of size $25 \times 12 \times 0.6$ cm, 30–100 μl serum in the slot, and 10–12 volts/cm for 2 h. Two buffers were used:

(a) For the gel, 50 mmol/l Tris in 5 mmol/l hydrochloric acid (6·05 g Tris and 5 ml 1 mol/l hydrochloric acid per litre), pH 8·8. The gel pH is 8·6.

(b) For the bridge, 300 mmol/l Tris in 50 mmol/l hydrochloric acid (36·3 g Tris and 50 ml 1 mol/l hydrochloric acid per litre), pH 8·6.

Another very satisfactory buffer is that of Bodman (1960). The stock solution contains 60·5 g Tris, 4·6 g boric acid, and 6·0 g EDTA per litre of solution. Dilute 1 to 10 for the gel and 1 to 5 for the bridge.

Latner and Skillen (1961) stained with a solution containing 300 mmol Tris/l in 220 mmol/l hydrochloric acid, pH 7·4, 2 parts, and 500 mmol/l sodium lactate, 1 part. This keeps well at 5 °C. To an amount sufficient to cover the gel (about 15 ml) add 10 mg NAD^+, 4 mg MTT (p. 491), 0·25 mg PMS (p. 491) and 5 mg sodium cyanide. The amounts of these constituents are not critical, different workers have used quantities varying widely, but the lactate molarity should not exceed 500 mmol/l since inhibition of LD–1 and LD–2 occurs with higher concentrations. Stain for an hour away from light.

Van der Helm *et al.* (1962) carried out agar gel electrophoresis on a microscope slide, running for 30 min at 140 V and applying 8 μl in a 5 mm slit. For staining they incubated at 37 °C for 2 h in a mixture of 3·6 ml solution A and 0·1 ml B containing 4 mg NAD^+ added just before use.

Solution A, pH 7·4, 1 ml sodium lactate solution (700 g/l), 1·87 g Na_2HPO_4, $2H_2O$, 0·272 g KH_2PO_4, 25 mg Nitro Blue Tetrazolium, 50 mg sodium cyanide, and water to 90 ml. Keep at 4 °C.

Solution B, PMS 1 mg/ml in water. Keep at 4 °C in a dark bottle.

Place the slide upside down on two colourless matches on a glass plate and run the above mixture from a pipette under the agar. Less than 4 ml is needed. After incubating wash the slide with water, fix with ethanol–acetic acid–water, 70/5/25 v/v, and dry while covered with filter paper.

Notes.

1. A more recent method (McKenzie and Henderson, 1983) uses thin-film agarose electrophoresis, again with lactate as substrate. The NADH is measured using a fluorescent recording densitometer.

2. Several kits for the separation of LD isoenzymes are available commercially.

3. Quantitative measurement of isoenzyme activity by densitometry is of doubtful validity since the conditions chosen will be sub-optimal for some of the isoenzymes. This is not too great a disadvantage if one is examining changes in the proportions of LD–1 and LD–2 as they have similar optimal conditions.

Immunoinhibition. LD–1 can be assayed as the residual activity after precipitation of all the other isoenzymes. In the Isomune-LD Test (Roche Products Limited) goat antiserum to LD–5 is added to the patient's serum and allowed to act for 5 min with all isoenzymes containing the M-subunit. Anti-goat gamma-globulin bound to an inert polymer is then added and incubated for 5 min. Insoluble complexes with the M-containing isoenzymes are removed by centrifugation, LD–1 remaining in the supernatant fluid. The assay is precise, easy to perform and results are available quickly if needed.

Heat Stability. LD–1 is more heat resistant than LD–5 and Latner and Skillen (1963) used a heat stability index, the ratio of the activity after heating at 60 °C for 1 h to that of untreated serum. There is a tendency for the index to increase as total LD activity increases. See also Wroblewski and Gregory (1961).

Use of Other Substrates. *Hydroxybutyrate Dehydrogenase (α-HBD)*. LD catalyses the reversible reduction of other α-oxo acids besides pyruvate. Elliot and Wilkinson (1961) studied its action on 2-oxobutyrate:

$$CH_3CH_2.CO.COO^- + NADH + H^+ \rightleftharpoons CH_3CH_2.CH(OH).COO^- + NAD^+$$

The technique used phosphate buffer (65·4 mmol/l) at pH 7·4, 2-oxobutyrate (3·3 mmol/l) as substrate instead of pyruvate, and 0·13 mmol/l NADH.

To differentiate the activity from that against pyruvate, Elliot and Wilkinson termed it 'α-hydroxybutyrate dehydrogenase'. For this they found the reference range to be 56 to 125 U/l at 25 °C (mean ± SD, 90 ± 19) and also used the ratio of the LD/α-HBD activities. This they found to be 1·18 to 1·60 in normal persons.

The conditions selected by Elliot and Wilkinson (1961) were devised so as to give the greatest discrimination between LD–1 and LD–5. The assay is sub-optimal for LD–1 and this was aggravated when the assay was performed at higher temperatures. As a result, 'optimised' procedures using higher substrate concentrations have been developed for use at higher temperatures (Shaw and Gray, 1974; Ellis and Goldberg, 1971). The Association of Clinical Biochemists (1980) proposed an assay using the sub-optimal concentration of 3·3 mmol/l originally used by Elliot and Wilkinson (1961) but changed the pH to 7·2 to give optimal conditions at 30 °C. The NADH concentration was increased to 0·2 mmol/l to extend the linear range of the assay. These various modified assays have been compared with regard to the best discrimination between the isoenzymes of LD (Leung and Henderson, 1981), using isoenzyme activities obtained by thin-layer agarose electrophoresis as reference. It was decided that the Association of Clinical Biochemists (1980) method correlated best with LD–1 activity.

Glycerate Dehydrogenase (GD). This name was given by McQueen *et al.* (1972) to the activity measured with hydroxypyruvate as substrate instead of pyruvate. At 37 °C and using substrate conditions optimised for that temperature, they found the following reference ranges: GD, 300 to 850 U/l; LD, 240 to 525 U/l; α-HBD, 80 to 440 U/l.

Behaviour Towards Inhibitors. Emerson and Wilkinson (1965) studied the inhibition of serum LD by potassium oxalate, 20 μmol/l, and urea, 2 mol/l. They modified the method of Wroblewski and LaDue (1955) by adding either 100 μl of

6 mmol/l oxalate or 1·0 ml of 6 mol/l urea to the mixture of serum, buffer and coenzyme about 30 min before adding the substrate. Normal persons gave a mean percentage inhibition (and SD) with oxalate of 61 (3·5) and with urea 52 (6). LD–1 and LD–2 were much more affected by oxalate than LD–4 and LD–5, while the reverse was true for urea.

Clinical Usefulness of Isoenzyme Methods

Atypical LD isoenzymes are sometimes seen in the serum of patients with cancer and in the tumours themselves. Tumours, however, are usually richest in LD–3, 4 and 5 (Latner, 1964) as might be expected from their greater reliance on anaerobic glycolysis but such findings have not proved to be clinically helpful.

In general, a lesion of a particular organ results in a serum isoenzyme pattern more closely resembling that of the organ concerned. There is a marked increase in the proportion of LD–1 in the serum in myocardial infarction, and of LD–5 in liver disease, findings which may be seen even when the total LD activity is not raised. In myocardial infarction, serum LD–1 activity exceeds that of LD–2, the reverse of normal proportions. For this diagnosis the demonstration of increased amounts of LD–1 and LD–2 is, however, adequate. For this reason many of the techniques outlined above have concentrated on the detection of increased LD–1 activity. Thus Latner and Skillen (1963) found that their heat stability index was almost always greater than 0·5 in myocardial infarction, a figure rarely exceeded in other conditions.

Elliot and Wilkinson (1961) found their LD/α-HBD ratio to be below 1·18 in most cases of myocardial infarction and above 1·60 in liver disease. In acute liver disease it was frequently above 2·0, in chronic liver disease and in obstructive jaundice usually between 1·6 and 2·0. Thus α-HBD activity is a more sensitive index of myocardial infarction than LD and frequently remains increased for a longer time. They found that the average number of days (SD in parentheses) during which increased activity of various enzymes was detectable was: AST, 4·3 (2·7); LD, 8·0 (1·6); α-HBD, 13·3 (3·3). In hepatitis, while total LD activity increases considerably, α-HBD stays normal or only shows a small increase; in chronic liver disease and obstructive jaundice it remains normal or even becomes subnormal.

McQueen *et al.* (1972) compared the activities of CK, AST, LD, α-HBD, GD and ALT in a group of 38 patients with unequivocal evidence of myocardial infarction and obtained mean increases, expressed as a multiple of URL, of:

Enzyme	Time (hours)				
	0–12	13–24	24–48	49–72	73–96
CK	3·65	6·00	3·90	2·30	1·10
AST	2·50	4·10	3·65	1·60	1·10
LD	1·60	2·75	3·30	2·20	1·95
HBD	1·55	2·75	3·30	2·20	2·00
GD	1·35	2·35	2·95	2·00	1·85
ALT	0·60	1·00	0·95	0·70	0·75

Emerson and Wilkinson (1965) using oxalate and urea inhibition methods found that the mean percentage inhibition with oxalate was reduced from 61 (SD,

3·5) to 39 (15) in liver disease and increased to 72 (4) in heart disease. The reverse was seen with the figures using urea inhibition. The normal result of 52 (SD, 6) was increased to 78 (9·5) in liver disease and reduced to 31 (12) in heart disease.

Foo *et al.* (1981) examined a variety of techniques for their ability to discriminate between patients with liver and heart disease. The techniques tested were LD–1 activity after immunoprecipitation, LD–1 activity by electrophoresis and the activities of α-HBD, urea-stable LD and heat-stable LD. The last three were measured using the Association of Clinical Biochemists Proposed Methods (1980). LD–1 activity after immunoprecipitation correlated well with LD–1 activity determined by electrophoresis and gave the best differentiation between patient groups. This was followed by heat-stable LD and LD measured by electrophoresis. Urea-stable LD and α-HBD gave less discrimination.

PHOSPHATASES
(Alkaline phosphatase: Orthophosphoric monoester phosphohydrolase, 3.1.3.1; Acid phosphatase: Orthophosphoric monoester phosphohydrolase, 3.1.3.2)

Phosphatases are enzymes which catalyse the splitting off of phosphoric acid from monophosphoric esters. Two types are commonly estimated in serum, a mixture of alkaline phosphatases with maximum activity at about pH 10, and acid phosphatases, maximum activity between pH 5 and 6. The activity is due to a mixture of isoenzymes from various organs.

ALKALINE PHOSPHATASES

Purified alkaline phosphatases from different sources exhibit three types of activity; hydrolytic (1), phosphotransferase (2) and pyrophosphatase (3):

$$
\begin{array}{l}
\overset{\displaystyle O^-}{\underset{\displaystyle O^-}{R-O-\overset{|}{\underset{|}{P}}=O}} + H-OH \rightleftharpoons R-OH + \overset{\displaystyle O^-}{\underset{\displaystyle O^-}{HO-\overset{|}{\underset{|}{P}}=O}} \qquad (1)
\end{array}
$$

$$
\begin{array}{l}
\overset{\displaystyle O^-}{\underset{\displaystyle O^-}{R-O-\overset{|}{\underset{|}{P}}=O}} + R'-OH \rightleftharpoons R-OH + \overset{\displaystyle O^-}{\underset{\displaystyle O^-}{R'-O-\overset{|}{\underset{|}{P}}=O}} \qquad (2)
\end{array}
$$

$$
\begin{array}{l}
\overset{\displaystyle O^- \quad O^-}{\underset{\displaystyle O^- \quad O^-}{R-O-\overset{|}{\underset{|}{P}}-O-\overset{|}{\underset{|}{P}}-O-R'}} + H-OH \rightleftharpoons \overset{\displaystyle O^-}{\underset{\displaystyle O^-}{R-O-\overset{|}{\underset{|}{P}}=O}} + \overset{\displaystyle O^-}{\underset{\displaystyle O^-}{R'-O-\overset{|}{\underset{|}{P}}=O}} \qquad (3)
\end{array}
$$

Alkaline phosphatases are present in most tissues, the richest sources being osteoblasts in the bone, bile canaliculi in the liver, small intestinal epithelium, proximal tubules in the kidney, the placenta, and the breasts during lactation. In all these sites it seems to be involved in the transport of phosphate across cell membranes. The alkaline phosphatase of normal serum in adults appears to be mainly derived from the liver with a small, variable intestinal component. The relatively small amounts and the diffuse nature of the bone band on electrophoresis led to reports that the bone isoenzyme is virtually absent. Heat-inactivation studies, however, suggest that a substantial part of the normal adult alkaline phosphatase is a phosphatase of presumed bone origin. The contribution from bone is greater in infancy, childhood and adolescence. During pregnancy some placental enzyme is present.

Alkaline phosphatase requires metal ions: Mg^{2+}, Zn^{2+} and, to a lesser extent, Mn^{2+} and Co^{2+}. Magnesium is essential for stability and for maximum catalytic activity. Zinc, which is essential for catalysis, can also inhibit the enzyme by binding to the magnesium site, its affinity for which is ten times greater than that of magnesium. An optimal Mg^{2+}/Zn^{2+} ratio is required for maximum activity. The enzyme is inhibited by Cu^{2+}, Hg^{2+}, by EDTA which removes the Mg^{2+} ions and by some amino acids of which L-phenylalanine has been used in distinguishing the enzymes from different sources (see p. 540).

Determination of Serum Alkaline Phosphatase Activity

Alkaline phosphatase activity has been measured by many methods differing in substrate, buffer type, buffer concentration, temperature of incubation and unit of measurement. This discussion deals mainly with more recent methods. The previous edition contained a brief historical review. For a detailed review of the subject see McComb *et al.* (1979).

Substrates. The substances used as substrate include β-glycerophosphate (Bodansky, 1932), disodium phenylphosphate (King and Armstrong, 1934), 2-naphthyl phosphate (Seligman *et al.*, 1951), 1-naphthylphosphate (Babson and Read, 1959) and phenolphthalein mono- and di-phosphates (Babson *et al.*, 1966 and Huggins and Talalay, 1945 respectively). All required further reactions or a change in pH to measure the products. Methods using β-glycerophosphate and the earlier phenylphosphate methods involved protein precipitation. In 1946, Bessey *et al.* published a method using 4-nitrophenylphosphate (NPP) which overcame both difficulties. The product, 4-nitrophenol, could be measured directly. Pure substrate, however, was not readily obtained and the method was not widely adopted in the UK.

All these substances have different activities as enzyme–substrate complexes so that coupled with the different colour intensity ($\Delta\varepsilon_{max}$) of the products the sensitivity varies widely. Table 22.2 shows some characteristics of several of these substrates when reacting with alkaline phosphatase from different sources. Although phenyl phosphate and 2-naphthyl phosphate are hydrolysed most rapidly their low $\Delta\varepsilon_{max}$ makes them less sensitive than NPP. In the case of the phthaleins their relatively low molar activities makes them less sensitive than NPP in spite of their high $\Delta\varepsilon_{max}$.

In 2-amino-2-methyl-1-propanol buffer, NPP shows minimal bias towards the individual isoenzymes normally found in human serum. This, together with the sensitivity shown in Table 22.2 and the ability to monitor the reaction continuously has made NPP the preferred substrate.

Buffers. The barbiturate buffers, pH 7·4 to 9·0, used initially required lengthy incubation periods; the introduction of bicarbonate-carbonate buffer pH 10·0 doubled the rate of reaction allowing the period of incubation to be reduced to 15 min. Glycine-sodium hydroxide, pH 9·0, was used by Huggins and Talalay (1945) and by Bessey *et al.* (1946) at pH 10·3 in their method using NPP as substrate. In all these the reaction was according to equation (1) opposite. None introduced a structure capable of stimulating the alkaline phosphatase to act as a phosphorylating enzyme. The situation changed with the introduction of amino alcohols as buffers by Lowry *et al.* (1954) who, although not recommending it as

TABLE 22.2
Reactions of Substrates with Alkaline Phosphatases from Different Sources
(Bowers et al., 1967)

| Substrate | $\Delta\varepsilon_{max}$ × 10^{-3} | Wavelength (nm) | Relative molar activity | | | Relative sensitivity* |
			Calf mucosa	Human serum	Human liver	Human liver
4-Nitrophenyl phosphate	18·8	404	100	100	100	100
Phenyl phosphate	1·6	288	167	94	119	10
1-Naphthyl phosphate	5·4	334	126	104	116	34
2-Naphthyl phosphate	2·4	347	140	109	114	14
Phenolphthalein monophosphate	22·0	555	50	33	28	33
Thymolphthalein monophosphate	26·0	595	7	—	23	32

In 750 mmol/l 2-amino-2-methyl-1-propanol, pH 10·15 at 30 °C

*Ratio of $\Delta\varepsilon_{max}$ of substrate to that of NPP multiplied by relative molar activity.

the buffer of choice, used 2-amino-2-methyl-1-propanol. Wilson *et al.* (1964) studied the use of Tris and attributed the increased activity obtained to transphosphorylation in which the net transfer of phosphate from substrate to the hydroxyl group of the buffer is a more rapid reaction than transfer to water (hydrolysis). For significant transphosphorylation to occur, the phosphate acceptor must contain a hydroxyl group and either a second hydroxyl group or an amine. McComb and Bowers (1972) studied 23 buffers in a continuous monitoring method using NPP as substrate. Some appear in Table 22.3. At a low

TABLE 22.3

Activity of Alkaline Phosphatase with Various Buffers at Low and High Concentrations
(McComb and Bowers, 1972)

Buffer	Structural formula	pK_a	Activity (U/l) at pH 10·15 Final concentration of buffer	
			45 mmol/l	900 mmol/l
2-Ethylaminoethanol (EAE)	$C_2H_5.NH.CH_2.CH_2OH$	9·9	140	375
Diethanolamine (DEA)	$CH_2.CH_2OH$ NH $CH_2.CH_2OH$	8·7	106	280
2-Methylaminoethanol	$CH_3.NH.CH_2.CH_2OH$	9·6	129	222
2-Dimethylaminoethanol	CH_3 $N.CH_2.CH_2OH$ CH_3	9·2	95	179
2-Isopropylaminoethanol	CH_3 $CH.NH.CH_2.CH_2OH$ CH_3	9·7	121	144
Tris	CH_2OH $H_2NC.CH_2OH$ CH_2OH	7·8	53	117
2-Amino-2-methyl-1-propanol (2A2M1P)	CH_3 $H_2N.C.CH_2OH$ CH_3	9·3	104	104
Diethylamine	$C_2H_5.NH.C_2H_5$	10·9	102	96
2-Amino-2-methyl-1,3-propanediol	NH_2 $HO.CH_2.C.CH_2OH$ CH_3	8·6	78	99
Sodium carbonate–sodium bicarbonate		9·9	90	45
3-Aminopropanol	$H_2N.CH_2.CH_2.CH_2OH$	9·4	89	30
Triethanolamine	$CH_2.CH_2OH$ $N.CH_2.CH_2OH$ $CH_2.CH_2OH$	7·6	36	74
Propylamine	$CH_3.CH_2.CH_2.NH_2$	10·6	75	27
Ethanolamine	$H_2N.CH_2.CH_2OH$	8·8	57	18
Ammonium hydroxide		9·3	46	3

buffer concentration, 45 mmol/l, reaction (1) is favoured while at 900 mmol/l there is some contribution from (2). The highest activity among the non-transphosphorylating buffers is with diethylamine. That the hydroxyl group is involved in the activation of the phosphatase is evident when activity with diethylamine, ethylaminoethanol and diethanolamine is compared. The first six buffers show a marked increase in enzyme activity paralleling the increased buffer concentration presumably due to transphosphorylation. The first five all have a substituted amino group separated from the hydroxyl by two carbon atoms, but this is not the sole determinant. While ethanolamine has only a low activity, substitution in the amine group or on the carbon to which it is attached gives compounds in most cases with greater activity than with non-phosphorylating buffers. Such increased activity suggests the removal of an inhibiting action of the primary amine group. Comparison of the three non-phosphorylating buffers, ammonium hydroxide, propylamine and diethylamine, shows that progressive substitution with alkyl residues clears the inhibition at 45 mmol/l, a difference accentuated at higher concentrations.

With all the various factors involved, choice of the most satisfactory buffer is not easy. Carbonate–bicarbonate has a low buffering capacity at concentrations at which activity is at a maximum, which is also the case with glycine used in some methods. DEA and 2A2M1P have a lower substrate concentration optimum than EAE or carbonate–bicarbonate which is an advantage with NPP as substrate because at higher concentrations of buffer there is a higher initial absorbance and more non-enzymatic hydrolysis occurs. Carbonate–bicarbonate buffer supports less activity for the same amount of enzyme than either DEA or 2A2M1P and although it may be adequate for many purposes it is less suitable for measuring the low activities of isoenzymes following heat or chemical inactivation. Thus DEA and 2A2M1P are preferred. However, the increased sensitivity with DEA is so great that one has to decrease the analytical range or use such small sample volumes that pipetting errors become significant. Maximum activity in DEA buffer is not achieved until a concentration of 1·8 mol/l, which results in an increase in viscosity sufficient to cause measurement errors. For this reason sub-optimal concentrations of DEA are used. This is not necessary with 2A2M1P since maximum activity is obtained at 0·9 mol/l and a concentration of 0·35 mol/l gives approximately 95 % maximum activity. This lower concentration has the additional advantage of less competition between substrate and buffer for their specific sites on the enzyme, thus decreasing substrate requirement. The pK for DEA buffer is 8·7 at 30 °C whereas that for 2A2M1P is 9·7, much nearer to the pH of the reaction mixture. As already stated, NPP shows minimal bias towards the various isoenzymes when 2A2M1P is used; the bias is much more pronounced with DEA. For these reasons 2A2M1P has become the buffer of choice.

Both DEA and 2A2M1P preparations can contain impurities acting as inhibitors. DEA solutions can contain monoethanolamine (MEA), a potent inhibitor of alkaline phosphatase. It has been suggested that batches of DEA should be screened by gas chromatography for the presence of MEA. Solutions of 2A2M1P may contain 5-amino-3-azo-2,2,5-trimethylhexanol which inactivates the enzyme by binding Zn^{2+} ions essential for activity. This inhibition can be avoided by screening the 2A2M1P for the impurity or by using a metal-ion buffer which will provide the enzyme with Zn^{2+} ions if these are sequestered by the inhibitor. The latter approach is recommended by the Expert Panel on Enzymes of the IFCC (IFCC, 1983b). The highly alkaline pH of the buffer can inactivate the enzyme so it is recommended that the reaction be started by the addition of the serum to keep to a minimum the exposure of the sample to alkaline conditions.

Recommended Methods

With such a variety of available substrates and buffers standardisation between laboratories has been difficult to achieve. This also applies to the various national bodies who have made recommendations (see Moss *et al.*, 1971; Bretaudière *et al.*, 1977; IFCC., 1983b). Moss *et al.* (1971) suggested the use of a phenylphosphate method, however this substrate is not suitable for continuous monitoring. The use of NPP is mandatory if continuous monitoring is used and NPP is universal in recommended methods published since 1972. For details of some recommended methods the reader is referred to Bretaudière *et al.* (1977) and IFCC (1983b). See also IFCC (1978) and Tietz *et al.* (1983) for systematic discussion of the considerations concerning the measurement of enzyme activity in serum.

Bowers and McComb (1966) and Hausamen *et al.* (1967) investigated continuous monitoring methods using NPP as substrate but chose different buffers, the former 2A2M1P, the latter DEA. The latter has been recommended by the German and Scandinavian Societies but the former has found more favour in the rest of Europe and the USA. A tentative reference method (Bowers and McComb, 1975) requires quality control of the reagents and rigorous standardisation at all stages in their preparation. As an example of this approach, which merits wider use, their method is given here.

Continuous Monitoring Method of Bowers and McComb (1975)

Reagents.
1. 2-Amino-2-methyl-l-propanol buffer, 890 mmol/l, pH 10·33 at 30 °C. Warm the 2A2M1P to 30–35 °C until completely liquefied. Weigh exactly 78·5 g directly into a litre volumetric flask, add 500 ml deionised water and mix. Add 200 ml hydrochloric acid 1·000 mol/l from a 200 ml volumetric flask with at least one rinse. Dilute to nearly a litre, allow to come to room temperature (25 ± 1 °C), adjust to the mark and mix. This buffer has a pH of 10·33 (range 10·31 to 10·35) at 30 °C. Protected from atmospheric carbon dioxide, it is stable for one month when stored at room temperature.
2. Magnesium solution, 1·5 mmol/l. Dissolve 30·0 mg $MgCl_2$, $6H_2O$ in water and make to 100 ml. This keeps indefinitely.
3. Substrate, NPP, 225 mmol/l in the magnesium solution. For each ml substrate solution dissolve 83·5 mg NPP disodium salt, hexahydrate (mol. wt. 371) in 1 ml reagent (2). Prepare freshly. It is then stable at room temperature in neutral or slightly alkaline solution for 8 h. The pH should be between 8 and 9.
4. Stock standard 4-nitrophenol, 1 mmol/l. Dissolve 139·1 mg high purity 4-nitrophenol in water, dilute to a litre and mix. Stored in the dark this can be used for many months.

Technique. To 2·70 ml buffer add 100 µl serum using a 'to contain' pipette and wash out thoroughly. Alternatively, use an automatic dilutor. Place the tube in a 30 °C water bath for 5 min and allow to come to temperature. Warm the substrate to 30 °C and to start the reaction add exactly 200 µl to the buffer sample and mix thoroughly. Transfer immediately to a preheated 10 mm cuvette and place in the temperature-controlled compartment of the spectrophotometer. Record the absorbance continuously at 402·5 nm or at intervals of 30 s for 5 min against a blank prepared from 2·80 ml buffer and 200 µl substrate. Calculate the rate of change per minute.

Calculation. Serum alkaline phosphatase activity $(U/l) = \Delta A_{402.5}/min$ $\times 1.592 \times 10^3$, when the total volume used is 3·0 ml and the molar absorbance of 4-nitrophenol in 2A2M1P buffer, pH 10 at 30 °C, is 18 800 for the instrument used (see note (3) below).

Notes. Bowers and McComb (1975) give full specifications for the purity of the reagents by spectrophotometric readings under standard conditions. Conversely, if reagents of known purity are used these solutions can be used to check the wavelength and photometric accuracy of the spectrophotometer, as indicated in Chapter 7 (p. 150).

1. NPP. Measured in a quartz cuvette in an instrument as described in Chapter 7 (p. 149) the molar absorbance in 10 mmol/l sodium hydroxide at 25 °C and 311 nm is 9 850. To check and correct for this so as to allow for variations in the water of crystallisation of different batches add 200 µl 225 mmol/l NPP substrate (reagent (3)) to about 200 ml water in a 500 ml volumetric flask, mix and add 5·0 ml 1·0 mol/l sodium hydroxide, mix well and make to the mark with water. Read against a blank of 10 mmol/l sodium hydroxide in a 1·0 cm cell at 311 nm and 25 °C. After correcting for the blank the absorbance should be 0·885 ± 0·010. To adjust, dilute with magnesium chloride solution or weigh in more substrate until the required reading is obtained, then use the adjusted amounts for preparing future substrate with this batch of reagent.

2. The slight yellow colour of the substrate solution is due to free 4-nitrophenol which should be less than 0·1 % expressed as a molar fraction of 4-nitrophenol in NPP. To check mix equal volumes of substrate (reagent (3)) and 20 mmol/l sodium hydroxide. If the absorbance of this mixture read at 415 nm in a 1 cm cuvette is less than 1·7 it meets this requirement.

   The inorganic phosphate concentration determined by one of the usual methods should also be less than 1 % on a molar basis.

3. The molar absorbance of 4-nitrophenol at 401·0 nm at 25 °C in a 1 cm cuvette when dissolved in 10 mmol/l sodium hydroxide is 18 400. To prepare 4-nitrophenol of the required purity recrystallise from boiling water as described in Chapter 7 (p. 150). Pipette 20·0 ml stock 1 mmol/l 4-nitrophenol solution (reagent (4)) into a 500 ml volumetric flask and dilute to the mark with 10 mmol/l sodium hydroxide, mix well and read at 401 nm against a reagent blank of 10 mmol/l sodium hydroxide. This should read 0·736. For the use of this solution in checking spectrophotometer wavelength and accuracy see p. 150.

4. The molar absorbance of 4-nitrophenol in 2A2M1P buffer, pH 10·3 and 30 °C is 18 800. To check prepare 500 ml buffer as described for reagent (1) and remove 50 ml for use as a blank. Transfer 20 ml 4-nitrophenol stock standard (reagent (4)) at 25 ± 1 °C to the volumetric flask using a class A volumetric pipette. Dilute to the mark with water and mix well. The absorbance of this solution read at 402·5 nm against the buffer blank in a 1·0 cm cell at 30 °C should be 0·750. If the reading R differs more than 1 % from this, multiply the observed value by 0·750/R in calculating the activity.

Reference Values and Units

As the units for a method vary with the conditions of the reaction such as type of substrate and its concentration, the type of buffer, pH, temperature and concentration of activator, it will be evident that for alkaline phosphatase there will be quite a number of normal ranges, comparison of which even when converted to U/l will not be easy. The classical King–Armstrong (1934) method gave a normal range of 22 to 92 U/l. Hausamen *et al.* (1967) working at 25 °C found a range of 61 to 171 U/l but Bowers and McComb (1975) found the lower range of 7 to 127 U/l at the higher temperature of 30 °C. Laboratories are recommended to develop reference ranges for the populations they serve. The alkaline phosphatase activity in the serum of apparently healthy individuals is positively skewed and this should be considered in the selection of the method used to calculate the reference range. Before calculation of the ranges, the population should be subdivided to take account of the major age- and sex-related differences in alkaline phosphatase.

The alkaline phosphatase activity in serum increases during the first few months of life to reach a level up to 2·5 times the URL for adults. This level is maintained throughout childhood. With the onset of the adolescent growth spurt there is a gradual rise in alkaline phosphatase activity followed by a fall to adult levels towards the beginning of the third decade. This process starts at approximately 11 years old in females and is completed by the age of 20. The changes occur later in males and they do not reach adult levels till well after the age of 20. During puberty, peak alkaline phosphatase activities show a better correlation with sex-maturity ratings than with chronological age.

Alkaline phosphatase activity in maternal serum rises during normal pregnancy because of the presence of the placental isoenzyme. Typical rises are up to approximately 1·5 times the URL for non-pregnant females although levels up to 12 times this level have been reported in apparently normal pregnancy. The activity may remain elevated in the serum for one month after delivery.

In contrast to the relatively wide variation in alkaline phosphatase activity in serum of normal individuals it would appear that the intra-individual variation is very small once adult levels have been reached.

Analytical Performance of Alkaline Phosphatase Methods

Bowers and McComb (1975) quoted a between-batch CV of 4·6 % at activities between 65 and 150 U/l in their laboratory using the manual method described on p. 533. This could be improved using automated equipment. Lohff *et al.* (1982) showed a CV of less than 5 % between-batch intra-laboratory imprecision at three different levels with a number of different analysers. Inspection of the results from external quality assessment schemes suggests that the performance achieved is more instrument-dependent than method-dependent.

INTERPRETATION

As discussed, there are several different reference ranges even between methods producing results in U/l. Abnormalities of results will be expressed as multiples of the URL.

Increase in alkaline phosphatase activity occurs mainly in bone disease and in diseases of the liver and biliary tract. For the latter see p. 745. In bone disease, the activity is increased when osteoblasts are more actively laying down osteoid. It therefore occurs when bone regeneration is taking place or is being attempted. It is not related directly to osteoclastic activity and no increase in alkaline phosphatase is found when there is bone destruction unless there is simultaneous formation of new bone or osteoid tissue. Thus there is a marked increase in rickets, in which osteoid is produced in excess but is poorly calcified, the increase roughly paralleling the severity of the condition. Values up to 8 times URL may be found. There is usually an increase in osteomalacia, not usually so marked as that in children. Levels up to 20 times URL have been seen in Asian patients with osteomalacia in the UK. In malabsorptive conditions the impaired absorption of vitamin D and calcium leads to bone changes and to a moderate increase to between 2 and 5 times URL. In osteitis deformans (Paget's disease) the very high figures which may be reached are a reasonable index of the activity of the disease process. When activities greater than 15 times URL occur, they are thought by some workers to suggest the development of osteogenic sarcoma, a known complication of Paget's disease, although Poretta *et al.* (1957) disagree. Treatment of Paget's disease with mithramycin, sodium etidronate or calcitonin causes a fall in alkaline phosphatase levels and discontinuation of therapy results in a return to pre-treatment levels. In some patients on calcitonin therapy, the values rise in spite of continuing medication and persisting clinical remission. Thus alkaline phosphatase values do not correlate well with clinical improvement during treatment.

Most patients with primary hyperparathyroidism have normal alkaline phosphatase levels. In hyperparathyroidism with bony involvement, bone destruction is more extensive than bone regeneration so that the increase in alkaline phosphatase activity is usually between the top of the reference range and 5 times the URL. Normal levels may be found even with bone involvement.

In osteoporosis, bone formation rates at the time of diagnosis are generally thought to be normal. In accordance with this belief, alkaline phosphatase levels in osteoporosis are either normal or only slightly elevated. The presence of a significantly raised alkaline phosphatase suggests a disorder other than osteoporosis.

In bone tumours the findings are variable, depending on the amount of new bone being formed. Marked increases may be found in osteogenic sarcoma, a malignant tumour of osteoblasts, but in other cases normal or near normal results are obtained. In patients with secondary deposits in bone appreciable increases may occur. This is particularly the case in carcinoma of the prostate, while small increases may sometimes be seen in cancer of the breast, thyroid, pancreas or stomach. In multiple myeloma in which the lesion is almost purely destructive, alkaline phosphatase is usually within normal limits, never with more than a very small increase.

In summary, the estimation of serum alkaline phosphatase activity alone is of limited value in bone disease. For differential diagnosis it is necessary to take the findings in conjunction with those for other constituents of serum such as calcium, inorganic phosphate and proteins.

A 'transient hyperphosphataemia of infancy' with alkaline phosphatase activity up to 30 times the URL for adults has been reported in children less than 3 years old. It disappears within 2 months of being detected and has been seen in children with no radiological or biochemical evidence of bone or liver disease. The increased activity appears to be derived from bone in some cases; in others, the enzyme may be an excessively sialylated liver isoenzyme. There is no consistent pattern of symptoms in these children although several have presented with abdominal pain, diarrhoea or vomiting.

A decrease in serum alkaline phosphatase activity has been reported in severe anaemia, in scurvy, in kwashiorkor and in arrested growth in children with cretinism and achondroplasia. Hypophosphatasia has also been recognised as a congenital defect inherited as an autosomal recessive, usually first recognised in childhood but occasionally presenting in adults. Bone changes are similar to those seen in rickets. Serum alkaline phosphatase may be below the lower limit of the normal adult range but in children with their higher normal range, values below the mid-point of the adult normal range may be significant. A feature of the condition is the presence of an increased amount of phosphoryl ethanolamine (PEA) in the urine and plasma of patients and of their parents. The origin of this increase is not clear. Also increased is the excretion of pyrophosphate. Rasmussen (1968) studied the renal clearance of PEA and showed that this varied directly with plasma concentration and approached the creatinine clearance in homozygotes with the highest values for plasma PEA. Hypercalciuria and hypercalcaemia are also sometimes present. For an account of this condition see Rasmussen (1983).

Changes in the alkaline phosphatase result are often associated with drug therapy. Mostly an increased value is found but SH-compounds are said to reduce the result as does azathioprine in some cases (but see below). Most increases either follow as a result of cholestasis induced by the drug or as a consequence of hepatocellular toxicity. Many drugs have been implicated in both processes. Examples of drugs producing a cholestatic increase are androgens, anabolic steroids, oestrogens, sulphonamides, phenothiazines, tricyclic anti-depressants, monoamine oxidase inhibitors, antibiotics, diuretics, anticoagulants and immunosuppressants such as azathioprine. This formidable list, including many of the drugs used in modern medicine, has to be supplemented by hepatotoxic drugs which include aspirin, paracetamol, antibiotics such as chlortetracycline, gentamicin and lincomycin, cyclophosphamide, halothane, methylthiouracil and several antidepressants. An increase in the bone enzyme occurs in children on long-term anticonvulsant therapy and such drugs produce increases in alkaline phosphatase figures in adults also. Small increases in the activity of this enzyme in hospital patients must therefore always be considered in the light of drug treatment.

The assay of 5'-nucleotidase activity in serum has been used in cases in which the serum alkaline phosphatase is increased. An increase is found in diseases of the liver and biliary tract roughly parallel to those in the serum alkaline phosphatase. These are therefore highest in post-hepatic obstructive jaundice, frequently over 3 times the URL. Only small increases are seen in hepatic jaundice, e.g. in infective hepatitis and also in the later stages of cirrhosis. On the other hand, in bone diseases in which the alkaline phosphatase is increased, such as Paget's disease, 5'-nucleotidase usually remains within normal limits; if there is an increase it is only slight. The determination was used to help in distinguishing the source of an increase in serum alkaline phosphatase but has been superseded by the separation of alkaline phosphatase isoenzymes (see the 5th edition of this book for details of the determination).

Isoenzymes of Alkaline Phosphatase

Several electrophoretic techniques have been used to separate and distinguish the isoenzymes of alkaline phosphatase. Although electrophoresis cannot be used as the sole indicator of the origin of a raised alkaline phosphatase activity, only electrophoresis will reveal the presence of an abnormal band. Unfortunately, currently available electrophoretic media do not completely separate the two most clinically relevant isoenzymes, bone and liver.

Starch gel, cellulose acetate, agar, agarose and polyacrylamide gel have been used. Starch gel gives good resolution of some bands and can be used for phenotyping the placental isoenzyme. However, the separation of bone and liver is not as good as in polyacrylamide gel and the technique is cumbersome for routine use. Although cellulose acetate does not have the molecular sieving effect, electro-endosmosis improves resolution and it is commonly used because of the relative simplicity of the method and wide availability of suitable equipment (see Karmen *et al.*, 1984). The method used in the author's laboratory is given below. Polyacrylamide gel electrophoresis is the preferred technique as the separation of bone and liver bands is clearer, particularly on vertical slab gels. Five per cent gels are generally used since below this concentration there is inadequate resolution of bone and liver isoenzymes while with gels above 7% the liver and placental bands tend to run together. Agar gel electrophoresis is suitable for separation of the major isoenzymes if care is taken with the selection of the batch of agar. Much of the seminal work of Wieme (1959) was carried out using agar gel. Agarose is now replacing agar for this purpose and is readily available in commercially-prepared thin films.

The electrophoretic mobility of the isoenzymes is affected by the medium used. Liver alkaline phosphatase normally runs as an alpha-2 band, bone runs in the alpha-2/beta region as does placental alkaline phosphatase which must be differentiated by heat inactivation studies. Intestinal isoenzyme is usually found in the beta-2/gamma region. In cholestatic disorders, however, there is an extra band which has been termed the 'biliary', 'fast liver' or 'alpha-1 liver' band. This activity appears to be associated with other membrane-bound enzyme activities in a high molecular mass complex. This biliary band is seen in the alpha-1 region on non-sieving media such as agar and cellulose acetate but remains at the origin with starch and polyacrylamide.

Method of Smith *et al.* (1968, modified) Using Polyacrylamide Gel Electrophoresis

This is the preferred technique. The Shandon equipment for disc electrophoresis on polyacrylamide gel columns is used.

Reagents.
1. Tris-borate buffer, pH 9·5. Dissolve 45·5 g Tris in 900 ml water, add boric acid to pH 9·5 and make to 1 l with water. Store at 2 to 4 °C in the dark.
2. Tris-borate-TEMED buffer, pH 9·5. Prepare and store as for reagent (1) except that 1·2 ml TEMED (see p. 77) is added before the boric acid.
3. Gel monomer. Dissolve 19 g acrylamide and 1 g bisacrylamide in water and make to 100 ml. Store as reagent (1).
4. Ammonium persulphate solution, 2 g/l. Prepare 100 ml and store as reagent (1) but renew every 2 weeks.
5. Sucrose solution, 200 g/l.
6. Enzyme location buffer. Dissolve 3·74 g boric acid and 2·04 g $MgCl_2,6H_2O$ in 900 ml water, adjust to pH 9·7 with potassium hydroxide and dilute to 1 l.
7. Substrate solution. Dissolve 200 mg 2-naphthyl phosphate in 100 ml reagent (6).
8. Enzyme incubation mixture. Prepare just before use by adding Fast Blue BB diazonium salt to reagent (7) using 1 mg per ml substrate. Add a few mg charcoal, shake and filter.

Technique. The gel is cast to a height of 6.5 cm in glass tubes, permanently siliconised with dichlor-dimethylsilane, sold for use with the electrophoresis equipment. Warm appropriate volumes of reagents (2), (3) and (4) to room temperature. Mix one volume each of reagents (2) and (3) with two volumes reagent (4). Pour into the glass tubes to the correct height and cover with 20 μl water. Use the gel within a few hours of completion of polymerisation which takes 30 min. Place the tubes in the equipment and add *cold* reagent (1) to both electrode vessels just before use.

For sera with normal alkaline phosphatase values mix 1 volume serum with 2 volumes sucrose solution and apply 20 μl to the top of the gel. For raised enzyme values, dilute appropriately with the sucrose solution. On one column use a sample prepared similarly from a control serum containing a trace of bromophenol blue (BPB). Adjust the current to 1 mA per gel (90 V) for 5 min so that the BPB band penetrates a few mm into the gel. Increase the current to 3 mA per gel (270 V) to bring the BPB band to the bottom of the tube in 30 to 40 min. Remove the tubes from the apparatus.

Place 5 ml fresh reagent 8 in a suitable small test tube. Rim a gel in its tube, transfer the gel to the incubation mixture so that it is fully immersed and keep at room temperature in the dark for 1 h. Transfer the gel to distilled water and allow to destain overnight. Examine the bands by eye or in a scanner.

Method of Siede and Seiffert (1977, modified) Using Cellulose Acetate

This method takes advantage of electro-endosmosis and uses a fixation technique to avoid elution and diffusion of the enzyme during incubation and staining.

Reagents.
1. Stock barbitone buffer, 0·15 mmol/l, pH 8·6. Dissolve 4·6 g barbitone and 25·8 g sodium barbitone in 900 ml of water and make to 1 litre with distilled water.
2. Working barbitone buffer, 0·075 mmol/l, pH 8·6. Dilute stock buffer 1:1 with distilled water. Check and adjust pH as necessary.
3. Lead acetate, 125 g/l.
4. Fixative. Mix 30 ml lead acetate solution and 70 ml absolute ethanol.
5. Saturated sodium acetate.
6. Tris buffer, 1·0 mmol/l. Dissolve 12·1 g Tris(hydroxymethyl)aminomethane and make up to 100 ml with distilled water.
7. Magnesium chloride, 123 mmol/l. Dissolve 250 mg of $MgCl_2$, $6H_2O$ in 100 ml distilled water.
8. Dye solution. Dissolve 0·1 g Fast Blue VB salt in 10 ml dimethylformamide. Filter and use within two weeks. Store in the dark.
9. Incubation mixture. Dissolve 30 mg sodium naphthyl-1-phosphate in a mixture of 0·5 ml magnesium chloride solution, 2·5 ml Tris buffer and 22·5 ml saturated sodium acetate. Adjust to pH 10·2. Prepare immediately before use.
10. Staining mixture. Mix 1·0 ml Tris buffer, 1·0 ml dye solution and 100 ml distilled water.
11. Cellulose Acetate Membranes. Sepharose III (Gelman Instrument Company).

Technique. Prepare the electrophoresis tank with working barbitone buffer. Soak the cellulose acetate membrane in working barbitone buffer, blot quickly and position in the tank. Apply 0·4 μl of sample to the membrane about 1 cm from the centre of the strip on the cathodal side. Pass a constant current of 1·16 mA/cm. The voltage should be 260–300 V and will drop to 160–190 V during the run.

Remove the membranes and place in fixative solution for 10 min, agitating occasionally. Line the bottom of a tray with filter paper and saturate this with substrate solution. Place the membranes face down on the filter paper and cover with another layer of filter paper saturated with substrate solution. Incubate at 37 °C for 2 h after covering the tray with a glass plate, clingfilm or similar material. After incubation place each membrane in a covered staining bath containing 100 ml staining mixture. Examine the bands as soon as they appear. This takes 5 to 10 min.

Identification of the bands is made easier if a portion of the specimen is incubated at 56 °C for 10 min. This should then be run on the same strip as the untreated sample with bone and liver controls.

INTERPRETATION

Serum from healthy adults usually contains more than one isoenzyme. The predominant activity is derived from the liver isoenzyme but there is also a variable amount of bone, and in about 25% of normal individuals, some intestinal isoenzyme. The intestinal isoenzyme is more probable in individuals of B or O blood groups who are secretor-positive. The concentration of this isoenzyme is increased in a variety of diseases but is not invariably present in particular conditions. This means that no firm diagnostic interpretation can be made when the isoenzyme is found in increased amounts. It is important to be aware of the presence of increased levels of intestinal isoenzyme to be able to identify correctly the origin of a raised alkaline phosphatase activity.

It has been shown that after treatment with neuraminidase the mobility of the alkaline phosphatases from all sources except the small intestine is reduced. This enzyme removes a terminal sialic acid group which is either missing from the small intestinal enzyme molecule or is buried in the three dimensional structure (Fishman and Ghosh, 1967).

Electrophoresis may reveal the presence of abnormal bands not seen in normal serum. The biliary band has already been mentioned. Other bands with some of the characteristics of placental isoenzyme, as judged by inhibitor and heat-inactivation studies, have been found in patients with various types of cancer. Space does not allow a discussion of this topic and the reader is referred to Briere (1979).

Effect of Inhibitors

Heat Stability. The placental enzyme is much the most stable towards heat. Whereas those from liver, bone and kidney are completely inhibited and the small intestinal one almost completely so in 30 min at 56 °C, the placental isoenzyme is stable after 30 min at 70 °C. The thermal stabilities of bone and liver isoenzymes are slightly different. After accurately timed incubation at 56 °C, the residual activity can be used to calculate the proportion of each isoenzyme contributing to the total activity. Moss and Whitby (1975) measured the residual activity after incubating the sample for 15 and 25 min at 56 °C. By using the thermal inactivation curve of each sample they could take into account the variation in heat stability between specimens. Each specimen has different heat stability characteristics because the rate of inactivation of isoenzymes is affected by pH, protein concentration and the concentration of substrates and cofactors.

Heat inactivation prior to electrophoresis can be used to help to identify bands.

Urea. Bahr and Wilkinson (1967) showed that 2 mol/l urea inhibited the bone enzyme almost completely, the kidney 80%, liver 70%, small intestine 40%, and placental less than 25%, (see also Horne *et al.*, 1968; Birkett *et al.*, 1967).

L-**Phenylalanine**. L-Phenylalanine 5 mmol/l, inhibits the small intestinal and placental enzymes but not those from liver, bone and kidney. Eaton and Moss (1968) showed that pyrophosphatase activity was also affected.

Levamisole, a broad spectrum anti-helminthic, has the converse inhibitory effects. The intestinal and placental isoenzymes are insensitive and liver, bone and kidney isoenzymes are inhibited by 50% at a levamisole concentration of 10 μmol/l (Van Belle, 1976).

A number of other substances specifically inhibit purified human alkaline phosphatase isoenzymes. It has proven difficult to identify the components of a mixture of isoenzymes in serum using these techniques. Most laboratories would fractionate the alkaline phosphatase by electrophoresis and then use inhibitors or heat inactivation to help to identify the bands. Pledger *et al.* (1982) used L-phenylalanine amide to inhibit placental alkaline phosphatase to allow the assay of the other components in serum from pregnant patients.

For a review of alkaline phosphatase isoenzymes see Moss (1982b).

ACID PHOSPHATASE

The prostate after puberty is the organ with by far the highest concentration of acid phosphatase. The red cells also contain a significant amount, also there is some in the leucocytes and platelets, and small amounts in bone (osteoclasts), liver, kidney, spleen and pancreas. The small amount of acid phosphatase activity in the blood plasma in adult females and children is non-prostatic but in post-pubertal males a small proportion may be prostatic. The non-prostatic part is thought to be derived from the platelets and red cells and possibly from the liver.

Determination of Serum Acid Phosphatase

A variety of substrates has been used for the determination of serum acid phosphatase activity. Gutman and Gutman (1938; 1940) first adapted the original King–Armstrong method for alkaline phosphatase. Subsequently most of the substrates proposed for alkaline phosphatase were tried for acid phosphatase. As the clinical value of the determination has been almost entirely concerned with increases in serum prostatic acid phosphatase in adult males much attention has been given to excluding, as far as possible, the activity of the non-prostatic portion. This has been done in two ways, firstly by finding the substrate most nearly specific for the prostatic enzyme, that is with the greatest relative activity for this fraction, and secondly, to find an inhibitor which inhibits one or more of the types of acid phosphatase present.

Babson *et al.* (1959) showed that l-naphthyl phosphate was more specific than previous substrates, which included phenyl phosphate, NPP, β-glycerophosphate, and phenolphthalein monophosphate. They used it in a modified method (Babson and Phillips, 1966), but it is now known to be affected by platelet acid phosphatase. Sodium thymolphthalein monophosphate was found by Roy *et al.* (1971) to be more specific for the prostatic enzyme than other substrates in common use. Ewen and Spitzer (1976) investigated the method further and introduced modifications claimed to increase the sensitivity threefold compared with the original method.

Several inhibitors have been used in an effort to inhibit selectively acid phosphatases from different sources which may be present in serum. These have included L(+)-tartrate and fluoride which inhibit the prostatic enzyme leaving the red cell enzyme relatively unaffected. Formaldehyde and cupric ions have the reverse effect and ethanol inactivates both red cell and prostatic acid phosphatases. Of these inhibitors, tartrate is now the most commonly used and the 'tartrate-labile' serum acid phosphatase is taken as corresponding to the prostatic fraction. However, the inhibition of a significant part of the acid phosphatase in the serum of prepubertal males and females by tartrate suggests that the inhibition is not absolutely specific for prostatic acid phosphatase.

Platelet acid phosphatase contributes much of the non-prostatic activity to the tartrate-labile fraction. In an attempt to avoid this problem some workers have substituted heparinised plasma for serum but this causes turbidity in some methods. Haemolysis and prolonged storage of cells should be avoided because of the contribution from red cell phosphatase. The *in vitro* instability of the prostatic enzyme can also cause errors. Acid phosphatase is stable at pH 5–7 but loses activity at the higher pH of stored separated serum. It is advisable to acidify the serum with 3·3 mol/l acetic acid (10 μl/ml serum). The acidified specimen is then stable for several days at room temperature. Doe *et al.* (1965) added 18 mg disodium citrate/ml of serum to stabilise the activity for several days at room temperature or 4 °C. Stabiliser tablets are commercially available.

With the advent of methods using monoclonal antibodies for the immunological determination of prostatic acid phosphatase it was hoped that the problems of specificity and instability would be overcome. It was also hoped that these assays would improve the performance of the assay in detecting early cancer of the prostate. Several forms of immunoassay have been used including radioimmunoassay, immunoradiometric assay, enzyme immunoassay and conventional catalytic assay following the precipitation of the prostatic fraction. With most of these assays, except the last-mentioned, the instability problem has been largely overcome. There is no convincing evidence that the immunoassays are more specific than the measurement of tartate-labile acid phosphatase for the detection of cancer of the prostate and even those workers who feel that the immunoassays are more sensitive agree that this leads to no marked advantage in the early diagnosis or the follow-up of prostatic cancer (Cooper *et al.*, 1981; Davies and Griffiths, 1982; Mensink *et al.*, 1983; Pontes, 1983; Samuell *et al.*, 1984). An evaluation of kits for the immunological determination of prostatic acid phosphatase has been published by the Department of Health and Social Security (Pendower and Rosalki, 1985; Code STB3A/85/21). There seems little advantage in using an immunoassay particularly since they are more expensive and may be more time-consuming. In view of this an activity assay is recommended.

The most commonly used methods for serum acid phosphatase are those using either thymolphthalein monophosphate or 1-naphthyl phosphate as substrate. The latter is usually a continuous monitoring version of the method of Babson and Read (1959) such as that devised by Hillmann (1971). The 1-naphthol released is coupled with Fast Red TR (the stabilised diazonium salt of 4-chloro-*o*-toluidine) to produce a coloured compound which is read at 405 nm. There has been criticism of the use of continuous monitoring methods for acid phosphatase since, because of the low activity, the absorbance change per minute is very small in specimens with normal activity. Examples of two-point and continuous monitoring assays are given below.

Method Using Sodium Thymolphthalein Monophosphate
(Ewen and Spitzer, 1976)

Reagents.
1. Acetate buffer, 5 mol/l, pH 5·4 at 25 °C. Dilute 28·9 ml glacial acetic acid to 100 ml with water and add sodium acetate solution containing 680 g of the trihydrate/l until the pH is 5·4 at 25 °C.

2. Brij 35 solution. Dilute the 300 g/l solution obtainable from BDH Chemicals Limited to give a solution containing 3·24 g/l.
3. Substrate buffer reagent. Dissolve 74·7 mg disodium thymolphthalein monophosphate (17·7% water) in 50 ml Brij 35 solution, add 1·92 g sodium acetate (CH_3. COONa, $3H_2O$), mix and when dissolved adjust the pH to 5·4 (25 °C) with 100 mmol/l hydrochloric acid and dilute to 100 ml. Keep in the refrigerator and discard if the blank value increases.
4. Alkaline solution for colour development, sodium carbonate 1·0 mol/l in 1·0 mol/l sodium hydroxide (106 g anhydrous sodium carbonate and 40 g sodium hydroxide/l). For the working solution dilute 1 to 10.
5. Thymolphthalein stock standard, 3 mmol/l. Dissolve 129·3 mg thymolphthalein (mol. wt. 431) in propanol–water (70/30 v/v) and make to 100 ml with this.

Technique. After centrifuging the blood add 0·5 ml serum to a tube containing dry acetate buffer prepared by pipetting 25 µl of the buffer, evaporating to dryness at 60 °C and storing stoppered until required. Shake to dissolve the salts and keep frozen if not to be assayed on the same day. For the determination measure 550 µl substrate buffer reagent into each of two tubes. Bring one (the test) to 37 °C and add 50 µl specimen, mix, and incubate for 30 min, then add 1 ml working alkaline solution to this and to the second tube (the control).

For a standard curve prepare a set of dilutions of the stock standards as follows:

Serum acid phosphatase activity (U/l)	10	20	30	40	50	60	70	80
Stock thymolphthalein solution (ml)	0·1	0·2	0·3	0·4	0·5	0·6	0·7	0·8
Propanol–water (70/30 v/v) (ml)	0·9	0·8	0·7	0·6	0·5	0·4	0·3	0·2

Add 50 µl of each of these to 1·0 ml working alkali reagent and 550 µl buffer–substrate reagent. Read the standards, test and control against a propanol–water blank, at 590 nm.

Calculation. This is as follows for the standard 50 U/l:

$$\text{Serum acid phosphatase activity (U/l)} = \frac{\text{Reading of unknown} - \text{Reading of control}}{\text{Reading of standard}} \times 50$$

The *normal range* is given as 0·5 to 1·9 U/l (mean ± 2SD).

Continuous Monitoring Method Using 1-Naphthyl Hydrogen Phosphate
(Association of Clinical Biochemists, 1980; Hillmann, 1971)

Reagents.
1. Sodium 1-naphthyl hydrogen phosphate (mol. wt.246·1). Store in a desiccator at −20 °C.
2. Citrate buffer (0·2 mol/l) pH 5·5 at 20 °C. Dissolve 42 g (0·2 mol) citric acid ($C_6H_8O_7$, H_2O) in 800 ml water. Add 40 ml sodium hydroxide (7·5 mol/l), mix and adjust to pH 5·5 with further acid or alkali if required. Make up to 1 litre. The solution is stable for 6 months at 4 °C if kept free from bacteria. The pH of the buffer increases by 0·004 per °C rise in temperature.

3. Fast Red TR salt (mol. wt. 440·9). A product yielding low serum and reagent blanks is best. Test by adding 0·2 ml of a normal serum to 2 ml of a solution of 30 mg Fast Red TR salt in 10 ml citrate buffer. Incubate at 30 °C for 5 min. If the absorbance is greater than 0·020 at 405 nm and greater than 0·005 at 550 nm the product should not be used.

4. Substrate buffer reagent. Dissolve 0·98 g sodium 1-naphthyl hydrogen phosphate in 20 ml citrate buffer. The solution is stable for 4 days at 4 °C.

5. Dye Reagent. Dissolve 70 mg Fast Red TR salt in 20 ml citrate buffer. The solution is stable for 4 days at 4 °C.

6. Sodium (+) tartrate solution (1·31 mol/l). Dissolve 7·5 g disodium (+) tartrate ($(CHOH.COO)_2Na_2$, $2H_2O$; mol. wt. 230) in 20 ml water and make up to 25 ml. The solution is stable for 6 months at 4 °C if kept free from bacteria.

Technique. Add 0·2 ml serum and 0·2 ml tartrate solution to 2·0 ml dye reagent and mix. Prepare a blank tube by mixing 2·0 ml dye reagent and 0·4 ml water. Warm to 30 °C and add 0·2 ml substrate solution. Mix and read the absorbance at 550 nm for 5 min in a spectrophotometer thermostatted at 30 °C. Take readings at 1 min intervals. Plot the absorbances as a function of time and draw the best straight line through the points. Calculate the changes in absorbance per minute for both test and blank tubes.

Calculation. The molar absorption coefficient of the reaction product is 11 100 at 550 nm. Thus from the formula given on p. 495.

Serum acid phosphatase activity (U/l at 30 °C)

$$= (\Delta A/min_{test} - \Delta A/min_{blank}) \times \frac{1000}{\text{Volume of serum used (ml)}}$$

$$\times \frac{\text{Total volume in the cuvette (ml)}}{11 \cdot 1}$$

$$= (\Delta A/min_{test} - \Delta A/min_{blank}) \times \frac{1000}{0 \cdot 2} \times \frac{2 \cdot 6}{11 \cdot 1}$$

$$= (\Delta A/min_{test} - \Delta A/min_{blank}) \times 1170$$

Reference Range. Tartrate-labile acid phosphatase up to 4 U/l.

Notes.

1. The above method can be modified to give total acid phosphatase activity by replacing the tartrate by an equal volume of water.

2. The method may be applied directly to serum with activities up to 100 U/l and is suitable for manual or automated techniques. Heparinised plasma should not be used since this causes turbidity.

3. Earlier methods using Fast Red TR recommended 405 nm as the wavelength. However, there is significant interference at this wavelength as a result of a side reaction between serum and the diazo salt and this is minimised by measurement at 550 nm.

4. Bilirubin reacts with Fast Red TR under the conditions of the assay and serum bilirubin levels greater than 50 μmol/l produce an apparent reduction in enzyme activity. A substrate-initiated reaction such as that given above overcomes this problem by allowing the reaction between bilirubin and Fast Red TR to go to completion before substrate is added.

INTERPRETATION

The determination of serum acid phosphatase is mostly used to detect prostatic carcinoma and to monitor its treatment. The tumour invades local pelvic tissues and frequently metastasises to bone. Increases in serum total acid phosphatase values are uncommon in the early stages of the disease but are more frequent and of greater degree when skeletal involvement is established. Early studies of tartrate-labile acid phosphatase suggested increased sensitivity for earlier detection of the disease (Fishman *et al.*, 1953) but subsequent studies failed to support these observations. Nevertheless the use of inhibitors to improve the specificity of the assay is widespread. Increases are rare in cases of benign prostatic hypertrophy. Examples of the diagnostic limitations of the test were shown by Herbert (1946) and Sullivan *et al.* (1942) using disodium phenyl phosphate to measure total acid phosphatase. In cases of prostatic carcinoma without bone metastases, Sullivan found no abnormal levels of acid phosphatase while Herbert detected raised levels in only 26% of cases. Skeletal involvement increased the numbers of abnormal results to 83% and 73% in the studies of Herbert and Sullivan respectively. Doubt has been cast on early reports of small transient increases in acid phosphatase in acute urinary retention and following prostatic palpation or massage. Although it is agreed that such increases may occur with prostatic palpation in prostatic carcinoma and benign prostatic hypertrophy, this is unlikely to occur with the palpation of a normal gland. Bodansky has noted elevations in serum acid phosphatase which appear to be related to the use of catheters or the formation of faecal impactions (Bodansky, 1972). Other conditions producing small increases in total acid phosphatase include Paget's disease and hyperparathyroidism, in both of which osteoclastic activity is increased, Gaucher's disease when splenomegaly is marked and some cases of breast carcinoma (Bodansky, 1972).

The rate of growth of prostatic carcinoma cells is frequently hormone-dependent and is inhibited, at least initially, by the synthetic oestrogen, stilboestrol. The stimulant effect of testosterone can be reduced by orchidectomy. An effective response to such treatment is shown by a fall in serum acid phosphatase activity and the test is helpful in assessing progress. The relationship is not always clear; see, e.g. Bodansky (1972). Moderately increased activity of serum *alkaline* phosphatase is common with prostatic bony secondaries. This often rises further after successful treatment during bone healing, and then falls. Determination of both phosphatases can therefore be helpful in monitoring any therapeutic response.

REFERENCES

Amador E., Wacker W. E. C. (1965). In *Methods of Biochemical Analysis*, Vol 13. (Glick D., ed) p. 274. New York, London: Academic Press.
Ammann R., Bühler H., Häcki W., Schmid M. (1982). *Lancet*; **1**: 1312.
Association of Clinical Biochemists. (1980). *News Sheet* 202, Supplement. Association of Clinical Biochemists, London.
Babson A. L., Grelly S. J., Coleman C. M., Phillips G. E. (1966). *Clin. Chem*; **12**: 482.
Babson A. L., Phillips G. E. (1966). *Clin. Chim. Acta*; **13**: 264.
Babson A. L., Read P. A. (1959). *Amer. J. Clin. Pathol*; **32**: 88.
Babson A. L., Read P. A., Phillips G. E. (1959). *Amer. J. Clin. Pathol*; **32**: 83.
Bahr M., Wilkinson J. H. (1967). *Clin. Chim. Acta*; **17**: 367.
Bais R., Edwards J. B. (1982). *CRC Crit. Rev. Clin. Lab. Sci*; **16**: 291.
Bergmeyer H. U. (1973). *Z. Klin. Chem. Klin, Biochem*; **11**: 39.
Bergmeyer H. U., Scheibe P., Wahlefeld A. W. (1978). *Clin. Chem*; **24**: 58.
Bernstein R. E. (1963). *Clin. Chim. Acta*; **8**: 158.
Bessey O. A., Lowry O. H., Brock M. J. (1946). *J. Biol. Chem*; **164**: 321.

Beutler E. (1983). In *The Metabolic Basis of Inherited Disease*, 5th ed. (Stanbury J. B., *et al.* eds) p. 1629. New York: McGraw-Hill.

Beutler E., Mitchell M. (1968). *Blood*; 32: 816.

Birkett D. J., *et al.* (1967). *Arch. Biochem. Biophys*; 121: 470.

Bodansky A. (1932). *J. Biol. Chem*; 99: 197.

Bodansky O. (1972). *Adv. Clin. Chem*; 15: 44.

Bodman J. (1960). In *Chromatographic and Electrophoretic Techniques*, 2nd ed., Vol. II. (Smith I., ed) p 96. London: William Heinemann Medical Books.

Bourne J. G., Collier H. O., Somers G. F. (1952). *Lancet*; 1: 1225.

Bowers G. N. Jr. (1972). In *Panel Discussion: International Seminar and Workshop on Enzymology*. (Tietz M. W., Weinstock A., eds). *Clin. Chem*; 18: 1024.

Bowers G. N. Jr., Kelley M. L., McComb R. B. (1967). *Clin. Chem*; 14: 606.

Bowers G. N. Jr., McComb R. B. (1966). *Clin. Chem*; 12: 70.

Bowers G. N. Jr., McComb R. B. (1975). *Clin. Chem*; 21: 1988.

Bretaudière J-P., *et al.* (1977). *Clin. Chem*; 23: 2263.

Briere R. O. (1979). *CRC Crit. Rev. Clin. Lab. Sci*; 13: 1.

Briggs G. E., Haldane J. B. S. (1925). *Biochem. J*; 19: 338.

Brown S. S., *et al.* (1981). *Adv. Clin. Chem*; 22: 1.

Brown S. S., Price E. M. (1975). *Clin. Chem*; 21: 1041.

Campbell A. K., Holt M. R., Patel A. (1985). In *Recent Advances in Clinical Biochemistry*, Vol. 3. (Price C. P., Alberti, K. G. M., eds) p. 1. Edinburgh: Churchill Livingstone.

Cho H. W., Meltzer H. Y. (1979). *Amer. J. Clin. Pathol*; 71: 75.

Cleland W. W. (1963). *Biochim. Biophys. Acta*; 67: 104.

Cooper E. H., *et al.* (1981). *Clin. Chim. Acta*; 113: 27.

Dacie J. V., Lewis S. M. (1975). *Practical Haematology*, 5th ed., p. 311. London: Churchill Livingstone.

Dale G., Latner A. L. (1968). *Lancet*; 1: 847.

Davies R. O., Marton A. V., Kalow W. (1960). *Can. J. Biochem. Physiol*; 38: 545.

Davies S. N., Griffiths J. C. (1982). *Clin. Chim. Acta*; 122: 29.

Degenaar G. P., Thijssen C., Van Der Wal G. (1976). *Clin. Chim. Acta*; 67: 79.

Demetriou J. A., Drewes P. A., Gin J. B. (1974). In *Clinical Chemistry, Principles and Technics*. (Henry R. J., Cannon D. C., Winkelman J. W., eds) p. 815. New York: Harper and Row.

Department of Health and Social Security, Scientific and Technical Branch, No. 7/82 (1982). *Comparative Evaluation of Creatine Kinase Kits*. London: HMSO.

De Ritis F., Coltori M., Giusti G. (1958). *Lancet*; 2: 214.

De Ritis F., Coltori M., Giusti G. (1972). *Lancet*; 1: 685.

Dietz A. A., Rubinstein H. M., Lubrano T. (1973). *Clin. Chem*; 19: 1309.

Dinwoodie A. J. (1964). *Proc. Ass. Clin. Biochem*; 4: 156.

Dixon M., Webb E. C. (1964). *Enzymes*, 2nd ed. London: Longman.

Dobosz I. (1974). *Clin. Chim. Acta*; 50: 301.

Doe R. P., Millinger G. T., Seal U. S. (1965). *Clin. Chem*; 11: 948.

Doran G. R., Wilkinson J. H. (1971). *Clin. Chim. Acta*; 35: 115.

Duggan P. F. (1979). *Clin. Chem*; 25: 348.

Dybkaer R., Jørgensen K. (1967). *Quantities and Units in Clinical Chemistry*. Including Recommendations (1966) of the Commission on Clinical Chemistry of International Union of Pure and Applied Chemistry and of the International Federation for Clinical Chemistry. Copenhagen: Munksgaard.

Eaton R. H., Moss D. W. (1968). *Enzymologia*; 35: 31.

Elliot B. A., Wilkinson J. H. (1961). *Lancet*; 1: 698.

Ellis G., Goldberg D. M. (1971). *Amer. J. Clin. Pathol*; 56: 627.

Emerson P. M., Wilkinson J. H. (1965). *J. Clin. Pathol*; 18: 803.

Evans R. T., Gray P. W. S., Lehmann H., Silk E. (1952). *Lancet*; 1: 1229.

Evans R. T., Wardell J. (1984). *J. Med. Genet*; 21: 99.

Ewen L. M., Spitzer R. W. (1976). *Clin. Chem*; 22: 627.

Felber J-P. (1973). *Metabolism*; 22: 1089.

Fenton J. J., *et al.* (1984). *Clin. Chem*; 30: 1399.

Fishman W. H., *et al.* (1953). *J. Clin. Invest*; **32**: 1034.
Fishman W. H., Ghosh N. K. (1967). *Adv. Clin. Chem*; **10**: 255.
Florkin M., Stotz E. H., eds. (1973). *Comprehensive Biochemistry*, 3rd ed., Vol. 13. Enzyme Nomenclature. Amsterdam, London, New York: Elsevier.
Foo A. Y., Nemesánsky E., Rosalki S. B. (1981). *Ann. Clin. Biochem*; **18**: 232.
Garry P. J., *et al.* (1976). *J. Med. Genet*; **13**: 38.
Gerhardt W., Kofoed B., Westlund L., Parlu B. (1974). *Scand. J. Clin. Lab. Invest*; **33**: Suppl, 139. Quality Control of NADH.
Gitlin N. (1982). *Amer. J. Gastroenterol*; **77**: 2.
Good N. W., *et al.* (1966). *Biochemistry*; **5**: 467.
Gorus F., Schram E. (1979). *Clin. Chem*; **25**: 512.
Grannis G. F. (1976). *Amer. J. Clin. Pathol*; **66**: 206.
Grannis G. F. (1977). *Amer. J. Clin. Pathol*; **68**: 142.
Griffiths P. D. (1986). *Ann. Clin. Biochem*; **23**: 238.
Gutman A. B., Gutman E. B. (1940). *J. Biol. Chem*; **136**: 201.
Gutman E. B., Gutman A. B. (1938). *J. Clin. Invest*; **17**: 473.
Haeckel R., Hørder M., Zender R. (1982). *IFCC News*, No. 32, p. 8.
Hargreaves T. (1968). *The Liver and Bile Metabolism*. New York: Appleton Century Crofts.
Hargreaves T. (1970). *J. Clin. Pathol*; **23**: Suppl. 3 (*Ass. Clin. Path.*): 1.
Harris H., Hopkinson D. A., Robson E. B. (1962). *Nature*; **196**: 1296.
Harris H., Robson E. B. (1963). *Biochim. Biophys. Acta*; **73**: 649.
Harris H., Whittaker M. (1961). *Nature*; **191**: 496.
Hausamen T-U., Helger R., Rick W., Gros W. (1967). *Clin. Chim. Acta*; **15**: 241.
Herbert F. K. (1946). *Quart. J. Med*; NS **15**: 221.
Hess B., Walter S. I. (1960). *Klin. Wchschr*; **38**: 1080.
Hess B., Walter S. I. (1961). *Ann. N. Y. Acad. Sci*; **94**: 890.
Hillmann G. (1971). *Z. Klin. Chem. Klin. Biochem*; **3**: 273.
Horne M., Cornish C. J., Posen S. (1968). *J. Lab. Clin. Med*; **72**: 903.
Huggins C., Talalay P. (1945). *J. Biol. Chem*; **159**: 399.
Innes R. K. R., Strömme J. H. (1973). *Brit. J. Anaesth*; **45**: 185.
International Committee for Standardisation in Haematology. (1977). *Br. J. Haematol*; **35**: 331; (1979); **43**: 469.
International Federation of Clinical Chemistry. Expert Panel on Enzymes. Part 1. IFCC. (1978). General Considerations. (1979). *Clin. Chim. Acta*; **98**: F163–F174.
   Part 2. IFCC. (1975). Method for Aspartate Aminotransferase. (1976). *Clin. Chim. Acta*; **70**: F19–F42.
   Part 3. IFCC. (1979). Method for Alanine Aminotransferase. (1980). *Clin. Chim. Acta*; **105**: F147–F172.
   Part 4. IFCC (1983). Method for Gammaglutamyltransferase. (1983a). *Clin. Chim. Acta*; **135**: F315–F338.
   Part 5. IFCC (1983). Method for Alkaline Phosphatase. (1983b). *Clin. Chim. Acta*; **135**: F339–F367.
International Union of Biochemistry. (1961). *Report of the Commission on Enzymes*. London: Pergamon Press. (1964). *Enzyme Nomenclature*. Amsterdam, London: Elsevier.
International Union of Pure and Applied Chemistry—International Union of Biochemistry, Commission on Biochemical Nomenclature. (1976). In (1977). *J. Biol. Chem*; **252**: 5939.
Ishii H., Okuno F., Shigeta, Y. and Tsuchiya M. (1978). *Curr. Alcohol*; **5**: 101.
Jockers-Wretou E., Pfleiderer G. (1975). *Clin. Chim. Acta*; **58**: 223.
Kalow W., Davies R. O. (1958). *Biochem. Pharmacol*; **1**: 183.
Kalow W., Genest K. (1957). *Can. J. Biochem. Physiol*; **35**: 239.
Kalow W., Lindsay H. A. (1955). *Can. J. Biochem. Physiol*; **33**: 568.
Karmen A. (1955). *J. Clin. Invest*; **33**: 131.
Karmen C., *et al.* (1984). *J. Clin. Path*; **37**: 212.
King J. (1959). *J. Med. Lab. Tech*; **16**: 265.
King E. J., Armstrong A. R. (1934). *Can. Med. Ass. J*; **31**: 376.

King J., Griffin D. (1973). *Brit. J. Anaesth*; **45**: 450.

King J., Morgan H. G. (1970). *J. Clin. Pathol*; **23**: 730.

King J., Morgan H. G. (1971). *J. Clin. Pathol*; **24**: 182.

King J., Waind A. P. B. (1961). *Brit. Med. J*; **1**: 166.

Kornberg A., Horecker B. L. (1955). In *Methods in Enzymology*, Vol. 1, p. 323. New York, London: Academic Press.

Landon J., Carney J., Langley D. (1977). *Ann. Clin. Biochem*; **14**: 90.

Lang H., Würzburg U. (1982). *Clin. Chem*; **28**: 1439.

Latner A. L. (1964). *Proc. Ass. Clin. Biochem*; **3**: 120.

Latner A. L., Skillen A. W. (1961). *Lancet*; **2**: 1286.

Latner A. L., Skillen A. W. (1963). *Proc. Ass. Clin. Biochem*; **2**: 100.

Latner A. L., Skillen A. W. (1968). *Isoenzymes in Biology and Medicine*, p. 167. New York, London: Academic Press.

Laursen T. (1959). *Scand. J. Clin. Lab. Invest*; **11**: 134.

Lehmann H., Liddell J. (1969). *Brit. J. Anaesth*; **41**: 235.

Leung F. Y., Henderson A. R. (1981). *Clin. Chim. Acta*; **115**: 145.

Liddell J., Lehmann H., Davies D. (1963). *Acta Genet*; **13**: 95.

Lineweaver H., Burk D. (1934). *J. Amer. Chem. Soc*; **56**: 658.

Lohff M. R., *et al.* (1982). *Amer. J. Clin. Pathol*; **78**: 634 (suppl.).

London J. W., Shaw L. M., Fetterolf D., Garfinkel D. (1975). *Clin. Chem*; **21**: 1939.

Lowry O. H., *et al.* (1954). *J. Biol. Chem*; **207**: 19.

Lum G. (1979). *Clin. Chem*; **25**: 873.

Martinek R. G. (1972): *Clin. Chim. Acta*; **40**: 91.

Martinez-Carrion M., Barber B., Pazoles P. (1977). *Biochim. Biophys. Acta*; **482**: 323.

Matloff D. S., Selinger M. J., Kaplan M. M. (1980). *Gastroenterology*; **78**: 1389.

McComb R. B., Bowers G. N. Jr. (1972). *Clin. Chem*; **18**: 97.

McComb R. B., Bowers G. N., Posen S. (1979). *Alkaline Phosphatase*; New York: Plenum.

McKenzie D., Henderson A. R. (1983). *Clin. Chem*; **29**: 189.

McQueen M. J., Garland I. W. C., Morgan H. G. (1972). *Clin. Chem*; **18**: 275.

Mensink H. J. A., Marrink J., Hindriks F. R., van Zanten A. K. (1983). *J. Urol*; **129**: 1136.

Mercer D. W. (1976). *Clin. Chem*; **22**: 552.

Michaelis H., Menten M. L. (1913). *Biochem. Z*; **49**: 333.

Morin L. G. (1977). *Clin. Chem*; **23**: 646.

Moss D. W. (1972). *Clin. Chem*; **18**: 1449.

Moss D. W. (1982a). *Isoenzymes*. London: Chapman and Hall.

Moss D. W. (1982b). *Clin. Chem*; **28**: 2007.

Moss D. W., Baron D. N., Walker P. G., Wilkinson J. H. (1971). *J. Clin. Pathol*; **24**: 740.

Moss D. W., Whitby L. G. (1975). *Clin. Chim. Acta*; **61**: 63.

Nealon D. A., Pettit S. M., Henderson A. R. (1981). *Clin. Chem*; **27**: 402.

Nemesánszky E., Lott J. A. (1985). *Clin. Chem*; **31**: 797.

Orlowski M. A., Meister A. (1965). *Biochim. Biophys. Acta*; **73**: 679.

Park H. R., Geitner H. R., Fritsche H. A. (1984). *Clin. Chem*; **30**: 1010.

Penn R., Worthington D. J. (1983). *Brit. Med. J*; **286**: 531.

Pledger D. R., *et al.* (1982). *Clin. Chim. Acta*; **122**: 71.

Plowman K. M. (1972). *Enzyme Kinetics*. New York: McGraw-Hill.

Pontes J. E. (1983). *J. Urol*; **130**: 1037.

Poretta C. A., Dahlin D. C., Jones J. M. (1957). *J. Bone Joint Surg*; **39**A: 1314.

Price E. M., Brown S. S. (1975). *Clin. Biochem*; **8**: 384.

Rasmussen H. (1968). *Danish Med. Bull*; **15**: 1.

Rasmussen H. (1983). In *The Metabolic Basis of Inherited Disease*, 5th ed. (Stanbury, J. B., *et al.*, eds) p. 1497. New York: McGraw Hill.

Rautela G. P., Snee R. D., Miller W. K. (1979). *Clin. Chem*; **25**: 1954.

Rej R. (1980). *Clin. Chem*; **26**: 1694.

Rej R., Bretaudière J-P., Graffunder B. (1981). *Clin. Chem*; **27**: 535.

Richterich R., Schafroth P., Aebi H. (1963). *Clin. Chim. Acta*; **8**: 178.

Rosalki S. B. (1975). *Adv. Clin. Chem*; **17**: 53.

Rosalki S. B. (1980). *Ann. Clin. Biochem*; **17**: 74.

Rosalki S. B., Nemesánszky E., Foo A. Y. (1981). *Ann. Clin. Biochem*; **18**: 25.
Rosalki S. B., Tarlow D. (1974). *Clin. Chem*; **20**: 1121.
Roy A. V., Brower M. E., Hayden J. E. (1971). *Clin. Chem*; **17**: 1093.
Rubinstein H. M., *et al.* (1970). *J. Clin. Invest*; **49**: 479.
Rubinstein H. M., Dietz A. A., Lubrano T. (1978). *J. Med. Genet*; **15**: 27.
Rubinstein H. M., Dietz A. A., Lubrano T., Garry P. J. (1976). *J. Med. Genet*; **13**: 43.
Salgó L., Szabó A. (1982). *Clin. Chim. Acta*; **126**: 9.
Samuell C. T., Morgans B. T., O'Donoghue E. P. N. (1984). *Brit. J. Urol*; **56**: 208.
Scandinavian Committee on Enzymes, Scandinavian Society for Clinical Chemistry and Clinical Physiology.
SCE. (1974). *Scand. J. Clin. Lab. Invest*; **33**: 291.
SCE. (1976). *Scand. J. Clin. Lab. Invest*; **36**: 119.
SCE. (1979). *Scand. J. Clin. Lab. Invest*; **39**: 1.
SCE. (1981). *Scand. J. Clin. Lab. Invest*; **41**: 107.
Schiele F., *et al.* (1981). *Clin. Chim. Acta*; **112**: 187.
Seligman A. M., *et al.* (1951). *J. Biol. Chem*; **190**: 7.
Shaw L. M., Gray J. (1974). *Clin. Chem*; **20**: 494.
Siede W. H., Seiffert U. B. (1977). *Clin. Chem*; **23**: 28.
Silk E., King J., Whittaker M. (1979). *Ann. Clin. Biochem*; **16**: 57.
Smith I., Lightstone P. J., Perry J. D. (1968). *Clin. Chim. Acta*; **19**: 499.
Strömme J. H., Bjornstad P., Eldjarn L. (1976). *Scand. J. Clin. Lab. Invest*; **36**: 505.
Sullivan T. J., Gutman E. B., Gutman A. B. (1942). *J. Urol*; **48**: 426.
Szasz G., Gerhardt W., Gruber W. (1978). *Clin. Chem*; **24**: 1557.
Tarkkanen P., *et al.* (1979). *Clin. Chem*; **25**: 1644.
Tietz N. W., *et al.* (1983). *Clin. Chem*; **29**: 751.
Tsung S. H. (1976). *Clin. Chem*; **22**: 173.
Turner J. M., *et al.* (1985). *Ann. Clin. Biochem*; **22**: 175.
Turner J. M., Hall R. A., Whittaker M., Kricka L. J. (1984). *Ann. Clin. Biochem*; **21**: 363.
Van Belle H. (1976). *Clin. Chem*; **22**: 972.
Van der Helm H. J. (1961). *Lancet*; **2**: 108.
Van der Helm H. J., Zondag H. A., Hartog, H. A. Ph., Van der Kovi M. W. (1962). *Clin. Chim. Acta*; **7**: 540.
Weber H. (1966). *Deut. Med. Wschr*; **91**: 1927.
Wenham P. R., Horn D. B., Smith. A. F. (1985). *Clin. Chem*; **31**: 569.
Whitaker J. F. (1969). *Clin. Chim. Acta*; **24**: 23.
Whitehead T. P., Kricka L. J., Carter T. J. N., Thorpe G. H. G. (1979). *Clin. Chem*; **25**: 1531.
Whittaker M. (1968). *Acta Genet*; **18**: 556.
Wieme, R. J. (1959). *Clin. Chim. Acta*; **4**, 317.
Wilkinson J. H. (1970). *Isoenzymes*, 2nd ed. London: Chapman and Hall.
Wilkinson J. H. (1976). *The Principles and Practice of Diagnostic Enzymology*. London: Arnold.
Wilson J. B., Dayan K., Cyr K. (1964). *J. Biol. Chem*; **239**: 4182.
Wimmer M. C., Artiss J. D., Zak B. (1985). *Clin. Chem*; **31**: 1616.
Wong J. T. (1975). *Kinetics of Enzyme Mechanisms*. New York, London: Academic Press.
Wroblewski F. (1958). *Adv. Clin. Chem*; **1**: 340.
Wroblewski F., Gregory K. F. (1961). *Ann. N. Y. Acad. Sci*; **94**: 912.
Wroblewski F., LaDue J. S. (1955). *Proc. Soc. Exp. Biol. Med*; **90**: 210.
Wu A. H. B., Bowers G. N. (1982). *Clin. Chem*; **28**: 2017.

23

ELECTROLYTES AND ACID–BASE DISTURBANCES

BODY FLUIDS AND THEIR COMPOSITION

The volume of total body water (TBW) for a 70 kg man is 42 l, i.e. 60% of the body weight. Although there are variations between individuals, for any given person the TBW remains constant. Traditionally, TBW is divided into two main compartments, intracellular fluid (ICF) 28 l, and extracellular fluid (ECF) 14 l, the latter being further subdivided into interstitial fluid (IF) 11 l, and plasma 3 l. Transcellular fluid (TF) can be considered as a component of ECF (e.g. gastrointestinal tract secretions 500 ml and cerebrospinal fluid, 100 ml). This model, while having practical value is of dubious validity for ICF, which of necessity has to be considered as a bag containing solvent and solute without regard to structure. Of particular importance, is that the ICF is inaccessible directly, and volume determinations have to be inferred.

Body fluid compartments are usually estimated indirectly by determining the volume of distribution of an injected substance, often radioactively labelled, by a dilution technique (p. 229). By a suitable choice of substance, TBW, ECF and plasma volumes can be measured. The ICF volume is then calculated as the difference between TBW and ECF, while interstitial fluid volume is the difference between ECF and plasma. TBW and plasma volumes are fairly satisfactorily determined using tritiated water (T_2O) and radio-iodinated human serum albumin respectively. The determination of ECF volume is more problematic as the distribution volumes of substances which were thought to leave the circulation but not to enter the cells vary appreciably. Thus inulin, mannitol and $^{35}SO_4^{2-}$ give much lower results than thiocyanate, $^{82}Br^-$ and $^{38}Cl^-$; sucrose results are intermediate. It is possible that the larger molecules such as inulin penetrate some parts of the ECF slowly and with difficulty, a problem more easily overcome by the smaller inorganic ions. In clinical practice, only the plasma volume is measured directly, though acute changes in weight (greater than 500 g/day) can be used to estimate overall fluid loss or gain if a weighing bed is available. ECF volume is estimated clinically by means of the jugular venous pressure, pulse rate, blood pressure, skin turgor, etc., while biochemically, serum urea, haematocrit, plasma protein concentration and the composition of urine can be used. The importance of the fluid balance chart cannot be over emphasised.

The composition of the body fluids varies. Plasma is accessible for direct analysis; the composition of other fluids is derived indirectly. Interstitial fluid is similar to an ultrafiltrate of plasma. In both these fluids the predominant cation is Na^+ (140 mmol/l) while K^+ (4·5 mmol/l), Ca^{2+} (1·2 mmol/l) and Mg^{2+} (0·7 mmol/l) are present in much lower concentrations. The predominant anions are Cl^- (100 mmol/l), and HCO_3^- (26 mmol/l); organic ions (3 mmol/l), phosphate (1 mmol/l) and sulphate (0·5 mmol/l) are minor components. Plasma proteins are also anions. The marked difference in protein concentration between IF and plasma results in minor differences in the concentrations of (mainly) Na^+ and Cl^- due to the Donnan equilibrium. The composition of ICF is less precisely known, but is markedly different. The figures, as mmol/kg water, for cations are approximately: K^+, 165; Mg^{2+}, 14; Na^+, 12; while Ca^{2+} is present in very low concentrations. For the smaller anions the order is phosphates, 60; HCO_3^-, 10, SO_4^{2-} 10; organic anions, 5; while Cl^- is virtually absent. About half of the total calcium in plasma is in the ionic form and it is thought that about 30% of magnesium in plasma and ICF is complexed or protein-bound. ICF anions of particular importance are polyvalent proteins and phosphate esters which cannot diffuse across cell membranes (Flear *et al.*, 1981). Their concentrations are determined by net synthesis and degradation—energy-requiring (ATP-dependent) processes. The major cation covering these anions is K^+. The difference between ICF and ECF $[Na^+]$ is maintained by the activity of an ATP-dependent 'sodium pump' in the cell membrane which constantly extrudes Na^+ against a concentration gradient. Pump failure, as in the 'sick cell syndrome', results in Na^+ moving into cells and a rise in plasma $[K^+]$.

For any fluid the sum of the electrical charges on the cations equals that on the anions. Formerly, stress was laid on this aspect by considering concentrations in mEq/l. Difficulties arise with substances such as proteins and phosphates, both organic and inorganic, as their valency varies with pH and is often not known precisely. Accepting that electroneutrality occurs, estimates of equivalent weight can be made if the mass composition of a fluid is known. It is often more informative to consider concentrations of the various components in mmol/l as this leads to fewer assumptions, although there are problems with protein mixtures when a mean molecular weight has to be assumed.

THE REGULATION OF BODY FLUID VOLUMES

All cells whether in health or disease behave as perfect osmometers, i.e. water moves freely across cell membranes and the cell volumes alter such that isosmolality between ECF and ICF is preserved (Wynn, 1957). Thus if the major ECF cation is Na^+ and the major ICF cation is K^+ the following relationships should hold between the osmolality of plasma (Os_P) and of TBW (Os_{TBW}) (Edelman *et al.*, 1958):

$$Os_P = Os_{TBW} \propto [Na_P^+] \propto \frac{Na_e + K_e}{TBW}$$

where $[Na_P^+]$ is the plasma sodium concentration and Na_e, K_e are exchangeable sodium and potassium. Experimentally it has been shown (Edelman *et al.*, 1958) that

$$[Na_P^+] = 1\cdot11 \frac{(Na_e^+ + K_e^+)}{TBW} - 25\cdot6$$

The important features to note are that Os_P and $[Na_P^+]$ are dependent upon the variables Na_e, TBW and K_e, the last being in part dependent upon the concentration of non-diffusible anions.

Tonicity. Although the terms tonicity and osmolality are often used interchangeably there is a clear distinction. Osmolality is a physical property dependent upon the total number of solute particles present in a solution whether or not they penetrate cell membranes. Tonicity, or 'effective osmolality', is a physiological property dependent upon the selectively permeable characteristics of particular cell membranes. A solution is referred to as isotonic if it causes no alteration in cell volume. The body's homœostatic mechanisms respond to changes in tonicity rather than osmolality.

Cell membranes can be considered to be impermeable to the major determinants of body fluid osmolality such as Na$^+$ and Cl$^-$ in ECF, and K$^+$, protein and phosphate in ICF. Erythrocytes do not change volume if placed in NaCl (150 mmol/l, 300 mosmol/kg approximately). The NaCl solution is referred to as iso-osmolal and isotonic with plasma. Erythrocytes swell if suspended in a more dilute sodium chloride solution and shrink if suspended in a more concentrated solution because of the transmembrane osmotic gradients induced. The former solution is both hypo-osmolal and hypotonic; the latter is both hyperosmolal and hypertonic. Similarly, if erythrocytes are suspended in any other solution containing 300 mosmol/kg of impermeant solute, the solution is both iso-osmolal and isotonic. If erythrocytes are suspended in solutions of permeant solute, e.g. urea (300 mosmol/kg), solute enters the cells followed by solvent resulting in an increased cell volume. These solutions though iso-osmolal are hypotonic.

In vivo under steady state conditions, permeant solutes such as urea and ethanol are distributed throughout TBW. These solutes contribute to total osmolality but not to tonicity as they cause no transmembrane osmotic gradient.

Calculated tonicity. Although tonicity cannot be measured, it can be estimated;

plasma tonicity = measured plasma osmolality − plasma [urea] mmol/l.

If any other permeant solute is present (e.g. ethanol) it should be included in the calculation.

The Renal Excretion of Water

In health, osmolality is maintained within narrow limits (280 to 290 mosmol/kg) by the regulation of water input monitored by the thirst centres and the adjustment of water loss by the kidney under the control of antidiuretic hormone (ADH, vasopressin), a nonapeptide secreted by the posterior pituitary gland. Although about 120 ml of glomerular filtrate is normally formed each minute, only about 1 ml/min appears in the urine so that over 99% of the water is reabsorbed. With variations of water intake, the kidney has the ability to regulate the urine flow rate over the maximal range of 0·2 to 20 ml/min so that even in the most marked diuresis, water reabsorption is still over 84%. The details of the way in which water is handled in the different parts of the nephron are now clarified (Fig. 23.1). Water is never actively reabsorbed but passes from the lumen to the interstitium by a process of passive diffusion along an osmotic gradient. This osmotic gradient is largely created by Na$^+$ which is actively extruded at various sites in the nephron. Certain regions may, however, be impermeable to water and in this case any reabsorption of Na$^+$ results in reduction of the osmolality of the luminal fluid.

In the proximal convoluted tubule the greater part of the Na$^+$ is actively reabsorbed with Cl$^-$ and water following passively. The fluid emerging from the proximal tubule is iso-osmolar with glomerular filtrate although its composition is very different. About 30 ml/min enters the descending limb of the loop of Henle which passes down into the medulla. The medullary interstitial fluid is hyperosmolar, particularly near the renal papillae. Water passes out and the luminal fluid becomes hyperosmolar. The ascending limb of the loop of Henle is thick and impermeable to water, but actively reabsorbs Na$^+$. The emerging fluid is now hypo-osmolar and remains so as it enters the first part of the distal tubule usually at a rate of 24 ml/min. The walls of the later part of the distal tubule and of the collecting ducts are variably permeable to water. The permeability is

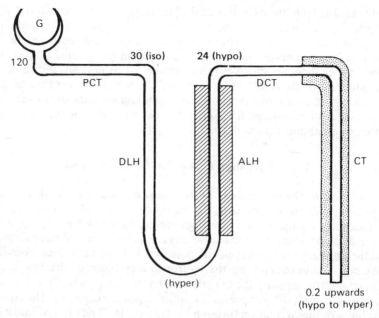

Fig. 23.1. Diagrammatic Representation of the Reabsorption of Water by the Nephron. G, glomerulus; PCT, proximal convoluted tubule; DLH, descending limb, loop of Henle; ALH, ascending limb, loop of Henle; DCT, distal convoluted tubule; CT, collecting tubule. The figures are flow rates in ml/min. The osmolality is indicated in parentheses by: iso, iso-osmolar; hypo, hypo-osmolar; hyper, hyperosmolar. The cross-hatched zone is impermeable to water and the stippled area has variable permeability determined by the plasma [ADH].

dependent on the plasma ADH concentration. In the absence of ADH the walls of the collecting ducts are virtually impermeable to water so that the hypo-osmolar fluid in the distal tubule remains hypo-osmolar. The osmolality may be further reduced by the active reabsorption of Na$^+$ at the end of the distal tubules and in the collecting tubules. At maximal plasma ADH concentrations, water leaves the distal tubule and enters the interstitial fluid of the cortex which is iso-osmolar. In the collecting tubule during its course to the tip of the renal papilla, water will pass into the interstitial fluid of increasing osmolality so that a hyperosmolar urine emerges. This mechanism thus regulates the final water excretion by the kidney and thereby alters the osmolality of the plasma and other body fluids.

The Control of ADH Secretion

An increase in tonicity causes the sensation of thirst and the secretion of ADH, mediated by osmoreceptors in the hypothalamus. A rise in plasma osmolality due to increased [Na$^+$] stimulates ADH secretion and water is retained. Other substances such as urea and glucose which enter the osmoreceptor cells provoke a lesser response or no ADH response (Baylis, 1983). Hypotonicity abolishes thirst, the secretion of ADH ceases and a diuresis ensues. The extra water lost in the hypo-osmolar urine results in a rise in the osmolality of body fluids. The secretion of ADH is stimulated by other factors, most importantly vagal nerve impulses, probably arising from the right side of the heart and the great veins (often loosely called 'volume receptors'), which occur when the blood volume falls by about 7 %. While the responses to osmolality changes are rapid and sensitive, the hypothalamic centres are rather insensitive to changes in the volume of body fluids. Thus whenever there are changes in the *amount* of osmotically active solute in body fluids, particularly of Na^+, there will be a volume readjustment with minimal changes in osmolality, provided hypothalamic control is operative. In the first stages of pathological changes, the *concentration* of these solutes will therefore be maintained near normal.

Fluid Exchange Across the Capillary Wall

The regulation of the interchange of fluid between plasma and IF in health is dependent on the *oncotic pressure*, the osmolality of the plasma colloids. Small molecules and ions diffuse easily through the capillary wall but larger molecules, such as plasma proteins, do so to a lesser degree. The differential osmotic pressure across the capillary wall is the oncotic pressure. This attracts water from IF into plasma but is counteracted by the hydrostatic pressure of the blood. At the arterial end of the capillary the net effect is that fluid leaves the blood vessel but this partly returns at the low pressure venous end of the capillary. The balance of fluid returns to the circulation through the lymphatics. The total colloid osmotic pressure is less than 1 mosmol/kg or about 0·3 % of the total osmolality. Expressed in hydrostatic terms, it is about 25 mmHg, a figure intermediate between arteriolar and venous hydrostatic pressures. Over half the oncotic pressure is due to plasma albumin so that the level of this protein is an important factor for fluid exchange. Hypoalbuminaemia is one factor which allows accumulation of IF and the development of oedema.

An important regulator of plasma volume is the renin-angiotensin-aldosterone system. Renin is stored in the granular cells of the juxtaglomerular apparatus in the kidney which is close to the afferent arteriole of the renal glomerulus and is sensitive to the degree of stretching of the arteriolar wall. If the blood volume should contract, this stretch diminishes and renin is released into the circulation. Renin secretion is also regulated by the carotid sinus baroreceptors, circulating catecholamines and perhaps Na^+ flux in the macula densa. Renin is an enzyme which converts the plasma protein, angiotensinogen, into the decapeptide angiotensin I, which is subsequently cleaved to angiotensin II, an octapeptide, by an angiotensin-converting enzyme present in the lung endothelium. Angiotensin II stimulates thirst and has a constrictive effect on most arterioles thereby increasing the blood pressure. It also directly stimulates the adrenal cortex to secrete aldosterone which results in the renal retention of Na^+ and water and excretion of K^+ in the distal convoluted tubule. This retention expands the ECF volume and, usually, the plasma volume. Once this is achieved, renin release is suppressed, i.e. there is negative feedback. In health, plasma volume regulation maintains IF volume. In pathological states, the Na^+ and water retained may leave the plasma and accumulate in the interstitial space, the condition recognised clinically as oedema.

WATER METABOLISM

Typical figures for water turnover each day are shown in Table 23.1 for a healthy adult in a temperate climate. Metabolic water is derived from the oxidation of

TABLE 23.1

Typical Figures for Water Balance in the Adult (ml/24 h)

Input		Output	
Beverages	1500	Lungs	400
Water in food	600	Skin-insensible loss	400
		-sweat	100
Metabolic water	400	Faeces	100
		Urine	1500
Total	2500	Total	2500

hydrogen and depends on the rate of metabolism and the fuel metabolised. For instance, 100 g fat provides 110 ml, a similar quantity of carbohydrate or protein produces only about 60 ml. Water production is markedly increased in hyper-catabolic states. Expired air is saturated with water vapour at 37 °C and the exact loss will depend on the lung ventilation rate and the humidity of inspired air. Skin losses are as water vapour not normally noticed by the subject (insensible-loss) and sweat which is small in amount in temperate conditions. An increase in body temperature of 1°C increases insensible loss by about 250 ml/24 h. The normal colon removes most of the water from the 8 l of gastrointestinal secretions produced daily. If water intake ceases, then skin and lung losses continue and the kidney produces a maximally concentrated urine. When required to excrete an average osmolar load, the normal kidney will still excrete at least 500 ml urine daily making the obligatory water loss 1·5 l/24 h or about 3·5 % of TBW.

Water Excretion. The osmotic gradient achieved by the kidney is the ratio of the urinary osmolality (U_{osm}) to the plasma osmolality (P_{osm}). This ratio is 1 if the urine is iso-osmolar but can rise to 4 or more (U_{osm} 1200 to 1400 mosmol/kg) under the influence of ADH. In a marked diuresis the ratio may fall to 0·1 with U_{osm} approaching 40 mosmol/kg, although in most cases it is rarely below 50 mosmol/kg. An increase in plasma osmolality of 1 mosmol/kg results in the urine osmolality increasing by approximately 100 mosmol/kg. The *osmolar clearance*, C_{osm}, may be defined in the usual way (see p. 767) as

$$C_{osm} = \frac{U_{osm} \times V}{P_{osm}}$$

C_{osm} represents the volume of water needed to excrete the urinary solutes at the same osmolality as that of plasma. When the urine is iso-osmolar, that is U_{osm} equals P_{osm}, C_{osm} equals V, the volume of urine produced per minute. If a greater urine volume is passed, the urine is hypo-osmolar and the extra water excretion is referred to as the *free water clearance*, usually abbreviated C_{H_2O}. Under such circumstances

$$V = C_{osm} + C_{H_2O}$$

or

$$C_{H_2O} = V - C_{osm} = V\left\{ 1 - \frac{U_{osm}}{P_{osm}} \right\}$$

In a moderate water diuresis C_{H_2O} may vary from 10 to 15 ml/min, and at maximal diuresis may reach 18 ml/min.

Under conditions where a hyperosmolar urine is produced, extra water is reabsorbed by the collecting tubules and the free water clearance becomes negative. This negative value is usually quoted as a positive result with the abbreviation $T^c_{H_2O}$ the tubular capacity for the reabsorption of water, but the units are still ml/min. Thus

$$V = C_{osm} - T^c_{H_2O}$$

or

$$T^c_{H_2O} = C_{osm} - V = V \left\{ \frac{U_{osm}}{P_{osm}} - 1 \right\}$$

Under most conditions when a hyperosmolar urine is passed, $T^c_{H_2O}$ equals about 1 ml/min but may reach a maximal value of about 5 ml/min at very high loads of solute excretion. As C_{H_2O} is appreciably greater than $T^c_{H_2O}$ it follows that ADH is most important in preventing excretion of an unduly dilute urine and that the ability to produce hyperosmolar urine is a less important adaptation.

Effect of Varying Osmolar Load for Excretion. The wide range of urinary osmolality is only seen if a relatively small osmotic load (U_{osm}. V) is excreted. In an adult consuming a diet of 100 g protein/24 h this is around 900 mosmol/24 h and mainly consists of urea 500 mmol/24 h derived from protein catabolism and the Na^+, K^+ and Cl^- in excess of the body's requirements. It can be as low as 200 mosmol/24 h on a low protein, low electrolyte diet. An increased osmotic load occurs if salt intake is increased, in glycosuria, and when there is marked protein catabolism with the formation of urea. The greater osmotic pressure exerted by these substances in the luminal fluid limits the passive transfer of water to the interstitium thereby reducing the degree of hyperosmolality achieved. It also offsets the effect of any Na^+ reabsorption at water-impermeable sites of the nephron thereby preventing a very hypo-osmolar urine from being excreted. As U_{osm}. V increases, so does C_{osm} thus increasing V. The diuresis observed is referred to as an *osmotic diuresis*. Such a state can be produced by the infusion of an osmotically active substance such as mannitol which is not subject to tubular processes after its filtration at the glomerulus. During an osmotic diuresis the flow rate through the nephron is markedly increased allowing less time for the reabsorption of various substances. An important effect occurs with Na^+ which is normally reabsorbed to about 99·5 % in the tubules. Even if this is only lowered to 99 % during the diuresis, it represents a doubling of the amount of Na^+ excreted. Such a Na^+ diuresis is important in certain pathological states, e.g. uncontrolled diabetes mellitus.

SODIUM, POTASSIUM AND CHLORIDE METABOLISM

The body content of Na^+ for a 70 kg adult, as determined by cadaver analysis, is about 4200 mmol. The exchangeable sodium (Na_e) determined by isotope dilution methods (p. 229) is about 3000 mmol (i.e. 70–75 % of the total) of which the greater part (1800 mmol) is in ECF. About 200 mmol is in ICF and 1000 mmol in bone in equilibrium with ECF.

The exchangeable potassium (K_e) content of the body is about 3200 mmol for a 70 kg man (95 % of total). Although this figure is similar in magnitude to that for Na_e, the distribution is quite different—70 % in the skeletal muscle, 10 % in the skin and only 5 % in the ECF. Bone K^+ content is considerably less than bone Na^+. Thus muscle provides the main body store of K^+ which falls with age as muscle mass diminishes. Another difference is that the main store is separated from the absorptive and excretory sites by the ECF, the K^+ concentration, $[K^+]$, of which is easily measurable but is not a direct indicator of the status of the total body K^+.

Plasma $[K^+]$ is influenced by ECF pH. A decrease in ECF pH results in H^+ moving into cells at the expense of K^+ which is extruded. The converse occurs when the ECF pH increases. Intracellular K^+ depletion results in an influx of H^+ producing ICF acidosis and ECF alkalosis. Plasma $[K^+]$ is also under hormonal influence. Insulin, the secretion of which is stimulated by hyperkalaemia, and adrenaline, acting via β_2 receptors, cause redistribution of K^+ from ECF to ICF. Aldosterone lowers plasma $[K^+]$ by increasing urinary K^+ excretion.

The daily balances of the common ions for a healthy adult in a temperate climate are shown in Table 23.2. Regulation of Na^+ balance is achieved in part by modification of the renal tubular handling of this ion by aldosterone. Very low values for urinary Na^+ excretion (1 mmol/24 h) can be obtained by this mechanism. Thus provided some food is being eaten, Na^+ deficiency occurs only if there are abnormal losses, Sodium retention is only likely if urinary Na^+ excretion is low. The regulation of K^+ balance is not so tightly controlled (or well understood) and there is an obligatory renal loss. Renal readjustments are less rapid for K^+ than Na^+ if intake is reduced abruptly.

TABLE 23.2

The Daily Intake and Output of Na^+, K^+ and Cl^- for a Healthy Adult (mmol).
(Whitby et al., 1984.)

Ion	Intake	Output		
		Urine	Faeces	Skin
Na^+	100–200	100–200	< 5	< 5
K^+	20–100	20–100	< 5	trace
Cl^-	100–200	100–200	< 5	< 5

The measurement of Cl^- is of secondary importance. Although it is the main anion of ECF, its concentration is affected by the concentration of other anions and of the main cations. The sum of Na^+ and K^+ concentrations on average exceeds those of Cl^- and HCO_3^- by 17 mmol/l, the so called 'anion gap'. This is due to the fact that other anions, especially protein and to a lesser extent phosphate, sulphate and organic acid anions such as lactate, exceed the other cations, mainly Ca^{2+} and Mg^{2+} by this amount. Calculation of the anion gap after measurement of the four principal electrolytes can then often give warning of some change, usually in anions. The calculation should be treated with caution as its total variance is the sum of the variances of each individual measurement. The practical value of the anion gap is the subject of dispute (Editorial, 1977; Zilva, 1977). A lower value than usual suggests hypoalbuminaemia while an increase is seen in the phosphate and sulphate retention of chronic renal failure, and in acidotic states associated with increased amounts of lactate or aceto-acetate. Further investigations can be planned as appropriate.

Plasma $[Cl^-]$ is also affected by changes in $[Na^+]$ and $[HCO_3^-]$. In hyponatraemia the $[Cl^-]$ is usually reduced by a similar amount unless there are acid–base disturbances which affect the $[HCO_3^-]$. Similarly, changes in $[HCO_3^-]$ without alteration of the $[Na^+]$ will affect $[Cl^-]$. An increased value is seen, e.g.

in metabolic acidosis in which the primary disturbance is loss of HCO_3^-. In chronic vomiting, very low $[Cl^-]$ down to about 50 mmol/l, is associated with severe hyponatraemia and a considerably raised plasma $[HCO_3^-]$.

METHODOLOGICAL CONSIDERATIONS

The Measurement of Osmolality

One mole of any substance contains the same number of particles (molecules, ions, etc.) which is Avogadro's number 6.061×10^{23}. One osmole is the mass of solute which when dissolved in one kg of pure water produces an osmotic pressure of 22.4 atm at NTP.

Molality $= n_a/w$ where n_a = moles of solute and w = mass of solvent. Thus molality = number of moles per unit mass of solvent (mol/kg of solvent).

Molarity $= n_a/v$ where v = volume of solution. Thus molarity = number of moles per unit volume of solution (mol/l).

The molality of a solution is unaffected by temperature as the mass of solvent is independent of temperature. The molarity, in contrast, alters with temperature as the volume of solvent is temperature-dependent.

When a solute is dissolved in water, four physico-chemical parameters alter. These *colligative properties* are an increase in osmotic pressure, an increase in boiling point, a decrease in vapour pressure and a decrease in freezing point. The effects on all four are related quantitatively and any one of them may be measured to allow the others to be calculated.

If n_a mol of a solute, a, is dissolved in n_w mol of water, the laws of physical chemistry state that in dilute solution the change in freezing point, Δt, from that of pure water is proportional to the mole fraction of a. Thus

$$\Delta t = k \frac{n_a}{n_a + n_w}$$

If the mass of water is w kg the equation can be rewritten as

$$\Delta t = k \frac{n_a/w}{(n_a + n_w)/w}$$

the term n_a/w is M_a, the molality of the solution with respect to a. In dilute solution, n_w will be much larger than n_a and $(n_a + n_w)$ will be virtually constant allowing simplification to

$$\Delta t = k_f . M_a$$

where k_f is referred to as the cryoscopic constant (or molal depression constant) and for water has the value $1.858\,°C$. Thus a solution of osmolality 300 mosmol/kg will depress the freezing point of water to -0.300×1.858 or $-0.557\,°C$.

The above equations apply well to dilute solutions of solutes such as mannitol which do not dissociate or associate in aqueous media. Many salts, however, dissociate to a varying degree into their constituent ions when dissolved in water. If n ions are produced when each molecule of salt dissociates fully, then

$$\text{Osmolality} = \phi . n . M_a$$

where M_a is the osmolality of undissociated salt and ϕ is a factor varying from 0 to 1 expressing the fractional dissociation under the conditions of measurement. For salts such as sodium chloride, the value of ϕ is about 0.93.

Turning to osmotic pressure, the relationship which is applicable to dilute solutions is

$$\Pi = M_a . RT$$

where Π is the osmotic pressure, R the gas constant and T the temperature in Kelvins, while M_a is as before. Again there is a linear relationship between molality and the colligative property, in this case osmotic pressure, and the pressure is 17 000 mmHg or 2·27 MPa for a 1 osmol/kg solution.

Likewise for the decrease in vapour pressure, Δp, the equation becomes,

$$\Delta p = p_w . M_a$$

where p_w is the vapour pressure of pure water. The fall is 0·3 mmHg or 40 Pa for a 1 osmol/kg solution.

Instrumentation. Osmotic pressure is usually measured by the depression of the freezing point of water, though one instrument measures the change in vapour pressure using electrical detection of the dew point. In the presence of volatile solutes, e.g. ethanol, this method is of doubtful validity (Weisberg, 1975). A colloid osmometer uses a semi-permeable membrane and a sensitive pressure transducer to measure colloid osmotic pressure.

The freezing point of the solution under test is measured using a thermistor, a device the resistance of which changes markedly with temperature. The resistance is measured using a Wheatstone bridge circuit and often the balancing potentiometer is linked to a digital display which gives the osmolality directly once the instrument has been calibrated with standard solutions. These are NaCl solutions of known composition, but due allowance has to be made for the value of ϕ. This is 0·944 at an osmolality of 100 mosmol/kg but falls with increasing osmolality to reach $0·910 \pm 0·001$ over the range 900 to 2000 mosmol/kg, thereafter rising again. These factors are incorporated into the stated osmolality of the manufacturer's standards but need to be used if standards are prepared from dried pure sodium chloride and water.

The freezing point osmometer consists of a thermostatic cooling bath (some instruments incorporate a solid state cooling block utilising the Peltier effect) into which the sample tube is lowered with the thermistor central in the fluid. Cooling occurs rapidly, and in the absence of any particulate matter in the sample, its temperature falls below freezing point without any ice crystals forming, i.e. the sample is supercooled. Crystallisation is initiated at a fixed low temperature by operating a vibrating wire immersed in the sample. This forms multiple small ice crystals on which further growth can take place. The conversion of water to ice is accompanied by the release of latent heat of fusion and the temperature rises until, under ideal operating conditions, the temperature curve reaches a plateau, where the latent heat effect is balanced by the continued abstraction of heat by the cooling bath (Fig. 23.2). The thermistor in the centre of the sample is surrounded by a mixture of fluid and ice crystals in equilibrium and the temperature (or osmolality readout) is taken at this stage. Later all the sample will freeze and its temperature falls towards that of the cooling bath.

Practical Problems. To obtain reproducible and accurate measurements of osmolality, certain errors should be avoided. Thermistor damage alters its resistance characteristics, also its position must be central in the sample tube. The temperature of the cooling bath is critical. If too high, supercooling is difficult and the plateau poorly defined. If too low, cooling is too rapid and prevents the plateau forming during crystallisation as the rate of heat removal is too great. Keep the sample containers clean and dry and avoid carry-over between samples.

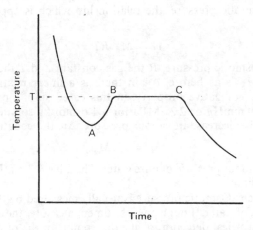

Fig. 23.2. Cooling Curve During Measurement of Osmolality.
At *A* the liquid sample is supercooled and crystallisation is initiated; the temperature rises to *B*. During the plateau *B – C* the mixture of liquid sample and ice crystals is at the freezing point, *T*.

Dry the thermistor and vibrator between samples and rinse and dry containers before re-use. Avoid rinsing with solvents such as acetone as traces remaining are osmotically active. Ensure that containers and samples are at room temperature before starting the cooling cycle. There is controversy concerning whether serum as well as plasma specimens are suitable. Redetzki *et al.* (1972) reported that only plasma should be used. Whichever type of specimen is used it is advisable to perform the analysis promptly and not to freeze and thaw the specimen. Avoid particulate matter in the samples as it may initiate ice crystal formation, preventing proper supercooling and adequate plateau formation.

Calculated osmolality is the predicted osmolality derived from the sum of molar concentrations using various formulae (Weisburg, 1975). For both plasma and urine this can be done if the molar concentrations of sodium, potassium, urea and glucose are known.

Calculated osmolality $= 2 \times 0.93$ ($[Na^+] + [K^+]) + [urea] + [glucose]$,

$$\text{Osmolal gap} = \text{observed osmolality} - \text{calculated osmolality}.$$

For most plasma specimens the calculated osmolality is close to 2 ($[Na^+] + [K^+]$). Its comparison with that actually determined is often helpful in pointing to the presence of some previously unsuspected osmotically active substance. Thus ethanol in a concentration of 800 mg/l, the legal limit for drivers of motor vehicles in the UK, contributes 17 mosmol/kg to the osmolality. Similarly in urine the finding that the osmolality is much greater than that predicted from Na^+, K^+ and urea concentrations may be an indication of the presence of glucose, alcohol or drugs.

Measurement of Specific Gravity

Before osmolality determinations became feasible as a routine laboratory procedure, the specific gravity of urine was used as an indirect index of its osmolality. This has the merit of simplicity of measurement. However, specific gravity is dependent on the *mass* concentration of urinary solutes while osmolality depends on *molecular* concentration. The relationship between the two is thus influenced by the composition of the solutes in urine. Thus although a specific gravity of 1·010 corresponds to an osmolality of 320 mosmol/kg on an average diet, this may vary over the range to 126 to 520 mosmol/kg if the composition of the diet is varied widely.

Use of a Urinometer. Weighted with mercury, this instrument floats in the urine; the calibration mark which corresponds to the surface level of the urine is read. The lower the specific gravity, the further the urinometer sinks. As it is usually calibrated at 15 °C, it should not be used for a warm, freshly-passed specimen. After cooling, correct for any temperature difference by adding 0·001 for every 3 ° above 15 °C or subtracting 0·001 for every 3 ° under. Make sure the urinometer clears the side of the vessel and avoid the presence of detergents in the collecting vessel which lower the surface tension and alter the reading.

The Refractometer. This requires only a drop of urine to measure its refractive index which is related to the specific gravity; directly calibrated instruments are available.

Note. Proteinuria increases the specific gravity. Subtract 0·003 for every g/l of urinary protein.

Determination of Sodium and Potassium

Flame Photometric Methods

The introduction of emission flame photometry into the clinical biochemistry laboratory was a major advance permitting the simple and rapid determination of $[Na^+]$ and $[K^+]$. Modern instruments (see Chapter 7, p. 164) incorporate an internal standard, often lithium, with simultaneous measurement of $[Na]$ and $[K]$ and electronic amplification of the flame signal. This permits greater dilution of the sample allowing a smaller volume to be used and also reduces the effect of protein on the viscosity of the diluted sample. Most manually operated instruments now incorporate an automatic dilutor and provide a digital readout of the results once the zero has been adjusted by aspirating water and the instrument has been calibrated using a single standard. The samples are then aspirated serially into the instrument and diluted by a lithium nitrate solution. The details of operation vary from one instrument to another and will not be described further here.

This type of flame photometer lends itself to operation in an automated mode. Some are linked to an automatic turntable on which the samples are loaded in plastic cups and are equipped with a printer for recording the results. This provides a convenient automated instrument for the rapid, simultaneous determination of $[Na^+]$ and $[K^+]$. Flame photometers are also often incorporated into multi-channel analysers either of the continuous flow or discrete types (see Chapter 8).

The analytical performance of these instruments varies somewhat. For plasma $[Na^+]$ the between-batch precision over several weeks is 1·8 mmol/l for internal standard instruments used in manual or discrete automated mode, but is about 1·5 mmol/l for continuous flow systems. A similar pattern is seen for plasma $[K^+]$ with precision figures of 0·10 mol/l for the first group and 0·09 mmol/l for continuous flow systems.

Determination of $[Na^+]$ and $[K^+]$ in urine is conveniently carried out by flame photometry but the $[K^+]$ is higher than in plasma and the $[Na^+]$ is more variable. Accordingly the calibration fluid usually has the composition, sodium, 100 and potassium, 100 mmol/l instead of sodium, 140 and potassium, 5 mmol/l used for plasma. Particularly concentrated urines may need dilution before analysis but this is unusal.

Determination of Sodium and Potassium in Erythrocytes. Some indication of the composition of ICF may be obtained by consideration of the composition of erythrocytes although these behave rather differently from skeletal muscle cells which constitute much of the ICF. However, the determination of concentrations within erythrocytes is possible using an ordinary heparinised blood sample and is much less troublesome for the patient than a muscle biopsy.

The $[Na^+]$ and $[K^+]$ are measured in plasma in the usual way and in whole blood after standardising the flame photometer with the same solution as is used for urine. The haematocrit of the sample needs to be measured. If X_p is the plasma concentration of the ion X, while X_b is the whole blood concentration and h is the haematocrit, then if X_c is the erythrocyte concentration of this ion, the following equation will apply to the amount of X in one litre of whole blood.

$$X_b = h \cdot X_c + (1 - h) \cdot X_p$$

and hence

$$X_c = X_p + (X_b - X_p)/h$$

This allows X_c to be calculated. For K^+, $(X_b - X_p)$ is positive but for Na^+ it is negative.

Determination of Plasma Chloride

Colorimetric Methods

Chloride ions form an undissociated but soluble salt, mercuric chloride, with mercuric ions and this provides a major principle on which Cl^- is determined. In the method of Schales and Schales (1941), plasma is titrated with mercuric nitrate in acid solution until free mercuric ions can be detected at the end-point using diphenylcarbazone.

$$Hg(NO_3)_2 + 2NaCl \rightarrow HgCl_2 \text{ (undissociated)} + 2NaNO_3$$

The method is modified to provide a colorimetric technique suitable for automated procedures by using an excess of the poorly dissociated mercuric thiocyanate as the primary reagent. In acid solution, this forms mercuric chloride leaving thiocyanate ions in solution which then react with a ferric salt. The colour produced by the red ferric thiocyanate is measured.

$$Hg(CNS)_2 \text{ [undissociated]} + 2Cl^- \rightarrow HgCl_2 \text{ [undissociated]} + 2CNS^-$$

$$3CNS^- + Fe^{3+} \rightarrow Fe(CNS)_3 \text{ [red]}$$

In order to avoid too intense a colour and to increase the sensitivity over the required analytical range, it is usual to include mercuric nitrate in the reagent. The Cl^- present converts this entirely to mercuric chloride (see equation above) and only the excess is available for colorimetric reaction.

Manual Method of Schales and Schales (1941)

Reagents.

1. Mercuric nitrate solution, approximately, 8·5 mmol/l. Dissolve 2·9 to 3·0 g $Hg(NO_3)_2$, H_2O in a few hundred ml water, add 20 ml 2 mol/l nitric acid and make to one litre with water. The amount of acid is critical, otherwise the end-point will not be so sharp.
2. Diphenylcarbazone indicator. Dissolve 100 mg in 100 ml ethanol, 950 ml/l. Store in the dark at 4 °C. The solution fades in light within a few days and cannot then be used. Prepare freshly once a month.
3. Standard chloride solution, 10 mmol/l. Dissolve 585 mg sodium chloride, dried at 120 °C, in water and make to one litre.

Technique. Add 0·2 ml plasma to 1·8 ml water followed by 60 μl of the indicator. Titrate with the mercuric nitrate solution using a microburette calibrated to 0·01 ml. Repeat the titration on 2 ml of the standard chloride solution; the expected titrant volume is about 2·3 ml. The end-point is better with protein-free solutions which give an intense violet-blue colour on adding the first drop of *excess* mercuric nitrate. Confusion may arise with protein-containing solutions as there is an *immediate* colour change to salmon-red quickly changing to deep violet. On adding more titrant this becomes pale yellow or colourless until a sharp change to pale violet denotes the end-point.

Calculation.

$$\text{Plasma chloride (mmol/l)} = \frac{\text{ml titrant needed for unknown}}{\text{ml titrant needed for standard}} \times 100$$

Note. The average between-batch precision for this method is 3·1 mmol/l and the results are on average about 0·7 mmol/l higher than those obtained using multi-channel analysers.

Coulometric Titration Methods

In the coulometric method a constant electric current is passed between two silver electrodes which dip into an acid buffer solution to which a known volume of plasma is added. According to the laws of electrochemistry, one mol Ag^+ is released from the anode by 96 487 coulombs (the Faraday constant). If the current is constant, the molar quantity of Ag^+ released is therefore directly proportional to time. The concentration of Ag^+ in the medium will remain low in the presence of Cl^- as insoluble AgCl is formed. This is usually held in suspension by gelatine added to the acid buffer. At the end-point of the titration, free Ag^+ appear in solution resulting in a sudden increase in potential between the two silver detecting electrodes. This sudden increase is used to switch off a timing circuit which had been activated when the Ag^+-generating current was switched on. The time elapsed is a measure of the $[Cl^-]$ in the sample and the relation can be made by a simple one adjustment of the current and the use of a fixed volume of sample. It is possible to add successive samples to the same reaction mixture and repeat the procedure thereby increasing the rate of throughput of samples. The average between-batch precision is 2·0 mmol/l. The results are, on average, 0·6 mmol/l lower than those obtained using multi-channel analysers. This method is convenient for urine $[Cl^-]$ measurement if required. Use the same volume of urine as plasma initially but repeat using a different volume if the result is particularly high or low.

Chloride Ion Selective Electrode

A portable instrument containing Ag/AgCl electrodes can be used for sweat [Cl^-] determination in the diagnosis of cystic fibrosis.

Ion-selective Electrodes

If a metal rod is placed in a solution of one of its salts (a half cell), it acquires an electrical potential. If two dissimilar metals are each dipped into solutions of their own salts, the difference in potential can be measured or calculated from the two half cells. A standard electrode is thus required against which the potential of all other electrodes can be compared. This is the standard hydrogen electrode. In its original form the electrode coated with platinum black is surrounded by hydrogen at atmospheric pressure. The electrode dips into a solution containing H^+ at unit activity, i.e. a molar solution of a strong acid. This electrode by definition has a potential of zero. When a similar electrode is dipped into acid of different concentration to act as the other half cell to a standard hydrogen electrode and they are connected by means of a bridge of KCl solution, the potential difference, E, is related to the hydrogen ion activity (a_{H^+}).

The difficulty of using the standard hydrogen electrode as the reference electrode for everyday use is obvious, but other secondary reference electrodes of known potential in relation to the standard hydrogen electrode are available. These consist of a metal in contact with a paste of its salt. The most commonly used is the calomel electrode consisting of mercury in contact with mercurous chloride (calomel) in paste form covered with a solution of KCl. The latter acts as part of the electrolyte bridge to the other electrode. It moistens a porous plug on the outer surface of the electrode. The electrical circuit is completed when the electrode is placed in a solution. The potential of a platinum wire in contact with the mercury varies with the [KCl] which may be 0.1 mol/l, 1.0 mol/l, or saturated, the last being the most common. The KCl solution must then be kept saturated for the electrode potential to remain constant.

The H^+ glass electrode is a special case of an ion-selective electrode (ISE) and such electrodes have now been developed for many ions in addition to H^+. An ion-selective membrane is required to separate the solution of unknown activity from the detecting system. The membrane may consist of: a special glass (as in the H^+ electrode); a disc of crystalline material, sometimes fused or pressed from the powder or cut from a single crystal (as in the solid state electrode); an organic ion-exchanger saturating a water-immiscible solvent held in a porous plug or immobilised in a gel or plastic; or a neutral carrier, e.g. the valinomycin K^+ electrode (as in liquid membrane electrodes). Each form of the electrode usually contains an Ag/AgCl detector electrode. The potential difference between this and a calomel or silver chloride reference electrode is measured, and as the reference electrode potential is constant any change that is generated at the ion-exchange membrane is also measured. (Developments in reference electrode technology may lead to the replacement of these by some form of solid state electrode.) If the unknown solution has a different concentration of the particular ion from that of the solution filling the electrode, ions migrate towards the lower concentration, thus changing the potential across the membrane. An equilibrium potential soon develops which just prevents further movement of ions. The number of ions transported across the membrane is so small that the change in sample concentration is infinitesimal.

The potential for a wide range of activity of the ion x is given by the Nernst equation.

$$E = E_0 + \frac{2 \cdot 303\, RT}{nF} \log a_x$$

where E = electrode potential recorded; E_0 = constant for the electrode system including reference electrodes; R = the universal or molar gas constant, $8 \cdot 31$ J/K; T = temperature (K); F = the Faraday, $96\,487$ coulombs; n = the number of charges on the ion, including sign; a = the activity of the ion x to which the electrode responds.

For a monovalent ion at 25 °C this expression becomes

$$E = E_0 + 0 \cdot 059\ 1 \times \log a_x$$

Thus for each 10-fold change of activity of a given ion the potential will change by $59 \cdot 1$ mV. This is the slope of the line when E (ordinate) is plotted against $\log a_x$ (abscissa). An alternative version of the equation is therefore

$$E = E_0 + S \cdot \log a_x$$

the slope (S) often being expressed as millivolts per decade, i.e. 10-fold change in activity of the ion. It is important to note that ISEs measure activity. Activity is related to the concentration by $a = fc$, where f is the activity coefficient and c the molal concentration.

In ideal solutions at infinite dilution, f is equal to unity. It is impossible to determine the activity of a single ion, but the mean activity coefficient of an electrolyte can be determined. For dilute aqueous solutions, Debye and Huckel predicted a theoretical relationship for a single ion at 25 °C

$$-\log f = 0 \cdot 51\, z^2 \sqrt{\mu}$$

Where μ is ionic strength and is defined by

$$\mu = \tfrac{1}{2} \Sigma m z^2$$

where m is molality and z is valence.

Thus the EMF generated is not strictly proportional to concentration but can be used for determination of concentration by careful calibration against standard solutions. As the Nernst equation shows, the slope S is positive for cations and negative for anions and is twice as great for monovalent than for divalent ions at a given temperature. Under ideal conditions at 25 °C for monovalent ions it is $59 \cdot 1$ mV/decade and for divalent ions, $29 \cdot 6$. In practice the selectivity of electrode response varies from this ideal and the slope decreases with ageing of the electrode. This decreased sensitivity is associated with reduced precision.

Electrodes are available in dip type as in the original pH glass electrodes, or flow-through type as in the modified Sanz electrode for blood pH measurements. Some ISE analysers are of the *direct reading* type, where the ion activity of the sample is measured directly. Others are *indirect reading* and incorporate a dilution step. This distinction is of importance and is discussed below. Electrodes are used to measure dissolved gases as in the determination of blood P_{CO_2}.

Glass Electrodes

Determination of pH. The most accurate method for the routine measurement of pH is the pH meter which utilises the glass electrode. The potential between a glass surface and the solution in which it is immersed varies with the pH of the solution. If a thin glass membrane separates two solutions of different pH, a potential difference is generated across the membrane. Ordinary soft glass has too great an electrical resistance for practical use. A suitable glass has the composition 6% CaO, 22% Na_2O, 72% SiO_2 and has the lowest melting point of any glass prepared from these materials. In the standard dip type of electrode the sensitive but fragile tip is fused to the stem of the electrode. The interior of the electrode usually contains hydrochloric acid of fixed concentration, usually 0·1 mol/l, into which dips a Ag/AgCl electrode of defined potential. Less often the electrode contains a buffer of pH 4 and a little quinhydrone into which dips a platinum wire. The resistance of the glass membrane is still too great for the potential difference to be measured simply, hence the transistor amplifiers used in contemporary pH meters. For a given glass electrode and reference calomel electrode at 25 °C,

$$pH = (E - K)/0·0591$$

where E is the measured potential and K a constant.

The response is linear with pH and the slope of the calibration line depends on the temperature but this can be allowed for electrically. As a result the calibration of the meter can be directly in pH units rather than mV. In practice the instrument is calibrated by immersion of the glass electrode in suitable buffers of known pH.

This glass electrode has several advantages: no chemical is added to the specimen, its potential is independent of the oxidation-reduction potential, it can be used in unbuffered solutions and it attains equilibrium rapidly. The most useful range is from pH 0 to 10 but this can be extended to pH 12 with careful calibration. Disadvantages are its fragility and its high resistance which increases the cost of the electronic part of the pH meter. The system, therefore, comprises the glass electrode in contact with the solution to be measured, the calomel reference electrode, a KCl bridge and the measuring device (Fig. 23.3). In the general purpose form both electrodes dip into the test solution, either separately or as a combined single unit. The KCl solution in the calomel electrode must be

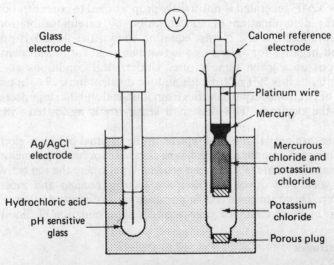

Fig. 23.3. System for Measuring pH Using a Glass Electrode and Calomel Electrode. (Reproduced by kind permission of Dr. J. P. Blackburn and the editor of 'Teach-In'.)

topped up at intervals to keep moist the porous plug through which contact is made with the sample. The uncontrolled leak of KCl through the porous plug of the calomel electrode can lead to variable junction potentials and instability, but if this leak is controlled and is less than 50 μl per day, a very stable and reproducible liquid junction potential is produced. The life of a properly maintained calomel electrode is several years. The fragile tip of the glass electrode must not be scratched; even when carefully used its life is variable and ageing occurs even on storage, leading to a less than theoretical response. The response must thus be checked with two buffers covering the required range. Most modern instruments incorporate a slope control to compensate for slight deterioration of the electrode as well as for temperature changes. A new electrode should be immersed for a period in hydrochloric acid (0·1 mol/l) before use to improve its stability. A deteriorating electrode may sometimes benefit from this treatment.

The determination of blood pH requires several extra refinements. The measuring system must be capable of providing a stable reading with a discrimination of 0·005 pH units. Readings are made under anaerobic conditions along with the measurement of P_{CO_2} and P_{O_2} on a microsample of blood (see p. 585).

The Sodium Electrode. The H^+ glass electrode shows activity towards other ions to a varying degree. Although not specific, the electrode can be made selective by choosing the conditions so that the activity of the ion in question far outweighs interference from other ions. The composition of glass typical for a H^+ electrode is compared with those showing greater activity for Na^+ or K^+ in Table 23.3. Although the silica concentration remains fairly constant for all three glasses, addition of CaO greatly increases sensitivity for H^+ in the pH glass electrode. After replacement of CaO by Al_2O_3 there is a greater sensitivity for K^+ than Na^+ but not sufficient to outweigh the greater $[Na^+]$ than $[K^+]$ in plasma. With the marked reduction in Na_2O and increase in Al_2O_3 the glass has a much greater sensitivity for Na^+ than K^+. Also considering the greater concentration of Na^+ than K^+ in plasma it is possible to use such electrodes for the determination of plasma $[Na^+]$. They are constructed in a manner similar to capillary pH electrodes so that the sample flows through the glass electrode. The glass electrode is similarly completed by an Ag/AgCl indicator electrode whose potential is measured against a calomel reference electrode.

The long-term between-batch precision of Na^+ electrodes is similar to that of an automated flame photometer system at 1·6 mmol/l. Table 23.3 shows that glass electrodes have insufficient selectivity for K^+ in the presence of Na^+ to permit the determination of plasma $[K^+]$ unless a correction is made for the $[Na^+]$ which has been measured simultaneously. This is of little practical use.

TABLE 23.3

Composition of Glass Membranes in Ion Selective Glass Electrodes

| Selected ion | Per cent composition | | | | Comments |
	SiO_2	CaO	Na_2O	Al_2O_3	
H^+	72	6	22	—	Also reacts to Na^+, K^+, NH_4^+, Ag^+
Na^+	71	—	11	18	Na^+/K^+ activity 2800
K^+	68	—	27	5	K^+/Na^+ activity 20

Liquid Ion-exchanger Membrane Electrodes

These electrodes contain a liquid ion-exchanger with a high activity for the ion being determined. The internal filling solution contains the ion in question, either saturated or at a fixed concentration, and is separated from the test solution by a porous plug or a membrane. The plug may be saturated with a water-immiscible liquid ion-exchanger or the membrane itself is made of a selective exchange material. The liquid ion-exchanger may be used as a saturated resin plug or be embedded in plastic. Whatever form the membrane takes, the inner filling liquid is in contact with a Ag/AgCl detector electrode whose potential is compared with a reference electrode in the usual manner. This type of electrode has found application in the determination of ionised calcium where the ion-exchanger is often the calcium salt of an alkyl phosphate or more recently a synthetic neutral carrier has been used.

Liquid Neutral Carrier Membrane Electrodes

These electrodes contain an ionophore which complexes selectively with the ion to be detected. The common type of K^+ electrode has a membrane of valinomycin, an antibiotic, as the ionophore and can be incorporated in a flow-through electrode. Recently synthetic ionophores have been used. As K^+ in the red cell is effectively retained by its membrane, it is possible to determine plasma $[K^+]$ using whole blood samples, an advantage for determinations under emergency conditions or for continuous monitoring.

Dissolved Gas Sensors

Gas molecules diffuse from the sample solution through a hydrophobic gas-permeable membrane and redissolve in a solution filling the sensor. At equilibrium the partial pressure of the gas in this solution and the sample are equal. The filling solution is a thin layer between the membrane and a pH electrode which measures the chemical change in the filling solution produced by the gas. The effective volume of the solution is very small which gives a rapid response while minimising the amount of gas exchanged with the sample. This system can be used with ammonia which increases the pH or CO_2, SO_2 or nitrogen oxides which decrease it. With a suitable filling solution such electrodes obey the Nernst equation over a very wide range. Thus for ammonia the response is linear for concentrations from 1 μmol/l to 100 mmol/l.

Following the introduction of the P_{CO_2} electrode the development of other dissolved gas electrodes was slow until the ammonium electrode came into use. Progress in details continues, particularly in reducing the response time which depends on the rate of gas diffusion. The newer membranes consist of a micro-porous plastic film and a hydrophobic matrix which are more permeable than the dense plastic films originally used.

The P_{CO_2} (Severinghaus) Electrode. This is essentially a pH electrode system containing a calomel and glass electrode (Fig. 23.4). The tip of the glass electrode is surrounded by a solution of bicarbonate (approximately 10 mmol/l) separated from the sample under test by a gas-permeable membrane. Carbon dioxide from the sample diffuses across the membrane and reacts with the bicarbonate altering its pH in accordance with the Henderson–Hasselbalch equation. This pH is measured by the glass electrode and is usually displayed directly as P_{CO_2} on a logarithmic scale.

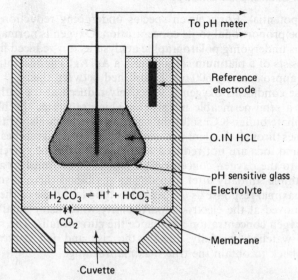

Fig. 23.4. Diagrammatic Representation of P_{CO_2} (Severinghaus) Electrode.
The reference electrode is a calomel electrode. (Reproduced by kind permission of Dr. J. P. Blackburn and the editor of 'Teach-In'.)

The P_{O_2} (Clark) Electrode

Although not strictly an ISE, it is convenient to include this electrode here. The electrode system is that used in the polarograph. In this instrument, the electrical potential difference is applied between two electrodes dipping in a solution (Fig. 23.5). If one of these is an electrode of known potential then the potential of the other electrode, usually the cathode, can be measured from the applied potential difference. Various substances in the solution may be capable of electrolytic reduction at the cathode, but they will usually differ in their oxidation–reduction potential and selective reduction can be achieved by altering

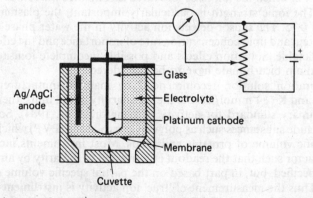

Fig. 23.5. Diagram of P_{O_2} Electrode.
The bulk of the cathode is sealed in glass but the tip is close to the membrane and is in contact with the electrolyte (phosphate buffer–KCl). (Reproduced by kind permission of Dr. J. P. Blackburn and the editor of 'Teach-In'.)

the cathode potential. For a given species undergoing reduction the current flowing will be proportional to its concentration. Oxygen is normally displaced from solutions undergoing polarographic analysis as it is reduced first. The Po_2 electrode consists of a platinum cathode and a Ag/AgCl anode with a potential difference of approximately 600 mV established between them.

Under these conditions oxygen is selectively reduced at the cathode. This is covered with a semi-permeable membrane which separates the blood sample from a phosphate buffer-KCl solution which is in contact also with the anode. Oxygen diffuses through the semi-permeable membrane and reaches the cathode. Other gases and ions are not reduced at this potential. The current flowing is proportional to the oxygen concentration (about 20 pA/mmHg) and hence to Po_2 in the sample. Initially after introducing the blood there is some delay in achieving a maximal response as oxygen takes time to diffuse to the cathode. As oxygen is removed at the electrode, particularly when using small volumes of blood, the oxygen concentration and hence the current falls. The reading must therefore be watched carefully. Ideally the rise and fall curves should be extrapolated back to obtain the true maximal reading.

Some Problems of Ion-selective Electrodes

Direct reading ISEs have many advantages. The common electrolytes such as Na^+ and K^+ can be measured quickly and conveniently on whole blood using small sample volumes. They are well suited to intensive care units, etc., because of the speed of analysis, and no requirement for centrifugation or inflammable gases. Some disadvantages are that the running costs are often higher than flame photometers, they are not so easily serviced by laboratory technical staff owing to their 'black box' nature and the use of whole blood may mask haemolysis.

The accuracy and calibration of direct reading ISEs is very problematic. Flame photometry, and most other methods of analysis for that matter, measures the mass of substance per unit volume (molarity) while ISEs attempt to measure activity. Different manufacturers' instruments give a considerable variability in readings. This is often in part due to the design of the instrument, particularly the residual liquid junction potentials and geometry. The latter is usually patented. The selectivity of ISEs for a particular ion is crucial in assessing performance.

The matrix in which the ion to be measured is contained influences the activity coefficient. The ionic strength is particularly important, the plasma f_{Na} being estimated at 0·75. The sensor detects ion activity in the water phase only. Thus variable protein and lipid concentrations are of importance and the effects are not wholly predictable. Solvation effects and possible incomplete ionisation of, for instance, sodium bicarbonate have to be considered.

The calibration solution recommended by many manufacturers is Na^+, 140 mmol/l and K^+, 4 mmol/l. Note the incongruity of the units, there being no accepted primary standard for activity (Covington *et al.*, 1984). Some manufacturers include substances such as polyvinylpyrrolidone (PVP) which simulates partial specific volume of proteins and lipids. Most instruments incorporate a correction factor such that the readout is converted to molarity by an algorithm, usually unspecified, but, in part based on the partial specific volume of proteins and lipids. Thus the measurement of 'true' ion activity is instrument-dependent and as a consequence the IFCC is currently investigating whether an international consensus concerning standardisation can be achieved. Broughton *et al.* (1985) have proposed that all direct reading ISEs should be adjusted to give the same values for Na^+ in plasma as those obtained by flame photometry at a total protein concentration of 70 g/l. Also, all quality control specimens used should have a similar protein concentration. With indirect reading ISEs (used mainly in multichannel analysers) the problems are not so severe. Dilution results in a much decreased concentration of the measured ion and near elimination of differing protein and lipid concentration effects. The values obtained in practice are close to those obtained by flame photometry and are reported as molarity.

When measuring Na^+ and K^+ in urine a dilution step is required. This is because the a_{K^+} commonly found in urine is outside the measuring range of the instrument and there is interference from any lipophilic organic anions present. Magnesium acetate is sometimes used as diluent as this has similar electrochemical properties to plasma, for which the instrument is designed.

DISORDERS OF BODY FLUIDS AND ELECTROLYTES

Water Depletion

This term describes loss of water from the body with little or no loss of solute and occurs whenever water balance is negative. If uncorrected, the water loss is distributed proportionately between ICF and ECF (2:1 approximately) which both become hypertonic. By the time water loss poses a threat to life, 10 litres or 15% of TBW have been lost. The ECF volume is preferentially maintained by renal Na^+ and water retention mediated by the renin-angiotensin-aldosterone mechanism. The plasma volume is further protected by the oncotic pressure of plasma proteins thereby minimising the effects on the circulatory system. Brain cells are partly able to maintain their volume by generating additional ICF solute. These idiogenic osmoles comprise Na^+, K^+ and Cl^- from the ECF and amino acids produced intracellularly.

Water depletion arises from an inadequate water intake, abnormal losses via the lungs and skin as in pyrexia, and abnormal renal losses–*polyuria*. Relative water depletion occurs if hypotonic fluid such as sweat is lost and not replaced. The initial symptom of severe thirst is followed by apathy, confusion and weakness leading to death in coma if water deprivation progresses. The tongue is shrunken, the mouth dry and 'dehydration fever' may be present although tissue turgor and the peripheral circulation are preserved initially. Oliguria with urine of high osmolality occurs unless the primary cause is polyuria. Most blood constituents are present in increased concentration but the most useful measurements are plasma osmolality and $[Na^+]$. The latter may exceed 180 mmol/l.

Correction of the abnormality requires either oral fluids or intravenous glucose solution, 50 g/l, which is isotonic but leaves water only, once the glucose has been metabolised. If ADH deficiency is the primary cause, DDAVP (an ADH analogue) should also be given. Progress is assessed by monitoring plasma $[Na^+]$, urinary volume and the quenching of thirst. The investigation of polyuria is discussed below (p. 577).

Water Overload

This occurs when water is retained in excess of solute, the kidney being unable to excrete the excess water. This is commonly seen in patients with chest infection, post-operatively or following more severe trauma or illness, particularly if isotonic glucose therapy is used. Water overload may occur in hypopituitarism as cortisol is required for proper water handling by the renal tubule. Rare causes of water overload are freshwater drowning, following colonic washouts using hypotonic fluid, during transurethral resection of the prostate gland and ectopic or appropriate ADH secretion.

Again the disordered water balance is shared by all body fluid compartments, and while some slight oedema may be present, the effects are mainly a consequence of increased brain volume. Nausea, lethargy, headaches and mental clouding may lead to convulsions, and finally, coma. The urine is dilute (not in ADH excess), of moderate volume and all plasma constituent concentrations are decreased. The plasma osmolality and [Na$^+$] are the most helpful investigations. Very low plasma [Na$^+$] is more often due to water overload than to Na$^+$ depletion; a normal [Na$^+$] effectively excludes water overload. In severe cases [Na$^+$] may be as low as 100 mmol/l. Many cases are preventable but if the condition is established it usually responds to restriction of fluid intake until the [Na$^+$] becomes normal. If cerebral symptoms require it, ICF volume can be reduced more rapidly by intravenous mannitol or hypertonic saline.

Saline Depletion

Saline depletion implies loss of approximately isotonic sodium-containing fluid and is the middle of a spectrum varying from pure water depletion to pure Na$^+$ depletion.

Loss of isotonic sodium-containing fluids is borne by the ECF the volume of which is reduced, although the plasma [Na$^+$] may alter only little in the early stages. In more marked saline depletion (about 3 l), some water is retained which minimises the reduction in ECF volume; the plasma [Na$^+$] then falls. Values below 125 mmol/l are uncommon in all but the most severe cases. In all patients the ECF volume is reduced and progressively affects the cardiovascular system causing hypotension (often postural), reduced cardiac output and reduced renal blood flow. The veins are collapsed, tissue turgor and intra-ocular pressure are reduced and circulatory shock is clinically apparent in more severe cases (6–7 l lost). In mild depletion, loss of energy, anorexia and muscle cramps following water drinking are the main effects.

'Heat exhaustion', 'sun stroke', and 'stoker's cramp' are terms describing inadequate Na$^+$ replacement following excessive sweating. More severe losses through the skin may occur following extensive burns. An important common cause is loss of alimentary secretions, either by pooling in an atonic gut as in paralytic ileus, or by such external losses as vomiting, repeated gastric aspirations, or watery diarrhoea. Repeated aspiration of effusions such as ascitic fluid may cause significant loss. Urinary losses arise during recovery from acute renal failure, in some cases of chronic renal failure, following relief of chronic urinary tract obstruction, in the rare crises of Addison's disease, during an osmotic diuresis and when extra anions are excreted as in diabetic ketoacidosis.

Urinary Na$^+$ excretion is low unless the kidney is the primary route of loss. Plasma [Na$^+$] may be misleading but some fall is usual. Plasma protein concentration, blood haemoglobin concentration and haematocrit values increase but the wide normal variation makes these investigations more suitable for following progress than for initial assessment. The diminished renal blood flow and consequent fall in glomerular filtration rate, leads to a rise in plasma creatinine concentration. The combination of a rather low plasma [Na$^+$] with increased urea and protein concentrations is in contrast to the changes in water retention when all are low.

Sodium replacement may be orally as added salt in mild depletion or as isotonic saline, 9 g/l NaCl, given intravenously in more severe cases until the abnormal biochemical findings and circulatory defects return to the patient's normal state. The overall deficit rarely exceeds 5 l of saline. Some patients show a mixture of pure water depletion and pure Na^+ depletion so that therapy in such cases requires a mixture of isotonic saline and isotonic glucose therapies.

Urine Analysis and Renal Disease

The urine concentrations of common analytes in hypovolaemia (pre-renal uraemia) and established acute renal failure are shown in Table 23.4. These figures are a useful guide taken in conjunction with the clinical findings. Sometimes there is some overlap. All the measurements can be done on 'spot' samples and 24 h urine collections usually add little additional information. The

TABLE 23.4

Differentiation of Pre-renal Uraemia (Hypovolaemia) from Established Acute Renal Failure (ARF)

	Pre-renal Uraemia	Established ARF
Urine osmolality (mosmol/kg)	> 500	< 400
Urine/plasma osmolality	> 1·5	< 1·1
Urine Na (mmol/l)	< 10	> 30
FENa	< 1	> 1
Urine urea (mmol/l)	> 250	< 150
Urine/plasma urea	> 10	< 10
Urine/plasma creatinine	> 10	< 10

Values for incipient ARF are intermediate

fractional excretion of sodium (FENa) has been claimed to be of greater diagnostic value (Espinel and Gregory, 1980);

$$FENa = \frac{\text{amount of } Na^+ \text{ excreted per min}}{\text{amount of } Na^+ \text{ filtered per min}} \times 100\%$$

which reduces to;

$$FENa = \frac{\text{urine } [Na^+]}{\text{plasma } [Na^+]} \times \frac{\text{plasma } [\text{creatinine}]}{\text{urine } [\text{creatinine}]} \times 100\%$$

Values greater than 1% are associated with acute renal failure and values less than 1% with pre-renal uraemia. Oken (1981) found the calculation of FENa to be of little additional help, particularly in those cases where the diagnosis was uncertain. A plasma creatinine concentration greater than 250 μmol/l is associated with a 90% chance of renal impairment (Morgan *et al.*, 1977).

Saline Excess

This results in expansion of the ECF volume with little alteration in $[Na^+]$. The expansion is mainly in the IF so that its normal sponge-like consistency is overloaded and free fluid moves under gravity to dependent parts to give the clinical signs of oedema. During the stage of increase in ECF volume, Na^+ balance is positive. The renal retention of Na^+ is mainly mediated by increased aldosterone secretion. Water retention may be due in part to increased ADH secretion.

The factors regulating the normal exchange of fluid at the capillary level between plasma, interstitial fluid and lymph have been discussed. Disturbance of this balance may arise in various ways, all of which produce either local or generalised oedema depending on whether the disorder is local or general. Thus increase in venous pressure as in congestive cardiac failure, reduction in oncotic pressure as a consequence of hypoalbuminaemia from any cause, obstruction to lymph flow, or increased capillary wall permeability as in inflammation all alter the balance. The first two are likely to be generalised, the last two are usually more local. If renal function is normal, those conditions leading to generalised oedema are accompanied, in the early stages at least, by a reduction in plasma volume which stimulates the renin-angiotensin-aldosterone system. Aldosterone aids Na^+ retention by the kidney, but this and the isotonic equivalent amount of water are mainly located in the IF. The plasma $[Na^+]$ is usually normal at this stage.

Many patients with oedema are treated by the administration of diuretic drugs. These potent agents interfere with tubular Na^+ reabsorption leading to increased Na^+ excretion. A common hazard with the use of diuretics is the development of hypokalaemia, probably as a consequence of increased entry of Na^+ into the distal tubule where it is exchanged for K^+. Hypokalaemia of mild degree is often seen in patients whose oedema is successfully controlled by drugs. In some cases of congestive cardiac failure the patient may develop resistance to diuretic therapy and remain oedematous with a low plasma $[K^+]$ usually in association with an increased plasma urea concentration. The uraemia is probably pre-renal and consequent upon reduced renal perfusion by the failing circulation. The cause of the hyponatraemia is uncertain but in some cases may be an effect of K^+ depletion.

Changes in Plasma Sodium Concentration

Plasma $[Na^+]$ determinations of themselves do not provide much information about body Na^+ content. In summary, *hyponatraemia* may result from Na^+ depletion, from water excess, from changes in body K^+ content and when there is an artefactual decrease of the $[Na^+]$ by an excess of lipids or protein. Plasma $[Na^+]$ is often lower in the hospital population than in healthy people (Payne and Levell, 1968) and this non-specific change is in most cases not an indication of Na^+ deficiency. The interpretation of hyponatraemia requires consideration of other plasma analytes and the clinical state of the patient.

Hypernatraemia is most commonly due to water depletion. Mild hypernatraemia occurs in primary aldosteronism and in some cases of Cushing's syndrome due to the Na^+-retaining action of the hormones. Hypernatraemia may occur in infants following excessive dietary salt consumption. The condition can occur in adults with renal impairment particularly if hypertonic saline solutions are given parenterally. Useful reviews of hyponatraemia and hypernatraemia are by Baylis (1980) and Gill and Flear (1985).

Changes in Plasma Potassium Concentration

These are often associated with Na$^+$, water and acid–base disturbances, all of which may affect plasma [K$^+$]. Thus attempts to assess the state of K$^+$ stores from plasma [K$^+$] may be misleading though it usually falls if K$^+$ balance becomes negative and rises during positive balance, especially with impaired renal excretion. Plasma [K$^+$] is also dependent upon K$^+$ redistribution from ECF to ICF and *vice versa* as described previously. Changes in plasma [K$^+$] are partly responsible for the signs and symptoms of disordered K$^+$ metabolism.

Hyperkalaemia. This, a plasma [K$^+$] in excess of 5·4 mmol/l, affects skeletal muscle very little, but has profound myocardial actions leading to arrhythmias including ventricular fibrillation, bradycardia and eventually cardiac arrest in diastole when the plasma [K$^+$] reaches 8 to 10 mmol/l. Hyperkalaemia is seen in acidotic states, in catabolic states, in acute and chronic renal failure, in the 'crises' of Addison's disease, in haemolytic disorders, in the 'sick cell' syndrome and following the use of K$^+$-sparing diuretics. In many cases the infusion of glucose and insulin rapidly lowers the plasma [K$^+$] to safer levels. For longer term control, reduction of dietary intake, the use of ion-exchange resins orally or renal dialysis may be required.

Artefactual causes of hyperkalaemia such as forearm exercise following tourniquet application, use of EDTA specimen tubes, haemolysis, refrigeration of the specimen before plasma separation and delay in plasma separation should all be considered. If serum is used for [K$^+$] analysis, thrombocytosis or leucocytosis of leukaemia may cause a spurious elevation. A rare cause of confusion is pseudohyperkalaemia due to abnormal K$^+$ leakage from erythrocytes *in vitro*.

Hypokalaemia. This, a plasma [K$^+$] below 3·6 mmol/l, is associated with varying degrees of muscle weakness, increased neuromuscular excitability, and disordered myocardial function—arrhythmia, tachycardia, flattening of T waves in the ECG. Such effects increase, the lower the plasma [K$^+$] falls, sometimes to below 1·0 mmol/l. Even lower values may result in cardiac arrest in systole. Loss of K$^+$ from the renal tubular cells affects their function as shown by decreased concentrating capacity, impaired handling of abnormal Na$^+$ loads and an increased excretion of H$^+$ leading to a metabolic alkalosis.

The causes of hypokalaemia are increased alimentary or renal losses, or redistribution of K$^+$ from ECF to ICF. Impaired intake is usually of less importance. Hypokalaemia can occur when K$^+$ moves into cells in anabolic states, when insulin and glucose therapy is used, in alkalosis, with high circulating levels of catecholamines or in the rare condition of familial periodic paralysis. The main cause of loss may be ascertained by measuring the urinary excretion of K$^+$ If this exceeds 20 mmol/l on a spot sample of urine when signs of K$^+$ deficiency are present, a renal loss is indicated.

Alimentary losses include protracted vomiting as in pyloric stenosis, watery diarrhoea from any cause, steatorrhoea, and the rather rare mucous-secreting villous papilloma of the colon or rectum. In some patients, excessive consumption of purgatives is the cause.

Renal losses are considered under several headings:

1. Renal excretion of K$^+$ lost from ICF as in wasting diseases, uncontrolled diabetes and acidosis.
2. Renal tubular disease affecting the excretion of K$^+$. This occurs in some cases of chronic pyelonephritis, during recovery from acute renal failure, in the Fanconi syndrome, in renal tubular acidosis, and nephrocalcinosis.
3. Normal renal tubules may be under abnormal control. Increased mineralo-

corticoid activity occurs in severe Cushing's syndrome (particularly the 'ectopic ACTH syndrome'), primary and secondary hyperaldosteronism and during therapy with liquorice extracts, particularly carbenoxolone. Diuretics reducing proximal tubular reabsorption of sodium increase the distal tubular exchange of K^+ for Na^+. A similar effect occurs in alkalosis where Na^+ exchange for H^+ is decreased leaving more for exchange with K^+.

Investigation of Primary Aldosteronism (Conn's Syndrome)

Primary aldosteronism is a rare but curable cause of hypertension due to an adrenal adenoma. Hypokalaemia occurs in about 80 % of patients. If absent, it is often helpful to measure plasma $[K^+]$ following 7 days on a high salt diet (200 mmol/24 h). This ensures adequate Na^+ delivery to the distal tubule and enhances K^+ exchange, which in the presence of excess aldosterone may 'unmask' hypokalaemia. Plasma $[K^+]$ rather than serum $[K^+]$ should be measured for the reasons cited above. The mainstay of diagnosis is measurement of plasma aldosterone concentration and plasma renin activity. Ideally, the patient should be receiving no medication; if this is impractical, diuretic therapy must be stopped for 3 weeks prior to aldosterone measurement. The plasma specimen must be taken in the early morning after overnight recumbency. Under *no* circumstances should the patient be allowed to sit or stand before the sample is taken. An aliquot can be stored at $-20\,°C$ for the analysis of renin activity in the event of an increased plasma aldosterone concentration being found. Primary aldosteronism is associated with decreased plasma renin activity in contrast to secondary aldosteronism when it is increased.

Primary aldosteronism is treated by surgical removal of an adenoma or by the drug spironolactone, an aldosterone antagonist.

Treatment of Potassium Depletion

Moderate K^+ depletion involving losses of less than 10 % of total K^+ is not uncommon and usually responds to dietary potassium supplements of 50 to 100 mmol daily, given preferably as effervescent tablets or in a slow-release form. More severe depletion may necessitate intravenous administration of KCl. The concentration in the infusion is usually less than 40 mmol/l and less than 15 mmol is given hourly unless glucose and insulin are given simultaneously. Preferably such treatment should be controlled by frequent monitoring of the plasma $[K^+]$.

Polyuria and Renal Disease

One of the earliest signs of impaired renal tubular function is a decreasing ability to secrete a concentrated urine. The defect is especially apparent if tubular function is affected more than glomerular function. With progressive destruction of nephrons the osmolar load has to be shared between fewer nephrons, even if glomerular and tubular function are affected equally, so that each deals with a load greater than normal. A state of relative osmotic diuresis ensues in which urea represents an important osmotically active substance. The ability to secrete a concentrated urine is more important than the secretion of a dilute urine but diluting capacity is also affected later in renal disease and for similar reasons to those mentioned for the concentrating ability. Thus with increasing failure of tubular function, the osmolality range of the urine narrows from that of 40 to

1400 mosmol/kg found in full health under extreme circumstances. Ultimately values in the range 320 to 350 mosmol/kg are found. This restriction of osmolality, *isosthenuria*, corresponds to the passage of urine the osmolality of which equals that of glomerular filtrate although its composition will be very different. This progressive loss of tubular concentrating ability occurs early in tubular dysfunction. By the time isosthenuria is reached, other renal function tests are abnormal and their further deterioration can be followed. A consequence of the fall in concentrating power is that an increased volume of urine is passed during the night (nocturia) so that the ratio of day to night urine volumes, normally over two in younger adults, falls towards one as renal tubular impairment progresses. Such a fall is also common in old age. For the comparison, collect urine from 0800 h to 2000 h for the day urine and 2000 h to 0800 h for the night specimen. It is normally the case that the osmolality of a 24 h urine is greater than that of plasma. Reduction in concentrating capacity will thus lead to a polyuria with the accompanying symptom of thirst.

The Investigation of Polyuria

Polyuria may arise because of a low concentration of ADH in the circulation, renal tubules that are unresponsive to circulating ADH, or an osmotic diuresis. The investigation of polyuria therefore requires an assessment of the mechanisms normally releasing ADH, a study of the effect of administered ADH and the search for any osmotically active excretory product.

Lack of ADH. The polyuria usually exceeds 5 l and occasionally reaches 20 l daily. In *cranial diabetes insipidus* there is an inability to secrete ADH. The polyuria is marked, constant and gives rise to thirst as a secondary symptom. A personality disorder usually in middle aged females, referred to as '*compulsive water drinking*', involves the primary intake of excessive quantities of fluid resulting in the suppression of ADH secretion. The water intake and hence the polyuria fluctuates from day to day. A similar effect is seen rarely in cerebral lesions affecting the thirst centre.

In diabetes insipidus there is a tendency for the plasma osmolality and [Na$^+$] to be increased above normal; the reverse is true in compulsive water drinkers. This simple observation may clarify the diagnosis in some patients but there is an overlap in the normal range so that further tests are then needed. The conditions are differentiated either by administering DDAVP or by attempting to elicit ADH secretion by water deprivation. Both procedures are not without risk so that careful supervision of the patient is necessary. Following the administration of DDAVP renal conservation of water occurs. In diabetes insipidus this is followed by the abolition of thirst which is a secondary phenomenon. In the compulsive water drinker, however, thirst and water intake continue with the possible development of water overload.

Alternatively, water intake can be withdrawn. In compulsive water drinking this is usually followed by the secretion of ADH and the passage of increasingly concentrated urine, usually reaching an osmolality greater than that seen after a single dose of DDAVP. In some long-standing cases however, medullary osmolality is so reduced below the normal hypertonic levels that the urinary response may be only partial. In diabetes insipidus, water withdrawal is accompanied by continuing polyuria with an increasing plasma osmolality. The urine osmolality may rise but remains less than that achieved by a single dose of DDAVP. The hazard is that the patient with diabetes insipidus may become markedly water depleted if the test is unduly prolonged.

Inadequate Renal Response to ADH. Both types of patient just described usually show a rapid rise in urinary osmolality after DDAVP administration. If no such response occurs the condition is referred to as *nephrogenic diabetes insipidus* which exists in congenital or acquired forms. The congenital variant may occur as an isolated renal tubular defect or in conjunction with other tubular defects in the Fanconi syndrome; both are familial. The affected subject may pass over 7 l of urine daily but water intake is increased to compensate for the polyuria, especially in adults.

The acquired type is seen in some patients with hypercalcaemia, nephrocalcinosis and increased calcium excretion in the urine. It is also associated with multiple myelomatosis. Patients with chronic hypokalaemia also show DDAVP-resistant polyuria and this may be present to a more marked degree in some cases of chronic renal failure. Tubular damage and a poor osmotic gradient in the medulla are contributory factors but in some cases primary polydipsia can be present also. Having demonstrated the nephrogenic nature of the polyuria, plasma urea, creatinine, calcium, protein and electrolyte concentrations should be measured. Determination of osmolar clearance and free water clearance may be helpful.

Osmotic Diuresis. This is the most common cause of polyuria and is seen in uncontrolled diabetes mellitus with heavy glycosuria. Urea produces an osmotic diuresis in patients consuming very high protein diets or with chronic renal failure. Some cases of chronic pyelonephritis of advanced degree have decreased tubular reabsorption of Na^+ with the excretion of large quantities of Na^+ and a consequent osmotic diuresis.

Water Deprivation Test (after Dashe *et al.*, 1963)

The patient is encouraged to drink overnight. A light breakfast is allowed without tea or coffee but there must be no smoking prior to or during the test. The test lasts 8 h (usually 0830 h–1630 h) during which no fluids are allowed though some dry food is permitted. The patient must be supervised throughout the test and weighed hourly. If more than 3 % of body weight is lost the test is discontinued. Urine is collected hourly (with no preservative) and the volumes recorded. The following timed specimens should be sent to the laboratory for osmolality determinations:

Plasma specimens—0900, 1200, 1500, 1600
Urine specimens—0830–0930, 1130–1230, 1430–1530, 1530–1630.

DDAVP Test (after Monson and Richards, 1978)

DDAVP (20 μg intranasally or 2 μg intramuscularly) is often given immediately on completion of the water deprivation test. Urine is collected each hour for 4 h for osmolality determination. The patient may drink water but no more than twice the volume excreted during the deprivation test is allowed for the next 24 h, due to the danger of water overload.

INTERPRETATION

According to Baylis and Gill (1984), the plasma osmolality does not exceed 295 mosmol/kg and the urine osmolality exceeds 750 mosmol/kg at some time during both tests in normal persons. The plasma osmolality exceeds 295 mosmol/kg in cranial and nephrogenic diabetes insipidus. In the former condition, the urine osmolality remains less than 300 mosmol/kg during water deprivation but exceeds 750 mosmol/kg following DDAVP administration. In nephrogenic diabetes insipidus the urine osmolality fails to exceed 750 mosmol/kg following DDAVP administration. Some patients show intermediate values. The adequacy of the test, primary polydipsia and partial defects should be considered in such cases.

ACIDS, BASES AND pH

The Brønsted–Lowry definition of acids and bases is generally accepted. According to this acids are substances (neutral molecules or ions) which donate H^+ (protons); bases substances which accept them. Bases are formed when an acid dissociates to give H^+. Thus:

Acids		Bases
HCl	$\rightleftharpoons$	$H^+ + Cl^-$
H_2CO_3	$\rightleftharpoons$	$H^+ + HCO_3^-$
HCO_3^-	$\rightleftharpoons$	$H^+ + CO_3^{2-}$
HPO_4^{2-}	$\rightleftharpoons$	$H^+ + PO_4^{3-}$
$H_2PO_4^-$	$\rightleftharpoons$	$H^+ + HPO_4^{2-}$
H_3PO_4	$\rightleftharpoons$	$H^+ + H_2PO_4^-$
NH_4^+	$\rightleftharpoons$	$H^+ + NH_3$
$H \cdot Protein$	$\rightleftharpoons$	$H^+ + Protein^-$
$H \cdot Protein^+$	$\rightleftharpoons$	$H^+ + Protein$
$H \cdot HbO_2$	$\rightleftharpoons$	$H^+ + HbO_2^-$
$H \cdot Hb$	$\rightleftharpoons$	$H^+ + Hb^-$

Some ions can act either as an acid or a base, for example HPO_4^{2-}. At body pH it acts as a base. Hydrogen ions do not exist free, but are accepted by a base. The water molecule acts in this way in aqueous solution (hydration) to form a hydroxonium ion, thus

$$H^+ + H_2O \rightleftharpoons H_3O^+$$

Water is another substance that can act either as an acid or a base. In forming the hydroxonium ion it acts as a base; in the following as an acid:

$$H_2O \rightleftharpoons H^+ + OH^-$$

The ionisation of water is written

$$H_2O + H_2O \rightleftharpoons H_3O^+ + OH^-$$

However, in clinical biochemistry it is satisfactory to use the term H^+ rather than hydroxonium ion and represent the ionisation of water by

$$H_2O \rightleftharpoons H^+ + OH^-$$

from which we have

$$\frac{[H^+][OH^-]}{[H_2O]} = K$$

[H_2O] is constant so [H^+] [OH^-] = K_w (ion product of water). At 25 °C this constant is 10^{-14} mol^2/l^2. At the neutral point [H^+] = [OH^-] so that each equals 10^{-7} mol/l or 100 nmol/l. When the [H^+] is greater than this the solution is acid, when less, alkaline. The term usually used to indicate the [H^+] is pH, its negative logarithm. Thus at neutrality this is 7 and the range covered on pH meters is from 0 to 14. pH is temperature-dependent.

The pH glass electrode responds logarithmically to a_{H^+} rather than [H^+]. Thus pH can be redefined as $-\log a_{H^+}$, and the above equation rewritten in terms of activity. However, the activity of individual ion species cannot be measured but only estimated. The modern definition of pH is defined operationally in terms of the method of measurement. A cell including a hydrogen electrode and a calomel reference electrode is used with a standard solution as near to $-\log a_{H^+}$ as can be estimated. For a concise and logical discussion see Bryan (1976).

Generally, the most convenient method of expressing [H^+] is pH. The range of pH in health is 7·36 to 7·42 and in disease from about 6·80 to 7·80, a 10-fold change in [H^+]. An alternative suggestion for this range is to express [H^+] in nmol/l, which emphasises the magnitude of changes in [H^+]. Thus when the pH changes from 7·4 to 7·0, the [H^+] increases by two-and-a-half times and falls to two-fifths from 7·4 to 7·8. These are greater changes than the body can tolerate for some cations, a fact which is not readily apparent from the figures for a change in pH.

The dissociation of an acid (HB) can be represented as

$$HB \underset{k_{-1}}{\overset{k_{+1}}{\rightleftharpoons}} H^+ + B^-$$

where k_{+1} and k_{-1} are the relevant kinetic constants.

Thus at equilibrium

$$[HB] K_a = [H^+][B^-]$$

where K_a is the acid dissociation constant. It follows that

$$[H^+] = K_a \frac{[HB]}{[B^-]}$$

This is the Henderson equation which was put into logarithmic form by Hasselbalch;

$$pH = pKa + \log \frac{[B^-]}{[HB]}$$

The negative logarithm to the base 10 of K_a, termed pK_a, is used to compare the strength of acids in aqueous solution. The smaller the pK_a the stronger the acid. When an acid is 50% ionised, i.e. [HB] is equal to [B^-], the pK_a is numerically equal to the pH of the solution. An indicator is a weak organic acid or base where ionisation is accompanied by a change in colour. An indicator is chosen for a particular titration point if its pK_a is approximately the pH of the equivalence point. Most indicators now in use are synthetic organic compounds, a series of which, given in the Appendix, cover the range from pH 1 to 13 in a series of overlapping ranges. The approximate pH of a solution can be quickly found by observing its reaction with an appropriate indicator.

Buffers

Buffers are solutions of weak acids (or bases) together with their conjugate bases (or acids) which diminish the change in pH which would otherwise occur from the addition of acid or base. The most common examples are solutions of weak acids with one of their salts. As the acid is only relatively slightly dissociated, there is an excess of anions (base) which can accept H^+ should these be added. When base is added, the undissociated acid can dissociate and donate H^+ to the added base. In these ways the added acid or base is neutralised with a much smaller change in $[H^+]$ and pH than would result if the same amount had been added to water. Assuming that the salt is completely ionised and that the ionisation of the weak acid is negligible, the Henderson–Hasselbalch equation;

$$pH = pK_a + \log \frac{[B^-]}{[HB]}$$

can be reformulated in a more convenient form;

$$pH = pK_a + \log \frac{[salt]}{[acid]}$$

The buffering capacity of such systems depends upon two factors: the concentration of the buffer and the pK_a. It is maximal when the salt and acid concentration are equal, i.e. the pH equals pK_a and is mainly effective over the pH range, $pK_a \pm 1$, corresponding to a change in the ratio of concentration of salt/acid from 10 to 0·1.

Hydrogen Ion Metabolism

The pH of ECF is 7·4 (7·36–7·42) while that of ICF is problematic to determine. Estimates of ICF pH have been made using microelectrodes, dimethyl-oxazolidinedione (DMO) and ^{31}P-nuclear magnetic resonance (see Cohen *et al.*, 1982 and Radda *et al.*, 1982 for reviews).

Hydrogen ions are produced following digestion of phospholipids, nucleic acids and proteins. The sulphur-containing amino acids derived from protein digestion are further metabolised with the production of sulphate and H^+. The acid produced can be thought of as a mixture of phosphoric and sulphuric acids (often colloquially referred to as fixed acids), and amounts to 70 mmol/24 h, though it may reach 150 mmol/24 h with a high protein diet.

Aerobic metabolism produces CO_2 (22 mol/24 h) and water (22 mol/24 h, equivalent to 400 ml). The CO_2 and water are catalytically converted by carbonic anhydrase in erythrocytes to carbonic acid which dissociates to yield H^+ and HCO_3^-.

$$CO_2 + H_2O \rightleftharpoons H_2CO_3 \rightleftharpoons H^+ + HCO_3^-$$

In health, there is no net production of H^+ by this mechanism as the reverse reaction rapidly takes place in the pulmonary circulation and the CO_2 (often colloquially called volatile acid) is excreted. The turnover of H^+ in the healthy adult is of the order of 150 mol/24 h (Newsholme and Leach, 1983). In health, the H^+ produced by intermediary metabolism are consumed by other metabolic processes with no net production.

A major example of H^+ turnover occurring in cells is:

$$ATP^{4-} + H_2O \rightarrow ADP^{3-} + HPO_4^{2-} + H^+$$

and

$$ADP^{3-} + HPO_4^{2-} + H^+ \rightarrow ATP^{4-} + H_2O$$

The anaerobic oxidation of glucose in such tissues as the optic nerve and erythrocytes produces lactate, which diffuses into ECF and is transported to the liver and kidney where it is metabolised by gluconeogenesis or other pathways., thus:

$$\text{glucose} \to 2 \text{ lactate}^- + 2 \text{ H}^+$$

and

$$2\text{H}^+ + 2 \text{ lactate}^- \to \text{glucose}$$

Similarly lipolysis in adipose tissue produces palmitate:

$$\text{tripalmitylglycerol} + 3\text{H}_2\text{O} \to \text{glycerol} + 3 \text{ palmitate}^- + 3\text{H}^+$$

and in the liver

$$\text{palmitate}^- + \text{H}^+ + 5\text{O}_2 \to 4 \text{ 3-hydroxybutyrate}^- + 4\text{H}^+$$

In health the small amount of 'ketone bodies' produced by the liver is readily metabolised, though on prolonged fasting the burden of H^+ in the body may be 150 mmol. However, it can be seen how in the unrestrained lipolysis of diabetic ketoacidosis the H^+ production may reach 350 mmol/24 h (Johnson and Alberti, 1983). It is not surprising that with such a large H^+ turnover the most common forms of acid–base disturbances are acidoses.

The H^+ produced by digestion are excreted by the kidney. About 4500 mmol of HCO_3^- are filtered by the glomeruli every 24 h. In the healthy adult eating a normal carnivorous diet, little or no HCO_3^- appears in the urine and the pH is acidic. Proximal renal tubular cells contain intracellular carbonic anhydrase. The H^+ produced (4500 mmol/24 h) by its catalytic action are secreted into the lumen and the HCO_3^- produced (4500 mmol/24 h) enter the systemic circulation. The secretion of H^+ is coupled to the reabsorption of Na^+ (4500 mmol/24 h) and electroneutrality preserved. The secreted $H^{+\cdot}$ reacts (catalytically assisted by carbonic anhydrase in the brush border) with filtered HCO_3^- to produce CO_2 and water. Much of the CO_2 back-diffuses into the renal tubular cells. This process results in no net H^+ excretion and is termed *bicarbonate reclamation*.

Only a small amount of HCO_3^- (10% of that filtered at the glomerulus) enters the distal tubule where further H^+ is secreted into the tubular lumen in response to the acid load. Some H^+ is buffered (mainly by HPO_4^{2-}) and accounts for the titratable acidity (30 mmol/24 h). The remainder is excreted as NH_4^+ (40 mmol/24 h), ammonia having been secreted by renal tubular cells. The stoichiometry of this latter process is debatable (Newsholme and Leach, 1983; McGilvery, 1983). For each H^+ excreted a HCO_3^- is *regenerated*. For each NH_4^+ excreted a Na^+ is retained. The major anion excreted is Cl^-.

Regulation of pH

The constancy of pH is maintained in the first instance by physiological buffers and later by the elimination of H^+ and CO_2. Buffers may be intracellular or extracellular. Intracellular buffers are known to be very important (Pitts, 1974) and consist mainly of protein and to a lesser extent bicarbonate and phosphates. Their role will not be further discussed, save for haemoglobin in erythrocytes. 'Bone buffering' is also of importance, particularly in chronic metabolic acidoses, H^+ displacing Ca^{2+} and Na^+ from the crystal lattice structure (Pitts, 1974).

1. **Physiological Buffers**. Three buffer systems are important.

Dihydrogenphosphate-monohydrogenphosphate. This system of pK_a 6·8, plays a very minor part in blood but is more important in the tissues and particularly in the urine for regulating pH.

$$\text{H}_2\text{PO}_4^- \rightleftharpoons \text{HPO}_4^{2-} + \text{H}^+$$

Protein buffers. In plasma these play a much smaller part than the bicarbonate system but in all cells (particularly erythrocytes) proteins form a most important buffering system. At the pH of blood the plasma proteins are anions acting as weak acids:

$$H \cdot Protein^{(n-1)-} \rightleftharpoons H^+ + Protein^{n-}$$

The imidazole ring of histidine has a pK_a of 6·0–7·0 (the exact value in a protein being dependent upon its micro-environment).

$$H^+ + N \qquad CH_2-CH-COO^- \rightleftharpoons HN^+ \qquad CH_2-CH-COO^-$$

The buffering properties of proteins are mainly dependent on histidine residues. Haemoglobin has a very high histidine content (36 residues/molecule) and is present in blood in high concentration (150 g/l). For these reasons it has a large buffering capacity. Oxyhaemoglobin is a stronger acid than (reduced) haemoglobin so when oxygen is released in tissues and CO_2 taken up, H^+ from the carbonic acid is buffered by the reduced haemoglobin and little change in pH results. The haemoglobin buffer system is of particular importance in hypercapnia. Haemoglobin also acts reversibly with carbonic acid giving an even weaker carbamino acid.

Carbonic acid-bicarbonate. The equilibrium of the first reaction is very much to the left, the concentration of dissolved CO_2 being some 600 times that of carbonic

$$(\text{dissolved } CO_2) + H_2O \overset{(1)}{\rightleftharpoons} H \cdot HCO_3 \overset{(2)}{\rightleftharpoons} H^+ + HCO_3^- \overset{(3)}{\rightleftharpoons} H^+ + CO_3^{2-}$$

acid at 37 °C. The contribution of reaction (3) is assumed to be negligible at physiological pHs. Thus the Henderson–Hasselbalch equation for this system may be written:

$$pH = pK_1 + \log \frac{[HCO_3^-]}{[\text{dissolved } CO_2]}$$

where pK_1 is the 'overall' first dissociation constant of H_2CO_3. Quantitatively it is easily the most important buffer system in plasma and also plays some part in the red cells. Although the pK_1 is 6·1, it is a particularly flexible buffer system system since an excess of CO_2 can be removed by the lungs and HCO_3^- excreted by the kidney.

2. Respiratory Control. Carbon dioxide is continuously produced in the tissues by aerobic metabolism. It diffuses into venous plasma along a pressure gradient and thence enters erythrocytes which contain the enzyme carbonic anhydrase catalysing the reaction:

$$(\text{dissolved } CO_2) + H_2O \rightleftharpoons H \cdot HCO_3 \rightleftharpoons H^+ + HCO_3^-$$

The H^+ produced is buffered by haemoglobin in the erythrocytes. The HCO_3^- formed, diffuses into the plasma down a concentration gradient; Cl^- moves in the opposite direction to maintain electroneutrality (chloride shift). The lung capillaries are in intimate contact with the alveoli. As blood passes through the lungs, CO_2 diffuses into the alveoli along a pressure gradient and the reactions described above are reversed.

Alveolar ventilation is influenced by pH and P_{CO_2}. A fall in pH or a rise in P_{CO_2} increases alveolar ventilation and excretion of CO_2, resulting in a fall in alveolar and arterial blood P_{CO_2}. The converse occurs following an increase in pH. These changes occur rapidly and take minutes to hours to become maximal. The P_{CO_2} of arterial blood is directly proportional to the CO_2 production rate and inversely proportional to alveolar ventilation.

3. Renal Control. A rise in P_{CO_2} or a fall in pH stimulates carbonic anhydrase activity, ammonia production and the consequent excretion of excess H^+ as described on p. 582. Ammonium ion excretion may reach 400 mmol/24 h. The excretion of NH_4^+ is extremely important in minimising losses of Na^+, and maintaining ECF volume and composition. The renal response in contrast to the respiratory response, takes about 5 days to become maximal.

Determination of the Parameters Affecting Acid–Base Balance

Variations in the carbonic acid-bicarbonate system are technically convenient to study and are frequently used in assessing acid–base disturbances. The three factors are related as follows:

$$pH = pK_1 + \log \frac{[HCO_3^-]}{[\text{dissolved } CO_2]}$$

where concentrations are in mmol/l, or

$$pH = pK_1 + \log \frac{[HCO_3^-]}{0.0301 \times P_{CO_2}}$$

where P_{CO_2} is the partial pressure of CO_2 in mmHg. For plasma, $pK_1 = 6.10$ (Robinson *et al.*, 1934), range 6.071 to 6.117. So if any two of these three quantities are known, the third can be calculated.

1. Blood pH

The principles of the glass H^+ electrode have been described (p. 565). The most accurate results are obtained using arterial whole blood collected with a small amount of heparin (up to 1 mg per ml) as anticoagulant, and read as soon as possible. The blood is best kept at 0 to 4 °C. Siggaard-Andersen (1961) showed that no significant change then occurred within 3 h. If the blood had to be kept at room temperature for this time he used 1 mg sodium fluoride per ml blood and found a variable error from +0.006 to −0.014 in pH.

The tendency is for the pH of plasma to become more alkaline than that of whole blood on keeping. Plasma separated from whole blood which has been cooled to room temperature and reheated to 38 °C has a pH 0.003 units per °C higher so that the average difference will be about 0.05 (Nunn, 1959). In addition to this effect there is also one of time. On standing, the pH of whole blood exposed to air changes slowly, in contrast the pH of plasma changes rapidly, rising to well over 8.0 in 45 min.

2. Blood P_{CO_2} (Respiratory Parameter)

This is the P_{CO_2} of arterial blood collected anaerobically and is expressed in mmHg (or kPa). It is related to the percentage of CO_2 in alveolar air or plasma.

$$P_{CO_2} = (\text{Barometric pressure} - \text{Water vapour pressure}) \times \frac{\% CO_2}{100}$$

At 37 °C the water vapour pressure at saturation is 47 mmHg (6·25 kPa). Thus at a barometric pressure of 750 mmHg (99·8 kPa), 5·7 % CO_2 corresponds to a P_{CO_2} of 40 mmHg (5·32 kPa). The [dissolved CO_2] in mmol/l can be obtained by multiplying the P_{CO_2} in mmHg by 0·030 1 (CO_2 solubility constant) or if in kPa by 0·226.

3. Metabolic Parameter

Several different quantities (all measured in mmol/l) are used.

(a) *The actual bicarbonate* concentration in plasma separated from blood taken anaerobically is not measured directly but can be calculated from the pH and P_{CO_2} using the Henderson–Hasselbalch equation.

(b) *Standard bicarbonate* (Jørgensen and Astrup, 1957; Astrup, 1959) is $[HCO_3^-]$ in plasma from whole blood which has been equilibrated at 37 °C at a P_{CO_2} of 40 mmHg (5·32 kPa) and with oxygen to give full saturation of haemoglobin. Plasma $[HCO_3^-]$ is influenced by changes in P_{CO_2} and the degree of oxygen saturation. Under these standard conditions the effect of altered respiration is eliminated. Changes in standard bicarbonate are thus due only to non-respiratory factors.

(c) *Base Excess* (BE) (Siggaard-Andersen and Engel, 1960; Mellengaard and Astrup, 1960; Siggaard-Andersen, 1964) is defined as the titratable base on titration to normal pH (7·40) at normal P_{CO_2} (40 mmHg or 5·32 kPa) and normal temperature (37 °C), and is expressed in mmol/l. It is positive if there is an actual excess of base or deficit of acid. On the other hand, if non-volatile acid has to be titrated to bring the blood to pH 7·40 at P_{CO_2} 40 mmHg (5·32 kPa), the BE is negative; there is an actual deficit of base or an excess of acid. It is unaffected by haemoglobin concentration.

4. Total Carbon Dioxide

Total carbon dioxide (often erroneously called bicarbonate) is that liberated from dissolved CO_2 and HCO_3^- present in plasma when blood is drawn anaerobically and not further treated. [Total CO_2] = $[HCO_3^-]$ + 0·0301 P_{CO_2} (mmHg). When [total CO_2] is to be determined the usual equation becomes:

$$pH = 6·10 + \log \frac{\text{Total } CO_2 - 0·0301\ P_{CO_2}}{0·0301\ P_{CO_2}}$$

The determination of [total CO_2] in venous blood without measurement of pH or P_{CO_2} is often performed, usually using automated equipment, often in multi-channel form. The analysis is performed on plasma which has not been separated anaerobically nor re-equilibrated with gas of known CO_2 content. The method relies on the colour change of an indicator in a carbonate–bicarbonate buffer following the release of CO_2 on acidification of the sample. Alternatively, this CO_2 can be measured by a P_{CO_2} electrode. The methods underestimate the original [total CO_2] by 2 to 3 mmol/l but have the advantage that arterial puncture is not required though the finding of an abnormal result may need to be followed by a fuller appraisal of acid–base status.

Use of the 'Blood Gas' Analyser

Most instruments used for acid–base measurement on blood incorporate a P_{O_2} electrode which makes a useful additional contribution to the study of respiratory and circulatory disturbances. In some instruments, a single blood sample is in contact with pH, P_{CO_2} and P_{O_2} electrodes simultaneously, in others the electrodes are in contact with separate sub-samples. In most instruments, capillary samples in addition to arterial blood samples are suitable. The sample volume required may be as low as 50 μl. A further refinement is the addition of a microprocessor which can calculate standard bicarbonate, actual bicarbonate, [total CO_2] and base excess. This can be combined with automatic calibration and washing cycles. The use of derived parameters is questionable (see p. 589) as they are dependent upon the applicability of the Henderson–Hasselbalch equation to real patients rather than blood specimens and the validity of the algorithms used by the manufacturer.

Calibration. The primary standards for pH measurements are phosphate buffers, pH 6·840 and pH 7·384 prepared to the US National Bureau of Standards' specifications. For P_{CO_2} the primary calibration standards are gas mixtures of known CO_2 content, often 5% and 10%. Their accuracy should be guaranteed by the manufacturer and may be checked by infrared spectroscopy. The gases must be humidified. P_{CO_2} is determined by the percentage composition, barometric pressure and vapour pressure of water (see p. 584).

The P_{O_2} electrode is also calibrated using two gases of known composition. An oxygen mixture of 12% or 20% is commonly used for the higher level and nitrogen (oxygen-free) for the other. Again the gases must be humidified and the P_{O_2} calculated. P_{O_2} electrodes respond differently to dissolved oxygen and gaseous oxygen (blood–gas difference). In general the more modern the instrument the smaller the blood–gas difference, but it can never be eliminated. It is due in part to the rate of gas diffusion across the membrane, the geometry of the electrode and the amount of oxygen consumed at the cathode. The value is approximately 2·5% at 100 mmHg but increases with P_{O_2}. When analysing specimens with a high P_{O_2} it is advisable to calibrate with a gas mixture close to the specimen value. The electrode response may not be linear at high values of P_{O_2} and the blood-gas difference is increased. If a tonometer is available it is possible to equilibrate whole blood with gases of known P_{O_2} and P_{CO_2} to provide the most physiological calibration materials. The blood–gas difference for a given P_{O_2} can thus be determined. In clinical practice, the blood-gas difference produces few problems. Care must be taken with the measurement of P_{O_2} in the presence of anaesthetic gases. Both halothane (Douglas *et al.*, 1978; Norden and Flynn, 1979) and nitrous oxide (Evans and Cameron, 1978) interfere with some P_{O_2} electrodes. Spuriously low P_{O_2} values may be observed in blood from patients with a high leucocyte count, perhaps due to fouling of the membrane (Chan *et al.*, 1984).

Precision. Studies can be performed using tonometered plasma or whole blood and commercially available equilibrated buffer solutions. Liquid materials are preferable as these are better for detecting faults in the electrode membrane or performance, temperature control, and in sample introduction technique. Commercial QC preparations are usually purchased in sealed ampoules with target values for pH, P_{CO_2} and P_{O_2}. Most are aqueous but some contain stroma-free human erythrocytes; neither are cheap. Their main drawback is that they do not mimic blood in respect of ionic strength, viscosity or temperature coefficient of the buffer and are usually single-phase containing no protein. They also have low oxygen affinity. Despite these problems, they provide useful day-to-day checks of precision.

The method of choice, where available, is tonometry. A single tonometer can be used to monitor the performance of a number of blood gas analysers, including those on extra-laboratory sites. Sterile frozen plasma can be used for pH studies after thawing an aliquot and equilibrating with a gas of constant P_{CO_2} (Bird and Henderson, 1971). Fresh whole blood can be similarly equilibrated with CO_2 and oxygen gas mixtures.

Minty and Nunn (1977) reported precision figures within one laboratory over a 12 week period giving SDs for serum of 0·011 for pH, 0·83 mmHg (0·11 kPa) for P_{O_2} and 1·2 mmHg (0·16 kPa) for P_{CO_2}. If the same blood sample was separately equilibrated with the same gas mixture in a tonometer in individual laboratories, the between-laboratory SDs were higher at 0·023 for pH, 5·4 mmHg (0·72 kPa) for P_{O_2} and 2·1 mmHg (0·28 kPa) for P_{CO_2}. Evans (1978) comparing different control materials over 3 weeks on a single instrument found the following SDs for a tonometered buffer solution: pH, 0·007; P_{O_2}, 2·8 mmHg (0·37 kPa); P_{CO_2}, 1·4 mmHg (0·19 kPa). If a commercial blood gas control preparation was used freshly daily, the SDs were a little higher but the accuracy of the measurements was in doubt while that of the tonometered buffer was satisfactory.

For indirect measurements of standard bicarbonate the precision will depend on the errors in pH and P_{CO_2} measurement. The achievable between-batch precision for the direct determination of plasma [total CO_2] is 1 mmol/l.

Notes.
1. *Use of capillary blood.* Under ordinary conditions capillary blood is similar to arterial. However, it cannot be assumed to be so in patients with a poor peripheral circulation. For satisfactory results a good flow of capillary blood is essential. If this cannot be obtained arterial blood must be used. If the patient's hand is cold, warm in warm water at 45 to 50 °C for at least 4 min. A falsely low pH is obtained if circulation is poor. Arterial blood is used from patients with hypothermia.
2. In hypothermia a correction can be made for the low body temperature. The measurements are made at 37 °C. Then if T is the actual body temperature:

$$\text{pH at } T °C = \text{pH at } 37 °C + 0·0146 (37 - T)$$

and

$$P_{CO_2} \text{ at } T °C = \text{anti-log} (\log P_{CO_2} \text{ at } 37 °C - 0·021 (37 - T)).$$

The appropriate calculation is uncertain (see Ashwood *et al.*, 1983 for a review). Blood gas analysers often calculate corrected pH, P_{CO_2} and P_{O_2} but different manufacturers use different algorithms. It is sensible to report results as measured, whatever the temperature of the patient, as the 'normal' values for such patients are unknown (Whitby *et al.*, 1984).
3. Exercise causes a profound change so that after activity a period of rest is necessary.
4. Blood must not be exposed to air. This can be avoided when collecting into capillary tubes as described above.
5. Fear and painful arterial puncture may induce hyperventilation.

ACID-BASE DISTURBANCES

Reference Intervals

Actual bicarbonate, 24 to 33 mmol/l.
Arterial P_{CO_2}, 34 to 45 mmHg (4·52 to 5·98 kPa) or 1·02 to 1·35 mmol/l.
Standard bicarbonate, 22·4 to 25·8 mmol/l.
Base excess of blood, −2·3 to 2·3 mmol/l.
pH 7·36 to 7·45.

Definitions

Acidaemia—a blood pH below the lower reference interval.

Alkalaemia—a blood pH above the upper reference interval.

Acidosis—an abnormal process which produces acidaemia or would do so if no compensation (secondary change) were to occur.

Alkalosis—an abnormal process which produces alkalaemia or would do so if no compensation were to occur.

These definitions make a clear distinction between acidaemia (or alkalaemia) which is a chemical description and acidosis (or alkalosis) which is a pathophysiological description without regard to blood pH (Campbell, 1984).

Types of Disturbance

Four *primary* acid–base disturbances are possible. An acidosis can result from either a primary increase in P_{CO_2} or a primary decrease in plasma $[HCO_3^-]$. Likewise, an alkalosis can result from either a primary increase in plasma $[HCO_3^-]$ or a primary decrease in P_{CO_2}. Primary changes in P_{CO_2} are due to alterations in ventilation resulting in acidosis or alkalosis and are described as *respiratory*. Primary changes in plasma $[HCO_3^-]$ resulting in acidosis or alkalosis are usually termed *metabolic*. Two or more primary changes may coexist; a *mixed* disturbance. The changes can be additive so that the acidosis or alkalosis has both a respiratory and a metabolic component. Some workers prefer the term non-respiratory since changes in $[HCO_3^-]$ due to renal insufficiency or to loss of gastrointestinal contents are not metabolic. The Henderson–Hasselbalch equation can be reformulated

$$pH \propto \log \frac{\text{Metabolic or non-respiratory parameter}}{\text{Respiratory parameter}}$$

Whenever a primary change occurs in one of these factors there is usually a (partial) compensatory change in the other. Thus a primary fall in $[HCO_3^-]$ is generally accompanied by a secondary fall in P_{CO_2} due to increased alveolar ventilation. A primary increase in plasma $[HCO_3^-]$ is followed by reduced ventilation thus increasing P_{CO_2} in the alveolar air and hence plasma. The change in ventilation is a direct consequence of the effect of pH on the respiratory centre. In this way a metabolic acidosis or alkalosis is, in varying degree, compensated by a change in the rate of respiration. Conversely, a primary disturbance of respiration may be partly compensated by a change in plasma $[HCO_3^-]$. Thus plasma $[HCO_3^-]$ rises in hypoventilation and falls in hyperventilation. The change in P_{CO_2} increases the renal tubular secretion of H^+ and regeneration of HCO_3^- (see p. 582). If the P_{CO_2} decreases, the tubular secretion of H^+ is reduced to such degree that there is insufficient to neutralise the HCO_3^- normally present in the glomerular filtrate, resulting in an alkaline urine. If the change is well compensated, blood pH remains within normal limits. However, as the primary disturbance becomes more severe, compensation is only partial and pH then becomes abnormal.

pH and P_{CO_2} are the only two directly measured parameters; all others are derived. The *respiratory parameter* is defined as P_{CO_2}. The *metabolic parameter* used is a matter of choice. The standard bicarbonate, BE and actual bicarbonate have all been used. Standard bicarbonate and BE have the advantage that they are independent of the P_{CO_2} but the disadvantage that they are derived from *in vitro* manipulations and may not reflect *in vivo* circumstances. Actual bicarbonate has the disadvantage that it is not independent of P_{CO_2} and so is not a 'true' metabolic parameter. In practice, this causes little confusion. The advantage is that it reflects *in vivo* circumstances. The Henderson–Hasselbalch equation is not always strictly applicable (see Howorth, 1975 for a full discussion) but in practice few problems arise (Hood and Campbell, 1982). Errors in derived parameters are in part dependent upon errors in measurement of pH and P_{CO_2} and also the method of calculation used. The latter is of particular importance when using automated blood gas analysers, as different instrument manufacturers use a variety of algorithms (Kofstad, 1981).

Alternative approaches to the evaluation of acid–base disturbances using *in vivo* data without recourse to derived parameters and the associated assumptions are available (Flenley, 1978; Stoker *et al.*, 1972), the most popular being that of Flenley (Fig. 23.6). Hydrogen ion concentration (or pH) is plotted against P_{CO_2} (or log P_{CO_2}). Results can be plotted on the chart and patient management followed by plotting subsequent results.

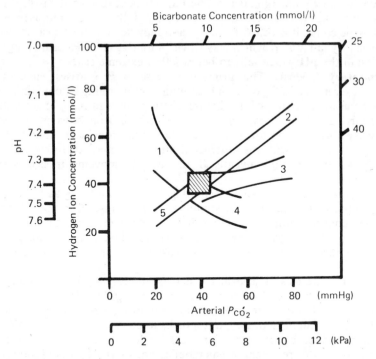

Fig. 23.6. Acid–Base Diagram (after Flenley, 1978).
Points are plotted on the diagram after determination of the two primary measurements, pH (or $[H^+]$) and P_{CO_2} of arterial blood. The bicarbonate concentration is obtained by extrapolation of a line joining the origin to this point. The shaded rectangle is that defined by the two reference ranges. The curved lines indicate the 95 % confidence limits of the pH/P_{CO_2} relationship in single disturbances of acid–base balance. The numbered areas correspond to: 1, metabolic acidosis; 2, acute respiratory acidosis; 3, chronic respiratory acidosis with compensation; 4, metabolic alkalosis; 5, respiratory alkalosis.

Description of Disturbances

Metabolic Acidosis. This primary decrease in $[HCO_3^-]$ arises either from increased production or decreased removal of acids (other than H_2CO_3) which deplete plasma $[HCO_3^-]$, or by loss of base (usually HCO_3^-) from the body. Common causes are diabetic ketoacidosis, mild ketoacidosis seen in starvation and lactic acidosis (see p. 593). Decreased elimination of H^+ occurs in acute or advanced chronic renal failure and renal tubular acidosis type I. Ingestion of NH_4Cl produces an acidosis since the ammonia is converted to urea, liberating H^+ which neutralises HCO_3^-.

Direct loss of HCO_3^- in secretions occurs in prolonged watery diarrhoea and in patients with an intestinal, biliary, or pancreatic fistula, and renal tubular acidosis type II. Acetazolamide, a carbonic anhydrase inhibitor, has a similar effect; so has chlorothiazide. Transplantation of the ureters into the lower part of the alimentary tract can produce a similar acidosis since Cl^- is more rapidly absorbed and hence replaces HCO_3^-.

Compensatory mechanisms include an early increase in pulmonary ventilation and, as a slower 'recovery' process, increased secretion of H^+ and ammonia by the kidneys. In an adequately compensated mild to moderate acidosis, the standard bicarbonate is usually between normal and 14 mmol/l with a fall in P_{CO_2} to between 30 and 25 mmHg (4·0 and 3·5 kPa) sufficient to keep the pH near to or within normal limits. In severe cases, the $[HCO_3^-]$ falls further until, as in diabetic and uraemic coma, it is below 6 mmol/l and may be almost unmeasurable. The compensatory fall in P_{CO_2} which may reach 14 mmHg (1·9 kPa) is no longer able to maintain the pH which falls to below 7·0 in extreme cases.

Respiratory Acidosis. This primary increase in P_{CO_2} arises when there is impaired excretion of CO_2 or from breathing or rebreathing air containing CO_2. It may occur in any chronic lung disease whether this is primary or secondary to some heart condition. Common causes are chronic bronchitis, emphysema or pulmonary fibrosis. It occurs in more acute form in bronchial asthma and in the unconscious patient with an obstructed airway. It may also develop, e.g. in myasthenia, and in poliomyelitis if the muscle movements necessary for respiration are affected.

The P_{CO_2} will not rise above 100 mmHg (13·3 kPa) as long as the patient is breathing room air because of the stimulus of hypoxia (see Campbell, 1965) but, if a higher concentration of oxygen is given, much higher values can be reached and survived. The compensatory increase in standard bicarbonate can reach 35 to 40 mmol/l and is accompanied by a fall in plasma Cl^- with the secretion of a more acid urine.

Metabolic Alkalosis. This primary increase in plasma $[HCO_3^-]$ is due to the accumulation of base or loss of acid other than H_2CO_3. This can occur with therapy such as HCO_3^- itself, but citrate (e.g. following massive blood transfusion with blood containing sodium citrate) or lactate are both oxidised to HCO_3^-. More marked disturbances occur if an excessive dose of $NaHCO_3$ has been given intravenously in the treatment of a metabolic acidosis. It may occur following loss of HCl by vomiting or by gastric aspiration. Potassium deficiency tends to produce an alkalosis by migration of H^+ into ICF.

The increase in standard bicarbonate can reach 45 to 50 mmol/l. There is usually some respiratory compensation with P_{CO_2} 45 to 55 mmHg (6·0 to 7·3 kPa). Very rarely full compensation with P_{CO_2} up to 70 mmHg (9·3 kPa) occurs in young persons. The pH can rise up to about 7·65 in the most severe cases.

Respiratory Alkalosis. This primary decrease in plasma P_{CO_2} is due to excessive ventilation. Hyperventilation occurs physiologically at high altitudes, the stimulus being oxygen lack but it can be produced by excessively rapid and deep respirations in normal persons. Clinically, it can be seen in patients with encephalitis, in hysterical attacks, in salicylate poisoning, in fever particularly in association with septicaemia, and in some cases of cerebral tumour. P_{CO_2} can fall to 20 mmHg (2·7 kPa) and pH rise to about 7·55; the compensatory fall in plasma $[HCO_3^-]$ can be between normal and about 18 mmol/l. The compensation is achieved by the passage of an alkaline urine. A sudden change in pulmonary ventilation is reflected quickly in a change in P_{CO_2}; the compensatory change in $[HCO_3^-]$ takes longer to occur. Thus in acute hysterical attacks the fall in P_{CO_2} is uncompensated and pH rises as the P_{CO_2} falls.

Tetany, which occurs when there is reduced ionised plasma calcium (see p. 610) may also develop in alkalosis and so may be found in patients with severer forms of metabolic or respiratory alkalosis. The proportion of ionised calcium falls as pH rises (Bull, 1955).

In the above four cases a compensatory change tends to counteract the primary change. However, the changes in both acidosis and alkalosis can be additive.

Combined Respiratory and Metabolic Acidosis. This may occur when there is profound circulatory failure leading to severe hypoxia. P_{CO_2} is increased because of the depressed respiration while formation of lactic acid in the tissues neutralises HCO_3^-. This occurs, e.g. following cardiac arrest, in severe barbiturate overdosage and in respiratory distress of the newborn.

Combined Respiratory and Metabolic Alkalosis. This may develop during the treatment of primary respiratory acidosis. Thus in severe bronchitis, in which P_{CO_2} is raised and a compensatory rise in HCO_3^- is present, removal of the excess CO_2 on a respirator can correct and reverse the change in P_{CO_2} while the more slowly changing HCO_3^- remains increased. In salicylate poisoning, respiration is stimulated so that P_{CO_2} falls while an accompanying primary metabolic acidosis produces a fall in HCO_3^-. The two changes may largely *counteract* each other leaving the pH little altered if at all. However, the salicylate may cause vomiting; then sufficient acid may be lost from the stomach to produce an alkalosis which has both a respiratory and metabolic component.

The Determination of Blood Lactate

The determination of lactate concentration by spectrophotometry using lactate dehydrogenase (LD) is simple and specific. LD converts lactate into pyruvate in the presence of nicotinamide adenine dinucleotide (NAD^+), under alkaline conditions. The amount of NADH formed is measured at 340 nm. The lactate and pyruvate are normally in equilibrium but the reaction is caused to proceed to pyruvate formation by an excess of NAD^+ and by converting pyruvate into its hydrazone using hydrazine. Instruments using immobilised enzymes coupled to a P_{O_2} electrode are now available. The blood can be collected with venous stasis but with the patient resting. In particular, muscular activity of the arm should be avoided (Braybrooke *et al.*, 1975). Any enzyme activity affecting pyruvate and lactate concentrations is avoided by immediate inactivation with perchloric acid. Plasma is suitable if fluoride/EDTA preservative is used.

Spectrophotometric Method Using Lactate Dehydrogenase

Reagents.

1. Glycine buffer, pH 9·0 (0·5 mol/l) containing hydrazine (0·4 mol/l). Dissolve 3·753 g glycine and 2·925 g NaCl in water and make up to 100 ml. Add 89 ml to 11 ml NaOH (0·5 mol/l) and add 5·20 g hydrazine sulphate. Adjust the pH if necessary with NaOH.
2. NAD^+ solution, 27 mmol/l, 20 mg in 1 ml.
3. LD solution containing 2 mg enzyme protein in 1 ml.
4. Perchloric acid. Dilute 5 ml of the 70 % acid to 100 ml with doubly distilled water.

Technique. Add 0·5 ml blood, immediately after collection, to 1 ml perchloric acid, mix well and centrifuge. Measure 200 μl supernatant fluid into a tube containing 2 ml buffer and 20 μl LD solution. Then add 200 μl NAD^+ solution, shake well to mix and keep at 25 °C in a water bath for 1 h. Read against a reagent blank, using perchloric acid instead of the supernatant, at 340 nm in 1 cm cells.

Calculation. Since the absorbance of a 1 mol/l solution of NADH is 6·30 and as the final volume of 2·42 ml contains 0·2 ml of supernatant, then if ΔA is the increase in absorbance

$$\text{Blood lactate (mmol/l)} = \frac{\Delta A}{6\cdot30} \times \frac{2\cdot42}{0\cdot2} \times F$$

where F is the dilution of the whole blood in the perchloric acid. Allowing for the water content and specific gravity of blood this factor is 2·85. Hence

$$\text{Blood lactate (mmol/l)} = \Delta A \times 5\cdot47$$

Notes

1. The amount of lactate in the reaction mixture should not exceed 0·2 μmol in order to preserve an appreciable excess of NAD^+. If necessary take a smaller volume of the supernatant fluid and adjust the calculation accordingly.
2. A standard lactic acid solution can be used to check the method.
3. A reagent kit is available from the Boehringer Corporation from whose leaflet the above method is taken.
4. Trichloracetic acid, 100 g in 1 l 0·5 mol/l HCl can be used instead of perchloric acid.
5. The supernatant fluid can be stored without change for at least 12 h at 40 °C.

INTERPRETATION

Lactate is derived exclusively from pyruvate in the presence of LD, hydrogen being supplied by NADH. The equilibrium is normally markedly in the direction of lactate with a lactate/pyruvate ratio of approximately 9, but is controlled by the ratio of NADH to NAD^+. During anaerobic glycolysis NADH is formed during the dehydrogenation of 3-phosphoglyceraldehyde to 3-phosphoglycerate and is usually reconverted into NAD^+ during oxidative phosphorylation. If this is less active or the rate of formation of NADH is increased then NAD^+ is regenerated by interaction of NADH with pyruvate whereby lactate is formed. Major factors in producing an increase in lactate are thus hypoxaemia and an increased rate of glycolysis.

In health, lactate is produced (1500 mmol/24 h) by resting muscle, erythrocytes and nervous tissue. The major sites of removal are the liver and kidney. In adults, arterial blood lactate in the completely resting state varies from 0·47 to 0·78 (mean

0·62) mmol/l but venous blood lactate taken under usual conditions varies from 0·76 to 1·25 (mean 1·00) mmol/l.

Hyperlactataemia unaccompanied by an acidosis is of little consequence. Blood lactate rises to 26 mmol/l following severe muscular exercise. Many definitions of lactic acidosis have been made (see Woods, 1971). Lactic acidosis is best considered as a primary metabolic acidosis (pH usually less than 7·25) with a blood lactate concentration greater than 5 mmol/l which is near the renal threshold (6·7 mmol/l). The disturbance may be due to increased H^+ and lactate production, to decreased H^+ and lactate removal, or a combination of both. It may be amplified by loss of base (lactate) in the urine. In abnormal conditions, values up to 26 mmol/l may be seen and can change rapidly. As lactate accumulates it replaces HCO_3^- producing an increased 'anion gap'. Confusion in diagnosis can occur because other primary metabolic acidoses, e.g. uraemic acidosis may co-exist.

Lactic acidosis Type A occurs in hypoxaemic states of either circulatory or respiratory origin. Large changes are seen in shock with peripheral circulatory failure or during operations with by-pass circulation and in their most severe form following cardiac arrest.

Lactic acidosis Type B occurs with a normal circulation and oxygenation of blood. It is associated with systemic disorders such as diabetes mellitus, severe infection, leukaemia, liver and renal disease. It also can be precipitated by drugs and poisons, e.g. ethanol, phenformin and salicylates. Some inherited disorders such as G6PD deficiency may be a cause.

In some cases of alkalosis, following $NaHCO_3$ infusion and particularly due to hyperventilation following salicylate poisoning, the liver is converted from an organ that utilises lactate (via gluconeogenesis and other pathways) to an organ that produces lactate (via glycolysis). Lactic acidosis has been extensively reviewed (Krebs *et al.*, 1975; Relman, 1978).

pH of Urine

This determination is best done on freshly voided urine using a pH meter. Less accurate results can be obtained with indicator papers. For most normal persons the pH varies from 5·2 to 6·8 but it is lower on a high meat diet and may be above 7·0 in vegetarians. In diabetic ketosis, the pH may be as low as 4·6. Urines which have been allowed to stand are easily infected with urease-producing organisms and the pH of such urines may be alkaline due to ammonia production. In generalised renal disease, even when glomerular filtration rate is markedly reduced, the urinary pH is still within normal limits although titratable acidity and NH_4^+ excretion are reduced. The measurement of urine pH on a random specimen of urine is of little clinical value.

Determination of Titratable Acidity

A suitable volume of fresh urine is titrated with NaOH (50 mmol/l) to pH 7·4 using a pH meter.

$$\text{Titratable acidity (mmol/24 h)} = \text{ml NaOH} \times \frac{\text{Volume 24 h urine}}{\text{Volume urine titrated}} \times \frac{50}{1000}$$

The normal titratable acidity is 15 to 40 mmol/24 h (mean 30). Values up to 150 mmol/24 h occur in severe diabetic acidosis. Titratable acidity is reduced in alkalosis and becomes zero when the urinary pH is 7·4 or more. In generalised renal disease and renal tubular acidosis titratable acidity is reduced.

Determination of Ammonia Using the Berthelot Reaction
(Henry, 1964)

Reagents.
1. Phenol–sodium nitroprusside solution, 50 g phenol and 0·25 g nitroprusside/l. Dilute 1 to 5 for use.
2. Sodium hydroxide-sodium hypochlorite, 25 g of the hydroxide and 2·1 g hypochlorite per litre. Dilute 1 to 5 for use.
   These two solutions keep at least two months in brown bottles if cold.
3. Standard solution of ammonium sulphate, 1·320 g/l ($\equiv$ 20 mmol/l NH_4^+).

Technique. Measure 2 ml phenol reagent into each of four test tubes. To one add 40 μl fresh urine diluted 5-fold (the test), to the second and third add 20 and 40 μl respectively of standard. The fourth tube serves as blank. To each add 2 ml alkaline hypochlorite, place in a bath at 55 °C for 3 min, then keep at 37 °C for 20 min. Remove, and if necessary dilute the test to bring to a satisfactory absorbance. Read test and standards against the blank at 630 nm.

Calculation. For the weaker standard and no further dilution of the test:

$$\text{Urinary } [NH_4^+] \text{ (mmol/24 h)} = \frac{\text{Reading of unknown}}{\text{Reading of standard}}$$

$$\times \frac{5}{40} \times 20 \times 20 \times \frac{\text{Volume 24 h urine (ml)}}{1\,000}$$

The normal NH_4^+ excretion is 25 to 60 (mean 40) mmol/24 h on an average diet, increasing if acid-forming foods are eaten and decreasing with an alkali-producing diet. Ammonium ion excretion is almost always higher than titratable acidity in normal urine. In diabetic acidosis, there is a marked increase up to 400 mmol/24 h. The NH_4^+ excretion may then form as much as 40% of the total urinary non-protein nitrogen. There is also an increase in the acidosis of starvation. In generalised renal disease, the mass of tubular cells is reduced as is H^+ secretion but NH_4^+ excretion is depressed relatively more. In renal tubular acidosis, the excretion of NH_4^+ is relatively well preserved. Urine which has been kept for a few hours without preservative is unsuitable for the determination as NH_3 is formed from urea by bacteria.

Short Test of the Tubular Ability to Excrete an Acid Load
(Wrong and Davies, 1959)

No restriction of activity or meals is necessary for the test. At 06.00 h the patient empties his/her bladder and the urine is discarded. Further urine samples are collected hourly until 16.00 h and saved separately. The samples should be stored on ice as collected and sent to the laboratory at the end of the test. At 08.00 h, NH_4Cl, 0·1 g/kg body weight, is given orally in hard gelatin capsules (*not* enteric-coated) over the space of an hour; it is important that the patient takes them over this period as otherwise the large dose will provoke nausea and vomiting. Venous blood is collected for plasma [total CO_2] at 08.00 h and noon in order to check that the NH_4Cl has produced an acidosis. The pH of all urine samples is measured. The $[NH_4^+]$ is measured in the urine collected prior to and in the pooled samples collected after the dose of NH_4Cl.

INTERPRETATION

Normal persons pass at least one specimen of urine with a pH of 5·3 or less and have an NH_4^+ excretion of 30 to 90 μmol/min. This excretion rate is reduced proportionately to any reduction in GFR. In most cases of chronic renal failure there is a systemic metabolic acidosis; the ability of the kidney to secrete a urine of low pH is unimpaired although the NH_4^+ excretion rate is much reduced.

In renal tubular acidosis (see below) type I, the urinary pH does not reach 5·3 or less during the test. The NH_4^+ excretion is usually normal unless there is an associated reduction in GFR or parenchymal renal damage. Patients with renal tubular acidosis type II are able to excrete an acid urine with a pH of 5·3 or less during the test. The test is of particular value in the investigation of the 'incomplete' form of type I.

Renal tubular acidosis is a metabolic acidosis accompanied by a decreased ability to secrete H^+. The cases of renal tubular acidosis have been divided into two main types (Wrong, 1967). In type I (distal tubular defect) there is a failure to generate H^+ in the distal tubule resulting in a diminished ability to acidify the urine and excrete titratable acidity and NH_4^+. The urinary pH usually remains greater than 6·0. Administration of $NaHCO_3$ does not alter the urinary pH. The pathogenesis of type I is uncertain (Wrong and Davies, 1959; Halperin, 1974; Muldowney, 1979).

In type II (proximal tubular defect) there is a reduced maximal ability to secrete H^+ (T_{mH+}) and reclaim HCO_3^-. This results in an increased fractional excretion of HCO_3^-, a reduction in the renal threshold for HCO_3^- and the attainment of a new steady state. Thus administration of $NaHCO_3$ to return the plasma $[HCO_3^-]$ to normal is followed by the excretion of HCO_3^- in the urine in excess of that neutralised by the secreted H^+. The condition has been called 'bicarbonate-losing renal disease' (Schwartz *et al.*, 1959) and is often accompanied by uraemia.

Both conditions result in a hypokalaemic, hyperchloraemic acidosis. The K^+ loss may be prolonged and severe, being augmented by hyperaldosteronism. Patients with type I, in contrast to type II, are prone to stone formation and nephrocalcinosis but respond to $NaHCO_3$ therapy. Hypokalaemia and nephrocalcinosis may result in a loss of concentrating ability and polyuria (p. 578). An 'incomplete' form of type I has been described in which the defect is insufficient to produce a systemic acidosis. Nephrocalcinosis is accompanied by a normal NH_4^+ excretion rate in the acidification test but the urinary pH fails to fall to 5·3 or less. The condition may progress to the complete form later. The defects in type II are often multiple, with an aminoaciduria, glycosuria and phosphate depletion.

BLOOD GASES AND RESPIRATORY FUNCTION

The **oxygen content** of blood is the volume of oxygen combined with haemoglobin plus that physically dissolved. It is dependent upon Po_2 and haemoglobin concentration. The units are ml oxygen, corrected to NTP, per litre blood. Dissolved oxygen accounts for less than 3% of the total and can be ignored for practical purposes. The normal value for arterial blood is about 190 ml/l while that for venous blood is about 140 ml/l.

Oxygen utilisation (%)

$$= \frac{\text{Arterial } O_2 \text{ content} - \text{venous } O_2 \text{ content}}{\text{Arterial } O_2 \text{ content}} \times 100$$

and using the above figures

$$= \frac{190 - 140}{190} \times 100 = 26$$

Oxygen capacity is the volume of oxygen which the blood contains at 37°C when fully saturated and is expressed in ml oxygen per litre of blood.

The **oxygen combining power** of blood is the volume of oxygen combined with fully saturated haemoglobin at 37 °C. It excludes the volume of oxygen in physical solution. It is also expressed in ml oxygen per litre of blood. Each gram of haemoglobin combines with a maximum of 1·34 ml of oxygen.

Oxygen saturation (So$_2$) is the actual oxygen combined with haemoglobin expressed as the percentage of the oxygen combining power. It is also the ratio of the oxygen content less the oxygen in physical solution to the oxygen capacity less the oxygen in physical solution, multiplied by 100.
Or

$$So_2 = \frac{[\text{oxyhaemoglobin}]}{[\text{deoxyhaemoglobin}] + [\text{oxyhaemoglobin}]} \times 100$$

Oxy- and deoxyhaemoglobin are measured by oximetry (see Dacie and Lewis, 1984) which is beyond the scope of this book. The value for So$_2$ in arterial blood is normally not less than 94 % while that for venous blood is usually in the range, 70 to 75%. When So$_2$ is plotted against Po$_2$ the resulting dissociation curve is sigmoid in shape (Fig. 23.7).

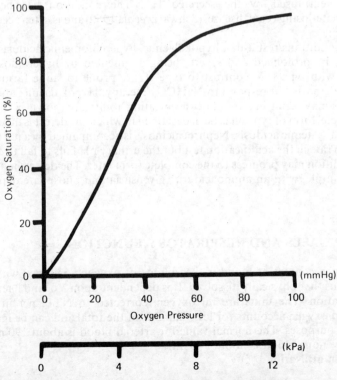

Fig. 23.7. The Oxygen Dissociation Curve.

Other information follows from examination of this curve. The potential oxygen supply to tissues is the cardiac output (l/min) multiplied by the oxygen content, e.g. 5×190 or $950 \, ml/min$. However, many tissues cannot tolerate a capillary P_{O_2} of less than $20 \, mmHg$, so they cannot remove the last 30% of oxygen (see curve) making almost $300 \, ml/min$ unavailable in practice. As the resting subject has an oxygen consumption of about $200 \, ml/min$, the S_{O_2} must be at least 40% in order to supply this. In practice, disturbed function of the brain and other vital organs begins to appear if the S_{O_2} falls below 50%. If anaemia is present (lower oxygen content) or cardiac output is impaired, poor tissue oxygenation will occur at even higher values of S_{O_2}.

The curve is shifted to the right by acidaemia (Bohr effect) or hypercapnia. 2,3-Diphosphoglycerate (DPG) is present in high concentration in erythrocytes. Acidaemia inhibits erythrocyte glycolysis and lowers the DPG concentration. Hypoxia causes a rise in DPG concentration. An increase in DPG concentration shifts the curve to the right by binding to the β-chains of deoxyhaemoglobin. An increase in temperature also shifts the curve to the right. Changes in pH, P_{CO_2}, DPG concentration and temperature in the opposite direction shift the curve to the left. The position of the curve can be defined by the P_{O_2} at 50% saturation (P_{50}) which is normally $27 \, mmHg$ ($3.59 \, kPa$). The measurement of P_{50} and the plotting of the dissociation curve (see Dacie and Lewis, 1984) are again beyond the scope of this book.

The partial pressure of oxygen (P_{O_2}) is given by:

$$P_{O_2} = (\text{Barometric pressure} - \text{Water vapour pressure}) \times \frac{\% O_2}{100}$$

The normal arterial P_{O_2} varies from 80 to $100 \, mmHg$ (10.7 to $13.3 \, kPa$), saturation being 95 to 98%. P_{O_2} gradually declines with age. The P_{O_2} of atmospheric air at a total pressure of $760 \, mmHg$ is about $150 \, mmHg$ ($20.0 \, kPa$). Alveolar air has a different composition following exchange of oxygen and carbon dioxide across the alveolar wall. The volume of carbon dioxide added is less than the oxygen loss as the respiratory quotient (RQ) is usually around 0.8. Thus:

$$\text{Alveolar } P_{O_2} = \text{inspired air } P_{O_2} - P_{CO_2}/RQ$$

This is known as the alveolar gas equation. At a normal P_{CO_2} of $40 \, mmHg$ ($5.32 \, kPa$) this corresponds to a P_{O_2} in alveolar air of $150-(40/0.8)$ or $100 \, mmHg$ ($13.3 \, kPa$). If the transfer factor is normal and the distribution of air and blood in the lungs is matched, the P_{O_2} of the blood leaving the alveoli is usually within $1 \, mmHg$ ($0.13 \, kPa$) of the alveolar P_{O_2} (West, 1966). The P_{O_2} of normal venous blood varies from 30 to $60 \, mmHg$ (4.0 to $8.0 \, kPa$).

Hypoxia

This is a general term for an insufficient availability of oxygen for normal tissue metabolic requirements. Tissue damage occurs when the S_{O_2} falls to 50% or the arterial P_{O_2} falls to about $30 \, mmHg$ ($4.0 \, kPa$). Death may occur at a P_{O_2} of $20 \, mmHg$, $2.7 \, kPa$ (Campbell, 1965). Four categories of hypoxia are recognised:

1. **Hypoxic**, in which oxygen capacity and (total) haemoglobin concentration are normal but the S_{O_2} is reduced to 90% or lower due to a decreased P_{O_2}. Severer forms are associated with cyanosis (see p. 598) and if persistent, a

secondary polycythaemia results. Hypoxic hypoxia is also termed hypoxaemia.

Hypoxaemia may be due to hypoventilation (associated with hypercapnia), ventilation perfusion inequality (see below), right to left shunts, or impaired alveolar-capillary diffusion.

2. **Anaemic**, in which there is a reduction in circulating haemoglobin available for oxygen carriage. The Po_2 is normal but the reduced oxygen capacity leads to oxygen deficiency in the tissues. It is seen in all varieties of anaemia and also when some of the haemoglobin has been converted into such derivatives as carboxyhaemoglobin, methaemoglobin or sulphaemoglobin (see pp. 659, 667).

3. **Stagnant or congestive**, in which there is poor tissue perfusion resulting in decreased oxygen delivery to the tissues. The arterial oxygen capacity and Po_2 are normal but the So_2 is markedly reduced, commonly producing cyanosis. It is common in chronic venous congestion especially associated with decompensated heart disease.

4. **Histotoxic**, in which tissue cells show a reduced oxygen uptake and utilisation as a consequence of poisoning, e.g. by cyanide.

Cyanosis is the term used to describe the bluish appearance of the skin and mucous membranes as a result of an increased amount of deoxyhaemoglobin (50 g/l or more) in the capillaries at the site of observation. This subjective impression is open to considerable observer error. Cyanosis may be due to central or peripheral causes. In *central cyanosis*, arterial Po_2 is reduced either as a result of deficient oxygenation in the lungs or in association with a congenital heart lesion which allows blood to by-pass the lungs through a right to left shunt. In *peripheral cyanosis* the arterial Po_2 is normal but there is a poor blood flow through the capillaries and the tissues look blue because of the consequently greater degree of oxygen extraction. Cyanosis is also seen in methaemoglobinaemia and sulphaemoglobinaemia (see p. 667); the Po_2 is normal. Carbon monoxide poisoning does not produce cyanosis as carboxyhaemoglobin is formed which is pink.

Hypercapnia (arterial Pco_2 greater than 50 mmHg (6·65 kPa)) may be due to hypoventilation or ventilation perfusion inequality.

INTERPRETATION

Respiratory failure is defined by an arterial Po_2 less than 60 mmHg (8·0 kPa). Two types are generally recognised: (1) hypoxaemia without hypercapnia and (2) hypoxaemia with hypercapnia. The former is sometimes called type I and the latter type II respiratory failure or, confusingly, ventilatory failure (Flenley, 1977).

The majority of lung alveoli are ventilated ($\dot{V}$) and perfused ($\dot{Q}$) such that the overall ventilation/perfusion ratio ($\dot{V}/\dot{Q}$) is close to unity. In disease, there may be $\dot{V}/\dot{Q}$ inequality such that some alveoli are adequately perfused but underventilated; conversely other alveoli may be underperfused but adequately ventilated. Both $\dot{V}$ and $\dot{Q}$ are measured in l/min. For a very high ratio the alveolar air composition approaches that of moist atmospheric air. In areas of lung with a very low ratio, the alveolar gas composition approximates to that of venous blood, e.g. Po_2, 40 mmHg (5·32 kPa); Pco_2, 46 mmHg (6·12 kPa). Where this wide variation exists, the low ratio areas lead to arterial hypoxaemia, not compensated for by the high ratio areas. The Po_2 falls but initially the Pco_2 does not rise and may even fall due to carbon dioxide removal being maintained in the high ratio areas. Eventually the Pco_2 may rise but is unlikely to rise above 100 mmHg

(13·3 kPa) if the patient is breathing atmospheric air as the alveolar Po_2 will then be only 25 mmHg (3·3 kPa), a potentially lethal level.

Carbon dioxide is more soluble than oxygen in water and diffuses across the alveolar–capillary membrane 20 times faster than oxygen. Thus in conditions where there is impaired diffusion across the alveolar–capillary membrane such as in pulmonary oedema, adult respiratory distress syndrome or fibrosing alveolitis, the initial result is again hypoxaemia without hypercapnia. Similar arterial gas pressures occur in right to left shunts where the arterial blood is an admixture of systemic and pulmonary venous blood.

Chronic bronchitis and emphysema are by far the most common causes of both type I and type II respiratory failure. Patients with a high $\dot{V}/Q$ are commonly called 'pink puffers' and those with a low $\dot{V}/Q$ 'blue bloaters' due to their appearances. Other causes of type I respiratory failure include pneumonia, bronchial asthma and cyanotic congenital heart disease. Type II respiratory failure occurs in primary hypoventilation. As indicated above type I respiratory failure may progress to type II respiratory failure.

REFERENCES

Ashwood E. R., Kost G., Kenny M. (1983). *Clin. Chem*; **29**: 1877.

Astrup P. (1959). In *Symposium on pH and Blood Gas Measurement*. (Woolmer R. F., ed) p. 81. London: Churchill Livingstone.

Baylis P. H. (1980). *Clin. Endocrinol. Metab*; **9**: 625.

Baylis P. H. (1983). *Clin. Endocrinol. Metab*; **12**: 747.

Baylis P. H., Gill G. V. (1984). *Clin. Endocrinol. Metab*; **13**: 295.

Bird B., Henderson F. A. (1971). *Brit. J. Anaesth*; **43**: 592.

Braybrooke J., Lloyd B., Natrass M., Alberti K. G. M. M. (1975). *Ann. Clin. Biochem*; **12**: 252.

Broughton P. M. G., Smith S. C. H., Buckley B. M. (1985). *Clin. Chem*; **31**: 1765.

Bryan W. P. (1976). *Biochem. Education*; **4**: 49.

Bull G. H. (1955). *Lancet*; **1**: 732.

Campbell E. J. M. (1965). *Brit. Med. J*; **1**: 1451.

Campbell E. J. M. (1984). In *Clinical Physiology*. 5th ed. (Campbell E. J. M., *et al.* eds) Chapter 5. Oxford: Blackwell Scientific Publications.

Chan B. Y., Pang C. P., Swaminathan R. (1984). *Clin. Chem*; **30**: 1429.

Cohen R. D., *et al.* (1982). In *Metabolic Acidosis*. (Ciba Foundation Symposium 87) p. 20. London: Pitman.

Covington A. K., Boink A. B. T. J., Maas A. H. J. (1984). In *Ionized Calcium, Sodium and Potassium by Ion-selective Electrodes*. (Maas A. H. J., Kofstad J., Siggaard-Andersen O., Kokholm G., eds). Vol. 5, p. 229. Copenhagen: Private Press.

Dacie J. V., Lewis S. M. (1984). *Practical Haematology*. 6th ed. Edinburgh: Churchill Livingstone.

Dashe A. M., *et al.* (1963). *J. Amer. Med. Assoc*; **185**: 699.

Douglas I. H. S., McKenzie P. J., Ledingham. I. McA., Smith G. (1978). *Lancet*; **2**: 1370.

Edelman I. S., Leibman J., O'Meara M. P., Birkenfeld L. W. (1958). *J. Clin. Invest*; **37**: 1236.

Editorial. (1977). *Lancet*; **1**: 785.

Espinel C. H., Gregory A. W. (1980). *Clin. Nephrol*; **13**: 73.

Evans J. R. (1978). *Ann. Clin. Biochem*; **15**: 168.

Evans M. C., Cameron I. R. (1978). *Lancet*; **2**: 1371.

Flear C. T. G., Gill V. G., Burn J. (1981). *Lancet*; **2**: 26.

Flenley D. C. (1978). *Br. J. Hosp. Med*; **20**: 384.

Gill G. V., Flear C. T. G. (1985). In *Recent Advances in Clinical Biochemistry*. (Price C. P., Alberti K. G. M., eds) p. 149. Edinburgh: Churchill Livingstone.

Halperin M. L. (1974). *Ann. Roy. Coll. Phys. Surg. Can*; **7**: 103.

Henry R. J. (1964). *Clinical Chemistry, Principles and Technics.* p. 329. New York: Harper and Row.
Hood I., Campbell E. J. M. (1982). *New Engl. J. Med*; **306**: 864.
Howorth P. J. N. (1975). *Brit. J. Dis. Chest*; **69**: 75.
Johnsen D. G., Alberti K. G. M. M. (1983). *Clin. Endocrinol. Metab*; **12**: 267.
Jørgensen K., Astrup P. (1957). *Scand. J. Clin. Lab. Invest*; **12**: 187.
Kofstad J. (1981). In *Blood pH, Carbon Dioxide, Oxygen and Calcium-ion.* (Siggaard-Anderson O., ed) Vol. 1. p. 83. Copenhagen: Private Press.
Krebs H. A., Woods H. F., Alberti K. G. M. M. (1975). *Essays Med. Biochem*; **1**: 81.
McGilvery R. W. (1983). *Biochemistry, a Functional Approach*, 3rd ed., Chapter 38. Philadelphia: W. B. Saunders.
Mellengaard K., Astrup P. (1960). *Scand. J. Clin. Lab. Invest*; **12**: 187.
Minty B. D., Nunn J. F. (1977). *Ann. Clin. Biochem*; **14**: 245.
Monson J. P., Richards P. (1978). *Brit. Med. J*; **1**: 24.
Morgan D. B., Carver M. E., Payne R. B. (1977). *Br. Med. J*; **2**: 929.
Muldowney F. P. (1979). In *Renal Disease*, 4th ed. (Black D. A. K., Jones N. F., eds) Chapter 19. Oxford: Blackwell Scientific Publications.
Newsholme E. A., Leech A. R. (1983). *Biochemistry for the Medical Sciences*, Chapter 13. New York: John Wiley and Sons.
Norden A. G. W., Flynn F. V. (1979). *Clin. Chim. Acta*; **99**: 229.
Nunn J. F. (1959). In *Symposium on pH and Blood Gas Measurements.* (Woolmer R. F., ed) p. 64. London: Churchill Livingstone.
Oken D. E. (1981). *Amer. J. Med*; **71**: 916.
Payne R. B., Levell M. J. (1968). *Clin. Chem*; **14**: 172.
Pitts R. F. (1974). *Physiology of the Kidney and Body Fluids*, 3rd ed. Chapter 10. Chicago: Year Book Medical Publishers.
Radda G. K., Gadian D. G., Ross B. D. (1982). In *Metabolic Acidosis.* (Ciba Foundation 87) p. 36. London: Pitman.
Redetzki H. M., Hughes J. R., Redetzki J. E. (1972). *Proc. Soc. Exp. Biol. Med*; **139**: 315.
Relman A. S. (1978). In *Acid-Base and Potassium Homeostasis.* (Brenner B. M., Stein J. H., eds) Chapter 3. Edinburgh: Churchill Livingstone.
Robinson H. W., Price J. W., Cullen G. E. (1934). *J. Biol. Chem*; **160**: 7.
Schales O., Schales S. S. (1941). *J. Biol. Chem*; **140**: 879.
Schwartz W. B., Hall P. W., Harp R. M., Relman A. S. (1959). *J. Clin. Invest*; **38**: 39.
Siggaard-Andersen O. (1961). *Scand. J. Clin. Lab. Invest*; **13**: 196.
Siggaard-Andersen O. (1964). In *The Acid-Base Status of the Blood*, 2nd ed. Copenhagen: Munksgaard.
Siggaard-Andersen O., Engel K. (1960). *Scand. J. Clin. Lab. Invest*; **12**: 178.
Stoker J. B., Kappangoda C. T., Grimshaw V. A., Linden R. J. (1972). *Clin. Sci*; **42**: 455.
Weisberg H. F. (1975). *Clin. Chem*; **21**: 1182.
West J. B. (1966). In *A Symposium on Oxygen Measurements in Blood and Tissues.* (Payne J. P., Hill D. W., eds) p. 13. London: Churchill Livingstone.
Whitby L. G., Percy-Robb I. W., Smith A. F. (1984). *Lecture Notes on Clinical Chemistry*, 3rd ed. Oxford: Blackwell Scientific Publications.
Woods H. F. (1971). *Brit. J. Hosp. Med*; **6**: 688.
Wrong O. (1967). *Bulletin Post Graduate Committee in Medicine*, University of Sydney; **23**: 233.
Wrong O., Davies H. E. F. (1959). *Quart. J. Med*; **28**: 259.
Wynn V. (1957). *Lancet*; **2**: 1212.
Zilva J. F. (1977). *Lancet*; **1**: 948.

24

CALCIUM, MAGNESIUM AND PHOSPHATE

CALCIUM

Calcium is the most plentiful cation in the body which contains 25 to 35 mol (1·0 to 1·4 kg) in the adult. Over 98 % is in the bones and teeth, the former providing a large reserve which can be drawn on as required. The small part of body calcium present in plasma and other extracellular fluids (27 mmol or 1·1 g) is, however, vitally important for normal neuromuscular transmission and glandular secretion, and for the activity of enzyme systems, particularly those involved in blood coagulation. There is very little calcium in red blood cells and intracellular fluids.

Plasma calcium is composed of a protein-bound fraction which is non-diffusible but is in equilibrium with a diffusible part, most of which is ionised except for a small amount complexed with salts of organic acids such as citrate as well as bicarbonate. Although the total plasma calcium level varies little in health, the body's homeostatic mechanisms are primarily directed towards maintaining a constant ionised calcium concentration, which is the biologically active fraction. Three hormones are involved. They are *parathyroid hormone* (PTH), a polypeptide produced by the parathyroid glands, *calcitonin*, a polypeptide produced by the parafollicular or C-cells of the thyroid, and 1,25-dihydroxycholecalciferol (DHCC, dihydroxy-vitamin D_3) produced from cholecalciferol (vitamin D_3) by 25-hydroxylation in the liver followed by 1α-hydroxylation in the kidney. As DHCC is active at sites remote from its point of production it is regarded as a hormone.

Calcium Metabolism

The circulating calcium concentration is regulated at three sites: bone, kidney and gut, the last two controlling exchange with the external environment. An average dietary daily intake is 25 mmol and a further 5 mmol enters the gut in various secretions. A typical daily absorption from the gut is 10 mmol, leaving 20 mmol to be excreted in the faeces. The daily net absorption of 5 mmol corresponds to the daily loss in the urine when an individual is in calcium balance.

Exchange of calcium between bone and extracellular fluid is quantitatively much larger than the amounts handled by kidney or gut and three processes are involved in a dynamic equilibrium: ionic exchange, bone formation and bone resorption. Bone mineral is deposited as minute crystals closely linked to the collagen fibres of osteoid, the uncalcified bone matrix. These small crystals have a large surface area in relation to their mass and this surface is bathed by interstitial fluid. Bone mineral is mainly hydroxyapatite ($3Ca_3(PO_4)_2 . Ca(OH)_2$) arranged as a lattice of Ca^{2+}, PO_4^{3-} and OH^- ions. Such ions in the lattice surface exchange rapidly with identical ions in the surrounding fluid, but it is possible for other ions of similar radius to replace one of the ions of hydroxyapatite. This occurs rapidly with the lattice surface and more slowly with deeper parts of the lattice. Thus Na^+ and H_3O^+ can replace Ca^{2+} as can Mg^{2+}, Sr^{2+} and Pb^{2+}. The skeleton thus contains quite a lot of sodium (p. 556) and contributes to the regulation of acid–base balance (Chapter 23, p. 582). Lead poisoning involves deposition in the skeleton and later release (p. 656). The rapid ionic exchange of bone Ca^{2+} and extracellular fluid Ca^{2+} is quickly corrected if disturbed and is able to maintain a plasma calcium concentration of about 1·5 mmol/l. Increases above this depend on hormonal control.

Bone is constantly being remodelled even after growth ceases. Osteoclast cells in bone are responsible for destruction and mobilisation of calcium and phosphate, whereas bone production involves osteoblasts in osteoid formation and calcification. The rate of bone turnover depends on the rate of differentiation of the stem cells covering the bone surfaces (periosteal and endosteal) into osteoblasts and osteoclasts. In the normal adult, the activity of these two cell types is balanced. Bone growth implies relatively greater osteoblastic activity, while bone resorption occurs if osteoclastic activity predominates. A useful biochemical marker of osteoblastic activity is the production of the bone isoenzyme of alkaline phosphatase (p. 535).

Normally, plasma ionised calcium concentration is regulated by a negative feedback mechanism. If the level falls, PTH is released and, in the presence of adequate DHCC, stimulates osteoclastic activity, thereby releasing calcium from bone to replenish the deficit. Should plasma ionic calcium rise above normal, PTH release is suppressed, diminishing osteoclastic activity. The importance of calcitonin in man is uncertain, but its action on osteoclasts is opposed to that of PTH.

On an average diet, about 30 to 35 % of the calcium intake is absorbed in the small intestine, both passively and under the influence of DHCC, which binds to a specific receptor in the cytosol of the intestinal cells. It seems that receptor-bound DHCC is rapidly transferred to the nucleus where it stimulates messenger RNA coding for calcium (and phosphorus) transport proteins which facilitate movement of calcium from the intestinal lumen, across the brush border, possibly via the mitochondria, before expulsion at the basal lateral membrane. This latter process requires the presence of sodium ions (De Luca, 1980).

DHCC is therefore the main influencing factor in the entry of calcium into the body, assuming a normal diet. PTH acts only indirectly by stimulating 1α-hydroxylation and hence DHCC synthesis in the kidney. The pH of the intestinal contents is also influential, an acid pH favouring absorption. The extent of fat absorption (see p. 697) and dietary factors, such as the calcium to phosphorus ratio and the presence of phytate, can also have effects on absorption.

Over 200 mmol of calcium is filtered daily by the glomeruli and active tubular reabsorption recovers up to 98 %. The amount excreted depends partly on the filtered load, increasing in hypercalcaemia and falling in hypocalcaemia. PTH increases tubular reabsorption of calcium and diminishes that of phosphate. There is evidence that DHCC also stimulates reabsorption of calcium and phosphate in the distal tubules; calcitonin has the opposite effect.

The processes involved in calcium metabolism are represented diagrammatically in Fig. 24.1 and the subject is reviewed in more detail by Woodhead (1983). Clinical aspects of calcium homeostasis are discussed by Agus *et al.* (1982).

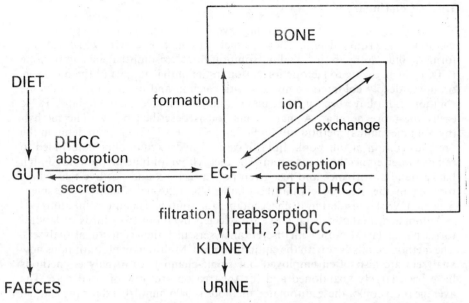

Fig. 24.1. Calcium Metabolism.

Determination of Total Serum Calcium

Early methods for measurement of total serum calcium involved precipitation as oxalate followed by titrimetric quantitation. Current methods fall into two main groups: atomic absorption spectrophotometry and techniques depending on the ability of calcium ions to form coloured or fluorescent complexes with certain organic compounds. For a detailed review, see Gosling (1986).

Titrimetric Methods

Compounds such as those mentioned above were first used as indicators to detect end-points in complexometric titrations with such calcium-complexing agents as ethylenediamine tetraacetate (EDTA) or ethylene glycol bis-(2-aminoethyl ether) tetraacetate (EGTA). These agents have a high affinity for calcium, that of EGTA being greater than that of EDTA, but both suffer some interference from magnesium. The end-point is recognised by the indicator failing to undergo further colour change when all the calcium has been drawn from it by the complexing agent.

EGTA has a slight advantage over EDTA in that, owing to its greater affinity for calcium, it can be used to measure calcium in samples anticoagulated with EDTA or in patients receiving EDTA infusions. A commercial system, the Corning 940 Calcium Analyzer, uses EGTA in an automatic titrator with end-point detection by fluorimetry using calcein as indicator. The fluorescence of the calcium–calcein complex is diminished as calcium is removed by the EGTA. Full details of these titrimetric methods are given in the previous edition of this book.

Direct Colorimetry

Two organic substances have found favour in recent years in colorimetric methods for serum calcium. They are methylthymol blue, with which calcium forms a blue complex in alkaline solution, and cresolphthalein complexone (CPC) which, owing to lactone formation in the phthalein part of the molecule, produces deeply coloured complexes with calcium and magnesium in alkaline solution. Both have been used in manual and automated methods but CPC is easily the more popular. A manual method is described below. The methylthymol blue manual method of Gindler and King (1972) is given in detail in the previous edition of this book. In both cases, 8-hydroxyquinoline is included to remove interference by magnesium. The methylthymol blue method has a high background absorbance and has given poor precision and positive bias which resulted in the steering committee of the UK External Quality Assessment Scheme (1983) considering it unacceptable for routine calcium estimations.

Automated methods using CPC are selected by about two-thirds of laboratories, particularly for use with discrete analysers, including centrifugal analysers. The method details vary with the equipment used. Multi-channel continuous flow analysers are also often employed but single-channel AutoAnalyzer methods have been largely abandoned and for this reason are now omitted here. The average precision of these automated methods is 0·06 mmol/l and for the manual method 0·09 mmol/l.

Methods using Cresolphthalein Complexone

In early CPC methods, calcium was precipitated from serum as the oxalate, which was then converted to carbonate by heat before complexing the calcium with CPC (Stern and Lewis, 1957). In the first AutoAnalyzer methods, Kessler and Wolfman (1964) diluted serum with acid to split the calcium–protein complex, dialysed the calcium into an acid recipient stream and added CPC before developing the colour using diethylamine as base. There have been several subsequent modifications, including incorporation of 8-hydroxyquinoline into the reagents. Manual methods using these reagents directly on serum have not been entirely successful because of interference from protein, but Baginski et al. (1973) described a modified CPC reagent suitable for use with small samples, requiring only 20 μl serum.

Manual Micro-determination (Baginski et al., 1973).

Serum or plasma is treated directly with a CPC reagent containing dimethyl sulphoxide and 8-hydroxyquinoline. After adding diethylamine the colour is read at 575 nm.

  Reagents.
  1. Cresolphthalein complexone. Add 1 ml concentrated hydrochloric acid to 40 mg CPC in a 50 ml beaker. Swirl until dissolved. The solution may appear opalescent but no particles should be present. The addition of a few drops of water may facilitate wetting. Wash the solution into a litre volumetric flask with 50 ml dimethyl sulphoxide. Add 2·5 g 8-hydroxyquinoline and wash down the neck of the flask with a further 50 ml dimethyl sulphoxide. Mix thoroughly until dissolved and add water to the mark.

2. Diethylamine buffer solution. Dissolve 500 mg potassium cyanide in water, add 40 ml diethylamine and dilute to a litre with water. Store in a polythene bottle.
3. Ethylene glycol bis-(2-aminoethyl ether) tetraacetic acid (EGTA), 5 g/l in water.
4. Stock standard calcium solution, 12·5 mmol/l. Add to 1·25 g of 'Analytical Reagent' grade calcium carbonate previously dried at 105 °C for 24 h, 100 ml water followed by 7 ml concentrated hydrochloric acid, stand to dissolve, make up to 1 litre and mix well.
5. Stock standard magnesium solution, 40 mmol/l. Add 8·12 g of 'Analytical Reagent' grade magnesium chloride, $MgCl_2$, $6H_2O$, to 500 ml water in a litre volumetric flask, make up to the mark with water and mix well.
6. Working calcium standard, 2·5 mmol/l, containing magnesium, 0·8 mmol/l. Dilute 20 ml stock calcium solution and 2 ml stock magnesium solution to 100 ml with water. Mix thoroughly.

Technique. Pipette 20 μl serum into a plastic colorimeter cuvette and 20 μl standard into another, preferably in duplicate. To each, add 1 ml CPC reagent and mix. To a further cuvette, add 1 ml reagent for a blank. To each, then add 1 ml diethylamine reagent and mix thoroughly with a plastic paddle. Read tests and standards against the blank at 575 nm. In the case of turbid or lipaemic sera, add 20 μl EGTA solution to the test and blank and re-read. Any difference between them is subtracted from the previous reading.

Calculation.

$$\text{Serum calcium (mmol/l)} = \frac{\text{Reading of unknown}}{\text{Reading of standard}} \times 2\text{·}50$$

Notes.
1. Reagents keep well at room temperature although the blank reading may increase after several weeks with slight reduction in sensitivity.
2. The standard should give an absorbance of about 0·55. This high sensitivity makes cleanliness of pipettes and reaction cuvettes essential.
3. Further simplification of the procedure can be achieved by mixing the two reagents in equal volumes immediately before use and adding 2 ml of the mixed reagent to each reaction tube.
4. The response should be linear from 1·25 mmol/l to at least 3·75 mmol/l.
5. Jaundice and haemolysis do not cause serious interference.
6. Baginski *et al.* (1973) did not use magnesium in their standard solution, but magnesium at normal concentrations increases the reading at 575 nm by about 0·03 and results are consistently high compared with more specific methods, if magnesium is not included.

Determination of Serum and Urinary Calcium and Magnesium Using Atomic Absorption Spectrophotometry

Measurement of calcium can be performed with great accuracy by isotope dilution-mass spectrometry, and Cali *et al.* (1973) developed an atomic absorption reference method, based on that of Pybus *et al.* (1970), which they assessed against the isotope technique. An independent assessment was performed and some revision suggested by Pickup *et al.* (1974). This reference method was not intended to be suitable for routine use, but to be useful for assigning values to control material and as a method against which others could be compared.

For routine use, many atomic absorption methods have been described and the details vary depending on the make and model of instrument employed. The main problems are variable interference by protein and inhibition of absorption by phosphate and sulphate which form poorly volatile calcium salts. Some workers have precipitated proteins before measurement of calcium by atomic absorption techniques, but this is no longer considered necessary and dilution of the sample with a solution of lanthanum chloride in hydrochloric acid is usually sufficient to remove protein interference and to suppress inhibition by phosphate, as the lanthanum combines with phosphate and leaves calcium in the easily dissociated chloride form.

Specimens diluted with lanthanum chloride solution are sprayed directly into an air-acetylene flame. With modern instruments a dilution of 1 in 50 usually affords adequate sensitivity and resonance lines at 422·7 nm for calcium and 285·2 nm for magnesium are obtained from a combined calcium and magnesium lamp.

According to Pybus *et al.* (1970), a pH of below 2·5 is necessary for lanthanum to suppress phosphate interference adequately and they added hydrochloric acid to give an acidity of 50 mmol/l. However, some workers ignore this and simply use aqueous lanthanum chloride solution. A lanthanum concentration of 10 mmol/l in the diluent was found to be sufficient to cope with phosphate concentrations up to about 16 mmol/l when using sample dilutions of 1 in 50 (Pybus *et al.*, 1970), but higher phosphate concentrations may be encountered in urine and other workers have used more concentrated lanthanum solutions up to 50 mmol/l. It is important to use a lanthanum preparation that is low in calcium impurities. BDH 'Spectrosol' reagent is marketed for this purpose and is available as an aqueous solution of lanthanum chloride, i.e. not acidified.

Manufacturers of atomic absorption spectrophotometers provide detailed instructions and specific application sheets for the use of their instruments and reference should be made to these for procedural information and specific method details. Atomic absorption methods, usually non-automated, are routinely used by about 4% of laboratories and have a satisfactory average precision of 0·05 mmol/l.

Collection of Blood for Total Calcium Estimation. In order to avoid changes in plasma protein concentration, do not employ stasis during blood collection. The blood should either be allowed to clot or anti-coagulated with lithium heparin. Citrate, oxalate and EDTA should not normally be used as they will cause differing degrees of interference depending on the method of estimation employed.

Determination of Ionised Calcium

That the 'free' or 'ionised' calcium is the physiologically active fraction was first shown by McLean and Hastings (1934, 1935) in their work on the contraction of frog heart muscle. About 50% of plasma calcium is ionised, 40% is bound to protein (mainly albumin) and the remaining 10% is complexed with bicarbonate, citrate and other organic ions. Of the ionised fraction, less than one-third is 'biologically active' in that the rest is rendered inactive by electrostatic forces of other electrolytes in the plasma.

Techniques Using Ion-selective Electrodes

The principle of the action of ion-selective electrodes was outlined in Chapter 23 (p. 564). Electrodes responsive to calcium began to be introduced in the late 1960s.

The calcium electrode is commonly of the liquid ion-exchange type, consisting of the calcium salt of an alkyl phosphate dissolved in di-*n*-octylphenyl phosphonate supported in an inert matrix such as PVC. The electrode has sufficient selectivity over magnesium, sodium, potassium and zinc to be useful for serum calcium estimation, but it is not completely specific for calcium. There are now several dedicated instruments available for the measurement of ionised calcium using temperature-controlled flow-through electrodes.

Factors Influencing the Measurement of Ionised Calcium. Several factors are known to affect the determination.

Ionic strength. Electrodes respond to the activity of the ionised calcium in serum according to the Nernst equation, but this is influenced by the ionic strength of the solution and, when calibrating electrodes of this type, it is usual to do so with standards containing salts at normal serum levels. A change in ionic strength of 10 mmol/l is said to affect results by about 1·2 % (Siggaard-Andersen *et al.*, 1980).

Temperature. Protein-binding of calcium increases slightly with increasing temperature and instruments are usually controlled to perform measurements at 37 °C. However, correction to the temperature of the patient, e.g. in cases of hypothermia, is unlikely to yield very different results.

pH. This is an important influencing factor in ionised calcium measurement, an increase in pH causing a lowering of the ionised fraction. It is best to collect and handle blood specimens anaerobically so that the ionic calcium is measured at the pH of the patient. If this is not possible and loss of carbon dioxide has occurred, the plasma or serum can be equilibrated to a normal P_{CO_2}, the ionised calcium measured and then a correction applied to express the result at a standard pH of 7·40. Several of the current instruments have the facility for simultaneous pH measurement and can accept serum, plasma or whole blood samples, although the electrode response can be affected by the haematocrit (Fogh-Andersen *et al.*, 1978). It must be remembered, however, that it is the ionised calcium at the actual pH of the patient that has physiological importance. Control of the patient's pH during blood sampling is also necessary and hyperventilation by the patient should be avoided.

Anticoagulants. Most anticoagulants bind calcium and are, therefore, unsuitable for use in specimens being subjected to ionised calcium measurement. Heparin can be used, but even this binds some calcium and one solution to the problem entailed using heparin in accurately determined concentration in whole blood so as to produce a negative error that would be balanced by the positive error caused by red cells at the electrode. Alternatively, very low concentrations of heparin can be employed, but this is associated with a risk of coagulation. Another method involves addition of calcium to the heparin to give a calcium ion activity similar to that of normal plasma, thus eliminating bias for specimens in the normal range but introducing a small positive bias for samples with low ionised calcium levels and a negative bias for those with high levels. A further complication is that heparin from different sources differs in the amount of calcium that must be added.

Protein. With some electrode systems, protein in the sample can bind to the calcium carrier in the membrane and trypsin and ethanolamine have been added to standards to decontaminate the membrane. As these agents themselves bind some calcium, results are affected and the procedure has met with disapproval by some workers (Robertson, 1976), although Worth *et al.* (1981) suggested the addition of calcium gluconate to the triethanolamine to overcome the problem. An alternative approach is to prevent electrode contamination by covering the tip with a cellophane membrane (Christiansen, 1975).

Despite considerable improvements in electrode systems for ionised calcium measurement, there is still a degree of uncertainty about the technique, partly because of the influencing factors referred to above and partly because of poor agreement between reference ranges derived by different groups of workers using different electrode systems. The clinical value of the measurement will be discussed later.

Ultrafiltrable Calcium. Measurement of ultrafiltrable calcium has been used to give an approximate estimate of the ionised fraction, as it comprises all those fractions not bound to protein, i.e. it includes that complexed with organic ions in addition to the ionic form. The technique involves forcing plasma through an ultrafiltration membrane. It is influenced by pH and temperature and is rather tedious and has now largely been superseded by ion-selective electrode techniques.

Calculated Ionised Calcium. Many formulae have been derived for the purpose of calculating ionised calcium concentration from actual total calcium, albumin and total protein concentrations. That of Pottgen and Davis (1976) was given in the previous edition of this book and the subject is discussed in detail by Vanstapel and Lissens (1984).

Adjustment of Total Serum Calcium for Variations in Serum Protein Concentration

As about 40% of serum calcium is bound to protein and as variations in protein concentration, particularly of albumin, are common in hospital patients, some adjustment of the total calcium figure is advisable to attain meaningful results. Venous occlusion by tourniquet during collection of blood samples can also result in altered protein concentration.

Various formulae have been proposed for this adjustment. Moore (1970) showed that about 81% of protein-bound calcium is attached to albumin and so most calculations in current use are based on albumin concentration. Orrell (1971) investigated the relationship between total calcium by an AutoAnalyzer cresolphthalein complexone method and albumin by a bromocresol green method and suggested a formula correcting to an albumin concentration of 34 g/l. Payne *et al.* (1973) derived an alternative formula correcting to an albumin concentration of 40 g/l and this was supported (Editorial, 1977) as the following formula:

Adjusted calcium (mmol/l) =

Measured calcium (mmol/l) − 0·02[albumin (g/l) − 40]

or + 0·02[40 − albumin (g/l)]

Strictly, such correction formulae should be derived by each laboratory using its own analytical methods, because different techniques for calcium and albumin estimation may produce some variation in the relationship.

Despite general acceptance of this approach, Phillips and Pain (1977) criticised the use of average regression lines on the grounds that there are wide individual variations, saying that a subject's own regression line had to be determined by sampling blood for calcium and albumin before and after occlusion with a tourniquet, which would result in changes in albumin and consequently calcium concentrations. They also stressed that such corrections could not be applied for changes of albumin in the nephrotic syndrome as abnormal binding of calcium to globulins occurs. In fact, adjustments of this kind are unlikely to be reliable in any subject with grossly abnormal plasma proteins involving globulin changes, because correction formulae tend to assume a normal globulin concentration. Furthermore, with very low albumin levels, methods such as bromocresol green tend to overestimate the albumin concentration and correction may also be invalid in this situation.

. INTERPRETATION

Improvements in precision of methods for total serum calcium estimation have resulted in quoted normal ranges becoming narrower. After a retrospective study over a year and including 1371 hospital patients, Hooper (1975) suggested a reference range of 2·15 to 2·60 mmol/l for in-patients and 2·25 to 2·65 mmol/l for out-patients. These figures reflect lower plasma albumin levels in in-patients and are in fairly close agreement with other studies of this sort. A very large study in Australia (Sinton *et al.*, 1986) subdivided reference ranges according to sex and age group, and Payne *et al.* (1986) have demonstrated 'clustering' of serum calcium (and magnesium) concentrations in siblings, suggesting that families may have narrower reference intervals than the general population and that abnormalities in an individual might be more readily detected by comparison with levels in his or her siblings than by comparison with the population ranges.

Fluctuations in plasma albumin owing to physiological or pathological changes, or to stasis with associated water redistribution during blood sampling, will produce changes in total serum calcium concentration. Even the postural changes associated with confinement to bed cause sufficient fluid redistribution to lower the plasma albumin level and are partly responsible for the lower reference range for in-patients compared with that for out-patients.

The normal range for serum ionised calcium, measured by ion-selective electrode, is approximately 1·15 to 1·30 mmol/l, but different studies have produced quite widely differing ranges and each laboratory should establish its own. It does seem, however, that values in late pregnancy tend to fall a little, whereas cord blood and neonates show a tendency towards higher levels than normal adults (Siggaard-Andersen *et al.*, 1980).

Ionised calcium determination has both advantages and disadvantages compared with total calcium. Posture and venous occlusion have much less effect than on total calcium, but ventilation of the patient has to be normal and sampling should preferably be anaerobic. The concentration of ionised calcium is usually roughly proportional to total serum calcium, but in some circumstances total calcium may not reflect the true calcium status. For example, transfusions of large amounts of blood containing acid–citrate–dextrose, as in open heart surgery, can cause a fall in ionised calcium without affecting total calcium. In acid–base disorders, the fraction of ionised calcium is altered owing to the effect of pH on the equilibrium. In this case, careful interpretation of ionised calcium results is necessary taking into account whether it is the patient's current ionised calcium status that is important or the calcium status at a more normal pH. In some patients suffering from hyperparathyroidism, total calcium is sometimes within accepted normal limits when ionised calcium is increased, suggesting that the latter may be diagnostically superior.

Menopausal women tend to exhibit a rise in total serum calcium and Marshall *et al.* (1982) were able to show that most of this rise could be accounted for by an increase in the ionised fraction.

The level of total serum calcium may be affected by deficient intestinal absorption of calcium, by changes in bone metabolism, by altered renal excretion and by alterations in plasma proteins. In the last case, the physiologically active, ionised fraction is unaffected. DHCC, the active form of vitamin D, stimulates active transport of calcium and phosphate from the small intestine to the blood. It functions, together with PTH, to mobilise calcium and phosphate from bone and may also stimulate renal reabsorption of calcium, as does PTH. In addition, PTH stimulates 1α-hydroxylation of 25-hydroxy vitamin D_3 in the kidney. Calcitonin has an opposing effect on serum calcium by suppressing mobilisation from bone. Although increased PTH activity mobilises both calcium and phosphate from bone, its effect on the kidney is to retain calcium and increase phosphate excretion, resulting in an increase in plasma calcium and a decrease in plasma phosphate concentrations.

Hypocalcaemia. A reduction in serum calcium affecting the ionised fraction is one of the causes of tetany. There is a region of latent tetany down to about 2·0 mmol/l; between 2·0 and 1·75 mmol/l abnormal reflexes can be demonstrated (Trousseau and Chvostek signs) and below 1·75 mmol/l carpopedal spasms may occur. Some of the lowest serum calcium values are found in hypoparathyroidism, which may arise spontaneously (idiopathic hypoparathyroidism) but occurs more commonly following surgical removal of parathyroid tissue, e.g. during thyroidectomy, and levels may occasionally fall below 1·25 mmol/l.

Diseases in which calcium absorption is impaired do not usually show such low values as the tendency to hypocalcaemia stimulates PTH production. This secondary hyperparathyroidism maintains a more normal calcium level. Hence in rickets, the more characteristic abnormality is a low serum inorganic phosphate. Serum calcium may be just within normal limits or not more than 0·25 mmol/l below the lower limit of normal and symptoms of tetany are rarely present. A greater fall in serum calcium is more often seen in the adult form of rickets, osteomalacia. In more generalised malabsorption, such as occurs in coeliac disease, idiopathic steatorrhoea, tropical sprue and following surgical resection of the small intestine, serum calcium is often moderately reduced, usually in association with a low plasma protein concentration, but severe cases can show considerable falls.

In the nephrotic syndrome, in which plasma albumin is reduced, calcium is also low, but the ionised fraction is unaffected so there is no significant biological effect. The high serum inorganic phosphate of advanced renal failure (p. 787) is sometimes accompanied by a marked decrease in serum calcium, down to perhaps 1·5 mmol/l, as a consequence of poor renal production of DHCC. The co-existing acidosis usually prevents tetany, although occasionally symptoms are seen. Often secondary hyperparathyroidism develops and the high serum inorganic phosphate is then accompanied by a normal or only slightly low serum calcium.

A fall in serum calcium, sometimes severe, can occur a day or two after an attack of acute pancreatitis or after a massive transfusion of citrated blood. Rare causes of hypocalcaemia include ethylene glycol intoxication, in which tissue deposition of calcium oxalate occurs. Calcium phosphate precipitation in soft tissues can have a similar effect in cases of acute hyperphosphataemia after phosphate enemas, laxative abuse or cell lysis consequent upon cytotoxic therapy in, e.g. leukaemia. Loop diuretics such as frusemide may exacerbate hypocalcaemia in susceptible subjects owing to the renal calcium-wasting effect of these drugs.

It has been claimed that chronic anticonvulsant therapy can lead to hypocalcaemia as a result of induction of hepatic enzymes that catabolise 25-hydroxy vitamin D but, although low serum calcium does occur in some of these patients, not everyone agrees with this explanation of the phenomenon.

Neonatal hypocalcaemia, presenting as convulsions, occurs in some babies in whom artificial feeding has been established with phosphate-rich cow's milk and also in the infants of some mothers who have diabetes, osteomalacia or hyperparathyroidism. Very high plasma magnesium levels after intravenous infusion of magnesium salts have been shown to be associated with hypocalcaemia and may have a suppressing effect on PTH secretion (Cholst *et al.*, 1984). Paradoxically, hypomagnesaemia can also cause hypocalcaemia by limiting PTH secretion or decreasing bone response to PTH.

Hypercalcaemia. Very high serum calcium figures may be found in primary hyperparathyroidism. Occasionally up to 5·0 mmol/l, they are mostly between the upper limit of normal and 3·75 mmol/l. Most cases are caused by a single parathyroid adenoma, but occasionally, parathyroid carcinoma, hyperplasia or multiple adenomata are present. The condition may be accompanied by other endocrine disorders. Although most of the calcium increase is due to mobilisation from bone, skeletal disease (osteitis fibrosa cystica) is uncommon. A more common finding is renal stones associated with the hypercalciuria, and calcium deposition in the kidney tissue, nephrocalcinosis, with secondary renal damage. Other presenting features of the hypercalcaemia include anorexia, nausea, constipation, abdominal pain and pancreatitis. More recently, milder cases without clinical symptoms are regularly discovered as a consequence of biochemical screening procedures.

In secondary hyperparathyroidism, diffuse hyperplasia of all parathyroid glands occurs as a result of chronic stimulation by the hypocalcaemic state primarily present. In some long-standing cases, one or more of the hyperplastic glands may become adenomatous and behave in an autonomous fashion with no feedback control. The patient becomes hypercalcaemic and the condition is known as tertiary hyperparathyroidism.

In elderly populations, malignancy is the most common cause of hypercalcaemia. Tumours of the lung and breast, especially those of the squamous cell type, have a high association with hypercalcaemia, whereas anaplastic or oat-cell types are rarely linked (Mundy *et al.*, 1984). About 20 to 30% of patients with myeloma have hypercalcaemia at some stage, particularly if dehydrated or when the condition is advanced. The cause of the hypercalcaemia in malignancy is increased bone resorption either caused by metastases or by humoral factors produced by the tumour cells.

Hypercalcaemia may develop in patients with Paget's disease of bone, especially if they are immobilised. The source is again bone, and similar increased bone resorption is seen in some cases of hyperthyroidism. Increased calcium absorption from the gut leading to hypercalcaemia occurs in excessive vitamin D therapy and in some cases of sarcoidosis who show increased sensitivity to vitamin D. This is also thought to be important in idiopathic hypercalcaemia of infancy. Increased intestinal absorption also occurs in the milk-alkali syndrome. In patients given thiazide diuretics, hypercalcaemia is a complication if there is some pre-existing increased bone resorption. Familial hypocalciuric hypercalcaemia is discussed later (p. 613) and requires differentiation from primary hyperparathyroidism.

A scheme for investigating the hypercalcaemic patient has been proposed by Jamieson (1985) and management has been discussed by Selby *et al.* (1984). Treatment usually depends on the severity of the hypercalcaemia and on the cause. Oral phosphate or glucocorticoids have been used to inhibit calcium absorption from the gut and steroids have an additional suppressing effect on the hypercalcaemia of malignancy. Sodium EDTA infusion produces rapid lowering of plasma calcium but is nephrotoxic. Calcitonin has been used, as has mithramycin, a cytotoxic antibiotic with specific action against osteoclasts but with a serious side-effect of bone-marrow suppression. Hydration by saline infusion is often beneficial together with frusemide therapy, which produces a calcium diuresis. A new group of drugs that shows promise is the diphosphonates, which are able to suppress osteoclast activity.

Calcium Excretion

Determination of Urinary Calcium

Atomic absorption spectrophotometry is the most suitable technique for urinary calcium but cresolphthalein complexone methods can also be employed. Urines (24 h) should be collected into vessels containing acid, e.g. 100 ml 1 mol/l hydrochloric acid, to prevent precipitation of calcium salts.

Determination of Faecal Calcium

Dry the faeces, weigh and ash a portion of about 1 g in a crucible in an electric furnace. Dissolve the ash in dilute acid and determine the calcium by the method in use for urine.

INTERPRETATION

Most of the calcium excreted from the body is in the faeces. The quantity varies considerably depending on the diet but in an adult may average about 20 mmol/24 h. Urinary calcium excretion is influenced by diet to a lesser extent and, on an average diet, amounts to between 2·5 and 7·5 mmol/24 h. On a low daily intake of 3·75 mmol, the upper limit of urinary excretion would be about 3·85 mmol/24 h (McGeown, 1961).

In general, urinary calcium output is low when serum calcium is low, and urinary excretion normally balances intestinal absorption. Hence, urinary calcium output falls in diseases associated with defective absorption, such as vitamin D deficiency, whereas faecal calcium tends to be high if intake is normal. This illustrates that faecal calcium measurement is really only of value in careful studies of calcium balance when accurate knowledge of intake and output are required.

When plasma ionised calcium is high there is an associated elevation of urinary calcium. Thus, in many patients with hyperparathyroidism, between 7·5 and 17·5 mmol/24 h may be lost. Sometimes, however, normal values do occur, especially if some renal impairment is present. Increased calcium excretion can occur in hyperthyroidism, hypervitaminosis D, sarcoidosis, multiple myeloma and in subjects who form renal stones.

Osteomalacia usually results primarily from inadequate intestinal absorption but can sometimes be caused by excessive urinary excretion, as in renal tubular acidosis, when neutral or alkaline urine, low in ammonia but high in sodium, potassium and calcium, is passed. There is associated hyperchloraemic acidosis which enhances loss of calcium from bone.

Drugs reported to increase urinary calcium excretion include cholestyramine, loop diuretics such as frusemide, and steroids.

There is a condition, first described by Foley *et al.* (1972) and known as *familial benign hypercalcaemia* or *familial hypocalciuric hypercalcaemia*, that can be mistaken for hyperparathyroidism if it is not realised that urinary calcium excretion is inappropriately low (less than 5 mmol/24 h) for the plasma calcium level. Recognition of this condition, which is of autosomal dominant inheritance, is of considerable importance because surgical intervention is contra-indicated as subtotal parathyroidectomy has usually failed to correct the hypercalcaemia (Davies *et al.*, 1981; Paterson and Gunn, 1981). The calcium excretion index (Ca_E), described below, may be helpful in making the necessary differential diagnosis.

Calcium Excretion Index

The calcium excretion index was introduced by Nordin *et al.* (1967) and is a measure of calcium excretion independent of the influence of glomerular filtration rate, being expressed as mmol/l of glomerular filtrate.

$$Ca_E = \frac{U_{Ca} \times P_{Cr}}{U_{Cr}}$$

where U and P refer to urine and plasma concentrations of calcium (Ca) or creatinine (Cr) in mmol/l.

The test can be performed on a 4 h urine specimen collected while the patient is fasting. A blood sample must also be collected during this period, for the estimation of plasma creatinine. The normal range in SI units is about 0·0125 to 0·0375 mmol/l. The index is increased in hyperparathyroidism and in other types of hypercalcaemia, but in familial hypocalciuric hypercalcaemia it is normal.

Calcium Balance Tests

In these tests, which are only occasionally carried out, the patient is placed on a diet of known calcium content and, after allowing at least three days to become adjusted, collection of 24 h urine specimens is begun and continued for several days, e.g. 3 to 5. For collection of faeces over this period see p. 318. The calcium content of the urine and faeces is then determined and the daily excretion compared with the known intake. Reliable collection of specimens is, however, difficult under ordinary hospital conditions.

A normal diet may contain about 20 mmol of calcium per day. On this a normal person should be in a state of calcium balance with intake and output about the same. If more calcium is excreted than is taken in, the patient is said to have a negative balance and *vice versa*. A patient on a diet containing only 2·5 mmol per day will normally excrete about 6·25 mmol daily since a state of balance is not reached until about 12·5 mmol is being taken. With such a low intake a negative calcium balance can be said to exist when more than 6·25 mmol is excreted daily and a positive balance when the excretion is less than this. This low-intake form of the test is preferable as it is less subject to errors in performance.

MAGNESIUM

The body contains about 1 mol of magnesium and most of it is in bone and soft tissues such as liver, kidney and muscle with only about 1% in extracellular fluid. Of that present in the extracellular fluid, 20 to 30 % is protein-bound and most of the remainder is in the free ionised form. On an average daily intake of about 15 mmol, between 25 and 60 % is absorbed, mainly in the jejunum. Absorption is inhibited by excess calcium or phosphate and does not require vitamin D. In the kidney, there is active reabsorption and the kidney is the main regulator of serum concentration, 90 to 95 % being reabsorbed from glomerular filtrate, but this is influenced by dietary intake and serum concentration. Hypercalcaemia inhibits magnesium reabsorption and the evidence suggests that calcium and magnesium reabsorption are similarly affected by PTH and calcitonin. Aldosterone increases renal excretion of potassium and magnesium.

Magnesium is essential for normal nerve and muscle function and is an activator of various enzymes such as alkaline and acid phosphatases, creatine kinase, leucine aminopeptidase and carboxylase.

Determination of Serum Magnesium

Early, outdated methods involved removal of calcium and precipitation of magnesium as the phosphate or 8-hydroxyquinoline complex before determination, sometimes by complexometric titration. Alternatively, the latter complex was measured fluorimetrically in ethanolic solution. Colorimetric methods used the coloured magnesium complexes of titan yellow or methyl thymol blue. Emission flame photometry was also tried.

Currently, atomic absorption photometry is the method of choice and the only other method in common use is the colorimetric one using either the Mann-Yoe dye or, more often, Calmagite (1-azonaphthalene-3-sulphonic acid-1'-(2-methylbenzene)), now popular for both automated and manual use.

Recently, Tabata et al. (1985) described a reaction-rate method based on the activation of hexokinase by magnesium ions. They linked this via glucose-6-phosphate dehydrogenase to an $NADP^+/NADPH$ reaction and measured the production of NADPH at 340 nm. Good correlation with atomic absorption values was claimed for this method.

Atomic Absorption Method

See the method for determining calcium and magnesium (p. 605). The average between-batch precision for the manual technique is 0·06 mmol/l.

Colorimetric Method Using Calmagite (Gindler and Heth, 1971; Khayam-Bashi et al., 1977)

Magnesium reacts with the blue dye, Calmagite, in alkaline solution to form a red complex. Protein interference and dye precipitation are avoided by including the 9-ethylene-oxide adduct of p-nonylphenol (Bion NE9) and polyvinylpyrrolidone (Bion PVP). Calcium interference is avoided by preferential combination with EGTA and heavy metal interference is prevented by cyanide.

  Reagents.
  1. Dye reagent. This contains 60 mg Calmagite, 28 g potassium chloride, 1·08 g Bion NE9 and 10 g Bion PVP per litre. It is obtainable ready prepared as Magnesium Rapid Stat Dye Reagent (Product No. 455084; Pierce Chemical Co) and is stable at room temperature for 2 years.

2. Base reagent. This contains 2 g potassium cyanide, 15·8 g potassium hydroxide and 450 mg EGTA per litre. It is obtainable ready prepared as Magnesium Rapid Stat Base Reagent (Product No. 455043, Pierce Chemical Co) and is stable at room temperature for 2 years.
3. Working reagent. Prepare freshly each day by mixing one volume of reagent (2) with 10 volumes of reagent (1). The mixture is stable for 24 h.
4. Standard magnesium solution, 10 mmol/l. For the stock solution dissolve 2·033 g MgCl$_2$, 6H$_2$O or 2·463 g MgSO$_4$, 7H$_2$O in water and make to a litre.
5. Working standards, 1 and 3 mmol/l. Dilute the stock standard 1 to 10 and 3 to 10.

Technique. Place 50 μl serum in a test tube and add 5 ml working reagent. Similarly treat 50 μl of the standards. Mix and allow to stand for 20 min before reading in a spectophotometer at 532 nm using the working reagent as blank. The colour is stable for several hours. Beer's Law is obeyed up to at least 2 mmol/l.

Calculation.

$$\text{Serum magnesium (mmol/l)} = \frac{\text{Reading of unknown}}{\text{Reading of lower standard}} \times 1 \cdot 0$$

Notes.

1. The method is unaffected by citrate used as an anticoagulant.
2. The 3 mmol/l standard can be used to check the extent of linearity and to give an approximate result if the serum figure is high.
3. The average between-batch precision is 0·08 mmol/l and the results are on average 0·01 mmol/l higher than those obtained by the atomic absorption method.

INTERPRETATION

Normal ranges for serum magnesium are rather dependent on the method of analysis but 0·7 to 1·0 mmol/l is appropriate for atomic absorption methods.

Increased serum magnesium concentration can occur in the oliguric phase of acute renal failure, in dehydration and in chronic renal failure. In these circumstances, it behaves in a similar way to potassium and this is also seen in Addison's disease and during the development of diabetic ketoacidosis. Hypermagnesaemia is associated with depression of central and peripheral nervous activity.

Magnesium deficiency is usually associated with *low serum magnesium* levels. It can occur because of impaired intake, increased faecal loss, increased urinary loss, or altered balance between intracellular and extracellular fluids. The last is seen during insulin treatment of diabetic ketoacidosis. It may be a factor in causing a slight reduction of serum magnesium in diabetic subjects compared with non-diabetics but there is no difference in tissue magnesium levels (Levin *et al.*, 1981).

Hypomagnesaemia may be accompanied by tetany, unrelieved by calcium administration; by muscle twitching and tremors with mental irritability, hallucinations and aggressiveness (as in delirium tremens); by convulsions and by eventual death if severe. It also causes hypocalcaemia unresponsive to PTH or vitamin D but corrected by magnesium replenishment, which also corrects the other manifestations. Nephrocalcinosis with possible progressive renal damage also occurs.

Impaired intake of magnesium is seen especially in kwashiorkor, to some extent in alcoholism, and in prolonged intravenous nutrition without magnesium supplements. *Increased faecal losses*, usually accompanied by diminished urinary magnesium excretion, occur in malabsorption and steatorrhoea, in persistent diarrhoea, vomiting or gastric suction, and in some cases of laxative abuse, or ingestion of increased amounts of calcium salts.

Renal losses, normally about 5 mmol/24 h, when increased may be considered under several headings:

1. *Inherited tubular disorders* may involve magnesium alone but more often are associated with impaired handling of potassium or hydrogen ion, as in renal tubular acidosis.
2. *Hormonal influences* are seen in primary hyperaldosteronism, with concomitant potassium loss, in Bartter's syndrome and in some cases of hyperthyroidism.
3. *Tubular cell damage* leading to impaired conservation is associated with aminoglycoside (e.g. gentamicin) and cisplatin therapy. Losses also occur during the diuretic phase of acute renal failure.
4. *Decreased reabsorption* affecting magnesium and potassium is seen in prolonged diuretic therapy and is sometimes important in patients coming to open heart surgery.
5. *Increased filtered load* with appropriate increased renal excretion occurs following tissue mobilisation as in starvation, injury, early diabetic ketoacidosis and acute pancreatitis. Mobilisation from bone occurs in primary hyperparathyroidism but this usually matches the increased renal excretion and hypomagnesaemia is uncommon. This may occur, however, after removal of the adenoma and be associated with refractory hypocalcaemia which only disappears after treatment of the magnesium deficiency. Hypomagnesaemia may be a factor in post-operative tetany in these patients.

PHOSPHATE

The body contains about 17 mol of phosphorus of which 87% is present in bones, the remainder being found in cells and soft tissues, i.e. more widely distributed than is calcium. Phosphorus is a constituent of many important biological compounds, e.g. some proteins, some lipids, nucleic acids and some coenzymes. It also plays a part in acid–base regulation, particularly by the kidneys (see p. 582).

Phosphorus in the blood may be classified thus:

1. Inorganic phosphorus, present as $H_2PO_4^-$ and HPO_4^{2-}.
2. Organic or ester phosphorus, e.g. glycerophosphates, nucleotide phosphate, hexose phosphate.
3. Lipid phosphorus, lecithin, cephalin, sphingomyelin.
4. A small amount of residual phosphorus.

Red cells are richer in phosphorus than is plasma, mainly because they contain more ester phosphates.

Dietary intake of phosphate is about 32 to 64 mmol per day and approximately 80% is absorbed, mainly in the jejunum under the influence of vitamin D. There is also some secretion of phosphate into the intestine resulting in an amount equivalent to 30 to 40% of the intake being excreted in the faeces. The kidney is the primary regulator of plasma phosphate concentration, PTH being the main influence leading to decreased tubular reabsorption with some contribution from 1,25-DHCC. Normally, 85 to 90% of filtered phosphate is reabsorbed.

Mobilisation of phosphate from bone is not a major factor influencing plasma phosphate. For a review of phosphate homeostasis see Stoff (1982).

Determination of Inorganic Phosphate

Most methods have used the reaction between phosphate and an acid molybdate reagent. The hexavalent molybdenum of the phosphomolybdic acid formed absorbs light at 340 nm and can be reduced to molybdenum blue, whereas the reducing agent has negligible effect on the uncomplexed molybdic acid. A variety of reducing agents has been used including 1,2,4-aminonaphthol-sulphonic acid (Fiske and Subbarow, 1925) and stannous chloride (Kuttner and Lichtenstein, 1930). The latter has enjoyed considerable popularity especially in automated continuous-flow methods where precise timing minimises problems associated with the rather unstable colour which is formed. Hurst (1964) improved the reagent· by inclusion of hydrazine. Another reagent, *p*-methylaminophenol sulphate (Metol, Elon) was introduced by Gomori (1942) and is more stable, easier to prepare, less affected by the amount of acid present and unaffected by oxalate, citrate or fluoride in the sample. However, it is less sensitive than the other methods mentioned above. In 1963, Dryer and Routh introduced 4-aminodiphenylamine (semidine) hydrochloride. Their method was subsequently modified by Garber and Miller (1983) to eliminate occasional interferences related to the protein precipitation step and sometimes to the presence of endogenous ascorbic acid.

Robinson *et al.* (1971) developed an automated continuous-flow method that needs no reducing agent. The sample was diluted with and dialysed into dilute sulphuric acid, then coupled with a molybdovanadate reagent to form a yellow complex and read at 403 nm. This, however, is a much less sensitive method.

Itayi and Ui (1966) introduced a new technique in which phosphate produces a colour change from yellow-brown to green in a molybdic acid-malachite green solution but this is little used now.

Most of the early methods involved protein removal, either by trichloracetic acid precipitation in manual methods or dialysis in continuous flow methods, but techniques operating in the presence of protein following the addition of various stabilisers are now the most frequently used, particularly in conjunction with discrete and centrifugal analysers. Continuous flow methods remain popular but usually in multi-channel configuration and for this reason, the single channel AutoAnalyzer method given in the last edition of this book has now been omitted.

Methods using phosphomolybdate formation are far more popular than those involving phosphomolybdovanadate while among the former, reduction methods and those employing direct measurement at 340 nm find roughly equal favour. In general, however, the current selection of analytical methods for phosphate in regular use probably shows more variation than for any other common analyte measured in clinical biochemistry laboratories.

Analytical performance varies. The average between-batch precision is least (0·030 mmol/l) for continuous flow methods using phosphomolybdate, either with reduction or 340 nm measurement, but deteriorates (0·045 mmol/l) with use of phosphomolybdovanadate. Non-protein-precipitation methods employing phosphomolybdate in automated equipment, although convenient, show rather worse precision (0·045 mmol/l), again with little difference between reduction and 340 nm techniques. Manual methods have, as usual, rather poorer precision but those with protein precipitation and phosphomolybdate reduction are best

(0·050 mmol/l) with deterioration if measured at 340 nm (0·065 mmol/l) or if protein is not precipitated (0·075 mmol/l) or if phosphomolybdovanadate is used (0·070 mmol/l). For these reasons we have retained a traditional manual method of the first type.

Method of Gomori (1942)

Reagents.

1. Trichloracetic acid solution, 100 g/l in water.
2. Sulphuric acid, 5 mol/l. Add 450 ml concentrated acid slowly while cooling to 1300 ml water. Dilute some of this 1 to 10 and titrate with 1 mol/l sodium hydroxide, and make any necessary adjustment to the original solution.
3. Ammonium molybdate solution. Dissolve 7·5 g in about 200 ml water, add 100 ml of the 5 mol/l sulphuric acid and make to 400 ml with wather.
4. Metol (*p*-methylaminophenol sulphate) solution, 1 g in 100 ml sodium bisulphite solution, 30 g/l.
5. Stock standard phosphate solution, 20 mmol/l. Dissolve 1·36 g potassium dihydrogen phosphate (KH_2PO_4) in about 300 ml water and make to 500 ml.
6. Working standard phosphate solution, 2 mmol/l. Dilute the stock solution 1 to 10 with water.

Technique. Add 0·8 ml serum to 7·2 ml trichloracetic acid, mix well and filter or centrifuge. Set up three tubes containing respectively 5 ml (= 0·5 ml serum) of the filtrate (the unknown), 0·5 ml standard plus 4·5 ml trichloracetic acid (the standard), and 5 ml trichloracetic acid (the blank). To each add 1 ml ammonium molybdate solution and 1 ml metol. Allow to stand 30 min and read at 680 nm against the blank.

Calculation.

$$\text{Serum inorganic phosphate (mmol/l)} = \frac{\text{Reading of unknown}}{\text{Reading of standard}} \times 2\cdot0$$

To prepare a standard curve set up the following tubes:

Serum phosphate (mmol/l)	0	0·4	0·8	1·2	1·6	2·0	2·4	2·8
Working standard (ml)	0	0·1	0·2	0·3	0·4	0·5	0·6	0·7
Trichloracetic acid (ml)	5·0	4·9	4·8	4·7	4·6	4·5	4·4	4·3

Add 1 ml molybdate solution and 1 ml metol, stand 30 min and read at 680 nm.

Note. Inorganic phosphate determination should be performed on serum or plasma separated from the cells soon after withdrawing the blood as ester phosphates in red cells are hydrolysed with formation of inorganic phosphate, causing the serum concentration to rise.

INTERPRETATION

In adults, the normal range for serum inorganic phosphate is approximately 0·8 to 1·5 mmol/l. In children it is higher ranging from about 1·3 to 1·9 mmol/l, being highest in the neonate and falling slowly with increasing age until adult levels are reached. However, it is important to realise that serum phosphate concentrations may vary during a normal day owing to redistribution between cells and extracellular fluid influenced by carbohydrate intake and insulin secretion, which tend to lower serum phosphate levels. Ideally therefore, blood for phosphate estimation should be collected when the patient is fasting.

An increasing serum phosphate is found in chronic nephritis, progressing with increasing renal failure and reaching levels around 6·4 mmol/l when uraemic coma is present. In hypoparathyroidism only a moderate increase occurs up to about 2·6 mmol/l in association with a low serum calcium. Elevated serum phosphate concentrations also occur in cases of vitamin D excess.

A decrease in serum phosphate usually occurs in rickets or osteomalacia, caused in part by secondary hyperparathyroidism. PTH activity in primary hyperparathyroidism may also cause low serum phosphate levels in some patients, but this is not as noticeable as the elevation in serum calcium, and if renal impairment is present, this tends to favour an increase in phosphate. In other conditions affecting bone, serum phosphate is usually normal.

Hypophosphataemia may result from increased urinary phosphate loss caused by a disorder of tubular reabsorption as in some cases of the Fanconi syndrome. Some drugs, such as antacids containing aluminium and magnesium hydroxides, bind both dietary and secreted intestinal phosphate resulting in negative balance.

Many cases of hypophosphataemia result from an acute shift of phosphate into the cells, often after intravenous glucose administration which results in formation of phosphorylated hexose intermediates. Insulin therapy has a similar effect. This is particularly noticeable during treatment of diabetic ketoacidosis when some phosphate depletion probably exists. In some cases, phosphate uptake by liver and muscle cells may be at the expense of the erythrocyte, leading to decreased red cell 2,3-diphosphoglycerate which causes an increase in the oxygen affinity of haemoglobin and can result in tissue hypoxia. This possibility must also be borne in mind during the course of parenteral nutrition when very low serum phosphate levels may occur, requiring phosphate supplements to be added to infusion fluids.

Phosphate Excretion

Determination of Inorganic Phosphate in Urine

With a suitable dilution, usually 1 in 10 unless the urine is already very dilute, any of the methods for serum can be used.

INTERPRETATION

Urinary phosphate excretion is more influenced by diet than is the case with calcium because a higher proportion of phosphate intake is absorbed from the gut. On average, the daily excretion is about 32 mmol and over 96% of the total phosphorus compounds is inorganic, present mostly as a mixture of HPO_4^{2-} and $H_2PO_4^-$, the proportion varying with the urinary pH. Dihydrogen salts are acidic and monohydrogen alkaline. Dihydrogen salts of calcium and magnesium are more soluble than monohydrogen forms so that the latter precipitate more readily if the urine becomes alkaline. Such precipitation does not necessarily indicate increased phosphate excretion and can occur in patients taking aspirin, acetazolamide, steroids or diuretics. In osteomalacia, phosphate excretion is low because of poor intestinal absorption and treatment with vitamin D leads to an increase.

Increased PTH, as in hyperparathyroidism, causes phosphaturia and increased phosphate clearance. The opposite occurs in hypoparathyroidism. Several attempts have been made to utilise this phenomenon for the diagnosis of hyperparathyroidism by calculating the ratio of phosphate clearance to creatinine clearance (C_P/C_{Cr}), which is a measure of the proportion of the filtered phosphate that has not been reabsorbed in the tubule and has been lost in the urine. This can be expressed as follows:

$$\frac{C_P}{C_{Cr}} = \frac{U_P V/P_P}{U_{Cr} V/P_{Cr}} = \frac{P_{Cr} \cdot U_P}{P_P \cdot U_{Cr}}$$

where P and U refer to plasma and urinary concentrations and so the expression is independent of urine volume. In normal persons, the ratio is less than 0·15 and elevated values are often found in hyperparathyroidism. The percentage tubular reabsorbed phosphate (TRP) can also be calculated from it:

$$TRP = (1 - C_P/C_{Cr}) \times 100$$

The normal range for this is usually regarded as 84 to 95 % and reduced values occur in hyperparathyroidism. However, these indices can be influenced by dietary phosphate intake owing to its effect on serum phosphate and Nordin and Fraser (1960) attempted to eliminate this problem by the use of a Phosphate Excretion Index (PEI). The calculation of this was subsequently modified by Fraser and MacIntyre (1970). Their formula has been adapted below to accommodate serum inorganic phosphate in SI units.

$$PEI = (C_P/C_{Cr}) - (0·155 \times \text{Serum inorganic phosphate (mmol/l)} - 0·05)$$

Normal values for this are $-0·12$ to $+0·12$ and most cases of hyperparathyroidism have a high index.

It has been claimed by Walton and Bijvoet (1975) that the above indices fail to reflect accurately the activity of renal tubular phosphate reabsorption because they are influenced either by glomerular filtration rate or by net inflow of phosphate into extracellular fluid. They consider the renal threshold phosphate concentration (TmP/GFR) to be superior in this respect and have published a nomogram to calculate this when serum inorganic phosphate concentration and either TRP or C_P/C_{Cr} is known. After an overnight fast, a urine sample is collected over about 1 to 2 h together with a single blood sample. These are used to determine serum inorganic phosphate and TRP. The normal range for TmP/GFR in SI units is 0·80 to 1·35 mmol/l. Low values are found in hyperparathyroidism.

Faecal Phosphorus

Faecal phosphorus is both organic and inorganic. Since an estimation would only be done in metabolic studies, total phosphorus must be determined. Dry the faeces, powder well, weigh about 1 g and ash in an electric furnace at about 400 °C, rather below red heat. Dissolve the ash in 25 ml trichloracetic acid solution (200 g/l), filter into a 200 ml flask, washing in with further acid up to 25 ml and then make to the mark with water. Take 1 ml of this and estimate the phosphate as described above (p. 618).

On an adequate intake of phosphorus, about 32 to 64 mmol daily, intake and output balance with about two-thirds in the urine and one-third in the faeces.

REFERENCES

Agus Z. S., Wasserstein A., Goldfarb S. (1982). *Amer. J. Med*; **72**: 473.
Baginski E. S., Marie S. S., Clark W. L., Zak B. (1973). *Clin. Chim. Acta*; **46**: 49.

Cali J. P., Bowers G. N. Jr., Young D. S. (1973). *Clin. Chem*; **19**: 1208.
Cholst I. N., *et al.* (1984). *New Engl. J. Med*; **310**: 1221.
Christiansen T. F. (1975). *Scand. J. Clin. Lab. Invest*; **35**: Suppl. 143, 56.
Davies M., *et al.* (1981). *Brit. Med. J*; **282**: 1023.
De Luca H. F. (1980). *Clinics in Endocrinol. Metab*; **9**: No. 1, 3.
Dryer R. L., Routh J. I. (1963). *Stand. Methods Clin. Chem*; **4**: 191.
Editorial. (1977). *Brit. Med. J*; **1**: 598.
Fiske C. H., Subbarow Y. (1925). *J. Biol. Chem*; **66**: 375.
Fogh-Andersen N., Christiansen T. F., Komarmy L., Siggaard-Andersen O. (1978). *Clin. Chem*; **24**: 1545.
Foley T. P., Harrison H. C., Arnaud C. D., Harrison H. E. (1972). *J. Pediatrics*; **81**: 1060.
Fraser R., MacIntyre I. (1970). In *Biochemical Disorders in Human Disease*. (Thompson R.H.S., Wootton I.D.P., eds). London: Churchill Livingstone.
Garber C. C., Miller R. C. (1983). *Clin. Chem*; **29**: 184.
Gindler E. M., Heth D. A. (1971). *Clin. Chem*; **17**: 662.
Gindler E. M., King J. D. (1972). *Amer. J. Clin. Path*; **58**: 376.
Gomori G. (1942). *J. Lab. Clin. Med*; **27**: 955.
Gosling P. (1986). *Ann. Clin. Biochem*; **23**: 146.
Hooper J. (1975). *Ann. Clin. Biochem*; **12**: 255.
Hurst R. D. (1964). *Can. J. Biochem*; **42**: 287.
Itayi K., Ui M. (1966). *Clin. Chim. Acta*; **14**: 361.
Jamieson M. J. (1985). *Brit. Med. J*; **290**: 378.
Kessler G., Wolfman M. (1964). *Clin. Chem*; **10**: 686.
Khayam-Bashi H., Liu T. Z., Walter V. (1977). *Clin. Chem*; **23**: 289.
Kuttner T., Lichtenstein L. (1930). *J. Biol. Chem*; **86**: 671.
Levin G. E., Mather H. M., Pilkington T. R. E. (1981). *Diabetologia*; **21**: 131.
McGeown M. G. (1961). *Proc. Ass. Clin. Biochem*; **1**: 46.
McLean F. C., Hastings A. B. (1934). *J. Biol. Chem*; **107**: 337.
McLean F. C., Hastings A. B. (1935). *J. Biol. Chem*; **108**: 285.
Marshall R. W., Francis R. M., Hodgkinson A. (1982). *Clin. Chim. Acta*; **122**: 283.
Moore E. W. (1970). *J. Clin. Invest*; **49**: 318.
Mundy G. R., *et al.* (1984). *New Engl. J. Med*; **310**: 1718.
Nordin B. E. C., Fraser R. (1960). *Lancet*; **1**: 947.
Nordin B. E. C., Hodgkinson A., Peacock M. (1967). *Clin. Orthopaed. Related Res*; **52**: 292.
Orrell D. H. (1971). *Clin. Chim. Acta*; **35**: 483.
Paterson C. R., Gunn A. (1981). *Lancet*; **2**: 61.
Payne R. B., Jones D. P., Walker A. P., Evans R. T. (1986). *Clin. Chem*; **32**: 349.
Payne R. B., Little A. J., Williams R. B., Milner J. R. (1973). *Brit. Med. J*; **4**: 643.
Phillips P., Pain R. (1977). *Brit. Med. J*; **1**: 1473.
Pickup J. F., Jackson M. J., Price E. M., Brown S. S. (1974). *Clin. Chem*; **20**: 1324.
Pottgen P., Davies E. R. (1976). *Clin. Chem*; **22**: 1752.
Pybus J., Feldman F. J., Bowers G. N. Jr. (1970). *Clin. Chem*; **16**: 998.
Robertson W. G. (1976). *Ann. Clin. Biochem*; **13**: 540.
Robinson R., Rougham M. E., Wagstaff D. F. (1971). *Ann. Clin. Biochem*; **8**: 168.
Selby P. C., Peacock M., Marshall D. H. (1984). *Brit. J. Hosp. Med*; **31**: 186.
Siggaard-Andersen O., Thode J., Wandrup J. (1980). *IFCC, EPpH Workshop*, Copenhagen, AS79, p. 163.
Sinton T. J., Cowley D. M., Bryant S. J. (1986). *Clin. Chem*; **32**: 76.
Stern Y., Lewis W. H. P. (1957). *Clin. Chim. Acta*; **2**: 576.
Stoff J. S. (1982). *Amer. J. Med*; **72**: 489.
Tabata M., Kido T., Totani M., Murachi T. (1985). *Clin. Chem*; **31**: 703.
Vanstapel F. J., Lissens W. D. (1984). *Ann. Clin. Biochem*; **21**: 339.
Walton R. J., Bijvoet O. L. M. (1975). *Lancet*; **2**: 309.
Woodhead J. S. (1983). In *Biochemical Aspects of Human Disease* (Elkeles R. S., Tavill A. S., eds) p. 217. Oxford: Blackwell Scientific Publications.
Worth G. K., *et al.* (1981). *Clin. Chim. Acta*; **114**: 283.

25

IRON, COPPER AND ZINC

IRON

The body contains about 50 mg of iron per kilogram in the adult male and 40 mg per kilogram in the female (Finch and Huebers, 1982). Of this about three-quarters is physiologically active and the remaining quarter is storage iron. Most of the iron is present in the form of haem compounds, 90% as haemoglobin and about 10% as myoglobin with less than 1% as the various haem enzymes such as cytochromes and peroxidase. Small quantities are present in plasma bound to transferrin and there are non-haem enzymes containing iron, frequently in combination with sulphur (e.g. aconitase and xanthine oxidase).

Storage iron, present mainly in the reticulo-endothelial system—liver, bone marrow and spleen—is in two forms, ferritin and haemosiderin, and amounts to about 100–1000 mg in the adult. Ferritin consists of 24 polypeptide units, each of approximately 20 000 mol. wt., forming a sphere within which iron is stored in a polynuclear complex of hydrous ferric oxide phosphate. This soluble iron storage compound has been found in all cells of the body and each molecule contains on average 2000 atoms of iron. Haemosiderin is formed as ferritin stores increase and is an aggregated form of ferritin, in which the protein moiety is partially degraded and iron may comprise up to 50% of the deposit which stains blue with potassium ferrocyanide.

Iron in food is present mainly as organic chelates with ferric iron and its availability is dependent on the type of food. In the presence of acid (below pH 4) and reducing agents (e.g. ascorbic acid) iron is released and reduced to the ferrous, Fe(II), form in which it is absorbed mainly in the duodenum and upper jejunum. The absorptive process is controlled by the body's need for iron but the precise mechanism is still unclear. Sloughing of intestinal cells containing ferritin and actual excretion of mucosal iron may be important as well as decreased absorption (Bjorn-Rasmussen, 1983). Absorbed iron is released to plasma as Fe(III) bound to transferrin and transported as such to sites of storage or utilisation.

Less than 100 μg of iron is excreted in the urine per day and a little is lost in desquamated epithelium from the skin. These losses, together with absorbed iron which ultimately finds its way into faeces, give a total loss of not more than 1 mg. Faecal iron which is in the range 6 to 16 mg per day is thus very largely unabsorbed iron. Women, as a result of menstruation and pregnancy, have a greater average daily loss.

For reviews of iron absorption and metabolism see Bothwell et al. (1979), Jacobs and Worwood (1980), Aisen and Listowsky (1980), Finch and Huebers (1982) and Bjorn-Rasmussen (1983).

Determination of Serum Iron

It is only the ability of iron to form complexes with high absorption coefficients that permits its spectrophotometric analysis in serum. Organic chelating agents, usually containing the group $-N=C-C=N-$, are employed to form Fe(II) complexes and the choice of chromogen is largely determined by the absorption coefficient, solubility in water and cost. Examples are sulphonated bathophenanthroline (molar absorptivity 22 100) tripyridyl-s-triazine (TPTZ molar absorptivity 22 000) and another substituted triazine, ferrozine (molar absorptivity 27 900).

All spectrophotometric methods involve initial release of Fe(III) from transferrin by acidification (usually by hydrochloric acid) and reduction to Fe(II) by a reducing agent such as ascorbic acid (Sanford, 1963), thioglycollic acid (Giovanello and Peters, 1963) or hydrazine (Henry *et al.*, 1958). Reduction is largely achieved by acid alone due to the reducing nature of fresh serum but in stored serum, reduction may be incomplete in the absence of added reducing agent and coprecipitation of Fe(III) with protein may occur as a result (Ryall and Fielding, 1970).

Manual methods may be divided into those employing protein precipitation and those employing direct reaction of serum with chromogen. Trichloracetic acid is the usual protein precipitant and addition of reducing agent after deproteinisation removes the risk of releasing haemoglobin iron (ICSH Iron Panel, 1972). When precipitation is not employed, blank readings must be taken on a second tube or on the same tube prior to addition of chromogen to allow for interference by bilirubin, haemoglobin or turbidity. The advantages of the direct method are simplicity, smaller sample volume and reduced risk of contamination by extraneous iron. Ionic detergents have been employed to maximise sample clarity and Martinek (1973) has recommended Triton X–100 (iso-octylphenoxypolyethoxy ethanol) as the most satisfactory, but problems with stored or highly pigmented samples are occasionally reported when a direct method is used (Horak *et al.*, 1975). Direct methods are, however, widely used in automated discrete systems with satisfactory results.

Method Using Bathophenanthroline Sulphonate

In 1978 the International Committee for Standardisation in Hematology (ICSH) proposed a method using sulphonated bathophenanthroline which is soluble in water and used a single reagent containing acid, protein precipitant and reducing agent.

Reagents.

1. Protein precipitant. Dissolve 100 g trichloracetic acid in 700 ml water, add 30 ml thioglycollic acid and 86 ml concentrated hydrochloric acid and make up to 1 litre. Stored in a dark bottle this is stable for about 2 months.
2. Colour reagent. Dissolve 204 g sodium acetate trihydrate in 800 ml water, add 250 mg bathophenanthroline sulphonate and make up to 1 litre. Stored in a dark bottle the reagent is stable for 2 weeks at least.
3. Standard solution of iron, 2 mmol/l. Dissolve 556 mg ferrous sulphate $FeSO_4, 7H_2O$ in water, add 1 ml concentrated sulphuric acid and make to a litre. Alternatively use a solution of ferrous ammonium sulphate $(NH_4)_2SO_4, FeSO_4, 6H_2O$, 784 mg/l.
4. Working standard, 40 μmol/l. Dilute 2 ml of the stock solution to 100 ml.

Technique. To 2 ml serum add 2 ml protein precipitant solution, mix thoroughly and stand for 5 min. At the same time add 2 ml of precipitant to 2 ml water and 2 ml working standard as blank and standard respectively. Treat as the test. Centrifuge until optically clear. To 2 ml of supernatant add 2 ml colour reagent, mix and stand for at least 5 min. Read against a distilled water blank at 535 nm.

Calculation.

$$\text{Serum iron } (\mu\text{mol/l}) = \frac{\text{Reading of unknown} - \text{Reading of blank}}{\text{Reading of standard} - \text{Reading of blank}} \times 40$$

The reading of the blank should not exceed 0·015 when read against water using a cuvette with a 1 cm light path.

Notes. The method can be used routinely with 1 ml of serum and 1 ml of chromogen solution. The average between-batch precision is 2·5 μmol/l. Persijn *et al.* (1971) used ferrozine in a similar manual method.

Determination with AutoAnalyzer

Methods using the AutoAnalyzer have been available for some time but initially lacked sensitivity. Ferrozine (3-(2-pyridyl)-5,6-bis (phenyl-4-sulphonic acid)-1,2,4-triazine, disodium salt) has become widely used as a reagent of high sensitivity and low cost, but suffers interference from copper. To avoid this a specific copper-chelating agent, neocuproine, may be used. Dialysis of charged particles can be influenced by Donnan equilibrium effects and there may be lack of comparability between samples and aqueous standards caused by the higher protein concentration of the serum. This can be reduced by addition of neutral salt to the serum diluent (Babson and Kleinman, 1967) though the problem may not be entirely removed (Lestas and Tan, 1972). Jones and Deadman (1973) avoided dialysis and protein precipitation in an AutoAnalyzer II method.

Dialysis is retained but with serum-based calibration in the major AutoAnalyzer II method given here (Fig. 25.1) which is also employed on the SMAC. The serum samples (60 per hour) are added to the acid diluent stream. The donor stream now containing free Fe(II) is dialysed against the colour reagent. Finally, addition of sodium acetate to the recipient stream produces an appropriate pH for the formation of the red ferrozine complex which is estimated at 560 nm in a 15 mm light path cell. (Technicon method SF4–0025 FL–4.)

Reagents.
1. Acid diluent. To 34·8 g sodium chloride and 1 g neocuproine hydrochloride add about 500 ml distilled water and mix to dissolve. Add 9 ml concentrated hydrochloric acid (35·4 %) and make to 1 litre. For use, dissolve 2 g ascorbic acid in 200 ml of this reagent. Stored in the refrigerator it is stable for 2 weeks.
2. Colour reagent. Dissolve 350 mg Ferrozine in approximately 500 ml distilled water, add 9 ml concentrated hydrochloric acid (35·4 %) and dilute to 1 litre with distilled water.
3. Sodium acetate solution. Dissolve 82 g anhydrous sodium acetate in about 800 ml distilled water and then make to 1 litre.
4. Standard. This is a good quality calibrated control serum.

Technique. Set up the manifold as in Fig. 25.1. Pump the reagents until a steady base line is achieved. Place the samples in the sample tray with the standard at every tenth position to check for drift, having loaded an initial two or three standards. Adjust the peak height for these initially and at intervals later if

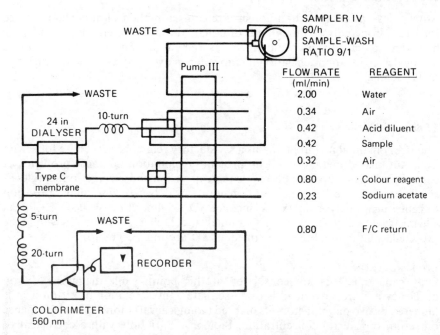

Fig. 25.1. AutoAnalyzer II Diagram for the Determination of Iron.

drift is present. After the analyses are completed wash the system with water containing 1 ml/l of 'Tween 20' containing 200 ml Tween/l.

Other Automated Methods

Of the fully automated methods, centrifugal analysis or the use of a discrete analyser are the most widely used techniques, employing modifications of manual non-precipitation methods. For example, the Roche Iron test utilises 4·5 mol/l guanidine hydrochloride in sodium acetate buffer (pH 5·0) and ascorbic acid to release Fe(II) which is complexed with ferrozine and the absorbance measured at 562 nm. A serum blank must be read.

The Determination of Serum Iron Using Atomic Absorption Spectrophotometry

The conventional methods involving chelation of iron and extraction into methyl isobutyl ketone (Zettner *et al.*, 1966) or initial protein precipitation (Olsen and Hamlin, 1969) are prone to contamination and tedious for routine use. Small samples of undiluted serum can be aspirated directly to the flame (Sebastiani *et al.*, 1973; Manning, 1975) and the height or area of absorption peaks recorded but even slight haemolysis precludes analysis as haemoglobin iron is measured. Matrix effects are also important in this method and calibration is by means of serum unless prior protein precipitation is used. The concept of flow injection analysis (Chapter 8, p. 196), in which small volumes of neat sample are injected into a continuously flowing non-segmented stream of water, may be combined with atomic absorption spectrophotometry in a manner applicable in the routine laboratory (Rocks *et al.*, 1983). This method employed deproteinised serum.

Atomic absorption spectrophotometry remains a method of minor importance for serum iron analysis, though it is of potential use as a reference method. It is, however, a practicable procedure for measurement of high levels of iron in urine during desferrioxamine chelation therapy of iron overload, as in the treatment of thalassaemia.

Choice of Methods

The ICSH manual method remains a satisfactory reference procedure for serum iron. Automated methods with no protein precipitation minimise problems of contamination and are capable of adequate precision and accuracy on samples as small as 100 μl. The AutoAnalyzer II method is widely used with similar precision to centrifugal analyser methods (median SD 1·5 μmol/l on Wellcome Clinical Chemistry Quality Control Programme) and higher precision, as would be expected, than manual methods (median SD around 2·5 μmol/l).

INTERPRETATION

Only general factors are considered at this point, while diagnosis of iron deficiency and iron overload is discussed later. Interpretation of serum iron is hindered by two major factors: its marked biological variation and its dependence on serum transferrin concentration. Biological variation, with a coefficient of variation within individuals of 30% over a few days, is approximately six times greater than likely analytical precision (Dallmann, 1984). This is partly due to a circadian variation which results in higher serum iron concentrations in the morning, and sampling is recommended at between 9.00 and 10.00 am. Biological variation is said to be less in iron deficiency but there is little documentary evidence for this (Dallmann, 1984).

A consensus of reports suggests a normal range for serum iron in the adult of 10–35 μmol/l. Some workers have found serum iron in women and men to be almost identical despite smaller iron stores in women (Bothwell *et al.*, 1979b; Klein *et al.*, 1969) but others have found a slightly higher serum iron in men with a range of 13–35 μmol/l. Serum iron is decreased in the latter half of pregnancy and during menstruation; the newborn infant has a serum iron of 27–39 μmol/l but it falls quickly in the first hours to less than 18 μmol/l and is about 10 μmol/l at 3–6 months, slowly rising to adult levels by the third to seventh year. In aged individuals, the serum iron concentration tends to be lower than in middle life. Serum iron is increased in conditions of reduced erythropoeisis (aplastic anaemia) or ineffective erythropoeisis (pernicious anaemia, thalassaemia) and it is also raised by release of storage ferritin in hepatic necrosis. Various drugs alter serum iron concentration. A decrease occurs with aspirin in large doses and with allopurinol which may cause a 40% fall within a week of starting therapy. Cholestyramine impairs iron absorption. The administration of intravenous iron dextran can result in elevated serum iron concentrations for prolonged periods due to its slow removal from the blood.

Under normal circumstances serum iron does not rise significantly after meals even if the meal is supplemented with iron (Milder *et al.*, 1978), but a temporary rise is observed after administration of iron in the fasting state or in an iron-depleted individual after a meal containing readily available iron. This has been used to assess iron absorption in iron deficiency anaemia by administering 600 mg of ferrous succinate after an overnight fast. There should be a 3-fold increase if absorption is normal. Practically no iron is excreted in health.

Iron Binding Capacity

Plasma iron is firmly bound by the β-globulin transferrin. Estimates of the mol. wt vary but the most reliable value to date is 81 000 (MacGillivray *et al.*, 1977) including 6% carbohydrate. The molecule is a single chain and its most characteristic feature is the strong association of metal combining function with · anion binding. The anion is usually carbonate or bicarbonate and strong binding of either the two cations or two anions is not possible in the absence of the other. Transfer of iron to reticulocytes involves the binding of transferrin to the reticulocyte membrane.

Transferrin exists in plasma as a mixture of apotransferrin and the mono- and diferric forms. Full saturation corresponds to the binding of two Fe(III) atoms to each transferrin molecule and transferrin may thus be measured as total iron binding capacity (TIBC), 1 μmol of transferrin corresponding to 2 μmol of iron.

As the iron protein complex is red an increase of this red colour as iron is added to serum gives a measure of the unsaturated iron binding capacity of the serum (UIBC). The sum of this and the serum iron gives the total iron binding capacity (TIBC).

Three other major methods are available for measurement of transferrin or TIBC:

1. Add an excess of iron to saturate the transferrin and allow equilibration to occur. Remove the excess unbound iron with an anion exchange resin (Peters *et al.*, 1956; Lehman and Kaplan, 1971) or magnesium carbonate (Ramsay, 1957, 1958) and determine the serum iron by one of the above techniques to give the TIBC. The use of magnesium carbonate is the most common method for measuring TIBC at present.
2. Add an excess but known amount of iron and determine the iron unbound to protein. At an alkaline pH this can be separated from the bound fraction by dialysis or more simply by using a reagent which will react with unbound iron. The difference between the two amounts of iron is that taken up by the protein and therefore the UIBC.
3. Transferrin can be determined directly by immunological methods using the Mancini radial immunodiffusion method, electroimmunoassay (the Laurell rocket technique), or immunonephelometric or immunoturbidimetric assays.

Total Iron Binding Capacity Using Magnesium Carbonate Adsorption

Reagents.
1. Ferric chloride solution, 5 μg iron per ml in hydrochloric acid, 5 mmol/l. Prepare a stock solution containing 240 mg $FeCl_3$, $6H_2O$ per 100 ml of 0·5 mol/l hydrochloric acid. Dilute this 1 to 100 with water as required to give the saturating solution.
2. Magnesium carbonate, 'light' for adsorption. Each batch should be tested for adsorptive properties by substituting water for serum in the TIBC method. Analysis of the supernatant should show no iron.

Technique. To 1 volume serum add 2 volumes ferric chloride solution, the volume used depending on the amount of supernatant required for the subsequent iron determination. With the manual bathophenanthroline method above, 1 ml of serum is required. Cover and mix. After 5 min add approximately 100 mg magnesium carbonate per ml of iron solution. Re-cover with parafilm and mix thoroughly at 10 min intervals for up to 30 min. Martinek (1973) avoids mixing continuously and prefers thorough mixing 4 or 5 times during 15 min. Mixing may continue beyond 15 min but never as long as 60 min. Centrifuge at high speed for 10 min and analyse the supernatant for iron. For the ICSH method and AutoAnalyzer techniques the result is multiplied by 3 to allow for the dilution with ferric chloride solution. This method is used for the iron binding capacity determination in the manual method of Martinek (1973) and the automated methods of Klein *et al.* (1969), Kunesh and Small (1970), and the AutoAnalyzer II procedure. Yee and Zin (1971) used ferric ammonium citrate instead of ferric chloride.

Determination of Unsaturated Iron Binding Capacity

O'Malley *et al.* (1970) used TPTZ and Tris buffer, pH 9, to estimate unbound iron in their manual procedure. Tris buffer at alkaline pH has also been used in manual (Persijn *et al.*, 1971) and direct automated (Hunteler *et al.*, 1972) methods. The most comprehensive automated system for iron and UIBC is that of Friedman and Cheek (1971) in which iron is determined on one channel using dialysis and bathophenanthroline sulphonate at pH 4·65. At the same time, on a dual channel system, excess iron is determined using a direct method with glycine buffer at pH 8·5 on one channel while the second channel determines individual blanks.

Notes. Techniques utilising addition of excess iron and subsequent removal of free iron by adsorption involve three assumptions. These are that the added iron binds quantitatively with transferrin, that the adsorbent removes no iron from combination with transferrin and that the excess iron is removed quantitatively. An excellent review of factors involved is given by Bothwell *et al.* (1979c) and is briefly described here. The first two assumptions have, under appropriate conditions, been shown to be true using radioisotopic iron methods though removal of water from plasma by resin or magnesium carbonate may produce apparent recoveries of bound iron of greater than 100%. The quantitative removal of saturating iron by adsorbent is not entirely valid and increasing values for TIBC may be obtained with increasing quantities of saturating iron.

These factors indicate that care must be taken to ensure reproducible conditions for the saturating and adsorption procedures otherwise imprecision may result. Despite this, in practice the SD of TIBC methods is approximately twice that of the method used to measure iron alone (p. 624), suggesting that the CV% of the two techniques is comparable.

Tsung *et al.* (1975) found good agreement between immunological transferrin measurement and conventional manual (Ramsay, 1958) and continuous flow methods (Yee and Zin, 1971) for TIBC. However, results were 20% higher using a radioisotopic method for UIBC as had been found by Van der Heul *et al.* (1972). This may be attributable to exchange of unbound iron in the saturating solution with transferrin-bound iron rather than the binding of saturating iron to non-transferrin globulins as was originally proposed. Immunological techniques, especially with the availability of automated solution methods (Blom and Hjorn, 1976; Spencer and Price, 1980), have a theoretical and practical advantage (small volumes of serum and total automation) but suffer at present from lack of uniformity in calibration material (Bandi *et al.*, 1985).

INTERPRETATION
The adult normal range for TIBC is found to be slightly wider in women than men, approximately 45–70 μmol/l in men and 40–80 μmol/l in women (Davies *et*

al., 1952; Bothwell *et al.*, 1979a; Milman and Cohn, 1984). Analytical and biological variations are of similar magnitude with a CV of approximately 5–6% between days (Dallman, 1984). At birth, serum concentrations of transferrin are lower (TIBC, 40 μmol/l) and increase to reach adult values by about 2 years, then increasing further so that the 2·5 to 97·5 centile range for 4–13 year old children is 60–94 μmol/l (Milman and Cohn, 1984).

Serum TIBC rises substantially in the second half of pregnancy to about 90 μmol/l in the eighth month. Oral contraceptives may have a similar effect depending on oestrogen content. With old age there is a tendency for TIBC to decline. Transferrin is a negative acute phase reactant, thus any cause of trauma, inflammation or infection is associated with decreased concentrations of TIBC, as of course, are protein-losing conditions such as the nephrotic syndrome. Glucocorticoids or ACTH cause a fall in serum transferrin. A TIBC of 60 μmol/l corresponds to 2·43 g/l of transferrin assuming a molecular weight of 81 000 for transferrin.

Serum Ferritin

Concentrations of serum ferritin are closely related to the amount of storage iron. In approximate terms, 1 μg/l ferritin represents 8–10 mg of storage iron (Finch and Huebers, 1982) though, particularly in children, a weight-related value of 1 μg/l ferritin for 140 μg/kg of storage iron is preferable. This appears to apply between 15 and 500 μg/l serum ferritin. The circulating ferritin is apoferritin, containing little or no iron except in cases of acute release of storage ferritin from the liver due to cell necrosis.

Determination of Serum Ferritin

The first practicable assay of serum ferritin, a one site immunoradiometric assay (IRMA) was described by Addison *et al.* (1972), and a two site IRMA was later described by Miles *et al.* (1974). Increasing use is now being made of enzyme linked immunosorbent assay (ELISA) techniques employing ferritin antibodies labelled with horseradish peroxidase or alkaline phosphatase. Radioimmuno-assay (RIA) has also been used.

The IRMAs are potentially more sensitive than RIA which may be near its sensitivity limit at the point of interest for iron deficiency (around 10 μg/l) and sensitivity limits are improving for ELISA methods. The shape of the dose–response curve for labelled antibody methods is such that two ferritin concentrations may correspond to one recorded number of counts per minute (the high dose hook) and analysis may be required at two different dilutions to be sure the ascending part of the standard curve is being used. It is necessary to prepare ferritin (from liver or spleen) for use in calibration and there are standard methods for this, involving ultracentrifugation or precipitation of ferritin using cadmium sulphate; a reference ferritin preparation is available. Jacobs and Worwood (1984) have reviewed methods for assay of serum ferritin.

Erythrocyte Protoporphyrin

When iron is unavailable in sufficient quantity for incorporation to haem in the developing reticulocyte (as in iron deficiency) or when its incorporation is impaired (as in lead toxicity) protoporphyrin IX accumulates and remains in the mature red cell until its destruction. Erythrocyte protoporphyrin is increased in certain rare disorders of porphyrin metabolism but this does not preclude its use for diagnosis of iron deficiency. Its determination is discussed in the next Chapter (p. 654).

The Diagnosis of Iron Deficiency and Iron Overload

Iron Deficiency

The traditional diagnosis of iron deficiency anaemia rests on the finding of a microcytic hypochromic anaemia. This does not appear until storage iron has disappeared and is an advanced stage of a gradual process. However, in many cases the study of haematological indices together with clinical findings and a therapeutic trial of iron will obviate the requirement for analysis of serum iron or related substances.

Diagnostic difficulties arise if the anaemia of chronic disease is suspected as this may cause mild microcytosis. The problem is compounded if there is suspicion of an underlying iron deficiency. A further area of difficulty is latent iron deficiency in which haematological changes in peripheral blood have not manifested themselves, but iron stores are exhausted. The single most useful test is serum ferritin. In otherwise healthy subjects with iron deficiency, serum ferritin concentrations are less than 15 μg/l. Retesting after iron therapy should not be carried out until 2 weeks after cessation of therapy to allow a reliable indication of iron stores (Worwood, 1982). Acute infection or inflammation causes a rise in serum ferritin and iron-deficient patients with no stainable marrow iron may have serum ferritin concentrations of 50–100 μg/l. The test remains useful in this difficult condition as a patient with normal iron stores and inflammation would have a markedly higher serum ferritin. Serum ferritin is high in the newborn but decreases later and concentrations below 15 μg/l may be found although this, like the lowered values in pregnancy, may be a reflection of high erythroid activity and latent iron deficiency.

Serum iron alone is not a useful test. Combined with assessment of TIBC to give percentage transferrin saturation its use increases as iron deficiency lowers serum iron concentration and increases TIBC and a transferrin saturation of less than 15% usually indicates inadequate iron stores. Inflammation and infection depress both serum iron and TIBC but not necessarily in parallel, and saturation may fall below 15% with adequate iron stores. For unequivocal indication of iron deficiency the saturation should be less than 15% and the TIBC should be elevated.

In iron-replete 4 year old children, the 2·5th centile for transferrin saturation is 3% so that the test is able to indicate satisfactory iron stores if transferrin saturation is high, but a low value has a very poor predictive value for iron deficiency (Milman and Cohn, 1984). Erythrocyte protoporphyrin reflects the unavailability of iron for erythropoiesis and is increased in iron deficiency to values of greater than 700 μg/l of red cells (Piomelli *et al.*, 1976) but may also be increased when iron release from the reticulo-endothelial system is impaired as in inflammatory disease or infection.

Iron deficiency is difficult to diagnose after trauma or surgery as serum iron and TIBC are depressed and serum ferritin increased in the acute phase in the absence of postoperative complications (Mohammed *et al.*, 1983). For detailed consideration of the factors involved in diagnosis of iron deficiency the reader is referred to reviews and papers by Dallman (1977), Finch and Huebers (1982), Jacobs and Worwood (1984), Milman and Cohn (1984), Piomelli *et al.* (1976).

Iron Overload

Two major disorders lead to parenchymal (as opposed to reticulo-endothelial) accumulation of iron. These are conditions producing high erythropoeitic rates (thalassaemia, sideroblastic anaemia) with concurrent excessive iron absorption, and the genetically determined idiopathic haemochromatosis (IHC) (Finch, 1982). In these conditions serum ferritin is greatly increased, in IHC to between 1 and 10 mg/l in established disease. But the use of serum ferritin in assessing minor degrees of iron overload is controversial (Worwood, 1982) and a rise in serum iron and transferrin saturation may often occur before increase in serum ferritin concentration. A transferrin saturation of more than 60 % and an increased serum ferritin make increased iron stores very likely and normal values for both reduce the likelihood of IHC to almost zero (Gollan, 1983).

The use of laboratory tests to aid diagnosis of iron deficiency or overload is a subject requiring the cooperation of haematologists, clinicians and biochemists if the appropriate tests are to be made available and unnecessary, expensive and misleading investigations are to be avoided.

COPPER

The body contains about 100 mg (1·6 mmol) of copper, widely distributed in various tissues but with the highest concentrations in liver and brain. The copper in plasma exists largely in the form of ceruloplasmin, a metalloprotein of molecular weight 132 000 containing 6 atoms of copper per molecule (Ryder, 1971) and 7–8 % carbohydrate. Ceruloplasmin copper constitutes 90–95 % of serum copper, most of the remainder of plasma copper being albumin bound, with 1–2 % associated with amino acids.

Ceruloplasmin has a number of potential functions, mostly of uncertain importance (Frieden and Hsieh, 1976). It is an oxidase (previously called copper oxidase, now ferroxidase I) able to oxidise Fe(II) on its release from the hepatocyte permitting the formation of the Fe(III)-transferrin complex, and providing a possible molecular link between copper and iron metabolism. Removal of Fe(II) may also have an important protective function by reducing formation of superoxide ion in plasma and this activity could link with its nature as an acute phase reactant, increasing in concentration after trauma, inflammation or infection. Finally, ceruloplasmin may act as an important vehicle of copper transport to the tissues, in particular to cytochrome c oxidase (Hsieh and Frieden, 1975).

Copper is a constituent of a number of enzymes other than ceruloplasmin, most of them involved in electron transfer or oxygen binding. Examples are cytochrome c oxidase, superoxide dismutase and lysyl oxidase (important in biosynthesis of connective tissue). Connective tissue abnormalities of blood vessels and bone are prominent in copper deficiency. The recommended daily dietary allowance for copper is about 2·5 mg (40 μmol) and this intake is often exceeded on a normal diet, though bio-availability varies and the presence of other metal ions may inhibit absorption. In neonates, the intake is much less as milk (cow's milk in particular) is relatively poor in copper. About one to two-thirds of ingested copper is absorbed in the small intestine probably by a mechanism closely related to that for zinc. After transport across the brush border, copper and zinc may pass from the intracellular pool to combine with plasma albumin in the portal blood, or remain in the enterocyte bound to intestinal metallothionein (Cousins, 1985). Absorption is impaired in conditions of mucosal damage.

Copper is excreted primarily in bile, thus faeces contain both unabsorbed and excreted copper. The copper concentration in urine is very low. For reviews of copper metabolism and copper proteins the reader is referred to Aspin and Sass-Kortsak (1981), Walravens (1980), Sandstead (1981) and Cousins (1985).

Determination of Serum Copper and Ceruloplasmin

Colorimetric methods for the determination of serum copper have been superseded by atomic absorption spectrophotometry. As this method is also used for analysis of serum zinc and many factors are common to both methods they are discussed together below.

Ceruloplasmin

Serum ceruloplasmin is now usually determined by immunological methods. Radial immunodiffusion (Mancini technique) is the most common procedure, but electroimmunoassay (Laurell rockets) can also be used. Light scattering immunoassay procedures are quite feasible, but the small numbers tested in most centres may not justify this approach.

Enzymatic determination of ceruloplasmin as an oxidase (see the 5th edition of this book) is potentially less precise than immunological methods which also have the potential advantage of calibration against reference preparations (WHO, 1978; Nakamura et al., 1981).

INTERPRETATION
A satisfactory normal range for serum copper is 12–25 μmol/l though there have been marked interlaboratory differences (Versieck and Cornelius, 1980). Most authors find no difference between concentrations in men and women. Normal serum ceruloplasmin concentration ranges from 200 to 500 mg/l in adults. Except in Wilson's disease ceruloplasmin accounts for approximately 95% of serum copper (1 μmol/l copper is equivalent to 22 mg/l ceruloplasmin) and changes in serum copper and ceruloplasmin concentration with age and disease are thus parallel (Neumann and Sass-Kortsak, 1967).

Neonatal serum ceruloplasmin concentration is low (mean 100 mg/l, copper 4·5 μmol/l (Shaw, 1980)), and increases to reach adult levels around 6 months to 1 year. Hypocupraemia is rare and may be caused by copper deficiency (due to an inadequate diet or impaired absorption) or by decreased ceruloplasmin (due to inadequate synthesis or increased loss).

Copper deficiency has been recognised increasingly frequently in humans, especially in infants and those receiving synthetic oral or intravenous feeding. The most common presenting features are anaemia, neutropenia or, less often, bone changes resembling those seen in scurvy. Predisposing factors are prematurity (resulting in low liver copper stores at birth (Shaw, 1980)) and gastrointestinal disturbance. Serum copper is low in the two inherited disorders of copper metabolism, Menkes' disease and Wilson's disease (Danks, 1983). Menkes' disease is an X-linked recessive condition in which copper concentration in serum is low and many features are consistent with defective synthesis of copper enzymes due to copper deficiency (though the most common feature of copper deficiency, anaemia, is absent). Intestinal mucosal copper is high and a block appears to occur at this stage, although the situation is complex (Walravens, 1980). Intravenous administration of copper causes increased ceruloplasmin synthesis and a normal serum copper, but this does not have therapeutic application. Clinical findings are characteristic and the disease is rapidly lethal; laboratory investigation is required only infrequently. Excessive protein loss, e.g. in nephrotic syndrome, decreases serum copper due to loss of ceruloplasmin.

Hypocupraemia is thus a rare but often significant finding; on the contrary, a high serum copper concentration is fairly common, but a secondary finding of little diagnostic importance. Ceruloplasmin is an acute phase reactant and serum copper is raised by trauma, or inflammation, and also by oestrogens as in pregnancy (when it reaches twice the normal adult value) or oral contraceptive therapy (Shaw, 1980). Increased dietary copper is rarely a cause of increased serum copper as biliary excretion is adequate to maintain homeostasis. When biliary excretion is impaired, as in primary biliary cirrhosis or longstanding bile duct obstruction serum copper concentrations rise substantially. Malignancy often causes increased serum copper and ceruloplasmin, notably in Hodgkin's disease, but this is insufficiently specific for diagnostic use, though it may be of value in following treatment.

Determination of Urinary Copper

Great care must be taken in collection of urinary copper samples to avoid contamination. Plastic collection bottles should be washed in dilute acid (nitric or hydrochloric) as should any plastic vessel used for initial collection of the urine before transfer to the bottle.

Urinary copper is measured by atomic absorption spectrophotometry. Dawson *et al.* (1968) employed undiluted urine but found significant suppression of the copper absorption by inorganic salts present in the urine. This interference was not concentration-dependent and they compensated for it by loading standards with a mixture of salts. Meret and Henkin (1971) utilised the same method as for serum, diluting the urine 10-fold in water.

Lack of sensitivity is a problem in analysis of urinary copper at normal concentrations but the absence of a protein matrix effect allows use of lower dilutions. The direct injection of boluses of undiluted urine (see p. 625) is also more practicable than it is for serum. The problems associated with ionic interference must be assessed for a particular method and instrument as described later.

INTERPRETATION

Urinary copper excretion is somewhat variable, but in most cases is between 0·3 and 0·6 μmol/24 h (Aspin and Sass-Kortsak, 1981), although Dawson *et al.* (1968) reported 0·3–1·0 μmol/24 h and Meret and Henkin (1971) 0·15–1·8 μmol/24 h. An elevated urinary copper (more than 4 μmol/24 h, normal less than 0·6 μmol/24 h) is virtually pathognomonic of Wilson's disease in the absence of liver or renal disease, especially if the excretion rises to greater than 20 μmol/24 h on penicillamine treatment (excretion on penicillamine less than 13 μmol/24 h in normals). In this test, 1 g of penicillamine is given in 2 or 4 equal daily doses, However, cirrhosis due to other causes is also associated with increased 'free' copper and copper excretion. Fortunately, in hepatic cirrhosis not associated with Wilson's disease, serum copper and ceruloplasmin concentrations are high in contrast to the low values in Wilson's disease. Urinary excretion is not raised presymptomatically.

Wilson's disease, which is inherited in an autosomal recessive fashion, may present primarily as a neurological or hepatic problem or a combination of the two and the symptoms are those of copper toxicity. The neurological presentation is more common in adults and the hepatic in children, but the disease is rarely manifest before 8 years of age. Treatment is very successful in the neurological form and, if started early enough, may be life-saving in the hepatic presentation so it is important to consider this diagnosis in all patients with neurological disease relatable to the basal ganglia or with hepatic cirrhosis of unknown cause. The basic defect appears to be in biliary excretion of copper which thus accumulates in the liver and then in other organs, particularly brain and kidney. In addition, copper incorporation into ceruloplasmin is grossly impaired. As a consequence serum copper and ceruloplasmin are usually low (86% of patients have a ceruloplasmin less than 100 mg/l) though they may be low normal, particularly in liver disease. The proportion of 'free' or non-ceruloplasmin-bound copper is greater than usual (i.e. more than 10% of total serum copper) and sometimes very much greater. Imprecision in the determinations of serum copper and ceruloplasmin must, however, be taken into account in interpreting the apparent concentration of 'free' copper. The excessive 'free' copper is associated with tissue toxicity and increased urinary copper excretion.

ZINC

The body contains an average of approximately 2 g (30 mmol) of zinc in the adult, the highest concentration being found in the prostate with bone, muscle, liver and kidney containing about 50 μg/kg (Sandstead, 1981). There are numerous zinc-containing enzymes, e.g. alkaline phosphatase, DNA polymerase, pyruvate carboxylase and alcohol dehydrogenase. The ubiquity of zinc-dependent enzymes helps to explain why zinc deficiency has been associated with a wide range of symptoms such as growth failure, delayed sexual maturation, congenital malformation, skin rashes, susceptibility to infection, delayed wound healing and impaired taste (Aggett and Harries, 1979; Walravens, 1980; Gordon *et al.*, 1981; Sandstead, 1981). Marginal deficiency may be comparatively common, especially in those receiving low quality diets and an adequate laboratory test to detect mild zinc deficiency would be of value. Such a test is not, however, readily available (Solomons, 1979a).

The average daily intake of zinc in the adult is 13 mg (200 μmol) and absorption, mainly in the upper small intestine, is homeostatically controlled. The availability of dietary zinc is affected by the nature of the food (decreased by dietary fibre and phytate, increased by meat products) and there is an antagonistic effect of ferrous iron on zinc absorption (Meadows *et al.*, 1983; Solomons *et al.*, 1979b). After mucosal uptake (by an enzyme or carrier-mediated process), some zinc binds to metallothionein in intestinal mucosal cells. The synthesis of metallothionein is stimulated by zinc, and this cysteine-rich protein probably acts to limit zinc (and copper) entry into the portal blood.

In plasma approximately 80% of zinc is bound to albumin and 20% to globulin, almost exclusively α_2-macroglobulin (Foote and Delves, 1983) with only 2% non-protein bound.

Faeces contain zinc from gastrointestinal secretions as well as sloughed intestinal cells and unabsorbed dietary zinc and this is the main route of excretion. As a result, diarrhoea is an important cause of increased zinc loss. Urinary losses of zinc account for about 300–600 μg/24 h and sweat losses can be of similar magnitude in hotter weather. Urinary zinc losses are increased in cirrhosis of the liver (Halsted and Smith, 1970) and intravenous administration of amino acids (Main *et al.*, 1982).

A genetic deficiency disease, acrodermatitis enteropathica, has been described in which zinc malabsorption occurs after weaning from breast milk and results in severe zinc deficiency which is fatal if untreated but responds well to pharmacological doses of zinc. A facilitator of zinc absorption appears to be deficient in the affected child but present in breast milk and this has been postulated to be picolinic acid. For further details of zinc in health and disease the reader is referred to the reviews cited above and in addition to that of Cousins (1985).

Measurement of Serum Zinc and Copper by Atomic Absorption Spectrophotometry

All reagents, containers and procedures should be considered as potential sources of contamination when copper and zinc are being analysed (Reimold and Besch, 1978; Versieck 1984) but zinc poses the greater problems. Each individual laboratory should assess the various procedural steps of its own method in this respect.

The Sample

Conventional plastic disposable syringes are adequate for blood collection but the specimen should be placed in a polypropylene tube with a polythene cap to minimise contamination. Rubber stoppers are a rich source of zinc and cap liners can be a source of zinc or copper contamination. Standard Vacutainer tubes are inappropriate for trace metal analysis (Helman *et al.*, 1971) but 'low metal' Vacutainer tubes are better (Reimold and Besch, 1978). Clotting was said to release zinc from platelets and cause serum to have a higher zinc concentration than plasma (Foley *et al.*, 1968) but Kiilerich *et al.* (1981) showed this to be an artefact and equivalent serum and plasma specimens to have indistinguishable zinc concentrations. Batches of heparin should be checked if plasma is used as it contains variable quantities of zinc though very little copper (Sansoni and Iyengar, 1980).

Sample and Standard Treatment and Matrix Effects

Early methods employed extraction of zinc and copper into organic solvents, or use of very low dilutions of serum to make up for the poor sensitivity of apparatus at the time. This is no longer necessary, but a choice must still be made between use of a highly diluted sample which minimises matrix effects and interference, or a low dilution which maximises sensitivity. This is particularly so for copper which gives absorbances approximately half those of zinc at the same concentration. Protein affects viscosity and surface tension and these in turn affect aspiration rate and aerosol formation in the spray chamber. The effect of viscosity on aspiration rate is mainly determined by the diameter of the capillary (Reinhold *et al.*, 1968; Winefordner and Latz, 1961). Size distribution of droplets in the aerosol determines the proportion of sample entering the flame.

Inorganic ions, in particular sodium or its salts, may interfere by suppressing the ionisation of zinc or copper, by emission, or by scattering of the incident light. These effects are highly dependent on the flame conditions and will vary with gas pressure, the position of the light path in the flame, aspiration rate (and thus flame temperature) and the geometry of the nebulising system (Reinhold *et al.*, 1968; Winefordner and Latz, 1961). As a consequence different authors have frequently disagreed on the importance of particular matrix effects and their conclusions as to the best method have been different. It is necessary that individual laboratories should assess the main factors on their own instrument and with their own procedures rather than accepting literature reports as transferable. Any significant matrix effects must be reproduced in the standards to obtain accuracy.

Sample Dilution

The aspiration rate of a one in ten dilution of serum in water is very similar to that of water itself (Momcilovic *et al.*, 1975) and standards may be prepared in simple aqueous solution (Meret and Henkin, 1971). Dawson *et al.* (1968, 1969) used a higher dilution of one in twenty for both serum zinc and copper and the diluent in this case was hydrochloric acid 100 mmol/l. Under these conditions no difference was found in serum concentration of zinc or copper as determined by wet-ashing techniques or by simple one in twenty dilution and the organic matrix was considered to have no effect at this dilution. Meret and Henkin (1971) utilised 6% butanol as diluent (one part serum in ten of diluent) and achieved a 30% increase in sensitivity compared to the use of water only. This effect is due to decreased viscosity and differences in droplet formation and the technique is widely used, especially for serum copper (Taylor and Bryant, 1981).

A serum dilution of one in five improves sensitivity, but usually results in significantly slower aspiration rates compared to simple aqueous solution. The aqueous standards may be replaced by ones made up in 5% glycerol to give comparable viscosity (Smith *et al.*, 1979) and in this case the slope of the standard curve matches exactly that of a series of serum specimens of known zinc concentration (Butrimovitz and Purdy, 1977). Dextran has been used instead of glycerol (Hackley *et al.*, 1968) but the limitation of any viscosity adaptation is that viscosity is not the sole cause of different absorbances obtained from serum and aqueous standards of the same concentration and like any other addition it is a further possible cause of contamination.

If protein is precipitated the effect of the protein matrix is removed. Olsen and Hamlin (1969) recommended the use of trichloracetic acid and heating to release all the zinc, but Kelson and Shamberger (1978) used one part of serum to three parts of trichloracetic acid (67 g/l) with no heat treatment and obtained results more accurate and higher than those using a one in ten aqueous dilution of serum. (The standard curve was, however, not linear using standards made up in trichloracetic acid.) Volume changes on precipitation were not the cause of this difference, nor was difference in aspiration rate, and the postulated interfering factor was not removed from serum by dialysis. The precipitation method is not commonly used, however, as it is tedious and prone to contamination.

The main inorganic interference is due to sodium and a variety of effects has been reported. Prasad *et al.* (1965) found sodium to depress the absorbance of zinc solutions, whereas Henkin (1971) found enhancement and Smith *et al.* (1979) found no effect. Most workers have not noted problems with copper analysis (interferences are in general less severe at longer wavelengths) but Meret and Henkin (1971) reported up to 50 % increase in absorbance of copper solutions in the presence of sodium at concentrations greater than 125 mmol/l. It is clear that individual laboratories must make their own decision in this respect. If sodium causes interference it must be included in standards or possibly allowed for by background correction, a means whereby the absorbance of light from a continuous deuterium arc source is used to compensate for non-specific absorbance in the analytical beam from the hollow cathode lamp (p. 171).

In the analysis of zinc, Momčilović *et al.* (1975) compared standards made up in water, 150 mmol/l sodium chloride, a synthetic serum containing other ionic species but not protein, and nitric acid (10 g/l). When measuring zinc concentration in serum to which zinc had been added, use of dilute nitric acid gave recoveries of 100 % whereas water gave 110 % and saline and synthetic serum gave 92 % recovery. The effects of nitric acid were considered to balance fortuitously the matrix effects in serum when diluted one in ten with water.

Equipment

Published methods differ in many other respects, e.g. the washing procedure for glassware or the means of preparation of standards. It is recommended that glassware is soaked for 24 h in acid: nitric or hydrochloric have been used at several concentrations, e.g. 0·1 mol/l nitric acid (Momčilović *et al.*, 1975) or 6 mol/l hydrochloric acid (Kelson and Shamberger, 1978). Additional washing with a solution of EDTA may be carried out (Smith *et al.*, 1979). Plastics in general are not acid-washed, or, if so, in dilute nitric acid (50 g/l nitric acid; Dawson, 1968) as strong nitric acid may expose zinc binding sites. Some authors use 'ageing' of glassware in the concentration of standard in which it is to be used, as glassware may remove zinc as well as add it to solutions (Dawson, 1968; Meret and Henkin, 1971). Standards may be made by dissolution of pure zinc in hydrochloric acid, or zinc or copper in nitric acid. Alternatively, commercially prepared standards may be used with appropriate dilutions. Copper is estimated at a wavelength of 324·7 nm and zinc at 213·9 nm, and both employ a lean flame of acetylene and air.

Analytical Performance

Accuracy is often assessed by comparison with a method of standard additions and also by recovery experiments. It is subject to the matrix and interference problems described above, and reliable assayed quality control material is not readily available. Precision between days for zinc analysis is such that the CV may be as low as 2–4 % (Kelson and Shamberger, 1978; Reimold and Besch, 1978) and similar precision is obtainable with copper. Baseline drift may be a significant problem at the scale expansion used with higher dilutions of serum and the cause of imprecision for zinc is probably more often contamination than is the case with copper (Taylor and Bryant, 1981). Careful standardisation of procedures and close attention to detail is necessary. The checking of linearity and the slope of the standard curve (Reimold and Besch, 1978) is a useful form of quality control. The results of an external quality assessment scheme have been reported (Taylor and Bryant, 1981).

Choice of Method for Serum Zinc and Copper

The choice of method and procedural details will depend on the equipment used and relative importance placed on frequently contradictory literature reports. An outline method is described.

Standard. Use atomic absorption standards (BDH Chemicals), 1 g/l, for both copper and zinc. Prepare a mixed stock standard of 1 mmol/l each of copper and zinc by pipetting 6·37 ml of copper standard and 6·54 ml of zinc standard to an acid-washed 100 ml volumetric flask. Make to 100 ml with high quality deionised water. Store in a plastic bottle. Prepare working standards of 10, 20 and 30 μmol/l by diluting 1, 2 and 3 ml of mixed stock standard to 100 ml in volumetric flasks, possibly incorporating sodium chloride at a concentration of 150 mmol/l if the instrumentation and conditions require this. Store in plastic bottles and remake all standards every 2 weeks or whenever control values or linearity indicate problems have developed.

Samples. Dilute samples and standards one in ten in water. The dilution is best performed using an automatic dilutor and, if sample volume permits, in duplicate. For analysis of both trace metals 4 ml of diluted serum is adequate. Linearity of the standard curve should be checked, together with the actual absorbance of standards, and two serum controls at different concentrations should be incorporated.

Other Modifications

Weinstock and Uhlemann (1981) used a method of *direct injection* whereby 100 μl of undiluted serum was inserted into a funnel and aspirated directly to the spray chamber with boluses of water in between to prevent clogging of the burner. As matrix effects are not simply a matter of viscosity, standardisation employed a serum previously calibrated by the method of standard additions rather than a 'viscosity adapted' aqueous standard. These authors describe a method for copper but similar procedures for zinc have been described (Manning, 1975 and Makino and Takahara, 1981). Concentrations are determined by recorded heights of absorbance peaks measured using a chart recorder or peak integrator. The technique combines use of small sample volumes with high sensitivity.

A related technique is that of *flow injection analysis* (p. 196) which has been applied by Rocks *et al.* (1982) to zinc and copper analysis of undiluted serum by atomic absorption spectrophotometry. The advantages are small sample size and sensitivity combined with rapid sample throughput and low contamination risk. *Electrothermal atomisation* involves the direct application of samples to a graphite furnace in which they are ashed and vapourised without the use of a flame. Very small samples are required and the method is very sensitive but the technique requires special apparatus and makes strict demands as regards reproducible sample application, avoidance of contamination and compensation for non-atomic absorption.

INTERPRETATION OF SERUM ZINC

Normal adult ranges are laboratory dependent with the mean varying from 13–17 μmol/l (Sandstead, 1981) but most recent reports give an adult range of approximately 10–22 μmol/l (Versieck and Cornelius, 1980), with children having similar values to adults. Lower serum zinc concentrations in infants are probably associated with inadequate intake. There is diurnal variation resulting in higher concentrations in the morning than in the afternoon (Hetland and Brubakk,

1973) and this is probably associated with meals. Haemolysis increases serum zinc due to the high red cell concentration of carbonic anhydrase, a zinc metallo-enzyme. Serum zinc concentration is decreased in late pregnancy. Increased concentrations of serum zinc are rarely found except in parenteral nutrition with excessive supplementation of zinc.

Interpretation of serum zinc is hampered by the many factors other than zinc nutrition that affect its concentration. These include hypoalbuminaemia, trauma, stress, inflammation and infection. The subject is too extensive for discussion here and the reader is referred to the excellent review by Solomons (1979a) and the general reviews of zinc metabolism referred to above. Because of the poor specificity of serum zinc as an indicator of zinc deficiency many other approaches have been proposed, such as measurement of leucocyte zinc (Patrick and Dervish, 1984), hair zinc (Laker, 1982; Hambidge, 1982) and changes in metalloenzyme activities on zinc therapy (Danks, 1981), but the single most effective test remains a therapeutic trial of zinc in association with careful clinical assessment (Aggett and Harries, 1979; Solomons, 1979a).

REFERENCES

Addison G. M., *et al.* (1972). *J. Clin. Pathol*; **25**: 326.

Aggett P. J., Harries J. T. (1979). *Arch. Dis. Childh*; **54**: 909.

Aisen P., Listowsky I. (1980). *Ann. Rev. Biochem*; **49**: 357.

Aspin N., Sass-Kortsak A. (1981). In *Disorders of Mineral Metabolism*, Vol. I. (Bronner T., Coburn J. W., eds) p. 59. New York: Academic Press.

Babson A. L., Kleinman N. M. (1967). *Clin. Chem*; **13**: 163.

Bandi Z. L., Schoen I., Bee D. E. (1985). *Clin Chem*; **31**: 1601.

Bjorn-Rasmussen E. (1983). *Lancet*; **1**: 914.

Blom M., Hjorn N. (1976). *Clin. Chem*; **22**: 657.

Bothwell T. H., Charlton R. W., Cook J. D., Finch C. A. (1979). *Iron Metabolism in Man.* Oxford: Blackwell Scientific Publications. (a) p. 295, (b) p. 297, (c) p. 367.

Butrimovitz G. P., Purdy W. C. (1977). *Anal. Chim. Acta*; **94**: 63.

Cousins R. J. (1985). *Physiol. Rev*; **65**: 238.

Dallman P. R. (1977). *J. Pediatr*; **90**: 678.

Dallman P. R. (1984). *Amer. J. Clin. Nutr*; **39**: 937.

Danks D. M. (1981). *Amer. J. Clin. Nutr*; **34**: 278.

Danks D. M. (1983). In *The Metabolic Basis of Inherited Disease.* (Stanbury J. B., *et al.*, eds) p. 1251. New York: McGraw-Hill.

Davies G., Levin B., Oberholtzer V. G. (1952). *J. Clin. Pathol*; **5**: 312.

Dawson J. B., Ellis D. J., Newton-John H. (1968). *Clin. Chim. Acta*; **21**: 33.

Dawson J. B., Walker B. E. (1969). *Clin. Chim. Acta*; **26**: 465.

Finch C. A. (1982). *New Engl. J. Med*; **307**: 1702.

Finch C. A., Huebers H. (1982). *New Engl. J. Med*; **306**: 1520.

Foley B., *et al.* (1968). *Exper. Biol. Med*; **128**: 265.

Foote J. W., Delves H. T. (1983). *Analyst*; **108**: 492.

Frieden E., Hsieh H. S. (1976). *Adv. Enzymol*; **44**: 187.

Friedman H. S., Cheek C. S. (1971). *Clin. Chim. Acta*; **31**: 315.

Giovanello T. J., Peters T. Jr. (1963). *Standard Methods of Clinical Chemistry.* (Seligson D., ed); **4**: 523. New York: Academic Press.

Gollan J. L. (1983). *Gastroenterol*; **84**: 418.

Gordon E. F., Gordon R. C., Passal D. B. (1981). *J. Pediatr*; **99**: 341.

Hackley B. M., Smith J. C. Jr., Halsted J. A. (1968). *Clin. Chem*; **14**: 1.

Halsted J. A., Smith J. C. Jr. (1970). *Lancet*; **1**: 322.

Hambidge K. M. (1982). *Amer. J. Clin. Nutr*; **36**: 943.

Helman E. Z., Wallick D. K., Reingold I. M. (1971). *Clin. Chem*; **17**: 61.

Henkin R. I. (1971). In *Newer Trace Elements in Nutrition.* (Mertz W., Comatzer N. E., eds) p. 255. New York: Marcel Dekker.

Henry R. J., Sobel C., Chiamori N. (1958). *Clin. Chim. Acta*; **3**: 523.

Hetland O., Brubakk E. (1973). *Scand. J. Clin. Lab. Invest*; **32**: 225.

Horak E., Hohnadel D. C., Sunderman F. W. (1975). *Ann. Clin. Lab. Sci*; **5**: 303.

Hsieh H. S., Frieden E. (1975). *Biochem. Biophys. Research Commun*; **67**: 1326.

Hunteler J. L. A., Van der Slik W., Persijn J.-P. (1972) *Clin. Chim. Acta*; **37**: 391.

International Committee for Standardisation in Hematology (ICSH) (Iron Panel). (1972). *Modern Concepts in Haematology.* (Izak G., Lewis S. M., eds) p. 69. New York, London: Academic Press.

ICSH (Iron Panel). (1978). *Brit. J. Haematol*; **38**: 291.

Jacobs A., Worwood M. eds. (1980). *Iron in Biochemistry and Medicine II.* New York, London: Academic Press.

Jacobs A., Worwood M. (1984). Broadsheet 111. Association of Clinical Pathologists, London.

Jones J., Deadman N. M. (1973). *Clin. Chim. Acta*; **48**: 367.

Kelson J. R., Shamberger R. J. (1978). *Clin Chem*; **24**: 240.

Kiilerich S., Christensen M. S., Naestoft J., Christianson C., (1981). *Clin. Chim. Acta*; **114**: 117.

Klein B., Lucas L. B., Searcy R. L. (1969). *Clin. Chim. Acta*; **26**: 517.

Kunesh J. P., Small J. L. (1970). *Clin. Chem*; **16**: 148.

Laker M. (1982). *Lancet*; **2**: 260.

Lehman P. H., Kaplan A. (1971). *Clin. Chem*; **17**: 941.

Lestas A. N., Tan M. P. B. (1972). *J. Clin. Pathol*; **25**: 545.

MacGillivray R. T. A., Mendez E., Brew K. (1977). *Proteins of Iron Metabolism.* (Brown E. B., Aisen P., Fielding J., Crichton P. R., eds) p. 133. New York: Grune and Stratton.

Main A. H. N., *et al.* (1982). *Gut*; **23**: 984.

Makino T., Takahara K. (1981). *Clin. Chem*; **27**: 1445.

Manning D. C. (1975). *Atomic Absorption Newsletter*; **14**: 99.

Martinek R. G. (1973). *Clin. Chim. Acta*; **43**: 73.

Meadows N. J., *et al.* (1983). *Brit. Med. J*; **287**: 1013.

Meret S., Henkin K. I. (1971). *Clin. Chem*; **17**: 369.

Milder M. S., Cook J. D., Finch C. A. (1978). *Acta Haematologica*; **60**: 65.

Miles L. E. M., Lipschitz D. A., Bieber C. P., Cook J. D. (1974). *Anal. Biochem*; **61**: 209.

Milman N., Cohn J. (1984). *Eur. J. Paediatr*; **143**: 96.

Mohammed R., *et al.* (1983). *Brit. J. Surg*; **70**: 161.

Momčilović B., Belonje B., Shah B. G. (1975). *Clin. Chem*; **21**: 588.

Nakamura R. M., *et al.* (1981). *Pathology*; **35**: 377.

Neumann P. Z., Sass-Kortsak A. (1967). *J. Clin. Invest*; **46**: 646.

Olsen A. D., Hamlin W. B. (1969). *Clin. Chem*; **15**: 458.

O'Malley J. A., Hassan A., Shiley J., Traynor H. (1970). *Clin. Chem*; **16**: 92.

Patrick J., Dervish C. (1984). *CRC Critical Rev. Clin. Lab. Sci*; **20**: 95.

Persijn J.-P., Van der Slik W., Riethorst A. (1971). *Clin. Chim. Acta*; **35**: 91.

Peters T., Giovanello T. J., Apt L., Ross J. F. (1956). *J. Lab. Clin. Med*; **48**: 280.

Piomelli S., Brickman A., Carlow E. (1976). *Pediatrics*; **57**: 136.

Prasad A. S., Obereleas D., Halsted J. A. (1965). *J. Lab. Clin. Med*; **66**: 508.

Ramsay W. N. M. (1957). *Clin. Chim. Acta*; **2**: 214.

Ramsay W. N. M. (1958). *Advances in Clinical Chemistry.* (Sobotka H., Stewart C. P., eds); **1**: 1. New York: Academic Press.

Reimold E. W., Besch D. J. (1978). *Clin. Chem*; **24**: 675.

Reinhold J. G., Pascoe E., Kfoury G. A. (1968). *Anal. Biochem*; **25**: 557.

Rocks B. F., Sherwood R. A., Turner Z. J., Riley C. (1983). *Ann. Clin. Biochem*; **20**: 72.

Rocks B. F., Sherwood R. A., Bayford L. M., Riley C. (1982). *Ann. Clin. Biochem*; **19**: 338.

Ryall R., Fielding J. (1970). *Clin. Chim. Acta*; **28**: 193.

Ryder L. (1971). *FEBS Lett*; **18**: 321.

Sandstead H. H. (1981). In *Disorders of Mineral Metabolism*, Vol. I. (Bronner T., Coburn J. W., eds) p. 93. New York, London: Academic Press.

Sanford R. (1963). *J. Clin. Pathol*; **16**: 174.

Sansoni B., Iyengar G. V. (1980). In *Elemental Analysis of Biological Materials*, Techn. Report Series No. 197, (Int. Atom. Energy Agency), Vienna, p. 57.

Sebastiani E., Ohls K., Riemer G. (1973). *Z. Anal. Chem*; **264**: 105.

Shaw J. C. L. (1980). *Arch. Dis. Childh*; **134**: 74.

Smith J. C., Butrimowitz G. P., Purdy W. C. (1979). *Clin. Chem*; **25**: 1487.

Solomons N. W. (1979a). *Amer. J. Clin. Nutr*; **32**: 856.

Solomons N. W., Jacob R. A., Pineda O., Viteri F. E. (1979b). *J. Lab. Clin. Med*; **94**: 335.

Spencer K., Price C. P. (1980). *Centrifugal Analysers in Clinical Chemistry*. (Price C. P. and Spencer K., eds) p. 457. Eastbourne: Praeger.

Taylor A., Bryant T. N. (1981). *Clin. Chim. Acta*; **110**: 83.

Tsung S. H., Rosenthal W. A., Milewski K. A. (1975). *Clin. Chem*; **21**: 1063.

Versieck J. (1984). *Trace Elements in Medicine*; **1**: 2.

Versieck J., Cornelius R. (1980). *Anal. Chim. Acta*; **116**: 217.

Van der Heul C., Van Eijek H. G., Wiltink W. F., Leijnse B. (1972). *Clin. Chim. Acta*; **38**: 347.

Walravens P. A. (1980). *Clin. Chem*; **26**: 185.

Weinstock N., Uhlemann M. (1981). *Clin. Chem*; **27**: 1438.

WHO Expert Committee on Bio-standardisation (1978). Twenty-ninth Report, Techn. Report Series 626, Geneva pp. 19 and 147.

Winefordner J. D., Latz H. W. (1961). *Anal. Chem*; **33**: 1727.

Worwood M. (1982). *Clinics in Haematology*; **11**: 275.

Yee H. Y., Zin A. (1971). *Clin. Chem*; **17**: 950.

Zettner A., Silvia L. C., Capacho-Delgado L. (1966). *Amer. J. Clin. Pathol*; **45**: 533.

26

PORPHYRINS, HAEMOGLOBIN AND RELATED COMPOUNDS

PORPHYRINS

Porphyrins are metal-free cyclic tetrapyrroles. In combination with certain divalent metals they form important biological compounds such as haem (Fe), chlorophyll (Mg) and vitamin B_{12} (Co). The haem moeity is found in haemoglobin, myoglobin, the cytochromes, and such enzymes as catalase and peroxidase. Although the porphyrin molecule is essential for biological oxidation its clinical importance arises from the fact that deficiencies in the enzymes involved in haem synthesis lead to the cutaneous and neurological disorders called porphyrias.

Porphyrinogens consist of four pyrrole rings linked by four methylene bridges to form a rigid planar structure on which 8 side chains may be attached. Although four isomeric forms of the porphyrinogen, uroporphyrinogen, may be synthesised, only two (types 1 and 3) occur naturally (Fig. 26.4, p. 645). Porphyrinogens are irreversibly oxidised to porphyrins. The loss of 6 H atoms gives a molecule with a conjugated double bond system which absorbs light in the visible region. Porphyrins are thus coloured, porphyrinogens are not. The 3 different side chains of protoporphyrin allow 11 isomeric forms, of which only protoporphyrin 9 occurs naturally. It combines with ferrous iron to form the metallo-porphyrin, haem (Fig. 26.4, p. 645).

Two systems of nomenclature exist. In the original described by Fischer the 'porphins' have their rings labelled A, B, C and D while the methylene bridges are labelled α, β, γ and δ. The more recent system recommended by IUPAC involves the sequential labelling of each carbon atom such that the methylene bridges are numbered 5, 10, 15 and 20.

Synthesis of Porphyrins

The biosynthetic pathway is outlined in Fig. 26.1. It is important to note that, except for protoporphyrin, the metabolic precursors of haem are porphyrinogens.

Initially 4-aminolaevulinic acid (ALA) is formed by the condensation of succinyl-coenzyme A with glycine via an unstable intermediate 1-amino-2-oxoadipic acid (Fig. 26.2). The reaction is catalysed by ALA synthase (EC 2.3.1.37), the primary rate-limiting enzyme of haem synthesis. This enzyme is bound to the inner mitochondrial membrane and requires pyridoxal phosphate as a co-factor. The activity of the enzyme is inhibited by haem, ALA and sulphydryl compounds but increased by drugs such as the barbiturates and sulphonamides. It is believed that haem acts directly to inhibit ALA synthase and also acts as a co-repressor at the gene level (Fig. 26.3).

The next stage of synthesis occurs in the cytoplasm where two molecules of ALA condense to form porphobilinogen (PBG), a monopyrrole. This reaction is

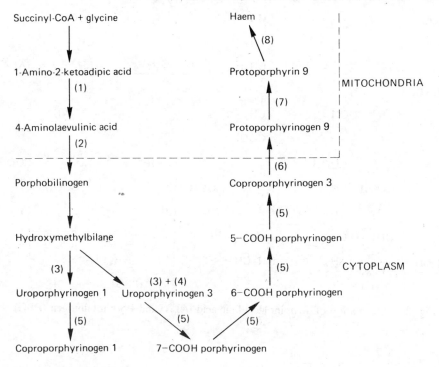

Fig. 26.1. Haem Synthesis.

catalysed by PBG synthase (EC 4.2.1.24), also called **ALA** dehydratase, which requires sulphydryl compounds and 5 to 6 atoms of zinc per mole of enzyme for full activity.

Four molecules of PBG are linked together through the 1-aminomethyl side chains to form the porphyrinogen ring (Figs. 26.1 and 26.4). The initial porphyrinogens formed are uroporphyrinogen 1 and uroporphyrinogen 3. The latter has the side chains of the D ring reversed (Fig. 26.4). Two cytoplasmic enzymes are involved in this stage of the synthesis. The first, PBG deaminase (EC 4.3.1.8) acting alone produces only uroporphyrinogen 1. The second enzyme, uroporphyrinogen 3 cosynthase, acting in combination with PBG deaminase produces uroporphyrinogen 3. It is believed that an intermediate linear tetrapyrrole, hydroxymethylbilane is produced which spontaneously forms the ring structure.

The four acetate groups in both isomeric forms of uroporphyrinogen are converted to methyl groups by the enzyme uroporphyrinogen decarboxylase (EC 4.1.1.37) forming the four carboxylate-containing compound, coproporp-

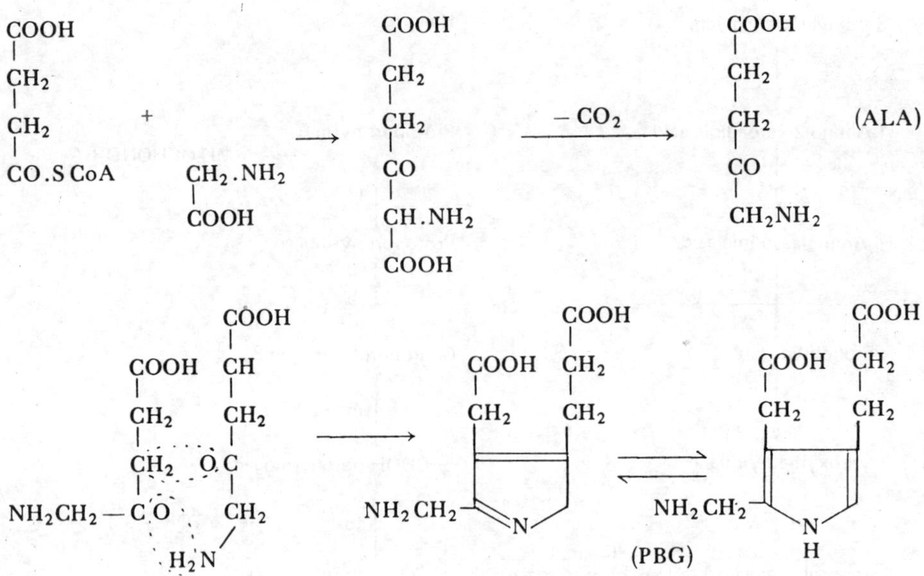

COOH   COOH   COOH

$\mid$ $\mid$ $\mid$

CH_2 CH_2 CH_2

$\mid$ $\mid$ $-CO_2$ $\mid$

CH_2 $+$ $\longrightarrow$ CH_2 $\longrightarrow$ CH_2 (ALA)

$\mid$ $\mid$ $\mid$

$CO.S\,CoA$ $CH_2.NH_2$ CO CO

           $\mid$ $\mid$ $\mid$

           COOH $CH.NH_2$ CH_2NH_2

                     $\mid$

                     COOH

Fig. 26.2. Formation of 4-Aminolaevulinic acid (ALA) and Porphobilinogen (PBG).

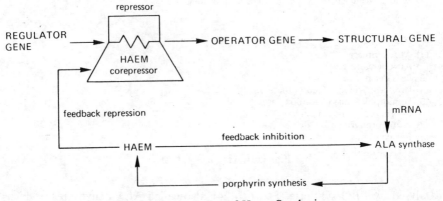

Fig. 26.3. Regulation of Haem Synthesis.

phyrinogen. Normally porphyrinogens of the 3 series predominate over the isomer 1 series and are more rapidly decarboxylated. The hepta-, hexa- and penta-carboxylate-containing porphyrinogens are formed as intermediates in these decarboxylations.

Only coproporphyrinogen 3 can be further metabolised to haem within the mitochondria. This involves the conversion of two propionate side chains to ethyl groups followed by hydroxylation and finally dehydration to form vinyl groups. The enzyme required for this reaction is coproporphyrinogen oxidase and uses molecular oxygen and S-adenosylmethionine as the hydride acceptor. This produces protoporphyrinogen 9 within the mitochondria. If the mitochondria are damaged, this enzyme may leak out into the cytoplasm and act upon the coproporphyrinogen precursors to form isocoproporphyrinogen. This would

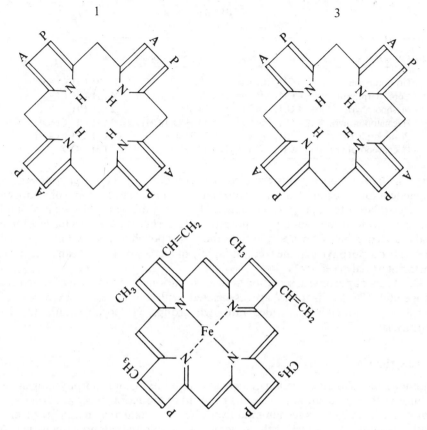

Fig. 26.4. Uroporphyrinogens 1 and 3 (above) and Haem (below). A = $-CH_2 \cdot COOH$, P = $-CH_2 \cdot CH_2 \cdot COOH$.

explain the unique finding of isocoproporphyrin in the urine and faeces of patients with porphyria cutanea tarda (see p. 647).

Protoporphyrinogen 9 is converted by the enzyme protoporphyrinogen oxidase to protoporphyrin 9. Insertion of a molecule of ferrous iron into the centre of the protoporphyrin 9 by the enzyme ferrochelatase (EC 4.99.1.1) produces haem. Haem moves out of the mitochondria and binds to the microsomes prior to haematoprotein synthesis. Haem can bind to many proteins but within the cell binds most avidly to ligandin. In the plasma, haem can bind to haemopexin and albumin.

For convenience the relationship between the various porphyrins is summarised in Table 26.1.

Porphyrin Metabolism and its Disorders

Various porphyrins and porphyrinogens are normal excretory products. In fact the names uroporphyrin and coproporphyrin are derived from their initial isolation from urine and faeces respectively. The substances of the isomer 1 series, the minor pathway in the normal state, are not convertible to haem and form 60 to

TABLE 26.1

Structures of Various Porphyrins

Porphyrin	Side Chains			
Uroporphyrin	$4\,CH_2COOH$			$4\,CH_2CH_2COOH$
Coproporphyrin	$4\,CH_3$			$4\,CH_2CH_2COOH$
Mesoporphyrin	$4\,CH_3$	$2\,C_2H_5$		$2\,CH_2CH_2COOH$
Haematoporphyrin	$4\,CH_3$	$2\,CH(OH)CH_3$		$2\,CH_2CH_2COOH$
Protoporphyrin	$4\,CH_3$	$2\,CH{=}CH_2$		$2\,CH_2CH_2COOH$
Isocoproporphyrin	$3\,CH_3$	$CH{=}CH_2$	$3\,C_2H_5$	CH_2COOH

80% of the total porphyrins excreted. The solubility of the porphyrinogens is dependent on the number of carboxylate residues. Thus uroporphyrinogen (8 carboxylates) to coproporphyrinogen (4 carboxylates) are water-soluble and are excreted in urine, while protoporphyrin (2 carboxylates) is water-insoluble and excreted in bile. Coproporphyrin is the major porphyrin present in urine and faeces. Protoporphyrin in the faeces is largely of dietary origin but can arise from gastrointestinal bleeding.

Disorders of porphyrin secretion are seen in various diseases most of which are congenital. These disorders are associated with an increased excretion of porphyrins and may be divided into two groups; (1) porphyrinuria (2) the porphyrias.

Porphyrinuria

This term refers to the excretion of increased amounts of coproporphyrinogens as a consequence of acquired disease or as a result of the action of certain drugs and poisons. Notably this is seen in mild liver disease, certain anaemias, pyrexia and lead poisoning. Drugs such as the anticonvulsants and the sulphonamides, which increase the activity of ALA synthase and hence haem synthesis, may also lead to porphyrinuria. Increased haem synthesis increases coproporphyrin 1 formation as a side-product. Interference in the conversion of coproporphyrinogen 3 to haem increases its excretion in the urine.

Porphyrias

The porphyrias are a group of characteristic congenital (or, less commonly, acquired) diseases caused by a deficiency of one or more of the enzymes of haem synthesis. These porphyrias may be classified on pathological (hepatic or erythropoietic), clinical (acute or chronic) or aetiological (congenital or acquired) grounds.

A few simple rules will simplify the diagnostic clinical and biochemical features of the porphyrias.

1. Haem exerts negative feedback control over ALA synthase activity (see p. 644). Thus any reduction of haem synthesis (e.g. due to an enzyme deficiency) will increase mitochondrial ALA synthase activity and increase the flux through the haem synthetic pathway. An increase in ALA synthase activity may be the only evidence of latent porphyria.

2. Enzyme deficiencies leading to an accumulation of the early precursors (ALA and PBG) will produce an acute clinical disorder with abdominal pain, neuropathy, hypertension and/or psychosis. These symptoms may be related to the neurotoxic effect of ALA, PBG and their metabolites (notably

the presence of 2,4-dimethyl-3-ethyl pyrrole reported by Irvine and Wetterberg, 1972). Peripheral and central demyelination and axonal degeneration (Gibson and Goldberg, 1956; Albers *et al.*, 1978) have been observed, while ALA has been shown to inhibit sodium/potassium ATPase (Becker *et al.*, 1971). As a corollary, patients with the above symptoms but no increase in urinary ALA and PBG excretion do not have acute porphyria.

3. Diseases causing an accumulation of the later precursors will present as dermatological disorders. Porphyrins in the skin absorb ultraviolet light energy causing photosensitivity, blistering, ulceration and scarring.

4. Except for erythropoietic porphyria (autosomal recessive), all the congenital porphyrias have an autosomal dominant pattern of inheritance.

5. Although the abnormality in most of the porphyrias is inherited, some other initiating factor is required to produce symptoms. These include drugs, alcohol, sunlight or even the natural hormonal changes occurring at puberty.

1. Hepatic Porphyria

Increased synthesis occurs in the liver.

(a) **Acute Intermittent Porphyria (Pyrroloporphyria or Swedish-type Porphyria).** Typically this presents with severe acute attacks in which the passage of 'port-wine' coloured urine is associated with neurological and abdominal symptoms. The dark urine is thought to be in part due to porphobilin, possibly a dipyrrylmethane, formed spontaneously from PBG. Severe abdominal pain with vomiting and constipation may mimic other acute intra-abdominal conditions. Neurological disturbances include peripheral neuropathy with pain and muscular weakness, bulbar damage which may imperil respiration, and mental disturbances simulating a psychosis. It usually appears in the third decade of life. The attacks vary in severity and may be rapidly fatal or may be milder and more chronic. They can be precipitated by drugs, e.g. barbiturates, sulphonamides, oestrogens (including oral contraceptives), griseofulvin, chloroquine, glutethimide and methyldopa. Photosensitivity is not seen. The highest incidence is in Scandinavia, about 1 in 10 000 population in Sweden, but in Lapland it may be as high as 1 in 1000. There is evidence that the enzyme change is a partial deficiency of liver and red cell PBG deaminase leading to an accumulation of porphyrin precursors (ALA and PBG).

(b) **Porphyria Variegata (Protocoproporphyria or South African-type Porphyria).** In addition to the acute abdominal and neurological attacks, chronic photosensitivity is common especially in males. Precipitating factors are similar to those for acute intermittent porphyria. The highest incidence is in white South Africans (1 in 400) especially in Cape Province (1 in 250). The majority of affected cases are recognised as descendants of two Dutch settlers who married in 1688 (Dean, 1963). There is believed to be a deficiency of protoporphyrinogen oxidase (or ferrochelatase) in this condition.

(c) **Hereditary Coproporphyria** (Goldberg *et al.*, 1967). This disorder also presents in acute attacks during which large quantities of coproporphyrin 3 appear in the urine. In addition to increased ALA synthase activity, it is suggested that there is a block in the conversion of coproporphyrinogen 3 to protoporphyrin due to coproporphyrinogen oxidase deficiency.

(d) **Porphyria Cutanea Tarda (Symptomatic Porphyria).** In this acquired condition (Waldenström, 1935, 1937), secondary to liver disease and strongly associated with alcoholism, photosensitivity usually develops later in life. There is increased urinary excretion of uroporphyrin with varying quantities of the 7-

COOH to 4-COOH porphyrins. Characteristic of this disease is the presence of isocoproporphyrin. There is a hereditary component with an associated deficiency of uroporphyrinogen decarboxylase.

2. Erythropoietic Porphyria

The defect is in the red cell precursors in the bone marrow. Two variants are known but both are uncommon.

(a) **Erythropoietic Porphyria (Congenital Porphyria, Gunther's (1911) Disease, *Pink-tooth Disease*).** The probable defect is in uroporphyrinogen 3 cosynthase leading to increased formation of uroporphyrinogen 1 in the bone marrow. It is inherited as an autosomal recessive character. Homozygotes are very uncommon, less than 100 being recorded. Features appear in infancy and continue in chronic form throughout life which is not unduly shortened. Uroporphyrin 1 accumulates in bones and teeth, while its presence in the skin causes marked photosensitivity. Urinary and faecal porphyrins of series 1 are increased markedly but there is also an increase in series 3. It has been suggested that the primary fault may be lack of a repressor gene with considerable increase in synthetase activity. The isomerase may then be rate-limiting diverting most of the synthetic activity into series 1 but increasing series 3 output also. Red cell uroporphyrin and coproporphyrin are also increased and a haemolytic anaemia with splenomegaly is usual. Hypertrichosis and erythrodontia are common findings.

(b) **Erythropoietic Protoporphyria** (Magnus *et al.*, 1961; Rimington and Cripps, 1965). In this autosomal dominant condition there is a deficiency of the enzyme ferrochelatase causing an overproduction of protoporphyrin which accumulates in red cells and their precursors and can be demonstrated by its intense red fluorescence. Protoporphyrin excretion in the faeces is increased and its precursor, coproporphyrin 3, is increased in urine and faeces.

The main clinical feature is intolerance to sunlight present from infancy. There is often little to find on examination but older patients complain of severe itching and pain on exposure to light.

TESTS USED IN THE INVESTIGATION OF DISORDERS OF PORPHYRIN METABOLISM

Preservation of Samples

Urine. Twenty-four hour samples are preferable to avoid problems caused by diurnal variation. Sodium bicarbonate (10 g) should be added as a preservative and the sample should be protected from light.

Faeces. Specimens are stable for two days at room temperature and may be stored at $-20\,°C$ for several months.

Blood. Lithium heparin or EDTA-anticoagulated blood may be used. Samples are stable at $4\,°C$ for up to 10 days if kept protected from light.

Qualitative Tests

Tests for Porphobilinogen in Urine

PBG, like urobilinogen, gives a red compound with Ehrlich's aldehyde reagent. This is used as a simple test for markedly increased PBG excretion.

Differential Extraction (Watson and Schwartz, 1941; Rimington, 1958a). Mix equal volumes of fresh urine and Ehrlich's reagent (0·7 g *p*-dimethylaminobenzaldehyde, 150 ml concentrated hydrochloric acid and 100 ml water). Allow to stand for 3 min. To this, add saturated aqueous sodium acetate solution (2 volumes) and leave 3 min. Add a few ml chloroform and shake thoroughly. PBG forms a red compound which, unlike that formed by urobilinogen, is insoluble in chloroform. Any red colour remaining in the aqueous phase after a second extraction with chloroform constitutes a positive test for PBG and is highly suggestive of acute porphyria.

Notes.
1. The sodium acetate must be saturated to bring the urobilinogen completely into the chloroform.
2. Rimington *et al.* (1956) used a modified Ehrlich's reagent prepared by dissolving 15 g *p*-dimethylaminobenzaldehyde in 65·6 ml concentrated hydrochloric acid and 194·4 ml glacial acetic acid.
3. Rimington (1958a) extracted into an amyl alcohol/benzyl alcohol mixture (3/1, v/v) which he found gave a more complete removal of the coloured complex due to urobilinogen.

Method of With (1970). With found that excess of Ehrlich's reagent suppressed the colour due to urobilinogen thereby permitting a simpler test. Add 1 drop only of urine to 1 ml Ehrlich's reagent (*p*-dimethylaminobenzaldehyde 20 g/l in hydrochloric acid, 6 mol/l). Urines containing over 45 μmol/l (10 mg/l) of PBG give a clear rose-red colour. Urobilinogen in concentrations up to 350 μmol/l (200 mg/l) gives a yellow or orange colour only and is readily differentiated.

The use of the Urobilistix text (Ames Company) is not satisfactory, as it gives false negative results owing to its insensitivity (Kanis, 1973).

Tests for Porphyrins in Urine and Faeces

Spectroscopic Examination. Porphyrins show characteristic absorption spectra (Table 26.3, p. 661). In porphyrinuria the porphyrin levels are rarely sufficiently elevated for the urine to appear red in colour. On the other hand, with the greatly increased PBG and porphyrin excretion in the acute episodes in some porphyrias it is usually dark reddish-brown, partly due to porphobilin formed on standing. Spectroscopic examination of the urine in acute intermittent porphyria shows the zinc-uroporphyrin absorption spectrum with bands at 577 and 541 nm and general absorption below 500 nm. These may be confused with the bands of oxyhaemoglobin, but acidification with hydrochloric acid to 10 % (w/v) splits the zinc complex, and develops the characteristic acid porphyrin spectrum with bands at 597 and 553 nm. Also the urine will give a negative test for blood unless haemoglobin derivatives are present.

Ultraviolet Fluorescence. The porphyrins excreted in erythropoietic porphyria are usually free so that examination of untreated urine shows a red fluorescence in ultraviolet light. The fluoresence of the zinc uroporphyrin complex in acute intermittent porphyria or porphyria cutanea tarda is weak compared with porphyria variegata. The PBG present in acute intermittent porphyria may mask the fluorescence due to porphyrins. In porphyrinuria, the amount excreted is so small that fluorescence cannot be seen unless the porphyrin is extracted into a suitable organic solvent and so concentrated. A suitable source of ultraviolet light is a 100 W Mercra lamp.

Extraction of porphyrins. Both copro- and uroporphyrins can be extracted from acidified urine or faeces by amyl alcohol. Shake urine acidified with acetic acid with a quarter of its volume of amyl alcohol. No fluorescence should be seen with normal urines when the extract is looked at in ultraviolet light (Rimington, 1958a). For faeces, disperse a small fragment in 2 ml of a mixture of equal parts of amyl alcohol, glacial acetic acid and ether. A pink fluorescence indicates the excretion of excessive amounts of porphyrins or chlorophyll. Add 2 ml hydrochloric acid, 1·5 mol/l, and shake. The porphyrins are extracted into the lower acid layer (Dean, 1971). With (1969) prefers TLC separation on talc as a screening test, carrying out the separation on microscope slides in 10 to 15 min.

Tests for Protoporphyrin in Red Cells

Add 2 drops of blood to 2·5 ml ether–acetic acid (5/1, v/v), mix well, decant and add 0·5 ml hydrochloric acid, 3 mol/l. A red fluorescence in ultraviolet light is seen in the lower acid layer.

A rapid method for diagnosing patients with erythropoietic porphyria, erythropoietic protoporphyria and lead intoxication is to examine a blood smear made on a glass slide using a fluorescence microscope with a dark field condenser. The erythrocytes are illuminated with blue-violet light (360–420 nm). Erythrocytes from patients with erythropoietic protoporphyria exhibit a transient fluorescence lasting about 5–20 s while those from patients with erythropoietic porphyria fluoresce for up to 3 min. The fluorescence seen in lead intoxication lasts only a few seconds.

Screening Tests for the Detection of Persons at Risk

The three inherited hepatic porphyrias may result in serious illness following administration of commonly used drugs. Screening tests are important in the detection of *asymptomatic cases* either in the general population in areas where the gene frequency is comparatively high or in the investigation of relatives of a proven case. In acute intermittent porphyria, the test for PBG in urine is usually positive whereas urinary or faecal porphyrins are only slightly increased, if at all. In asymptomatic porphyria variegata, PBG is absent from the urine, urinary porphyrins are only slightly increased but faecal porphyrin excretion is markedly increased, and the same is true for hereditary coproporphyria.

Quantitative Tests

Determination of 4-Aminolaevulinic Acid

ALA can be separated from PBG and from porphyrins by adsorbing these on Dowex-2 ion-exchange resin and then adsorbing the ALA on Dowex-50. After eluting, ALA is condensed with acetylacetone to form a monopyrrolic compound which, like PBG but unlike ALA, reacts with Ehrlich's reagent (Mauzerall and Granick, 1956; Goldberg *et al.*, 1967).

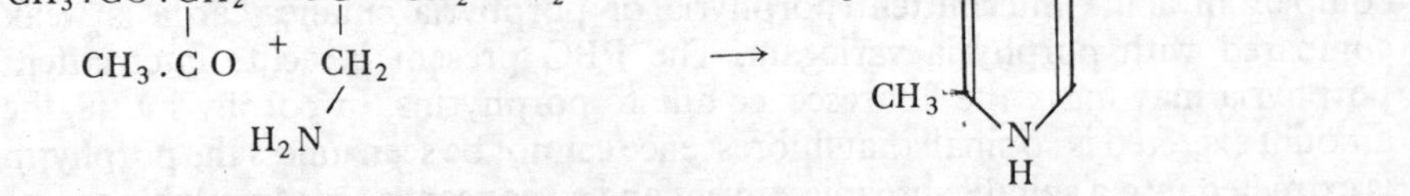

$$CH_3.CO.CH_2 \quad OC-CH_2.CH_2.COOH$$
$$| \qquad\qquad + \qquad |$$
$$CH_3.CO \qquad CH_2$$
$$\diagup$$
$$H_2N$$

$\longrightarrow$

$$CH_3.CO \underline{\qquad\qquad} CH_2.CH_2.COOH$$

$$CH_3 \diagdown \underset{H}{\overset{}{N}}\diagup$$

Fig. 26.5. Determination of 4-Aminolaevulinic Acid.

Reagents.
1. Dowex 2 × 8, 200 to 400 mesh.
2. Dowex 50 × 8, 200 to 400 mesh.
3. Sodium acetate solutions, 3, 1 and 0·5 mol/l (408, 136 and 68 g of trihydrate/l solution respectively).
4. Silver nitrate solution. Dissolve a small quantity of silver nitrate in 50 ml water and add 1 ml nitric acid.
5. Sodium hydroxide, 2 mol/l.
6. Hydrochloric acid, 4 mol/l, 2 mol/l and 1 mol/l.
7. Acetylacetone.
8. Acetate buffer, pH 4·6. Dissolve 54 ml glacial acetic acid and 136 g sodium acetate (the trihydrate) in about 500 ml water and dilute to a litre.
9. Ehrlich's reagent. Dissolve 1 g *p*-dimethylaminobenzaldehyde in about 30 ml glacial acetic acid and 8 ml perchloric acid, sp.gr. 1·54. Make to 50 ml with more glacial acetic acid. Prepare on the same day it is to be used.

Technique. *Preparation of the ion-exchange resins.* (a) Dowex 2 × 8. To remove finer particles stir the resin in water, stand 1 to 2 h, decant and repeat until a clear supernatant is obtained. Use a tube 30 cm × 0·7 cm with an indentation 10 cm from the bottom above which a plug of glass wool is fitted. Add enough of a slurry of the resin to give a column of height 2·0 ± 0·1 cm when it has settled. A flow rate of about 0·3 ml/min is obtained. Wash the column with 3 mol/l sodium acetate. Test the eluate with silver nitrate and continue washing until chloride-free. Then wash free of acetate with double distilled water. The column is then ready.

(b) Dowex 50 × 8. Wash free from finer particles as above. To convert to the sodium form allow to stand overnight in sodium hydroxide. Prepare the column as above then wash until neutral with water and reconvert to the acid form. Treat with one volume of 4 mol/l hydrochloric acid, then successively with six volumes each of the 2 mol/l acid, 1 mol/l acid and water.

The columns can be kept in twice their volume of distilled water.

Determination. Apply 1 ml urine to the Dowex 2 × 8 column. Wash twice with 2 ml distilled water, then apply the combined eluates to the Dowex 50 × 8 column and wash with 16 ml water to remove urea. To elute the ALA, first add 3 ml 0·5 mol/l sodium acetate. This should produce a decrease in colour for only three-quarters of the length of the column. After allowing to drain, elute the ALA with 7 ml 1 mol/l acetate into a 10 ml stoppered graduated tube, add 0·2 ml acetylacetone, make to 10 ml with the acetate buffer and place in a boiling water bath for 10 min. Cool to room temperature, then add 2 ml Ehrlich's reagent. Mix, and read the resulting colour 15 min later at 555 nm against a blank of 0·5 mol/l sodium acetate treated in the same way as the eluate.

Calculation

Urinary ALA (μmol/l) = Absorbance of the unknown × 3·58

Note. PBG can be eluted from the 2 × 8 column with 2 ml of 1 mol/l acetic acid, and 2 ml of 0·2 mol/l acetic acid. Make eluates to 10 ml with water and mix 2 ml with 2 ml of ordinary Ehrlich's reagent (2 g *p*-dimethylaminobenzaldehyde in 100 ml 6 mol/l hydrochloric acid). Read after 4 min against distilled water treated in the same way. Then:

Urinary PBG (μmol/l) = Absorbance of unknown × 200

Normal Values. The usual range of ALA excretion is less than 50 μmol/24 h.

Determination of Porphobilinogen

Reagents.
1. Ehrlich's reagent. Dissolve 2 g p-dimethylaminobenzaldehyde in 50 ml concentrated hydrochloric acid and make to 100 ml with water.
2. Acid blank. Dilute 50 ml concentrated hydrochloric acid to 100 ml with water.

Technique. Dilute fresh urine with water so as to bring the concentration of PBG to below 50 μmol/l. To those familiar with it, the qualitative test above can give a rough indication of the dilution required. To 2 ml diluted urine, add 2 ml Ehrlich's reagent and to another 2 ml add 2 ml acid blank. Mix and read the test from 30 s onwards at 552 nm in a spectrophotometer, noting the maximum absorbance reached in the next 2 min.

Calculation.

$$\text{Urinary PBG } (\mu\text{mol/l}) = A_{max} \times \text{dilution factor} \times 62$$

Note. On standing PBG oxidises to porphobilin and, especially in acid solution, undergoes spontaneous conversion to uroporphyrin. Freshly passed urine should be used. Standing also forms inhibitors of the colour reaction. These are not troublesome if the resin column method is used.

Normal Values. The normal excretion of PBG is up to 30 μmol/24 h.

Determination of Porphyrins

Ether-soluble porphyrins and porphyrinogens (oxidised to the porphyrin by shaking with a weak iodine solution), which include all except uroporphyrins, can be extracted directly from urine with ether after acidification or from faeces, bile or serum, with mixtures of ether and acetic acid. In urine, these are coproporphyrins, in faeces, coproporphyrin and protoporphyrin. After removal of the ether-soluble porphyrins the uroporphyrin remaining has been concentrated by adsorption on to calcium phosphate and then eluted with 1 mol/l hydrochloric acid (Sveinsson *et al*., 1949), extracted into ethyl acetate at pH 3·0 to 3·2 (Dressel *et al*., 1956) or with cyclohexanone at pH 1·5 (Kennedy, 1956; Rimington, 1958b). In this way urinary coproporphyrin and uroporphyrin can be determined separately. Faecal coproporphyrin and protoporphyrin can be separated by extraction into 100 mmol/l and 1·4 mol/l hydrochloric acid respectively. In all cases, spectrophotometric quantitation is used.

Determination of Urinary Coproporphyrins and Uroporphyrins (Rimington, 1958b; Moore, 1983)

Reagents.
1. Glacial acetic acid.
2. Ether, peroxide-free.
3. Cyclohexanone, technical grade redistilled *in vacuo*.
4. Sodium acetate solution, 30 g of the trihydrate/l.
5. Iodine solution 50 mg/l. Prepare freshly by diluting 1 ml of a solution of iodine in ethanol, 10 g/l, to 200 ml with water.
6. Hydrochloric acid 50 g/l. Dilute 120 ml concentrated acid to a litre with water.
7. Concentrated hydrochloric acid.

Technique. (a) *Coproporphyrin*. Measure 25 ml urine into a separating funnel. This volume is suitable for normal urines. Use smaller volumes down to

2 ml for those containing increased amounts. In such cases make to 25 ml with water. Acidify with 2·5 ml acetic acid and shake for about a minute with 50 ml ether. Run off the aqueous lower phase and re-extract with 50 ml ether. Combine the ether extracts and wash with 20 ml volumes sodium acetate until the liquid wash shows no red fluorescence. Extract the combined washings twice with an equal volume of ether and add the aqueous layer to the extracted urine. Combine all ether extracts and wash first with 50 ml iodine, then with about 25 ml distilled water. Then extract the coproporphyrin from the ether by shaking with 2 ml volumes of hydrochloric acid (reagent (6)) until no red fluorescence can be seen in the extract when examined in ultraviolet light. Measure the volume of the combined acid extracts, centrifuge to clear, and read in a spectrophotometer at about 401 nm (the peak of the Soret band) and at 380 and 430 nm so that the Allen correction formula can be used for background material.

Calculation. Urinary coproporphyrin (nmol/specimen)

$$= (2A_{401} - (A_{430} + A_{380})) \times 1284 \times \frac{\text{Volume of final acid extract}}{\text{Volume of urine taken}}$$

$$\times \text{Volume of urine specimen}$$

(b) *Uroporphyrin*. Take the combined urine and aqueous washings obtained above and make to pH 1·5 with concentrated hydrochloric acid. Extract twice with half their volume of cyclohexanone. Shake thoroughly but without forming an emulsion to permit a clear separation on standing. Add 2 volumes of ether to the pooled cyclohexanone extracts and extract the uroporphyrin from this by shaking with about 2 ml volumes of hydrochloric acid (reagent (6)) as above until the extract shows no red fluorescence. Again measure the volume of the combined extracts and read at about 405 nm (the peak of the Soret band) and at 380 and 430 nm. The calculation is the same as for coproporphyrin except that a factor of 1276 is used instead of 1284.

Normal values. The daily urinary excretion of porphyrins, including the non-fluorescent porphyrinogens, is 0 to 400 nmol. This is mainly coproporphyrin (0 to 300 nmol) but includes 0 to 100 nmol uroporphyrin. Mean values about 30 nmol higher have been reported for men than for women. The uroporphyrins are mainly series 1, as are about two-thirds of the coproporphyrins.

Determination of Faecal Coproporphyrins and Protoporphyrin

Reagents. As above excluding cyclohexanone.

8. Hydrochloric acid, 100 mmol/l.

Technique. Weigh two approximately half-gram samples of the well-mixed faeces, one into a weighing bottle, the other into a stoppered centrifuge tube. Place the weighing bottle in an oven at 105 °C and dry to a constant weight to obtain the water content of the faeces. Add 2 ml acetic acid to the sample in the centrifuge tube, mix well with the faeces, then shake with 20 ml ether. Centrifuge and transfer the ether layer to a 250 ml measuring cylinder. Repeat until no red fluorescence shows in the extract. Note the total volume of extract. Transfer the whole, or a suitable portion, to a separating funnel, wash twice with 25 ml sodium acetate, re-extract the combined sodium acetate washes with 25 ml ether, return this to the original ether extract, and shake the combined ether extracts, first with about one fifth its volume of iodine then with 25 ml water.

Extract the *coproporphyrin* as described above for urine with 2 ml volumes of hydrochloric acid (reagent (8)) and read similarly.

Calculation. Faecal coproporphyrin (nmol/g dry weight)

$$= (2A_{401} - (A_{430} + A_{380})) \times 1.12 \times \frac{\text{Volume of final acid extract}}{\text{Weight of faeces extracted}}$$

$$\times \frac{\text{Wet weight of faeces}}{\text{Dry weight of faeces}} \times \frac{\text{Volume of ether extract}}{\text{Volume of ether extract used}}$$

Extract *protoporphyrin* from the ether extract after removing the coproporphyrin, in the same way, using stronger hydrochloric acid (reagent (6), p. 652). The calculation is the same except that the factor is 2·02 instead of 1·12 and reading is at about 407 nm (the peak of the Soret Band) and at 380 and 430 nm.

The fluorescence still remaining in the ether extract is due to chlorophyll pigments.

Normal values. Coproporphyrin in faeces may reach 80 nmol/g dried weight, that is about 20 μmol/24 h. Other porphyrins, mainly protoporphyrin, are much more influenced by the diet, particularly the amount of meat, and may exceed coproporphyrin in amount.

Red Cell Coproporphyrin and Protoporphyrin (Rimington, 1971; Moore, 1983)

The porphyrins and haem are extracted into ethyl acetate/acetic acid and coproporphyrin and protoporphyrin back-extracted with strong hydrochloric acid. After neutralisation, extraction into ether and differential extraction with hydrochloric acid separates coproporphyrin from protoporphyrin as for faecal analysis.

Reagents. Reagents (1), (4), (6), (7) and (8) as for urinary and faecal porphyrins.
  9. Ethyl acetate/acetic acid mixture. Add 4 volumes peroxide-free analytical grade ethyl acetate to 1 volume glacial acetic acid.
 10. Hydrochloric acid, 150 g/l, Dilute 360 ml reagent (7) to 1 litre with water.
 11. Sodium chloride solution, 9 g/l.
 12. Sodium acetate solution, saturated.
 13. Sodium acetate trihydrate.

Technique. To 20 ml fresh venous blood add 0·1 ml heparin (500 units) and centrifuge for 30 min at 3 000 rpm in a graduated tube. Remove the plasma, resuspend the cells in 2 volumes of saline and recentrifuge for 20 min. Remove the supernatant, repeat and note volume of packed cells. Transfer to a beaker with a little saline and add 15 volumes of ethyl acetate/acetic acid slowly with stirring, rinsing the centrifuge tube with the solvent. Store in the dark for at least 1 h and preferably overnight.

Filter the precipitated protein through a sintered glass funnel, wash the residue twice with a little of the same solvent and transfer all extracts to a separating funnel. Wash twice with half volumes of saturated sodium acetate solution, re-extracting the washings with a little ethyl acetate which is returned to the organic phase. Wash once with a half volume of sodium acetate (reagent (4)) and then extract the porphyrins with three or four 10 ml quantities of strong hydrochloric acid (reagent (10)), collecting the extracts in a separating funnel. Add solid sodium acetate until no longer acid to Congo Red paper and extract twice with 50 ml ether. Wash the combined ether extracts with a little water.

Extract the *coproporphyrin* into hydrochloric acid (reagent (8)) and measure spectrophotometrically as for faecal coproporphyrin. Repeat using stronger acid (reagent (6)) as for faecal *protoporphyrin* and read as before.

Calculation. Red cell coproporphyrin (nmol/l)

$$= (2A_{401} - (A_{430} + A_{380})) \times 1120 \times \frac{\text{Volume of final acid extract}}{\text{Volume of packed red cells}}$$

Red cell protoporphyrin (nmol/l)

$$= (2A_{407} - (A_{430} + A_{380})) \times 2020 \times \frac{\text{Volume of final acid extract}}{\text{Volume of packed cells}}$$

Note. Some uroporphyrin is present in the precipitated protein and can be extracted by washing two or three times with ammonia (sp. gr. 0·88, diluted 10-fold). The washings mixed with the saturated sodium acetate washings are then treated as for urinary uroporphyrin.

Normal values. The usual range for coproporphyrin (mostly 3) is 0 to 64 nmol/l and 0 to 657 nmol/l for protoporphyrin. There is a significant sex difference for protoporphyrin, the mean figure for females is approximately 50 % higher than for males.

Chromatographic Separation of Porphyrins

Three chromatographic methods are available for separation of porphyrins namely paper, thin-layer and column chromatography (Moore, 1983).

1. Paper Chromatography. Free acid porphyrins are separated on the basis of the number of side-chain carboxyl groups, those with the least number tending to migrate fastest. Whatman No. 1 paper is used with 2,6-lutidine and water (5:2 v/v) as the mobile phase. The atmosphere within the chromatographic tank is saturated with 2,6-lutidine, water and 7 mol/l ammonium hydroxide. The chromatographs are run for 12 h at room temperature, dried and examined for fluorescence under ultraviolet light.

2. Thin-layer Chromatography (TLC). Silica TLC plates are activated by heating for 1 h at 120 °C. The porphyrin samples are esterified with 10 volumes of concentrated sulphuric acid–methanol (5:95 v/v), neutralised with 50 g/l ammonium hydroxide solution and extracted twice with chloroform. The esterified porphyrins are washed with distilled water and dried using anhydrous sodium sulphate. The mobile phase consists of carbon tetrachloride–dichloromethane–ethyl acetate–ethyl propionate (2/2/1/1 v/v). After drying the plate, the porphyrin fluorescence may be enhanced by a factor of 10 by dipping in a solution of dodecane–hexadecane–chloroform (1/1/18 v/v).

3. Column Chromatography. In recent years, high pressure liquid chromatography has been developed to provide sensitive and specific methods for the measurement of porphyrins. Many systems are available using either normal or reverse-phase with porphyrin or porphyrin esters as the sample. The method of Lim and Peters (1984) provides a simple method for estimating all porphyrins in their type 1 or 3 isomers. They use a reverse-phase system with a SAS-Hypersil column (Shandon) and have a gradient system of solvent A: 10 % acetonitrile in 1 mol/l ammonium acetate pH 5·16; solvent B: 10 % acetonitrile in methanol. There is a linear gradient from 0 to 65 % B in 30 min followed by isocratic elution at 65 % B for 10 min.

INTERPRETATION

The concentrations of porphyrins (quantitative and semi-quantitative assays) are as important as the pattern of porphyrin excretion in the diagnosis of the porphyrias. There are many conditions where porphyrin concentrations are increased in body fluids, particularly urine (porphyrinuria), and these are distinct from the congenital porphyrias. The diagnosis of most porphyrias will be made on the pattern of porphyrin excretion as determined by TLC or HPLC and confirmed by specific enzyme activity determinations (Elder, 1983).

In the *porphyrinurias* the urinary coproporphyrin excretion shows a small increase which rarely exceeds 1700 nmol/24 h in liver disease and alcoholism (mainly 3), in haemolytic anaemias, polycythaemia and fevers (mainly 1). Increases (mainly 3) up to 3500 nmol/24 h are seen in leukaemias and Hodgkin's disease. In some cases of Hodgkin's disease, carcinomatosis and cirrhosis increased excretion of PBG and even of uroporphyrin is also seen. Urinary coproporphyrin increases are also apparent in toxic manifestations of excessive barbiturate or gold intake, and in poisoning by arsenic, benzene and chlorinated hydrocarbons.

Determination of urinary coproporphyrin is useful in lead poisoning (Kench *et al.*, 1942) and as an additional control of the hazard in industry. The amount (mainly 3) excreted in acute lead poisoning may rise to 15 to 35 μmol/24 h and appears to be a rough guide to the severity of the condition. In severe cases, the excretion of coproporphyrin 1 also increases (Kench *et al.*, 1952). There is also an increased excretion of PBG and especially of ALA which may be increased 100-fold in acute severe poisoning. Uroporphyrin excretion is only infrequently increased even when the increase in coproporphyrin is marked. Red cell porphyrins are increased to 1000 to 3000 nmol/l in lead poisoning with even higher figures in acute lead intoxication.

For the *porphyrias* the excretion of porphyrins and precursors varies between types and also between acute attacks and remissions. Amounts vary greatly but a guide to these and patterns of excretion appears in Table 26.2.

For *acute intermittent porphyria* during remission, ALA excretion varies from normal up to 600 μmol/24 h but PBG excretion is more often increased, up to 800 μmol/24 h. During an acute attack, the amounts increase further, up to 2000 μmol/24 h for ALA and several thousand μmol/24 h for PBG. The urinary porphyrins may be slightly increased in remission, uroporphyrin more so than coproporphyrin. During an attack a considerably increased excretion of uroporphyrin and coproporphyrin occurs, an excretion considerably greater than in the porphyrinurias and with a preponderance of uroporphyrin. Most of the porphyrins and porphobilin form on standing. (The uroporphyrin is mainly isomer 1 in fresh urine but if the urine is heated, a marked increase in uroporphyrin 3 occurs, presumably by condensation of PBG.) Faecal porphyrins are normal or only slightly increased during remissions in the order protoporphyrin > coproporphyrin > uroporphyrin. During attacks, however, faecal porphyrin excretion increases, particularly uroporphyrin.

In *porphyria variegata*, ALA and PBG excretion is normal in remission but variably increased during acute attacks to the ranges seen in acute intermittent porphyria. Urinary porphyrins are relatively normal in remission but increase during attacks. In this disease, coproporphyrin is increased more than uroporphyrin (unlike acute intermittent porphyria). They are mainly type 3 isomers. The major abnormality is in the faecal porphyrins and even in remission there is markedly increased excretion which increases further during attacks. Protoporphyrin excretion is increased more than coproporphyrin while uroporphyrin excretion remains relatively normal (Dean and Barnes, 1959; Marver and Schmid, 1972; Miyagi *et al.*, 1971; Lim and Peters, 1984).

TABLE 26.2
Pattern of Porphyrin Excretion in the Porphyrias

Porphyria	Isomer Type	Red Blood Cells			Plasma			Urine				Faeces		
		Uro	Copro	Proto	Uro	Copro	Proto	ALA	PBG	Uro	Copro	Uro	Copro	Proto
Erythropoietic porphyria	1	↑↑↑	↑↑	↑	↑	↑				↑↑	↑	↑--	↑↑	↑
Erythropoietic protoporphyria	3		↑--	↑↑↑			↑						↑	↑↑↑
Acute intermittent porphyria	3							↑↑	↑↑↑	↑↑↑	↑↑		↑	
Porphyria variegata	3							↑	↑	↑	↑↑↑		↑↑	↑↑↑
Hereditary coproporphyria	3*							↑	↑	↑--	↑↑↑↑		↑↑↑↑	
Porphyria cutanea tarda	3							↑↑	↑↑	↑↑↑**	↑↑	↑↑	↑↑***	↑--

* approx 95% Type 3 isomer.
** 65% type 1/35% type 3. 7-COOH porphyrin 98% type 3 isomer (characteristic of this disease)
*** Isocoproporphyrin + 7-COOH porphyrins also present (characteristic of this disease)

In *hereditary coproporphyria* (Goldberg et al., 1967) urinary excretion of the monopyrroles is similar to porphyria variegata. The urinary and faecal excretion of the porphyrins is mainly composed of coproporphyrin, approximately 98% of which is isomer 3, and this always exceeds the excretion of protoporphyrin.

In *porphyria cutanea tarda* (Waldenström, 1935, 1937) the excretion of ALA and PBG is normal. Urinary porphyrins, especially uroporphyrin, are increased, with a characteristic excretion pattern of 65/35% types 1 and 3 isomers respectively. A special feature is the presence of porphyrins intermediate in structure between uroporphyrin (8 COOH groups) and coproporphyrin (4 COOH groups). The product with 7 COOH groups accounts for 25% of urinary porphyrins and is almost entirely type 3. Uroporphyrin is about 60% and coproporphyrin about 9% of the total excretion. Porphyrins with 5 or 6 COOH groups are present in amounts of 3% each. In addition, isocoproporphyrin is found. These products may be identified by TLC or HPLC. Faecal porphyrin excretion is variable but both uroporphyrin and coproporphyrin can be markedly increased up to several hundred nmol/g dry weight. Isocoproporphyrin and the porphyrins intermediate between uro- and coproporphyrin are also found in the faeces.

A feature of *erythropoietic porphyria* is that the porphyrins are excreted in the free form and not as the zinc complexes characteristic of the hepatic porphyrias. The excretion of ALA and PBG is normal. Urinary porphyrins, mainly of type 1, are considerably increased. Faecal porphyrin excretion is also increased, sometimes markedly so for coproporphyrin. Red cell uroporphyrin and, to a lesser extent, coproporphyrin concentrations are markedly increased, while those of protoporphyrin may be only slightly elevated.

In *erythropoietic protoporphyria*, the major abnormality is a marked increase in the red cell protoporphyrin concentration. Faecal excretion of protoporphyrin is also greatly increased with lesser increases in coproporphyrin.

For recent reviews of porphyrias and porphyrins see Goldberg and Moore (1980), Pathak and West (1982), Rimington (1985) and Blake et al. (1985).

HAEMOGLOBIN AND RELATED CHROMOPROTEINS

The major end product of porphyrin synthesis is haem in which the iron is in the form of Fe(II). The iron atom is linked to the four nitrogen atoms of protoporphyrin such that the planar configuration is maintained. In haemoglobin, four haem units are linked to four polypeptide chains, the product having a mol. wt. of approximately 68 000. Combination of one haem with a single polypeptide gives the related pigment myoglobin, present in muscle tissue. Haemoglobin and myoglobin combine with oxygen in a reversible fashion giving rise to their important role as respiratory pigments. One molecule of oxygen is taken up for each atom of iron such that 1 mol haemoglobin combines with 4 mol oxygen to give 1·36 ml oxygen/g haemoglobin at NTP. During the formation of oxyhaemoglobin the iron remains in the Fe(II) state. The oxygen molecule is linked directly to the iron by linking of two unpaired electrons of the haem group with those of the oxygen molecule. Oxyhaemoglobin has no unpaired electrons and is therefore diamagnetic while haemoglobin and oxygen both show paramagnetism. Oxidation of the iron to the Fe(III) state yields the related pigments methaemoglobin and metmyoglobin in which the prosthetic group is now referred to as haemin. Both haem and haemin can occur in combination with other proteins, e.g. methaemalbumin. Furthermore, there are a large number of genetic variants of the polypeptide chains known which combine with haem to produce abnormal haemoglobins some of which show disordered function (haemoglobinopathies). The structure and function of haemoglobin and details of the haemoglobinopathies may be found in the 5th edition of this book and in standard textbooks of haematology (Williams *et al.*, 1977; Dacie and Lewis, 1984).

Occurrence of Haemoglobin and Related Pigments in Cells, Plasma and Urine

Haemoglobin is an intracorpuscular pigment and does not normally occur in appreciable amounts in plasma (less than 10 mg/l). However, since it is not easy in practice to obtain serum or plasma completely free from haemolysis, faint bands of oxyhaemoglobin can often be seen on careful spectroscopic examination of these fluids. With careless technique gross haemolysis may occur. It is important to bear this in mind when examining blood in cases where intravascular haemolysis is suspected. Haemoglobin released from the cells is bound to a group of glycoproteins known as the haptoglobins (see Chapter 19, p. 423) and the complex formed is rapidly removed by the reticulo-endothelial system. Removal of the complex greatly exceeds hepatic synthesis of the haptoglobins so that the measurement of low levels of haptoglobin is a valuable aid in the diagnosis of haemolysis. When the binding capacity of the haptoglobins is exceeded (40–160 mg haemoglobin/dl), free haemoglobin is found in the plasma. Free haemoglobin has a renal threshold of approximately 1·5 g/l and therefore appears in urine in conditions in which there is appreciable intravascular haemolysis.

Methaemoglobin is haemoglobin in which the iron atom is in the Fe(III) state. Methaemoglobin is present in erythrocytes (less than 0·5 g/dl) where it is formed during glycolysis and constantly reconverted to haemoglobin. Increased amounts of methaemoglobin cause a shift of the oxygen dissociation curve (Fig. 23.7, p. 596) to the left so that the tissues receive less oxygen. Methaemoglobin is liberated from the cells during intravascular haemolysis and can be filtered by the glomeruli in the same way as haemoglobin. Haemoglobin may also be converted into methaemoglobin after it has been passed in the urine. Methaemoglobin may thus be found in cells, plasma and urine. Pathological increases in the amount of methaemoglobin may be due to drugs which enhance the synthesis of met-haemoglobin or depress the reconversion of methaemoglobin to haemoglobin. A decreased rate of conversion of methaemoglobin to haemoglobin occurs in the congenital methaemoglobinaemias.

Methaemoglobin, formed by the action of oxidising agents, contains Fe(III) as haemin which has one fewer electron than haem. Thus it no longer binds oxygen but forms a brown hydroxide or red cyanide, cyanmethaemoglobin. The former gives a characteristic hue to urine and blood which contain it in abnormal amounts. Reducing agents such as ammonium sulphide or sodium dithionite reconvert methaemoglobin to haemoglobin by converting iron to the ferrous state.

Sulphaemoglobin contains one more sulphur atom than normal haemoglobin and appears to be a product of the reaction of a haemoglobin–hydrogen peroxide complex with hydrogen sulphide. The iron is in the ferrous state but will not bind oxygen although it still binds carbon monoxide (to form carboxysulphaemo-globin). Sulphaemoglobin is not reconverted to haemoglobin *in vivo* and remains in the red cell unless haemolysis occurs. In plasma and urine, it is probable that those factors which convert haemoglobin to methaemoglobin will also produce sulphaemoglobin if hydrogen sulphide is present.

Carboxyhaemoglobin is formed by the action of carbon monoxide on haemoglobin and oxyhaemoglobin by virtue of the fact that haemoglobin has a higher affinity for carbon monoxide than for oxygen (200 times). However, once the patient stops breathing carbon monoxide or when blood is exposed to oxygen, oxyhaemoglobin is reformed. Breathing normal air will eliminate 50% of the carbon monoxide in the blood within 3 h whereas breathing oxygen or hyperbaric oxygen will produce the same result in 15 min.

Methaemalbumin formed by linkage of haemin and plasma albumin, is found in plasma, but is not filtered by the glomeruli and so does not appear in the urine. Serum or plasma containing an appreciable amount of methaemalbumin has a characteristic muddy brown colour. Methaemalbumin is found in the plasma in acute intravascular haemolysis when the binding capacity of the haptoglobins is exceeded, and in acute haemorrhagic pancreatitis. In the latter condition, methaemalbumin appears after approximately 10 h and reaches a peak in 3 to 5 days.

Myoglobin comprises approximately 3% of the muscle protein. It has a mol. wt. of 17 000 being composed of 152 amino acids and containing one iron atom in the ferrous form. Abnormal forms have been found in juvenile muscular dystrophy and some types of dermatomyositis but these do not contribute to defective muscle action. Plasma levels are increased in many forms of muscle injury ranging from exercise to myocardial infarction but because of the relatively small size of the molecule it is rapidly cleared by the kidney and appears in the urine. Increased levels of myoglobin may lead to renal damage. Myoglobin forms a series of derivatives similar to oxy, carboxy, and methaemoglobin (Table 26.3).

Haemin is haem in which the iron has been oxidised to the ferric form. It is a dark powder, insoluble in water, but soluble in alkalies to form haematin and in acids to give acid haemin. The dark colour of altered blood in haematemesis is due to acid haemin.

The Identification of the Pigments

With the exception perhaps of carboxyhaemoglobin, quantification of these pigments is rarely necessary in clinical practice. Qualitative assessment of these pigments is achieved by using a combination of spectroscopy with a study of the effect of a variety of reducing agents.

Hartridge's Reversion Spectroscope (Hartridge, 1912, 1922)

This instrument was designed to allow rapid differentiation of bands of only slightly different wavelengths. Two spectra of the substance are formed alongside each other with one reversed. One of these can be moved so that any band of one spectrum can be aligned with the same band of the other. Then if a solution containing a substance with a band of wavelength only slightly different from this is placed in the instrument, the two bands will no longer be in line since they will each have moved slightly in opposite directions. There is a scale which gives an indication of the wavelength of the bands.

Recording Spectrophotometer

The availability of the recording spectrophotometer (Chapter 7, p. 142) has relegated the reversion spectroscope to a secondary role. An appropriate dilution

TABLE 26.3
Wavelengths of Absorption Maxima of Haemoglobin and Derivatives (nm)

	α	β	γ	δ
Haemoglobin	555	430		
Oxyhaemoglobin	577	541	413	
Carboxyhaemoglobin	570	535	418	
Methaemoglobin	630	500	406	
Alkaline methaemoglobin	600	577	540	411
Sulphaemoglobin	618	577	541	
Methaemalbumin	623–624	540	501	
Cyanmethaemoglobin	540	414		
Haemalbumin	558	529		
Acid haemin (in glacial acetic acid)	632	540	510	400
Alkaline haemin, haematin (in NaOH)	580			
Myoglobin	560	434		
Oxymyoglobin	582	542	418	
Carboxymyoglobin	578	540	424	
Metmyoglobin	632	500	413	
Alkaline metmyoglobin	586	540	413	
Cyanmetmyoglobin	543	424		
Deuteroporphyrin*	591		548	404
Corproporphyrin*	593·5	(574)	550·5	401
Uroporphyrin*	597	(577)	553·5	405
Zinc uroporphyrin	577	541		
Protoporphyrin*	602·5	582	557·2	407
Urobilin	490			
Zinc urobilin	506·5			

* In 6 mol/l HCl

of blood, serum (or urine) is scanned using water (or normal urine) in the reference cuvette. The absorption peaks of the test solution and of authentic compounds are superimposed on the same chart for direct comparison. The method also makes quantitative measurements possible.

Details of the characteristic spectra are shown in Fig. 26.6 (p. 662) and Table 26.3. The most intense absorption peak, occurring between 400 and 420 nm is termed the Soret band. Bands are termed α, β, γ, δ in that order from the red end of the spectrum.

The α and β bands in the yellow and the green are particularly characteristic of *oxyhaemoglobin*, which has a third band in the violet which is not so easily seen. The α band is narrower and more intense than the β.

Haemoglobin shows a broad, not very intense band, centred between the α and β bands of oxyhaemoglobin, covering the whole of the space between them and part of the bands themselves. *Carboxyhaemoglobin* has α and β bands similar to those of oxyhaemoglobin but displaced slightly towards the violet end of the spectrum. *Methaemoglobin, sulphaemoglobin* and, in serum, *methaemalbumin*, all show a narrow band of relatively weak intensity in the red. In spectroscopic examination of blood very careful observation should be made for such a band. Its presence may sometimes be overlooked, in the case of the first two, unless blood only moderately diluted is used or a deep layer of blood diluted 1 in 50 observed, when only the α band in the red will be seen. As deep a layer of serum as possible should be used when looking for methaemalbumin. Table 26.3 above

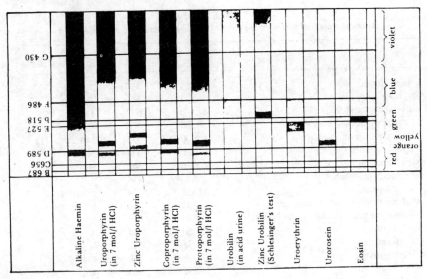

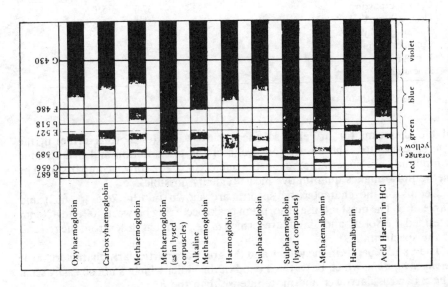

Fig. 26.6. Absorption Spectra of Haemoglobin and its Derivatives.

shows that the position of this band in the red is slightly different in the three cases. Differentiation is also possible because of their different behaviour towards reducing agents. The spectrum of *haemalbumin* is characterised by two bands in the yellow green, the α band situated between the two characteristic bands of oxyhaemoglobin being very much more intense than the β which is rather faint. The α band is also considerably more intense than that of oxyhaemoglobin.

Myoglobin and its derivatives give spectra similar to those of the corresponding derivatives of haemoglobin (Table 26.3 p. 661), except that the bands are displaced a little towards the red (Bywaters *et al.*, 1941).

Since the pigments in some cases may be either intracorpuscular or extracorpuscular, it may be of interest to study both whole blood and plasma.

The Hartridge Reversion Spectroscope is particularly useful in distinguishing between carboxyhaemoglobin and oxyhaemoglobin, and for contrasting the α bands of methaemoglobin, and sulphaemoglobin. In the former case place normal blood, suitably diluted, in the instrument and align the α bands of the two •spectra of oxyhaemoglobin. Then replace with the blood under test for carboxyhaemoglobin. If this is present the two α bands will be displaced a little to the violet and will no longer coincide. A specimen containing carboxyhaemoglobin can be prepared by bubbling carbon monoxide through normal blood and ; the α-bands compared with the α-bands of the specimen being tested.

To contrast the α bands of methaemoglobin and sulphaemoglobin oxidise a suitable dilution of blood with a crystal of potassium ferricyanide. Methaemoglobin is formed. Place in the instrument and adjust so that the bands in the red are aligned. Then substitute the blood under test. If it contains methaemoglobin the bands are still in line but are not if sulphaemoglobin is present or, using plasma or serum, if methaemalbumin is present. A solution containing sulphaemoglobin can be prepared by adding to 10 ml of normal blood diluted 1 in 100, 0·1 ml of phenylhydrazine hydrochloride solution (1 g/l) and 1 drop of water saturated with hydrogen sulphide. If methaemalbumin is introduced its α band will overlap neither of these prepared solutions of methaemoglobin or sulphaemoglobin. It may also be noted that when carbon monoxide is passed into a solution of sulphaemoglobin its α band moves towards the violet whereas that of methaemoglobin is not affected.

Alternatively, direct recording of the spectra will give similar information particularly if the spectra of the unknown and of the reference substances are recorded by superimposition.

Action of Reducing Substances

In most cases it is possible to identify a blood pigment by a combination of spectroscopic examination with study of the effect of reducing agents. The blood is first observed carefully at different dilutions. If no band in the red is seen then methaemoglobin and sulphaemoglobin can be reported as not detected. In the case of apparent absence of methaemalbumin in serum or plasma, Schumm's test should be performed as haemalbumin has a spectral absorption band much more intense than any of the bands of methaemalbumin. Use the following reducing agents:

Ammonium sulphide reduces methaemoglobin and oxyhaemoglobin to reduced haemoglobin, so that the α band in the spectrum of methaemoglobin is removed. Carboxyhaemoglobin and sulphaemoglobin are not affected. If the presence of methaemalbumin is being investigated, reduction of plasma or serum is carried out. This is *Schumm's test*. Place some serum or plasma in a test tube, cover with ether and add one tenth its volume of concentrated ammonium sulphide solution. Examine spectroscopically looking particularly for the α band intermediate between the α and β bands of oxyhaemoglobin. Neither oxyhaemoglobin nor methaemoglobin give such a band when treated in this way.

Sodium dithionite, $Na_2S_2O_4$, added in solid form reduces methaemoglobin but not carboxy- and sulphaemoglobin. It also converts oxyhaemoglobin to haemoglobin, and reduces methaemalbumin to haemalbumin.

Action of Alkalies and Cyanide

One to two drops of ammonia added to 3 to 5 ml of the diluted blood convert methaemoglobin to alkaline methaemoglobin, which has no band in the red (see Table 26.3, p. 661; Fig. 26.6, p. 662). Sulphaemoglobin is unaffected. Oxyhaemoglobin and carboxyhaemoglobin behave differently when equal volumes of blood and 6 mol/l sodium hydroxide are mixed. Oxyhaemoglobin turns brown whereas carboxyhaemoglobin is unaffected.

The addition of a few drops of sodium cyanide solution (50 g/l) converts oxyhaemoglobin and methaemoglobin to cyanmethaemoglobin whereas sulphaemoglobin is unaffected.

Quantitative Determination of Haemoglobin and Carboxyhaemoglobin

Several methods exist to determine haemoglobin and related pigments (Dacie and Lewis, 1984). The clinical biochemist will rarely have need for any quantitative methods other than those for haemoglobin, myoglobin and carboxyhaemoglobin. Methods for glycosylated haemoglobin, useful in the long term management of diabetes mellitus, are given in Chapter 16, p. 341.

Blood Haemoglobin

Techniques used to determine haemoglobin have measured it as oxyhaemoglobin, carboxyhaemoglobin, cyanmethaemoglobin, acid and alkaline haemin, by its oxygen capacity and by its iron content. The cyanmethaemoglobin technique is now recommended as the standard method (International Committee for Standardization in Hematology, 1965; British Standards Institution, 1966).

Cyanmethaemoglobin Method for Haemoglobin

The haemoglobin is treated with a reagent containing potassium ferricyanide, potassium cyanide and potassium dihydrogen phosphate. The ferricyanide forms methaemoglobin which is converted to cyanmethaemoglobin by the cyanide.

Reagents.
1. Ferricyanide-cyanide reagent (van Kampen and Zijlstra, 1961). Dissolve 200 mg potassium ferricyanide, 50 mg potassium cyanide and 140 mg potassium dihydrogen phosphate in water and add 1 ml Nonidet P40 (Shell Chemical Company, London) or 0·5 ml of Sterox SE (Hartman-Leddon Company, Philadelphia) and make to a litre with water. The last two are colourless surface-active reagents. Check the pH which should be etween 7·0 and 7·4. The reagent keeps for several months in a dark polythene bottle between 4 and 20 °C. It should not be frozen.
2. Cyanmethaemoglobin standard. The International Committee for Standardization in Hematology (1967) adopted specifications using a mol. wt. for haemoglobin of 64 458 and a millimolar absorption coefficient of 44·0. These are used in a British Standard (BS 3985 : 1966). Standard solutions based on this are available commercially in sealed ampoules, sterile and without suspended particles. Kept in the dark between 4 and 10 °C, the colour remains unchanged until the date stated. The equivalent haemoglobin concentration is given on the label. A typical value is 60 mg/dl.

Technique. Add 20 μl blood to 4·0 or 5·0 ml of the reagent. Stand at least 4 min and read against a reagent blank at 540 nm. Read the standard in the same way.

Use a fresh ampoule of the standard each day and keep in the dark during the day of use. Then

$$\text{Blood haemoglobin (g/dl)} = \frac{\text{Reading of unknown}}{\text{Reading of standard}}$$

$$\times \text{ Dilution factor } \times \frac{\text{Concentration of standard (mg/dl)}}{1000}$$

The dilution factor is 201 or 251 according to whether 4·0 or 5·0 ml of reagent is used.

A standard curve can be prepared by suitably diluting the standard with the reagent.

Note. Haemoglobin, oxyhaemoglobin, methaemoglobin and carboxyhaemoglobin are all measured. Only sulphaemoglobin remains unchanged. At 540 nm it has an absorption equal to 78% of that of cyanmethaemoglobin. Carboxyhaemoglobin is however converted only slowly requiring 3 h or the use of a reagent containing more potassium ferricyanide (Taylor and Miller, 1965).

Normal Range. The following figures (g/dl) are given by Dacie and Lewis (1984)

Men	13·0–18·0
Women	11·5–16·5
Infants, at birth	13·5–19·5
Children one year	11·0–13·0
10 to 12 years	11·5–14·5

Blood Carboxyhaemoglobin

It is of extreme importance that the sample is collected correctly. Carboxyhaemoglobin rapidly dissociates in the presence of air and is photolabile. It is recommended that samples are collected under oil and kept in the dark prior to assay.

Method of Whitehead and Worthington (1961)

Heat inactivation under strictly controlled conditions completely precipitates oxyhaemoglobin while approximately 80% of the carboxyhaemoglobin remains in solution.

Reagents.
1. Sodium acetate solution. Dissolve 40·8 g CH_3COONa, $3H_2O$ in water and make to 100 ml.
2. Acetic acid. Dilute 28 ml glacial acetic acid to 100 ml with water.
3. Sodium chloride solution 9 g/l.

Technique. Dilute 1 ml whole blood with 9 ml saline in a centrifuge tube and centrifuge for 5 min. Remove the supernatant fluid as completely as possible. Repeat the washing with a further 9 ml saline and again remove the supernatant fluid. Add 4·5 ml water and mix well. Place 1 ml of this solution in a 15 × 1·2 cm test tube. Pour the remainder into a conical flask and bubble carbon monoxide through for 1 min while shaking well. Transfer 1 ml of treated blood to a similar test tube. To both tubes add with mixing, first 3 ml sodium acetate solution then 0·75 ml acetic acid.

Place the tubes in a water bath at 57 to 57·5 °C for exactly 8 min. Cool and filter through 7 cm Whatman No. 1 papers. Centrifuging prior to filtration will decrease the time required for this stage. Read at 555 nm. Dilute the 100% carboxyhaemoglobin specimen 1 in 10 before reading and, if necessary, dilute the test solution sufficiently to give about the same reading.

Calculation. Blood carboxyhaemoglobin (%)

$$= \frac{\text{Reading of unknown} \times \text{Dilution factor}}{\text{Reading of 100 per cent control} \times 10} \times 100$$

Normal range. Less than 1%.

Note. If the red cells are not washed, results are about 1·5% too high, so that washing need not be carried out if such a degree of accuracy is not required.

CO-Oximeter

This instrument is a dedicated spectrophotometer designed to measure at four wavelengths simultaneously and at constant temperature. Dilution, calibration and calculation of results are performed automatically under microprocessor control. The instrument measures total haemoglobin and the percentages of oxyhaemoglobin, methaemoglobin and carboxyhaemoglobin in blood. Sulphaemoglobin has a similar absorbance spectrum and may interfere with these measurements. These instruments provide rapid results and are a convenient means of measuring the oxygen availability of compromised patients.

Plasma and Urinary Myoglobin

The measurement of myoglobin in plasma and urine is important in two areas, namely in the diagnosis of myocardial infarction and in those conditions where gross muscle trauma may release sufficient myoglobin to cause renal damage. A variety of chemical and immunochemical methods has been reported ranging from complement fixation (Kagen *et al.*, 1975) to high performance liquid chromatography (Bowie *et al.*, 1985). Several radioimmunoassay kits are available particularly in the USA where assay of myoglobin is used in the diagnosis of myocardial infarction. A rapid latex agglutination method available from Hoechst, designed to measure myoglobin in plasma (Bachem *et al.*, 1983), is noteworthy as it is readily adapted to measure myoglobin levels in urine (semi-quantitative), an area which has proved troublesome in the past.

Haemoglobin and Related Chromoproteins

INTERPRETATION

Haemoglobin is normally confined to the corpuscles but may be present free in the plasma, haemoglobinaemia, when there is appreciable intravascular haemolysis. Levels of less than 100 mg/l occur in sickle cell disease and thalassaemia. Concentrations over 300 mg/l occur in the severe haemolytic anaemia of malaria known as blackwater fever, in septicaemia due to haemolytic streptococcus, as a result of transfusion with incompatible blood, in the paroxysmal haemoglobinurias, whether due to cold, severe exercise (march haemoglobinuria), or nocturnal haemoglobinuria, or from the action of chemicals such as the sulphonamides, phenylhydrazine and arsenicals.

Haemoglobin does not appear in the plasma in normal persons. When haemolysis occurs haemoglobin is bound by the plasma haptoglobins and only when these have been saturated is free haemoglobin excreted in the urine. The determination of plasma haptoglobin can be useful in some conditions in which haemolysis is occurring. The combination can be regarded as a mechanism protecting the kidney from the harmful effects of free haemoglobin.

Haemoglobin free in the plasma is partly excreted as haemoglobin in the urine and is partly converted into methaemalbumin prior to conversion to bilirubin.

Methaemoglobin. The blood of normal persons usually contains between 0·01 to 0·5 g/dl methaemoglobin. Methaemoglobin in a concentration above 5 g/dl results in clinically detectable cyanosis. In disease, it is usually formed from haemoglobin inside the corpuscles but may be present in the plasma if haemolysis then occurs. Methaemoglobin may be formed from haemoglobin in the acute haemolytic anaemias mentioned above or produced by the action of various drugs such as aspirin, nitrites and sulphonamides. It is found in the urine only if free in the plasma. Congenital methaemoglobinaemias in which methaemoglobin forms up to 40% of the haemoglobin are relatively rare. These appear to be due either to a defect in NADH diaphorase (methaemoglobin reductase) or NADPH diaphorase in the red cells with impaired ability to keep the haemoglobin in the ferrous state, or to a reduced rate of synthesis of reduced glutathione. Methaemoglobin levels are increased also in haemoglobin M disease, in which the abnormality may be in the alpha or beta chain of the globin part of the molecule. It is noteworthy that fetal haemoglobin is more easily oxidised than adult haemoglobin.

Sulphaemoglobin is not detectable in normal blood and arises similarly by the action of drugs such as the sulphonamides, nitrates, sulphur compounds and aniline derivatives. It was found fairly frequently in the blood of patients taking mixed phenacetin, aspirin and codeine tablets. Sulphaemoglobin is usually intracorpuscular and once formed in the erythrocytes it persists until the cells are destroyed at the end of their natural life span by the reticuloendothelial system. If levels reach 3% of the total haemoglobin, cyanosis occurs. Although said to be liberated into the plasma occasionally, when sulphaemoglobinuria would be expected to occur, this is uncommon.

Carboxyhaemoglobin is present in the blood of heavy smokers in concentrations up to 9% of the haemoglobin but it is of most importance in suspected carbon monoxide poisoning. Haemoglobin has a much greater affinity for carbon monoxide than for oxygen (about 200 times greater). If air is breathed containing carbon monoxide in one two-hundredth the concentration of oxygen, i.e. a concentration of about 0·1% of carbon monoxide, 50% of the haemoglobin is converted to carboxyhaemoglobin and will produce marked symptoms within about 1 h. With 0·2% in the air, death may occur within a few hours. Town gas contains less carbon monoxide than formerly and in many areas has been replaced by natural gas but carbon monoxide poisoning is still a hazard in circumstances where carbonaceous matter is incompletely combusted. A car engine running in a closed garage or a solid fuel stove with a cracked vent in a poorly ventilated room are more common causes than coal gas poisoning now.

In a person with a normal haemoglobin content symptoms begin to appear when there is about 20% saturation of the haemoglobin with carbon monoxide. There may be a feeling of lassitude with some headache. Above this point, symptoms steadily worsen, the headaches become more severe, with increasing feeling of fatigue. Muscular weakness, giddiness, fainting and shortness of breath are very marked at 50% saturation. Unconsciousness supervenes between 50 and 70% with death following soon if exposure to the gas continues. Death follows quickly when 80% saturation is reached.

Methaemalbumin. The normal range for this pigment in plasma is up to 6 mg/l, expressed as haematin. The route of excretion is via the bile. An increased concentration indicates that intravascular haemolysis has occurred with liberation of haemoglobin into the plasma. Haemin is formed during the course of its conversion to bilirubin, and links with plasma albumin to form methaemalbumin. Methaemalbumin is not formed when there is increased breakdown of haemoglobin in the reticulo-endothelial system. Methaemalbuminaemia is occasionally found in malaria and in many other acute haemolytic anaemias and in pernicious anaemia. An increase is characteristically seen in patients with acute haemorrhagic pancreatitis (Northam *et al.*, 1963, 1965; Winstone, 1965) following tryptic digestion of the haemorrhagic exudate. If there is associated liver disease then the levels of methaemalbumin may be higher due to reduced clearance in the bile.

Myoglobin is excreted in the urine following accidents in which muscles are crushed and after extensive burns and severe electric shock. It is released from muscles in malignant hyperthermia following anaesthesia and from the myocardium following infarction. It also occurs as a primary form in paroxysmal myoglobinuria after exercise. Myoglobinuria may be mistaken visually for haemoglobinuria but can be distinguished by immunochemical methods, differential precipitation and by careful spectroscopy (Table 26·3, p. 661). Red blood cells are not present but the urine deposit contains casts which are stained with this brown pigment. Myoglobin is believed to be responsible for the tubular damage and blockage which often results in renal failure (Schulze, 1982). It is not surprising in view of the relatively small molecular weight, that myoglobin is not found in the plasma. It is not bound to haptoglobins and is filtered too quickly by the glomeruli.

REFERENCES

Albers J. W., Robertson W. C., Daube J. R. (1978). *Muscle and Nerve*; **1**: 292.
Bachem M. G., *et al.* (1983). *Dtsch. Med. Wschr*; **108**: 1190.
Becker D., Viljoen D., Kramer S. (1971). *Biochim. Biophys. Acta*; **225**: 26.
Blake D., McManus J., Ratnaike S., Campbell D. (1985). *Clin. Biochem. Revs*; **6**: 52.
Bowie L. J., Kinney R. S., Hoppe J. F. (1985). *Clin. Chem*; **31**: 944.
British Standards Institution, *Specification for Cyanmethaemoglobin Solution for Photometric Haemoglobinometry*, British Standard 3985; 1966, British Standards House, 2, Park Street, London W.1.
Bywaters E. G. L., Delory G. E., Rimington C., Smiles J. (1941). *Biochem. J*; **35**: 1164.
Dacie J. V., Lewis S. M. (1984). *Practical Haematology*, 6th ed. London: Churchill Livingstone.
Dean G. (1963). *The Porphyrias*. London: Pitman.
Dean G. (1971). *Lancet*; **1**: 86.
Dean G., Barnes H. D. (1959). *S. African Med. J*; **33**: 274.
Dressel S. I. B., Rimington C., Tooth B. E. (1956). *Scand. J. Clin. Lab. Invest*; **8**: 73.
Elder G. H. (1983). *Brit. J. Dermatol*; **108**: 729.
Gibson J. B., Goldberg A. (1956). *J. Path. Bact*; **71**: 495.
Goldberg A., Moore M. R. (1980). The Porphyrias. *Clinics in Haematology*. Philadelphia: W. B. Saunders Company Ltd.
Goldberg A., Rimington C., Lochhead A. C. (1967). *Lancet*; **1**: 632.
Gunther H. (1911). *Deut. Arch. Klin. Med*; **105**: 89.
Hartridge H. (1912). *J. Physiol*; **44**: 1.
Hartridge H. (1922). *J. Physiol*; **57**: 47.
International Committee for Standardization in Hematology (1965). *J. Clin. Path*; **18**: 353.
International Committee for Standardization in Hematology (1967). *Brit. J. Haematol*; **13**: Suppl. 71.

Irvine D. G., Wetterberg L. (1972). *Lancet*; **2**: 1201.

Kagen L., *et al.* (1975). *Amer. J. Med*; **58**: 177.

Kanis J. A. (1973). *Lancet*; **1**: 1511.

Kench J. E., Gillam A. E., Lane R. E. (1942). *Biochem. J*; **36**: 384.

Kench J. E., Lane R. E., Varley H. (1952). *Brit. J. Ind. Med*; **9**: 133.

Kennedy G. Y. (1956). *Scand. J. Clin. Lab. Invest*; **8**: 79.

Lim C. K., Peters T. J. (1984). *Clin. Chim. Acta*; **139**: 55.

Magnus I. A., Jarrett A., Prankerd T. A. J., Rimington C. (1961). *Lancet*; **2**: 448.

Marver H. S., Schmid R. (1972). In *The Metabolic Basis of Inherited Disease*, 3rd ed. (Stanbury J. B., Wyngaarden J. B., Frederickson D. S., eds) p. 1087. New York: McGraw-Hill.

Mauzerall D., Granick S. (1956). *J. Biol. Chem*; **219**: 435.

Miyagi K., Cardinal C., Bossenmaier I., Watson C. J. (1971). *J. Lab. Clin. Med*; **78**: 683.

Moore M. R. (1983). Broadsheet 109. Association of Clinical Pathologists, London.

Northam B. E., Rowe D. S., Winstone N. E. (1963). *Lancet*; **1**: 348.

Northam B. E., Winstone N. E., Banwell J. G. (1965). In *Recent Advances in Gastroenterology*. (Badenoch J., Brook N. B., eds) p. 354. London: Churchill Livingstone.

Pathak M. A., West J. D. (1982). *Acta Dermatovener (Stockholm)*, Suppl; **100**: 91.

Rimington C. (1958). (a) Broadsheet 20, (b) Broadsheet 21, Association of Clinical Pathologists, London.

Rimington C. (1971). Broadsheet 70, Association of Clinical Pathologists, London.

Rimington C. (1985). *Scand. J. Clin. Lab. Invest*; **45**: 291.

Rimington C., Cripps D. J. (1965). *Lancet*; **1**: 624.

Rimington C., Krol S., Tooth B. (1956). *Scand. J. Clin. Lab. Invest*; **8**: 251.

Schulze V. E. (1982). *Postgraduate Medicine*; **72**: 145.

Sveinsson S. L., Rimington C., Barnes H. D. (1949). *Scand. J. Clin. Lab. Invest*; **1**: 2.

Taylor J. D., Miller J. D. M. (1965). *Amer. J. Clin. Path*; **43**: 265.

Van Kampen E. J., Zijlstra W. G. (1961). *Clin. Chim. Acta*; **6**: 538.

Waldenström J. (1935). *Deut. Arch. Klin. Med*; **178**: 38.

Waldenström J. (1937). *Acta Med. Scand*, suppl; **82**: 1.

Watson C. J., Schwartz S. (1941). *Proc. Soc. Exp. Biol. Med*; **47**: 393.

Whitehead T. P., Worthington S. (1961). *Clin. Chim. Acta*; **6**: 356.

Williams W. J., Beutler E., Erslew A. J., Rundles R. W. (1977). *Hematology*, 2nd ed. New York: McGraw-Hill.

Winstone N. E. (1965). *Brit. J. Surg*; **52**: 804.

With T. K. (1969). *J. Chromatog*; **42**: 389.

With T. K. (1970). *Lancet*; **2**: 1187.

27

GASTROINTESTINAL TRACT FUNCTION TESTS

GASTRIC FUNCTION

Two important constituents of gastric juice are hydrochloric acid, secreted by the parietal cells at a concentration of 155 mmol/l, and pepsinogen, secreted by the chief cells. The acid converts pepsinogen to pepsin and provides the right milieu for its proteolytic activity which is maximal at pH 1·6 to 2·3. Pepsinogen activation is also auto-catalysed by pepsin. A third component, secreted by the parietal cells, is intrinsic factor, a mucoprotein required for the absorption of cobalamin. Gastric mucus and bicarbonate are secreted by the columnar cells on the surface of the gastric epithelium. In addition to mucoprotein and bicarbonate, mucus contains the blood group substances A, B, or H, which are polysaccharides of mol. wt. 2 to 3×10^5. They may all act in concert to protect the gastric epithelium from the acid in the lumen.

Stimulation of Gastric Secretion

Secretion occurs in two phases:

1. *The cephalic phase*, in response to sensory and psychic factors such as sight, taste, smell and even the thought of food, produces hydrochloric acid and pepsinogen. The secretory stimulus is through the vagus nerves. Insulin, by causing hypoglycaemia, causes vagal stimulation and hence secretion.
2. *The gastric phase* results from the presence of food in the stomach. Gastric distension stimulates secretion of acid and pepsinogen and increases gastric motility by local reflexes resulting in vagal stimulation. This vagal activity releases acetylcholine which liberates the hormone *gastrin* from the pyloric mucosa. Food components, especially protein, may also act locally as stimulants of gastric secretion. Gastrin, which is thought to reach the target cells by diffusion, increases motility and acts on the parietal and chief cells to increase the output of hydrochloric acid and pepsinogen.

Human gastrin exists in a variety of molecular forms, the two most important of which are a 17 amino acid polypeptide, G17, and a 34 amino acid polypeptide, G34 (Hansky, 1984). The amino acid chain of G17 is (pyro) Glu–Gly–Pro–Trp–Leu–(Glu)$_5$–Ala–Tyr–Gly–Trp–Met–Asp–Phe–(CONH$_2$). G17 and G34 exist in two forms depending on whether the phenol group on Tyr is unconjugated (G17I and G34I) or sulphated (G17II and G34II). The four C-terminal amino acids are common to all species and are the active part of the molecule. They are available in the synthetic polypeptide pentagastrin (ICI Limited), the N-terminal end being blocked by butyloxycarbonyl-β-alanine: butyloxycarbonyl-β-alanine-Trp-Met-Asp-Phe(CONH$_2$). The same four terminal amino acids are present in cholecystokinin-pancreozymin (CCK-PZ). G17 appears to be the most important form with about seven times more biological activity than G34, but has a shorter half-life so that G34 accounts for most of the circulating fasting gastrin.

Histamine, a powerful stimulant of acid secretion, also acts as a gastrin-releasing substance.

Inhibition of Gastric Secretion

After the need for gastric secretion has passed there is a return to the basal condition. The entry of fat and digestion products of protein into the duodenum stimulates the release of secretin and CCK-PZ which have an inhibitory effect on gastric secretion. There may also be a separate inhibitory hormone, gastric inhibitory peptide (enterogastrone), released from the small intestine.

Tests of Gastric Function

While the earliest tests used food as the means of stimulation and later tests used histamine, the stimulant of choice is pentagastrin. This has a potent and predictable influence on acid secretion and an almost complete freedom from side-effects even when given in doses which stimulate maximally. Those reported are transient vasomotor effects, mild nausea or abdominal discomfort, and are less apparent with a single dose of pentagastrin than with continuous infusion. (See Wormsley *et al.*, 1966; Johnston and Jepson, 1967; Multicentre Pilot Study, 1967; Multicentre Study, 1967, 1969; Konturek and Lankosz, 1967.)

The Pentagastrin Test

This involves the maximal stimulation of the stomach after a period of assessment of the basal secretion rate and measures the total parietal cell mass. All the juice secreted over a known period must be collected.

Technique. After a period of 12 h without food or drink insert the largest nasogastric tube which can be passed comfortably through one nostril. Site the tube radiologically with the tip in the gastric antrum and attach it to the face with an adhesive strip. Without radiological confirmation of the siting, results are less reliable. Place the patient in a semi-recumbent position and then empty the stomach as completely as possible with a hand syringe. This specimen is the 'fasting contents'. Collect the next two 15 min specimens to give the basal secretion, then give a subcutaneous injection of pentagastrin in a dose of 6 μg/kg body weight and collect four accurately timed 15 min specimens. A suction pump with an interrupter should be used for these aspirations, the negative pressure never exceeding 50 mmHg. Interrupt the suction mechanically every minute or manually at 5 min intervals. Blow air down the tube every 5 min to prevent the tube from becoming blocked.

Measure the volume, the pH using a glass electrode, and the acid content of these six specimens and qualitatively test or inspect them and the fasting contents for blood and bile pigments. To determine the acid content titrate 5 or 10 ml with sodium hydroxide, 100 mmol/l, either to pH 7·4 using a glass electrode, or to an end-point with phenol red.

Calculation. Tabulate the results as follows:

		Volume of Specimen (ml)	Time of Collection (min)	Output of acid (mmol/h)
Basal secretion	1			
	2			
Post-stimulation	1			
	2			
	3			
	4			

Where: Acid output in mmol/h

$$= \frac{\text{ml sodium hydroxide}}{\text{ml gastric juice titrated}} \times \frac{\text{volume of specimen in ml}}{\text{period of collection in min}} \times 6$$

Note the mean of the two basal secretions and the maximal acid secretion rate after pentagastrin.

Notes.

1. A dose of 6 μg/kg gives maximal secretion (Multicentre Pilot Study, 1967). This can be given either as one dose subcutaneously or by intravenous infusion in isotonic saline over a period of 1 h. The results are very similar but the latter may give more side-effects.
2. Various authors have expressed the output in different ways, e.g. mmol secreted 15 to 45 min after stimulation, the highest output (mmol) in two successive 15 min periods, mmol secreted in the whole hour after stimulation. These all correlate well.
3. After subcutaneous injection the maximal response is usually between 30 and 60 min but with intravenous injection a plateau is reached after about 30 min.
4. Since the secretion rate is being measured, correct measurements of the total volume of secretion, the time of collection and the acid concentration of *all* the juice secreted by the stomach are essential. Hence the need for rigorous attention to details in carrying out the test.

INTERPRETATION

Nowadays, with the widespread use of endoscopy and high quality radiology, tests of gastric secretory function are infrequently employed in the diagnosis of peptic ulcer disease. The main indications for performing a pentagastrin test are in the diagnosis of the Zollinger–Ellison syndrome (caused by a gastrin-producing tumour) and pernicious anaemia and in the assessment of gastric secretion after gastric surgery.

The normal basal secretion rate is 1 to 2·5 mmol/h and the maximal secretion approximately 20 to 40 mmol/h. In patients with duodenal ulcer the range, 15 to 83 mmol/h, mean 43, overlaps that found in non-ulcer patients, 0·7 to 49·6 mmol/h, mean 16·7. Values above 40 mmol/h suggest duodenal ulcer. The Zollinger–Ellison syndrome is characterised by a high basal secretion, usually above 10 mmol/h, often with little or no increase in secretion after giving pentagastrin. The test is of little value in gastric ulcer. In cancer of the stomach, true achlorhydria is found in about 50% of cases, and hypochlorhydria in about

25%. Output of acid is also reduced transiently in acute gastritis, and permanently in chronic gastritis.

Achlorhydria is present when the pH is not below 6·0. In pernicious anaemia, the basic change is gastric mucosal atrophy with lack of intrinsic factor and, in the great majority of cases, achlorhydria. Some young persons with pernicious anaemia, however, have been found to have a good acid secretion (Mollin *et al.*, 1955; Lambert *et al.*, 1961).

Testing gastric secretory function after gastric surgery may reveal residual antral activity.

The Insulin Stimulation Test

Insulin-induced hypoglycaemia is a potent stimulus of acid secretion, attributable to central stimulation of the vagus, provided a sufficiently low plasma glucose, preferably below 2·5 mmol/l, is produced. This stimulation test is best limited to patients with recurrent ulceration after a vagotomy which was probably incomplete. It is not without hazard, and is not recommended as a general test of gastric function.

Technique. Carry out the test in the morning after a night's fast. Position a nasogastric tube as for the pentagastrin test (preferably under radiological control) so that the tip of the tube lies in the antrum of the stomach or in the stomach remnant. Collect four 15 min specimens of basal secretion, preferably by continuous aspiration, then give insulin intravenously, 0·2 units/kg body weight, and collect eight 15 min specimens. Take blood for glucose determination immediately before, then 30 and 45 min after giving the insulin. Patients rarely develop symptoms sufficiently severe to require treatment with glucose but this should be available. Measure the volume and pH of the specimens and determine the acid in the same way as for the pentagastrin test.

INTERPRETATION

In patients before vagotomy, there is a marked and prolonged rise in acid to over 100 mmol/l. After a successful vagotomy, there is no response so that only fluctuations in the basal secretion should occur; when there is no acid in the basal secretion any increase should not exceed 10 mmol H^+/l and when there is, it should not be more than 20 mmol/l. Increases greater than this suggest incomplete section of the vagus.

Notes.
1. The degree of stimulation of acid secretion is related to the degree of hypoglycaemia achieved and hence to the dose of insulin. The dose recommended above is designed to give near maximal stimulation.
2. Brooke (1949) suggested that a single test at least 6 months after vagotomy is sufficient. Although lack of acid secretion when the plasma glucose falls below 2·5 mmol/l cannot be taken as certain evidence that all the vagal fibres have been cut, it is usually so.

Pepsinogen

Pepsinogen from extracts of human gastric mucosa has been separated into seven distinct fractions by agar gel electrophoresis (Samloff, 1969). They have been numbered 1 to 7 in decreasing order of electrophoretic mobility. Fractions 1 to 5 inclusive have been grouped immunologically into pepsinogen I (PGI) and fractions 6 and 7 into pepsinogen II (PGII).

Plasma PGI, measured by radioimmunoassay, has been advocated as a non-invasive marker of gastric secretory function but is not thought to offer any significant advantages over the measurement of total pepsinogen in most cases (Hirschowitz, 1984). The latter determination is now performed rarely. Details are given in the 5th edition of this book.

Plasma PGI measured by radioimmunoassay tends to be very low in patients with pernicious anaemia but total pepsinogen activity is not decreased as greatly because PGII activity persists undiminished. PGI may also show a proportionately greater elevation in plasma from patients with the Zollinger–Ellison syndrome compared with the increase in total activity.

Gastrin

Gastrin is released from the pyloric mucosa by a variety of stimuli: peptides, amino acids and calcium in the lumen; vagal activity; blood-borne substances such as calcium, catecholamines and bombesin. Gastrin release is inhibited by decreasing the pH of the fluid bathing the antrum, beginning at pH 3·0 and reaching a maximum at pH 1·0 or less. Intravenous injection of somatostatin, calcitonin, vasoactive intestinal peptide, glucagon or secretin inhibits gastrin release but these responses may be pharmacological rather than physiological.

Gastrinoma is the most common cause of hypergastrinaemia, hyperacidity and peptic ulceration. This triad, first described in 1955, is known as the Zollinger–Ellison syndrome. The clinical features are persistent duodenal ulceration unresponsive to treatment and, more uncommonly, diarrhoea and steatorrhoea. The latter is due to the excess acid in the lumen inactivating pancreatic enzymes such as lipase, and damaging the small bowel mucosa.

Approximately 20% of gastrinoma patients form part of the multiple endocrine adenomatosis, Type I, syndrome. Hyperparathyroidism with hypercalcaemia is the most common associated endocrine abnormality, followed by insulinoma and pituitary chromophobe adenoma. The most common site for the tumour is the pancreas but 3 to 15% are found in the duodenum. They are often small, multiple and malignant with metastatic disease being found in 20 to 40% of patients at presentation.

Diagnosis is best made by measuring serum fasting gastrin levels; gastric acid-secreting studies are usually unnecessary if peptic ulceration is present.

Determination of Gastrin. Radioimmunoassay is the most common and sensitive means of measuring gastrin. Methods normally employ antibodies which are more specific against the C-terminus of gastrin and yet have low affinity for CCK-PZ which shares the same four C-terminal amino acids. The antibodies should measure both the sulphated and non-sulphated forms of the quick-acting G17 and the slower-acting G34 gastrins.

The patient should fast for at least 10 h before the sample is taken. Collect 10 ml blood into a heparin tube containing 1 ml Trasylol (to reduce proteolysis) and mix. Separate the plasma and cool to $-20\,°C$ within 15 min of venepuncture. Discard the sample if haemolysis is visible. Plasma gastrin is stable for several weeks at $-20\,°C$. Some methods require a serum sample similarly frozen.

INTERPRETATION

In normal subjects and in patients with common duodenal ulcers the fasting gastrin level has a skewed distribution with a modal value of 10 pmol/l. The mean is 20 pmol/l and 95% of all values lie below 50 pmol/l.

An increase to above 100 pmol/l in a patient with the clinical features of the Zollinger–Ellison syndrome is almost always diagnostic, provided that acid secretion is high-normal or raised. Hypergastrinaemia also occurs in patients where acid secretion is prevented or reduced. This is because the negative feedback mechanism for inhibiting gastrin release (i.e. acid in the antrum) is inoperative; 75% of patients with pernicious anaemia have achlorhydria with associated high gastrin levels. Patients receiving H2-receptor antagonists have hypergastrinaemia, as do those with conditions such as chronic gastritis and gastric carcinoma because of lower acid concentrations in the antrum. Patients with an intact antrum who have had massive resection of the small bowel may also have high gastrin levels. Vagotomy causes hypergastrinaemia and an increased gastrin response to food. As gastrin is normally destroyed in the kidney, many patients with chronic renal disease have raised gastrin levels.

Several provocative tests have been used to investigate those patients who have suggestive clinical symptoms of the Zollinger–Ellison syndrome but who do not have strikingly raised gastrin figures. Intravenous infusion of calcium for 3–4 h normally results in a small increase in serum gastrin but there is a dramatic rise in the Zollinger–Ellison syndrome. Injection of secretin (1–2 clinical units/kg of GIH-Karolinska secretin) decreases circulating gastrin levels in normal subjects and those with antral G-cell hyperplasia or retained antrum, but a paradoxical and often dramatic increase is found in patients with gastrinoma.

Other Gut Peptides

In addition to gastrin, the determination of other peptide hormones produced by the gastrointestinal mucosa may be helpful in certain pathological conditions. These hormones include pancreatic polypeptide, CCK-PZ, gastric inhibitory peptide, secretin, motilin, neurotensin and enteroglucagon. Their measurement is now almost always performed by immunoassay techniques. For reviews on the physiology and pathology of the gut peptides see Bloom and Polak (1980), Rehfeld (1981) and Bloom (1986).

PANCREATIC FUNCTION

Changes in the internal and external secretions of the pancreas may be found in pancreatic disease either separately or together.

Conditions in which only the internal secretions, insulin and glucagon, are affected have already been considered (Chapter 16, p. 333). Glycosuria with hyperglycaemia is sometimes found during an attack of acute pancreatitis. Considerable recovery of insulin secretion occurs in most cases but occasionally a permanent diabetes mellitus is produced. Diabetes is also likely to be present in carcinoma of the pancreas and in the later stages of chronic pancreatitis. However, tests in pancreatic disease are mostly concerned with the external secretion of the organ.

External Secretion of the Pancreas

The external secretion entering the duodenum is made up of two components under different hormonal control. One, inorganic, is mainly an aqueous solution of sodium bicarbonate, stimulated by secretin, a hormone elaborated in the duodenal mucosa in response to the presence of acid chyme in the duodenum. The main cations are sodium and potassium present in equivalent concentrations to those in plasma, with small amounts of calcium, magnesium and zinc. During a continuous infusion of secretin, there is an increased flow of pancreatic juice with bicarbonate concentrations reaching about 127 mmol/l. Chloride concentration varies inversely with that of bicarbonate, the sum of the two approximating to 155 mmol/l.

The other secretion, which is organic, is stimulated by CCK-PZ secreted by the duodenal and jejunal mucosa in response to the presence of the products of digestion in the intestine, the most powerful stimulants of which are essential amino acids and long chain fatty acids. This stimulates an outflow of enzymes which includes:

1. α-**Amylase** (EC 3.2.1.1: α-1,4-glucan-4-glucanohydrolase) an endo-α-1, 4-glucosidase which hydrolyses randomly α-1,4-glucoside links in the two components of starch, amylose and amylopectin. Activated by chloride ions, it has a pH optimum around 7·0 to 7·2, and mol.wt. 50 000.
2. **Lipase** (EC 3.1.1.3: triacylglycerol acyl-hydrolase) acts on emulsified triglycerides containing acids with chains over 12 C long. Unlike other esterases it only acts at an oil-water interface. The optimal pH ranges between 7·0 and 9·0 varying with different substrates. In the presence of bile salts, stepwise hydrolysis occurs to fatty acids, di- and monoglycerides. Fatty acids at the 1 and 3 positions are preferentially attacked but since fatty acids on the 2 position tend to isomerise to 1 or 3 if these are vacant, intermediate products include 1,3-diglyceride and 1-monoglyceride as well as the 1,2-di- and 2-monoglycerides.
3. **Peptidases** which include the endopeptidases *trypsin* (EC 3.4.21.4) and *chymotrypsin* (EC 3.4.21.1) secreted in the inactive forms trypsinogen and chymotrypsinogen. The former is initially activated by enterokinase secreted by the small intestine but later, trypsin activates both precursors. Also present are the exopeptidases, procarboxypeptidases A and B activated by trypsin to the *carboxypeptidases*, which split peptide bonds at the carboxyl ends of the peptide chains.
4. Also present in the pancreatic secretion are ribonuclease and desoxyribonuclease, cholesterol esterase and phospholipase.

The effect of CCK-PZ on water and bicarbonate output is slight but in addition to stimulating enzyme secretion it causes contraction of the gall bladder with passage of bile into the duodenum thereby aiding the action of pancreatic lipase. Both actions reside in the same molecule.

Secretin and CCK-PZ are straight chain polypeptides. Secretin with 27 amino acids and a C-terminal amide group has a structure with some similarities to that of glucagon while CCK-PZ with 33 amino acids has the same C-terminal tetrapeptide as gastrin. While CCK-PZ acts on the acinar cells, secretin acts mainly on the duct cells and the centroacinar cells, those cells of the duct draining the acinus penetrating into the central part of the acinus. In addition to its action on the stomach gastrin also stimulates secretin production but has little effect of gall bladder contraction. While the hormonal stimuli predominate, there is also a cephalic and gastric stimulation of pancreatic secretion acting through the vagus. The gastric effect is partly due to gastrin secreted as a result of antral distension.

Tests in Pancreatic Disease

The pancreas can be studied *directly* by estimating the output of fluid, bicarbonate and enzymes obtained by duodenal intubation following stimulation of the pancreas by secretin and CCK-PZ or by a test meal and *indirectly* by procedures which can be divided into the following groups:

1. **Determination of Enzymes in Serum and Urine**. In acute pancreatitis, enzymes from damaged cells pass into the blood in considerable amounts. In other pancreatic disorders this may occur to a lesser extent if the pancreatic ducts are obstructed either by fibrous tissue formation, tumour or calculus. Such rises are diminished by destruction of acinar tissue but even then may be revealed by pancreatic stimulation.

2. **Evidence of Impaired Digestion**. This may be obtained by determination of the average daily faecal excretion of fat. However, increases not only occur when digestion is impaired but also when absorption is defective. The test is not helpful in the diagnosis of pancreatic disease, but helps to assess the progress of established pancreatic disorders. The determination of faecal enzymes, particularly chymotrypsin, has been used as an index of their pancreatic output.

Tubeless pancreatic function tests which measure the products of digestion by pancreatic enzymes of certain labelled substrates have been increasingly used. In these tests, one of the products of digestion or its metabolites can be readily measured in the urine. Decreased excretion indicates impaired digestion.

3. **Evidence of Disordered Carbohydrate Metabolism**. This may be obtained from the glucose tolerance test and indicates that the pancreatic lesion has also involved the endocrine tissue of the pancreas.

4. **Demonstration of an Associated Abnormality**. Some pancreatic disorders are associated with hyperlipidaemia or hypercalcaemia. In fibrocystic disease affecting the pancreas, a high concentration of sodium and chloride ions in sweat is usually demonstrable. Some familial types of pancreatitis are associated with aminoacidurias.

5. **Visual Procedures**. These include radiographic methods such as endoscopic retrograde cholangiopancreatography (ERCP), ultrasonic scanning and computed tomography scanning.

Some of the indirect tests have the advantage that they are quick and simple and in severe acute, and in the later stages of chronic, pancreatitis can give much of the information required. However, in the earlier stages of chronic pancreatitis and carcinoma of the pancreas examination of duodenal contents after appropriate stimulation may be more successful in showing the presence of some impairment of pancreatic function. For a review of pancreatic function tests see Gowenlock (1977).

Tests Based on the Determination of Enzymes in Serum and Urine

A study of the diagnostic sensitivity and specificity of enzyme assays used in acute pancreatitis (Steinberg *et al.*, 1985) showed that of the methods studied (serum amylase, isoamylase, lipase and trypsinogen), amylase was as good as any. Bouchier (1985) also concluded that the ease of measurement of amylase in serum makes this the initial assay of choice. Isoamylase measurement would only be indicated if it was essential to show that an elevated amylase activity was of pancreatic origin.

Determination of Serum Amylase (EC 3.2.1.1)

Traditional Methods. Early techniques used starch (variable mixture of amylose and amylopectin) or amylose as substrates and either measured the amount of reducing sugars produced in a fixed time (*saccharogenic methods*) or the amount of polysaccharide remaining by its colour reaction with iodine (*amyloclastic or iodometric methods*). Examples of both techniques appear in the 5th edition of this book. The properties of starch substrates vary with the starch source and the method of preparing it in colloidal solution and native starch substrates have now been almost completely superseded.

Chromolytic Methods. These employ modified starches in which the polysaccharide is covalently linked to a dye. Amylase activity releases oligosaccharides linked to the dye and these are measured colorimetrically. Some substrates are water-insoluble but release coloured products into the reaction mixture making separation simple. Examples are Phadebas (Pharmacia), Cibachron blue bonded to starch by epoxide links, and Amylochrome (Roche), a similar product based on amylose. The water-soluble substance DyAmyl (Warner) is Reactone Red-2B bonded to amylopectin and the unhydrolysed material has to be precipitated before colorimetry. Chromolytic methods are simple and show zero-order kinetics over a wide range of enzyme activity. Over 75 % of laboratories using a manual amylase method now use a chromolytic technique and Phadebas is by far the most popular procedure.

Methods using Oligosaccharide Substrates. Simple oligosaccharide substrates provide better defined products and well characterised kinetics. They have been particularly used with reaction rate methods on discrete analysers, including centrifugal analysers. Two types of substrate are in common use: simple oligosaccharides such as maltopentaose (5 glucose units) and maltotetraose (4 glucose units) or oligosaccharides in which a 4-nitrophenyl (4NP) group is covalently attached to the reducing end of the molecule. 4NP-maltoheptaoside (4NP-7G) with 7 glucose units, and 4NP-maltohexa- and pentaosides together (4NP-6/5G) with 6 and 5 glucose units, are the usual substrates. In all methods using oligosaccharides the assay employs other linked enzyme reactions.

Maltopentaose is cleaved by amylase to maltotriose and maltose. In the Dupont aca method, these products are split to 5 glucose molecules per initial molecule of substrate by the enzyme maltase (α-glucosidase, EC 3.2.1.20) and the glucose is measured using a hexokinase method (p. 326) allowing the rate of formation of NADH to be followed at 340 nm. The substrate maltotetraose is cleaved to two maltose units and in the Beckman DS method the reaction sequence becomes:

Maltose + P_i → Glucose + Glucose-1-P   maltose phosphorylase (EC 2.4.1.8)

Glucose-1-P → Glucose-6-P   phosphoglucomutase (EC 2.7.5.1)

Glucose-6-P + $NADP^+$ → 6-P-Gluconolactone + $NADPH + H^+$

The last reaction uses glucose-6-phosphate dehydrogenase (EC 1.1.1.49) and the rate of production of NADPH is followed at 340 nm.

The 4NP-substrates release 4-nitrophenol during the reaction and this is measured at 405 nm in a kinetic method. Amylase splits such substrates into smaller oligosaccharides and smaller 4NP-oligosaccharides. These are further hydrolysed by maltase present in the reagents. With 4NP-7G rather more than 30 % of the cleavages achieved by amylase eventually result in 4-nitrophenol release. The figure for 4NP-6/5G is 88 %. The 4-NP oligosaccharide methods are probably the best currently available (Foo and Rosalki, 1986).

Other Methods. The only other favoured at present is a reaction-rate turbidimetric technique (Astra) in which amylase activity is measured by its ability to disintegrate starch molecules into smaller, soluble oligosaccharides and dextrins with much reduced light-scattering properties.

Amylase Units. The different substrates result in different enzyme activities even when expressed in U/l. The Somogyi unit, still sometimes encountered, was based on a saccharogenic method and corresponded to the formation of reducing sugars with the reducing capacity of 1 mg glucose during 30 min incubation under defined conditions at 40 °C. This corresponds to 1·85 U.

Chromolytic methods are usually calibrated by comparison with a reference saccharogenic method. The factor may differ depending on the enzyme activity and source (Ali, 1974; Hamlin and Schwede, 1974). Methods using oligosaccharides as substrates give results directly in U/l but consideration must be given to the molar relation between the product measured and the substrate. Thus for the methods outlined above, the relationships are: maltopentaose (five NADH), maltotetraose (two NADPH), 4NP-7G (approx. 0·33 4-nitrophenol) and 4NP-6/5G (approx. 0·88 4-nitrophenol).

The turnover rate is by far the highest for 4NP-7G, with the Astra turbidimetric and maltotetraose methods very much lower. In an intermediate position and closely similar are maltopentaose, 4NP-6/5G, Phadebas, Amylochrome and DyAmyl. Direct comparison of units is thus difficult and reference ranges are required for each method.

Performance of Amylase Methods. As expected the analytical variation for automated methods is lower than for manual techniques. External quality assurance schemes suggest that the between-day CV for the various automated methods in common use is 3 to 5 %. Among the manual methods, the Phadebas technique has the lowest CV at about 7·5 %. Average figures for the CV between laboratories using the same method is 9 % for automated techniques and 11 % for the Phadebas method.

Determination of Amylase by the Phadebas Method. Full instructions are given by the manufacturer (Pharmacia) and should be followed. They are not repeated here.

Notes.
1. Good results require the use of a spectrophotometer correctly adjusted (pp. 147–150) with a band width of 2 nm or less.
2. The distribution curve for precision performance in different laboratories is skewed towards higher results indicating poor technique in some cases. For better precision it is preferable to separate the particles of unaltered substrate by centrifugation rather than filtration.

Determination of Urinary Amylase

The molecular size of circulating amylase is sufficiently small to permit some excretion in the urine under normal conditions. The renal clearance of amylase is on average 2·1 ml/min or 1·1 to 4·1 % of the creatinine clearance. The figures are, however, somewhat influenced by the analytical method used for amylase. Urinary clearance ratio studies do not require a timed collection of urine but this is required if excretion rates of amylase or urinary amylase concentration are to be measured. Timed collections over 2 or 24 h have usually been used.

It is usually convenient to use the same amylase method that is in use for serum amylase. A dilution of the urine 2 to 4-fold with sodium chloride solution, 9 g/l is usually advisable.

A *urinary test strip* for amylase, Rapignost-Amylase (Hoechst), has been developed which allows rapid semi-quantitative assessment of urinary amylase excretion. Holdsworth *et al.* (1984) found 24 positive results in 61 patients presenting to a casualty department and claimed a sensitivity of 100% and a specificity of 78% in the detection of pancreatic disease. However, 19 of the positive tests were from patients already known to have acute pancreatitis and if these are excluded, the specificity falls to 33%. False negative results have been reported by Steele and Lee (1985) and it appears that the test is only positive when the serum amylase activity has risen to four times the upper reference limit (URL). This cut-off level is probably too high and the test strip is probably best used only in situations where serum amylase measurements are unavailable.

Serum and Urinary Amylase

INTERPRETATION

The reference range depends on the analytical method selected. The range is slightly higher for females than males and is also subject to ethnic influences. The URL is increased appreciably in Asians and West Indians compared with Caucasians (Tsianos *et al.*, 1982) and this should be borne in mind when investigating patients.

Amylase occurs in the salivary glands and Fallopian tubes as well as in the pancreas and these different isoamylases show slightly different properties. Variations in urinary amylase reflect alterations in serum amylase so long as renal function is normal. Pancreatic isoamylase, however, has a higher clearance than salivary isoamylase and this may be diagnostically helpful. In renal failure the clearance of amylase is reduced and serum amylase figures are increased while urinary amylase excretion is normal. The increase does not usually exceed twice the URL (Waller and Ralston, 1971).

Considerable increases in serum amylase can occur in acute pancreatitis reaching levels of 5 to 33 × URL at 24 to 48 h after onset of the attack with a correspondingly large increase in urinary amylase. In not all cases is the rise so obvious. The increase reflects the absorption of enzyme liberated from damaged acinar cells but the magnitude and duration of the serum changes are not always related to the extent of the damage (Trapnell, 1972). The rise starts within an hour of onset of pain and usually returns to normal in 4 to 8 days being partly removed by renal excretion. The fall in urinary amylase is somewhat slower, perhaps due to the greater clearance of the pancreatic isoenzyme, and the return to normal may take up to a week longer than for serum amylase. Serum amylase levels which remain high or which increase again later suggest the formation of a pseudocyst of the pancreas (Ebbesen and Schonebeck, 1967).

In carcinoma of the pancreas or chronic pancreatitis, the slow destruction of acinar cells fails to increase serum amylase but increases are seen in serum and urinary amylase during exacerbations of relapsing chronic pancreatitis. Extensive destruction of acinar tissue in the later stages of these diseases fails to reduce serum amylase levels which are usually normal even after total pancreatectomy. Partial obstruction of the pancreatic duct system by fibrous tissue or tumour is, however, an important factor in causing regurgitation of secretions and an increase in serum amylase. Such increases rarely exceed 1·3 × URL, are diminished with progressive acinar destruction, and are most easily demonstrated if the pancreas is stimulated (see 'evocative' test later). Duct obstruction also occurs at the ampulla either by an impacted gall stone or as a consequence of spasm of the sphincter of Oddi after morphine or pethidine. The increases following such drugs can be marked and may not return to normal for 24 h. Increases in serum amylase to over 5·5 × URL occur in biliary tract disease without pancreatitis (Vestrup *et al.*, 1974).

In such acute intra-abdominal conditions as small intestinal obstruction, acute peritonitis, perforated peptic ulcer and mesenteric thrombosis, reabsorption of pancreatic amylase from the splanchnic area produces modest increases in serum amylase, usually to less that 3 × URL. Greater increases (sometimes exceeding 10 × URL) occur in afferent loop obstruction, a late complication of gastrectomy (McGowan and Wills, 1964).

Amylase of Fallopian tube origin may cause increases of serum amylase up to 3 × URL in tubal pregnancy, especially if rupture occurs (Kelley, 1957). Serum amylase, but not lipase, is often increased in diabetic ketoacidotic coma and increases in serum amylase of both pancreatic and salivary origin are relatively common in small degree in post-operative surgical patients. Increases comparable with those in acute pancreatitis without increases in serum lipase occur in acute parotitis usually due to mumps but also following parotid surgery or irradiation. Some lung tumours and ovarian tumours secrete amylase causing increases in the serum enzyme activity to 50 × URL. Associated pleural effusions in such malignancies contain even higher activities.

There may thus be an appreciable overlap in both the serum and urinary amylase figures in pancreatic and extra-pancreatic disorders. Determination of serum lipase may aid differential diagnosis in some cases but other ancillary investigations may be necessary.

Macroamylaseaemia. Normal circulating amylase has a mol. wt. of about 50 000 (4·4 S) as judged from gel filtration studies. In macroamylaseaemia, a condition described in several variant forms (see review by Gowenlock, 1977), circulating amylase has an increased molecular size resulting in reduced clearance, increased serum amylase concentration and reduced urinary amylase excretion. A few cases show villous atrophy and malabsorption but the majority are symptom-free. The abnormal amylase is usually in the molecular size range 5 to 11 S but may vary from near normal to 19 S. This arises by binding of either pancreatic or salivary amylase to a circulating protein. The differentiation of macroamylaseaemia from the increased serum amylase in, for example, acute pancreatitis is most simply made by determination of the urinary amylase which will be increased if the amylase is of the usual molecular weight.

Amylase Isoenzymes

There are two biochemically and genetically distinct groups of α-amylases found in human tissues. They are designated the salivary and pancreatic isoenzymes (S and P) but whereas P amylase appears to be only of pancreatic origin, S amylase is associated with the Fallopian tube and certain tumours as well as with the salivary glands. They are thought to be the products of two genes (Amy 1 and Amy 2 respectively) with multiple alleles at each locus (Merritt and Karn, 1977).

Isoelectric focusing of salivary gland extracts shows 5 to 6 distinct isoamylases and extracts of pancreatic gland have 6 to 8 isoamylases (Rosenmund and Kaczmarek, 1976; Royse and Jensen, 1984). Neuraminidase treatment reduces the number of S isoamylases to three and the P isoamylases to four. The number of isoamylases in serum varies with the individual and with the technique used. Not all the isoamylases found in gland extracts occur in serum and isoelectric focusing usually reveals 3 to 7 isoamylases (Rosenmund and Kaczmarek, 1976). Agarose gel electrophoresis separates between 7 and 9 bands (Leclerc and Forest, 1982; Royse and Jensen, 1984). These have been designated, from the cathode to the anode, P1a, P1b, P2 (major), S1, P3, S2 (major), P4, S3 and S4. Different patterns are found in different individuals and change in disease states. P2, S2 is the most common normal pattern but various combinations of P1, P2, S2 and S3 are also seen. The isoamylase P3 is not found in normal sera.

Determination. Three main methods have been used.

Electrophoresis on cellulose acetate or agarose and subsequent staining using a Phadebas suspension (Leclerc and Forest, 1983; Royse and Jensen, 1984) is relatively slow and requires skill. It does not lend itself to emergency situations but has the advantage that the P3 isoenzyme can be detected and quantitated by densitometry.

The use of selective inhibitors of S amylase prepared from wheat germ has found wider acceptance, especially as an emergency procedure. P amylase activity is then measured by conventional colorimetric means (O'Donnell *et al.*, 1977; Tietz and Shuey, 1984). A commercial kit is available (Pharmacia isoamylase kit). The inhibitor is not fully selective and about 20 % of P amylase activity is also lost. The technique does not detect the presence of the P3 isoamylase. Serum standards must be of human origin because of the relative insensitivity of animal amylases to the inhibitor. The precision of the test is rather poor (Tsianos *et al.*, 1985).

Antibodies have been developed which are specific for S and P isoamylases allowing radioimmunoassay methods to be used (Jalali *et al.*, 1985). Alternatively, precipitation of S amylase by specific monoclonal antibodies allows its removal and later determination of P amylases by conventional means (Gerber *et al.*, 1985; Mifflin *et al.*, 1985).

INTERPRETATION

Estimates of the relative activity of P and S isoamylases in normal serum depend somewhat on the analytical method used. Electrophoresis (Royse and Jensen, 1984) followed by amylase determination in the various fractions using a Phadebas method gave the following reference intervals: P1b, 0–21; P2, 25–114; P3, 0–8; S2, 24–123; S3, 0–18 U/l in 14 apparently healthy adults. Using wheat germ inhibition followed by determination using the Phadebas method, O'Donnell *et al.* (1977) found reference intervals for P amylase of 37–162 U/l in males and 52–175 U/l in females; for S amylase the ranges were 9–172 U/l for males and 9–196 U/l for females. Immunological precipitation of S amylase and quantitation of P amylase using maltotetraose as substrate (Mifflin *et al.*, 1985) gave reference intervals of 11–50 U/l for P amylase and 18–79 U/l for S amylase. There is a tendency for S amylase to predominate over P amylase and this is more obvious in 'ethnic' hyperamylaseaemia where the increase is mainly attributable to the S amylase (Tsianos *et al.*, 1982, 1985).

Marked increases of P amylase occur in acute pancreatitis and, to a lesser degree, in exacerbations of relapsing pancreatitis. The isoamylase P3 occurs in patients with acute pancreatitis (Legaz and Kenny, 1976) and seems to be the most sensitive index of this condition. P3 may be derived from P2 by proteolytic attack by pancreatic peptidases. During an attack of acute pancreatitis, P3 appears and increases after the increase in P2. It also remains longer in the serum, possibly due to a lower clearance rate, and is detectable after serum lipase has returned to normal (Leclerc and Forest, 1983).

An increase in P amylase does not necessarily indicate acute pancreatitis as it is also seen after reabsorption of P amylase in perforated peptic ulcer, intestinal obstruction, peritonitis and mesenteric thrombosis as well as after administration of morphine. A decrease in P amylase is characteristic of destruction of pancreatic acinar tissue leading to pancreatic insufficiency. The total amylase activity may remain within conventional limits.

Increases in S amylase of marked degree are associated with mumps parotitis, but again are not specific as they are also seen in ectopic pregnancy and in association with some lung and ovarian tumours. Many of the cases of post-operative hyperamylaseaemia show an increase in S amylase predominantly. Macroamylaseaemia is usually associated with increased S amylase activity in the macromolecular complex. In contrast, the retention of amylases in renal insufficiency affects both S and P amylases.

The place of isoamylase measurement has yet to be clarified. In patients presenting with acute abdominal pain, measurement of P amylase is best reserved as a confirmatory test for those patients with an increased total amylase activity (Steinberg *et al.*, 1985; Tietz *et al.*, 1986). Isoamylase investigations are sometimes helpful in the investigation of patients with symptomless, unexpected hyperamylasaemia.

Use of Serum Lipase

This enzyme will only be considered briefly as many laboratories have now discontinued the investigation. Analytical methods for lipase preferably use a long chain triglyceride as substrate and olive oil or triolein are convenient. There are difficulties in preparing a stable oil emulsion and the reaction rate tends to fall with long incubation times. A method requiring 3 h incubation is given in the 5th edition of this book. There may be advantages in adding colipase to the assay system.

In many patients with pancreatic disease, changes in amylase and lipase are roughly parallel. Diagnostic accuracy is improved by measuring both enzymes (Lifton *et al.*, 1974; Schultis *et al.*, 1969) when the enzyme increases are small or when measurements are made some days after an acute attack of pancreatitis as the fall in lipase is slower than that of amylase. Lipase activity increases in those non-pancreatic conditions where pancreatic amylase rises, e.g. perforated peptic ulcer, morphine administration and chronic renal insufficiency. Obvious dissociation occurs if the amylase is of extra-pancreatic origin or if there is macroamylaseaemia.

Determination of Serum Enzymes after Stimulation of the Pancreas

Attempts have been made to detect chronic pancreatic disorders by measuring changes in serum pancreatic enzymes after stimulating pancreatic secretion submaximally. Normally there is no increase; entry of enzymes into the circulation is interpreted as obstruction to the flow of pancreatic juice in the presence of moderate or normal acinar function.

Such an 'evocative test' (Burton *et al.*, 1960b) using secretin and CCK-PZ as stimulants may usefully be combined with duodenal intubation studies. After collecting a resting blood sample, secretin is administered and 30 min later a second blood sample is taken and CCK-PZ is then given. Further blood samples are collected 1, 2, 4 and 24 h after the secretin dose. In normal subjects, serum enzyme levels increase little, but increases to above the URL can occur in chronic pancreatitis and carcinoma of the pancreas. The rise in lipase is sometimes more marked.

In more advanced pancreatic disease, acinar destruction obliterates the response but by then there is often sufficient islet tissue loss to produce an abnormal oral glucose tolerance test. An abnormal evocative test or glucose tolerance test is found in 86 % of cases of chronic pancreatitis or pancreatic cancer (Howat, 1970). The evocative test is not specific for pancreatic disease and a positive response may occur in disease of the liver or biliary tract or in the presence of enlarged retroperitoneal glands. It should be performed in combination with the examination of duodenal contents following pancreatic stimulation.

Examination of Duodenal Contents Following Pancreatic Stimulation

The poor serum enzyme responses in more advanced disease arise from acinar cell destruction. This destruction, or pancreatic duct obstruction, will reduce the flow of pancreatic secretions which can be collected after duodenal intubation. The duodenal contents normally contain pancreatic juice, bile, saliva and gastric secretions with some components from the duodenal mucosa. Measurements are made following stimulation by pancreatic hormones either given parenterally or after their physiological release from the duodenal mucosa.

Such tests are now mainly used to investigate patients who have borderline results for other pancreatic tests, or as a research procedure. They require skilled and experienced personnel to perform the intubation, collect the correct specimens, carry out the analyses and interpret the results.

Stimulation Using Exogenous Hormones

Although admixture of biliary and pancreatic secretions cannot be avoided, contamination with salivary and gastric secretions can be minimised by using a double lumen tube with one part 25 cm longer than the other positioned, under radiological control, so that the shorter tube ends at the pyloric antrum and the other in the third part of the duodenum. Continuous aspiration up both tubes permits recovery of uncontaminated duodenal contents from the longer tube. Other workers use two separate tubes similarly located.

The hormones used are obtained either from Boots (Nottingham, England) or the Karolinska Institute's Gastrointestinal Hormone Laboratory (GIH) marketed by Vitrum (Stockholm, Sweden). Boots secretin and CCK-PZ are assayed in Crick, Harper, Raper units (CHRU), GIH secretin is assayed in clinical units (CU) and their CCK-PZ in Ivy units (IU). For secretin, one CU is equivalent to two CHRU (Gutierrez and Baron, 1972) while for CCK-PZ one IU equals about 4 CHRU. The doses used may give sub-maximal (Burton *et al.*, 1960a) or maximal responses. The latter are better achieved using continuous intravenous infusion of hormones.

The many different test procedures, for details of which see Gowenlock (1977), give different responses. Not all authors have measured the same components of duodenal juice and results have been expressed in different ways.

Examination of Specimens

Collect the duodenal juice in containers chilled in ice. At the end of a collection period measure the volume and preserve from proteolytic attack either by adding an equal volume of glycerol and storing at 4 °C (Burton *et al.*, 1960a) or by adding Trasylol (Hanscom *et al.*, 1967). If the former is used, express the results in terms of the amount in the undiluted juice.

It is usual to measure the volume and to determine bicarbonate, one or more enzymes (usually amylase and trypsin) and, sometimes, bilirubin. The normal responses quoted in the original publications depend on the analytical methods used, some of which are now obsolete. If more modern methods are substituted, the results of the new and old methods should be compared on a variety of specimens in order to determine the appropriate conversion factor or, preferably, the normal range should be redetermined using the new methods.

Determination of Bicarbonate. A gasometric procedure is probably the best but equipment may not be readily available in which case indirect titration with acid is convenient.

To 5 ml duodenal juice add 10 ml 100 mmol/l hydrochloric acid in a small beaker, boil to expel carbon dioxide, cool and titrate with 100 mmol/l sodium hydroxide solution using phenolphthalein as indicator. Alternatively, titrate to pH 7·0 electrometrically. The difference in the volumes of standard acid and alkali used in ml × 20 gives the bicarbonate concentration (mmol/l) in the juice used.

Determination of Bilirubin. The concentration varies from 0 to 1000 μmol/l. Any of the usual methods for bilirubin can be used, particularly if preliminary dilution with sodium chloride solution (9 g/l) is required. If undiluted specimens are used, check the pH of the reaction mixture to ensure that the bicarbonate content has not altered this from its expected value and adjust if necessary.

Determination of Amylase. The amylase concentration in duodenal juice may be 1000 times greater than that in serum, especially following hormonal stimulation. Considerable but accurate dilution is needed before one of the methods for serum amylase can be employed. The diluent may be sodium chloride solution (9 g/l) or a polyvinylpyrrolidone solution (50 mg/l) if the Phadebas technique is used.

Determination of Lipase. Again dilution up to 1 in 100 will be needed before using the lipase method employed for serum. The preferred diluent is sodium chloride solution (9 g/l) containing albumin (0·5 g/l).

Determination of Trypsin. Most methods use specific synthetic substrates: *p*-toluenesulphonyl-L-arginine methyl ester (TAME), *N*-α-benzoyl-L-arginine ethyl ester (BAEE) or *N*-α-benzoyl-D,L-arginine *p*-nitroanilide (BAPNA). For the first two, the rate of formation of carboxyl groups is measured and for the last, the rate of release of *p*-nitroaniline is measured at 405 nm. The method given here (Wiggins, 1967) measures the rate of acid formation from BAEE at pH 8·2.

Reagents.
1. Sodium hydroxide solution, 40 mmol/l.
2. Sodium barbitone solution, 10 g/l.
3. BAEE substrate. To 10 ml reagent (2), add 90 ml water and 0·5 g BAEE. Bring to 25 °C and adjust to pH 9·0.
4. Acetate buffer, pH 5·8, 50 mmol/l. Dissolve 6·8 g CH_3COONa, $3H_2O$ in water, add 0·5 g calcium chloride and make to one litre. Adjust to pH 5·8 with a drop or two of strong acetic acid.

Technique. Mix 1 ml duodenal contents with 9 ml acetate buffer and bring to 25 °C. Place a small magnet in a glass vial, 2·5 cm diameter, 7·5 cm high, and mount it on the plate of a magnetic stirrer, preferably in a vessel containing water at 25 °C. Add 5 ml substrate to the vial, insert a small glass electrode system connected to a sensitive pH meter, start the stirrer and add 1 ml diluted juice. The starting pH, about 8·5, falls. When it reaches 8·0, add 100 μl sodium hydroxide and start a stopwatch. The pH rises to about 8·4 and falls as acid is liberated. Note the time to reach pH 8·0. Often this takes less than 4 min. If longer than 10 min, repeat using a 1 in 5 dilution of the juice.

Calculation. As 4 μmol of alkali is added and then neutralised

$$\text{Activity of enzyme} = 4/\text{time (min) } \mu\text{mol/min or U}$$

$$\text{Enzyme concentration (U/l)} = \text{activity} \times \text{dilution} \times 1000$$

Notes.
1. If the incubation time exceeds 10 min with the 1 in 5 dilution, report as less than 2000 U/l.
2. An automatic titrator can be used to record the rate of addition of alkali to maintain the pH at 8·25 in unbuffered solution. Use 5 ml BAEE solution (5 g/l in water) add 0·5 ml undiluted juice and titrate with sodium hydroxide, 100 mmol/l, at 25 °C. After an initial period of 30 s record the volume of alkali added over 2 min. Then activity equals volume (μl) × 100 U/l. The method is linear up to 40 000 U/l.

INTERPRETATION

Not all authors find that the addition of CCK-PZ to secretin gives useful extra information but the majority feel that the undoubted extra secretion of enzymes is worthwhile. Different enzymes are favoured by various investigators, but amylase, and a proteolytic enzyme (trypsin or chymotrypsin) are probably best. There is no agreement on the best method of expressing the results of the test. The use of rate of secretion rather than concentration seems preferable but some also relate these to body weight. It is also not determined whether maximal or submaximal stimulation gives the better discrimination between normal and pathological states.

These variations result in different figures for normal subjects and results of different authors cannot be compared directly. Comparison of results from cases of suspected pancreatic disease can only be made with the results for normal subjects found under identical conditions of stimulation and analytical methods. As the distribution curves for the outputs of bicarbonate and enzymes are skewed, allowance for this must be made in defining the lower limit of normal. When all these factors are taken into account there is a fair measure of agreement concerning the findings in various disorders. For a review see Gowenlock (1977).

Shortly after an attack of acute pancreatitis, bicarbonate and enzyme outputs are depressed but these return to normal, or even temporarily supranormal, levels as the pancreas recovers fully which is usually the case. Persistent reduction implies permanent damage and the possibility of a progressive disorder. This recovery of function differentiates relapsing acute pancreatitis from relapsing chronic pancreatitis in which impairment is apparent between the attacks. If the duct is obstructed by a simple stricture, a stone or carcinoma, the volume response to secretin is diminished. Provided acinar destruction is not marked, the maximal concentration of bicarbonate remains normal but its secretion rate is diminished. In the early stages of carcinoma the reduced output of enzymes following CCK-PZ is more marked than the bicarbonate fall just described and enzyme output may be unaffected by a stricture or stone. If acinar destruction predominates as in chronic pancreatitis the volume response to secretin is initially normal but the maximal bicarbonate concentration and hence output is reduced. Enzyme output is preserved until later and this dissociation is suggestive of chronic pancreatitis. However, progression of any pancreatic disease eventually results in depression of outputs of both bicarbonate and enzymes often of marked degree with the development of a pancreatic steatorrhoea.

Changes may occur in non-pancreatic disorders. The bicarbonate output following secretin is increased in duodenal ulcer and in cases of gall bladder disease, following cholecystectomy, and, especially, in cirrhosis and haemochromatosis.

Indirect Stimulation of the Pancreas

Tests using exogenous hormones developed alongside simpler tests using more physiological stimuli. Duodenal contents are removed using a single lumen tube without regard to gastric emptying or completeness of recovery following an oral test meal. Lundh (1962) used dried milk, vegetable oil and glucose and continuously collected four 30 min samples, analysing these for trypsin. The test meal liberates secretin and CCK-PZ from the duodenal mucosa and pancreatic stimulation results.

Method of Carrying out the Lundh Test (Cook *et al.*, 1967)

The patient, who should have fasted overnight, swallows a 12 Fr gauge radio-opaque tube with a small bag containing mercury at the tip. There are four holes in the terminal 6 cm. The tube is passed through the nose and usually enters the duodenum within an hour. Check radiologically and adjust the tip to lie at the duodeno-jejunal flexure. For a patient with a Polya gastrectomy pass the tube well past the stoma.

The test meal consists of 18 g corn or soya bean oil, 15 g dried milk protein (Casilan) and 40 g glucose, homogenised in hot water and made to 300 ml. After drinking this the patient reclines on the bed. Place the end of the tube in a measuring cylinder, chilled on ice and placed 80 cm below the duodenum. Collect the duodenal contents by siphonage over 2 h. If necessary, aspirate gently at first to start the flow and check regularly that the flow is unobstructed.

The specimen is mixed and analysed for trypsin by the BAEE method but can, if necessary, be stored at $-20\,^\circ$C for up to 4 weeks before analysis.

Normal Range. The distribution of trypsin concentration in normals and patients with no evidence of pancreatic disease is log-normal. In order to calculate the range as mean $\pm$ 2SD, preliminary logarithmic transformation is needed. Mottaleb *et al.* (1973) found this range in 235 patients to be 7000 to 38 000 (mean 16 800) U/l. Cook *et al.* (1967) recorded the lower limit as 9500 U/l. The figures in the former paper are erroneously reported as U/l but are actually in U/ml and have been corrected here.

INTERPRETATION

Published series of results (James, 1973; Mottaleb *et al.*, 1973) demonstrate reduced trypsin concentrations (positive test) in about 90% of cases of chronic pancreatitis but in only 79% of cases of pancreatic carcinoma, the most definite results being for tumours in the head of the organ. Differentiation between carcinoma and chronic pancreatitis and recovery following acute pancreatitis can be studied. Although markedly positive tests occur in pancreatic steatorrhoea about one quarter of patients with coeliac disease show a less markedly positive test as a consequence of diminished hormone release from the flat mucosa. Positive tests may also occur at times in diabetic patients with long-standing insulin deficiency, in cases of duodenal ulcer and following Billroth II gastrectomy. The latter is attributed to delayed emptying of the afferent loop.

The test has the merit of greater simplicity than the tests using exogenous stimulation but its discriminatory power is somewhat less.

Tubeless Pancreatic Function Tests

While procedures employing intubation and stimulation of the pancreas with the subsequent examination of the pancreatic secretions have been widely used with success they are expensive, invasive tests requiring skilled operators. Non-invasive tests suitable as an out-patient procedure are obviously attractive (Lankisch and Lambeke, 1984) and two have been specially studied: the *N*-benzoyl-L-tyrosyl-*p*-aminobenzoic acid (BT PABA or Bentiromide) test (Imondi *et al.*, 1972) and the pancreolauryl test (Barry *et al.*, 1982; Boyd *et al.*, 1982). The principle of these tests is to give the patient by mouth a substance which is specifically cleaved by pancreatic enzyme action in the gut lumen. One of the products is absorbed, metabolised, excreted in the urine and then measured. The amount excreted is a measure of pancreatic enzyme activity.

The BT PABA test has been the more extensively studied and has been modified to overcome some of its initial drawbacks. Orally administered BT PABA is specifically cleaved by chymotrypsin to *N*-benzoyl-L-tyrosine and *p*-aminobenzoic acid (PABA) which is absorbed and metabolised in the liver. The metabolites are excreted in the urine. Mitchell *et al.* (1978) tried to overcome the problems of malabsorption and impaired hepatic metabolism or renal excretion of PABA in some patients, and thereby improve the sensitivity of the test, by using a PABA excretion index (PEI). The percentage excretion of PABA released from BT PABA is compared with that following a separate dose of free PABA. However, this requires two urine collections on separate days and assumes that PABA is handled identically on both occasions. If a small amount of ^{14}C-labelled PABA is incorporated in the administered BT PABA, the PEI can be calculated on a single day from the percentage of radioactivity excreted in the urine (Kay *et al.*, 1983). The urinary PABA is measured by a modification of the colorimetric method of Bratton and Marshall (1939).

PABA Test of Kay *et al.* (1983)

Reagents.
1. Casein—light white.
2. Fruit syrup, for flavouring.
3. Sodium *N*-benzoyl-L-tyrosyl-*p*-aminobenzoate (BT PABA) as pentahydrate, mol. wt. 471·5 (Fluka).
4. ^{14}C-PABA stock solution, 250 μCi in 20 ml distilled water. The radioactive PABA is labelled in the COOH group and is available from Amersham International.

Technique. Homogenise 25 g casein, 10 ml fruit syrup and 450 ml water and stand to allow any froth to subside. This may take up to 4 h. In a 500 ml volumetric flask, dissolve 500 mg BT PABA in approximately 20 ml water. Add 400 μl (5 μCi) of the stock ^{14}C-PABA solution followed by the flavoured casein solution and make up to 500 ml with water. Mix well and remove 2·0 ml for counting.

The patient must be fasted overnight and all pancreatic supplements and all but the most essential drugs must be discontinued for 24 h before starting the test. The patient empties the bladder before starting the test; a portion of the urine is retained. The patient drinks the total contents of the volumetric flask within a 5 min period; all urine passed within the next 6 h is collected, during which time the patient is allowed water but not food. After 6 h the patient may eat and drink normally but urine collection continues for the next 18 h.

The three urine collections, pre-test, 0–6 h and 6–24 h are sent to the laboratory for determination of PABA and for scintillation counting.

Method for the Determination of PABA (Bratton and Marshall, 1939, modified)

PABA, released from its metabolites by alkaline hydrolysis, is diazotised and after removal of nitrous acid with sulphamate, is coupled with naphthyl-ethylenediamine to give an azo-dye which is measured colorimetrically.

Reagents.
1. Stock PABA solution, 1·46 mmol/l. Dissolve 20 mg pure PABA in water and make to 100 ml.
2. Working PABA standard, 14·6 μmol/l. Dilute the stock solution 1 to 100 with water.
3. Sodium hydroxide solution, 5 mol/l.
4. Hydrochloric acid, 6 mol/l.
5. Hydrochloric acid, 1·2 mol/l.
6. Sodium nitrite solution, 14·5 mmol/l. Dissolve 100 mg sodium nitrite in water and make up to 100 ml. Prepare freshly daily.
7. Ammonium sulphamate solution, 4·4 mmol/l. Dissolve 5·0 g ammonium sulphamate in water and make up to one litre.
8. Naphthylethylenediamine solution, 3·9 mmol/l. Dissolve 1·0 g of the hydro-chloride in water and make up to one litre.

Technique. Dilute duplicate 0·1 ml amounts of each of the three urine samples to 10 ml with water. Treat the working PABA standard as a diluted urine. Set up two borosilicate glass tubes for each urine and the standard, one designated as 'test' and the other as 'blank'. To each tube add 2·5 ml diluted urine or working standard, followed by 0·5 ml reagent (3). Place all the tubes in a boiling water bath for 90 min with the tubes loosely capped with marbles to prevent excessive evaporation. Cool and then add 0·5 ml reagent (4) to each tube to neutralise.

To each of the tubes marked 'test', add 0·5 ml reagent (5), 250 μl reagent (6), 250 μl reagent (7), 250 μl reagent (8) at 4 min intervals, mixing after each addition. To the 'blank' tubes add reagents (5) to (7) but substitute 250 μl water for reagent (8). After 20 min at room temperature read all tubes at 550 nm against a water blank.

Calculation. Recovery of PABA (%) =

$$\frac{\text{Absorbance (sample 'test'} - \text{sample 'blank')}}{\text{Absorbance (standard 'test'} - \text{standard 'blank')}} \times \text{urine sample volume (ml)} \times$$

$$\frac{100}{1000} \times 14\cdot6 \times \frac{471\cdot5}{500} \times \frac{100}{1000}$$

$$= \frac{\text{Absorbance (sample 'test'} - \text{sample 'blank')}}{\text{Absorbance (standard 'test'} - \text{standard 'blank')}} \times \text{urine volume} \times 0\cdot138.$$

Determination of ^{14}C-PABA

Reagents.
1. Trichloracetic acid, 50 g/l in water.
2. Glacial acetic acid.

Technique. To duplicate 1·0 ml quantities of the test meal add 3 ml trichloracetic acid. After 10 min, centrifuge at 3000 g and remove the supernatant fluid. Treat this and the urine samples in the same way by adding 0·5 ml amounts in duplicate to separate counting vials. Add 0·5 ml water, one drop of glacial acetic acid and scintillation fluid and measure the radioactivity using a beta counter.

Calculation. Recovery of ^{14}C-PABA (%)

$$= \frac{\text{count rate of test} \times \text{urine volume (ml)}}{\text{count rate of supernatant} \times 4 \times 500}$$

For the 0–6 h urine collection the PEI $= \dfrac{\% \text{ recovery of PABA}}{\% \text{ recovery of } ^{14}\text{C-PABA}}$

Notes.
1. A colour developing in the pre-test urine suggests drug interference. Drugs known to interfere include paracetamol, benzocaine, chloramphenicol, sulphonamides and xylocaine. Foods such as prunes and cranberries also give a colour reaction (Braganza *et al.*, 1983; Heyman, 1985).
2. Some workers measure the plasma PABA concentration, maximal at 2–3 h after BT PABA ingestion, and find it as discriminatory as the PEI (Weizman *et al.*, 1985).
3. The original Bratton–Marshall procedure used acid hydrolysis of the urine to deconjugate the aromatic amino group in PABA for diazotisation but such hydrolysis also causes some decarboxylation with altered colour equivalent of the product. This is avoided by alkaline hydrolysis (Braganza *et al.*, 1983).
4. Other methods for PABA determination have been investigated with the aim of avoiding interferences associated with the colorimetric method. They include fluorimetry (Lobley *et al.*, 1985) and HPLC (Ito *et al.*, 1982; Berg *et al.*, 1985; Bradbury *et al.*, 1985). Bradbury *et al.* (1985) used anthranilic acid, the *o*-isomer of PABA instead of ^{14}C-PABA to calculate the PEI and Berg *et al.* (1986) used *p*-aminosalicylic acid to avoid exposure to radioisotopes.
5. The recovery of PABA and ^{14}C-PABA in the combined 0–6 and 6–24 h urine collections can be used to identify interferences occurring during the test. A normal PEI but low 24 h recoveries (less than 80%) of both labelled and unlabelled PABA suggests incomplete ingestion of the meal, incomplete urine collection, or malabsorption. An abnormal PEI with apparent recoveries of more than 100% suggest interference from drugs or foodstuffs. Radioactivity from previous ^{75}Se scans of the pancreas will also interfere with the ^{14}C counting.

INTERPRETATION

The PEI is a useful screening measurement in cases of suspected chronic pancreatitis. It correlates well with the Lundh test meal (Kay *et al.*, 1983). The test has a sensitivity around 75% and a specificity of around 85%. Patients with chronic pancreatitis who have a normal PEI also tend to have normal duodenal intubation tests (Braganza *et al.*, 1983). The BT PABA test is useful in distinguishing patients with pancreatic exocrine insufficiency. The effectiveness of pancreatic enzyme replacement therapy can be monitored using this test (Heyman, 1985). False negative results may occur with bacterial overgrowth when bacterial enzymes may cleave the molecule.

A normal PEI suggests that the patient does not have chronic pancreatic disease or at least not in a sufficiently advanced form to reduce the exocrine secretion to less than 5–10% of normal. An abnormal result suggests further investigation is required (such as ultrasound scanning etc.) to separate the true from the false positives.

Faecal Enzyme Studies

Inadequate secretion of pancreatic enzymes should diminish their faecal excretion. Most studies have used the proteolytic enzymes, trypsin and chymotrypsin. These are normally partly adsorbed onto the small intestinal mucosa and undergo further inactivation in the colon so that the transit rate through the intestinal tract may be as important as the amount secreted. If the transit time is reduced by purgation over half the enzyme secreted appears in the faeces (Sale *et al.*, 1974).

Early methods for faecal enzymes used gelatin as substrate for the mixture of trypsin and chymotrypsin. More recently, specific substrates have been used to study the excretion of trypsin (using TAME) and chymotrypsin (using acetyltyrosine ethyl ester, ATEE) separately. The methods involve incubation with faecal homogenate and determination of the rate of acid liberation using an automatic titrator or measurement of the decrease in pH using a pH meter (Robinson *et al.*, 1975). Chymotrypsin excretion has proved more reliable than that of trypsin and for minor degrees of impaired excretion timed collections are claimed to give better discrimination.

A screening test for cystic fibrosis in the newborn has been described (Crossley *et al.*, 1977; Robinson and Elliott, 1976) in which stool samples are smeared onto a specially prepared card and sent to the laboratory where the enzyme activity in the faeces is measured.

Quantitative Method for Faecal Trypsin and Chymotrypsin (Robinson *et al.*, 1975)

The acid liberated by the action of trypsin or chymotrypsin on TAME and ATEE respectively is measured using a sensitive pH meter.

Trypsin Reagents.
1. Tris buffer, 5 mmol/l, pH 8·2; 0·354 g Tris-HCl, 0·334 g Tris, 2·34 g sodium chloride and 2·94 g calcium chloride dihydrate are made up to 1 litre with water.
2. Substrate, 2·075 g TAME in 50 ml of reagent (1).
3. Stock standard, crystalline trypsin, 1 mg/ml in reagent (1).
4. Calibration standards. Dilute the stock standard daily 1:1 (500 μg/ml), 1:10 (100 μg/ml) and 1:100 (10 μg/ml) with reagent (1).
5. Stool samples. Homogenise stool samples with isotonic saline (1 g wet weight/10 ml saline)

Technique. Place 2 ml sample homogenate (or 2 ml working standards), 5·5 ml Tris buffer and 2·5 ml TAME solution in a 25 ml beaker on a magnetic stirrer (a small paper clip can conveniently be used as a disposable stirring bar). Adjust the pH of the solution with either 0·2 mol/l HCl or NaOH to just above pH 8·2 using a pH meter, and then record the time for the pH to drop from pH 8·2 to 8·1 using a stopwatch. Readjust the pH and make a duplicate timing.

Chymotrypsin Reagents.

1. Tris buffer, 3 mmol/l, pH 7·8; 0·532 g Tris-HCl, 0·198 g Tris, 2·925 g sodium chloride and 0·735 g calcium chloride dihydrate are made up to 1 litre with water.
2. Substrate, 0·454 g ATEE dissolved in 25 ml methanol diluted to 1 litre with reagent (1).
3. Stock standard, crystalline chymotrypsin, 1 mg/ml in reagent (1).
4. Calibration standards. Dilute the stock standard daily 1:1, 1:10 and 1:100 with reagent (1).
5. Stool samples. Prepare as for trypsin assay.

Technique. Place 2 ml sample homogenate (or 2 ml working standards), 3 ml Tris buffer, and 5 ml ATEE solution in a 25 ml beaker and proceed as for the trypsin assay but time the pH fall from 7·8 to 7·7.

Calculation. Construct a calibration plot on log–log paper of enzyme concentration (μg/g stool) as a function of time (in seconds) for a pH drop of 0·1. Enzyme concentration can be read directly from the graph.

Notes.

1. Store the buffer solutions at 37 °C and the stock enzyme solutions at 4 °C.
2. Enzyme activity in stool samples appears generally to be reasonably stable but tryptic activity occasionally falls if the sample is not frozen soon after collection. If stored frozen they are stable for 2 months.
3. The second time taken for the pH to fall by 0·1 unit is often greater than the first result (i.e. lower enzyme activity) in stools from patients with cystic fibrosis. This phenomenon may be due to inhibition of the enzyme activity by undigested food present in these stools.
4. Pancreatic supplements should be stopped for at least 3 days prior to stool sampling.
5. The method can also be used to measure enzyme activity in duodenal juice of children with cystic fibrosis. Dilute aspirates 1:10 with isotonic saline.

INTERPRETATION

This quantitative method is better suited than semi-quantitative methods for studying minor degrees of pancreatic insufficiency. Stools from a reference population with no indication of pancreatic disease have trypsin activities ranging from 34–1250 μg/g (mean 229 μg/g) and chymotrypsin activities ranging from 159–746 μg/g (mean 338 μg/g). Normal babies have values ranging from 37–730 μg/g (mean 152 μg/g) for trypsin and 67–1092 μg/g (mean 411 μg/g) for chymotrypsin. In cystic fibrosis, trypsin activities range from 4–30 μg/g (mean 17 μg/g) and chymotrypsin 6–39 μg/g (mean 18 μg/g) so there is reasonable discrimination between the reference populations and such patients for trypsin and good discrimination for chymotrypsin. The stool enzyme activity of obligate heterozygote parents of children with cystic fibrosis is not statistically different from the reference population.

There is a correlation between the faecal chymotrypsin output and the pancreatic secretion of bicarbonate and enzymes (Ammann, 1969; Sale *et al.*, 1974). Faecal studies can aid in selection of cases for duodenal intubation studies and are useful in assessing the progress of the disease. Normal chymotrypsin excretion indicates no significant defect in pancreatic exocrine secretion and normal values in steatorrhoea exclude pancreatic steatorrhoea. Occasionally, falsely low results can occur in steatorrhoea from increased buffering action of faecal components or increased destruction of enzymes by the increased intestinal flora.

Faecal Fat

This is an important index of impaired digestion and hence absorption of fat and is discussed later in this chapter.

Other Investigations in Pancreatic Disease

These are used either to assess established disease or to demonstrate an associated abnormality. In acute haemorrhagic pancreatitis, absorption of digested haemoglobin from the necrotic area results in methaemalbuminaemia. The serum calcium level often falls after a severe attack of acute pancreatitis but as the maximal fall occurs between the fifth and eighth day it is not helpful in the early stages.

Relapsing pancreatitis is a complication of hypercalcaemia and this should be investigated. Other cases are associated with a hyperlipidaemia of Types I, IV or V. In familial relapsing pancreatitis starting in childhood, some cases are associated with increased urinary excretion of arginine, cystine and lysine or of glycine and lysine and chromatography of urine is useful in these cases.

An important cause of familial chronic pancreatitis is cystic fibrosis and in this disorder the abnormal excretion of sodium in the sweat should be investigated. Heeley and Watson (1983) have reviewed biochemical tests which are used to investigate cystic fibrosis. Di Sant'Agnese *et al.* (1953) showed that the sodium chloride content of sweat is higher in children with cystic fibrosis than in normal children. The finding has been repeatedly confirmed but the difference is much less apparent at low rates of sweat secretion. Sweating has been stimulated by heating or injection of mecholyl but the most satisfactory method is to stimulate with pilocarpine passed into the skin by an electric current—iontophoresis. Provided conditions are carefully regulated (Schwarz *et al.*, 1968), the technique is safe and errors are reduced to a minimum. The sweat secreted from the stimulated skin is collected on filter paper avoiding loss of water by evaporation and after elution the sodium and potassium content is determined.

Procedure for Sweat Test (after Schwarz *et al.*, 1968)

Cut sheets of filter paper (Whatman No. 541, unwashed) into pieces 1.5×2 cm, handling with forceps throughout. Place one piece in each of a series of small plastic weighing bottles, approximately 10 ml volume, and weigh each to the nearest 0·5 mg. Prepare similar stacks of at least 10 pieces of the same size of the same paper for iontophoresis. Store in plastic wallets without weighing. Prepare lengths (10 cm) of adhesive plastic tape (5 cm wide). The tape should be capable of being stretched. Material sold for sealing containers to be stored in deep-freeze chests is convenient. With forceps, attach a piece of washed and dried x-ray film backing, 1.5×2 cm, to the adhesive surface so that its shorter edge coincides with the centre of the longer edge of the adhesive tape.

The iontophoresis equipment provides direct current from four 9 V dry batteries in series. The circuit incorporates a fixed resistance of 2.7 kΩ and a variable resistance of 0 to 50 kΩ to limit the maximal current entering the skin. The anode is a carbon plate slightly smaller than 1.5×2 cm. The cathode is connected to a copper strip embedded in a paper towel moistened with a dilute solution of magnesium chloride and wrapped firmly round the upper part of the arm to be tested.

Wash the ventral surface of the forearm with gauze moistened with distilled water. Dip the stack of filter paper in pilocarpine nitrate solution (4 g/l) and blot off excess solution. Place the stack on the forearm skin and strap the anode over it. Switch on the current and after keeping at 0·2 mA for 30 s, increase gradually to 1 to 1·3 mA and maintain for 6 min adjusting the resistance as necessary to avoid increase of current above this range.

Remove the electrodes and filter paper stack. Wipe the upper arm and stimulated area with tissues wetted with distilled water. Dry the upper arm and wipe the stimulated area with dry filter paper (No. 541). Immediately on removing the paper, apply the adhesive tape with the film covering the stimulated area. With forceps, insert a weighed filter paper between the skin and the x-ray film and seal the edge with adhesive tape (2·5 cm wide) avoiding touching the skin with the fingers. At a secretion rate of 7 to 8 mg in 5 min the paper will appear uniformly damp after 10 to 15 min. Collection should cease at this point. At higher secretion rates the collection period will be shorter. Peel back the sealing strip at the edge, remove the paper with forceps, transfer with minimal delay to the weighing bottle and close the cap. Note the time, insert a second piece of filter paper, reseal with the tape and repeat the collection. With good sweat secretion rates, four collections may be completed in 20 min.

Reweigh each bottle to the nearest 0·5 mg and calculate the weight of sweat secreted. Elute the electrolytes with distilled water so that a dilution of approximately 200-fold is made. This is best done by attaching the paper strip to a filter paper wick immersed in a bath of distilled water in such a way that the strip to be eluted hangs vertically with its lower end over a weighed plastic bottle. Slow elution, over about 2 h, gives quantitative recovery of electrolytes. Reweigh the bottle to determine the weight of water and determine the sodium and potassium content in the flame photometer in the usual way, standardising with aqueous solutions. The chloride content should also be determined, coulometry being the most convenient method. Calculate the concentration of the electrolytes in the sweat as collected.

Notes.
1. Careful adherence to detail will avoid skin blistering or pain.
2. Avoid delay in transfer of the paper from skin to bottle. The evaporation rate may be as high as 0·1 mg/s.
3. If the sweating rate is less than 1 mg/min the test is unsatisfactory.
4. Some filter papers contain significant amounts of sodium. Whatman 541 papers contain negligible amounts.
5. A non-heated capillary sweat collection system (Macroduct, ChemLab Instruments Ltd, Essex) is available which obviates the need of absorption of the sweat onto filter papers. The osmolality of the sweat collected can then also be measured (Carter *et al.*, 1984).

INTERPRETATION

Green *et al.* (1985) retrospectively reviewing 1183 sweat test results reported that the following criteria are consistent with cystic fibrosis: (1) sweat sodium greater than 60 mmol/l, (2) sweat chloride greater than 70 mmol/l, (3) sweat chloride greater than sweat sodium, (4) sum of sweat sodium and chloride greater than 140 mmol/l. In borderline cases a sweat potassium above 30 mmol/l also indicates cystic fibrosis. If the Macroduct system has been used and the sweat osmolality measured then a sweat osmolality above 220 mmol/kg is suggestive of cystic fibrosis.

The results are more clear cut in young children (less than 1 year) and for older subjects an adequate secretion rate is especially important in making a diagnosis. The diagnosis should never be made on results from the sweat test alone but should be considered with clinical findings and laboratory evidence of pancreatic insufficiency (Green *et al.*, 1985).

INTESTINAL FUNCTION

The small intestine, averaging about 700 cm in length, stretches from the pylorus to the ileocaecal valve and is divided for descriptive purposes into three parts. Firstly, the duodenum, about 25 cm long and 4·5 cm in diameter extends from the pylorus to the duodeno-jejunal flexure. The pancreatic and common bile ducts open into it at the ampulla of Vater. The next part, the jejunum, is about 260 cm long and 4 cm in diameter and merges gradually into the last part, the ileum, some 400 cm long and 3·5 cm in diameter. The wall of the small intestine consists of four layers. The innermost layer is the mucosa which is in contact with the luminal contents. The mucosa rests on the submucosa, a layer rich in blood vessels and lymphatics. This is surrounded by a muscular layer containing smooth muscle. The outer surface is covered over most of its area by the peritoneum which is prolonged to cover both surfaces of a thin sheet, the mesentery, in which run the blood vessels and lymphatics. The arterial supply comes from branches of the superior mesenteric artery, the venous drainage leads into the portal vein which takes blood from the intestine to the liver. The lymphatics drain into the cisterna chyli which ascends to form the thoracic duct. Lymph draining from the intestine flows up this duct which eventually empties into large veins at the root of the neck.

The mucosa is thrown into folds from which numerous tiny finger-like villi protrude. These are about 600 μm long and 130 μm diameter so that 20 to 40 occupy one mm^2 in the jejunum. Ileal villi are less numerous as are the folds in the mucosa. Between the bases of the villi lie the crypts of Lieberkühn from which arise the columnar epithelial cells covering the surface of the villi. These cells are constantly being formed in the crypts, move up the villus and are eventually shed from its tip. The central core of the villus contains a projection of the submucosa with blood capillaries and a central lacteal or lymph vessel. Many of the epithelial cells have an absorptive function. The luminal surface, known as the brush border is composed of fine rod-like projections, 1 μm high and 0·12 μm wide. Several enzymes are located in these microvilli which form the absorptive surface. Other surface cells secrete mucus which besides its lubricant action also forms a protective layer and contains the immunoglobulin, IgA, characteristic of surface secretions.

The main functions of the small intestine are: (a) to allow the enzymatic breakdown of the larger molecules of dietary components such as fats, proteins and polysaccharides which occurs mainly within the lumen, (b) to complete digestion by breakdown of smaller molecules derived by these preliminary digestive processes, a process occurring mainly in the brush border and (c) to absorb the final products of digestion. Most of the luminal digestion depends on pancreatic enzymes which attack the products of digestion produced by preliminary action of salivary amylase and gastric pepsin. For this purpose the duodenal and upper jejunal mucosal cells release enterokinase which converts trypsinogen to the active enzyme trypsin by removing a terminal hexapeptide.

Trypsin is an important activator of other proteolytic enzyme precursors. The brush-border enzymes include maltase, isomaltase, sucrase, lactase and γ-amylase, concerned with carbohydrate digestion, and the aminopeptidases and several dipeptidases involved in oligopeptide digestion.

Absorption from the Small Intestine

This is of two types, *active* requiring energy and a transport mechanism allowing absorption against a concentration gradient, and *passive* when diffusion occurs only in accord with a concentration difference. Passive diffusion can occur alongside active transport if a marked concentration gradient exists but the latter permits much more rapid absorption and thereby reduces the concentration difference.

Absorption of most constituents is largely complete in the jejunum and duodenum but the ileum is capable of absorption if, for example, the transit rate is increased. Vitamin B_{12} and bile salts, however, are actively absorbed only in the terminal ileum.

Absorption of Carbohydrates

Dietary carbohydrate is mainly starch, sucrose and lactose, with small amounts of glucose and fructose. Starch is digested by pancreatic amylase in the duodenum and upper jejunum to glucose, maltose, isomaltose and short oligosaccharides. Further digestion occurs in the brush border. Remaining oligosaccharides are attacked by γ-amylase; maltose and isomaltose are split by maltase and isomaltase to glucose. Sucrase hydrolyses sucrose to glucose and fructose while lactase produces glucose and galactose from lactose. Isomaltase and sucrase are also active against maltose. The final products in the brush border are mainly glucose with smaller quantities of fructose and galactose. Glucose and galactose are actively absorbed, the transport mechanism being sodium-dependent. The sodium is absorbed with the monosaccharide and then extruded by the sodium pump requiring ATP as energy source. There may be sodium-independent transport systems for monosaccharides derived from disaccharides but they are not properly characterised in man. Fructose is absorbed passively but the concentration gradient is increased by partial conversion of fructose into glucose within the mucosal cell. Passive absorption is also the method for xylose. All monosaccharides are absorbed into the blood capillaries and hence into the portal vein.

Absorption of Fats

In the presence of bile salts and colipase, fats are emulsified to small droplets which are attacked by pancreatic lipase forming diglycerides, 2-monoglycerides and fatty acids. Bile salts also form loose aggregations of molecules, micelles, which take up considerable quantities of lecithin, lysolecithin, monoglycerides and fatty acids. These larger micelles can then incorporate cholesterol, diglycerides and residual triglycerides within their structure producing an expanded micelle which is still some 10^6 times smaller in volume than the original emulsified fat droplet. Their dimensions are such that they can pass between the microvilli to reach the absorptive sites. This process mainly refers to long chain triglycerides. For medium and short chain triglycerides, the micellar structures formed with bile salts are attacked by esterases and the fatty acids released are sufficiently water-soluble to reach the mucosal cell in solution.

The micelles containing long chain triglyceride derivatives are thought to release their lipid for passive diffusion into the cell. The bile salts may form additional large micelles but are eventually reabsorbed in the ileum. Monoglycerides and fatty acids absorbed are resynthesised into diglycerides and these together with any absorbed as such are then converted into triglycerides. The triglycerides are combined with apolipoprotein B in the mucosal cell to form the chylomicrons (Chapter 21, p. 454) which pass from the mucosal cell into the lacteals and hence to the thoracic duct. The medium and short chain triglycerides are mainly absorbed as the fatty acids and glycerol which are water-soluble, passing into the blood capillaries and then to the portal vein.

Absorption of Proteins

The digestion of protein, which begins in the stomach, mainly takes place in the lumen of the small intestine by the action of pancreatic enzymes to produce a mixture of amino acids, dipeptides and oligopeptides. Further digestion occurs in the brush border of the mucosal cells by the action of dipeptidases and of aminopeptidases which attack the peptide bond at the amino end of the oligopeptides. These enzymes are responsible for final breakdown to amino acids. The absorption of amino acids is an active process requiring transport mechanisms which are similar to those responsible for the renal tubular reabsorption of amino acids. Some direct absorption of dipeptides and oligopeptides occurs by a different mechanism facilitating the absorption of the products of protein digestion. The dipeptides and oligopeptides are then hydrolysed intracellularly. For both mechanisms, mostly the amino acids and any residual small peptides pass into the blood capillaries of the villus and hence into the portal vein (see Silk, 1974).

In the newborn, mucosal cells are more permeable to larger molecules allowing the absorption of intact maternal antibodies from the colostral milk which contains a protease inhibitor to protect them from proteolytic enzymes. Persistence of permeability to large molecules may be the basis of allergic responses to food proteins.

Absorption of Other Nutrients

Vitamins. The fat-soluble vitamins, A, D, E and K, are absorbed with fat in the micelles and so their absorption depends on the normal digestion and uptake of fat. Water-soluble vitamins apart from vitamin B_{12} and ascorbic acid are passively absorbed in the jejunum. Vitamin B_{12} absorption depends on the simultaneous presence within the lumen of intrinsic factor, secreted by the stomach, and on the existence of a specific absorption mechanism, located only in the terminal ileum. Ascorbic acid is mainly absorbed in the ileum (Rose, 1980).

Minerals. The absorption of *calcium, magnesium* and *iron* takes place in the duodenum and upper jejunum by active processes. Calcium absorption requires the presence of 1,25-dihydroxy-cholecalciferol, the active form of vitamin D, and is impaired if fat absorption or the activation of vitamin D are defective. Calcium absorption is also facilitated by lactose. Calcium and magnesium form insoluble salts with fatty acids or phytic acid, a polyphosphate component of cereals, and excess of these impairs absorption. Some iron appears to be retained in the mucosal cells and is later lost in the faeces when the mucosal cells are shed. Iron in Fe(II) form is more rapidly absorbed than Fe(III). Gastric secretion of acid increases iron absorption and pancreatic secretion inhibits it. Increased absorption is thus seen in chronic pancreatitis. Iron absorption is also interfered with by phytic acid which forms an insoluble iron salt. The entry of iron into the mucosal cell is controlled by a sensitive mechanism, controlled by the body's requirements (p. 622). The iron is transported across the cell bound to ferritin and released into the plasma as the complex with transferrin.

Sodium, potassium and *chloride* are present in the diet and considerable quantities enter the alimentary tract in the various secretions. These electrolytes are absorbed by two routes, across the mucosal epithelial cells or between them. In the jejunum where the tight junctions between the cells are leaky the latter mechanism is more important. Further down the alimentary tract where the junctions are tighter, most sodium and chloride is absorbed by a double exchange process, sodium for hydrogen and chloride for bicarbonate. The average daily volume of secretions into the alimentary tract is 7 litres. Some reabsorption occurs in the ileum but the daily output into the caecum is about 2 litres with average concentrations (mmol/l) of: sodium, 130; potassium, 16; chloride, 110. Considerable further active reabsorption takes place in the colon. A part of the sodium reabsorption occurs in exchange for potassium excretion. These reabsorptive mechanisms are efficient and daily faecal losses average between 100 and 200 ml water, 5 to 10 mmol Na and 10 to 15 mmol K. Their faecal excretion does not vary much with different dietary intakes. Regulation of the balance of these ions and water is predominantly the function of the kidney not the intestine.

Disordered Function of the Gastrointestinal Tract—Malabsorption

Many disorders affect gastrointestinal function leading to defective absorption of nutrients. The disorder may be relatively specific for a particular substance; others affect the absorption of a wide range of nutrients to a varying degree, a condition sometimes referred to as the 'malabsorption syndrome'. Classification of the causes can be made in various ways and the one used here is not fully comprehensive. It serves to illustrate the wide range of disorders and their consequences.

1. **Disordered Gastric Function**
   A. Defective secretion of intrinsic factor leading to defective absorption of vitamin B_{12} (Chapter 35, p. 922).
   B. Post-gastrectomy malabsorption probably involves several factors and affects the absorption of a range of nutrients including fat.
2. **Defective Digestion**
   A. **Defective luminal digestion.** This involves digestion of the major nutrients in the lumen of the duodenum and upper jejunum.
      (i) *Deficient bile salt secretion:* this is seen in extra-hepatic biliary obstruction, hepatic cirrhosis, and when the entero-hepatic circulation of bile salts is interfered with. The main effect is on the emulsification and hence absorption of fat and associated vitamins.
      (ii) *Deficient pancreatic enzyme secretion:* this is seen in chronic pancreatitis, cystic fibrosis and carcinoma of the pancreas where the disease is extensive. A rare inherited disorder is congenital trypsinogen deficiency (Morris and Fisher, 1967). In most cases of pancreatic insufficiency the defect of digestion involves protein and starch as well as fat. Their absorption and that of fat soluble vitamins is affected.
      (iii) *Inhibition of pancreatic enzymes* may occur when there is excessive gastric secretion of acid especially in the Zollinger–Ellison syndrome.

B. **Defective brush-border digestion**.
   (i) *Disaccharidase deficiencies* affect the digestion and absorption of specific disaccharides. Secondary effects on the absorption of other nutrients can result.
   (ii) *Secondary deficiency of enzyme synthesis* as in kwashiorkor or severe deficiency of dietary protein intake may involve several brush-border enzymes and also reduces the rate of pancreatic enzyme production.

3. **Defective Intestinal Absorption**
   A. **Congenital defects of the intestinal mucosa**, e.g. glucose transport defect, amino acid transport defects, abetalipoproteinaemia. The defect primarily is selective for a particular nutrient. In abetalipoproteinaemia, the defect interferes with the absorption of fats and of fat-soluble vitamins.
   B. **Lesions of the intestinal mucosa.** These include the most common and most important cause of malabsorption namely gluten-induced enteropathy (idiopathic steatorrhoea, coeliac disease, sprue). The disorder involves the impaired absorption of a wide range of nutrients. A similar spectrum occurs in tropical sprue resulting from infestation or infection of the upper gut. Various infiltrative lesions can occasionally affect the small intestinal mucosa; these include scleroderma, amyloidosis, leukaemia, lymphosarcoma and Hodgkin's disease. Inflammatory disease of the terminal ileum, in particular Crohn's disease, can interfere seriously with the absorption of vitamin B_{12} and the reabsorption of bile salts. The latter defect results in disordered fat digestion and absorption.
   C. **Small intestinal resection.** The effect depends on the extent and site of resection. Loss of jejunum can be compensated for by increased ileal reabsorption if not excessive but loss of the terminal ileum permanently affects vitamin B_{12} and bile salt reabsorption. If the resection is extensive the absorption of all nutrients can be involved.
   D. **Bacterial contamination of the small intestine.** This can occur in stagnant areas, the drainage of which is poor as in jejunal diverticulosis, 'blind-loops' created surgically, and as a consequence of strictures, fistulae or anastamoses. Several nutrients can be involved.
   E. **Iatrogenic malabsorption.** Neomycin, triparanol, phenindione, mefenamic acid, phenolphthalein and colchicine all have toxic effects but the mechanism varies. Radiation may damage the intestinal mucosa. The defect often involves fat absorption but other nutrients are sometimes involved.
   F. **Endocrine disorders**. Addison's disease, hypothyroidism, carcinoid tumour and diabetes mellitus may result in disordered absorption.
   G. **Lesions of vessels.** Arterial disorders (mesenteric artery occlusion), venous congestion (congestive cardiac failure, constrictive pericarditis) and lymph vessel abnormalities (Whipple's disease, intestinal lymphangiectasia) interfere with normal capillary and lacteal function.
   H. **Parasitic infections of the gut.** Strongyloides, hookworm and *Dibothriocephalus latus* infestations cause malabsorption but are uncommon in Britain where *Giardia lamblia* is the most common parasite involved. The defect is mainly of fat absorption.

Tests used in the Diagnosis of Malabsorption

Investigation should attempt to establish the degree and extent of malabsorption and the cause of the disorder. The tests used have mainly involved fats, carbohydrates and proteins. Fat digestion and absorption, being complex, is often the first to be disturbed. The resultant increase in the faecal fat, *steatorrhoea*, is present in generalised malabsorption and in many cases involving a more limited disturbance. The fat balance test is the most generally useful test and gives an indication of the degree of malabsorption. Tests studying the absorption of other fats or fat-soluble vitamins or the extent of hydrolysis of faecal triglycerides have proved less satisfactory for differentiating defective digestion of fat from its defective absorption. For this a study of the absorption of carbohydrate, especially xylose is preferable.

Tests involving carbohydrates have mainly used disaccharides or monosaccharides. Disaccharides have been applied to the investigation of defective brush-border digestion, while monosaccharides are used to test the absorptive capacity of the jejunum, no further digestion being required in their case. The xylose tolerance test has proved the most useful.

Tests involving proteins and amino acids have been less used. Defective luminal digestion of protein and defective absorption of amino acids can lead to an increase in faecal nitrogen and eventual reduction in the concentrations of various serum proteins. These changes may also be seen in protein-losing enteropathy and intestinal lymphangiectasia. Investigation of the defective absorption of other nutrients may sometimes be helpful. Disordered vitamin absorption is considered in Chapter 35 (p. 894). Defective absorption of elements such as iron, calcium, sodium and potassium can result in altered serum levels.

Malabsorption due to impaired digestion secondary to pancreatic disease can be investigated using pancreatic function tests. Extra-hepatic biliary obstruction leading to defective fat digestion requires the addition of liver function tests (Chapter 28, p. 715) to the list of investigations. The various endocrine disorders are also considered in other chapters.

Radiological techniques are helpful for the demonstration of disordered structure of the intestine or its associated vessels. Bacteriological examination may reveal colonisation of the upper small intestine. Histological examination of a portion of the jejunal mucosa obtained by per-oral biopsy using the Crosby capsule may reveal characteristic flattening of the villi with loss of absorptive surface, important in the diagnosis of gluten-induced enteropathy.

Determination of the Fat Content of Faeces

Fat in faeces is present in three forms:

1. *Neutral fat*, the triglycerides of long chain fatty acids derived from dietary fat which has escaped absorption, or from intestinal secretions. The latter are the main source in health but in steatorrhoea, excess fat is of dietary origin.
2. *Fatty acids*, produced by luminal hydrolysis of neutral fat by pancreatic lipase and by bacterial enzyme action.
3. *Soaps*, the sodium, potassium and calcium salts of fatty acids.

Analyses of total fat content are carried out on faecal homogenates. Alkaline hydrolysis (saponification) of neutral fats produces glycerol and soaps. The latter are also formed from any fatty acid initially present. After acidification, the fatty acids are extracted into light petroleum and quantitated by titration. Such faecal fat determinations may be used in conjunction with a fat balance test.

Determination of Total Faecal Fat—Fat Balance Test

The total fat content is determined by the method of van de Kamer *et al.* (1949) as modified by Anderson *et al.* (1952). If a fat balance study is needed, the patient is put on a known daily fat intake between 50 and 100 g; often 70 g is used.

Reagents.

1. Ethanolic potassium hydroxide; 30 g potassium hydroxide and 4 ml amyl alcohol made up to 1 litre with ethanol.
2. Hydrochloric acid. Dilute 330 ml concentrated acid to 1 litre with water.
3. Light petroleum, b.p. 40 to 60 °C.
4. Ethanolic sodium hydroxide, 100 mmol/l. Dilute aqueous sodium hydroxide, 1 mol/l, one part to ten with ethanol.

Technique. For the balance study begin the faecal collection after the patient : has been taking the diet for 2 to 3 days. In any case the collection should be at least three days but may be extended if the stool appearance suggests only moderate steatorrhoea. Chill the faeces until collection is complete. Prepare a suspension of the total faecal collection in water, 1 to 2 litres according to the faecal bulk. This is best done using a sealed homogeniser (Silverson Machines Limited) to avoid spraying faecal homogenate. Avoid introducing air into the mixture as this causes fat to rise to the surface making representative sampling difficult.

Measure a portion of homogenate (20 ml is convenient) into a 250 ml ground glass stoppered conical flask, add 95 ml ethanolic potassium hydroxide and heat for 20 min on a steam bath. Cool, add 30 ml hydrochloric acid and then 50 ml light petroleum. Stopper the flask and extract the fatty acids by shaking well for 1 min. Allow the phases to separate, remove 20 ml of the upper layer and titrate with reagent (4) using phenolphthalein or thymol blue as indicator.

Calculation. For the quantities used

$$\text{Total faecal fatty acids (mmol/day)} = \frac{0 \cdot 1 \times n \times 50 \times V}{d \times 20 \times 20} = \frac{nV}{80d}$$

where n = titration figure (ml),
V = total volume of faecal suspension (ml),
d = number of days faeces collected.

To convert to g/day (W) multiply by 0·284. Then if the fat intake is known,

$$\text{Percentage fat absorption} = \frac{(\text{Daily fat intake (g)} - W) \times 100}{\text{Daily fat intake (g)}}$$

Notes.

1. Successive 3 day collections can be used if the first period gives equivocal results.
2. Faecal marker dyes have been used to define the beginning and end of the collection periods. Incomplete collection of faeces is occasionally allowed for by giving a known weight (0·5 to 1 g) of chromium sesquioxide orally each day. It is excreted unchanged allowing the faecal fatty acids to be expressed in terms of this reference base. A simpler technique, which minimises faecal handling, involves the use of radio-opaque pellets (Simpson *et al.*, 1979). Such methods add to the complexity of the test but can be useful in borderline cases. However, extending the collection will usually suffice.
3. If liquid paraffin has been taken and excreted it will be extracted but not titrated.

4. This method may underestimate any medium chain triglycerides present in the faeces of patients taking such dietary supplements as the resultant fatty acids are less soluble in light petroleum.

INTERPRETATION

On an ordinary ward diet of about 70 g fat daily, the daily fat excretion is 1·7 to 28 mmol but the range is reduced to 1·7 to 16 mmol for a 3 day collection period. The normal absorption result is at least 90 % and is usually 95 to 97 %. Cooke *et al.* (1946) gave figures of 95 ± 4 % on a 50 g fat intake and similar figures are obtained when this is increased to 100 g. If the absorption is between 85 and 90 %, the period of collection should be extended.

An *increased amount of fat* in the faeces, *steatorrhoea,* is found in several conditions. The typical steatorrhoeic stool is bulky (volume 250 to 2000 ml/24 h, instead of less than 200), pale, greasy, malodorous and frothy. The colour is due to the increased fat content; if particularly high, the surface of a drying stool may develop a sheen akin to aluminium paint. The frothy nature arises from bacterial fermentation of unabsorbed carbohydrate, while bacterial degradation of fats to short chain fatty acids accounts for the odour. The stools float readily in water and are often difficult to flush away, partly because of their gas content as well as the fat. Although such features are usual, some bulky steatorrhoeic stools have a relatively normal appearance. Copious, watery, fat-rich stools are seen in severe steatorrhoea.

In general, *pancreatic steatorrhoea* is more severe and the stools have a higher fat concentration (Bo-Linn and Fordtran, 1984) than in defective absorption of fat. The daily excretion may amount to 70 to 180 mmol with an average fat absorption of about 50 % (range, 15 to 85). In extrahepatic obstructive jaundice, the lack of bile salts reduces pancreatic lipase action and *biliary steatorrhoea* results. The fat findings are again similar but now the lack of bilirubin, and hence urobilin, results in much paler stools than in other types of steatorrhoea—the 'putty-like' or clay-coloured' stool.

In steatorrhoea due to defective intestinal absorption or bacterial overgrowth, excretion is often less severe. The daily excretion is usually in the range 35–70 mmol with an average fat absorption of 72 % (range, 31 to 91). Defective absorption of a wide range of other nutrients than fat is more characteristic of gluten-sensitive enteropathy. Other tests of small intestinal function are therefore needed.

Other Tests of Fat Absorption

The difficulties and unpleasantness of faecal fat determinations have prompted the development of other tests. Some use radioactive fats, others measure plasma lipid substances after absorption. A general problem with the latter is that plasma changes depend not only on the rate of absorption but on the rate of removal by peripheral tissues. However, they have been advocated as screening tests in suspected fat malabsorption to reduce the number of faecal fat estimations performed or when collection of faeces is difficult as in children and some elderly patients. Various fat loads have been used, some more palatable than others. The butter fat test meal (Bentley *et al.*, 1975) is convenient and palatable.

A breath test for fat absorption using ^{14}C-labelled triglyceride has been developed (Newcomer *et al.*, 1979) and compared with other tests of fat malabsorption (West *et al.*, 1981). A positive breath test has a predictive value of 94 % on comparison with faecal fat analysis (Theodossi and Gazzard, 1984). The test is only performed in a few centres at present and, because it requires expensive isotopes and a scintillation counter, may be slow to be adopted widely.

Several tests have used ^{131}I-triolein in which measurements have been made on blood, faeces or urine, while comparison of the absorption of ^{131}I-labelled oleic acid and triolein was investigated for the differentiation between maldigestion and malabsorption. These tests have proved to be less reliable than faecal fat determinations and are now rarely used.

Absorption tests which study plasma changes after oral ingestion of various nutrients have included vitamin A or β-carotene given as such or the measurement of chylomicrons or total fatty acid concentration after fat intake. Such tests have not been generally accepted possibly because the rate of clearance from the plasma varies sufficiently to make them insensitive.

Butter Fat Test Meal (Bentley *et al.*, 1975)

A meal of buttered toast is eaten by the fasted subject. Blood samples are taken before and 2 h after the meal and the serum chylomicron content is measured using the Thorp micronephelometer (Stone and Thorp, 1966).

Technique. The patient must fast (apart from clear fluids) for 12–14 h. A fasting blood sample is taken and the serum separated. The meal consists of unsweetened orange juice (50 ml), two slices of buttered toast (0·5 g pure butter per kg body weight) and unsweetened tea or coffee with milk if desired. A second blood sample is taken 2 h later and the serum is separated.

Dilute the sera 1:10 with saline (0·9 g/l) and measure the Light Scattering Intensity (LSI) in the Thorp micronephelometer (Scientific Furnishings, Macclesfield). Deduct the LSI value of the fasted sample from the 2 h sample to give an index of the rise in blood lipids following the meal.

Notes.
1. Pure butter only should be used; margarine or 'blends' are unsuitable.
2. Nephelometric measurements of the diluted serum are performed before and after ultrafiltration using a pore size which excludes chylomicrons. The LSI is the difference in the instrumental readings and is an index of the triglycerides present as chylomicrons. The figure should be low in the fasted sample.

INTERPRETATION

Bentley *et al.* (1975) studied this test in 106 subjects (44 controls, 62 patients with gastrointestinal disease, 36 of whom had no evidence of malabsorption) on whom 3-day faecal fat estimations were also carried out. Of the 15 patients with abnormal faecal fat losses (more than 18 mmol/day), 14 showed a rise in LSI of less than 20 units, suggesting poor absorption. Rises of less than 20 were found in several other patients with gastrointestinal diseases and in 8 out of 15 patients with malabsorption and normal fat losses in the faeces. The correlation is thus not good.

For children, Robards (1975) used a higher dose of fat, 1 g/kg, in the more convenient form of a milk feed, supplemented with double cream as required, and given with cereal. He found a good correlation between the rise in LSI and small intestinal morphology in those children suspected of having coeliac disease. The test was unhelpful in children who had recurrent diarrhoea and gastroenteritis.

The test is probably best reserved for infants and young children but may have a place when faecal collection is difficult as in the confused, incontinent elderly patient.

Oxalate Excretion. Oxalate is the end product of several biochemical pathways and rare genetic variants are known which lead to oxalate overproduction. The increased urinary oxalate excretion which results is also seen after increased intake of oxalate or its precursors in pyridoxine deficiency, but the most common cause of hyperoxaluria is the increased colonic absorption of oxalate associated with various gastrointestinal disorders, particularly those in which there is fat malabsorption (Laker, 1983). The possible mechanisms for this increased absorption are preferential binding of calcium by unabsorbed fatty acids in the colonic lumen, thus enhancing oxalate solubility, or increased permeability of the colonic mucosa as a consequence of fatty acids and bile salts present in the lumen. Hyperoxaluria increases the risk of urinary calculus formation and calcium oxalate is the most common constituent of these calculi (Chapter 29, p. 757).

The measurement of urinary oxalate is thus important in the recognition and treatment of patients with hyperoxaluria. The many methods used include titrimetric, colorimetric, fluorimetric, GLC, HPLC, isotachophoretic and enzymatic techniques (Laker, 1983). Of these the most promising for a busy clinical biochemistry laboratory are enzymatic.

The first enzymatic methods used oxalate decarboxylase (EC 4.1.1.2) which catalyses the reaction

$$(COOH)_2 \rightarrow CO_2 + HCOOH$$

Various techniques have been used to measure the carbon dioxide liberated (Laker, 1983) but more recently the formate produced has been measured (Chalmers and Cowley, 1984; Urdal, 1984) using formate dehydrogenase (EC 1.2.1.2). The two enzymes have widely differing pH optima (3 and 7 respectively) and therefore have to be added sequentially but this should not be a problem if a modern discrete analyser is available. A major advantage is that common urinary constituents do not interfere with the activity of the enzyme; an exception is ascorbate which acts as a competitive inhibitor at certain concentrations (Rofe *et al.*, 1985). Unprocessed urine can be used directly although many of the methods have used some pretreatment. The main disadvantage is the time taken to perform the assay.

An alternative enzyme is oxalate oxidase (EC 1.2.3.4) which catalyses the reaction

$$(COOH)_2 \rightarrow 2\ CO_2 + H_2O_2$$

The liberated carbon dioxide may be measured and since twice as much is released as in the decarboxylase method, oxalate oxidase methods are potentially more sensitive. More commonly the hydrogen peroxide has been measured by a linked peroxidase-chromophore reaction. This is available in commercial kit form (Sigma). Oxalate oxidase is inhibited by such urinary constituents as nitrate (Goldsack *et al.*, 1984) but the effect can be partially overcome by incubating the reaction mixture for 45 min instead of 20 min. A further source of error, common to *all* oxalate methods, is the rapid conversion at alkaline pH of ascorbate to oxalate (Mazzani *et al.*, 1984; Chalmers *et al.*, 1985). Urine samples should therefore either be collected into acid or acidified to pH 4·5 to 5 as soon as possible after collection. Specific removal of ascorbate by ascorbate oxidase before starting the assay is advantageous.

INTERPRETATION

Crider and Curran (1984) using an oxalate oxidase method reported urinary oxalate values of 0·056–0·349 mmol/24 h in 64 men and 0·032–0·246 mmol/24 h in

42 women. The range found in 12 children was 0·103–0·302 mmol/24 h. The review by Laker (1983) lists reference ranges reported using various methods; the range for enzyme methods was 0·138–0·451 mmol/24 h for adults.

The literature accompanying the Sigma kit quotes urinary oxalate values of 0·39–2·58 mmol/24 h in cases of primary hyperoxaluria. Oxalate excretion in patients with intestinal disease is generally increased with figures of 2·2 mmol/24 h being reported in patients with extensive ileal resection (Laker, 1983).

Tests of Carbohydrate Absorption or Digestion

Disaccharidase Deficiencies

Defective digestion of disaccharides in the brush-border of the jejunum can be investigated by administering a standard dose of the disaccharide and studying the plasma glucose response. Thus lactase deficiency can be demonstrated by the poor plasma glucose rise following oral ingestion of 50 g lactose. Deficiency of maltase and sucrase are similarly studied using 50 g of maltose or sucrose. Normally the blood glucose level rises by about 2·7 mmol/l but in deficiency states by less than 1·1 mmol/l.

The flattened glucose response curve is differentiated from the similar curve resulting from defective glucose absorption by demonstrating, in true disaccharidase deficiency, a normal glucose tolerance curve following 50 g of a mixture of equal parts of the appropriate monosaccharides. Disaccharide tolerance tests are abnormal in gluten-sensitive enteropathy only if the total absorptive and digestive area is markedly reduced. Temporary disaccharidase deficiency is also present in severe protein-calorie malnutrition or after severe debilitating disorders.

The most common disaccharidase deficiency is that of lactase. This is occasionally found in infants as a congenital abnormality but is much more common in adults as an acquired deficiency. The adult incidence shows marked variation with race. In many parts of the world, lactase deficiency occurs in 80% of the population but in Northern European races the proportion may be less than 20%. A distinction must be noted between lactase deficiency and lactose intolerance. Many people with low levels of lactase can tolerate lactose-containing foods. Isomaltase-sucrase deficiency is much rarer and appears to be congenital. Symptoms appear on adding sucrose or starch to the diet. In disaccharidase deficiency states, the particular disaccharide passes into the colon and is attacked by bacteria with the formation of lactic acid and carbon dioxide. The passage of watery, frothy acid stools is often apparent especially in infants. In such cases the pH of the freshly-passed stool is often less than 5. The disaccharide involved may be present in varying amounts but may at times be almost totally fermented. The adult colon is more capable of reabsorption of the acid products of fermentation and fewer changes are apparent in the faeces passed.

Assay of jejunal disaccharidases in small per-oral biopsy specimens has been carried out (Dahlqvist, 1965, 1968) and affords definitive proof of specific enzyme deficiency. See also Crane (1960), Dawson (1965), Prader and Auricchio (1965) and Dahlqvist (1962).

Hydrogen Breath Test

Carbohydrate not absorbed from the small intestine is fermented by anaerobic bacteria in the colon forming hydrogen which diffuses throughout the body. It can be measured in the breath by an electrochemical detector specific for hydrogen (Bartlett *et al.*, 1980). A 50 g load of disaccharide such as lactose is administered to the patient and the breath hydrogen monitored. A marked increase in hydrogen excretion (greater than 0·5 ml/min) occurs if the lactose reaches the colonic bacteria. False positive results can occur in cases of bacterial overgrowth of the small intestine or with rapid transit through the small intestine. False negative results have been reported in patients whose colonic bacteria cannot produce hydrogen gas. This can occur after a course of antibiotics. This investigation is a useful screening test before definitive jejunal biopsy for enzyme estimation is performed.

Test of Monosaccharide Absorption—Xylose Excretion Test

The absorption of monosaccharides given orally is unaffected by deficiencies of enzymes digesting carbohydrates. Apart from the rare congenital deficiency of the glucose transport system, disordered absorption is a consequence of an impaired absorptive surface area. The test is mainly used in gluten-sensitive enteropathy and is an index of jejunal function. The use of glucose as the monosaccharide is not ideal as extra-intestinal factors determine the shape of the glucose tolerance curve as, e.g., the tendency towards a diabetic type of curve in pancreatic steatorrhoea. In many cases, however, a flattened absorption curve starting at a normal fasting level is obtained.

D-Xylose, a pentose not normally present in the blood in significant amounts, is preferable. When given by mouth it is absorbed by the jejunum and is partly metabolised to fructose-6-phosphate in the liver. Xylose entering the systemic circulation is excreted in the urine, there being no renal threshold for it. Provided renal function is normal, xylose appears rapidly. The investigation requires either urinary or plasma determination of xylose.

Carry out the test after the patient has been fasting overnight and has emptied the bladder completely. Originally, 25 g xylose dissolved in 250 ml water was given orally, followed immediately by 250 ml water. For young children 1·1 g/kg, up to 25 g, has been given. This quantity is unpleasant to take and rather expensive, so some workers prefer a dose of 5 g. After giving the xylose, collect all the urine passed during the next 5 h, emptying the bladder at the end of this period. Determine the xylose content of this specimen. Clearly the results will be unreliable if renal function is not normal. A blood sample may also be taken at 1 h.

Methods for analysing xylose in serum and urine include gas chromatography (Johnson *et al.*, 1984), and colorimetric assays using phloroglucinol (Johnson *et al.*, 1984) or *p*-bromoaniline (Roe and Rice, 1948). The latter has been the most commonly used.

Determination of Xylose (Roe and Rice, 1948; Goodhart and Kingston, 1969)

A pink colour is given on heating with *p*-bromoaniline.
   Reagents.
   1. Zinc sulphate solution, 50 g $ZnSO_4$, $7H_2O/l$.
   2. Barium hydroxide, 150 mmol/l.
   3. *p*-Bromoaniline reagent. Prepare a saturated solution of thiourea in glacial acetic acid by shaking 4 g per 100 ml and decanting. Dissolve 2 g *p*-bromoaniline in 100 ml of this.
   4. Stock standard solution, 200 mg xylose in 100 ml saturated benzoic acid solution.

5. Standard solutions for use. Dilute the stock standard 1 to 10 and 1 to 20 with saturated benzoic acid solution. These contain 200 and 100 mg/l.

Technique.

1. *Urine.* Dilute the urine to 1 litre. Then dilute further 1:40 if 25 g xylose was given or 1:10 if 5 g was used. Measure 1 ml diluted urine and 5 ml *p*-bromoaniline reagent into each of two test tubes. Place one tube, the test, in a water bath at 55 °C for 40 min, then cool and leave in the dark for 70 min. Read the pink colour of the test against the other tube as blank at 520 nm. At the same time treat the standard solutions in the same way, reading each standard against its own blank.

Then with the standard containing 200 mg/l

$$\text{Xylose excretion (g)} = \frac{\text{Reading of unknown}}{\text{Reading of standard}} \times n$$

where n = 2 for the 5 g dose and n = 8 for the 25 g dose

2. *Blood.* Deproteinise using 1 volume blood, 7 volumes water and 1 volume each of zinc sulphate and barium hydroxide. Filter or centrifuge and use 1 ml filtrate or centrifugate instead of 1 ml diluted urine as above.

Using the xylose standard containing 100 mg/l

$$\text{Blood xylose (mg/l)} = \frac{\text{Reading of unknown}}{\text{Reading of standard}} \times 1000$$

For the concentration in mmol/l divide this result by 150.

INTERPRETATION

If 25 g xylose are given, normal persons excrete more than 4 g in the 5 h period. Except in persons above 65 years old, lower results indicate some degree of malabsorption; for the older patient an excretion below 3 g can be taken as abnormal. If renal function is normal, a blood xylose above 250 mg/l should be found. Low urine volumes, especially if below 100 ml may lead to unreliable results. With the 5 g dose at least 1·2 g xylose should be excreted in 5 h. On the whole, this is the more satisfactory dose. Even in malabsorption the output after an 8 h collection period is similar to that in the normal. The more rapid absorption from the normal jejunum is apparent if a 2 h urine collection period is used. The ratio of the excretion at 2 h to the total excretion at 5 h is normally greater than 0·5 and may be the most sensitive indicator of minor degrees of malabsorption.

Heaney *et al.* (1978) showed that the best discrimination was achieved with the 1 h serum xylose measurement corrected to a constant body surface area. Their reference range was 0·65 to 1·33 mmol/l for values corrected to 1·73 m² and the incidence of false negatives and false positives was found to be 4·8 and 2·2% respectively. A normal serum and urine result have a predictive accuracy of 100%, in excluding jejunal disease (Theodossi and Gazzard, 1984).

Tests of Protein and Amino Acid Absorption and Excretion

Normally one quarter of the daily turnover of plasma proteins is due to their loss into the jejunum. This mainly involves albumin, up to 4 g daily, which is digested and reabsorbed during its passage along the intestine. In pancreatic disease with diminished secretion of proteolytic enzymes, this digestion and that of dietary protein is reduced and the patient may go into negative nitrogen balance as a consequence of the increased faecal nitrogen loss which may approach one third of the dietary nitrogen intake in the most severe cases. Disordered absorption of the products of normal protein digestion may also occur and is a feature of gluten-sensitive enteropathy. Both factors result in defective transfer of amino acids into the circulation, diminution of the amino acid pool and impaired synthesis of plasma proteins. The determination of total protein or albumin in plasma is useful in assessing the disordered protein metabolism.

Protein-losing Enteropathy

In this condition, entry of protein into the intestine is increased and may involve other proteins besides albumin. Depending on the site and degree of protein loss, the further digestion and reabsorption may be incomplete with increase in faecal nitrogen loss. In any case, the loss of proteins from the circulation results in hypoproteinaemia. For a review of protein-losing enteropathy see Waldmann (1970).

Moderate losses of protein may complicate the sprue syndrome, colitis or giant rugal hypertrophy of the stomach. Greater losses occur in multiple polyposis of the colon, in lymphatic obstruction of the small intestine (congenital lymphangiectasia, Whipple's disease), in severe venous obstruction as in constrictive pericarditis and in inflammatory disorders, particularly Crohn's disease. Altered immunological function of the gut can also result in protein loss as in hypogammaglobulinaemia and infantile intestinal allergies.

The investigation of the condition involves the demonstration of hypo-proteinaemia, particularly hypoalbuminaemia, in the absence of proteinuria and in the presence of adequate protein intake. Investigation of faecal nitrogen may be helpful but a normal result does not exclude the disorder. Radioactive methods have been more informative. The increased radioactivity of faeces and the decreased activity in plasma can be measured following an intravenous injection of ^{51}Cr-labelled albumin, ^{131}I-labelled albumin, ^{67}Cu-labelled ceruloplasmin or ^{131}I-labelled polyvinylpyrrolidone (PVP). ^{51}Cr-labelled albumin is probably the most favoured method as the ^{51}Cr is not reabsorbed. Normally less than 1% of the injected dose is lost in the faeces but this may exceed 30% in protein-losing enteropathy.

Another approach has been to estimate the levels of α_1-antitrypsin in the faeces, the rationale being that α_1-antitrypsin lost into the gut will resist digestion by proteolytic enzymes unlike other plasma proteins (Meyers *et al.*, 1985).

Tests Using Other Substances

The absorption of a wide range of substances has been shown to be defective in gluten-sensitive enteropathy. This is usually assessed either by demonstrating a reduced concentration of the substance in question in the plasma, e.g. iron, calcium, or by demonstrating a consequence of the malabsorption, e.g. the megaloblastic anaemia of folate deficiency. Many of these nutrients are absorbed in the jejunum.

Disease of the terminal ileal region will not be detected by such methods if absorption occurs normally before this area is reached. The most convenient substance in this case is vitamin B_{12}, the absorption of which is conveniently followed by administering the radioactively-labelled vitamin, if necessary in combination with intrinsic factor if gastric mucosal atrophy is suspected. For a review of vitamin B_{12} absorption in various conditions see Toskes and Deren (1973).

The bile acid breath test has been employed in terminal ileal disease. Conjugated bile salts pass unabsorbed into the colon where bacteria degrade them releasing glycine and the unconjugated bile salt. If the glycine moiety of glycocholic acid is labelled with ^{14}C then the radioactivity can be subsequently measured in the breath as $^{14}CO_2$.

For a general review of various aspects of steatorrhoea see Cooke and Asquith (1974) and Strober (1976) and for tubeless tests of small intestinal function see Laker and Bartlett (1985).

Tests for Bacterial Overgrowth

Normal gastric secretion and the mechanical cleansing effect of peristalsis prevent bacterial proliferation in the small intestine. However, if there is stasis for any reason, overgrowth of organisms may occur which can result in malabsorption, especially of vitamin B_{12}. The bacteria often manufacture and release folate so patients with overgrowth can be B_{12}-deficient with high levels of folate. Steatorrhoea occurs in one third of such patients, probably as a result of altered bile salt metabolism. D-Xylose can be metabolised by the bacteria and a low urinary xylose excretion after loading is seen thereby affecting interpretation of the xylose absorption test.

Aspiration and culture of duodenal contents has been used to assess overgrowth but is an uncomfortable procedure requiring a skilled operator. In the hydrogen breath test using glucose as the carbohydrate source, early release of hydrogen suggests either rapid transport to the colon or bacterial overgrowth in the ileum. Metz et al. (1976) combined results from the hydrogen breath test and a $[^{14}C]$glycocholate breath test to detect 11 out of 12 patients with bacterial overgrowth. Other tests have been employed: the Schilling test, urinary indican excretion, determination of intestinal unconjugated bile acids or free fatty acids— none are really satisfactory. Theodossi and Gazzard (1984) conclude that there is no satisfactory chemical test for bacterial overgrowth and 'a therapeutic trial with various antibiotics remains the best option in difficult cases'.

Tests for Occult Blood in Faeces

Tests to detect blood in faeces in amounts or forms not observable on inspection, i.e. occult blood, are important in the diagnosis and treatment of lesions of the alimentary tract. Tests using benzidine or o-tolidine are no longer used as both chemicals are potentially carcinogenic. Many alternative substances have been tried but none has gained universal acceptance (see review by Simon, 1985 in relation to colorectal cancer).

The amount of blood 'normally' lost in the faeces is debatable but 2–3 ml daily is usually accepted. This blood results from bleeding in the mouth, especially the gums, from minor abrasions in the gastrointestinal tract and from anal lesions such as haemorrhoids. The presence of haemoglobin and myoglobin and their breakdown products in food, especially meat and meat products, and of peroxidases of plant and bacterial origin may interfere depending on the method used to detect the 'blood'. A meat-free diet for 2–3 days before the test, although inconvenient, is said to improve the specificity of the guaiac-based 'Haemoccult' method. False positives due to plant peroxidases have been avoided by boiling the faecal suspension before testing, a procedure which denatures some of the haemoglobin and myoglobin. Specific inhibitors to plant peroxidases may be useful in future. Iron salts are also a possible source of error and it is best to stop iron therapy a few days before doing a guaiac-based test. Large doses of ascorbic acid also interfere with the guaiac-peroxidase reaction so patients should not take vitamin C immediately before and during the sampling period.

It is clearly desirable to have a test which is not so sensitive that positive results are given by the amount of blood present in the faeces of normal persons taking an ordinary diet (foods very rich in haemoglobin are easily excluded). A target sensitivity is that the test should be negative when less than 10 ml of blood per day is present, and very strongly positive when bleeding gives the characteristic black, tarry-looking stools which can be produced by giving 50–80 ml of blood per day. No entirely satisfactory test is available and there are always both false positives and false negatives. The tests in current use fall into 3 main categories: (1) oxidation of guaiac or other chromogen, (2) quantitative assay (Schwartz *et al.*, 1983) based on the conversion of non-fluorescing haem to fluorescing porphyrins, (3) immunochemical techniques (Barrows *et al.*, 1978). A quantitative spectrophotometric method has also been described (Welch and Young, 1983).

The fluorimetric assay and the immunochemical techniques look promising but have yet to be shown to offer better discrimination than the guaiac-based method in screening for colorectal cancer (Peterson and Fordtran, 1985; Armitage *et al.*, 1985). Developments of these more specific methods may improve their discrimination and make them the methods of choice in the future.

Guaiac is the least sensitive of the chromogens which can still be used. The sensitivity can be adjusted to a limited extent and so methods which are designed to screen for blood from the lower intestinal tract will be less sensitive than those which are adjusted to detect blood loss from the upper intestinal tract as well. Problems arise because of the variable quality of the guaiacum available. However when used in a commercial kit form it has found widespread use. The kit which has become the most popular is the Haemoccult, particularly for screening for colorectal cancer (Armitage *et al.*, 1985).

Haemoccult Kit (Smith Kline and French)

The kit consists of three slides, each of which contains two windows of guaiac impregnated paper. A thin smear of a specimen of faeces taken either on the ward or by the patient at home is applied to two windows using an applicator. The procedure is repeated with two subsequent bowel movements with the remaining two slides. The labelled folder can be developed immediately or sent to the laboratory by post if desired. In either case, a developing solution (hydrogen peroxide) is added to the faeces. Any blue colour developing at 30 s in any of the 6 windows is a positive test.

The sensitivity of the test increases if the dried out faeces are rehydrated prior to testing. This will obviously increase the number of false positives (and true positives) in any screening studies.

INTERPRETATION

A positive test indicates that blood has been introduced at some point between the mouth and the anus. If the test is being used in the diagnosis and treatment of gastric or intestinal diseases it is obviously necessary to exclude the possibility that blood has been introduced higher up or lower down the alimentary tract. The effect of haemorrhoids is particularly important. In such cases the blood can sometimes be seen as streaks of fresh blood on the surface of the stool. Inspection for such streaks should always be made. If there is doubt that a streak is really blood it can be examined microscopically. In the presence of such blood, further tests are valueless. Possible contamination with blood from the nose, throat, mouth or menstrual flow should also be borne in mind. A little bleeding may occur when a tube or endoscope is passed for diagnostic purposes and false positive results may be obtained during the next 2 or 3 days.

When bleeding is severe the stools are dark in colour (melaena) but in lesser loss the colour is unaffected. Oxyhaemoglobin is converted to haematin and porphyrins as it passes through the intestine; only haematin gives positive tests with the guaiac and immunological methods. If bleeding is from a lesion low down in the alimentary tract, oxyhaemoglobin may be still recognisable in the faeces by spectroscopic examination of the supernatant fluid from a centrifuged suspension.

The examination is mainly used in the diagnosis and treatment of ulcers or malignancy of the stomach, duodenum, small and large intestine. In addition, positive tests may be obtained in gastritis and in such haemorrhagic diseases as purpura and scurvy. A positive test affords no information as to the type of lesion present. Bleeding may be intermittent so that the test is often carried out at intervals. It is also sensible to do the test on three successive days when, if a patient is on a meat-free diet, the last specimen is unlikely to be affected by dietary components. In ulceration of the stomach and duodenum, the test may provide useful information with regard to the cessation of bleeding. Perhaps the most common use for the test has been in screening for colorectal cancer. The prevalence of this tumour in Western societies and the ability to prolong survival with early tumour detection has led to many screening trials with varying degrees of success. Simon (1985) considers that screening 'remains an appealing but unproven concept'. Future technological developments such as immunological and fluorimetric assays may well increase the predictive value of occult blood tests to acceptable levels. Carefully controlled trials of these more expensive tests in comparison with the cheaper guaiac-based tests are awaited.

Faecal Pigments

The normal colour of faeces is influenced by their urobilin content and by the kind of food or drugs taken.

Normal stools in the neonate are yellow due to their bilirubin content, once the dark green meconium has been passed. Occasionally greenish stools are seen due to the presence of biliverdin but as the normal colonic flora becomes established the stool colour becomes brown due to the formation of urobilin. Normal adult stools do not contain bilirubin or biliverdin unless there is rapid transit through the intestine; the colour then varies from brownish-yellow to green. Urobilin is formed from urobilinogen by oxygen so that on exposure to air, faeces darken in colour particularly on the surface.

Obstructive jaundice leads to absence of bile pigments in the intestine and poor fat digestion. The resultant stools are usually described as 'clay-coloured'. Steatorrhoea, especially the pancreatic variety, also produces pale stools but without jaundice. In contrast, in haemolytic jaundice the increased breakdown of haemoglobin and increased formation of bilirubin results in increased excretion of urobilin and the stools are darker coloured. When blood is present, faeces may be coloured all shades from brownish-red to black. The darker colours occur in cases where the haemorrhage is high in the alimentary tract, as in gastric or duodenal ulcer. Blood from the rectum or anal canal may be present as streaks of fresh blood on the surface of the stool.

A high residue diet gives light coloured stools while a mainly meat, low residue intake gives darker, brown ones. Undigested foodstuffs may colour the faeces: reddish-brown in the case of carrots, greenish in the case of vegetables rich in chlorophyll such as spinach, greyish or purple after eating anthocyanin-rich fruits such as bilberries.

Drugs may influence faecal colour. Broad spectrum antibiotics greatly diminish the colonic flora and there is a return to the yellow, bilirubin-containing stools seen in the neonate. Iron salts give dark, almost black faeces also seen after giving bismuth subnitrate which is converted to the black suboxide. Following a barium meal, whitish-coloured stools due to a high content of barium sulphate are found.

REFERENCES

Ali R. (1974). *Clin. Chem*; **20**: 91.
Ammann R. (1969). *Schweiz. Med. Woch*; **99**: 504.
Anderson C. M., et al. (1952). *Lancet*; **1**: 836.
Armitage N., et al. (1985). *Brit. J. Cancer*; **51**: 799.
Barrows G. H., Burton R. M., Jarrett D. D. (1978). *Amer. J. Clin. Pathol*; **69**: 342.
Barry R. E., Barry R., Ene M. D., Parker G. (1982). *Lancet*; **2**: 742.
Bartlett K., Eastham E., Dobson J. (1980). *Clin. Chim. Acta*; **108**: 189.
Bentley S. J., Eastham R. D., Lane R. F. (1975). *J. Clin. Path*; **28**: 80.
Berg J. D., et al. (1986). *Clin. Chem*; **32**: 1010.
Berg J. D., Chesner I., Lawson N. (1985). *Ann. Clin. Biochem*; **22**: 586.
Bloom S. R. (1986). *Medicine International*; **2**: 1040.
Bloom S. R., Polak J. M. (1980). *Adv. Clin. Chem*; **21**: 177.
Bo-Linn G. W., Fordtran J. S. (1984). *Gastroenterology*; **87**: 319.
Bouchier I. A. D. (1985). *Brit. Med. J*; **291**: 1669.
Boyd E. J. S. et al. (1982). *J. Clin. Pathol*; **35**: 1240.
Bradbury W. H., et al. (1985). *Gut*; **26**: PA 134, Abstract P128.
Braganza J. M., Kay G. H., Tetlow V. A., Herman J. H. (1983). *Clin. Chim. Acta*; **130**: 339.
Bratton A. C., Marshall E. K. (1939). *Analyt. Chem*; **128**: 537.
Brooke B. N. (1949). *Lancet*; **2**: 1167.
Burton P., et al. (1960a). *Gut*; **1**: 111.
Burton P., et al. (1960b). *Gut*; **1**: 125.
Carter E. P., Barrett A. D., Heeley A. F., Kuzemko J. A. (1984). *Arch. Dis. Childh*; **59**: 919.
Chalmers A. H., Cowley D. M. (1984). *Clin. Chem*; **30**: 1891.
Chalmers A. H., Cowley D. M., McWhinney B. C. (1985). *Clin. Chem*; **31**: 1703.
Cook H. B., Lennard-Jones J. E., Sherif S. M., Wiggins H. S. (1967). *Gut*; **8**: 408.
Cooke W. T., Asquith P. (1974). *Clinics in Gastroenterology*; **3**: 1–238.
Cooke W. T., et al. (1946). *Quart. J. Med*; N.S. **15**: 141.
Crane R. K. (1960). *Physiol. Rev*; **40**: 789.
Crider Q. E., Curran D. S. (1984). *Clin. Biochem*; **17**: 351.
Crossley J. R., Berryman C. C., Elliott R. B. (1977). *Lancet*; **2**: 1093.
Dahlqvist A. (1962). *Scand. J. Clin. Lab. Invest*; **14**: 145.
Dahlqvist A. (1965). In *Enzymes in Clinical Chemistry*. (Ruysen R., Vandendressche L., eds) p. 136. Amsterdam: Elsevier.
Dahlqvist A. (1968). *Analyt. Biochem*; **22**: 99.
Dawson A. M. (1965). *Abs. World Medicine*; **38**: 361.

Di Sant'Agnese P. A., Darling R. C., Perera G. A., Shea E. (1953). *Pediatrics*; **12**: 549.
Ebbesen K. E., Schonebeck J. (1967). *Acta Chir. Scand*; **133**: 61.
Foo A. Y., Rosalki S. B. (1986). *Ann. Clin. Biochem*; **23**: 624.
Gerber M., et al. (1985). *Clin. Chem*; **31**: 1331.
Goldsack K. L., Ginman R. F. A., Wright J. M. (1984). *Clin. Chem*; **30**: 813.
Goodhart J. M., Kingston G. R. (1969). *J. Clin. Path*; **22**: 621.
Gowenlock A. H. (1977). *Ann. Clin. Biochem*; **14**: 61.
Green A., Dodds P., Pennock C. (1985). *Ann. Clin. Biochem*; **22**: 171.
Gutierrez L. V., Baron J. H. (1972). *Gut*; **13**: 721.
Hamlin L. R., Schwede K. (1974). *Clin. Chem*; **20**: 96.
Hanscom D. H., Jacobson B. M., Littman A. (1967). *Ann. Int. Med*; **66**: 721.
Hansky J. (1984). *Postgrad. Med. J*; **60**: 767.
Heaney M. R., Culank L. S., Montgomery R. D., Sammons H. G. (1978). *Gastroenterology*; **75**: 393.
Heeley A. F., Watson D. (1983). *Clin. Chem*; **29**: 2011.
Heyman M. B. (1985). *Gastroenterology*; **89**: 685.
Hirschowitz B. I. (1984). *Postgrad. Med. J*; **60**: 743.
Holdsworth P. J., et al. (1984). *Brit. J. Surg*; **71**: 958.
Howat H. T. (1970). In *Biochemical Disorders in Human Disease*, 3rd ed. (Thompson R. H. S., Wootton I. D. P., eds) p. 703. London: Churchill Livingstone.
Imondi A. R., Stradley R. P., Wohlgemuth R. (1972). *Gut*; **13**: 726.
Ito S., et al. (1982). *Clin. Chem*; **28**: 323.
Jalali M. T., Laing I., Gowenlock A. H., Braganza J. M. (1985). *Clin. Chim. Acta*; **150**: 237.
James O. (1973). *Gut*; **14**: 582.
Johnson S. L., Bliss M., Mayersohn M., Conrad K. A. (1984). *Clin. Chem*; **30**: 1571.
Johnston D., Jepson K. (1967). *Lancet*; **2**: 585.
Kamer J. H. van de, Huinick H. ten B., Weijers H. A. (1949). *J. Biol. Chem*; **177**: 347.
Kay G. H., Tetlow V. A., Braganza J. M. (1983). *Clin. Chem*; **128**: 115.
Kelley M. L., Jr. (1957). *J. Amer. Med. Assoc*; **164**: 406.
Konturek S. J., Lankosz J. (1967). *Scand. J. Gastroenterol*; **2**: 112.
Laker M. F. (1983). *Adv. Clin. Chem*; **23**: 259.
Laker M. F., Bartlett K. (1985). In *Recent Advances in Clinical Biochemistry*, Vol. 3. (Price C. P., Alberti K. G. M. M., eds) p. 195. London: Churchill Livingstone.
Lambert H. P., Prankerd A. J., Smellie J. M. (1961). *Quart. J. Med*; **30**: 71.
Lankisch P. G., Lembeke B. (1984). *Clinics in Gastroenterology*; **13**, 717.
Leclerc P., Forest J. (1982). *Clin. Chem*; **28**: 37.
Leclerc P., Forest J. (1983). *Clin. Chem*; **29**: 1020.
Legaz M. E., Kenny M. A. (1976). *Clin. Chem*; **22**: 57.
Lifton L. J., Slickers K. A., Pragay D. A., Katz L. A. (1974). *J. Amer. Med. Assoc*; **229**: 47.
Lobley R. W., Holmes R., Pemberton P. W. (1985). *Clin. Sci*; **69**: Suppl. 12, 64P.
Lundh H. (1962). *Gastroenterology*; **42**: 275.
Mazzani B. C., Teubner J. K., Ryall R. L. (1984). *Clin. Chem*; **30**: 1339.
McGowan G. K., Wills M. R. (1964). *Brit. Med. J*; **2**: 189.
Merritt A. D., Karn R. C. (1977). *Adv. Human Genet*; **8**: 185.
Metz G., et al. (1976). *Lancet*; **1**: 668.
Meyers S., et al. (1985). *Gastroenterology*; **89**: 13.
Mifflin T. E., Benjamin D. C., Bruns D. E. (1985). *Clin. Chem*; **31**: 1283.
Mitchell C. J., et al. (1978). *Gut*; **19**: A973.
Mollin D. L., Baker S. T., Doniach I. (1955). *Brit. J. Haematol*; **1**: 278.
Morris M. D., Fisher O. A. (1967). *Amer. J. Dis. Childh*; **114**: 203.
Mottaleb A., et al. (1973). *Gut*; **14**: 835.
Multicentre Pilot Study. (1967). *Lancet*; **1**: 291.
Multicentre Study. (1967). *Lancet*; **2**: 534.
Multicentre Study. (1969), *Lancet*; **1**: 341.
Newcomer, A. D., et al. (1979). *Gastroenterology*; **76**: 6.
O'Donnell M. P., Fitzgerald C., McFeeney K. F. (1977). *Clin. Chem*; **23**: 560.
Peterson W. L., Ford an J. S. (1985). *New Engl. J. Med*; **312**: 1448.

Prader A., Auricchio S. (1965). *Ann. Rev. Med*; **10**: 345.

Rehfeld J. F. (1981). In *Recent Advances in Clinical Biochemistry*, Vol. 2. (Price C. P. Alberti, K. G. M. M., eds) p. 129. London: Churchill Livingstone.

Robards M. F. (1975). *Arch. Dis. Childh*; **50**: 631.

Robinson P. G., Elliott R. B. (1976). *Arch. Dis. Childh*; **51**: 301.

Robinson P. G., Smith P. A., Elliott R. B. (1975). *Clin. Chim. Acta*; **62**: 225.

Roe J. H., Rice E. W. (1948). *J. Biol. Chem*; **173**: 507.

Rofe A. M., Pholenz S. M., Bais R., Conyers R. A. J. (1985). *Clin. Chem*; **31**: 1574.

Rose R. C. (1980). *Ann. Rev. Physiol*; **42**: 157.

Rosenmund H., Kaczmarek M. J. (1976). *Clin. Chim. Acta*; **71**: 185.

Royse V. L., Jensen D. M. (1984). *Clin. Chem*; **30**: 387.

Sale J. K., Goldberg D. M., Thjodleifsson B., Wormsley K. G. (1974). *Gut*; **15**: 132.

Samloff I. M. (1969). *Gastroenterology*; **57**: 659.

Schultis K., Wagner E., Vossköhler E. (1969). *Schweiz. Med. Woch*; **99**: 603.

Schwartz S., Dahl J., Ellefson M., Ahlquist D. (1983). *Clin. Chem*; **29**: 2061.

Schwarz V., Sutcliffe C. H., Style P. P. (1968). *Arch. Dis. Childh*; **43**: 695.

Silk D. B. (1974). *Gut*; **15**: 494.

Simon J. B. (1985). *Gastroenterology*; **88**: 820.

Simpson F. G., Hall G. P., Kelleher J., Losowsky M. S. (1979). *Gut*; **20**: 581.

Steele R. J. C., Lee D. (1985). *Brit. J. Surg*; **72**: 501.

Steinberg, W. M., et al. (1985). *Ann. Int. Med*; **102**: 576.

Stone M. C., Thorp J. M. (1966). *Clin. Chim. Acta*; **14**: 812.

Strober W. (1976). *Clinics in Gastroenterology*; **5**: 427.

Theodossi A., Gazzard B. G. (1984). *Ann. Clin. Biochem*; **21**: 153.

Tietz N. W., Huona W. Y., Rauh D. F., Shuey D. F. (1986). *Clin. Chem*; **32**: 301.

Tietz N. W., Shuey D. F. (1984). *Clin. Chem*; **30**: 1227.

Toskes P. P., Deren J. J. (1973). *Gastroenterology*; **65**: 662.

Trapnell J. (1972). *Clinics in Gastroenterology*; **1**: 147.

Tsianos E. B., Jalali M. T., Braganza J. M., Gowenlock A. H. (1985). *Clin. Trials J*; **22**: 239.

Tsianos E. B., Jalali M. T., Gowenlock A. H., Braganza J. M. (1982). *Clin. Chim. Acta*; **124**: 13.

Urdal P. (1984). *Clin. Chem*; **30**: 911.

Vestrup J. A., Clay M. G., Bernstein M. (1974). *Clin. Chem*; **20**: 880.

Waldmann T. A. (1970). In *Modern Trends in Gastroenterology*, Vol. 3. (Card W. I., Creamer B., eds) p. 125. London: Butterworths.

Waller S. L., Ralston A. J. (1971). *Gut*; **12**: 878.

Weizman Z., et al. (1985). *Gastroenterology*; **89**: 596.

Welch C. L., Young D. S. (1983). *Clin. Chem*; **29**: 2022.

West P. S., Levin G. E., Griffin G. E., Maxwell J. O. (1981). *Brit. Med. J*; **282**: 1501.

Wiggins H. S. (1967). *Gut*; **8**: 415.

Wormsley K. G., Mahoney M. P., Ng M. (1966). *Lancet*; **1**: 993.

28

TESTS IN LIVER AND BILIARY TRACT DISEASE

Tests used in the study of patients with liver and biliary tract disease can be classified according to the function of the liver involved.

1. *Excretion*—particularly of bile pigments, bile salts and other organic anions, such as bromsulphthalein (BSP).
2. *Intermediary metabolism*—especially carbohydrates and amino acids.
3. *Synthesis*—mainly of proteins such as albumin and prothrombin.
4. *Detoxification*—usually of ammonia and antipyrine.

In addition, the increased activity of serum enzymes is used to indicate the pathological release of particular enzymes from damaged liver cells rather than to study a particular function.

This classification is incomplete but includes those tests which are most frequently used. For further general discussion see Jones and Berk (1982), Sherlock (1985), Schiff (1975) and Berk *et al.* (1985).

TESTS BASED ON THE EXCRETORY FUNCTION

Tests Involving Bile Pigments

Bilirubin Metabolism. Jaundice is due to an increase in the concentration of bilirubin in the blood and is a common symptom in liver or biliary tract disorders. The increase may be due to excessive production of bilirubin or a defect in its excretion. Bilirubin is formed from haemoglobin and other haems in the reticuloendothelial system (spleen, bone marrow and Kupffer cells of the liver). Ten to 25% arises from liver haems or ineffective erythropoiesis leading to early release of haemoglobin. The rest comes from senescent red cells. The α-methyne (–CH=) bridge of the protoporphyrin ring is oxidised to give carbon monoxide and biliverdin (Fig. 28.1). The central of the remaining three bridges (γ) is subsequently reduced to a methene bridge (–CH$_2$–) to give bilirubin which circulates bound to albumin. One mole of bilirubin is tightly bound per mole of albumin and further binding, not required physiologically, is weaker. Bilirubin is not water-soluble as such and the albumin binding aids transport in the watery plasma.

At the liver cell surface, bilirubin leaves the albumin and is taken into the liver cell by an easily saturated, carrier-mediated process and is then bound by two intracellular proteins, ligandin (Y protein) and Z protein. These act as storage and transport proteins. Ligandin is able to conjugate certain organic anions, notably BSP, with glutathione but this does not appear to occur with bilirubin. At the smooth endoplasmic reticulum (microsomes), UDP-glucuronyltransferase (EC 2.4.1.17) conjugates bilirubin forming mainly the diglucuronide with some monoglucuronide. Some conjugation with other carbohydrate moieties may occur. Another saturable, energy-dependent process transports conjugated

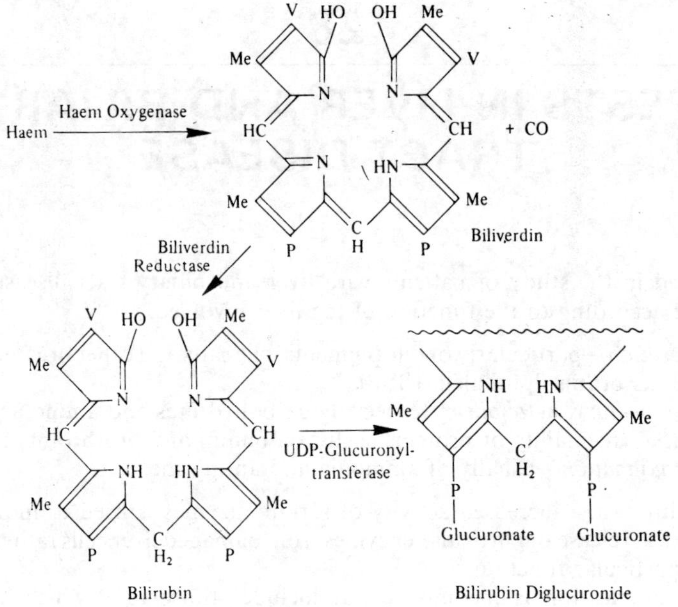

Fig. 28.1. The Formation and Conjugation of Bilirubin.
(Me = methyl, $-CH_3$; V = vinyl, $-CH=CH_2$; P = propionic acid residue, $-CH_2.CH_2.COOH$)

bilirubin and BSP, but not bile salts, across the canalicular membrane. This is the rate-limiting process in bilirubin metabolism and is very sensitive to liver damage.

The excreted bile passes to the gall bladder where it is stored and concentrated until the presence of food in the duodenum stimulates gall bladder contraction. The bile passes along the cystic duct and common bile duct to enter the duodenum by traversing the ampulla of Vater. Once in the small intestine, enterohepatic circulation of bilirubin is insignificant, except in the fetus where small intestinal β-glucuronidase deconjugates bilirubin allowing its reabsorption to occur. After birth, once the colonic bacterial flora is established, bacterial enzymes deconjugate the bilirubin glucuronide and reduce the bilirubin to 'urobilinogen', a general term for the products of a series of hydrogenations of the pyrrole rings and vinyl side chains, including d-urobilinogen, mesobilirubinogen and stercobilinogen. Most of these products are excreted in the faeces, where air oxidation converts some to 'urobilin', again a mixture of products. Some urobilinogen is reabsorbed from the gut into the portal vein, whereupon the majority is taken up by the liver and re-excreted into the bile. A small portion enters the systemic circulation and because of its water solubility some is excreted in the urine.

The urobilinogens (Fig. 28.2) have three methene bridges whereas the urobilins have a central methyne bridge. The urobilins are reddish orange in colour, show a distinct spectral absorption band, and form fluorescent zinc derivatives; in contrast, the urobilinogens are colourless but form a coloured derivative with Ehrlich's aldehyde reagent (pp. 648, 661, 662).

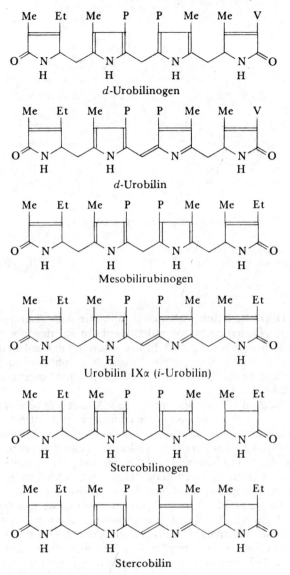

Fig. 28.2. Structural Formulae of Selected Urobilinogens and Urobilins. (Abbreviations as in Fig. 28.1 plus Et = ethyl, $-CH_2.CH_3$)

The Determination of Serum Bilirubin

Serum bilirubin is either measured by spectrophotometry of native bilirubin employing the absorption band at 450–475 nm or more usually by prior conversion to azobilirubin followed by spectrophotometry. Though not routinely used, high performance liquid chromatography (HPLC) of bilirubin allows analysis of mono- and diglucuronides of bilirubin as well as the unconjugated form.

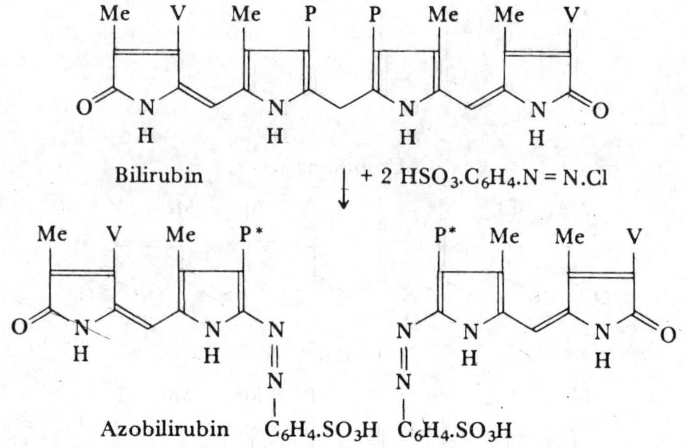

Fig. 28.3. The Formation of Azobilirubin.
(Abbreviations as in Fig. 28.1 plus $P^* = -CH_2.CH_2.COOR$ where $R = H$ or glucuronyl)

Use of the Diazo Reaction. Reaction of bilirubin with diazotised sulphanilic acid results in the formation of two molecules of azobilirubin, not quite identical (Fig. 28.3). Azobilirubin is red-purple in acid solution but in alkali it has a higher molar absorptivity and is blue-purple. Instead of sulphanilic acid, 2,4- or 2,5-dichloraniline may be used in a similar way, but the first reagent is preferred by over 80% of laboratories.

The direct addition of aqueous diazonium salt to serum results mainly in the reaction of the water-soluble conjugated bilirubin (the 'direct' reaction). To measure total bilirubin a further reagent, usually termed an 'accelerator', must be added. Originally, Van den Bergh and colleagues (Van den Bergh and Snapper, 1913; Van den Bergh and Muller, 1916) precipitated protein with ethanol which also acted as an accelerator when diazo reagent was added to the supernatant. However, appreciable quantities of bilirubin were lost on the protein precipitate and current methods avoid this form of protein removal. Methanol was employed by Malloy and Evelyn (1937) but a large sample dilution was required with consequent loss of sensitivity. Urea-benzoate (Powell, 1944), caffeine-benzoate (Jendrassik and Grof, 1938), dyphylline-acetate (Michaelsson, 1961) and Brij 35 (Colombo *et al.*, 1974) are more satisfactory as they permit the reaction of total bilirubin without protein precipitation and at a lesser dilution. Recently dimethyl sulphoxide has also been used but at present, caffeine or the related substance dyphylline are most commonly employed.

The addition of alkaline tartrate increases sensitivity by utilising the enhanced absorption of the chromogen in alkaline solution. In this case it is necessary to add ascorbic acid after the diazo reaction is completed in acid solution before making alkaline. This removes excess diazonium salt and avoids unwanted diazo-coupling. It should be emphasised that the terms 'direct-reacting' and 'indirect-reacting' bilirubin are related to but not completely synonymous with conjugated and unconjugated bilirubin (see also p. 723).

Diazo Methods in Current Use. Most laboratories use the diazo method on automated equipment; continuous flow methods, discrete analysers and centri-fugal techniques are all popular. It is not possible to give details of the use of the last two analysers here—methodological details are usually available from the manufacturers of the individual instruments. In the case of continuous flow analysers, the bilirubin channel is predominantly used in multi-channel form. As the single channel technique, an example of which appears in the 5th edition of this book, is now rarely used, it has been omitted on this occasion. Modern discrete analysers are increasingly using 2,5-dichlorophenyldiazonium salt which is more stable than diazotised sulphanilic acid. A detergent is used as an accelerator but direct bilirubin cannot be measured and falsely high results are possible with uraemic sera (Wahlefeld *et al.*, 1972). Among the manual methods, the alkaline diazo methods using sulphanilic acid are the most popular.

The preferred manual method remains that of Jendrassik and Grof (1938) as modified by Nosslin (1960), Michaelsson (1961) and Michaelsson *et al.* (1965). Jendrassik and Grof employed caffeine–sodium benzoate as accelerator, ascorbic acid to eliminate further coupling and alkaline tartrate addition before spectrophotometry, while Nosslin made modifications to give 'direct-reading' bilirubin as well. Michaelsson found that the omission of caffeine in the 'direct' method of Nosslin altered the azobilirubin absorbance relative to the standard which employed the total bilirubin conditions. Also ascorbic acid, not present in the blanks, gave some colour with the diazo reagent. Michaelsson therefore incorporated all the basic reagents in the final solution for each measurement (blank, total and 'direct' bilirubin) but varied the order of additions as appropriate. He used dyphylline, a more expensive reagent than caffeine, to avoid occasional problems of turbidity. Billing *et al.* (1971) co-ordinated these modifications and incorporated a calibration procedure.

Manual Method of Billing *et al.* (1971)

This is convenient for measuring total bilirubin but also has the option of measuring 'direct-acting' bilirubin as well.

Reagents.
1. Diazo reagent. Prepare freshly for use by mixing 10 ml solution A and 0·25 ml solution B.
   A. Sulphanilic acid, 5 g/l. Warm 5 g in about 500 ml water, add 15 ml concentrated hydrochloric acid, cool and make to a litre with water.
   B. Sodium nitrite solution, 5 g/l. Prepare 10 ml freshly daily.
2. Alkaline tartrate solution, 100 g sodium hydroxide and 350 g sodium potassium tartrate per litre.
3. Ascorbic acid solution, 40 g/l. Prepare daily the volume needed.
4. Dyphylline reagent. Dissolve in water at 40 °C, 50 g dyphylline (7-2′,3′-dihydroxypropyl theophylline) and 125 g sodium acetate trihydrate. Add 1 g EDTA, cool, and make to one litre with water.
5. Standard bilirubin solution, 200 μmol/l (see p. 722).

Technique. Dilute the serum 1 to 5 with water. To each of three test tubes add the reagents in the order given, mixing well after each addition.

Total	Direct	Blank
1·0 ml diluted serum	1·0 ml diluted serum	1·0 ml diluted serum
0·5 ml diazo reagent	0·5 ml diazo reagent	0·1 ml ascorbic acid
2·0 ml dyphylline	*Wait for* 10 min	0·5 ml diazo reagent
Wait for 10 min	0·1 ml ascorbic acid	2·0 ml dyphylline
0·1 ml ascorbic acid	*Immediately* add	1·5 ml alkaline tartrate
Immediately add	2·0 ml dyphylline and	
1·5 ml alkaline tartrate	1.5 ml alkaline tartrate	

Read immediately at 600 nm against water. Dilute the standard 1 to 5 with water and determine the total bilirubin.

Calculation.

$$\text{Serum bilirubin } (\mu\text{mol/l}) = \frac{\text{Reading of unknown} - \text{Reading of blank}}{\text{Reading of standard} - \text{Reading of blank}} \times 200$$

Notes.

1. If the bilirubin standard is not exactly 200 μmol/l, use the true concentration in the calculation instead of 200.
2. For high values, say over 200 μmol/l, use serum diluted 1 to 10; for low values use a dilution of 1 to 3.
3. Instead of dyphylline, caffeine-benzoate-acetate can be used. For this dissolve 75 g sodium benzoate in about 800 ml water at 60 °C, then add 50 g caffeine, 125 g sodium acetate trihydrate and 1 g EDTA. After cooling make to one litre and filter. This reagent is much cheaper but some batches of caffeine may produce turbidity.

Performance of Diazo Methods. The average between-batch coefficient of variation (CV) of the manual method given is 6% at a bilirubin level of 50 to 60 μmol/l. Figures for the methods of Powell (1944) and Evelyn and Malloy (1937) are nearer 8%. For the automated methods using sulphanilic acid and caffeine/dyphylline activation, the average performance with CV of 4% is similar for the various types of instrument. Those using other diazo reagents or other activators have a slightly higher CV, 5%. The relative accuracy of manual and automated methods using sulphanilic acid and caffeine/dyphylline is very similar but the use of other diazo reagents or activators produces figures on average about 1·5 to 2 μmol/l higher.

Spectrophotometric Determination of Native Bilirubin

Bilirubin in serum has an absorbance maximum between 450 and 475 nm. The shape of the absorption spectrum is slightly different for adult and infant bilirubin and different again for conjugated bilirubin. If a generally applicable method is required, the wavelength selected must minimise these differences. If the method is intended for use only with infant sera containing unconjugated bilirubin, the problems diminish. Oxyhaemoglobin, methaemoglobin, transferrin, carotenoids and turbidity also cause absorption at these wavelengths and, in theory, it is necessary to measure absorbances at several wavelengths and, by means of solving a series of simultaneous equations, eliminate the contributions of interfering substances. Again, restriction to infant bilirubin measurements removes the need to compensate for carotenoids.

In practice however, the results obtained by measuring the absorbance at two wavelengths only are similar to those employing more complex methods. The principal interfering substance is oxyhaemoglobin. Its contribution can be measured using the Soret band at 412–420 nm but the wavelength setting is critical at the sharp absorbance peak. The absorbance is much greater than at 460 nm, requiring differential dilution, and turbidity compensation is poor at this wavelength. The oxyhaemoglobin absorption peaks at 575–579 nm and 540 nm have absorbances equal to those at 455 and 453 nm respectively, allowing simple cancellation of the haemoglobin contribution, but unconjugated bilirubin has some absorbance at 540 nm. Hertz *et al.* (1974) compared a large series of published spectrophotometric methods and proposed 466 nm for bilirubin measurement (isosbestic for unconjugated infant bilirubin and conjugated bilirubin, with adult unconjugated bilirubin of similar absorbance) and 522 nm (isosbestic for oxyhaemoglobin and bilirubin) for compensation for interfering substances. Dilution was in borate buffer (dipotassium tetraborate, 100 mmol/l, pH 9·3) and readings were taken against borate blanks on a spectrophotometer checked regularly for wavelength and absorbance calibration. The formula then used was

$$\text{Total bilirubin } (\mu\text{mol/l}) = (21\cdot6 \times A_{466} - 27\cdot4 \times A_{522}) \times F$$

where F is the dilution factor and A is the absorbance at the wavelength stated. The results agreed well with those obtained with the Michaelsson *et al.* (1965) diazo method on human sera and on control materials. There was complete correction for oxyhaemoglobin and turbidity, good correction for transferrin and methaemoglobin and partial correction for carotenoids. No absorbance reading outside the range 0·05 to 1·0 was used and the steep portions of absorption spectra were avoided.

Several other methods have been reported. O'Brien and Ibott (1962) used 455 and 575 nm, Scott (1959) employed 454 and 574 nm; the diluents were phosphate buffer and saline respectively. The method of Hertz *et al.* (1974) has the advantage of proven compatability with an established diazo method and is potentially usable with samples other than paediatric ones.

Bilirubinometer. These principles have been used in the bilirubinometer (American Optical Corporation) for the direct determination of bilirubin in undiluted serum. The sample absorbance is measured simultaneously at 461 and 551 nm. The electrical balance of the two photometer circuits is achieved by adjustment of an optical wedge in the 551 nm light path. The wedge thickness varies logarithmically so that the bilirubin concentration scale is linear. Evans and Holton (1970) compared the bilirubinometer with a spectrophotometric method (O'Brien and Ibott, 1962) and a modified diazo method (Malloy and Evelyn, 1937). They found very good agreement with the former method but less good, although acceptable, agreement with the latter.

In contrast to the results with a spectrophotometric method, Stein *et al.* (1971) found that in the presence of increased amounts of haemoglobin, the bilirubinometer gave depressed results for bilirubin and at haemoglobin concentrations above 3 g/l this depression exceeded 10%. They also noted a lack of linearity at high bilirubin concentrations. Although Harkness *et al.* (1983) found the American Optical instrument to give lower values than the Michaelsson *et al.* (1965) method, 15% at 450 μmol/l and 5% at 210 μmol/l, they considered its use to be generally satisfactory as a 'side room' method.

All workers recommend that, although the instrument is very easy to use, it should be subject to frequent checks. Staff must be carefully trained if the instrument is used outside the laboratory's supervision. The problems of erroneously low results in haemolysed specimens and at high concentrations of bilirubin are significant in a method intended primarily for measuring neonatal bilirubin concentrations.

All these spectrophotometric methods are generally unsatisfactory at low bilirubin concentrations, particularly below 35 μmol/l, but the small sample volume (10 to 20 μl), simplicity of use and, given correct selection of wavelength, insensitivity to haemolysis make them especially valuable in jaundice of the newborn. However, it is important to ensure satisfactory accuracy and precision. Decisions involving exchange transfusion may be taken on either a single bilirubin value or on the rate of increase of serum bilirubin (Swyer, 1975); the former criterion requires an accurate measurement while the detection of an increase of 8 μmol l^{-1} h^{-1} over a period of a few hours requires a very precise method.

Calibration of Serum Bilirubin Measurement

The lack of common calibration materials is an important factor in inter-laboratory imprecision of paediatric bilirubin analysis (St John and Penberthy, 1979; Watkinson *et al.*, 1982) and also in analysis of adult samples. Difficulties in calibration arise from the following factors:

Calibration of Direct Spectrophotometric and Azobilirubin Methods.

1. Bilirubin is photolabile and readily oxidised, particularly in such organic solvents as chloroform. It is insoluble in aqueous solutions except in strong alkalies or in a protein matrix.
2. Difficulty in the preparation of pure bilirubin results in imprecise knowledge of its molar absorptivity which is usually taken to be $60\,700 \pm 800$ l cm^{-1} mol^{-1} at 453 nm.
3. Conjugated and unconjugated bilirubin have different absorption maxima, 463 and 453 nm respectively.
4. The spectrum of bilirubin is affected by the presence of protein and by the nature of the protein, e.g. animal or human, pure albumin or whole serum.
5. Both types of method may be used interchangeably for the same patient and a common calibrant is preferable. This may not be possible, however, unless the analytical methods are carefully selected.

Calibration of Azobilirubin Methods Only.

1. The results from some diazo methods depend on the nature of the protein present in the calibrant. This does not apply to the Michaelsson modification of the Jendrassik and Grof method (Doumas *et al.*, 1973).
2. Stable pure conjugated bilirubin preparations are not available. Thus an unconjugated bilirubin standard assayed by the 'total bilirubin' method has to be used to calibrate the 'direct bilirubin' method. This is unsatisfactory.

The use of HPLC overcomes the problems of impurity and of the different molecular species present, but doubts about the stability of bilirubin on the column and about the validity of possible derivatisation procedures detract from the use of HPLC as a reference method. The technique has, however, confirmed the presence of a fourth bilirubin fraction (δ-bilirubin) tightly bound to albumin which further complicates standardisation.

The problems of calibration of bilirubin assays have been reviewed by Turnell (1985). Solutions based on the use of lyophilised proteins are the most stable standard preparations, at least 3 years in the dark at room temperature. Such material, using human albumin and giving identical results with a diazo method (Michaelsson *et al.*, 1965) and a spectrophotometric method (Hertz *et al.*, 1974) should soon become available (Turnell, 1985). For preparation of a calibrant within the routine laboratory the procedure of Billing *et al.* (1971) based on that of Gadd (1966) is satisfactory.

Bilirubin Calibrant. Prepare a pool of non-icteric human serum, each sample of which has been frozen within 12 h of collection. Thaw, mix and centrifuge at 0 °C, or filter through glass wool to remove fibrin clots and other debris. Weigh 40 μmol (23·36 mg) bilirubin (ε $60\,700 \pm 800$ at 453 nm, BDH Chemicals) which has been dried in a desiccator for several days, placing it in a small stoppered tube.

Add 4 ml dimethylsulphoxide (DMSO) and dissolve by shaking and warming in water at 40 °C while keeping in a dim light. Then at once add 2·0 ml of this slowly, while mixing, to 40 ml of a pool of human serum which, after exposure to light, gives a diazo reaction equivalent to less than 3·5 μmol/l. Make up to 50 ml with the same serum. Should froth form, either add a trace of caprylic alcohol or touch the surface with a swab stick smeared with a trace of silicone grease. To calibrate this serum standard, which contains approximately 400 μmol/l, dilute 200 μl of the original DMSO solution (10 μmol/ml) to 250 ml with chloroform to give a solution containing 8 μmol/l. Read the absorbance using a 1 cm light path against a chloroform blank at 453 nm. This should read 0·486. Then

Serum bilirubin standard (μmol/l) =

$$\frac{400 \times \text{Reading of chloroform standard}}{0\cdot486} +$$

$$\text{Bilirubin concentration in pooled serum} \times \frac{96}{100}$$

A suitable range of standards can be prepared by diluting the above standard with the pooled serum, allowing for the bilirubin content of the pool. For use with each batch of tests, a standard of 200 μmol/l is suitable.

The standards can be most accurately calibrated to take into account the amount contributed by the serum pool bilirubin if several different dilutions are made. The absorbances of these different preparations, after the diazo reaction has been carried out, are plotted against the expected concentration assuming *no* bilirubin is present in the pooled serum. Extrapolation to zero absorbance gives a negative intercept on the concentration axis equal to the serum pool bilirubin concentration. An accurate calculation can then be made for the concentration in any bilirubin standard prepared.

The standards should be prepared in subdued light, dispensed into small cups and stored frozen in the dark. They are usable with any of the bilirubin methods discussed in this chapter.

Commercially assayed preparations are frequently used as secondary standards. A primary standard should be used to check new batches and to adjust the stated value if necessary in order to obtain adequate interlaboratory agreement. 'Correction' of stated values on the basis of a previous batch or from performance on an external quality assessment scheme are less satisfactory, error-prone procedures.

Conjugated Bilirubin and 'Direct-reacting' Bilirubin. It is necessary to use unconjugated bilirubin as a standard when measuring 'direct-reacting' bilirubin. This may lead to inaccuracies. Pure unconjugated bilirubin may give a colour in the 'direct' reaction, up to 10 % of the total bilirubin in some methods. Thus the terms, conjugated bilirubin and 'direct-reacting' bilirubin are not synonymous. Lo and Wu (1983) employed authentic bilirubin diglucuronide to show that, using the total bilirubin method described in this chapter and the unconjugated bilirubin standard, both unconjugated bilirubin and the diglucuronide were satisfactorily measured in an equivalent and additive fashion. However, the method for 'direct-reacting' bilirubin underestimated bilirubin diglucuronide, giving about 70 % of the equivalent concentration, and gave some reaction (2 to 6 %) with unconjugated bilirubin. The method also underestimated δ-bilirubin by 10 to 20 %.

Interference by Haemolysis. The presence of haemoglobin reduces the apparent bilirubin concentration as measured by various diazo methods; the reasons are incompletely understood. Michaelsson *et al.* (1965) found no such error with their modification of the Jendrassik and Grof method and considered that ascorbic acid eliminated haemoglobin interference in the total bilirubin method. Novros *et al.* (1979) found a modified Jendrassik and Grof method to give only 93% recovery of bilirubin in the presence of 5 g/l of haemoglobin. No haemoglobin effect was apparent when it was added to azobilirubin; the haemoglobin had to be present during diazo coupling. It was suggested that after splitting of bilirubin to form one azobilirubin molecule and a dipyrrole, the haemoglobin interfered with the formation of the second azobilirubin molecule. Caffeine may act to bind the haemoglobin and diminish the interference.

The interference of haemoglobin in spectrophotometry of native bilirubin was discussed earlier (p. 720).

HPLC Methods for Bilirubin

Two major methods have been used. Muraca and Blanckaert (1983) employed alkaline methanolysis and chloroform extraction to yield bilirubin and its mono- and dimethyl-esters (derived from mono- and di-conjugated bilirubin respectively). Ion-pair chromatography (p. 63) employing a methanolic tetrabutyl-ammonium phosphate gradient on a reverse-phase octodecyl-silica column and xanthobilirubinic acid methyl ester as internal standard was used by Scharschmidt *et al.* (1982). They showed serum conjugated bilirubin in obstructive disease to be about equally divided between the C-8 and C-12 monoglucuronides and the diglucuronide (about 30% each) but bilirubin in urine was excreted predominantly as the diglucuronide.

Lauff *et al.* (1981, 1983) were able to separate bilirubin fractions in serum by gradient elution on a reverse-phase column after removing globulins but not albumin. Fractions eluted, in reverse order, were unconjugated bilirubin (α), the monoglucuronide (β), diglucuronide (γ) and a fourth fraction (δ). This δ-bilirubin, previously described by Kuenzle *et al.* (1966) using an open column method, was bound to albumin by an alkali-stable link, possibly a covalent bonding of the monoglucuronide through its free carboxyl group. The δ-bilirubin is quantitatively important in all cases of conjugated hyperbilirubinaemia and actually predominates in the recovery phase of hepatitis; low concentrations occur in normal subjects and in patients with haemolytic disease (Weiss *et al.*, 1983; Wu, 1984). The ability to quantitate the unconjugated and various conjugated bilirubin fractions has proved disappointing for diagnostic purposes as overlap is too great between different clinical conditions.

INTERPRETATION OF SERUM BILIRUBIN RESULTS

Normal serum bilirubin concentrations follow an almost log normal distribution (Billing, 1981). The upper limit is often taken as 17 μmol/l but there is a sex difference with reported upper reference limits varying from 13·7 to 16·3 μmol/l in females and 20·5 to 24·0 μmol/l in males (Fevery *et al.*, 1981). Scharschmidt *et al.* (1982) found no conjugated bilirubin in normal serum but Muraca and Blanckaert (1983) reported up to 3·5% of the total bilirubin to be mono- or di-conjugated. For reasons discussed earlier, a 'direct-reading' fraction of up to 3 μmol/l may be found in normal subjects but an increase in this, even though total bilirubin is not increased, has been cited as a sensitive indicator of liver disease (Berk, 1981).

In jaundice the total bilirubin is increased and conjugated bilirubin may be present. The causes of jaundice are many and may be classified in several ways. The classification may be based on:

1. *The nature of the bile pigment*, i.e. unconjugated or conjugated bilirubin.
2. *The anatomical site of the disorder*, i.e. prehepatic, hepatic or posthepatic.
3. *The pathological cause of the disorder*, i.e. haemolysis, hepatocellular dysfunction, or obstruction to bile flow.
4. *The nature of the altered bilirubin metabolism.*
   (a) Jaundice due to the *retention* in the circulation of increased amounts of unconjugated bilirubin. This can arise from excessive production or defective handling in the liver cell.
   (b) Jaundice due to the *regurgitation* into the circulation of conjugated bilirubin which would normally pass along the biliary system. Cholestasis, the failure of normal amounts of bile to reach the duodenum, predisposes to regurgitation. Cholestasis arises from intrahepatic or extrahepatic (post-hepatic) obstruction of the bile ducts.

As more and more causes of jaundice have been discovered, the older 'anatomical' and 'pathological' classifications have become less satisfactory. The following discussion therefore considers two broad groups—retention and regurgitation jaundice with their subdivisions. The relationship of the various classifications together with some examples are shown in Table 28.1.

Retention Jaundice. This may arise from several prehepatic or hepatic causes but the common feature is an increase in serum unconjugated bilirubin without bilirubinuria. It is convenient to consider different subgroups separately.

Prehepatic or haemolytic jaundice. There is increased breakdown of haemoglobin to bilirubin at a rate exceeding the ability of the normal liver cell to remove it from the circulation. Excessive haemolysis may be due to (a) congenital abnormalities of the red cells such as spherocytosis, abnormal haemoglobins such as HbS, and enzyme defects such as glucose-6-phosphate dehydrogenase deficiency, (b) the effect of antibodies on previously normal cells as in acquired haemolytic anaemias, in haemolytic disease of the newborn and in incompatible blood transfusions, (c) the effect of drugs (e.g. methyldopa), chemicals (e.g. arsine) or organisms (e.g. *Plasmodium* spp., *Clostridium welchii*) on normal red cells.

Increased conversion of haemoglobin to bilirubin also occurs during resorption of haematomas and in ineffective erythropoiesis (e.g. pernicious anaemia).

Defective metabolism in the liver cell. This includes defective uptake by the hepatocyte, ineffective intracellular transport and defective conjugation at the microsomes.

Rifampicin can inhibit cell uptake of bilirubin while other drugs (novobiocin, primaquine) interfere at the conjugation stage. This group also includes the various forms of familial non-haemolytic jaundice, discussed later, and the temporary insufficiency of conjugating ability in the neonate producing the 'physiological' jaundice of the newborn. Interference with conjugation also occurs due to the presence of ill-defined factors in maternal serum (Lucey Driscoll syndrome) or milk during breast feeding of infants.

Regurgitation Jaundice. The defect may lie in the liver or in the biliary tree but conjugated bilirubin enters the circulation and appears in the urine. At the same time, as less bilirubin enters the intestine to be converted to urobilin, the stools may become pale.

Defective transport of conjugated bilirubin into the bile capillaries. This is impaired in the Dubin–Johnson and Rotor syndromes, variant forms of familial

TABLE 28.1
Classifications of Jaundice

Predominant plasma pigment	Anatomical	Cause		Examples
Unconjugated bilirubin (indirect Van den Bergh reaction)	Prehepatic	Haemolytic	**RETENTION** (a) Haemolytic	*Increased haemolysis:* haematoma absorption, abnormal red cells, antibodies, chemicals. *Ineffective erythropoiesis:* pernicious anaemia, thalassaemia minor, 'shunt' hyperbilirubinaemia
			(b) Non-haemolytic	*Impaired uptake:* rifampicin, Gilbert's syndrome. *Impaired glucuronyl transferase activity:* physiological jaundice of newborn, Gilbert's and Crigler–Najjar syndromes, drug interference
Conjugated bilirubin (direct Van den Bergh reaction)	Hepatic	Hepatocellular or Toxic and infective	**REGURGITATION** (a) Intrahepatic or Parenchymal	*Liver cell necrosis:* viral, drugs, poisons. *Impaired transfer to bile capillaries:* Dubin–Johnson and Rotor syndromes, drugs. *Intrahepatic cholestasis:* drugs, tumours or inflammation of bile ducts, primary biliary cirrhosis, intrahepatic cholestasis of pregnancy

Posthepatic	Obstructive	(b) Extrahepatic or Mechanical	*Extra-hepatic cholestasis:* within bile duct lumen gall stone atresia in bile duct wall tumour stricture outside bile duct carcinoma pancreas lymph node enlargement

non-haemolytic jaundice. Interference with transport is also seen in sensitivity to derivatives of testosterone substituted at C17, e.g. methyltestosterone, or to the contraceptive pill, especially the synthetic oestrogen component. A similar effect probably accounts for the occasional benign jaundice of late pregnancy.

A difficulty in transport occurs in cirrhotic nodules where the disorderly regeneration of hepatocytes prevents proper closely organised association with bile capillaries as occurs in the normal liver lobule.

Intrahepatic cholestasis. This includes disorders at the bile capillary level as in chlorpromazine sensitivity or at the level of the smaller bile ducts as in some forms of intrahepatic atresia, sclerosing cholangitis or bile duct carcinoma. Primary biliary cirrhosis also falls into this group.

Extrahepatic cholestasis. Also referred to as posthepatic or obstructive jaundice, this includes atresia of the main bile ducts as a congenital cause. Acquired causes are: a gall stone in the common bile duct or Ampulla of Vater, bile duct stricture following earlier surgery, and extrinsic tumours compressing the major bile ducts such as carcinoma of the head of the pancreas or secondary carcinoma in lymph glands surrounding the porta hepatis where the hepatic ducts emerge.

Mixed Retention and Regurgitation Jaundice. This is a consequence of liver cell necrosis and the proportion of retention to regurgitation may change during the course of the illness. Disordered uptake, transport and conjugation in badly damaged cells leads to retention jaundice. Direct regurgitation of conjugated bilirubin from the damaged cell may occur but this is aided by intrahepatic cholestasis at bile canalicular level either by blockage by bile thrombi or by compression by swollen liver cells. Examples of viral hepatitis causing this type of jaundice are hepatitis A (infective hepatitis), hepatitis B (serum hepatitis), non-A, non-B-hepatitis, infectious mononucleosis (glandular fever) and yellow fever. Drugs or poisons causing liver cell necrosis include cytotoxic drugs, paracetamol, iproniazid, tetracycline, alcohol, carbon tetrachloride and other halogenated hydrocarbons, and phosphorus.

The Familial Hyperbilirubinaemias. Several genetically determined disorders of bilirubin metabolism have been described, though most are uncommon. They are best considered in relation to the type of bilirubin circulating (Okolicsanyi, 1981).

Familial Unconjugated Hyperbilirubinaemia. About 5% of healthy blood donors have serum unconjugated bilirubin concentrations in the range 17–50 μmol/l unassociated with increased haemolysis or the stigmata of hepatocellular disease. The jaundice persists indefinitely and, though the level may fluctuate, there is no systematic increase over the years. The condition, though heterogeneous, is referred to as Gilbert's syndrome and is the most common form of jaundice. As the distribution of serum bilirubin concentrations in the normal population is approximately log normal, the distinction between a 'high normal' and Gilbert's syndrome is often unclear (Berk, 1981). In Gilbert's syndrome the serum bilirubin may rise to 85 μmol/l during an intercurrent infection, and it is also increased by fasting, a 400 kCal diet usually causes an increase of over 25 μmol/l compared to less than 18 μmol/l in normals, and rises after a nicotinic acid load, which increases red cell fragility and splenic sequestration. It is probably due in part to defective conjugation and as such the jaundice may be reduced by administration of phenobarbitone which induces the synthesis of glucuronyl transferase. Most liver function tests are normal but BSP retention may be increased. For further details see Fevery *et al.* (1981) and Billing (1983). In the Crigler–Najjar syndrome, jaundice is more severe and there is either absence

(Type I) or severe deficiency (Type II) of glucuronyl transferase activity. The enzyme is not detected in Type II but must presumably be present as phenobarbitone reduces jaundice. In Type I, a rare autosomal recessive condition, progressive retention jaundice commences soon after birth and results in kernicterus with a fatal outcome, but Type II, an autosomal dominant condition, is less severe and responsive to phenobarbitone therapy.

Familial Conjugated Hyperbilirubinaemia. These are rare disorders showing only a mild degree of jaundice. In the Dubin–Johnson Syndrome the conjugation step is normal but there is difficulty in transport into the bile capillaries leading to regurgitation jaundice. There is also accumulation of a brown pigment, lipofuscin, in the liver cells and a characteristic abnormality of BSP excretion. In the Rotor syndrome, there is a similar defect in bilirubin metabolism without the other features.

The importance of familial hyperbilirubinaemias of adult life lies in their differentiation from progressive forms of more serious liver disease, such as chronic hepatitis in which a mild jaundice is part of the clinical picture.

Neonatal Jaundice. Retention jaundice due to temporary insufficient glucuronyl transferase activity is a frequent and physiological occurrence in the neonate, especially if premature. The jaundice is usually maximal at around 5 days of age, but resolution is quicker if the baby is irradiated with blue-violet light which converts bilirubin to lumirubin. In Rhesus isoimmunisation, a haemolytic element increases the retention jaundice. This possibility should be investigated if the jaundice persists and other possibilities should also be considered. These include other causes of haemolysis, Crigler–Najjar syndrome, interference with bilirubin metabolism by breast feeding (try effect of cessation), hypothyroidism (usually excluded by screening) and, rarely, pyloric stenosis (Bleicher *et al.*, 1979). The monitoring of neonatal retention jaundice is directed towards deciding when to undertake exchange transfusion in order to avoid kernicterus. The likelihood of this is not only dependent on the bilirubin concentration and its rate of increase, but also on factors affecting the binding of bilirubin to albumin such as blood pH, and the concentrations of albumin itself and of free fatty acids and drugs such as salicylate.

If conjugated bilirubin is present then galactosaemia, tyrosinaemia, α_1-antitrypsin deficiency and cystic fibrosis need to be considered. Septicaemia is an important possible cause (Paton, 1984). The most important distinction is between biliary atresia and neonatal hepatitis and various biochemical tests have been suggested but found wanting. They include the serum concentrations of α-fetoprotein (Zeltzer *et al.*, 1974; Andres *et al.*, 1977; Zeltzer, 1978) and gamma-glutamyltranspeptidase (Wright and Christie, 1981). Early diagnosis is important as surgical intervention in biliary atresia has little chance of success if delayed beyond the sixth week of life. The Rose Bengal excretion test has been claimed to be a useful diagnostic procedure in this condition (Bouchier, 1982).

For a full account of neonatal jaundice and its monitoring see Odell (1980) and Isherwood and Fletcher (1985).

The Role of Serum Bilirubin Determinations. These are often used in conjunction with radiological, ultrasound and radioisotopic 'imaging' procedures and are complementary to them when assessing the jaundiced patient.

Bilirubin measurements are useful in sub-clinical jaundice where the demonstration of small increases up to 50 μmol/l is of diagnostic value particularly if conjugated and unconjugated fractions are measured. The latter is especially useful in investigating Gilbert's syndrome.

In clinical jaundice they allow the development and course of the jaundice to be followed giving a reliable, objective record of the degree of icterus and a more sensitive indication of change than does clinical observation. These measurements may also be used to assess the effects of treatment.

In pernicious anaemia and chronic haemolytic anaemia, the total serum bilirubin rarely exceeds 50 μmol/l but increases up to as high as 200 μmol/l during an acute haemolytic episode. Determination of serum bilirubin is particularly useful in neonatal jaundice. Facilities for the determination in paediatric samples should be available at all times.

In viral hepatitis and in liver damage due to drugs and poisons the serum bilirubin rises to a peak between 350 and 500 μmol/l and then steadily returns to normal if recovery ensues. It is unusual for the bilirubin not to be falling 4 to 5 weeks after the onset of jaundice though full return to normal may take some time.

In obstructive jaundice, particularly if this is due to tumour and the obstruction is complete, the serum bilirubin rises to about 400 μmol/l and then remains roughly constant. Partial obstruction with fluctuating bilirubin levels is more suggestive of gall-stone obstruction than tumour.

Tests for Bile Pigments in Urine

Bilirubin glucuronide or urobilinogen may be present. The former produces obvious visual changes in moderate amounts but sensitive tests may be needed when visual examination is uncertain. Urobilinogen, being colourless, is not apparent on inspection unless it has been converted on standing to urobilin which imparts an orange brown colour to the urine. This should not be confused with the presence of bilirubin.

Bilirubin. The concentration of bilirubin by initial absorption on to insoluble barium salts, formed by adding barium chloride to urine, provides a sensitive test for detecting bilirubinuria.

Fouchet's Test. Add a few ml barium chloride solution (100 g/l) to about 10 ml urine in a test tube. Filter, allowing to drain well. Spread the filter paper on another dry paper and add a drop or two of Fouchet's reagent. To prepare this, dissolve 25 g trichloracetic acid in 50 ml water, add 10 ml ferric chloride solution (100 g/l) and make to 100 ml with water. A greenish-blue colour due to an oxidation product of bilirubin is obtained if this is present.

Commercial products based on the diazo reaction are available in reagent strip form from the Ames Company and the Boehringer Corporation; a tablet test is also available from Ames.

Ictotest (Ames). The tablets contain 0·2 mg *p*-nitrobenzene diazonium *p*-toluenesulphonate, 100 mg sulphosalicylic acid, 10 to 20 mg sodium bicarbonate and 15 to 25 mg boric acid. Small square asbestos paper mats are provided. Place 5 drops of urine on one of these mats and place a tablet on the moistened area. Pipette 2 drops of water on to the tablet allowing a few seconds between drops. The appearance of a bluish-purple colour on the mat within 30 s constitutes a positive test for bilirubin; an orange or reddish colour is taken as a negative result.

Reagent strips (Ames). The Ictostix strip introduced originally had a test area of cellulose impregnated with stabilised diazotised 2,4-dichloraniline. The area is pale cream in colour when dry or pale yellow when moist and showing a negative result. It changes to various shades of brown when bilirubin is present. Although Ictostix is no longer available as a separate strip, this test area is incorporated into the multiple test strips, Multistix and Bili-Labstix. The strip is dipped into the urine and 20 s later is compared with colour blocks corresponding to about 0·2, 0·5 and 1 mg bilirubin/100 ml. In practice the colour change is difficult to judge and the sensitivity achieved is appreciably less than the Ictotest method. The same diazo salt but in a strongly acid medium has been introduced as a test area on the newer N-Multistix. A purple colour is produced which is more easily distinguished from the starting colour and the sensitivity has increased to be comparable with Ictotest, a lower level of 0·2 mg/100 ml being just detectable. The test is said to be specific for bilirubin as regards biological material but positives may be given by urines from patients taking phenothiazines, while metabolites of drugs such as phenazopyridine (Pyridium) may give a red colour.

Reagent strips (Boehringer). The test area contains the fluoroborate salt of diazotised 2,6-dichloraniline. The strip is dipped briefly into the urine and 30 s later the degree of any red-violet coloration is compared with colour blocks. Colours developing at the edge of the area only, or after 2 min, are disregarded. The sensitivity in our experience is equal to that of Ictotest. The specificity is similar to the Ames N-Multistix area.

In summary, the laboratory tests are the most sensitive but the commercial products have the advantage of convenience for tests performed outside the laboratory. All tests should be done on freshly voided urine as bilirubin is destroyed on standing, particularly when exposed to light.

INTERPRETATION

Bilirubin is found in the urine in cholestatic jaundice in which there is regurgitation of conjugated bilirubin which being water soluble and only loosely attached to plasma albumin passes into the urine. There is a low but variable threshold level for conjugated bilirubin below which bilirubinuria does not occur. Bilirubinuria may be found in the early stages of viral hepatitis before clinical jaundice has developed. The absence of urine bilirubin in the recovery phase of jaundice, long unexplained, is now interpretable on the basis of δ-bilirubin. This protein-bound species predominates in late jaundice due to its long half-life and is, of course, not filtered at the glomerulus.

Bilirubin is not normally present in *faeces* since bacteria in the intestine reduce it to urobilinogen. Some may be found if there is very rapid passage of material along the intestine. It is found in the stools of very young infants before the gut flora has developed and in the faeces of patients who are being treated with gut-sterilising antibiotics. Bilirubin may be detected by adding Fouchet's reagent to a faecal suspension. A green to blue colour is then obtained.

Urobilinogen. As mentioned earlier, this term includes a number of substances. Due to improvements in blood tests urobilinogens in urine or faeces are less frequently required in present laboratory practice. Fresh samples should be stipulated to avoid the necessity of testing for the oxidised urobilins. For determination of faecal urobilinogen and quantitative urine urobilinogen as well as all urobilin tests, the reader is referred to the 5th edition of this book.

The traditional test is the red colour given by *p*-dimethylaminobenzaldehyde (Ehrlich's aldehyde) in strongly acid solution. The reaction depends on the presence of a central methene group in the 'urobilinogens' (Fig. 28.2, p. 717). Other naturally occurring substances give positive reactions, particularly porphobilinogen and indican, while the drugs *p*-aminosalicylic acid, sulphonamides and the sulphonyl ureas also react.

For the laboratory test add to 10 ml freshly voided urine, 1 ml Ehrlich's aldehyde reagent prepared by dissolving 2 g of *p*-dimethylaminobenzaldehyde in

48 ml concentrated hydrochloric acid and 50 ml water. Allow to stand 3 to 5 min and note any colour produced. Normal urines give only a pink colour but a distinctly red colour suggests the presence of increased amounts of urobilinogen. Differential extraction procedures (p. 649) distinguish porphobilinogen. For a semiquantitative assessment dilute the coloured solution with water. No pink colour is apparent at a dilution of 1 in 20 in normal urines but persists up to dilutions of 1 in 100 or more if urobilinogen excretion is marked. To form a blank, hydrochloric acid (6 mol/l) may be added instead of Ehrlich's reagent as acidification of urine alters the colour substantially in some cases. Commercial reagent strips are available from Ames and Boehringer. These should be used on freshly voided, well-mixed urine collected in well-washed vessels. Centrifuge if turbid.

Reagent strips (*Ames*). The Urobilistix strips have the active Ehrlich's reagent, *p*-dimethylaminobenzaldehyde, stabilised in an acid buffer, in an absorbent area at the tip.

They are said not to react with porphobilinogen at concentrations usually present in the urine of patients with porphobilinogenuria. They react with *p*-aminosalicylic acid but not with haemoglobin.

Reagent strips (*Boehringer*). These rely on the coupling of *p*-methoxybenzene diazonium fluoroborate in acid solution on the test strip to give a red azo dye. The reaction is said to be specific for urobilinogen. Interference has only been seen with drugs such as phenazopyridine (Pyridium) which become red in acid.

INTERPRETATION

The urine urobilinogen is derived from that part of the urobilinogen reabsorbed from the intestine which is not excreted by the liver. The amount present thus depends both on the amount of bilirubin entering the intestine and on the ability of the liver to excrete the urobilinogen coming to it from the intestine. Urine urobilinogen tends to be raised a little in haemolytic jaundice since the liver is not able to excrete completely the increased quantity absorbed in the intestine. Amounts up to 17 μmol/24 h may be found so that positive qualitative tests for urobilinogen or urobilin may be obtained with negative tests for bilirubin, a characteristic of all forms of retention jaundice.

In extra-hepatic obstructive jaundice the complete, or almost complete, absence of bilirubin in the intestine, which usually occurs, is reflected in a very low urobilinogen, unless the obstruction is intermittent.

In viral hepatitis there is usually some bilirubin entering the intestine. Although the amount of urobilinogen absorbed may be less than in normal persons, the liver cell is relatively less able to excrete it, so allowing more to pass into the systemic circulation and to be excreted in the urine. Consequently, the very low values seen in obstructive jaundice are much less common in hepatitis. Increased excretion is likely during convalescence until recovery is complete. Similarly, in cirrhosis of the liver, although less urobilinogen is formed in the intestine, the impaired liver function often results in an appreciable increase in urine urobilinogen. This may be of diagnostic value for in such cases bilirubin may not be present in the urine. The investigation of urine urobilinogen is largely redundant in hepatitis or obstructive disease.

Other factors to be considered are that bacterial overgrowth in the small intestine increases the urinary excretion of urobilinogen as this substance then has access to a larger absorptive area. Urobilinogen excretion is decreased in acidic urines due to increased tubular reabsorption.

Bile Acids and Salts

Terminology is confusing because, although any bile acid may be readily converted to its sodium or potassium salt, the term 'bile salt' is used in physiology to refer only to such salts formed from bile acids which have first undergone conjugation.

Chemistry. The hepatocytes synthesise bile acids from cholesterol which is either newly synthesised in the liver or derived from plasma lipids. Such bile acid production is subject to negative feedback by the quantity of bile acids returning to the liver in the enterohepatic circulation.

Two primary bile acids are formed, cholic and chenodeoxycholic (Fig. 28.4), which are then conjugated with glycine or taurine via the carboxyl group at C-24 to form the corresponding bile salts, e.g. glycocholate. The ratio of glycine conjugates to those of taurine varies but averages three to one. Most of the bile salts entering the gut are reabsorbed in the terminal ileum. Some bacterial deconjugation may occur in the ileum but the small proportion of bile salts reaching the colon is completely deconjugated. In addition, the colonic anaerobes dehydroxylate the free bile acids, mainly at the 7α position to yield secondary bile acids of which the most important are deoxycholic and lithocholic acids (Fig. 28.4). Some secondary bile acids and the remaining primary bile acids are returned to the liver in the enterohepatic circulation and are then reconjugated without rehydroxylation. Lithocholic acid is sulphated at the C-3 position to a significant extent.

The stereochemistry of the bile salts is such that all the hydrophilic groups are on one face of the steroid nucleus and this gives them surfactant properties important in the formation of micelles with cholesterol and phospholipid in the gall bladder and additionally with dietary lipids in the jejunum.

The Enterohepatic Circulation. Some 10% of conjugated bile acids enter the duodenum continuously without storage in the gall bladder but most are ejected following gall bladder contraction when chyle enters the duodenum. Some passive reabsorption of deconjugated bile acids occurs in the ileum but 95% are absorbed in conjugated or unconjugated form by an active sodium-dependent process in the terminal ileum. Much of the remaining bile acid is reabsorbed in the colon and about 1 mmol is lost in the faeces daily. Both conjugated and unconjugated bile acids return to the liver via the portal vein, bound to albumin. The hepatocytes extract 60 to 90% in one pass, the higher figures being for conjugated forms (84–90% for glycocholate). This is much greater than the figure of 5% for one pass of bilirubin through the liver.

The uptake and passage across the hepatocyte and excretion of the bile salts into the bile capillaries is an example of an organic anion transport process similar to, but not identical with, that for bilirubin or BSP. The bile acid pool is about 7 mmol and it undergoes 6–10 cycles daily so that the flux across the liver is 40–70 mmol/24 h. The loss of 1 mmol daily in the faeces and 1 μmol daily in the urine are replaced by synthesis.

Serum Bile Acids

As a consequence of these chemical and physiological events, fasting serum contains conjugates of primary and secondary bile acids as well as some unconjugated bile acids. Serum concentrations increase after meals, peaking at about 90 min after eating. The clinical importance of serum bile acid measurement lies mainly in the effect of liver disease on the organic anion transport

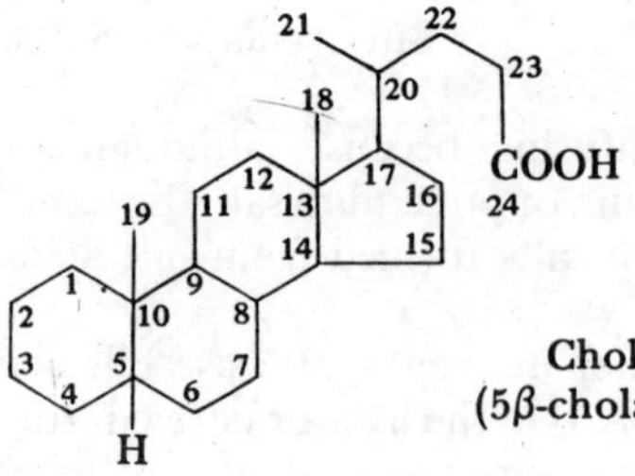

Cholanic acid
(5β-cholan-24-oic acid)

Primary Bile Acids

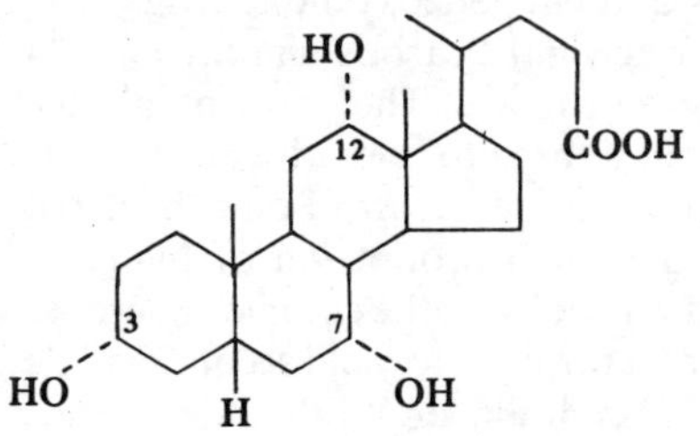

Cholic acid
(3α, 7α, 12α-trihydroxycholanic acid)

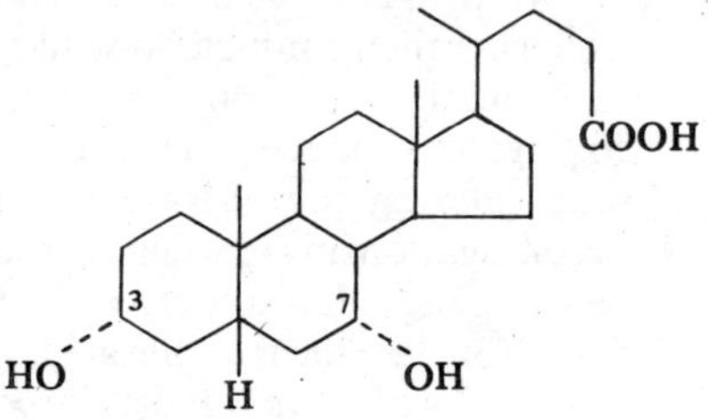

Chenodeoxycholic acid
(3α, 7α-dihydroxycholanic acid)

Secondary Bile Acids

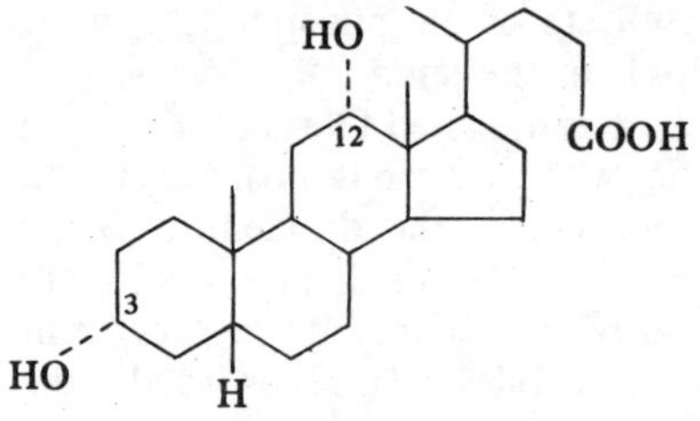

Deoxycholic acid
(3α, 12α-dihydroxycholanic acid)

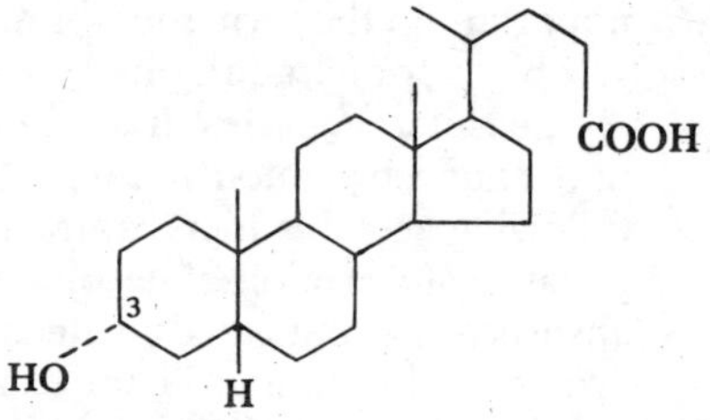

Lithocholic acid
(3α-hydroxycholanic acid)

Bile Salts Glycocholates   –CONHCH$_2$COOH

Taurocholates   –CONHCH$_2$CH$_2$SO$_3$H

Fig. 28.4. Structural Formulae of the Bile Acids and Salts.

process and the consequent ability to clear bile acids from the blood. Several other factors affect the concentration and pattern of serum bile acids, particularly deficient reabsorption in disease or absence of the distal ileum, and changes in the proportion of conjugated and unconjugated forms caused by bacterial over-growth of the small intestinal contents with consequent increase in ileal deconjugation.

Determination of Bile Acids in Serum

The number of bile acid species present and their low concentration in serum cause analytical problems and the results depend on the analytical procedure. Interpretation is also difficult, though potentially informative, because different species are extracted by the liver and absorbed by the intestine at different rates. At present, three main analytical methods are used.

Radioimmunoassay is very sensitive and requires no prior extraction of serum or derivatisation of the acids but it usually measures only conjugated forms and rarely the glycine and taurine conjugates separately. *Gas–liquid chromatography* (GLC), conventional or capillary, measures several species simultaneously but requires serum extraction, deconjugation of the acids and derivatisation. Preparative procedures which first separate the bile acids and their conjugates permit their later separate analysis. *Enzymatic methods* depend on the oxidation of the 3α-hydroxyl group to a 3-oxo group by 3α-hydroxysteroid dehydrogenase. The NADH produced at the same time is measured fluorimetrically. A bioluminescent method of NADH detection enhances the sensitivity. Enzymatic methods measure total bile acids as all possess the 3α-hydroxy group.

Radioimmunoassay of Serum Bile Acids. Radioimmunoassay (RIA) methods frequently measure glycocholic acid (Simmonds *et al.*, 1973; Miller *et al.*, 1981) but may also be used for other specific bile acid conjugates (e.g. of chenodeoxycholic acid) or primary bile acids as a group. Roda *et al.* (1980) compared two methods employing a ^{3}H-labelled tracer and four using a ^{125}I-labelled tracer. The former benefited from higher antibody affinity but sufficient sensitivity remained with the more convenient ^{125}I label. Miller *et al.* (1981) employed a cholylglycyltyrosine tracer iodinated using Chloramine T with subsequent Sephadex separation. The immunogen was coupled to bovine serum albumin and standards were prepared from ethanolic glycocholic acid. Anilinonaphthalenesulphonic acid in barbiturate buffer pH 6·8 releases glycocholate from protein, making extraction unnecessary. Polyethylene glycol was used to precipitate the antigen–antibody complex. The cross-reactivity was 7–17% for cholic, taurocholic and glycochenodeoxycholic acids, but was very low for all other bile acids and conjugates. A reference range of 0·0–1·29 μmol/l was found in the fasting state and comparison with a GLC method was satisfactory.

GLC Determination of Serum Bile Acids. GLC methods for bile acid analysis have been reported by Sandberg *et al.* (1965), Hofmann *et al.* (1970), Makino and Sjövall (1972), Ross (1977) and Setchell and Matsui (1983). Prior extraction of bile acids and conjugates, hydrolysis and subsequent formation of trimethylsilyl or trifluoroacetate derivatives is involved. Sandberg and colleagues used Amberlite ion-exchange resin followed by alumina chromatography to provide fractions for GLC. Setchell and Matsui employed reverse-phase bonded octadecylsilane cartridges (BondElut). Water was used to elute interfering substances and subsequently methanol eluted the bile acids and conjugates. Total non-sulphated bile acids were then measured by hydrolysing glycine and taurine conjugates using cholylglycine hydrolase. The unconjugated bile acids were extracted and separated on a Lipidex 10 000 column using methanol elution. After forming the methyl ester, trimethylsilyl ether derivatives, these were analysed by GLC using open glass capillary columns, wall-coated with OV-1. Alternatively, unconjugated and conjugated bile acids may be separated before the hydrolysis stage and derivatised separately before analysis. Such GLC techniques, possibly coupled with mass spectrometric detection, are mainly of specialised interest and should be regarded as supplements to, rather than replacements of, simpler methods.

Enzymatic Assay of Total Serum Bile Acids. This is a relatively simple procedure. In the method of Murphy *et al.* (1970), serum is pipetted into hot ethanol and the protein precipitate is further extracted with ethanol. The combined extracts containing the bile acids and their conjugates are evaporated to dryness. The residue is partitioned between alcohol and ether-heptane to remove neutral lipids and then further concentrated to give a 3-fold increase relative to the initial concentration in serum. The enzymatic oxidation is carried out with 3α-hydroxysteroid dehydrogenase from *Pseudomonas testosteroni* and the NADH so produced is measured fluorimetrically. The reaction is forced to completion by trapping the oxosteroid product with hydrazine. Full practical details are given in the 5th edition of this book.

Bile Acids in Urine. The detection and measurement of bile acids in urine is unsatisfactory and of less importance now that serum bile acid analysis is practicable. Colorimetric and thin-layer chromatographic methods are described in the previous edition of this book.

INTERPRETATION

The value of serum bile acid analysis is still a matter of debate but its main use appears to lie in the discrimination of mild liver disease and in the assessment of the progress of chronic liver disease.

Reference ranges (in μmol/l) are method-dependent: some examples are 0·6–4·7 (Sandberg *et al.*, 1965; GLC), 0·24–4·3 (Makino *et al.*, 1969; GLC), 0–4·7 for males and 1·0–8·2 for females (Murphy *et al.*, 1970; enzymatic), 0·3–1·5 for conjugated cholic acid and 0·4–2·5 for conjugated chenodeoxycholic acid (Roda *et al.*, 1980; RIA) and 0–1·29 for glycocholic acid (Miller *et al.*, 1981; RIA). Serum bile acids are found in higher concentrations in the neonate and in the last weeks of pregnancy and further study is needed in these groups.

An increased concentration of bile acids in non-fasting serum collected at 12·00 to 14·00 h was found to be a highly sensitive indicator of hepatobiliary disease but did not discriminate well between the different conditions causing this (Matsui *et al.*, 1982). A 2 h postprandial measurement was more sensitive than a basal, fasting one and probably superior to BSP retention at 45 min (Kaplowitz *et al.*, 1973). Discriminant analysis of serum bile acids and other conventional liver function tests showed no significant advantage of the former (Linnet and Andersen, 1983; Cravetto *et al.*, 1985). However, Lawrence *et al.* (1985) found bile acids to be more specific in diagnosis of occult liver disease as a cause of pruritus while Kishimoto *et al.* (1985) found that bile acids detected decompensation of liver cirrhosis earlier than other tests and 1–4 months before the onset of ascites.

Ratios of bile acid concentrations have found some favour. The ratio of trihydroxy to dihydroxy acids, mainly the cholic/chenodeoxycholic ratio, is affected by the greater depression of cholic acid synthesis in hepatocellular disease. In 80 % of hepatocellular lesions or cirrhosis, the ratio is less than one, but exceeds one in 80 % of cholestatic lesions. No distinction between intra- and extrahepatic cholestasis was possible (Javitt, 1975). Linnet and Andersen (1983) found the ratio to be the best discriminating factor in diagnosing parenchymal, obstructive or malignant liver disease. Bile acid measurements are normal in Gilbert's syndrome and unhelpful in the diagnosis of the Dubin–Johnson syndrome.

Serum concentrations of bile acids are affected not only by the ability of the liver to extract them from the blood but also by the efficiency of small intestinal absorption and by the effect of bacterial flora in the small intestine. The technical difficulties of analysis remain a problem, especially if there is a need to measure different bile acids or conjugates. For a comprehensive review of the value of bile acid measurement in man see Percy-Robb (1985).

The small quantity of faecal bile acids excreted in a 24 h period is a reflection of the rate of bile acid synthesis but measurement is laborious.

Tests Using Bromsulphthalein

The transport, conjugation and excretory abilities of the liver cell may also be tested by administration of a load of BSP or indocyanine green (ICG). This has the advantage that the load can be standardised, administered as a bolus or continuously, and the kinetics of changes in blood concentrations can be assessed. Similar procedures have occasionally been used with administered loads of bile acids or bilirubin.

BSP Metabolism. After intravenous injection, BSP binds largely to albumin and is taken up very little by extrahepatic tissues; its renal excretion accounts for about 2% of total excretion if the hepatic clearance is normal. The anion is taken up by the liver cell and is bound intracellularly to Z protein and to ligandin (Y protein) which also catalyses its conjugation with glutathione. The hepatic uptake and biliary excretion of BSP requires mechanisms common to bilirubin and ICG but different from those for bile acids (Goresky, 1965; Scharschmidt *et al.*, 1975). A significant proportion of BSP may be excreted unconjugated even in normals and the method of analysis does not distinguish between conjugated and unconjugated forms.

BSP Excretion Test

The simplest form of the test involves intravenous injection of a single bolus of a solution of BSP (50 g/l) and measurement of the serum concentration 45 min later. The dose is related to body weight (5 mg/kg) and is administered over 30 to 60 s. Assuming an average plasma volume an initial plasma concentration of approximately 100 mg/l is obtained. After 45 min, blood is taken from the other arm and the concentration of BSP calculated as a percentage of the initial concentration.

$$\text{Retention at 45 min } (\%) = \frac{\text{Serum concentration at 45 min (mg/l)}}{100} \times 100$$

Extravasation of BSP causes considerable pain so careful injection is imperative. Occasionally intravenous administration will cause anaphylactic shock and fatal results have been reported, usually with larger doses (Venger, 1961; Katz and Scarf, 1964).

Determination of BSP

BSP is purple in alkaline solution and colourless in acid. The difference in absorbance at 580 nm in acid and alkaline solutions is a measure of BSP.

Reagents.
1. Sodium hydroxide solution, 100 mmol/l.
2. Hydrochloric acid, 100 mmol/l.
3. Standard solution of BSP. Dissolve 100 mg BSP in water and make to 100 ml. Dilute 1 in 10 for use, giving a 100 mg/l solution.

Technique. To 0·5 ml serum add 2·5 ml water and 3·0 ml reagent (1). For the blank use 0·5 ml serum, 2·5 ml water and 3·0 ml reagent (2). Treat the standard in the same way. Mix and read all against water at 580 nm.

Calculation. Serum BSP (mg/l) =

$$\frac{\text{Reading of unknown in alkali} - \text{Reading of unknown in acid}}{\text{Reading of standard in alkali} - \text{Reading of standard in acid}} \times 100$$

For a standard curve to check linearity use 0·1, 0·2, 0·3, 0·4 and 0·5 ml of standard diluted to 3 ml with water and treat as for the test. These correspond to 20, 40, 60, 80 and 100 mg BSP/l.

It is usually assumed that the maximum BSP concentration reached is 100 mg/l. A rough check can be obtained by taking a 4 min specimen from the opposite arm to the injection site.

INTERPRETATION

In normals the retention of BSP at 45 min is less than 5% but somewhat higher values may be found in old age. Either cholestasis or impairment of liver cell function causes an increase in BSP retention and the test is very sensitive, being abnormal before the occurrence of jaundice. Indeed the test has little value in the presence of jaundice as it is very non-specific and not generally of diagnostic use in assessing the cause of the jaundice. The test may be used to detect mild impairment of hepatic function, or assess progress of anicteric cirrhosis, when BSP retention is increased. Occasionally, normal values are found in cirrhosis, possibly due to the increased volume of distribution consequent upon ascites. The reverse problem may be the cause of occasional high results in obesity when a large portion of the body mass used to calculate the BSP dose is not accessible to water-soluble species. Diminished hepatic blood flow in congestive cardiac failure without liver disease may prolong the retention of BSP. Haemolytic disease or conjugation defects such as Crigler–Najjar syndrome do not affect BSP retention but high results are usual in Gilbert's syndrome.

More Complex Treatment of BSP Excretion

More complex assessment depends on the use of mathematical modelling. This may take the form of curve fitting, concept fitting or biomathematics. Measurement of BSP at frequent intervals after a load defines a disappearance curve which may be 'fitted' by a mathematical equation, usually a multiple exponential of the form

$$c(t) = c_0 (ae^{-k_1 t} + be^{-k_2 t} + \ldots)$$

where, $c(t)$ = concentration at time t, k_1, etc. are rate constants and a, b, etc. are coefficients (parameters). The rate constants and parameters derived may or may not have any direct relation to physiological factors though it is often assumed that the number of parameters equals the number of compartments into which the dye passes. The disappearance curve for BSP can be fitted by the sum of two exponentials, the first (corresponding to 9–16% extraction per minute in normals) reflects mainly hepatic blood flow and hepatocellular uptake.

In the 'concept fitting' approach a model of BSP excretion is devised; for example

$$\text{plasma} \underset{g}{\overset{f}{\rightleftharpoons}} \text{liver} \overset{h}{\rightarrow} \text{bile}$$

Values for f, g and h may be obtained from plasma disappearance curves but the model is an oversimplification. Thus although f relates well to hepatic uptake, h relates to a number of processes including conjugation and excretion, and as such the value of the derived rates is limited.

The most sophisticated approach, that of biomathematics, attempts to represent each individual metabolic process mathematically and may be able to discern which of several possible pathways or processes are important in a complex physiological process and how they alter in pathology by calculation of rate constants and parameters associated with the various pathways.

An example of concept fitting is given below.

T_M **and** S **in Liver Disease.** Assume that BSP is not sequestered in any extravascular space, is not lost to urine and that it is transported to bile by a saturable process with a maximum rate T_M. Let us also assume that over a limited range of BSP concentration, the quantity of BSP stored in the liver is proportional to the serum concentration (proportionality constant S, storage capacity). At an infusion rate I_1 (greater than T_M) a constant rate of increase in plasma BSP concentration will be achieved $\left(\dfrac{\mathrm{d}C_P}{\mathrm{d}t}\right)_1$ and if the plasma volume is V_P then

$$I_1 = T_M + V_P\left(\frac{\mathrm{d}C_P}{\mathrm{d}t}\right)_1 + S\left(\frac{\mathrm{d}C_P}{\mathrm{d}t}\right)_1$$

and at a second infusion rate, I_2,

$$I_2 = T_M + V_P\left(\frac{\mathrm{d}C_P}{\mathrm{d}t}\right)_2 + S\left(\frac{\mathrm{d}C_P}{\mathrm{d}t}\right)_2$$

In practice BSP is infused for an hour at a rate approximately twice the expected T_M and in the second 30 min a constant increase in plasma concentration is achieved. The infusion rate is then decreased (I_2 approximately $0.3 \times I_1$) for 1 h and a constant decrease in plasma BSP concentration is achieved in the second half hour. Solution of simultaneous equations of the type shown above gives values for T_M and S. In normal subjects, T_M is approximately 8 mg/min and S is 6 mg l mg^{-1}. T_M agrees fairly well with direct measurements of BSP biliary excretion obtained by intubation.

In diffuse hepatic disease T_M and S are reduced, in obstruction T_M is reduced but S is normal. In Dubin–Johnson syndrome S is normal and T_M is less than 2 mg/min. In a conventional BSP excretion test, subjects with Dubin–Johnson syndrome have a normal 45 min value, but the serum concentration rises towards 90 min due to regurgitation. In the Rotor syndrome the reverse applies, and S is low but T_M approximately normal. Gilbert's syndrome does not follow a simple pattern and analysis, somewhat different from the above, has permitted distinction of three sub-groups, one with normal BSP excretion, one with decreased uptake and one with impairment after the stage of hepatic uptake.

For a fuller discussion of the factors involved in mathematical modelling and the potential value of such measurements in the study of liver function, see Carson and Jones (1979) and Jones and Berk (1982). In other than specialised centres, however, the main use of BSP excretion would appear to be in the assessment of moderate hepatic dysfunction and in the investigation of benign familial causes of jaundice.

TESTS BASED ON THE INTERMEDIARY METABOLIC FUNCTION

Tests of the ability of the liver to metabolise galactose to glucose or to remove amino acids from the plasma are of potential value in diagnosing liver cell dysfunction or in assessing the progress of chronic liver disease.

Galactose Elimination Tests

Galactose metabolism is confined to the liver and the rate-limiting step is the initial conversion to galactose-1-phosphate by galactokinase. The kinetics of this step depend on the rate of galactose delivery to the liver. The rate of utilisation of galactose, however expressed, is proportional to the functioning liver cell mass.

Tengstrom (1966, 1968) and Tengstrom *et al.* (1967) gave 350 mg galactose per kg body weight as a 25–30 % solution intravenously over 3 min and took capillary blood at 10 min intervals for 1 h after. Blood galactose concentrations fell according to first order kinetics and the half-life was determined by plotting the logarithm of the galactose concentration against time. This half-life was 12 ± 2.6 (SD) min in normals and was markedly longer in cirrhosis and infective hepatitis. A similar test has been shown to be relatively independent of hepatic blood flow, an important factor in cirrhosis (Tygstrup, 1966). Bircher (1983) used a higher dose, 500 mg/kg and found zero order elimination. He then calculated the initial galactose elimination capacity in $mg\,min^{-1}\,kg^{-1}$

Galactose can be measured in blood using galactose oxidase (de Verdier and Hjelm, 1962) in a manner equivalent to that for glucose using glucose oxidase. Alternatively, the production of NADH by the action of galactose dehydrogenase on galactose may be measured using commercial reagents (Boehringer).

Determination of Blood Galactose

Reagents.
1. Phosphate buffer, 200 mmol/l, pH 7·5.
2. Nicotinamide adenine dinucleotide, 13 mmol/l; the equivalent of 9 mg pure monohydrate per ml.
3. Galactose dehydrogenase, 5 mg/ml, (Boehringer).
4. Perchloric acid. Dilute 2·85 ml perchloric acid (sp. gr. 1·70) with water to 100 ml.

Technique. Add 200 μl fresh blood to 1 ml perchloric acid in a centrifuge tube, sucking up and down several times, and centrifuge. Pipette into a spectrophotometer cuvette, 3 ml buffer, 100 μl NAD$^+$ and 200 μl supernatant. Mix and read the absorbance (A_1) at 340 nm. Add 20 μl galactose dehydrogenase, mix, and when the reaction stops (30 to 40 min) again read the absorbance (A_2). To obtain the absorbance due to the enzyme (A_e) mix 3·3 ml buffer and 20 μl enzyme and read against the buffer.

Calculation.

$$\text{Blood galactose (mmol/l)} = (A_2 - A_1 - A_e) \times 15{\cdot}6$$

Serum Amino Acids in Liver Disease

An abnormal plasma amino acid profile is found in hepatic coma (Fischer *et al.*, 1974; Rosen *et al.*, 1977) with phenylalanine, tyrosine and methionine increased and the peripherally metabolised branched-chain amino acids, leucine, isoleucine and valine, reduced.

Phenylalanine, tyrosine and tryptophan figures correlate positively with blood ammonia after an ammonia load ($r = +0.758$) and negatively with galactose elimination capacity ($r = -0.657$) according to Zoli *et al.* (1981). The relationship to hepatocellular function is borne out by the decreased hepatic aromatic amino acid oxidase activity in cirrhosis (Nordlinger, 1979). The ratio of aromatic (phenylalanine and tyrosine) to branched-chain amino acids has shown some prognostic value in chronic active hepatitis (McCullough *et al.*, 1981). Both branched-chain and aromatic amino acids rise more after a protein load in cirrhotics than in normals (Marchesini *et al.*, 1983) as a result of a number of effects beside hepatic oxidase activity, including increased endogenous protein breakdown.

Apart from an automated colorimetric assay for methionine used in assessing the progress of acute liver failure (Collins *et al.*, 1978), analysis of plasma or serum amino acids is by ion-exchange chromatography or, more recently, by HPLC (Turnell and Cooper, 1982).

TESTS BASED ON THE SYNTHETIC FUNCTION

These have been almost entirely related to protein synthesis as the liver is the main source of plasma proteins, with the exception of immunoglobulins. Whereas obstructive jaundice, without liver cell damage, has little effect on serum protein concentrations, viral hepatitis, chronic active hepatitis and various forms of cirrhosis are associated with a fall in serum albumin and a rise in immunoglobulin concentrations in different degrees. Such changes were once assessed by a number of turbidity and flocculation tests which are no longer used. Concentrations of the different immunoglobulin fractions are affected differently in a number of liver disorders (p. 430) but the changes are seldom specific enough to be of great diagnostic value.

Plasma Proteins Synthesised in the Liver

Impaired hepatocellular function or decreased functional mass of liver results in decreased protein synthesis. The concentration of serum albumin may decrease as a result and its measurement has a well established role in this respect. Care in interpretation is necessary however, as variation in catabolic rate, distribution between intra- and extravascular spaces (especially with accumulation of extravascular fluid in ascites) and the role of renal or intestinal loss must be borne in mind. Rapid decreases in serum albumin can occur in the acute phase of reaction to trauma or infection and also in malignancy.

Serum albumin has a half-life of 16 days and responds slowly to altered conditions, especially in the recovery phase. Proteins with a shorter half-life (e.g. prealbumin, half-life 2 days) may respond more rapidly and sensitively to changes in liver function and prealbumin has been suggested as a liver function test (Hutchinson *et al.*, 1981; Teppo and Maury, 1983) though the problems outlined above with respect to interpretation of serum albumin still apply.

Fibrinogen is only decreased in severe liver failure, its concentration being increased in infection and other causes of acute phase reaction. Depressed synthesis of liver-produced clotting factors is of practical importance in treatment as well as diagnosis of liver disease. However, prothrombin synthesis is dependent on vitamin K availability as well as on adequate hepatocellular function. Purely obstructive conditions may depress vitamin K absorption due to inadequate entry of bile to the small intestine and an adequate supply of vitamin K must be assured by parenteral administration before a prolonged prothrombin time is attributed to liver cell damage. For a discussion of coagulation factors and their measurement see Biggs (1976) and Dacie and Lewis (1984).

Two specific proteins of use in diagnosis in liver disease are α-fetoprotein, frequently increased in primary hepatoma, and ceruloplasmin which is usually present in lower concentration in Wilson's disease (p. 634).

TESTS BASED ON THE DETOXIFICATION FUNCTION

The liver is involved in the removal of potentially hazardous substances from the body. These may be endogenous, e.g. ammonia, active hormones, or exogenous, chemicals and drugs. The metabolic changes often involve oxidation at the microsomes and conjugation with various substances to produce a more polar, water-soluble derivative suitable for excretion in the urine or in the bile. This function thus depends on the presence of an adequate functional mass of liver cells. An early test involved the conjugation of benzoate to form hippurate but currently only two substances are worthy of comment, ammonia and aminopyrine.

Blood Ammonia

Ammonia is present in high concentration in portal venous blood having been formed by bacterial action on nitrogenous material in the colon and then absorbed. It is also formed from glutamine in the kidney and from adenine in muscle. Ammonia reaching the liver is converted to urea but this process may be affected by liver cell damage or by the presence of shunts allowing portal blood to by-pass the liver.

Although ammonia is probably not the cause of hepatic encephalopathy, and its concentration in blood is not well correlated with the severity of coma, its measurement may be used to monitor deterioration or improvement in an individual with acute hepatic failure. Basal measurements, or those after an ammonia load, can be used to assess portocaval shunting in cirrhosis. After surgical portocaval anastomosis, blood ammonia can reflect the success of dietary or lactulose treatment on encephalopathic problems, should these occur.

The measurement of blood ammonia is useful in certain childhood diseases, notably acute illness in the very young which may be due to metabolic causes (p. 391), in particular urea cycle defects (Holton, 1982) and Reye's syndrome.

Determination of Ammonia in Blood and Plasma

Early methods employing diffusion in the Conway unit (Bessman, 1954) or colorimetric methods using the Berthelot reaction on a deproteinated supernatant (McCullough, 1967) have been largely superseded. Methods using ion-exchange resins are still employed (Dienst, 1961; Forman, 1964) but Gerron *et al.* (1976) using the Forman method found poor precision and accuracy and attributed these to five factors:

1. Pollution of the laboratory atmosphere or glassware by detergents containing ammonia.
2. Smoking by patients or staff. If the patient smokes one cigarette one hour before venepuncture, the plasma ammonia increases by 6 to 12 μmol/l. Smoking by staff releases ammonia into the atmosphere.
3. Delay, turbulence or the use of a heparin lock during venepuncture. An increase of 6 to 12 μmol/l results from the use of a heparin lock, or by drawing blood into a syringe followed by transfer to a tube containing anticoagulant, or by partial filling of an evacuated tube with subsequent admission of air.
4. Delay or allowing the plasma temperature to rise above 0 °C before mixing with the resin.
5. Delay in analysing the column eluate.

Stringent control of these factors improved analytical performance and some of them will be applicable to other methods.

Ammonia electrodes have been used, either based on an ammonium ion-selective electrode or on a glass pH electrode immersed in ammonium chloride solution and separated from the sample by an ammonia-permeable membrane. Currently, the enzymatic procedure is considered to be the method of choice. This involves the reaction:

$$\alpha\text{-Oxoglutarate} + NH_4^+ + NAD(P)H \xrightarrow{\text{GLDH}} \text{L-Glutamate} + NAD(P)^+ + H_2O$$

When there is an excess of enzyme, glutamate dehydrogenase, and NAD(P)H the reaction rate is dependent only on the concentration of ammonia and the equilibrium alters to favour glutamate formation. The amount of ammonia present is directly related to the rate of disappearance of NAD(P)H which may be followed spectrophotometrically (Muting *et al.*, 1968; Oreskes *et al.*, 1969) or fluorimetrically (Rubin and Knott, 1967). An end-point technique may also be used and a convenient kit for this is available from the Boehringer Corporation or Sigma. These commercial methods are recommended and the manufacturers' leaflets should be consulted for the full practical details.

The enzymatic procedure minimises technical problems of contamination from glassware, acidic solutions and release of ammonia from blood constituents. The rapid breakdown of nitrogenous substances in blood to release ammonia is delayed for up to 20 min by using heparin anticoagulation and placing the specimen in an ice bath. Leffler (1967) used an enzyme-inhibiting anticoagulant, the dipotassium salt of ethylene dinitrilotetracetate. Direct transfer of whole blood to a protein precipitant reduces this source of error in some methods and accounts for the frequent measurement of blood, rather than plasma, ammonia. Even then, glutamine may still release ammonia in the absence of enzymatic action.

INTERPRETATION
Measurement of ammonia in arterial blood is said to be more reliable than in venous blood due to the variable release of ammonia from peripheral muscle. Venous blood is, however, usually used and the Boehringer enzymatic kit method gives an upper reference limit of 50 μmol/l. Some methods have been reported to give a lower limit such as 35 μmol/l but slight increases are difficult to interpret due to the technical problems outlined earlier. Very significant increases in blood ammonia have been reported in acutely ill neonates without specific liver involvement (Beddis *et al.*, 1980).

An ammonia tolerance test has been used to assess the ability of the liver to deal with ammonia coming to it from the intestine (e.g. see Conn, 1961; Zoli *et al.*, 1981). This is carried out as follows. Fast the patient for 12 h before beginning the test, allowing only fluids during that time. Take a specimen of blood for ammonia determination, then give orally 10 g ammonium citrate dissolved in water flavoured with fruit juice. Determine the ammonia concentration in blood 30, 60, 120 and 180 min later. In patients with high initial results give only 5 g. In normal persons, blood ammonia increases little remaining within the reference range for the method. A marked rise to twice the initial value or more is seen in patients with cirrhosis and on occasion may exceed 200 μmol/l. Considerable increases occur if there is a collateral circulation (McDermott, 1959) and after portocaval anastomosis. The test has been used to show the presence and size of such a circulation or the patency of the surgical shunt. An occasional hazard is that a patient in prehepatic coma may deteriorate rapidly after the full dose of ammonium salt.

The Aminopyrine Breath Test

Aminopyrine is metabolised by the liver by *N*-demethylation to give carbon dioxide. Using [^{14}C]methyl-labelled aminopyrine, the appearance of $^{14}CO_2$ corresponds to the microsomal mixed function oxidase mass of rat liver (Lautenburg and Bircher, 1976). As a result, $^{14}CO_2$ excretion is reduced in parenchymal cell liver diseases such as cirrhosis, acute and chronic hepatitis, and neoplasia. Overlap of the values obtained limits diagnostic use but Schneider *et al.* (1980) found the test to predict short term survival, clinical improvement and histological severity more reliably than other conventional liver function tests.

After an overnight fast, 2 μCi of amino[^{14}C]pyrine and 2 mg unlabelled aminopyrine is administered orally. Breath, dried over calcium sulphate, is bubbled through a solution of 2 ml ethanol and 1 ml hyamine hydroxide, 1 mol/l, containing 2 drops of phenolphthalein. When the indicator colour changes, indicating the absorption of 1 mmol of carbon dioxide, the activity of $^{14}CO_2$ is measured in a scintillation counter. For further information and for the use of antipyrine as an alternative see Heppner and Vessell (1975), Vessell (1984) and Henry *et al.* (1985).

SERUM ENZYMES IN LIVER DISEASE AND JAUNDICE

The activity of hepatic enzymes in serum may be affected by their increased or decreased synthesis, release from damaged cells, release from extra-hepatic tissues and their disappearance rates from plasma. Several different enzymes have been studied.

Aminotransferases. Aspartate aminotransferase (AST, EC 2.6.1.1) and alanine aminotransferase (ALT, EC 2.6.1.2) increase in plasma activity in the presence of parenchymal liver cell damage. The increase is very great in viral and toxic hepatitis with ALT greater than AST. In alcoholic hepatitis and cirrhosis the ratio is often reversed and activities of both enzymes less elevated (De Ritis *et al.* 1972). These findings are related to the origin of the enzymes, which is cytoplasmic for ALT but both cytoplasmic and mitochondrial for AST. Return to normal values occurs in weeks or months after acute hepatitis and elevation beyond 6 months usually indicates development of chronic liver disease. Substantial increases occur in ischaemic liver damage due to myocardial infarction or congestive cardiac failure but return to normal may occur in a few days. Aminotransferases are often normal in chronic active hepatitis and cholestatic conditions may induce mild increases in serum activity. A number of other parenchymal enzymes may be measured (for example isocitrate dehydrogenase and glutamate dehydrogenase) but their measurement adds only marginally to the information gained from AST and ALT.

Alkaline Phosphatase. The isoenzyme of hepatic origin arises from the lining of bile canaliculi and also from sinusoidal surfaces of hepatocytes. The largest rises in serum activity occur in posthepatic obstruction and this is related in part to increased synthesis of the enzyme. Although there is some overlap, cholestasis associated with viral hepatitis usually causes lesser elevations than drug-induced cholestasis. Increased serum alkaline phosphatase activity is usually associated with jaundice, but infiltration due to sarcoid, tuberculosis, primary or secondary malignancies can cause an isolated increase in activity of the enzyme. Such an increase is also the earliest biochemical manifestation in primary biliary cirrhosis.

Other sources of alkaline phosphatase (bone, intestine or placenta) must be considered but, especially when elevations are moderate, difficulty of interpretation often makes isoenzyme analysis of marginal value except when a tumour-related placental alkaline phosphatase is involved, e.g. in cases of carcinoma of the bronchus. Unexplained increases in alkaline phosphatase activity are not uncommon, especially in infants (Lockitch *et al.*, 1984).

Gammaglutamyl Transpeptidase (GGT). This enzyme is increased in situations similar to those causing increased alkaline phosphatase and a normal value can be of use in identifying a non-hepatic origin for the latter. GGT is, however, very non-specific and is affected by induction of enzyme synthesis by alcohol and drugs such as the anticonvulsants, and also by release from damaged hepatocytes. These factors complicate its interpretation (Penn and Worthington, 1983).

Other Enzymes. Leucine aminopeptidase and 5'-nucleotidase activities are raised in obstructive biliary tract disease and may occasionally be of additional value. Cholinesterase is produced in the liver and then released normally into the circulation. The activity is reduced in liver cell dysfunction and has been used as a test of liver function in a similar fashion to serum albumin, prealbumin and prothrombin. The reduced activity may lead to prolongation of the effects of succinylcholine (p. 507).

The Use of Tests in Liver Disease

The various 'liver function tests' described measure different aspects of liver function, or are indices of liver cell damage rather than function; many may be affected by factors unrelated to the liver. Thus the hepatic blood flow affects some tests in the absence of cellular dysfunction, particularly those dependent on the capacity of the liver to extract species from the blood. Despite much interest, complex batteries of biochemical tests and discriminant analysis of the results have not become widely used. In part, this has been due to the development of other, non-biochemical methods of investigating the liver. These include the various 'imaging' techniques, the use of needle biopsy of the liver and immunological methods. For example the detection of antimitochondrial antibody is a useful early marker of primary biliary cirrhosis. Biochemical tests are therefore part of a spectrum of investigations available. For many purposes a limited range of biochemical tests suffices. Those generally regarded as helpful include the measurement of serum bilirubin (sometimes as conjugated and unconjugated fractions), enzymes, particularly alkaline phosphatase, AST, ALT and, in some cases, GGT, and such serum proteins as albumin, immunoglobulins and prothrombin.

The biochemical tests are used in three ways.

1. For the differential diagnosis of the various types of jaundice.
2. To assess the degree of liver damage in known liver disease, its alteration with time and its response to therapeutic measures.
3. In the diagnosis of subclinical impairment of liver function. This includes assessment of residual damage after apparent recovery from viral hepatitis; the screening of suspected cases during an epidemic of viral hepatitis; the screening of persons exposed to possible hepatotoxic substances in industry or to potentially hepatotoxic drugs; the monitoring of alcoholism.

1. *Differential diagnosis of jaundice.* Biochemical tests such as serum bilirubin and enzymes distinguish fairly well between haemolytic causes of jaundice, acute hepatitis and posthepatic obstruction. However, the distinction of greatest importance is that between extrahepatic cholestasis for which surgery is the usual course of action, and intrahepatic cholestasis for which medical treatment is appropriate and surgical intervention potentially life-threatening. Biochemical tests do not discriminate between these conditions unequivocally.

In recent years the refinement of 'imaging' techniques such as ultrasonography, percutaneous transhepatic cholangiography, endoscopic retrograde cholangio-pancreatography and computerised axial tomography have revolutionised the investigation of the more difficult problems. Such investigations are expensive in equipment and medical time and 75 % of cases may be diagnosed by the taking of a careful history, clinical examination and a few conventional biochemical tests of liver function (Bouchier, 1982).

Biochemical investigation can be particularly helpful in diagnosing benign familial causes of jaundice and, in so doing, avoiding excessive investigation for more serious liver disease. Thus in Gilbert's syndrome, increase in serum bilirubin on a low calorie intake, fall after phenobarbitone, normality of serum bile acids or occurrence of BSP retention will usually differentiate the condition from other causes of unconjugated hyperbilirubinaemia. The use of the BSP test to recognise the Dubin–Johnson syndrome was mentioned earlier.

2. *Assessing the extent of functional liver failure.* Galactose tests are particularly useful in the presence of jaundice as is the BSP test if cholestatic jaundice is absent. The aminopyrine breath test may also find increasing application. The fall in serum albumin and the rise in immunoglobulins give an indication of the severity of liver damage and are valuable in prognosis. Although liver function is severely impaired in widespread necrosis of liver cells, the reverse is not necessarily true. In advanced cirrhosis, increased activity of serum enzymes is often slight but considerable interference with function is shown by the marked increase in serum bile acids and urinary urobilinogen.

3. *Diagnosis of sub-clinical liver disease.* The liver has considerable functional reserve and regeneration capacity in chronic liver disease, e.g. alcoholic cirrhosis. The most sensitive indicator of impaired liver function varies as not all functions are affected equally at any particular stage. Several tests are preferable. In most cases jaundice is likely to be absent, so the BSP test can often be used and many workers consider this to be one of the most sensitive tests. If this, the serum bile acids and galactose tests are all normal it is unlikely that any other test would

prove to be abnormal. An exception is alcoholism in which GGT is a more sensitive index of liver changes (Rosalki *et al.,* 1970).

Serum ALT activity is very useful for screening suspects in the prodromal period during outbreaks of viral hepatitis.

REFERENCES

Andres J. M., *et al.* (1977). *J. Pediat;* **91**: 217.

Beddis I. R., Hughes E. A., Rosser E., Fenton J. C. B. (1980). *Arch. Dis. Childh;* **55**: 566.

Berk J. E., ed. (1985). *Bockus Gastroenterology,* Vol. 5, 4th ed. Philadelphia: Saunders.

Berk P. (1981). In *Familial Hyperbilirubinaemia.* (Okolicsanyi L., ed) p. 7. New York: John Wiley and Sons.

Bessman S. P. (1954). In *Advances in Clinical Chemistry,* Vol. 2. (Sobotka H., Stewart C. P., eds) p. 135. New York: Academic Press.

Biggs R., ed. (1976). *Human Blood Coagulation, Haemostasis and Thrombosis,* 2nd ed. Oxford: Blackwell Scientific Publications.

Billing B. H. (19o1). In *Familial Hyperbilirubinaemia.* (Okolicsanyi L., ed) p. 1. New York: John Wiley and Sons.

Billing B. H. (1983). *Postgrad. Med. J;* **59**: Suppl. 4, 19.

Billing B. H., Haslam R., Wald N. (1971). *Ann. Clin. Biochem;* **8**: 21.

Bircher J. (1983). *Semin. Liv. Dis;* **3**: 275.

Bleicher M. A., Reiner M. A., Rapaport S. A., Track N. S. (1979). *Pediat. Surg;* **14**: 527.

Bouchier I. A. D. (1982). *Brit. Med. J;* **283**: 1282.

Carson E. R., Jones E. A. (1979). *New Engl. J. Med;* **300**: 1016.

Collins D. J., Robinson R., Knell A. R. (1978). *Clin. Chim. Acta;* **88**: 277.

Colombo J. P., Peheim E., Kyburz S., Hoffmann J. P. (1974). *Clin. Chim. Acta;* **51**: 217.

Conn H. O. (1961). *Gastroenterology;* **41**: 97.

Cravetto C., *et al.* (1985). *Ann. Clin. Biochem;* **22**: 596.

Dacie J. V., Lewis S. M. (1984). *Practical Haematology;* 6th ed. London: Churchill Livingstone.

De Ritis F., Coltosti M., Giusti G. (1972). *Lancet;* **1**: 685.

Dienst S. G. (1961). *J. Lab. Clin. Med;* **49**: 779.

Doumas B. T., Perry B. W., Sasse E. A., Straumfjord J. V. (1973). *Clin. Chem;* **19**: 984.

Evans R. T., Holton J. B. (1970). *Ann. Clin. Biochem;* **7**: 104.

Fevery J., Muraca M., Verwilghen R. (1981). In *Familial Hyperbilirubinaemias.* (Okolicsanyi L., ed) p. 21. New York: John Wiley and Sons.

Fischer J. E., *et al.* (1974). *Amer. J. Surg;* **127**: 40.

Forman D. T. (1964). *Clin. Chem;* **10**: 497.

Gadd K. G. (1966). *J. Clin. Pathol;* **19**: 300.

Gerron G. G., *et al.* (1976). *Clin. Chem;* **22**: 663.

Goresky C. A. (1965). *Can. Med. Ass. J;* **92**: 851.

Harkness R. A., *et al.,* (1983). *Ann. Clin. Biochem;* **20**: 149.

Henry D. A., Kitchingman G., Langman M. (1985). *Dig. Dis. Sci;* **30**: 813.

Heppner G. W., Vessell E. S. (1975). *Ann. Int. Med;* **83**: 632.

Hertz H., Dybkaer R., Lauritzen M. (1974). *Scand. J. Clin. Lab. Invest;* **33**: 215.

Hofmann A. C., Schoenfield L. J., Kouke B. A., Poley J. R. (1970). In *Methods in Medical Research,* Vol. 12. (Olson, P. E., ed) p. 149. Chicago: Year Book Medical Publishers.

Holton J. B. (1982). *Ann. Clin. Biochem;* **19**: 389.

Hutchinson D., Halliwell R., Smith M., Parke D. (1981). *Clin. Chim. Acta;* **114**: 69.

Isherwood D. M., Fletcher K. A. (1985). *Ann. Clin. Biochem;* **22**: 109.

Javitt N. B. (1975). In *Diseases of the Liver,* 4th ed. (Schiff L., ed) p. 125. Philadelphia: Lippincott.

Jendrassik L., Grof P. (1938). *Biochem. Z;* **297**: 81.

Jones E. A., Berk P. D. (1982). In *Chemical Diagnosis of Disease.* (Brown, S. S., Mitchell, F. L., Young, D. S., eds) p. 525. Amsterdam: Elsevier.

Kaplowitz N., Kok E., Javitt N. B. (1973). *J. Amer. Med. Ass;* **225**: 292.

Katz W. A., Scarf M. (1964). *Amer. J. Med. Sci*; **248**: 545.

Kishimoto Y., Hijiya S., Takeda I. (1985). *Amer. J. Gastroent*; **80**: 136.

Kuenzle C. C., Sommerhelder M., Ruttner J. R., Maier C. (1966). *J. Lab. Clin. Med*; **67**: 282 and 294.

Lauff J. J., Kasper M. E., Ambrose R. T. (1981). *J. Chromat*; **226**: 391.

Lauff J. J., Kasper M. E., Ambrose R. T. (1983). *Clin. Chem*; **29**: 800.

Lautenburg B. H., Bircher J. (1976). *J. Pharmac. Exp. Ther*; **196**: 501.

Lawrence C. M., *et al.* (1985). *Ann. Clin. Biochem*; **22**: 232.

Leffler H. H. (1967). *Amer. J. Clin. Pathol*; **48**: 233.

Linnet K., Andersen J. R. (1983). *Clin. Chim. Acta*; **127**: 217.

Lo D. H., Wu T. W. (1983). *Clin. Chem*; **29**: 31.

Lockitch G., Pudek M. R., Halstead A. C. (1984). *J. Pediat*; **105**: 773.

Makino I., Nakagawa S., Mashino K. (1969). *Gastroenterology*; **56**: 1033.

Makino L., Sjövall J. (1972). *Anal. Letters*; **5**: 341.

Malloy H. T., Evelyn K. A. (1937). *J. Biol. Chem*; **119**: 481.

Marchesini G., *et al.* (1983). *Gastroenterology*; **85**: 283.

Matsui, A., *et al.* (1982). *J. Clin. Pathol*; **35**: 1011.

McCullough A. J., Czaja A. J., Jones J. D., Go W. (1981). *Gastroenterology*; **81**: 645.

McCullough H. (1967). *Clin. Chim. Acta*; **17**: 297.

McDermott W. V. (1959). *Surgical Forum*; **10**: 282.

Michaelsson M. (1961). *Scand. J. Clin. Lab. Invest*; **13**: Suppl. 56: 1.

Michaelsson M., Nosslin B., Sjohn S. (1965). *Pediatrics*; **35**: 925.

Miller P., Weiss S., Cornell M., Dockery J. (1981). *Clin. Chem*; **27**: 1698.

Muraca M., Blanckaert N. (1983). *Clin. Chem*; **29**: 1767.

Murphy G. M., Billing B. H., Baron D. N. (1970). *J. Clin. Pathol*; **23**: 594.

Muting D., *et al.* (1968). *Clin. Chim. Acta*; **19**: 391.

Nordlinger B. M. (1979). *J. Lab. Clin. Med*; **94**: 832.

Nosslin B. (1960). *Scand. J. Clin. Lab. Invest*; **12**: Suppl. 49, 1.

Novros J. S., Koch T. R., Knoblock E. C. (1979). *Clin. Chem*; **25**: 1891.

O'Brien D., Ibott F. A. (1962). *Laboratory Manual of Pediatric Micro and Ultramicro Biochemistry Techniques*, 3rd ed, p. 54. New York: Harper and Row.

Odell G. B. (1980). *Neonatal Hyperbilirubinaemia*, Monographs in Neonatology. Orlando, Florida: Grune and Stratton.

Okolicsanyi L., ed. (1981). *Familial Hyperbilirubinaemia*. New York: John Wiley and Sons.

Oreskes I., Hirsch C., Kupfer S. (1969). *Clin. Chim. Acta*; **26**: 185.

Paton A. (1984). *Brit. Med. J*; **289**: 857.

Penn R., Worthington D. J. (1983). *Brit. Med. J*; **286**: 531.

Percy-Robb I. W. (1985). In *Recent Advances in Clinical Biochemistry*. (Price C. P., Alberti K. G. G. M., eds). p. 125. Edinburgh: Churchill Livingstone.

Powell W. N. (1944). *Amer. J. Clin. Pathol*; **14**: 55.

Roda A., *et al.* (1980). *Clin. Chem*; **26**: 1677.

Rosalki S. B., Rau D., Lehmann D., Prentice M. (1970). *Ann. Clin. Biochem*; **7**: 143.

Rosen, M. H., Yoshimura N., Hodgman B. A., Fischer J. E. (1977). *Gastroenterology*; **72**: 843.

Ross, P. E. (1977). *Anal. Biochem*; **80**: 458.

Rubin M., Knott L. (1967). *Clin. Chim. Acta*; **18**: 409.

Sandberg D. H., Sjövall J., Sjövall K., Turner D. A. (1965). *J. Lipid Res*; **6**: 182.

Scharschmidt B. F., Waggoner J. G., Berk P. D. (1975). *J. Clin. Invest*; **56**: 1280.

Scharschmidt B. F., *et al.* (1982). *Gut*; **23**: 643.

Schiff L., ed. (1975). *Diseases of the Liver*, 4th ed. Philadelphia: Lippincott.

Schneider J. F., *et al.* (1980). *Gastroenterology*; **79**: 1145.

Scott P. (1959). Newsletter of Association of Clinical Biochemists, No. 24, p. 11., London.

Setchell K. D. R., Matsui A. (1983). *Clin. Chim. Acta*; **127**: 1.

Sherlock S. (1985). *Diseases of the Liver and Biliary System*, 7th ed. Oxford: Blackwell Scientific Publications.

Simmonds W. J., Korman M. G., Go V. L. W., Hoffman A. F. (1973). *Gastroenterology*; **65**: 705.

St. John A., Penberthy L. A. (1979). *J. Clin. Pathol*; **32**: 794.
Stein S. M., Keay A. J., Horn D. B. (1971). *Ann. Clin. Biochem*; **8**: 8.
Swyer P. R. (1975). *The Intensive Care of the Newly Born*, Monographs in Paediatrics, No. 6, Basle: Karger.
Tengstrom B. (1966). *Scand. J. Clin. Lab. Invest*; **18**: Suppl. 92: 132.
Tengstrom B. (1968). *Acta Med. Scand*; **175**: 506.
Tengstrom B., Hjelm M., de Verdier C. H., Werner I. (1967). *Amer. J. Dig. Dis*; **12**: 853.
Teppo A. M., Maury C. P. J. (1983). *Clin. Chim. Acta*; **129**: 279.
Turnell D. C. (1985). *Ann. Clin. Biochem*; **22**: 217.
Turnell D. C., Cooper J. D. H. (1982). *Clin. Chem*; **28**: 527.
Tygstrup N. (1966). *Scand. J. Clin. Lab. Invest*; **18**: Suppl. 92: 118.
Van den Bergh A., Muller P. (1916). *Biochem. Z*; **77**: 90.
Van den Bergh A., Snapper J. (1913). *Deut. Arch. Klin. Med*; **137**: 197.
Venger N. (1961). *J. Amer. Med. Ass*; **175**: 506.
de Verdier C. H., Hjelm M. (1962). *Clin. Chim. Acta*; **7**: 742. See also Hjelm M., Verdier C. H. (1976). In *Methods of Enzymatic Analysis*, 2nd English ed. (Bergmeyer H. U., ed) p. 1282. New York: Academic Press.
Vessell E. S. (1984). *Ann N. Y. Acad. Sci*; **428**: 293.
Wahlefeld A. W., Herz G., Bernt E. (1972). *Scand. J. Clin. Lab. Invest*; **29**, Suppl. 126: Abstr. 11.12.
Watkinson L. R., St. John A., Penberthy L. A. (1982). *J. Clin. Pathol*; **35**: 52.
Weiss J. S., *et al.* (1983). *New Engl. J. Med*; **309**: 147.
Wright K., Christie D. L. (1981). *Amer. J. Dis. Childh*; **135**: 134.
Wu T. W. (1984). *Clin. Biochem*; **17**: 221.
Zeltzer P. M. (1978). *J. Ped. Surg*; **13**: 381.
Zeltzer P. M., Neerhout R. C., Fonkalsrud E. W., Strehm E. R. (1974). *Lancet*; **1**: 373.
Zoli M., *et al.* (1981). *Scand. J. Gastroenterol*; **16**: 689.

29

URINARY ABNORMALITIES AND CALCULI–TESTS IN RENAL DISEASE

This chapter describes the deposits which may be formed in urine and considers the related topic of calculi. The investigation of pigmented urines by simple methods is discussed and finally the various tests of renal function and the findings in various forms of renal disease are considered in some detail.

URINARY DEPOSITS

These deposits may contain: crystalline or amorphous chemical substances; cells derived from the blood or various parts of the urinary tract; casts; organisms and foreign substances. Their microscopic examination is of diagnostic value. The urine should preferably be an early morning specimen collected in the same way as a 'mid-stream specimen' for bacteriological examination, directly into a clean container. Waxed paper cartons which can be sealed with a clip are convenient. Examine within an hour or so of collection or store at 4 °C for up to 24 h.

The constituents of urinary deposits may be derived from the kidney itself, or from the urinary and genital passages. They may form after the urine has been allowed to stand or may be contaminants entering during or after the collection process.

Chemical Substances

Inorganic substances present both physiologically and pathologically include calcium oxalate, calcium hydrogen phosphate, calcium carbonate, magnesium ammonium phosphate (triple phosphate) and magnesium phosphate. *Organic substances* are less often seen but the most common are uric acid and urates in the form of the ammonium, sodium, potassium, calcium or magnesium salts. Amino acids such as cystine, leucine and tyrosine are occasionally present as are drugs or their metabolites. Rare components of deposits include bilirubin, cholesterol, indigo and xanthine.

General points to note are the pH of the urine from which the deposit is obtained, and the solubility on heating or acidification. Thus phosphates and ammonium urate are usually deposited from alkaline urines while uric acid and other urates appear from acid urines. Calcium oxalate may be found in either. Uric acid and urates appear as the urine is cooled and redissolve on warming. Phosphates dissolve in cold dilute acetic acid, oxalates require dilute mineral acids but uric acid is unaffected by either in the cold. Uric acid and urates give a coloured deposit as do red cells.

Calcium Oxalate

Calcium oxalate is deposited from acid and alkaline urines. The crystals, commonly octahedral or envelope in shape, may sometimes be ellipsoidal, appearing as dumb-bells in side view (Fig. 29.1). Of variable size, they are usually smaller than other crystals. They are insoluble in acetic acid but dissolve in mineral acids. Calcium oxalate is a normal constituent of urine held in supersaturated solution. While usually deposited on standing, crystals may form in the urinary tract in a concentrated urine or if there is increased excretion of calcium, oxalate or both. Increased calcium excretion occurs in idiopathic hypercalciuria and in primary hyperparathyroidism. Some foods are rich in oxalate, particularly rhubarb and spinach, but over half of the average British dietary intake is drunk as tea (see also p. 704). Most of the excreted oxalate is derived from metabolism of ascorbate and amino acids, particularly glycine. Massive excretion with crystal formation occurs in the inherited metabolic disorder, primary hyperoxaluria (Williams and Smith, 1983).

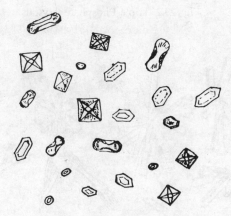

Fig. 29.1. Calcium Oxalate Crystals.

Phosphates

Magnesium ammonium phosphate is $MgNH_4PO_4$, $6H_2O$. Colourless triple phosphate crystals (Fig. 29.2) are of two types: prisms with oblique surfaces at the ends, the so-called coffin-lid type, which are more common than the feathery fern-like variety. They are typically found in alkaline urines when bacterial urease action has produced ammonium carbonate from urea. This may occur within an infected urinary tract or when the urine becomes contaminated after being passed.

Calcium hydrogen phosphate is usually found as crystals (Fig. 29.3) in the form of rosettes or star-shaped clusters, stellar phosphates. They are deposited from urine with pH varying from 6 to definitely alkaline and dissolve in acetic acid.

Other Inorganic Salts

Calcium carbonate occurs in amorphous form or sometimes as dumb-bell form crystals. Formation is facilitated in infected urine in which ammonium carbonate is formed. The deposits dissolve in acetic acid with evolution of carbon

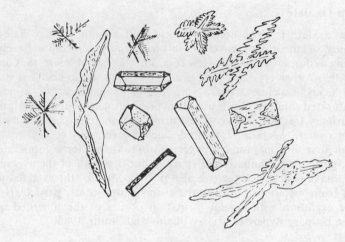

Fig. 29.2 Triple Phosphate Crystals.

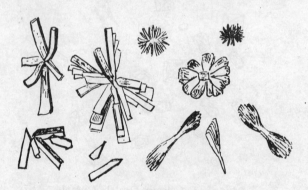

Fig. 29.3 Calcium Hydrogen Phosphate Crystals.

dioxide. *Calcium sulphate* crystals occur rarely and then usually in acid urines. *Magnesium phosphate* is occasionally seen as long rhombic plates in alkaline or weakly acid urines. Amorphous deposits of calcium and magnesium phosphates occur as granular white material soluble in acetic acid unlike the coloured amorphous urate deposits.

Organic Chemical Deposits

Uric Acid crystals are deposited from acid urines and incorporate urinary pigments to produce a very characteristic yellow to red-brown appearance. The crystals are very varied in form—rhombic prisms, rosettes, plates and barrel-shaped (Fig. 29.4). The crystals are insoluble in acid but dissolve in sodium hydroxide or on warming untreated urine to 60 °C. Uric acid crystals are found most frequently in the deposit from cooled, concentrated acidic urines but formation is more likely if urate excretion is pathologically increased.

Urates in the form of their ammonium, sodium, potassium, calcium and magnesium salts may be deposited. All except ammonium urate occur in acid

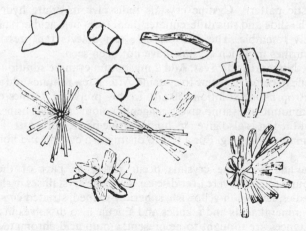

Fig. 29.4. Uric Acid Crystals.

urine. Most urates occur as an amorphous, coloured precipitate appearing as the urine cools and redissolving on warming. Occasionally urate crystals are seen. Monosodium urate may form stellar clusters similar to those of calcium hydrogen phosphate, from which they differ in solubility and pigmentation. Ammonium urate crystals, associated with infected urine, may show bizarre shapes but are often spiky spherical objects, 'thorn apple' crystals. Occasionally urate deposits are white but still have the characteristic property of redissolving on warming.

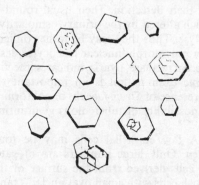

Fig. 29.5. Cystine Crystals.

Cystine crystals are seen as colourless hexagonal plates (Fig. 29.5) which dissolve in alkalies and mineral acids but not acetic acid. The urine, if not acid, should be made slightly so and then allowed to stand for a few hours before examination. The normal excretion of cystine ranges from 30 to 100 mg daily (Dent and Rose, 1951) rising to 0·5 to 1 g in cystinuria. This renal tubular defect (Chapter 18, p. 393) is characterised by poor reabsorption of cystine, arginine, ornithine and lysine and chromatographic examination of urine reveals the characteristic pattern. Cystine crystals redissolve in dilute hydrochloric acid added to the slide and this differentiates them from uric acid crystals which they occasionally resemble. The nitroprusside test detects the presence of excess cystine in urines in which crystals have not been seen.

Cyanide Nitroprusside Test. Add 2 ml sodium cyanide solution (100 g/l) to 3 to 5 ml urine to convert cystine to cysteine. After a few minutes add a few drops of sodium nitroprusside solution (50 g/l), freshly prepared. Urines containing an increased amount of cystine give a magenta colour, normal urines only a faint brown, but the test is also given by homocystine particularly after a loading dose of methionine, 100 mg/kg. For a test to distinguish cystine and homocystine see p. 383.

Leucine and Tyrosine crystals occur rarely as part of the generalised aminoaciduria seen in severe liver disease. Tyrosine crystallises in sheaves or tufts of fine needles, leucine in yellowish, spherical-shaped, striated crystals. Both are soluble in mineral acids and alkalies and leucine also dissolves in acetic acid. If these substances are thought to be present, amino acid chromatography of the urine should be done.

Other Substances. *Bilirubin* crystals are occasionally deposited from acid urines containing bile as tufts of fine needles or as rhombic plates, brown in colour which, unlike other deposits, are soluble in acetone. *Xanthine* crystals have been reported as small colourless rhombic plates but are extremely rare. They dissolve on heating or after adding dilute ammonia.

Cells

Red Blood Cells. In large numbers these colour the urine red. Smaller amounts produce a smoky appearance if the urine is swirled after standing. If present in numbers between 10 and 1000 per μl, microscopical examination is the most sensitive method for their detection. Their usual round biconcave appearance may, however, be much altered by the urinary osmolarity and they may shrink, swell or even haemolyse. Thus they may be rather difficult to recognise.

Leucocytes. A few polymorphonuclear leucocytes, less than 10 per μl, may occur in normal urine. An increase, pyuria, indicates infection of the urinary tract, for which microscopic examination is an important test. Pyuria is usually associated with the presence of *Strep. faecalis* or coliform bacilli in the urine and in their absence the possibility of tuberculous genitourinary disease should be considered.

Epithelial Cells. A few epithelial cells may be found in normal urine, particularly in women. Only large numbers are of pathological significance. Squamous epithelial cells derived from the surface of the bladder, urethra or vagina are large, flattish cells with small oval nuclei. Transitional epithelial cells originating from the prostate, bladder, ureter or renal pelvis are from two to three times the size of a leucocyte. Small round or polygonal cells, somewhat larger than a leucocyte are rare in normal urine and are of renal origin. Abnormal cells such as tumour cells may be present particularly if a bladder tumour is present.

Spermatozoa. Recognisable by their characteristic shape, these may be present in the urine for several hours after ejaculation of semen.

Organisms. Motile Gram-negative bacilli and chains of Gram-positive cocci, usually *Strep. faecalis*, are common in urinary tract infections. Occasionally fungi or yeasts are seen. The latter may be confused with erythrocytes under low power magnification.

Casts

Protein precipitating in a renal tubule forms a cast of its lumen and is then extruded, sometimes with damaged tubular cells attached, to appear in the urine. Classification is based on microscopic appearance (Fig. 29.6).

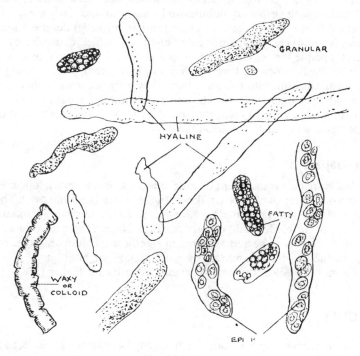

Fig. 29.6. Casts.

Hyaline Casts

These are the simplest and are composed of protein only. They have a pale, transparent, homogeneous, cylindrical structure and contain no cells. The length and width (average 25 μm) vary considerably. A few hyaline casts occur in normal urine, apparently protein-free on conventional testing. The number increases in normal people after exercise but many such casts are seen in the majority of cases of pathological proteinuria.

Erythrocyte and Leucocyte Casts

These contain red blood cells and leucocytes respectively, the cells being trapped as the cast forms. The number trapped varies. Erythrocyte casts imply renal haematuria and are seen, e.g. in acute glomerulonephritis and subacute bacterial endocarditis. Leucocyte casts are suggestive of pyelonephritis. Degeneration of the leucocytes may give the appearance of a granular cast.

Epithelial Casts

In tubular damage, the tubular epithelial cells may be shed with the cast. Usually the nuclei are preserved but degeneration may occur.

Granular casts contain granules of various sizes, arising from degenerating tubular cells. They should be distinguished from hyaline casts to which a few sediment granules have become attached. They are far less common in the urine of normal persons than are hyaline casts, and in appreciable numbers, their presence indicates tubular epithelial damage.

Fatty casts are epithelial casts in which the cells show severe fatty degeneration, with visible fat globules and some granules. They are not found in normal urine but only if there is severe tubular epithelial degeneration.

Waxy (colloid) casts are composed of highly refractile, yellowish material with a dullish, opaque lustre. They tend to split and crack and are shorter and wider than other casts probably because they originate from the collecting tubules. Their chemical composition is uncertain. They only occur when there are severe long-standing changes in the tubules and are common in renal amyloidosis. They stain with methyl violet, a characteristic of amyloid. Whilst acetic acid dissolves hyaline casts, waxy casts are insoluble.

Other Objects

Cylindroids are pale transparent threads of mucus, usually much longer than true casts and of varying thickness. Unlike casts, they often bend and twist. They occur occasionally in normal urine but are increased in number in inflammatory conditions of the bladder and urinary passages. *Artefacts* are introduced into the urine after it has been passed and are not significant. Examples are: hairs, fibres, bits of feathers, starch granules, oily globules and air bubbles.

For a more detailed account of urinary deposits see Haber (1981).

CALCULI

Of the stones, concretions or calculi which may be removed or excreted from the body, those from the urinary tract are the most common, but gall stones, salivary and pancreatic calculi are sometimes analysed, and have been included in this chapter for convenience.

Urinary Calculi

Formation. These may be found in any part of the urinary tract and vary considerably in size. Although certain factors favour the formation of stones, they do not explain the presence of all of them. Substances such as calcium oxalate and uric acid are known to be present in urine in a supersaturated state but are kept in solution by colloidal substances so there is always the potential for altered conditions to arise leading to the formation of crystals. Stone formation, however, requires a nucleus on to which the crystal is initially deposited and then continues to grow. Increased excretion of a substance is sometimes a factor as is decreased urinary volume leading to a concentrated urine. Hyperparathyroidism and hypervitaminosis D cause increased calcium excretion and may be accompanied by formation of calculi. In gout there is an increased excretion of uric acid. Hyperoxaluria is seen in inflammatory bowel disease.

Many stones originate on the surface of the renal papillae to which the crystals adhere initially. They may break off when still small and be passed through the urethra during an attack of renal colic. Larger fragments may lodge in the ureter or bladder. The presence of a calculus in the renal pelvis, ureter or bladder often interferes with the proper flow of urine. An important additional factor in causing such stasis is an associated anatomical abnormality of the ureter, bladder or urethra. A common example is prostatic hypertrophy which obstructs the passage of urine at the bladder neck. Stasis leads to more ready deposition of inorganic matter on the stone already present and it also predisposes to infection above the obstruction. Infected urines are usually alkaline due to urease-producing organisms and the ammonium and carbonate thus formed are incorporated into the stone. The deposition of calcium phosphate is also more rapid under these conditions. The stone may then grow rapidly, often shows stratification when cut across and may have a nucleus different from the superficial layers. Its shape will depend on its environment. In the renal pelvis it may fill the pelvic space and extend into its calyces to produce a 'stag-horn' calculus. The bladder stone is less restricted and assumes an ovoid shape. Untreated cases may produce bladder calculi up to 10 cm or more in diameter with a rough, coral-like surface.

Composition. Urinary calculi are composed of substances normally present in the urine, together with a certain amount of proteinaceous material. Occasionally foreign bodies form the nucleus. Substances found in calculi include uric acid, urates, calcium, magnesium, oxalate, phosphate, carbonate and cystine. The most common form of oxalate is as calcium oxalate, mainly $Ca(COO)_2,H_2O$ but some $Ca(COO)_2,2H_2O$ may be present. Calcium phosphate occurs most commonly as hydroxyapatite, $3Ca_3(PO_4)_2,Ca(OH)_2$, and to only a minor degree as brushite, $CaHPO_4,2H_2O$, whitlockite, $Ca_3(PO_4)_2$, or octocalcium phosphate, $Ca_8H_2(PO_4)_6,5H_2O$. Carbonate when present occurs as a carbonate-apatite, $3Ca_3(PO_4)_2,CaCO_3$. When magnesium occurs this is mainly as triple phosphate, $MgNH_4PO_4,6H_2O$, but newburyite, $MgHPO_4,3H_2O$, may be present as a minor component.

Xanthine calculi are very rare, while fibrin stones arise infrequently. It is unusual to find a stone composed of only one constituent unless it is very small. Stones of mixed composition with one substance often predominating are the rule (Hodgkinson *et al.*, 1969). Well over 90% of stones contain uric acid, urates, calcium oxalate or calcium phosphate with the last two predominating.

Calcium oxalate is found in the majority of small calculi, often mixed with a variable amount of phosphate. Oxalate stones have a rough crystalline surface and are among the hardest found so they are not easily crushed. Such crystalline stones form in the renal pelvis with oxalate as the chief anion. Further growth involves incorporation of calcium phosphate and some organic matter.

Phosphate calculi may contain either calcium phosphate or triple phosphate. The latter is associated with infected urine and its further deposition is apparent in large calculi. These are often rather soft and white with a striated cut surface and a nucleus of different texture.

Calcium carbonate is usually deposited on existing stones in infected urine and is present in varying amounts as a white soft surface layer.

Uric acid stones are usually brown in colour and are fairly hard with a varying surface structure. They are often small and multiple. Stones consisting almost entirely of uric acid are uncommon, many containing some added calcium phosphate.

Cystine stones are rare and are found in the inherited metabolic abnormality, cystinuria. They are usually fairly small and are smooth and waxy in appearance and to the touch, with a brownish-yellow or greenish colour.

Xanthine stones are even rarer and are associated with another metabolic abnormality, xanthinuria (Dent and Philpot, 1954, Holmes and Wyngaarden

1983). They are yellowish-brown in colour resembling uric acid calculi and sometimes contain uric acid also.

Fibrin calculi may form from blood clots. The fibrin is usually coated with calcium phosphate and may be seen as an obvious nucleus in cross section.

Foreign bodies of a remarkable variety have been removed from the bladder, sometimes as the centre of a calculus forming there.

Chemical Examination of Urinary Calculi

Wash the stone with water and dry in an incubator. Larger stones may consist of several layers so the stone should be cut in half and the cut surface examined. If possible, separate the layers and examine them separately. Very small stones are simply powdered. Make a note of the size, appearance and hardness of the stone.

Qualitative Analysis

Reagents.
1. Dilute hydrochloric acid, approx. 2 mol/l.
2. Dilute sulphuric acid, approx. 2 mol/l.
3. Concentrated nitric acid.
4. Acetic acid. Dilute 30 ml glacial acetic acid to 100 ml with water.
5. Potassium hydroxide solution, approx. 2 mol/l.
6. Concentrated ammonia solution (sp. gr. 0·88).
7. Dilute ammonia solution. Dilute reagent (6) 5-fold with water.
8. Ammonium molybdate solution, approx. 50 g/l. Prepare freshly.
9. Ammonium oxalate solution. Prepare a saturated solution.
10. Nessler's reagent (BDH Chemicals Limited).
11. Uric acid reagents (p. 358).
12. Sodium cyanide solution, 100 g/l.
13. Potassium permanganate solution, approx. 3 g/l.
14. Sodium nitroprusside solution, 50 g/l. Prepare freshly.
15. Sodium dithionite, solid.
16. Titan yellow (1 g/l in water) or Magneson II (4-*p*-nitrophenyl azo-1-naphthol, Hopkin & Williams; 1 g/l in sodium hydroxide, 10 g/l).
17. Ninhydrin solution (p. 371).

Technique. The following order of investigation is recommended. Since some stones are quite small it is necessary to become accustomed to working with very small quantities of material for each test.

1. **Heat a small amount of the powder in a small crucible**, or better, on a **small platinum lid** or foil. Since most calculi contain at least a small amount of organic matter there is always a little charring, but if the stone is almost entirely inorganic this will be small in amount and a greyish powder will be left. If the stone is organic as in uric acid and cystine stones it will burn away entirely or leave only a trace of ash. It is generally clear which is the case but with some mixed stones containing both inorganic and organic material it may not always be possible to recognise the presence of relatively small proportions of substances such as uric acid.

Watch carefully *for the presence of a flame.* Uric acid, ammonium urate and xanthine burn away without producing a flame, but cystine gives a pale blue flame with a rather sharp smell, while fibrin gives a yellow flame with a smell of burnt feathers.

A. *If the substance burns away completely* it contains only organic matter. Oxalate, phosphates and carbonates are absent. Proceed as follows:

2. **Test for Uric Acid and Ammonium Urate by the Murexide Test**. Add 2 or 3 drops of concentrated nitric acid to a small amount of the substance in a small evaporating dish or crucible and evaporate to dryness by heating on a water bath or very carefully over a small flame. The test is positive if a red or yellow residue is obtained which after being allowed to cool changes to a purplish-red on addition of a drop of dilute ammonium hydroxide.

Xanthine does not give a murexide test. It dissolves in nitric acid leaving a yellow residue which on addition of alkali changes to orange and to red on warming.

The uric acid reagents can also be used to test for uric acid. Dissolve a small portion of the stone in potassium hydroxide, add cyanide (or carbonate) and uric acid reagent. Uric acid gives a blue colour.

3. **Test for cystine** if the murexide test is negative. This would probably be suspected by the behaviour of the calculus on heating. Dissolve a small amount of the powdered stone in a few drops of concentrated ammonia solution and decant off any residue. Dilute part of the extract with 2 ml water, add 1 ml sodium cyanide, and, after standing 5 min, add a few drops of sodium nitroprusside solution. A deep magenta colour is given by cystine. Apply a drop of the ammonia solution to a filter paper, dry, and test with ninhydrin solution to confirm the presence of this amino acid. Finally, allow the remainder of the ammonia solution to evaporate off spontaneously on a watch glass. Hexagonal crystals of cystine will be deposited and can be examined microscopically (Fig. 29.5, p. 753).

4. **Fibrin** may occur as the nucleus of a stone usually in combination with altered blood pigments. Heat some of the suspected material with a little concentrated nitric acid for a minute. Cool, dilute with 2 volumes of water and pour potassium hydroxide down the side of the tube. The presence of a yellow or brown colour in the alkali layer, the xanthoproteic reaction, indicates protein is present. Test for altered haemoglobin by warming some of the original material with potassium hydroxide. Cool, add 1 ml of serum and a small quantity of sodium dithionite. Examine spectroscopically for the presence of haemalbumin (p. 661).

B. *If a deposit remains after heating on platinum*, inorganic material is present. Test as follows:

5. Add a little dilute hydrochloric acid to a portion of the original stone. An effervescence shows the presence of *carbonate*. The gas bubbles may be difficult to detect with the naked eye. Use a hand lens or examine under the microscope by carrying out the reaction under a cover slip (Hodgkinson, 1971).

6. After allowing the ash on the platinum to cool, test with dilute hydrochloric acid as in (5). Oxalates are converted into carbonates on heating, only prolonged heating decomposes carbonates. An effervescence shows the presence of *oxalate* or *carbonate*. No effervescence or a much weaker one in test (5) suggests the presence of *oxalate*. However the test is relatively insensitive and the following test is preferable particularly for small stones.

7. Heat a knife-point of the stone with 2 ml dilute sulphuric acid for 1 min. Allow to cool to 60 to 70 °C, then add dropwise, potassium permanganate solution. Prompt decolorisation with evolution of bubbles of carbon dioxide confirms the presence of *oxalate*.

8. Dissolve a little of the powdered stone in a few ml of concentrated nitric acid and then add an equal volume of ammonium molybdate solution. Heat to boiling.

If *phosphates* are present, a yellow precipitate of ammonium phosphomolybdate is obtained.

9. Heat about 100 mg of the stone with the potassium hydroxide solution and test for ammonia either by moist red litmus paper or by using Nessler's solution. Detection of ammonia shows the presence of *triple phosphate* or *ammonium urate*. Stones which are not well washed are often contaminated with ammoniacal urine. This can give a positive reaction with the very sensitive Nessler's reagent.

10. The presence of *calcium* and *magnesium* can be investigated as follows. Dissolve about 100 mg of the stone by heating with 2 ml dilute hydrochloric acid. Decant off from any residue, add 1 ml ammonium oxalate and enough concentrated ammonia until just alkaline. Readjust to pH 5 with acetic acid. A white precipitate of calcium oxalate shows the presence of *calcium*. Filter and to the filtrate add a few drops of Titan Yellow or Magneson followed by potassium hydroxide until strongly alkaline. The presence of *magnesium* is shown by a coloured flocculent precipitate of magnesium hydroxide which can be filtered off to leave a colourless filtrate. The colour is red for Titan Yellow and blue for Magneson.

Note. The fact that a deposit remains after heating does not exclude the presence of organic substances as the inorganic salts may have been deposited later on a stone initially largely organic. Therefore the tests for uric acid should be carried out as above.

Quantitative Analysis

It is sometimes necessary to obtain more precise information on the composition of a stone. A variety of physical techniques including X-ray diffraction, optical crystallography and infra-red spectroscopy have been employed but chemical analysis is the most convenient procedure. Hodgkinson (1971) uses the following procedure for stones suspected of containing calcium, magnesium, phosphate and oxalate.

Dissolve 20 mg powdered stone in 2 ml hydrochloric acid (equal parts, concentrated acid and water) and make up to exactly 10 ml with water. The concentration of calcium (mmol/g) is determined either by the cresolphthalein complexone method (p. 604) or by atomic absorption spectrometry (p. 605). Magnesium (mmol/g) is best determined by the latter technique also (p. 614). Phosphate (mmol/g) is determined by any of the standard methods (pp. 617, 618), oxalate by permanganate titration.

Determination of Oxalate in Stones (Hodgkinson, 1971)

Manganous ions are added to catalyse the oxidation of oxalate by hot permanganate. They also inhibit the oxidation of hydrochloric acid by permanganate especially if the temperature is above 70 °C.

Reagents.
1. Sulphuric acid, 1 mol/l.
2. Manganous sulphate solution, 50 g/l.
3. Potassium permanganate solution, 2 mmol/l.

Technique. Mix 1 ml of the hydrochloric acid solution of the stone with 2 ml sulphuric acid and add 1 drop manganous sulphate. Heat to 70 to 80 °C and titrate rapidly to a pink end-point with permanganate. Most stones give sharp end-points but uric acid and cystine react more slowly, giving a fading end-point.

The end-point should be taken as the persistence of a pink colour for a few seconds.

$$2KMnO_4 + 3H_2SO_4 + 5(COOH)_2 \rightarrow K_2SO_4 + 2MnSO_4 + 10CO_2 + 8H_2O$$

Calculation.

Oxalic acid (mmol/g calculus) = volume of permanganate (ml)

$$\times 2 \times \tfrac{5}{2} \times \tfrac{1}{2} = \text{volume of permanganate (ml)} \times 2\cdot5$$

Calculation of the Composition of a Stone (Hodgkinson, 1971).

The percentage composition of the stone is calculated on the assumption that the components are calcium oxalate, magnesium ammonium phosphate, and hydroxyapatite, as follows:

Calcium oxalate monohydrate = oxalic acid (mmol/g) × 14·6

Magnesium ammonium phosphate hexahydrate

$$= Mg \text{ (mmol/g)} \times 24\cdot5$$

Hydroxyapatite $(3Ca_3(PO_4)_2,Ca(OH)_2)$

$$= \{\text{total P (mmol/g)} - Mg(\text{mmol/g})\} \times 16\cdot7$$

The total calcium can be calculated from the content of calcium oxalate and hydroxyapatite and should agree with that determined experimentally. For many stones the above assumptions appear to be valid and account for between 80 and 90% of the total weight of the stone, the remainder being largely accounted for by protein and water (Hodgkinson *et al.*, 1969).

For further information on urolithiasis, see Chisholm and Williams (1982).

Gall Stones

Examination of gall stones may be required after their surgical removal. The substances found in them include cholesterol, bile pigments, calcium phosphate and calcium carbonate.

Gall stones may be single or multiple, large or small. Those containing calcium salts are radio-opaque. Single stones are uncommon but usually consist mainly of cholesterol and arise due to a disorder of the physico-chemical equilibrium which normally maintains cholesterol in micellar form in the bile. Sometimes several such stones occur. Their presence, however, predisposes to attacks of cholecystitis with formation of debris and impaired emptying of the gall bladder. Deposition of a mixture of cholesterol and bile pigments occurs on such debris and the resultant 'mixed' stones are the most common type. They are multiple, often with faceted surfaces due to tight packing in the gall bladder. Their content of calcium salts is variable. Whereas the cholesterol stones are often white or light coloured, mixed stones are usually quite dark.

Stones composed largely of *bile pigments* occur much less frequently but are associated with chronic haemolytic anaemia. They are usually multiple, very small, and may resemble grains of black sand. The pigment is mainly bilirubin present as calcium bilirubinate, but biliverdin and bilifuscin may be present.

Examination of Gall Stones

Wash with water, dry, and examine as follows:

1. Extract with ether. Powder the stone and heat some with successive small portions of ether in a test tube by inserting the tube in some warm water. Filter,

evaporate off the ether, dissolve the residue in ethanol and allow to crystallise. Typical rhomboid cholesterol crystals with notched corners are obtained if the crystallisation is done from ethanol. The Liebermann–Burchard reaction can be carried out. Dissolve a little of the residue, obtained on evaporating off the ether, in chloroform and add a mixture of acetic anhydride and sulphuric acid (in the proportion of 10 ml to 0·1 ml). A dark green colour develops rapidly.

2. Treat the residue remaining after ether extraction, with dilute hydrochloric acid (250 ml concentrated acid to a litre with water) to dissolve any inorganic salts and filter. Test the filtrate for phosphates with molybdate. Make some of the solution alkaline with ammonia and add acetic acid and ammonium oxalate solution. If calcium is present a precipitate of calcium oxalate is formed.

3. Test the precipitate remaining after treatment with hydrochloric acid, for bile pigments. Wash the material remaining on the filter paper with water, dry and extract with warm chloroform. Examine the chloroform extract for bilirubin using diazotised sulphanilic acid reagent (p. 719).

Pancreatic Calculi

Pancreatic calculi are usually found in association with chronic pancreatitis. They may be removed surgically or found at post-mortem. They vary in size, have a rough appearance and are mostly composed of inorganic material, mainly calcium carbonate and calcium phosphate, but there may be traces of magnesium salts. The presence of oxalates has been reported. Small amounts of protein and fats may be present.

They are investigated by the same scheme as for urinary calculi.

Salivary Calculi

Salivary calculi are usually formed in the parotid or submandibular ducts and are occasionally submitted for examination. Like pancreatic calculi they are usually composed of calcium phosphate and/or calcium carbonate with some organic matter and are examined in the same way.

URINARY PIGMENTS

The yellow colour of normal urine is attributed to *urochrome*, a substance of unknown composition with no characteristic absorption spectrum. It can be adsorbed onto charcoal and then eluted into alcohol from which it is obtained as a brown deposit. Small amounts of uroerythrin, urobilin, uroporphyrin and coproporphyrin may also contribute to the colour of normal urine.

Uroerythrin is the pink pigment adsorbed on to uric acid and urate deposits. It is soluble in ethanol, ether and chloroform and can be extracted using amyl alcohol in which it shows an absorption band in the green. Alkalies change its colour to green. While traces of *uroporphyrin* and *coproporphyrin* may be present they do not normally occur in sufficient quantity to be detected by spectroscopic examination or by ordinary tests. The colourless urobilinogen in urine is oxidised on standing to *urobilin*, but the small amount normally present contributes little to the colour. Another colourless substance, which is an indole derivative, is converted into *urorosein* if the urine is mixed with strong mineral acids. Like uroerythrin it can then be extracted into amyl alcohol and shows an absorption band in the green (p. 662).

The main determinant of the colour intensity of normal urine is the volume excreted daily. Very concentrated urines, recognised by their very high osmolality, may be so deeply coloured as to suggest the presence of abnormal pigments. The amount of urochrome excreted daily is independent of diet and is relatively constant for an individual. It is said to be increased if the rate of metabolism is increased and this substance is retained in the body in chronic renal failure thus contributing to the altered skin pigmentation in this condition.

Other pigments may also be increased in disease. A marked increase in urobilin excretion is seen in cirrhosis and in haemolytic anaemia to give the urine a characteristic brown colour. In acute hepatitis the urobilin increase is masked by the increase in bilirubin excretion. Indicanuria occurs if there is excessive bacterial degradation of tryptophan in the gut. Such urines are often deeper brown in colour and if they become ammoniacal on standing, some *indigo* may be formed. This can be extracted as a blue pigment into chloroform.

Abnormal Pigments

Of the pathological pigments, the greenish-yellow or brown of *bilirubin* (p. 730) is well known. Blood pigments which may be found in the urine (pp. 666–668) range from the red colour of *oxyhaemoglobin* to the brown of *methaemoglobin*. The presence of abnormal amounts of *porphyrins* (p. 649) gives a port wine colour which is often quite typical. Of the other pathological pigments, melanin and homogentisic acid only occur rarely.

Melanin in Urine

This type of pigment, never found in normal urine, occurs in patients with a malignant melanoma, usually when there are secondaries in the liver. The eye is a common site for such a tumour which may be removed and the secondaries, which are very slow growing, may not become apparent until years later. Freshly passed urines contain a colourless precursor, melanogen, which is oxidised to melanin when the urine is allowed to stand in contact with air. As melanin is dark brown or black, the urine slowly darkens, often from the surface downwards, taking as long as 24 h or more to become definitely noticeable. The tests used are for melanogen and so should be done on freshly passed urine.

Ferric Chloride Test. This is based on the oxidation by ferric chloride of melanogen to melanin.

Technique. To 5 ml urine add drop by drop an acid ferric chloride solution (100 g/l in 3 mol/l hydrochloric acid). The acid prevents the formation of ferric phosphate but the oxidation of melanogen results in a darkening in colour from varying shades of brown to black according to the amount of melanin formed.

Nitroprusside Test of Thormahlen.

Reagents.
1. Sodium nitroprusside solution. Prepare freshly before use by dissolving a few crystals in a few ml of water.
2. Acetic acid, 330 ml glacial acetic/l in water.
3. Sodium hydroxide, 400 g/l.

Technique. Add 3 or 4 drops of the nitroprusside solution to about 5 ml urine and make strongly alkaline with about 0·5 ml sodium hydroxide. Shake well to mix and make acid by adding a few ml of acetic acid. The presence of melanogen is shown by the development of a blue to blue-black colour. The actual colour seen depends on the colour of the original urine. If this was deep yellow the colour seen will be dark green. The less pigmented the urine, the bluer the colour produced.

This test is similar to the nitroprusside test for acetone and acetoacetic acid, when a reddish-purple colour is obtained. Creatinine gives a brown colour.

It is advisable to become familiar with the sort of colour which normal urines may give. This may be slightly brownish with a green tinge. Contrast a suspected positive with a normal control.

Other Tests. Other tests for melanogen are less satisfactory. If required, melanin can be precipitated from urine by methanol after oxidation of melanogen. Collect a 24 h specimen and evaporate to about a quarter of the original volume. Add 1 g potassium persulphate per 100 ml and after 2 h add an equal volume of methanol. Filter and wash in turn with water, methanol and ether.

Homogentisic Acid in Urine, Alkaptonuria

Metabolism of tyrosine (I) is defective in alkaptonuria due to congenital absence of homogentisate 1-2-dioxygenase (EC 1.13.11.5). The normal metabolic pathway is

where II is *p*-hydroxyphenylpyruvic acid, III is homogentisic acid and IV maleylacetoacetic acid. Homogentisate therefore accumulates in body fluids and is excreted in the urine causing the urine to darken on standing. The condition may first be noticed in infancy when the napkins are stained black. In later life most cartilage is stained black. This may give a bluish grey tinge to the nose and the pinna of the ear. The affected synovial cartilage is more easily damaged by mechanical forces than usually.

Homogentisic acid can be estimated by using the colour produced with ammonium molybdate and potassium dihydrogen phosphate using as standard a solution of hydroquinone similarly treated. Take 1 or 2 ml of urine, dilute to 15 ml with water, add 2 ml ammonium molybdate (20 g/l in 2·5 mol/l sulphuric acid) and 2 ml potassium dihydrogen phosphate solution (10 g/l) and dilute to 25 ml. Treat a hydroquinone standard (1 g/l) in the same way and compare the colours. One mg hydroquinone equals 0·79 mg homogentisic acid. If albumin is present in the urine it must first be removed.

Differentiation between melanogen and homogentisic acid. As many tests use the same reagents for both substances it is important to note their different behaviour in qualitative testing. The nitroprusside test for melanogen is not given by homogentisic acid so this test is useful for detecting the former.

Like melanogen, homogentisic acid is converted to dark polymeric products on standing, the colour appearing initially in the surface layer. If the urine is made alkaline when fresh, the dark colour appears within 30 seconds with homogentisic acid but no such acceleration occurs with melanogen. In the case of the latter, an acid medium increases the rate of darkening.

Urines containing homogentisic acid reduce alkaline copper solutions such as Benedict's. On boiling, a greenish-brown colour first results but on standing the typical yellow-brown precipitate of cuprous oxide is visible as with other reducing substances, but the supernatant is dark. This contrasts with the behaviour of melanogen which may give a greenish-black precipitate if an appreciable amount is present but otherwise shows little or no change. The reducing property of homogentisic acid is also demonstrated when a few drops of ammonia solution (100 ml sp. gr. 0·88 per litre in water) are added to a mixture of 0.5 ml urine and 5 ml silver nitrate (30 g/l) to form a black precipitate of silver. Indeed the black colour may develop without the addition of ammonia. Discard the product quickly and do not expose to sunlight to avoid producing explosive products.

On adding a few drops of ferric chloride solution (100 g/l) to a few ml of urine, in addition to the precipitation of ferric phosphate, a transient blue or green colour occurs with homogentisic acid. It is sometimes seen better if a more dilute ferric chloride solution is used. Melanogen gives a brown to black colour. A green colour with ferric chloride, fading in a few minutes, is given by the urine in *phenylketonuria* but such urine does not darken in air or have reducing properties.

Presence of Drugs, Dyes and Other Ingested Substances

Abnormally coloured urines may be due to ingested substances.

Foodstuffs. *Anthocyanins* form a group of the normal pigments of fruits and vegetables. In a small number of people they are found in the urine if appreciable quantities are ingested. Such anthocyaninuria is usually genetically determined and harmless. Deeply coloured foods such as beetroot, blackberries and bilberries are the usual source but large quantities of rhubarb may also produce a coloured urine. The colour of the urine superficially resembles haemoglobinuria but is pinker. The characteristic properties of the anthocyanins which are helpful in their identification are the failure to extract into amyl alcohol and the fact that they are indicators, being pinkish-red in acid and changing to yellow on adding alkali.

Natural or synthetic dyes added to the food may appear in the urine. *Riboflavin* taken in multiple vitamin preparations gives the urine a deeper amber colour with a greenish fluorescence. *Eosin* is used as a pink pigment in foodstuffs and gives the urine a characteristic green fluorescence. It is extracted by amyl alcohol and the extract shows an absorption band in the green (p. 662). In other cases, enquiries may reveal that coloured foods have been eaten.

Poisoning. Some toxic agents are associated with the appearance of haemoglobin, myoglobin or their derivatives in the urine. *Phenol* and *lysol* are now taken with suicidal intent much less frequently than in the past. In some cases the urine, instead of being darkened by haemoglobin derivatives, has a greenish tinge. Phenol and its conjugates with glucuronic acid and sulphuric acid are colourless but much of the phenol is oxidised to hydroquinone, pyrocatechol and higher oxidation products and these give the colour. Although tests may be done on the urine directly, it is better to acidify with sulphuric acid and then distil and test for phenols in the distillate. A white or yellowish precipitate is given with bromine water which forms tribromophenol. Colours are given with ferric chloride solution, blue with phenol and green with cresols. The phenolic glucuronides also reduce alkaline copper solutions.

Dyes used in Function Tests. There is usually a clear history of these being used. *Indocyanine green* colours the urine green. *Phenol red*, occasionally used, has indicator properties and is yellow in acid, turning red on adding alkali. *Bromsulphthalein* also acts as an indicator but is colourless at normal urinary pH. It imparts a purple colour if the urine becomes alkaline on standing.

Drugs. Colouring matter is often added to drugs by manufacturers for ready identification and may be excreted. *Methylene blue* imparts a green or greenish-blue colour to the urine. It is extracted by chloroform or amyl alcohol and the extract shows an absorption band in the red. *Indigo* may appear for similar reasons, is also extracted into chloroform and has a similar spectrum. They can be distinguished by reduction to the leuco base followed by attempted reoxidation (Harrison, 1947). Add a little glucose to 5 ml urine followed by 2 drops of 400 g/l sodium hydroxide. The green-blue colour should remain but disappears if the urine is boiled for a few minutes. Cool and shake with air when the blue colour is restored in the case of methylene blue but not indigo. It should be noted that methylene blue may also be added to foods. It is the most common cause of blue-green urines.

A variety of other drugs may either alter the colour of the urine or cause it to fluoresce, or react in the tests with ferric chloride or alkali used to investigate abnormal urinary pigments. *Tetracyclines* produce a yellower urine with a greenish fluorescence. *Methyldopa* darkens in alkaline conditions and gives a green colour with ferric chloride. *p-Aminosalicylic acid* and *aspirin* give purple colours with ferric chloride. *Phenolphthalein*, a purgative, behaves like bromsulphthalein (see above).

Unexpected colours, fluorescence or reaction with common reagents should always prompt careful enquiry into the drugs being taken by the patient. Sometimes examination of the drug will demonstrate the same finding. Where a metabolite is the cause, the urine of other patients taking the drug should be examined. Also, withdrawal of the drug, if warranted, should help to decide if a particular drug is responsible for the reactions observed.

Examination of Pigmented Urines.

Older books such as that of Harrison (1947) are often useful sources of information. Direct observation by an experienced person gives much useful information and a few tests are extremely helpful. These include spectroscopic examination of the urine and its amyl alcohol extract for characteristic absorption peaks; the behaviour of the colour to acid and alkali; the colour given with ferric chloride solution. If none of the pigments known to be present in pathological conditions is detected, the colour is almost certainly due to substances in the food or to drugs, though in the case of young children, chewing coloured articles may be responsible. Enquiry will often yield information about this.

RENAL FUNCTION

The formation of urine by the kidney involves two parts of the nephron. Firstly filtration occurs at the glomeruli, effected by the normal blood pressure as the blood passes through the capillary tufts in the glomeruli. The filtrate contains all plasma constituents except most of the protein (see p. 436) and those substances such as the lipids which are bound to plasma proteins. Subsequently, during the passage along the tubules, substances may be reabsorbed from, or sometimes secreted into, the glomerular filtrate. Generally those substances which the body needs are reabsorbed, allowing waste products, mostly nitrogenous, from the body's metabolic processes and surplus amounts of substances valuable to the body, to escape in the urine. Thus, e.g. almost all the water, sodium, chloride, glucose and amino acids are reabsorbed as are such proportions of potassium, calcium, magnesium and phosphate needed to maintain their concentration within the required limits.

There are three ways in which a substance can be handled by the kidney:

1. *Filtration at the glomeruli and (partial) reabsorption by the tubules.* This is by far the most common procedure. Such reabsorption may be either active, against concentration and osmotic gradients, or passive, when the tubular epithelium is permeable to a substance which has been absorbed less rapidly than water, so that its concentration becomes higher than in the plasma. An example of the latter is urea.
2. *Filtration at the glomeruli and secretion (and sometimes reabsorption) by the tubules.* Of physiological substances creatinine may in some circumstances be secreted by the tubules. Others, e.g. potassium and urate, are completely reabsorbed in the proximal tubules and are then actively secreted in the distal tubules. Several substances not normally present in the plasma are secreted by the tubules when injected into the blood.
3. *Filtration at the glomeruli without reabsorption or secretion in the tubules.* Several substances foreign to the body dealt with in this way have been used to study glomerular function since they enable the volume of glomerular filtrate formed per minute to be measured.

Renal function tests may be broadly divided into those which measure glomerular filtration and those which study tubular function. Disordered glomerular and tubular function may occur separately but in some cases both occur together. In both groups of tests some are suitable for routine clinical use and others are mostly used for more detailed investigation of individual cases and in research.

Clearance Studies

Many renal function tests involve the determination of various substances either in plasma or urine or both. Where both measurements are made it is possible to calculate a clearance (C), defined as

$$C = UV/P$$

where U and P are the concentrations of the substance concerned in urine and plasma respectively and V is the rate of urine flow in ml/min. If U and P are in the same units then C has the dimensions, ml/min. It represents the volume of plasma which would have to be completely cleared of the substance each minute in order to achieve an excretion rate per minute equal to UV. This calculation of clearance is independent of the mode of excretion of a substance by the kidney.

Clearance varies with body size and is proportional to the body area (A). Where this varies much from the normal in adults, and in all cases in children, the determined clearance is best corrected to a standard surface area of $1 \cdot 73$ m^2 by multiplying by $1 \cdot 73/A$. The value of A (m^2) can be calculated from the equation

(DuBois and DuBois, 1916)

$$\log A = 0{\cdot}425 \log W + 0{\cdot}725 \log H - 2{\cdot}144$$

where W is the body weight (kg) and H is the height (cm). Alternatively a nomogram may be used for children (Fig. 29.7) or adults (Fig. 29.8).

Although the formula for clearance is independent of the way the nephron handles a particular substance, the actual numerical value for the clearance of different substances varies considerably in a single individual. The clearance of a substance filtered at the glomeruli and neither reabsorbed nor secreted by the tubules gives the *glomerular filtration rate* (GFR) provided it is not metabolised in

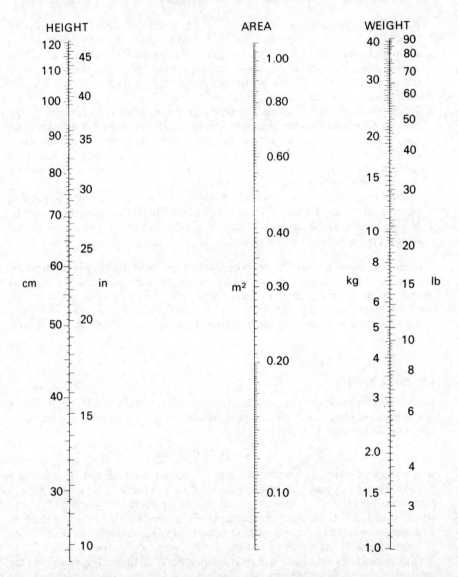

Fig. 29.7. Nomogram for Calculating Body Surface Area in Children from Height and Weight.

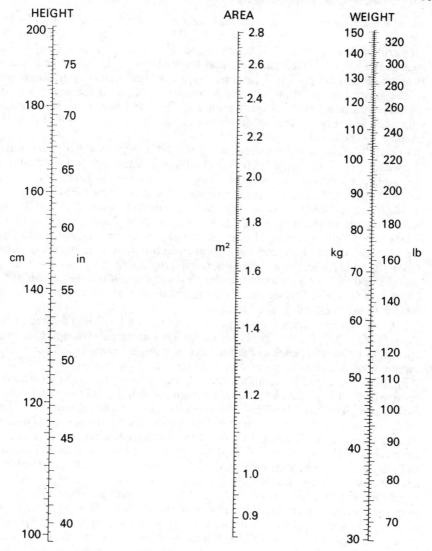

Fig. 29.8. Nomogram for Calculating Body Surface Area in Adults from Height and Weight.

the body, is not bound to plasma proteins and is not attacked by the tubular cells. When a substance is partly reabsorbed by the tubules, e.g. glucose, its clearance is less than the GFR and conversely, substances which are not reabsorbed but are also secreted by the tubules have clearances in excess of the GFR.

Our knowledge of renal physiology and pathology has been greatly advanced by information obtained from such clearance studies. For any substance the rate of excretion, UV, can be expressed as

$$UV \ (mg/min) = P \ (mg/ml) \times GFR \ (ml/min) \pm T \ (mg/min)$$

where P is its plasma concentration and T is the net tubular reabsorption (−) or secretion (+) rate. A substance testing GFR should only be filtered at the glomeruli and not further modified by the tubules, that is T should be zero. For such substances when their plasma concentration is varied, UV should be linearly related to P, and this line should, when extrapolated back, pass through the origin of the graph relating these two measurements. This is so for inulin and its clearance has been accepted as a measure of GFR and hence as a reference to which the clearance of other substances can be compared to assess how they are handled by the tubules.

For adults the normal inulin clearance is about 125 ml/min which is very nearly 70 ml min^{-1} m^{-2}. The range is 110 to 152 ml/min for men and 102 to 132 ml/min for women (Goldring and Chasis, 1944). For reasons of simplicity several radioisotope techniques have been proposed for measuring GFR. Prominent among these has been the use of ^{57}Co- or ^{58}Co-labelled vitamin B$_{12}$. A difficulty in this case arises from the fact that vitamin B$_{12}$ binds to plasma protein so that it is necessary to give a loading dose of the unlabelled vitamin prior to the test, a procedure which, however, does not appear entirely to remove errors (Foley *et al.*, 1966). ^{51}Cr-EDTA has been shown not to bind to plasma protein or to enter the red cells and to have a clearance similar to that of inulin (Garnett *et al.*, 1967; Chantler *et al.*, 1969). This seems to be the most satisfactory substance. The dose is very small and well below the toxic level.

Substances which are secreted by the tubules as well as being filtered at the glomeruli have a higher clearance than inulin. They are mainly foreign substances injected into the blood such as diodrast and *p*-aminohippurate. Such substances may be used in two ways to study renal function.

Firstly at low blood levels, about 10 to 20 mg/l, practically all the substance is removed from the plasma as it passes through the kidney. Only a small fraction passes through those parts of the kidney which are not functional nephrons. Then the clearance measures the *effective renal plasma flow*, that is the volume of plasma passing through the functional tissue of the kidney each minute. This can be converted into the *effective renal blood flow* if the haematocrit is known. Diodrast and *p*-aminohippurate clearances under such conditions are 600 to 700 ml/min (500 to 800 for men, 400 to 595 for women) so that the renal blood flow approximates to 1·1 l/min which is 20 to 25 % of the resting cardiac output. The *filtration fraction* is the ratio of the GFR to the renal plasma flow, e.g. the ratio of inulin and *p*-aminohippurate clearances, and represents the fraction of the plasma passing through the kidney which is filtered through the glomeruli. The normal range is 0·185 to 0·192 but figures are lower in acute glomerulonephritis and increased in hypertension.

Secondly, at higher concentrations of diodrast or *p*-aminohippurate the tubules are no longer able to clear the plasma completely as it passes through the kidney and the amount secreted by the tubules per minute ceases to increase. At such blood levels the rate of excretion is an index of the mass of functional tubular cells. The tubular secretion is the total rate of excretion less the amount filtered by the glomeruli, or

$$T_m = UV - P \times GFR$$

T_m has been termed the *tubular maximal capacity* for the substance under study. For *p*-aminohippurate, the average T_m is 76 mg/min (Goldring and Chasis, 1944).

If a substance is reabsorbed by the tubules, as is glucose, the *tubular maximal absorptive capacity*, T_m, can be measured similarly if a sufficiently high plasma level is achieved. At plasma glucose concentrations above 14 mmol/l when glycosuria is well established, the tubular reabsorptive capacity is saturated. Then T_m for glucose is the amount of glucose filtered each minute at the glomeruli less the excretion rate in the urine per minute or

$$T_m = P \times GFR - UV$$

The average value for T_m glucose is approximately 1·7 mmol/min.

The measurement of such indices of the renal handling of substances like inulin, *p*-aminohippurate and phenolsulphonephthalein (phenol red) is now performed so infrequently by hospital laboratories that details have been omitted from this edition, but can be found in the 5th edition of this book (pp. 1142–1149). The information obtained from earlier studies of these parameters forms the basis for our understanding of renal function in health and disease. In current practice, simpler tests of glomerular and tubular function are still performed and details of these are given.

CLINICAL TESTS OF RENAL FUNCTION

Many renal diseases are chronic and the biochemical changes which occur are therefore slow. Then the rate of excretion of a substance by the kidney must approximate to the normal rate and will remain so during a considerable part of the time the disease progresses, often until the terminal stages. This rate of excretion is UV and:

$$UV = \frac{UV}{P} \times P = C \times P = \text{constant}$$

This relationship between C and P (Fig. 29.9) is a set of rectangular hyperbolic curves corresponding to different values of UV. As a rule, this excretion rate for a substance equals its production rate in the body, plus any dietary intake. Under constant metabolic conditions, UV will thus be relatively constant.

Tests of Glomerular Function

A feature of renal disease is the gradual reduction in the clearance, but not excretion, of many substances, particularly those mainly handled by glomerular filtration. For such substances their clearance will depend on the GFR and Fig. 29.9 indicates that initially a marked fall in clearance may occur with only a slight rise in plasma concentration. Once GFR has been markedly reduced however, there may be considerable changes in plasma concentration, which will generally be high, with little change in clearance. Thus clearance determinations may be most helpful in the early stages of progressive renal disease while plasma determinations may be more sensitive when renal failure is advanced.

Commonly used tests of renal function involve measurements of urea or creatinine. Creatinine is not a component of the diet but is formed in the body at a relatively constant rate which is dependent upon the mass of muscle. Thus UV will be relatively constant for creatinine although it may fall slowly if muscle wasting develops over the years. The endogenous creatinine clearance has been much used as an approximate measure of GFR. Urea is derived from general protein metabolism. Both dietary protein and endogenous tissue protein contribute to the amount of urea produced but the former is often more important. Thus UV for urea can be modified by dietary means. The different

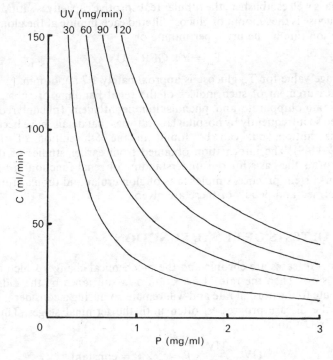

Fig. 29.9. The Relation Between the Clearance (C) and the Plasma Concentration (P) for any Substance in the Presence of Different Excretory Rates (UV).

curves in Fig. 29.9 correspond to different values of UV and hence to different protein intakes. Before creatinine determinations were technically quick and reliable much use was made of the urea clearance. As urea is always at least partially reabsorbed passively in the renal tubules its clearance cannot measure GFR but may bear a relatively constant ratio to it. When the urea clearance is low as in renal failure, the plasma urea concentration will vary considerably with the diet.

Determination of Plasma Urea and Creatinine

Determination of substances whose plasma concentration rises as GFR falls has mainly concentrated on urea and creatinine. Such determinations are often valuable in following the course of a progressive renal disorder and most laboratories are equipped to make the measurements. In the earlier stages of renal disease, clearance tests afford a more sensitive index of impaired function.

Urea Clearance Test

The passive tubular reabsorption of urea varies with urine flow rate, being lowest for high flow rates. At one time attempts were made to allow for this but they have been discontinued. The average urea clearance over a 24 h period can be measured by collecting a 24 h urine and taking a blood sample during this time. The clearance (C) is obtained from the plasma (P) and urine (U) urea concentrations after calculating V from the 24 h urine volume (ml) divided by 1440, the number of minutes in a day.

INTERPRETATION

The average 24 h urea clearance is relatively constant from day to day for an individual whose renal function is not altering rapidly. Figures for normal people lie in the range, 40 to 65 ml/min, appreciably lower than the GFR as even at very high urine flow rates, the tubules reabsorb about 40 % of the filtered urea. When glomerular function is steadily impaired by progressive renal disease, the urea clearance falls reaching 10 ml/min as renal failure becomes clinically apparent and falling further to 2 or 3 ml/min in terminal failure.

Endogenous Creatinine Clearance Test

For this test a 24 h urine specimen is collected and blood taken during the day. The time need not be exactly 24 h so long as it is accurately measured. The clearance is calculated as for the urea clearance.

INTERPRETATION

The endogenous creatinine clearance averages 120 ml/min (95 to 140) for men and 110 ml/min (85 to 125) for women, using an alkaline picrate method to measure creatinine. This is close to the GFR as measured by inulin clearance and has the advantage over urea clearance in that it varies little with urine flow rate. However, as the precision of plasma creatinine measurements at normal concentrations is rather poor, the calculated clearance is also rather imprecise but this improves as clearance falls. Creatinine clearances have proved moderately satisfactory in studying trends in renal function over a long period in the same patient with varying food and water intakes, but not all workers are convinced of the usefulness of this investigation (Payne, 1986).

The alkaline picrate method includes some non-creatinine chromogen but as there is less of this in urine than serum, the clearance found is less than the true clearance. However, this error offsets the effect of some tubular secretion of creatinine at normal or near normal concentrations of creatinine so the final result approaches the GFR. This is not so when the serum creatinine is increased by infusion or by renal disease and the clearance can then exceed inulin clearance by up to 40 % (Berlyne *et al.*, 1964).

Tests of Tubular Function

The composition of glomerular filtrate is modified by tubular reabsorption and secretion, to provide an important regulatory function for many body constituents. Renal damage reduces the functioning tubular mass and, if severe, seriously affects the regulatory function. Glomerular and tubular function are not always affected equally.

Tests of tubular function may involve an assessment of tubular handling of physiological substances, sometimes by imposing an extra load on the tubules to assess functional reserve which is normally considerable. Other tests involve the ability of the tubules to secrete foreign substances injected into the circulation and these were outlined earlier. Several tubular function tests still used in practice are discussed in relation to sodium, water and hydrogen ion metabolism in Chapter 23 (pp. 555, 577, 594).

BIOCHEMICAL FINDINGS IN DIFFERENT RENAL DISEASES

Knowledge of renal disease increased considerably with the introduction of the renal biopsy technique. Pathological processes in acquired renal disease may initially affect the glomeruli, the tubules or the blood vessels. *Glomerular disease* is classified into several types based on the changes seen on light or electron microscopy. Some changes are specific to the kidney but often the aetiology is obscure. Other changes arise from renal involvement in multi-system diseases. *Pyelonephritis* of various types affects the tubules initially while *vascular disorders* are often associated with hypertension. Hypertensive nephrosclerosis arises as a consequence of primary hypertension, but renal disease can itself cause secondary hypertension with the possibility of further renal damage.

These various renal diseases give rise to a smaller number of clinical syndromes, each of which may be associated with several different pathological processes in the kidney. As a disease progresses in a particular patient, the clinical syndrome may alter. Early classifications, based on the clinical features of renal disease, have been replaced by morphological classification, particularly for renal glomerular disease. Biochemical findings are more closely linked to the clinical syndromes and thus provide information complementary to histological studies. They give information about the severity and progress of the renal dysfunction rather than its cause or its effect on structure. An exception is renal tubular acidosis and other inherited tubular disorders.

Several clinical syndromes may be defined but may not be clearly separated. They are considered under seven headings later.

Outline Classification of Glomerular Disease

A brief outline is necessary to introduce current terminology. The glomerulus is a tuft of capillaries invaginated into the Bowman's capsule, composed of a single layer of epithelial cells continuous with the cells of the proximal convoluted tubule. These epithelial cells cover the capillary tuft. The afferent arteriole of the glomerulus divides into capillary loops supported by a small amount of connective tissue, the mesangium. The loops rejoin to form the efferent arteriole. The capillary walls are composed of endothelial cells and an important structure, the basement membrane (BM), 1·2 μm thick, lies between them and the epithelial cells of Bowman's capsule. These epithelial cells possess unique 'foot processes', delicate interdigitating prolongations of the cell which touch the BM leaving fine spaces between the processes. The endothelial layer is very thin, with gaps in the cytoplasm at intervals and it is this triple layer, endothelial cell, BM and epithelial cell, which is the selective filter during the first stage of urine formation. The filtrate passes into the space of Bowman's capsule and thence into the proximal tubule. These structures are shown diagrammatically in Fig. 29.10 and as seen by electron microscopy in Fig. 29.11.

For many glomerular disorders an abnormal immunological reaction occurs in the region of the BM. Complexes of an antigen and one or more immunoglobulins are detectable as deposits. In some cases this deposition is associated with activation of the multifactorial 'complement' system. The final products released by this process are responsible for a local inflammatory reaction—*glomerulonephritis*. Such an inflammatory reaction may result in the proliferation of epithelial, endothelial or mesangial cells or produce changes in the BM.

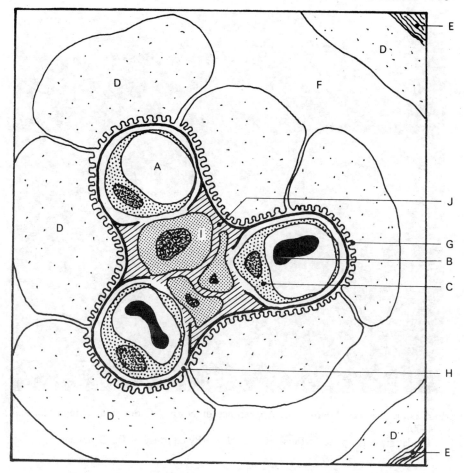

Fig. 29.10. Diagrammatic Representation of the Fine Structure of the Renal (Malpighian) Corpuscle Comprising the Glomerulus and Bowman's Capsule.
A—Lumen of glomerular capillary, B—Erythrocyte within capillary, C—Endothelial cell of capillary, D—Epithelial cells of Bowman's capsule, E—Connective tissue on outer surface of Bowman's capsule, F—Urinary space bounded by epithelial cells and communicating with the lumen of the proximal convoluted tubule, G—Foot processes of epithelial cell, H—Basement membrane, I—Mesangial cell, J—Mesangial matrix.

Selective filtration is provided by structures C, H, G and D which are interposed between the plasma and the urinary space.

The resulting abnormalities of structure in many cases involve most glomeruli to some degree, i.e. a diffuse disorder is present. Sometimes only a few glomeruli are affected while others are normal, i.e. the lesion is focal. The word 'segmental' refers to a change in part of a glomerulus; segmental lesions can affect many glomeruli. Some changes are reversible and healing occurs, in others the lesions become progressively worse at various rates. This is often referred to as *subacute or chronic glomerulonephritis* depending on the rate of progress. Such progress eventually involves destruction of a glomerulus and hence of its associated tubule. Progressive disorders lead to loss of nephrons and eventual renal failure.

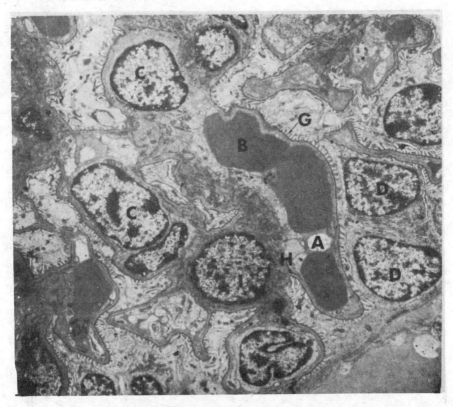

Fig. 29.11. Electron Microscopic Appearance of Normal Glomerulus (Magnification × 4000).
The letters correspond to those of Fig. 29.10. (By courtesy of Dr G. Williams.)

A. Primary Glomerular Disease

1. **Minimal Change (lipoid nephrosis, epithelial cell disease).** The structure is normal on light microscopy but the electron microscope shows fusion of foot processes of the epithelial cells. There is little evidence of immunological deposits. The disorder is most common in children, is potentially reversible, and is associated with increased glomerular permeability (Fig. 29.12).

2. **Membranous Nephropathy.** The BM is diffusely thickened with granular deposits on its epithelial surface. The deposits contain IgG and sometimes the third component of complement (C3, β_1-C-globulin). Spiky prolongations of BM separate these deposits. There is little inflammatory reaction and the aetiology is unknown. The glomerular filter becomes abnormally permeable and the disorder is usually slowly progressive. There is an increased incidence of renal vein thrombosis, probably a secondary complication.

3. **Focal Glomerulosclerosis (segmental or focal hyalinosis).** There is variation between glomeruli and for any glomerulus only a segment may be involved. Hyaline thickening occurs in the mesangium and capillary loops with granular deposits of immunoglobulins. Children are more often affected and the disorder is slowly progressive.

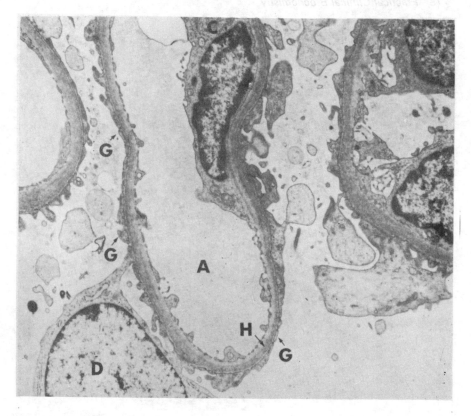

Fig. 29.12. Electron Microscopic Appearance of Glomerulus in Minimal Change Nephropathy (Magnification × 7 200).
The letters correspond to those of Fig. 29.10 and fusion of foot processes (G) is apparent. (By courtesy of Dr G. Williams.)

4. **Proliferative Glomerulonephritis (PGN)**. In these disorders an inflammatory reaction with cell proliferation is present. Classification depends on the cell type involved.

(a) *Active diffuse endothelial PGN* (acute exudative glomerulonephritis, post-streptococcal acute glomerulonephritis). Both endothelial and mesangial cells proliferate and polymorphs infiltrate into the glomeruli, i.e there is acute inflammation with glomerular ischaemia. Irregular granular deposits accumulate on the outer surface of the BM (Fig. 29.13). These are rich in IgG and C3. The disorder is most common in young adults and often reversible. Its usual association is with a streptococcal throat infection but malaria gives a similar picture.

(b) *Mesangial PGN* (lobular PGN, mesangial sclerosis). Mesangial cells proliferate with hyaline deposits of BM-like material in parts of the lobules. It again occurs in the younger patient, is usually static and interferes little with renal function. The aetiology is not known.

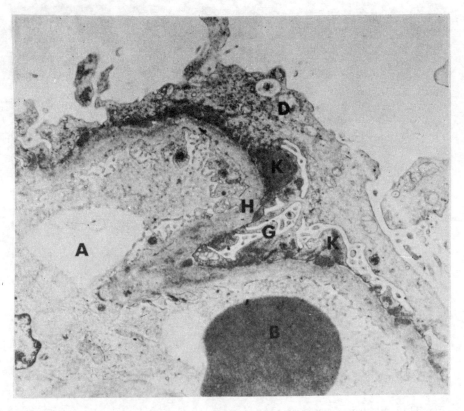

Fig. 29.13. Electron Microscopic Appearance of Glomerulus in Post-streptococcal Glomerulonephritis (Magnification × 9100).
The letters correspond to those of Fig. 29.10. There is deposition of immune complexes (K) on the epithelial border of the basement membrane. (By courtesy of Dr G. Williams.)

(c) *PGN with extensive epithelial 'crescents'*. There is marked proliferation of the epithelial cells of Bowman's capsule. Immunoglobulins, usually IgG in association with C3, are deposited all along the BM suggesting the formation of actual antibodies to this structure. The disorder, more common in the older patient, is rapidly progressive with early oliguria and renal failure. The aetiology is uncertain.

(d) *Mesangiocapillary PGN* (membranoproliferative glomerulonephritis, persistent hypocomplementaemic glomerulonephritis). Mesangial cells proliferate with increase in connective tissue fibrils in the mesangium. The BM is thickened especially on its inner surface with formation of extra fibrils in the endothelial cell. Immunoglobulins are deposited in these sites with considerable amounts of C3 reducing its circulating level. It is more common in young patients and is usually slowly progressive with associated renal hypertension.

(e) *Focal PGN*. Proliferation of mesangial or endothelial cells affects some glomeruli. It is potentially reversible and not usually progressive.

(f) *Unclassifiable and advanced glomerular sclerosis.* The later stages of the progressive lesions lead to extensive glomerular sclerosis with a common picture. At this stage of a diffuse disorder, detailed classification is not possible but renal failure is marked.

B. Glomerular Disease as Part of a Multi-system Disease

A variety of glomerular disorders of the patterns already described may occur in association with a disease process involving other parts of the body. Sometimes more specific changes occur in the glomeruli.

1. **Renal Amyloidosis.** Amyloidosis involves the deposition of the glycoprotein, amyloid, in relation to BMs in several organs. It may occur as a secondary complication of rheumatoid arthritis, multiple myeloma, chronic infection or as so-called primary amyloidosis. The effects are similar in both cases and in Britain primary and secondary types have a similar incidence. In the kidney, irregular clumps of hyaline amyloid are deposited on the inner surfaces of BMs in the glomeruli and in association with the renal tubules and blood vessels (Fig. 29.14). The glomeruli usually become abnormally permeable. The disorder is slowly

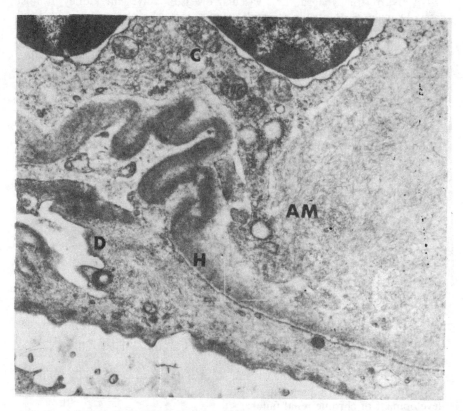

Fig. 29.14. Electron Microscopic Appearance of Glomerular Amyloidosis (Magnification × 17 500).
    The letters correspond to those of Fig. 29.10. There is a fibrillary deposit of amyloid (AM) between the endothelial cell and the basement membrane. (By courtesy of Dr G. Williams.)

progressive unless the primary disorder is curable. Some patients develop hypertension and some develop a secondary renal vein thrombosis which increases glomerular permeability further.

2. **Diabetic Nephropathy (Kimmelstiel–Wilson Syndrome)**. Nearly all diabetics show minor glomerular changes on electron microscopy. Typically a rounded, homogenous mass is found (20% of patients) but mesangial sclerosis, fibrin deposition on capillary loops and deposits on the Bowman's capsule also occur. The BM is thickened and the glomeruli are abnormally permeable. Thickening of the walls of the arterioles restricts the blood supply. Progressive damage to glomeruli results in renal impairment.

3. **Systemic Lupus Erythematosus (SLE, DLE)**. This multi-system disorder affects the kidney in about half the cases and produces a wide variety of glomerular changes ranging from mild focal lesions to diffuse PGN with extensive epithelial crescents. Immune deposits occur on the BM on the endothelial side. The antigen is DNA and the deposits usually contain IgG, often with C3 and sometimes with other immunoglobulins. The more diffuse lesions are often progressive, rapidly so if epithelial crescents are present. The affected glomeruli are abnormally permeable. The mild lesions may produce only slight symptoms.

4. **Polyarteritis Nodosa**. This vascular disease involves the kidney in most cases. Damage to the walls of small arteries and arterioles occurs with local fibrinoid necrosis and blockage of the vessel. If small renal arteries are involved this produces multiple small renal infarcts with recurrent haematuria. Hypertension may develop but renal function can be well preserved. A more serious variant involves glomerular arterioles producing PGN often with fibrinoid necrosis and epithelial crescent formation. In the latter case the disorder progresses rapidly.

5. **Henoch–Schönlein Purpura Syndrome**. This usually occurs in young children and renal involvement occurs in about half the cases. Usually this is a focal PGN with potential for recovery. Less often a diffuse PGN occurs and in the older patient this may be associated with epithelial crescent formation and a rapidly progressive course.

6. **Goodpasture's Syndrome**. The features of PGN with extensive epithelial crescents occur in combination with pulmonary haemorrhages. This serious syndrome is commonest in young adult males.

Disorders of Renal Tubules

Congenital Defects. Several of these are known and may involve a particular function as, e.g. renal tubular acidosis (p. 595), or cystinuria (p. 393) or several different functions may be affected together as in the Fanconi syndrome (pp. 337, 360, 386, 390, 575, 619). Some of these disorders are associated with structural abnormalities of the nephron itself. Others may lead to secondary effects such as nephrocalcinosis in renal tubular acidosis and stone formation in cystinuria. Further renal damage may then result. In a number of cases of the Fanconi syndrome there is progressive loss of renal functional tissue with the eventual development of chronic renal failure.

Acquired Disorders. These affect the tubules earlier than the glomeruli.

Acute pyelonephritis is an acute bacterial infection of the renal pelvis with retrograde spread along the distal tubules initially. The damage is potentially reversible as damaged tubules regenerate much more readily than damaged glomeruli. The disorder is common in pregnancy and in obstructive disorders of the lower urinary tract with superadded infection.

Chronic pyelonephritis is an important disorder whose aetiology is not fully understood. There is slowly progressive destruction of tubules with atrophy of the associated glomeruli. Remaining tubules are hypertrophied. In some cases recurrent urinary tract infection can be demonstrated and obstruction to urine flow increases the chance of developing the disorder. The disease usually affects the two kidneys unequally and is sometimes associated with the development of renal hypertension. In the absence of this complication the disease progresses slowly.

Impaired tubular function also occurs in potassium deficiency which may produce obvious degenerative changes in the tubular cells. Impaired medullary osmolality in compulsive water drinkers leads to poor concentrating ability.

Vascular Disorders

Multi-system disorders affecting the arteries have already been mentioned. The main other disorders affecting the vessels are hypertension, thrombosis and embolism. The arterioles are affected in hypertension. If this is not severe, as in benign hypertension, thickening of the walls of these vessels, as is seen in diabetic nephropathy, may impair glomerular blood supply increasing the slow rate of sclerosis of glomeruli which normally occurs with ageing. This usually produces little encroachment on the functional reserve of the kidney but may be an important factor if other renal disease is present. Malignant hypertension, a more severe disorder, is accompanied by fibrinoid necrosis of arterioles and small arteries as in polyarteritis nodosa and has similar consequences. Deterioration in renal function can then occur quickly.

Blockage of small renal arteries by emboli as, e.g. in subacute bacterial endocarditis produces small infarcts of the kidney with some loss of functional tissue and transient haematuria. Atheroma and thrombosis leading to partial occlusion of the main renal artery or one of its branches causes extensive renal ischaemia with impairment of function and the possibility of renal hypertension developing. Thrombosis of the renal vein has already been mentioned.

A reduction in blood pressure or renal blood flow as in shock is an important cause of renal damage with the development of acute renal failure. Depending on the severity and duration of the disordered blood supply the effect on kidney tissue varies from temporary glomerular shutdown through potentially reversible necrosis of varying degree to bilateral renal cortical necrosis where all nephrons are permanently destroyed.

Other Disorders of the Kidney

Renal calculi may produce intermittent haematuria or obstruction to urine flow with the likelihood of infection and pyelonephritis. *Tumours of the kidney* are usually either a nephroblastoma (Wilms' tumour) in young children or renal carcinoma (hypernephroma) in the adult. Local invasion destroys functional tissue and recurrent haematuria often occurs. The main hazard is the formation of extra-renal metastases. A number of *toxic substances* can affect the renal tubules. The effects may vary from a mild proteinuria of characteristic type as in cadmium poisoning to severe renal tubular necrosis with acute renal failure.

CLINICAL SYNDROMES

Asymptomatic Proteinuria

Proteinuria of mild to moderate degree is often discovered unexpectedly at a routine medical examination. The subject is covered in Chapter 20 (p. 436). Further investigations include assessment of its degree, constancy, and modification by posture. Constant proteinuria is usually indicative of renal disease. Tests of glomerular function, microscopic examination of the urine, measurement of the blood pressure and radiological examination of the kidneys and urinary tract help to decide whether significant renal damage is present.

Most renal diseases are accompanied by proteinuria. Usually urinary protein losses of less than one gram daily with no abnormal clinical or radiological findings and with normal renal function are associated with mild non-progressive renal diseases. However, proteinuria may be an indication of an early stage of a more serious and progressive kidney disease or of a multi-system disease. Repetition of the investigations at intervals enables deterioration in renal function or clinical state to be assessed. If the proteinuria is more marked this may eventually lead to the appearance of the nephrotic syndrome.

Recurrent Haematuria

As a manifestation of renal disease this is more common in children. It may arise post-renally but the presence of red cell casts in the urine indicates a renal origin for the haematuria. Radiological examination, cystoscopy and urine cytology help to differentiate renal parenchymal bleeding from that due to calculus formation and tumours of the pelvis, ureter, bladder or kidney itself. The usual renal function tests, tests for proteinuria and clinical examination are needed. If normal renal function exists with no proteinuria between attacks, normal blood pressure, and no structural changes in the urinary tract, recurrent haematuria is usually a benign disorder such as mesangial PGN. In some patients the symptom recurs over several years simultaneously with viral infections of the upper respiratory tract without change in renal function. In others, several members of the family may be similarly affected.

More serious disorders with progressive renal damage occur if proteinuria or hypertension is also present. Focal glomerulosclerosis may behave in this way as may the combination of hereditary haematuria and deafness (Alport's syndrome). The repetition of tests of glomerular function and urinary examination is therefore important for the proper investigation of recurrent haematuria.

Acute Nephritis

The most common form occurs in adolescents or young adults commencing suddenly one to three weeks following a haemolytic streptococcal infection, usually of the throat. This is active diffuse endothelial PGN representing a hypersensitivity reaction to a streptococcal protein and deposition of immune complexes with this in the glomeruli. A minority of cases have the histological features of mesangiocapillary PGN or PGN with extensive epithelial crescents, the latter sometimes being part of a multi-system disease such as SLE, polyarteritis nodosa or Goodpasture's syndrome. An acute nephritic presentation is also seen in Henoch-Schönlein purpura.

The clinical features are the rapid onset of general malaise, vomiting, oedema of the face and, sometimes, ankles. The urine output diminishes with the development of oliguria (less than 400 ml/day) or even anuria (less than 100 ml/day) in the more severe case. Haematuria is apparent. The patient is hypertensive with signs of left ventricular strain. The urine contains red cells and granular and red cell casts. Proteinuria of varying severity is present, the more marked degrees being associated with a poorer prognosis. The urine osmolality is high but the sodium concentration is often less than 40 mmol/l. Fibrin degradation products are often present.

The creatinine clearance is low as the glomeruli are acutely congested. Plasma urea is increased and the albumin concentration may be rather low during the oedematous stage. Changes in specific proteins may be helpful. The C3 component of complement is usually reduced but in Henoch-Schönlein purpura it is increased. A marked fall in C3 and C4 is suggestive of SLE. In the post-streptococcal type the anti-streptolysin O (ASO) titre is usually increased, unless antibiotics were given, but no marked changes in immunoglobulins occur. A considerable increase in IgG is suggestive of SLE and an increase in IgA is seen in Henoch-Schönlein syndrome. The presence of antinuclear antibodies or LE cells helps in the diagnosis of SLE.

In the usual post-streptococcal case the oliguria lasts for a few days only and the subsequent diuresis is accompanied by a rise in GFR, a fall in plasma urea and disappearance of the hypertension and oedema. The proteinuria and haematuria persist for much longer, often several months, before finally disappearing. The proteinuria may pass through an orthostatic phase. The plasma C3 level is usually back to normal within six weeks.

A few patients develop anuria and if this persists for more than a day or two the condition is described as acute renal failure (see p. 785). A few patients develop *subacute glomerulonephritis* characterised by continuing haematuria, heavy proteinuria often with development of the nephrotic syndrome, continuing oedema and hypertension and a fairly rapid deterioration in GFR with rising plasma urea. These patients enter the stage of terminal renal failure in a few weeks or months and the histological counterpart is marked epithelial crescent formation. This rapidly progressive course is more common in older patients, is often unrelated to a streptococcal infection, but may be a feature of multi-system disease.

Some patients run the slowly progressive course of *chronic glomerulonephritis.* There is apparent recovery with the exception of persisting proteinuria and occasional microscopic haematuria. The GFR slowly deteriorates with the eventual development of chronic renal failure and, often, renal hypertension. This downhill course can be followed by renal function tests and may take 10 to 30 years. Its histological counterpart is mesangiocapillary PGN. It is now thought probable that this differs from post-streptococcal nephritis. A particular biochemical feature in the plasma is that the reduction in C3 concentration persists unlike the typical post-streptococcal response.

Nephrotic Syndrome

The essential fault is increased glomerular permeability leading to marked proteinuria, of which albumin is a major component. If the rate of loss exceeds the synthetic capacity of the liver the serum albumin level falls and hypoproteinaemic oedema results. This combination of heavy proteinuria and oedema constitutes the nephrotic syndrome. A protein loss of 5 to 10 g/day is usually needed but in the young patient, liver synthesis may be rapid enough to compensate even at a loss of 10 g/day particularly on a high protein diet. In the elderly patient a daily loss of 3 g may be sufficient. Oedema does not usually occur until the serum albumin is less than 20 g/l and in severe cases this may fall to 10 g/l.

The reduction in colloid osmotic pressure allows fluid to move from the plasma into the interstitial fluid. This reduced plasma volume activates the renin-angiotensin-aldosterone system and the increased aldosterone output causes sodium retention by the distal tubules. Sodium retention is probably also aided by a reduced GFR. The retained salt and water accumulates in the interstitial fluid and gives rise to pitting oedema.

The degree of permeability of the affected glomeruli varies with the cause of the disease. In most cases the loss of IgG is sufficiently great to reduce its circulating concentration. The patients have a decreased resistance to infection.

Many patients with the nephrotic syndrome have hyperlipidaemia which develops at the same time as the hypoalbuminaemia. While there is usually an increase in cholesterol an increase in triglycerides may also be present and all lipoprotein fractions may be present in high concentration (pp. 463, 466). The appearance of the plasma varies from clear to milky as the triglyceride component increases. There is an increased formation of apolipoproteins in the liver as part of the general increase in the hepatic synthesis of proteins. The increased synthesis of lipoproteins is probably more important than any change in their removal (Cramp *et al.*, 1975).

Other features such as haematuria, hypertension and increase in plasma urea or creatinine are inconstant and depend on the cause of the nephrotic syndrome. In children the most common cause is minimal change glomerular disease in which the proteinuria is usually highly selective (p. 442) and potentially reversible by steroid therapy. There is no hypertension or renal failure. In adults this type accounts for about a quarter of those due to primary renal disease. This highly selective proteinuria is uncommon in all other causes of the nephrotic syndrome. The various forms of PGN account for rather more than half the cases of nephrotic syndrome in adults and for a minority of cases in children. Many of these disorders are progressive. Mesangiocapillary PGN and PGN with extensive epithelial crescents are accompanied by haematuria and hypertension and in the latter case by a raised plasma urea and rapid deterioration of renal function. Other causes of the nephrotic syndrome due to primary renal disease are the progressive disorders, membranous nephropathy and focal glomerulosclerosis; the latter is often accompanied by haematuria.

The nephrotic syndrome may be a manifestation of multi-system disease, in particular amyloidosis, diabetic nephropathy, SLE and multiple myeloma. Amyloidosis may be suggested by coincident chronic inflammatory disease and rectal or skin biopsy may show histological evidence of amyloid deposition. There is no generally satisfactory chemical test for amyloidosis in the intact patient. In some cases a monoclonal gammopathy may be demonstrable on serum electrophoresis (p. 430), or urine electrophoresis may reveal Bence–Jones proteinuria (p. 443). In diabetic nephropathy there is usually a history of long-standing diabetes often poorly controlled so that a high blood glucose and glycosuria are often present. SLE is accompanied by LE cells in the blood, DNA antibodies, reduced concentrations of C3 (also in mesangiocapillary PGN) and C4, and an increase in IgG. The latter is usually reduced in most other types of nephrotic syndrome. Multiple myeloma should be apparent from the presence of a monoclonal gammopathy on serum electrophoresis with an abnormal bone marrow picture and osteolytic lesions in the skeleton. Bence–Jones proteinuria is an inconstant feature. In addition the glomerular permeability often allows escape of the abnormal IgG or IgA into the urine. Urine electrophoresis may then give a complex pattern in which albumin, transferrin, abnormal immunoglobulin and Bence–Jones protein are prominent. In the majority of these varieties of nephrotic syndrome the renal component of the multi-system disease involves progressive glomerular damage. Renal vein thrombosis is rather rare, most often associated with amyloidosis or membranous nephropathy and may be apparent as a sudden increase in the severity of the proteinuria. Fibrin degradation products may also appear in the urine but these are also found in cases of nephrotic syndrome involving immune complex deposits in the glomeruli particularly membranous nephropathy, mesangiocapillary PGN and PGN with extensive crescents.

A feature of all the progressive disorders causing the nephrotic syndrome is destruction of glomeruli. Thus there is a progressive fall in GFR, an eventual rise in plasma urea and creatinine and a slow reduction in the proteinuria as the number of 'leaky' glomeruli diminishes. The proteinuria reaches a level where hepatic synthesis is adequate to increase the plasma albumin concentration. In this case the oedema will lessen and may vanish as the patient passes towards chronic renal failure.

During the oedematous phase a common finding is potassium deficiency with a low plasma potassium level. This may be a consequence of the hyperaldosteronism and the concurrent administration of diuretics.

Acute Renal Failure

Anuria is the important presenting symptom and an acute obstruction of the lower urinary tract should first be excluded as a cause. Some glomerular disorders causing acute or subacute renal failure have already been mentioned but are overshadowed in frequency of occurrence by the mixture of glomerular and, especially, tubular damage as a consequence of renal ischaemia (p. 781). The patient is often shocked and oliguria or anuria occurs early. The urinary sodium concentration is usually much higher than in the acute nephritic syndrome. In cases where excessive haemolysis or crush injuries of muscle are causative factors for the renal ischaemia the urine should be examined for haemoglobin or myoglobin (p. 438).

In cases where the renal ischaemia is short-lived little change may occur in plasma concentrations and the oliguria is transient. More severe damage produces a longer period of anuria. During this stage excretory products such as urea and creatinine accumulate in the plasma and should be monitored. The rate of increase of urea varies with the dietary intake of protein and endogenous protein catabolism. A rise of plasma urea to 33 mmol/l or to lower levels if the rate of increase is marked is often used as an indication for dialysis. At the same time changes in plasma potassium and in the degree of metabolic acidosis are measured. Dialysis is indicated if these approach dangerous levels. Continuing anuria is an indication of extensive, often irreversible, kidney damage but in milder cases as in renal tubular necrosis, a diuresis eventually commences.

In this diuretic phase the urine volume increases each day and a considerable polyuria may result eventually. Modification of the glomerular filtrate composition by the damaged tubules is initially ineffective and glycosuria and aminoaciduria may be demonstrated. The plasma urea and creatinine levels drop towards normal. A possible hazard occurs in excessive loss of electrolytes, particularly sodium and potassium, in the urine. If polyuria is marked, daily losses in the urine should be measured and plasma sodium and potassium determinations should be performed daily to help judge the need for their replacement to avoid serious deficiencies. The gradual healing of the tubules reduces the polyuria and the urine composition approaches normal during the later part of the diuretic phase.

Once recovery of tubular function has occurred in the late convalescent phase any irreversible glomerular damage and loss of nephrons is assessed by measuring the creatinine clearance.

For further information on acute renal failure see Chapman (1980).

Chronic Renal Failure

Many different renal diseases are progressive and involve the gradual destruction of nephrons. The glomerular disorders are more common causes than is chronic pyelonephritis or the pressure atrophy associated with hydronephrosis. A similar picture of chronic renal insufficiency is seen in all types and if the patient presents at this stage the nature of the original disease may not be determinable. The final outcome of progressive renal destruction is death in uraemic coma resulting from complex and marked biochemical changes in all body fluids. Such changes may be controlled by dietary measures initially but later, repeated dialysis or renal transplantation offers the only chance of survival. Biochemical tests assess the need for such measures and their efficiency.

A feature of the slowly failing kidney is that biochemical abnormalities in body fluids alter only slowly with time. It follows that the excretory function of the kidney must be adequate and that the remaining nephrons exert a normal regulatory influence (intact nephron hypothesis). The method whereby this is achieved depends on the way a particular substance is handled by the nephron.

Changes in plasma levels thus vary markedly for different substances. As described earlier (p. 769) the rate of excretion is the sum of the rate of production by glomerular filtration and the further modification by tubular activity. Using the usual symbols this is expressed by the equation

$$UV = P \times GFR - T_A + T_S$$

where $P \times GFR$ represents glomerular production, T_A the tubular reabsorption and T_S any tubular secretion. In slowly progressive renal failure UV remains relatively constant, unless it can be reduced by changes in the diet, while the GFR falls as nephrons are destroyed.

For *creatinine* where T_A and T_S are near zero, a fall in GFR by half is compensated for by a doubling in the plasma concentration. In advanced renal failure the GFR may be only 5% of normal and plasma creatinine levels may then be 20 times the normal. *Urea* is always partly passively reabsorbed by the tubules to an extent varying inversely with V. In renal failure there is a relative diuresis in each surviving nephron (p. 576) reducing this reabsorption thereby making T_A less. Thus the rise in plasma urea need not be so great for a given fall in GFR and when the GFR is 5% of the normal, P may be only 10 to 15 times the normal value. A further difference from creatinine is that diet affects the urea load to be excreted; it is reduced by a low protein diet helping to prevent excessive increases in the plasma urea.

In the case of *phosphate*, active tubular reabsorption (T_A) usually removes over two-thirds of that filtered at the glomerulus. A reduction in this reabsorption allows a smaller rise in P as GFR decreases. Thus in advanced renal failure the plasma phosphate concentration does not usually increase more than 5-fold.

For *potassium* or *urate* most of that filtered at the glomerulus is reabsorbed in the upper nephron, the excreted material being mainly derived by tubular secretion (T_S). The loss of nephrons reduces the tubular mass and hence the rate of excretion will depend on T_S. This has a limiting value for any degree of tubular damage and eventually retention occurs when the load requiring excretion exceeds this. Even so the rate of increase of plasma potassium or urate is only slow. Although the excretory load can be reduced by dietary alterations it is also possible that at the higher plasma level the filtered load per nephron exceeds the tubular reabsorptive capacity (T_A) thus increasing overall excretion. Furthermore there is increased colonic secretion of potassium and, probably, urate into the faeces.

The excretion of *hydrogen ion* is also dependent on the distal tubular mass. As this is reduced there is progressive difficulty in excreting the non-volatile acid produced during metabolism and even though the amount can be reduced by dietary protein restriction, eventually hydrogen ions will be retained and the buffer base in the plasma, including bicarbonate, will be reduced. As the first part of the hydrogen ions secreted by the tubules is normally used to react with bicarbonate, less is now needed for this purpose enabling hydrogen ions to escape from the body.

For *sodium*, only relatively small changes in plasma concentration are compatible with life. Normally about 99.5% of the filtered sodium is actively reabsorbed. In chronic renal failure the surviving nephrons are in a state of osmotic diuresis with reduction in sodium reabsorption. Other alterations in the active reabsorptive process may occur but it will be apparent that a reduction of reabsorption to 95% will increase the unabsorbed fraction from 0·5 to 5% permitting a 10-fold reduction in GFR to be fully compensated without change in plasma sodium concentration. Although the total amount of the sodium in the body is increased in oedematous renal disorders, the sodium concentration rarely rises. If anything there is a tendency in chronic renal failure to develop a low plasma sodium concentration when the sodium intake is poor.

Thus changes in plasma creatinine and to a lesser extent, plasma urea are useful in following the progress of renal disease while sudden changes often in association with similar changes in plasma potassium and the degree of metabolic acidosis indicate decompensation and the need for more vigorous therapy if death is to be avoided.

The kidney is responsible for the manufacture of particular substances and deficiency symptoms can arise in protracted renal failure. Thus the formation of 1,25-dihydroxycholecalciferol, the active metabolite of vitamin D, may be impaired with consequent poor intestinal absorption of *calcium* and defective calcification of bone. A low plasma calcium and increased plasma *alkaline phosphatase* levels are features of 'renal rickets'. In part, the low calcium level is compensated for by a secondary hyperparathyroidism. The increased circulating parathormone concentration produces the skeletal changes of osteitis fibrosa and perhaps those of osteosclerosis. The combination with the earlier changes is conveniently referred to as renal osteodystrophy. Very occasionally this parathyroid stimulation results in adenomatous hyperplasia of the glands, tertiary hyperparathyroidism, with the development of a raised plasma calcium concentration. The kidney also forms an erythropoietic factor which releases from a plasma globulin the substance, erythropoietin, important for the proper maturation of red cells. A feature of renal failure is a normochromic, normocytic anaemia in which both depressed formation and increased destruction of red cells are important factors. The serum iron concentration is usually low with a variable total iron binding capacity. Serum vitamin B_{12} concentration is increased but the reason is not clear. Serum folate levels are low probably reflecting poor dietary intake.

Lipid disturbances in chronic renal failure also occur but are by no means always present. The characteristic feature is *hypertriglyceridaemia* due to endogenous fat particles or VLDL (Chapter 21, p. 455). Plasma *cholesterol* and nonesterified fatty acids are usually normal. There appears to be increased synthesis of VLDL in the liver, possibly a consequence of carbohydrate intolerance. Decreased removal by lipoprotein lipase as a result of accumulated toxic products is a subsidiary factor. The disorder is not fully understood and the VLDL in chronic renal failure seems to contain an abnormally high cholesterol concentration. The condition is reviewed by Cramp *et al.* (1975). Carbohydrate intolerance can be demonstrated by an abnormal glucose tolerance curve. The reasons are not fully established but defective insulin production and interference with insulin by accumulated toxic metabolites have been suggested as the cause of impaired glucose uptake by cells. Growth hormone levels are often high perhaps as a consequence of protein malnutrition resulting from the low protein diets used in therapy.

For a detailed account of the biochemical disorders in chronic renal failure, see Wills (1971).

Renal Tubular Syndromes

Inborn functional defects of renal tubular function and tubular causes of polyuria have already been mentioned. Acquired diseases primarily affecting the tubules occur more commonly and although they may be progressive, the typical feature in the earlier stages is that tests of tubular function are affected more markedly than is the reduction in GFR. Often the kidneys are affected unequally and examination of the urine collected separately from the ureters during cystoscopy can give an indication of tubular function in each organ.

Such changes occur in chronic pyelonephritis and in urinary tract obstruction particularly if this is long-standing and bilateral. Impairment of concentration and dilution tests and a difficulty in conserving sodium are often seen. Sometimes the latter fault is especially emphasised leading to rapid sodium depletion and circulatory shock unless a high intake of sodium is maintained (Thorn *et al.*, 1944; Stanbury and Mahler, 1959). A similar but temporary fault is occasionally seen after correction of long-standing obstruction of the lower urinary tract which has produced bilateral hydronephrosis. In such patients repeated examination of plasma electrolytes and urea with assessment of daily urinary electrolyte losses are important in diagnosis and management.

For general reviews on renal disease and renal function tests, see Black and Jones (1979), Earley and Gottschalk (1979) and Brenner and Rector (1981).

REFERENCES

Berlyne G. M., Varley H., Nilwaragkiu S., Hoerne M. (1964). *Lancet*; **2**: 874.
Black D. A. K., Jones N. F., eds. (1979). *Renal Disease*, 4th ed. Oxford: Blackwell Scientific Publications.

Brenner B. M., Rector F. C. Jr. eds. (1981). *The Kidney*, 2nd ed. Philadelphia: W. B. Saunders.

Chantler G., Garnett E. S., Parsons V., Veall N. (1969). *Clin. Sci*; **37**: 169.

Chapman A., ed. (1980). *Acute Renal Failure*. Edinburgh: Churchill Livingstone.

Chisholm G. D., Williams D. I. eds. (1982). *Scientific Foundations of Urology*, 2nd ed., pp. 251–334. London: William Heinemann Medical Books.

Cramp D. G., Moorhead J. F., Wills M. R. (1975). *Lancet*; **1**: 672.

Dent C. E., Philpot G. R. (1954). *Lancet*; **1**: 182.

Dent C. E., Rose G. A. (1951). *Quart. J. Med*, NS; **20**: 205.

Du Bois D., Du Bois E. F. (1916). *Arch. Int. Med*; **17**: 863.

Earley L. E., Gottschalk C. W. eds. (1979). *Strauss and Welt's Diseases of the Kidney*, 3rd ed. Boston: Little Brown and Co.

Foley T. H., Jones N. F., Clapham W. F. (1966). *Lancet*; **2**: 86.

Garnett E. S., Parsons V., Veall N. (1967). *Lancet*; **1**: 818.

Goldring W., Chasis H. (1944). *Hypertension and Hypertensive Disease*. New York: The Commonwealth Fund.

Haber M. H. (1981). *A Textbook Atlas of Urinary Deposits*. Chicago: American Society of Clinical Pathologists Press.

Harrison G. A. (1947). *Chemical Methods in Clinical Medicine*, 3rd ed. London: Churchill Livingstone.

Hodgkinson A. (1971). *J. Clin. Pathol*; **24**: 147.

Hodgkinson A., Peacock M., Nicholson M. (1969). *Invest. Urol*; **6**: 549.

Holmes E. W., Wyngaarden J. B. (1983). In *The Metabolic Basis of Inherited Disease*, 5th ed. (Stanbury J. B. *et al.*, eds) p. 1192. New York: McGraw Hill.

Payne R. B. (1986). *Ann. Clin. Biochem*; **23**: 243.

Stanbury S. W., Mahler R. F. (1959). *Quart. J. Med*, NS; **28**: 425.

Thorn G. W., Kopf G. F., Clinton M. (1944). *New Engl. J. Med*; **231**: 76.

Williams H. E., Smith L. H. Jr. (1983). In *The Metabolic Basis of Inherited Disease*, 5th ed. (Stanbury J. B. *et al.*) p. 204. New York: McGraw Hill.

Wills M. R. (1971). *The Biochemical Consequences of Chronic Renal Failure*. Aylesbury: Harvey Miller and Metcalf.

30

THYROID FUNCTION TESTS

The biochemical assessment of thyroid function has continued to develop rapidly in the last decade as reliable methods for measuring total serum thyroid hormones have been refined and novel methods for serum thyrotrophin (TSH) and non-protein bound (free) concentrations of thyroid hormones introduced. These technical developments have improved the efficiency of diagnosis of thyroid dysfunction and improved understanding of its underlying pathophysiology. Current methods have largely replaced *in vivo* tests of thyroid function, such as radioiodine uptake, and *in vitro* tests such as protein-bound iodine (PBI), thyroid hormone binding capacity (e.g. triiodothyronine uptake) and measurement of thyroxine by competitive protein binding (CPB). The reader is referred to the 5th edition of this book for a description of these and other methods such as basal metabolic rate, serum cholesterol and creatine kinase in thyroid disease. This chapter considers some aspects of hypothalamic–pituitary–thyroid physiology, current methods for measuring thyroid-related hormones, interpretation of results, and concludes with a discussion on the choice of thyroid function tests suitable for the clinical laboratory.

PHYSIOLOGY

An understanding of the biosynthesis, secretion and transport of thyroid hormones, related aspects of iodine metabolism and control of the hypothalamic–pituitary–thyroid axis is an essential background for the investigation of thyroid function and is provided in standard texts (Hall *et al.*, 1980; Werner and Ingbar, 1986). Only aspects of particular relevance to the clinical biochemist are discussed here.

The thyroid follicular cells synthesise three major iodothyronines: thyroxine (T4, 3,5,3′,5′-tetraiodothyronine), triiodothyronine (T3, 3,5,3′-triiodothyronine) and reverse triiodothyronine (rT3, 3,3′,5′-triiodothyronine). T4 has been considered a prohormone since T3 is three to five times more biologically active and has a shorter half-life in blood (1 day) than T4 (7 days). T4 and T3 have indistinguishable effects on protein, carbohydrate and lipid metabolism and increase oxygen consumption, whereas rT3 is biologically inactive. Thyroid hormones are necessary for normal growth and development of many tissues including the nervous system in fetal and neonatal life. The thyroid secretes all the circulating T4 but only about 20% of T3 and 2·5% of rT3, the remainder of T3 and rT3 being derived from peripheral deiodination of T4 especially in the liver. The control of deiodination is poorly understood but is influenced by nutritional status, drugs and many pathological processes. Changes in the deiodination pathway of T4 to form either T3 or rT3 may be important in regulating the biological activity of thyroid hormones at tissue level.

Thyroid hormones are transported in plasma reversibly bound to thyroxine binding globulin (TBG), prealbumin (PA), and albumin (Hoffenberg and

Ramsden, 1983). TBG is the most specific binding protein, and has high avidity (higher for T4 than T3), but limited capacity (250–400 nmol T4/l plasma) and normally carries 70% of T4 and 75 to 80% of T3. PA has a lower avidity but higher capacity (approx. 3250 nmol T4/1) and normally carries about 20% of T4 and 10% of T3. Although only 25% of sites on TBG and 1% on PA are occupied by thyroid hormones, 99·97% of T4 and 99·7% of T3 circulate in protein-bound form. It is generally accepted that the free fractions (T4, approx. 20 pmol/l; T3, approx. 5 pmol/l) are responsible for biological activity and determine thyroid status. Within the cell, T3 is the active hormone. Some tissues (such as liver) utilise predominantly T3 derived from serum T3 whereas others (such as pituitary and brain) utilise, in addition, T3 derived from serum T4 by intracellular monodeiodination. Normally about half the nuclear binding sites for T3 in the liver are occupied compared with about 80% in the pituitary. Thus, the thyroid status of extra-pituitary tissues mainly reflects the plasma T3 concentration whereas in the pituitary it is determined by plasma T4 levels as well (Larsen *et al.*, 1981).

The production of thyroid hormones is controlled mainly by TSH secreted by thyrotrophs of the anterior pituitary. TSH is a glycoprotein (mol. wt. 28 000) composed of two dissimilar subunits, α and β. The α-subunit is common to the glycoprotein hormones HCG, FSH, and LH while the β-subunit differs. TSH release is controlled by two mechanisms: (1) directly at pituitary level by the negative-feedback action of non-protein bound T4 and T3 such that high levels inhibit and low levels stimulate, (2) hypothalamic factors modulate this negative feedback action. Thyrotrophin releasing hormone (TRH, L-pyroglutamyl-L-histidyl-L-prolineamide) is the major factor acting as the final common path by which the central nervous system influences TSH release, though others, such as dopamine and somatostatin, may also be involved. In certain pathological conditions, high concentrations of TRH also stimulate prolactin release. Circulating TSH levels show a circadian rhythm with peak levels in the early hours of the morning and trough levels in the late evening. How the circadian rhythm is controlled is not yet clear.

METHODS FOR THE MEASUREMENT OF CIRCULATING THYROID HORMONES

Total T4 and T3

Since the production of specific antibodies to T4 and T3 in the early 1970s (Chopra *et al.*, 1971), radioimmunoassay (RIA) has been the method of choice for total serum T4 and T3 for clinical purposes (Chopra, 1972; Larsen, 1972; Ratcliffe *et al.*, 1974b). RIA overcomes the major problems of PBI (iodine contamination, technical complexity and hazardous chemicals) and CPB methods (extraction, interference by non-esterified fatty acids). The assay of T4 and T3 in unextracted serum requires their displacement or release from serum binding proteins by agents such as 8-anilino-1-naphthalene sulphonic acid (ANS), or salicylate, and/or alkaline buffers such as barbitone, pH 8·6 or glycinate, pH 10·5. Total T4 and T3 are then measured by conventional, competitive, limited reagent immunoassay with separation of antibody-bound and free fractions and counting of the bound fraction. A wide range of 'in-house' and commercial methods is available, differing principally in the source of reagents, choice of displacing agent or phase separation.

Care in the selection of reagents, phase separation, and optimisation of the assay protocol are important factors in achieving satisfactory analytical performance. Antisera to thyroid hormones have been raised successfully in rabbits and sheep using T4 or T3 conjugated to bovine serum albumin (BSA) by the carbodiimide method and conventional immunisation protocols. Thyroglobulin should be avoided as carrier protein, since T3 antisera may cross-react significantly with T4. Antisera of relatively high avidity are required for T3 because it circulates at levels 50- to 100-fold less than T4. Cross-reaction of T4 antisera of up to 5 % with T3 is acceptable but T3 antisera should ideally cross-react less than 0·1 % with T4. Metabolites of T3 and T4 (e.g. triiodothyroacetic acid, TRIAC; tetraiodothyroacetic acid, TETRAC), and rT3 are unlikely to interfere significantly in the assays due to their low circulating levels.

T4 and T3 tracers labelled with ^{125}I of specific activity 40–60 mCi/mg (1·5–2·2 MBq/μg) and greater than 1000 mCi/mg (> 37 MBq/μg) respectively are available from commercial sources. The shelf-life of concentrated tracers in alkaline ethanolic solution stored at 4 °C is up to 8 weeks and is limited by radioactive decay rather than degradation.

T3 is more readily displaced from serum proteins than T4 because its affinity is at least an order of magnitude less than that of T4 at physiological pH. ANS is widely used as a displacing agent, effective concentrations being approximately 2 mg/ml serum for T3 and 10 mg/ml serum for T4 for sample volumes of 25–50 μl serum. The concentration of displacing agent should be selected experimentally to ensure quantitative hormone displacement without inhibiting the primary immunological reaction.

Standards. The assays are standardised with highly purified sodium salts of T4 and T3, which contain less than 1 % of other iodothyronines as assessed by HPLC and ultraviolet detection. The molar absorption coefficient of T4 is well defined (6200 l mol^{-1} cm^{-1} at 325 nm) but is less certain for T3. Hence standardisation of T4 can be based on spectrophotometry whereas for T3 it should be based on gravimetry after thorough desiccation in the dark for at least 48 h to remove the variable water of hydration (Malan *et al.*, 1983). Sodium salts of T3 and T4 dissolve in a small volume of ethanol to which has been added 0·5 ml of sodium hydroxide, 1 mol/l. Working standards are made in a human serum-based matrix in order to equalise non-specific serum effects in the RIA. Pooled human serum from donors individually tested for hepatitis B antigen and HIV antibody is treated with agarose-coated charcoal. The efficiency of removal of iodothyronines should be greater than 95 % as judged by the addition of trace amounts of ^{125}I-T4 or T3 to the serum pool. Each batch of iodothyronine-free serum must be tested for its suitability in RIA by comparing binding values in zero standard (B_0) and non-specific binding with those of a previous batch known to be satisfactory. Working standards covering the working range of the assay are prepared from a single batch of tested iodothyronine-free serum, subdivided into small volumes (e.g. 200 μl) in sealed tubes, and stored at -30 °C. Such standards are stable for at least 6 months. Suitable ranges of standard concentrations are 20–300 nmol T4/l and 0·5–10 nmol T3/l. New standards should not be prepared for each assay nor should standards be made by serial dilutions of a stock standard.

Phase Separation. Although methyl cellulose or dextran-coated charcoal has been used extensively for phase separation, it is less rugged in routine practice than polyethylene glycol (PEG)-assisted double-antibody methods for T4 (Ratcliffe *et al.*, 1974a). Precipitation of the bound fraction by PEG alone (13 % final concentration) is cheap and simple, though the relatively high concentrations are viscous and may be unsuitable for automated equipment. In addition, non-specific binding is relatively high. Double-antibody precipitation in liquid phase is slow requiring several hours for complete precipitation. More rapid alternatives include PEG-assisted double-antibody, in which a subprecipitating concentration of PEG is employed, and solid phase second-antibody methods. For T3 RIA, PEG alone is less satisfactory than PEG-assisted double-antibody or solid phase second-antibody techniques. All these methods involve centrifugation, avoided in commercial kits which employ either magnetisable solid phase to which antibody is coupled or antibody coated on the walls of tubes.

Assay Reproducibility. This should be assessed by including at least three internal quality control sera of human origin with clinically relevant thyroid hormone levels (e.g. T4, 50, 100, 150 nmol/l; T3, 1·5, 3·5, 5 nmol/l). Suitable sera are available commercially or can be prepared by pooling individual donations which have appropriate concentrations. Each individual serum must be negative for hepatitis B antigen and HIV antibody. A practical heat treatment procedure for pooled serum cannot be recommended unreservedly at the moment, though heating at 56 °C for 1 h is probably satisfactory for all except grossly infected sera.

Assay Bias. This is more difficult to assess since target values by independently validated methods are not available for thyroid hormones. Nevertheless, the UK External Quality Assessment Scheme (UKEQAS) has shown from recovery experiments that the all-laboratory trimmed mean (ALTM) for total T4 is a valid basis for assessing an individual laboratory's bias and variability of bias. The majority of laboratories in the UK achieve a bias of less than 5 % which is satisfactory for most clinical purposes. The reliability of the ALTM for total T3 is less well established because of method-related differences.

Reference Ranges. In most parts of the world, thyroid hormone concentrations are reported in molar SI units though traditional gravimetric units are still used. The conversion factors are: T4 in nmol/l × 0·0777 = T4 in μg/100 ml and T3 in nmol/l × 0·651 = T3 in ng/ml. In healthy, non-pregnant adults in iodine-replete areas, the reference range for T4 is approximately 50–150 nmol/l and for total T3, 1·0–3·0 nmol/l. The reference ranges increase throughout pregnancy as follows: first trimester-T4, 85–160 nmol/l and T3, 1·5–3·5 nmol/l; third trimester-T4, 85–195 nmol/l and T3, 2·0–4·0 nmol/l. In the neonate up to 5 days postpartum the reference range for T4 is 100–250 nmol/l and for T3, less than 0·5–3·2 nmol/l.

Free T4 and T3

Conventional methods for free thyroid hormones rely on equilibrium dialysis of serum to which has been added a trace amount of highly purified, labelled hormone. This allows the free fraction to be estimated, from which the absolute free hormone concentration can be calculated knowing the total hormone concentration. These methods are susceptible to impurities in the tracer and are imprecise (Ekins, 1979). Dialysis of serum in specially constructed dialysis chambers followed by direct RIA of thyroid hormones in the dialysate avoids the problems associated with tracer impurities (Ellis and Ekins, 1975; Giles, 1982). However, while dialysis/RIA is appropriate as a reference method, it is too complex for routine use. In recent years, several simpler and innovative approaches to the assay of free hormones in serum have become available (Ekins, 1983).

Two-stage Sequential Incubation Method. Introduction of a trace amount of thyroid hormone antibody into serum results in a fractional occupancy of binding sites which is closely related to the serum free hormone concentration at equilibrium. In practice, the first stage utilises a solid phase antibody after which serum is removed by washing. In the second stage, labelled hormone is added after which the solid phase is washed. The fraction of labelled hormone bound to solid phase is then inversely proportional to the free hormone concentration and can be quantitated by comparison with serum standards with known free hormone concentrations determined independently.

While this method is analytically valid, the sequential incubation and washing steps are inconvenient practically. A more severe problem is the vulnerability of such procedures to drift within assay and errors arising from variations in timing of incubation and wash stages. During the latter, unlabelled hormone may dissociate from antibody binding sites.

One-step Labelled-analogue Method. Concurrent incubation of reagents is possible if the tracer is a labelled analogue of the hormone which is able to bind to antibody but not to serum binding proteins. It is essential that the labelled analogue binds to an insignificant extent to serum proteins and that the amount of antibody introduced into the system is small (Gieseler *et al.*, 1986). Under those conditions, the proportion of label bound is inversely proportional to the free hormone concentration. Quantitation is achieved as described for the two-stage sequential incubation method. Labelled-analogue methods are widely available as commercial kits and are simple, quick and precise. However, there are reservations about their analytical validity which centre on the extent to which the labelled analogues interact with serum binding proteins such as albumin (Stockigt *et al.*, 1981; Stockigt *et al.*, 1983; Wilkins *et al.*, 1985). These effects suggest that labelled-analogue methods do not measure free hormones *per se* but are another type of free thyroid hormone index or FTI (Wilke, 1986).

In practice, labelled-analogue methods give results which correlate well with equilibrium dialysis methods in conditions in which altered TBG is the major abnormality. In such situations, these methods appear to be more reliable diagnostically than FTIs. However, they may not be reliable when there are changes in many serum constituents in more complex situations such as pregnancy, non-thyroidal illness and heparin therapy (Amino *et al.*, 1983; Csako *et al.*, 1986). Results by current labelled-analogue methods are artefactually raised in FDH (p. 798) due to binding of the analogue to the abnormal high affinity binding site on albumin and hence affected patients are at risk of misdiagnosis of hyperthyroidism (Byfield *et al.*, 1983). Unfortunately it is not possible to predict which samples are likely to give spurious results with labelled-analogue methods, and these are therefore unsuitable as sole first-line tests in assessing thyroid function (Alexander, 1986).

The analytical assessment of the validity of free hormone assays is not straightforward as formal recovery experiments are not possible. However dilution of sera over a limited range (e.g.10-fold) should not affect results significantly in a valid assay.

Thyrotrophin (TSH)

Radioimmunoassay

RIA has been the method of choice for clinical purposes for the last 15 years (Hall, 1972). RIAs for serum TSH have been gradually refined, simplified and made more rapid due to improvements in the quality of antisera and tracer TSH. Although RIA is adequate for distinguishing elevated from normal TSH levels, limitations of the technique have also become evident and provided a major impetus for the development of more sensitive, robust methods.

TSH RIA is based on established principles of limited reagent assays which have been applied generally to glycoprotein hormone assays. The many 'in-house' and commercial methods differ principally in their choice of incubation protocol and phase separation. The key to sensitive, specific, and reproducible TSH RIA lies in the selection of high quality reagents and optimised protocols (Raggatt *et al.*, 1985).

Antisera. These must be of high avidity, specificity and titre. Polyclonal antisera have been raised to highly purified, natural human TSH in guinea pigs, rabbits and sheep. Cross-reaction with structurally related glycoprotein hormones should be less than 1–2% with FSH, LH and their subunits and less than 0·1% with HCG in order to minimise the effects of high concentrations of FSH and LH found typically in post-menopausal women and HCG in pregnancy.

Labelled Hormone. Highly purified, natural, human TSH is iodinated with ^{125}I, usually by the conventional chloramine-T method though other methods (e.g. solid phase lactoperoxidase, *N*-bromosuccinimide) are also satisfactory. A specific activity of about 76 mCi/mg (2·8 MBq/μg), equivalent to one atom of carrier-free iodine per molecule TSH, is a reasonable compromise between immunoactivity, stability and count rate. Purification of the iodinated peptide by column chromatography on Sephadex G100 or Ultrogel ACA 54 is essential. The purified tracer is either stored at 4°C in phosphate buffer (50 mmol/l, pH 7·5) containing 1g/l BSA, or lyophilised and can be used for up to 10 weeks.

Standards. Assays should be standardised against the 2nd International Reference Preparation (IRP) human TSH (code 80/558) which replaced the 1st IRP in 1983. The 2nd IRP has an assigned value of 37 U/ampoule and contains less than 3% free α- or β-subunits and similar proportions of the five charge variants of TSH as the first IRP. It contains 2·5 IU LH and 0·14 IU FSH per ampoule by immunoassay. When other material is used as a secondary standard, it must be shown to have immunochemical identity with the second IRP in standard curves in the presence of TSH-free serum.

Matrix Effects. Most TSH RIAs are affected by the composition of the matrix used to reconstitute the standard material. It is the responsibility of the assayist to demonstrate that standards in his matrix yield valid quantitation. Working standards should be prepared in matrix selected to correct for non-specific serum effects in the RIA. The choice of matrix is often difficult. Potentially suitable materials include animal sera (e.g. horse), human sera from subjects whose TSH is suppressed with T3 (80 μg orally per day for 5–7 days), or from grossly thyrotoxic patients, normal human sera depleted of TSH by treatment with charcoal (> 98% must be removed), or by immunoadsorption with solid phase TSH antibody (though possible leakage of antibody into the serum must be checked by testing the binding of treated serum to tracer TSH). Each individual donation of human serum must be tested for hepatitis antigen and HIV antibody. Each batch of matrix must be assessed by comparison of zero antigen binding (B_0) with that in thyrotoxic or T3-suppressed sera, by parallelism of serial dilutions of test sera and standard in matrix, by quantitative recovery of added TSH from matrix and by comparison of values obtained on sera circulated in external quality assessment schemes which have reliable target values. Working standards prepared in TSH-free serum are stable in 250 μl portions stored at -30°C for at least 6 months. Serial dilutions of a stock standard should be avoided.

Phase Separation. This has traditionally been by double-antibody or PEG-assisted double-antibody methods for 'in-house' methods, but commercial kits often employ magnetic solid phase or coated-tube methods to avoid centrifugation. All TSH RIAs require extended incubation protocols and often delayed addition of tracer to maximise sensitivity. Overall assay time is usually at least 24 h and the most sensitive assays require up to 5 days.

General Comments. The major limitations of RIA identified by external quality assessment schemes are baseline insecurity (i.e. inability to identify as 'undetectable,' sera known to contain TSH levels below the limit of detection) and imprecision near the limit of detection. The fundamental problem is that RIA becomes susceptible to non-specific interference near to the limit of detection with loss of specificity and precision. Because of this, most RIAs cannot discriminate subnormal from normal levels reliably and it is therefore recommended that realistic detection limits are adopted in order to avoid misleading interpretation.

TSH RIAs are less precise than thyroid hormone assays. Even at elevated TSH concentrations the between-laboratory coefficient of variation is about 15% (compared to 5–10% for T4 and 10–15% for T3) and at euthyroid levels, the between-laboratory, between-assay coefficient of variation is often 30–40%. In the UKEQAS for TSH, 'in-house' methods generally show poor variability of bias suggesting that they are not rugged.

Immunometric Assays

Two-site immunometric assays for serum TSH offer potential solutions to the problems of sensitivity and precision at low levels discussed above. A wide variety of immunometric methods is now available commercially using monoclonal antibodies labelled either with radioiodine (IRMA) or non-isotopically (e.g time-resolved fluorescence, chemiluminescence, enzyme-amplified, enhanced chemiluminescence). Several of these methods have low detection limits (< 0·1 mU/l), extended working ranges (0·1 to more than 100 mU/l), brief assay times (up to 4 h) and are technically simple (Woodhead and Weeks, 1985).

The critical factors in achieving good performance in immunometric and RIAs differ. High antibody avidity is less crucial in immunometric assays though the antibodies must be carefully selected for compatibility and specificity (Soos *et al.*, 1984). One of the antibodies must be as specific for TSH as that required for RIA. Reproducible and complete separation of antibody-bound and free fractions is critical so that the background response in the absence of TSH is low, reflecting absence of non-specific binding of labelled antibody to the solid phase. Solid phases with high capacity for antibody are required such as walls of tubes, microtitre wells, particles (which may be magnetisable) or solid beads. Given a suitable solid phase, assay sensitivity is related to the specific activity of the tracer which can be higher with non-isotopic labels.

The best immunometric assays using monoclonal antibodies discriminate subnormal from normal TSH levels reliably, though significant method-related differences remain due in part to problems of standardisation. Immunometric assays are in general less susceptible to matrix effects so that standards may be prepared in diluent rather than TSH-free human serum.

An important advantage of high sensitivity TSH assays is the excellent correlation between basal TSH and the TSH response to TRH by RIA (Seth *et al.*, 1984). This suggests that basal TSH can replace the TRH test in the investigation of Graves' disease. The TRH test is still indicated, however, in the assessment of secondary hypothyroidism and the rare cases of TSH-dependent hyperthyroidism. Further information is required on the interpretation of subnormal TSH values in patients without Graves' disease, the effects of drugs, circadian rhythm, and TSH levels in toxic and non-toxic adenoma, and non-thyroidal illness. It remains to be established what sensitivity is really required for diagnostic application and how reliable these assays are in routine practice. Nevertheless, there is substantial evidence that a normal basal TSH value virtually excludes clinically important primary thyroid dysfunction.

Disadvantages of present immunometric assays include the cost of commercial kits and dedicated instrumentation required for non-isotopic assays. Depending upon arrangements for reimbursement, this may slow the rate at which the latter methods are adopted. While immunometric assays are generally relatively invulnerable to interfering factors, antibodies in test sera which bind to mouse IgG can give falsely elevated results. Such antibodies are present in about 6% of blood donors. Their effect can be simply abolished by including animal serum in the assay diluent. A theoretical problem may arise if the unique specificities of monoclonal immunometric assays distinguish between different molecular forms of TSH. Such isohormones occur both in the pituitary and circulation. Individual immunometric assays may thus recognise standard and endogenous TSH differently and even recognise differences between endogenous TSH iso-hormones in disease. It is not yet known whether this possibility is an important practical problem.

Assay Quality

Human quality control sera should be used with TSH levels at clinically important decision points. For RIA methods suitable values are 4, 10 and 20 mU/l; for more sensitive assays a control at about 0·5 mU/l should be added. It is important to assess continuously that patient samples with expected very low TSH (e.g. thyrotoxicosis, T3-suppressed) record count rates within the confidence limits of the zero calibrant.

The UKEQAS has shown that immunometric assays, but not RIA, give approximately quantitative recoveries at TSH levels within the euthyroid range. Most laboratories can achieve a bias of less than 10% though variability of bias is less satisfactory. Clinical requirements suggest that the maximum acceptable between-batch imprecision is between 10 and 25% depending on concentration. In healthy non-pregnant adults the TSH reference range, expressed in terms of second IRP human TSH units, is approximately 0·4–4·0 mU/l with a median of 1·5 mU/l for samples taken between 0900 and 1700 h. It should be noted that serum TSH levels have a circadian rhythm with peak values in the early hours of the morning and nadir values in late evening. However, the levels usually remain within conventional reference ranges during daytime sampling.

TRH Test

In the euthyroid subject, TRH given intravenously causes rapid release of TSH. The standard clinical test involves administering 200 μg TRH, dissolved in saline, intravenously as a bolus over a few seconds. Blood samples are taken for TSH analysis before, and 20 and 60 min after, the injection. TSH levels rise to between 5 and 25 mU/l at 20 min with an increment over basal values of at least 3mU/l, thereafter decreasing slightly at 60 min. The TSH response, which is related to oestrogens, is significantly greater in women than men. In hyperthyroid subjects, basal TSH levels are suppressed (< 0·1 mU/l) and there is little or no (≤ 1 mU/l) rise after TRH. In primary hypothyroidism, basal TSH levels are elevated and there is an exaggerated rise in TSH. In secondary hypothyroidism due to pituitary disease, basal TSH levels are low or low-normal and the TSH response is impaired. In hypothalamic disease, the TSH response tends to be delayed with the 60 min value higher than that at 20 min, but this trend is not sufficiently consistent for accurate discrimination of hypothalamic and pituitary disease. If sensitive TSH assays are available, TRH tests are not usually indicated in suspected hyperthyroidism and almost never in overt primary hypothyroidism, but are still required for the investigation of suspected hypothalamic–pituitary disease.

Screening for Familial Dysalbuminaemic Hyperthyroxinaemia (FDH)

The presence of abnormally high concentrations of inherited forms of albumin with increased affinity for T4 (and sometimes T3 and rT3), increases the total T4 concentration (Yabu *et al.*, 1985). FDH may be identified definitively by reverse-flow electrophoresis of serum equilibrated with tracer T4 (Lalloz *et al.*, 1983).

A simple screening procedure suitable for family studies or investigation of unexplained abnormal T4 levels is as follows (Stewart *et al.*, 1986). Test serum (10 μl) is incubated with 50 mmol/l phosphate buffer, pH 7·4 (1 ml) containing 0·5 g/l BSA, 1 nmol T4, and ^{125}I-T4 (10 000 c.p.m) for 2 h at 4 °C. The unlabelled T4 is present to saturate high affinity binding sites on TBG and pre-albumin and accentuate binding by the variant albumin. Dextran-coated charcoal (1 ml at 4 °C) is then added to adsorb the unbound tracer. After 15 min incubation, the tubes are centrifuged (10 min, 1000 *g*, 4 °C), the supernatant is aspirated, and the pellet counted. Typically, more than 50 % of tracer T4 is bound to serum proteins in FDH compared to less that 15 % in normal subjects and patients with increased TBG or autoantibodies binding T4.

Autoantibodies to T4 and T3

Autoantibodies to thyroglobulin which bind T4 and/or T3 may interfere in assays for total and free thyroid hormones. Depending on the method of separation employed, total hormone levels are increased or decreased. With PEG methods, spuriously low values are found whereas with double-antibody methods, levels are inappropriately high. Free hormone levels are variable depending on the specificity of the autoantibody in labelled-analogue methods (Pearce and Byfield, 1986).

Sera can be screened for the presence of these antibodies by incubating 50 μl test serum with tracer T4 (500 pg) or T3 (25 pg) in the presence of 8-ANS (100–400 μg/tube) in 50 mmol/l barbitone buffer, pH 8·6 for 1 h. Immunoglobulin-bound tracer is precipitated by addition of PEG (final concentration, 13 %). After 30 min incubation, assay tubes are centrifuged (1000 *g* for 15 min), the supernatant is decanted and the precipitate counted. Increased binding of tracer in the test sample compared to that in a control serum indicates the presence of autoantibodies. Binding in control sera is usually less than 10 % while a strongly positive serum will bind over 50 % of tracer.

INTERPRETATION OF THYROID FUNCTION TESTS

The interpretation of thyroid function tests in the untreated patient is usually straightforward. However, in patients with mild dysfunction, difficulties may arise particularly when complicated by extremes of age, intercurrent illness, pregnancy, drugs or abnormal serum thyroid hormone binding proteins. These effects will be considered in sections 1–5 below and the changes observed in thyroid disease in sections 6–9.

1. Age

At birth the serum T4 is elevated, free T4 normal, total and free T3 low and TSH normal, relative to adult non-pregnant values. Immediately after birth there is a rapid increase in serum TSH levels to about 80–90 mU/l. These levels decline sharply by 8 h postpartum then more slowly to approach adult levels by 5 days. Total T4 and T3 levels rise rapidly to peak at 24 h then decline, T3 more rapidly than T4 with both hormones remaining slightly above adult values by 5 days. After this major perturbation in thyroid function in the neonate, serum hormone levels decline very gradually to reach adult values by the end of the first decade.

There are no major sustained changes in serum hormone levels in adult life. Although abnormal thyroid function tests have been reported in the elderly (particularly low T3) these are probably associated with non-thyroidal illness. Decreased TSH responses to TRH are reported in elderly men but not women.

2. Pregnancy

There has been much uncertainty about changes in thyroid function during pregnancy, in part because some of the features of increased thyroid activity are usual clinical findings and in part due to analytical problems in measuring free thyroid hormones and TSH reliably. It is well-established that total thyroid hormone levels are commonly increased due to induction of TBG synthesis by high oestrogen levels. Measurement of free thyroid hormones by equilibrium dialysis/RIA indicates a slight rise in mean values in the first trimester, though levels remain within the non-pregnant euthyroid ranges. In subsequent trimesters, free hormone levels decline to low-normal or marginally subnormal levels. However, when measured by labelled-analogue methods, free hormone levels are subnormal in a significant proportion of pregnant subjects in the second and third trimesters (Gow *et al.*, 1985).

In contrast, basal serum TSH levels are slightly decreased in the first two trimesters, occasionally becoming undetectable. Thus, even sensitive TSH methods may have limited value in diagnosing hyperthyroidism in early pregnancy. Nevertheless, established cases of hyperthyroidism in pregnancy show markedly elevated free thyroid hormone levels by a variety of methods, and impaired TSH responses to TRH.

Significant changes in thyroid hormones occur commonly postpartum. Total hormone levels decline and there is a transient decrease in mean free thyroid hormones with a concomitant rise in serum TSH lasting several weeks, though overtly elevated values are uncommon. These changes may reflect the removal of factors which stimulate the maternal thyroid at term, with a compensatory increase in TSH release.

3. Non-thyroidal Illness

A wide spectrum of severe illness not primarily of thyroid origin can affect the control of thyroid hormone secretion, thyroid hormone binding proteins and extra-thyroidal metabolism of T4 (Wartofsky and Burman, 1982). Typically, severe illness (e.g. myocardial infarction, severe liver and renal disease, diabetic ketoacidosis) is associated with low total T3 levels (low T3 or 'sick euthyroid' syndrome) despite clinical euthyroidism. Total and free T4 levels are less affected and when subnormal, are associated with a grave prognosis. Free hormone levels have been reported as normal or subnormal and may be method-dependent. TSH levels and the TSH response to TRH usually remain normal but are occasionally subnormal. It is still unresolved whether these changes indicate tissue hypothyroidism or are a beneficial adaptation to illness. Present evidence does not suggest that thyroid hormone replacement is indicated. Because of these difficulties in interpretation, laboratory assessment of thyroid function should be postponed until the acute episode has resolved. Much confusion and unnecessary investigation has arisen from inappropriate requesting of thyroid function tests in ill, hospitalised patients in whom there is no clear clinical evidence of thyroid disease. When thyroid disease is life-threatening (as in thyroid storm or myxoedema coma) the diagnosis is based on clinical findings and treatment should be instituted before results of hormone measurement are known.

It should be noted that total starvation also causes progressive reduction in total and free T3 whereas T4, TSH and its response to TRH are unchanged. Serum rT3 levels increase in starvation and non-thyroidal illness due to decreased hormone clearance.

4. Drugs

Immunoassays for thyroid hormones are rarely interfered with directly by drugs, but drugs often alter thyroid hormone metabolism and thyroid hormone levels *in vivo* by a variety of mechanisms (Wenzel, 1981).

Altered TBG Concentration. Oestrogens (natural and synthetic) increase TBG concentrations and hence total T4 and T3 while free hormone and TSH levels remain normal. Anabolic steroids and androgens reduce TBG and hence total hormone levels.

Displacement of Thyroid Hormones from Binding Sites on TBG. Analgesics (salicylates, phenylbutazone) and anticonvulsants (e.g. diphenylhydantoin) decrease total T4 and T3 levels whereas free hormones and TSH are normal. The non-steroidal anti-inflammatory drug, fenclofenac, now no longer in use, was a very potent displacer of thyroid hormones from TBG resulting in subnormal total T4 and T3 levels, while free hormones are low-normal.

Inhibition of Thyroid Hormone Synthesis. Anti-thyroid drugs used therapeutically in hyperthyroidism (e.g. carbimazole, thiouracil, perchlorate) reduce total and free thyroid hormone levels as do many other drugs (e.g. iodide, lithium, sulphonamides, anti-TB drugs). TSH levels are variable depending upon the drug and whether the pituitary response is suppressed as commonly occurs for several weeks after drug treatment of hyperthyroidism.

Altered Thyroid Hormone Metabolism. Many drugs inhibit monodeiodination of T4 to T3 (e.g. β-blockers such as propranolol) giving increased T4 to T3 ratios, while others increase thyroid hormone clearance by inducing liver enzymes (e.g. diphenylhydantoin, phenobarbitone). The iodine-containing anti-anginal drug, amiodarone, has complex effects. It inhibits peripheral deiodination with consequent reduction of T3 levels, and may stimulate or suppress thyroid hormone synthesis due to release of variable amounts of iodine during drug metabolism.

Free Fatty Acids. Heparin given intravenously activates lipoprotein lipase which increases endogenous free fatty acids, high concentrations of which can interfere with certain free hormone measurements *in vitro*.

5. Abnormalities in Thyroid Hormone Binding Proteins

Congenital abnormalities in the concentration of circulating TBG are associated with abnormal total thyroid hormone levels but most subjects are euthyroid with free hormone levels in the normal reference ranges and normal basal TSH and TSH responses to TRH. FTIs calculated from thyroid hormone uptake tests fail to correct for extreme variations in TBG.

There are three types of *congenital TBG abnormality* inherited as a sex-linked codominant trait and resulting in elevation, reduction or absence of TBG. As with other X-linked abnormalities, males are more severely affected possessing only an abnormal X-chromosome, while females are heterozygous and have intermediate TBG concentrations. TBG abnormalities are due to altered concentrations of immunologically normal proteins.

Molecular variants of albumin, prealbumin and TBG, though uncommon, can produce significant abnormalities in thyroid function tests in clinically euthyroid subjects (Byfield *et al.*, 1983). *Variant pre-albumins* with increased affinity for T4 or variant TBGs with decreased affinity for T4 and T3 cause mildly elevated or reduced levels of total T4 respectively but normal free hormone values. *TBG variants* are common in certain ethnic groups, e.g. Australian Aboriginals, East African Asians.

Three distinct *genetic variants of albumin* are described with increased avidities for thyroid hormones and yield raised total thyroid hormone and FTI results. Types I and II give erroneously high values with labelled-analogue free T4 assays while free T3 levels are normal. In type III, both tests give falsely high values. These subjects with FDH are clinically euthyroid and have normal basal TSH and TSH responses to TRH. The true prevalence of variant albumins is not known but occurs sufficiently frequently to be an important cause of incorrect interpretation of apparently modestly elevated total and free hormone levels in routine practice.

The presence of T4 and/or T3 *autoantibodies* causes variable and unpredictable effects on total and free thyroid hormone levels. Autoantibodies occur in up to 1 % of routine samples tested and occur in euthyroid subjects without a history of thyroid disease. In all patients with abnormal thyroid hormone binding proteins, thyroid status is best assessed by basal TSH levels.

6. Hyperthyroidism

Hyperthyroidism is most commonly associated with autoimmune thyroid disease (Graves' disease) due to abnormal thyroid-stimulating immunoglobulins. Clinically the patient presents with a toxic diffuse or multinodular goitre with or without exophthalmos. In clinically overt cases, total and free thyroid hormone levels and FTI are markedly elevated while basal TSH levels are suppressed. Clinical hyperthyroidism may also occur with less obvious abnormalities of thyroid function tests, such as isolated T3 or T4 toxicosis. In T3 toxicosis, the patient is clinically hyperthyroid, total and free T3 levels are elevated while the total T4 level is normal and free T4 high normal. The TSH level is suppressed. This abnormality usually accounts for 5 % or less of cases of hyperthyroidism in iodine-replete regions but is more common in areas of iodine deficiency. Isolated T4 elevation causing thyrotoxicosis is rare whereas euthyroid hyperthyroxinaemia is relatively common (Rajatanavin and Braverman, 1983). Thus T4 toxicosis should not be diagnosed on the basis of biochemical findings alone. In ophthalmic Graves' disease, thyroid hormone levels are normal, and subnormal TSH levels may be the sole but not invariable finding.

A suppressed TSH level and impaired TSH response to TRH are constant features of all forms of hyperthyroidism except that due to a TSH-secreting pituitary tumour. A normal basal TSH level therefore excludes the diagnosis. However, it must be remembered that subnormal TSH levels and other abnormalities of thyroid function can occur in conditions other than hyperthyroidism, such as severe illness especially in the elderly, severe depression, hypopituitarism and following administration of drugs (e.g. glucocorticoids, dopamine).

Rarely, pituitary tumours secrete TSH and cause clinical hyperthyroidism (NIH Conference, 1981). TSH and α-subunit levels are modestly elevated as are total and free thyroid hormone levels. As in Graves' disease, TSH and T4 levels are unresponsive to TRH and suppression with T3. TSH levels are also inappropriately elevated when peripheral tissues are resistant to thyroid hormones but in this situation, the patient is clinically euthyroid despite elevated thyroid hormone levels and α-subunit levels are low.

Subnormal TSH levels with normal thyroid hormone levels can occur in patients without clinical evidence of thyroid dysfunction, intercurrent illness or drug treatment and may be classified as subclinical hyperthyroidism. A minority of such patients appear to represent an early stage of Graves' disease but the majority are associated with multinodular goitre with undetectable thyroid-stimulating antibodies but abnormal sensitivity to TSH. Neither the prevalence nor the rate at which subclinical hyperthyroidism progresses to overt hyperthyroidism is yet established.

In the first 3 to 6 months after surgery for hyperthyroidism, thyroid hormone levels are commonly subnormal, thereafter returning to the euthyroid range as pituitary TSH secretion recovers from suppression. Thyroid hormone replacement is not usually necessary during this self-limiting period of biochemical hypothyroidism. Similarly after radioiodine treatment, a temporary period of TSH suppression or isolated T3 elevation is not uncommon.

7. Hypothyroidism

Primary thyroid failure (*myxoedema*) is most commonly due to destructive autoimmune thyroid disease associated with high titres of thyroglobulin and/or microsomal antibodies. The thyroid gland is usually atrophic but may occasionally be goitrous (Hashimoto's thyroiditis). Typically, T4 levels are subnormal and basal TSH elevated, whereas T3 levels tend to be preserved as the failing thyroid secretes T3 preferentially. Elevated TSH levels are reversible when the thyroid failure is due to drugs, such as iodine-containing cough mixture or lithium.

Elevated TSH levels in the presence of normal thyroid hormone levels in clinically euthyroid subjects occur frequently in the general population and indicate *subclinical hypothyroidism*. The prevalence increases markedly with age in females such that about 10% of females aged over 45 years have raised basal TSH figures. Females with both increased TSH and raised anti-thyroid antibodies have about a 5% annual incidence of conversion to overt hypothyroidism and should be followed up at least annually. Whether such patients warrant treatment in the absence of clinical evidence of hypothyroidism is uncertain.

Primary hypothyroidism is a sufficiently frequent, long-term consequence of surgical or radioiodine treatment of thyrotoxicosis to necessitate regular follow up of such patients to identify those with subclinical hypothyroidism who are at increased risk of developing overt hypothyroidism. Patients with subclinical hypothyroidism merit annual thyroid function testing since their incidence of overt hypothyroidism is about 5 % whereas patients with normal TSH levels can be checked less frequently.

Congenital hypothyroidism occurs in about 1 in 4000 births in areas with adequate iodine intake. It is important to recognise this as soon as possible after birth since adequate thyroid function is necessary for normal skeletal and mental development if cretinism is to be avoided. Congenital hypothyroidism is usually due to thyroid aplasia (total absence of thyroid development) or dysplasia (in which some thyroid function is present). Since the biochemical hallmark is an elevated TSH, most developed countries have established screening programmes for neonatal hypothyroidism based on measuring TSH on filter paper blood spots taken between the first and second weeks of life. An elevated blood-spot TSH level should always be confirmed by serum TSH and thyroid hormone measurements. Early detection of congenital hypothyroidism enables treatment to be started within the first month of life and evidence so far suggests that timely therapy prevents major developmental abnormalities in early childhood, although it has still to be established whether subtle behavioural defects persist.

Very rarely, congenital hypothyroidism is associated with goitre due to an inborn error of thyroid hormone biosynthesis. The disorders include defects of iodine trapping, peroxidase deficiency coupling of iodotyrosines, dehalogenase deficiency and defective release of thyroid hormones. In presumed peroxidase deficiency, radioiodine is rapidly taken up by the thyroid but is not organified and can be discharged by perchlorate. Pendred's syndrome is characterised by partial organification defect, goitre and deafness.

In *central hypothyroidism* due to hypothalamic or pituitary disease, TSH levels are usually subnormal but may be low-normal and thyroid hormone levels only modestly reduced. The TSH response to TRH is typically impaired correlating well with basal TSH levels. Occasionally it is normal, possibly due to release of species of TSH with reduced biological but relatively normal immunological activity. Commonly, adrenal and gonadal function is also impaired and any deficiency in adrenal function should be corrected before implementing full thyroxine replacement to avoid precipitating an adrenal crisis.

8. Thyroxine Replacement

Clinically euthyroid patients stabilised on long-term thyroxine therapy for hypothyroidism due to primary thyroid failure or following radioiodine or surgical treatment for thyrotoxicosis commonly have marginally elevated total and free T4 levels, normal total and free T3 levels, while TSH values are normal or subnormal (Pearce and Himsworth, 1984). It is uncertain whether such patients are mildly over-replaced (as indicated by subnormal TSH levels) or not (as indicated by the normal T3 levels). Recent evidence suggests that peripheral tissues as well as the pituitary are overexposed to thyroid hormones as indicated by changes in sodium metabolism, hepatic enzyme activity in serum and systolic ejection time intervals (Beckett *et al.*, 1985). This suggests it would be logical to adjust thyroid hormone replacement to restore a normal TSH. However, there is little clinical evidence of significant tissue damage arising from conventional doses of T4 administered long-term, and it is questionable whether any measurements of thyroid-related hormones reliably distinguish euthyroid patients from those who are receiving inadequate or excessive replacement except in patients with gross abnormalities. It has been suggested therefore that routine biochemical monitoring of patients receiving thyroxine replacement has little clinical value, except to identify non-compliance (Fraser *et al.*, 1986).

9. Goitre

Thyroid function tests are useful in assessing thyroid status in patients with goitre, but do not distinguish the cause. The term 'non-toxic goitre' is applied to a benign, diffuse or multinodular enlargement of the thyroid not associated with apparent abnormal hormone secretion and occurring sporadically in a population. Conventionally it excludes the aetiologically defined causes of goitre (e.g. iodine deficiency, autoimmune, neoplastic, dyshormonogenetic, goitrogens). A small non-toxic goitre is common at puberty, especially in females, and usually regresses spontaneously. Thyroid function tests in non-toxic goitre are essentially normal though a proportion of patients with multinodular goitre have slightly decreased serum TSH and impaired TSH response to TRH implying a degree of thyroid autonomy.

CHOICE OF TESTS

A bewildering range of thyroid function tests is now available to the clinical laboratory. Since the last edition of this book, chemical methods for PBI and CPB methods for T4 have been superseded by RIAs for total T4 and T3, and FTIs have been challenged by direct methods for free thyroid hormones. RIAs of TSH used mainly to detect primary hypothyroidism and, in conjunction with the TRH test, to diagnose hyperthyroidism are being replaced by immunometric TSH assays. The indications for TRH tests have therefore been much reduced (e.g. investigation of hypothalamic–pituitary disease). In contrast, there has been little progress in developing simple tests for assessing the thyroid status of extra-pituitary tissues. Methods for thyroid-stimulating antibodies or thyrotrophin-binding-inhibiting immunoglobulins remain complex procedures more suitable for laboratories with a special interest in autoimmune thyroid disease.

The choice of tests requires consideration of both clinical and laboratory factors.

Clinical Factors

In general practice, the clinician needs to distinguish the relatively small number of patients who require further investigation from the many in whom thyroid dysfunction is unlikely but should be excluded. The test(s) should therefore be sensitive (i.e. few false negatives) and specific (i.e. few false positives). Currently, a sensitive TSH test best satisfies these requirements. In the hospital out-patient clinic, thyroid function tests should enable the clinician to diagnose hyper- and hypothyroidism, assess its severity, and determine the cause if possible. In addition, tests are required to assess thyroid function in patients with goitre or suspected ophthalmic Graves' disease and during pregnancy. Tests are needed to assess the adequacy of therapy (replacement T4 or anti-thyroid) and any effect on the thyroid in patients receiving drugs for non-thyroidal disease. In hospital patients, the assessment of thyroid function in seriously ill patients who are often receiving drugs presents additional problems.

It is perhaps not surprising that no single test or simple combination of tests can satisfy all these requirements. Formerly the main emphasis was placed on a measure of T4 (total T4 or FTI) supplemented as required with TSH (for suspected hypothyroidism) and total T3 and the TRH test (for suspected hyperthyroidism). Such a strategy allows accurate categorisation of thyroid status in most patients, with diagnostic uncertainty in less than 5% depending on case mix (Britton *et al.*, 1975). Currently there is much interest in assessing the role of direct methods for free thyroid hormones and sensitive TSH assays. Strategies based on either have been proposed as first-line tests. However, TSH assays have the important advantage of avoiding problems of interpretation generated by abnormal protein binding or drugs which affect the interaction of thyroid hormones with proteins, and are less misleading in non-thyroidal illness.

Laboratory Factors

Thyroid function tests must be technically simple, precise and unbiased, rapid and cheap. Total T4 and, to a lesser extent, total T3 assays satisfy these laboratory requirements. Free hormone assays using labelled-analogue methods are also simple, quick and precise but their analytical validity is uncertain. They are also relatively more expensive than total hormone assays, but probably no more expensive than thyroxine indices if one of the assays uses a commercial kit. The new generation of two-site immunometric TSH assays has the potential to meet the analytical criteria though an economic disadvantage for laboratories previously using 'in-house' RIA is the substantial extra revenue cost of commercial kits and instrumentation for non-isotopic methods. Furthermore, instrumentation for non-isotopic systems is often locked into a particular manufacturer's method. In contrast, laboratories using commercial RIAs can more readily change to IRMA as the revenue and instrumentation costs are similar for both types of assay.

Conclusion

So far there is insufficient clinical and laboratory experience with the newer analytical techniques to allow clear recommendations for the most cost-effective strategies of thyroid function testing for all circumstances. Overall however, there is accumulating evidence that increased reliance should be placed on a sensitive TSH assay early in investigation (Caldwell *et al.*, 1985). In untreated patients with possible thyroid dysfunction in general practice or in the out-patient setting, the demonstration of a normal TSH virtually excludes clinically significant thyroid dysfunction and additional tests are usually unnecessary. In more complex situations and for definitive diagnosis of thyroid disease, the TSH assay should be combined with some measure of T4. The choice of total T4, FTI, T4:TBG ratio or free T4 depends on local circumstances. Total T4 assays are widely available 'in-house', cheap and rugged but are affected by binding hormone concentration. Free T4 assays are diagnostically more useful than FTIs in primary TBG abnormalities but labelled-analogue methods are affected by changes in other serum proteins.

Assays for total or free T3 are required infrequently (e.g. diagnosis of T3 toxicosis) and are not indicated for investigating suspected hypothyroidism.

Assays for TBG, thyroid hormone antibodies and dysalbuminaemia are only required to clarify anomalous thyroid hormone results which might lead to inappropriate therapy and for family studies. In patients with non-thyroidal illness, thyroid function tests should be postponed until after the acute episode has resolved. In clinically euthyroid patients receiving conventional thyroxine replacement therapy, routine thyroid function tests are seldom helpful as the therapeutic implications of minor biochemical abnormalities are uncertain. With the availability of sensitive TSH assays, the TRH test is rarely required in suspected hyperthyroidism but is still indicated in the investigation of suspected secondary hypothyroidism.

REFERENCES

Alexander N. M. (1986). *Clin. Chem*; **32**: 417.

Amino N. *et al.* (1983). *Clin. Chem*; **29**: 321.

Beckett G. J. *et al.* (1985). *Brit. Med. J*; **291**: 427.

Britton K. E., Quinn V., Brown B. L., Ekins R. P. (1975). *Brit. Med. J*; **3**: 350.

Byfield P. G. H., Lalloz M. R. A., Pearce C. J., Himsworth R. L. (1983). *Clin. Endocrinol*; **19**: 277.

Caldwell G. *et al.* (1985). *Lancet*; **1**: 1117.

Chopra I. J. (1972). *J. Clin. Endocrinol. Metab*; **34**: 938.

Chopra I. J., Nelson J. C., Solomon D. H., Beall G. N. (1971). *J. Clin. Endocrinol. Metab*; **32**: 299.

Csako G., Zweig M. H., Benson C., Ruddel M. (1986). *Clin. Chem*; **32**: 108.

Ekins R. P. (1979). In *Free Thyroid Hormones*. (Ekins R., Faglia G., Pennisi F., Pinchera A., eds). p. 72. Amsterdam: Excerpta Medica.

Ekins R. P. (1983). In *Immunoassays for Clinical Chemistry*. (Corrie J. E. T., Hunter W. M., eds) p. 319. Edinburgh: Churchill Livingstone.

Ellis S., Ekins R. P. (1975). In *Radioimmunoassay in Clincial Biochemistry*. (Pasternak C. A., ed) p. 187. London: Heyden.

Fraser W. D. *et al.* (1986). *Brit. Med. J*; **293**: 808.

Gieseler D., Chodha P., Ekins R. (1986). *Clin. Chem*; **32**: 45.

Giles A. F. (1982). *Clin. Endocrinol*; **16**: 101.

Gow S. M. *et al.* (1985). *Clin. Chim. Acta*; **152**: 325.

Hall R. (1972). *Clin. Endocrinol*; **1**: 115.

Hall R., Anderson J., Smart G. A., Besser M., eds. (1980). *Fundamentals of Clinical Endocrinology*, 3rd ed. London: Pitman Medical.

Hoffenberg R., Ramsden D. B. (1983). *Clin. Sci*; **65**: 337.

Lalloz M. R. A., Byfield P. G. H., Himsworth R. L. (1983). *Clin. Endocrinol*; **18**: 11.

Larsen P. R. (1972). *J. Clin. Invest*; **51**: 1939.

Larsen P. R., Silva J. E., Kaplan M. M. (1981). *Endocr. Rev*; **2**: 87.

Malan P. G. *et al.* (1983). In *Immunoassays for Clinical Chemistry*. (Corrie J. E. T., Hunter W. M., eds) p. 48. Edinburgh: Churchill Livingstone.

NIH Conference (1981). *Ann. Int. Med*; **95**: 339.

Pearce C. J., Byfield P. G. H. (1986). *Ann. Clin. Biochem*; **23**: 230.

Pearce C. J., Himsworth R. L. (1984). *Brit. Med. J*; **288**: 693.

Raggatt P. R. *et al.* (1985). *Thyrotrophin: a review of performance and interpretation of clinical serum TSH assays in the UK*. Association of Clinical Biochemists, London.

Rajatanavin R., Braverman L. E. (1983). *J. Endocrinol. Invest*; **6**: 493.

Ratcliffe W. A., Challand G. S., Ratcliffe J. G. (1974a). *Ann. Clin. Biochem*; **11**: 224.

Ratcliffe W. A. *et al.* (1974b). *Clin. Endocrinol*; **3**: 481.

Seth J. *et al.* (1984). *Brit. Med. J*; **2**: 1334.

Soos M., Taylor S. J., Gard T., Siddle K. (1984). *J. Immunol. Meth*; **73**: 237.

Stewart M. F., Ratcliffe W. A., Roberts I. (1986). *Ann. Clin. Biochem*; **23**: 59.

Stockigt J. R. *et al.* (1981). *Clin. Endocrinol*; **15**: 313.

Stockigt J. R., Stevens V., White E. L., Barlow J. W. (1983). *Clin. Chem*; **29**: 1408.
Wartofsky L., Burman K. D. (1982). *Endocr. Rev*; **3**: 164.
Wenzel K. W. (1981). *Metabolism*; **30**: 717.
Werner S. C., Ingbar S. H. (1986). *The Thyroid*, 5th ed. Maryland: Harper and Row.
Wilke T. J. (1986). *Clin. Chem*; **32**: 585.
Wilkins T. A., Midgley J. E. M., Barron N. (1985). *Clin. Chem*; **31**: 1644.
Woodhead J. S., Weeks I. (1985). *Ann. Clin. Biochem*; **22**: 455.
Yabu Y. *et al.* (1985). *J. Clin. Endocrinol. Metab*; **60**: 451.

31

THE HYPOTHALAMIC–PITUITARY–ADRENOCORTICAL SYSTEM

STEROID CHEMISTRY

A basic knowledge of steroid chemistry is an essential prerequisite to understanding the physiology, pathology and analytical techniques for the measurement of this group of compounds. A brief review is given below and further details can be found in the 5th edition of this book and also in Gower (1979) and Makin (1984).

The parent compound of the steroid hormones is a tetracyclic hydrocarbon, cyclopentanoperhydrophenanthrene, $C_{17}H_{28}$ (Fig. 31.1). This nucleus is then modified by desaturation, the introduction of hydroxyl, carbonyl, aldehyde or methyl groups or by addition of a side chain of two carbon units in length at C-17 to produce the steroid hormones. The four-ring steroid structure is essentially flat and isomerism can occur at several carbon atoms. By convention, substituent groups can be orientated towards the reader 'β' or away 'α'. Important isomerisms of natural steroids occur at C-3, C-5 and C-20 while isomers at C-17 and C-20 are also found.

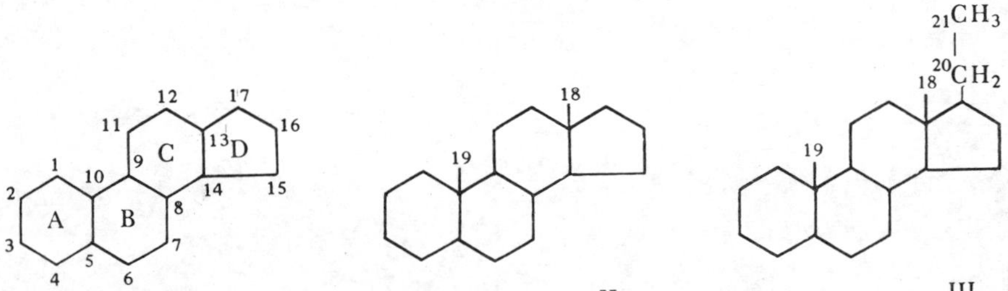

Fig. 31.1. Structures of Steroid Nuclei.
I, Cyclopentanoperhydrophenanthrene; II, androstane; III, pregnane. Oestrane is II without the C-19 methyl group.

Because of the large number of potential steroid molecules, nomenclature has caused considerable problems. The systematic nomenclature recommended by the International Union of Pure and Applied Chemistry, IUPAC (1969) is the accepted method but it is too cumbersome for use on a day-to-day basis. Therefore trivial names are used for the more common steroids. The most important steroids and their IUPAC names are given in Table 31.1. Abbreviations such as compound S, 17OHP, T, etc. can be confusing and are not recommended. The IUPAC nomenclature is based on the various parent nuclei (Fig. 31.1), pregnane (C_{21}) androstane (C_{19}) and oestrane (C_{18}). Substituents are indicated by abbreviations in the form of prefixes and suffixes. Only one prefix is permitted and the suffixes are given an agreed priority: alcohol, ketone, aldehyde, ester, lactone and acid. Another convention is sometimes used in trivial names to describe the position of a double bond in the molecule. Instead of the usual use of '-en(e)-' preceded by a number (Table 31.1), the symbol, Δ, with the number following in superscript form is used as a prefix. Thus DHA is a Δ^5-steroid and testosterone is referred to as a Δ^4-steroid.

TABLE 31.1
Accepted Trivial Names of Common Steroids

C_{21} *Steroids*	
Progesterone	4-pregnene-3,20-dione
Deoxycorticosterone	21-hydroxypregn-4-ene-3,20-dione
Corticosterone	11β,21-dihydroxypregn-4-ene-3,20-dione
Cortisol	11β,17α,21-trihydroxypregn-4-ene-3,20-dione
Cortisone	17α,21-dihydroxypregn-4-ene-3,11,20-trione
Aldosterone	11β,21-dihydroxypregn-4-ene-3,20-dione-18-al
C_{19} *Steroids*	
Dehydroepiandrosterone (DHA)	3β-hydroxyandrost-5-en-17-one
Testosterone	17β-hydroxyandrost-4-en-3-one
Dihydrotestosterone (DHT)	17β-hydroxy-5α-androstan-3-one
C_{18} *Steroids*	
Oestrone	3-hydroxyoestra-1,3,5(10)-trien-17-one
Oestradiol	3,17β-dihydroxyoestra-1,3,5(10)-triene
Oestriol	3,16α,17β-trihydroxyoestra-1,3,5(10)-triene

BIOSYNTHESIS OF STEROID HORMONES

The principal sites of steroid hormone biosynthesis are the adrenal cortex, gonads and placenta. Peripheral metabolism by other tissues is also involved in the conversion of some steroids to their active metabolites. A generalised pathway is shown in Fig. 31.2. The individual organs synthesising steroid hormones do not possess all the enzymes shown in this pathway and this regulates in part the steroids they can produce. In addition, alternative enzymes, isoenzymes and possible pathways for the synthesis of some steroids exist. Normally their activity is low but in patients with inborn errors of steroid biosynthesis or in tumours the activity of these alternative pathways can be considerably increased and this accounts for the many unusual steroids excreted in these conditions.

Steroids are synthesised from cholesterol which is usually exogenous; alternatively cholesterol can be synthesised *de novo* from acetate. Cholesterol is converted to pregnenolone by the enzyme 20,22-desmolase with the loss of the 6-C side chain. The action of various hydroxylases, dehydrogenases (reductases), 17,20-desmolase and A-ring aromatase converts pregnenolone to the active steroid hormones. Many of the enzymes of the steroid biosynthetic pathway involve cytochrome P 450s.

For details of steroid biosynthesis see Finkelstein and Shaefer (1979), Makin (1984) and Riad-Fahmy *et al.* (1979).

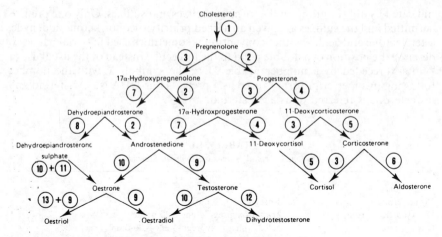

Fig. 31.2. Major Pathways of Steroid Biosynthesis.
The enzymes catalysing each step in the pathway are:

1. 20,22-Desmolase (complex)
2. 3β-Hydroxysteroid dehydrogenase
3. 17α-Hydroxylase
4. 21-Hydroxylase
5. 11β-Hydroxylase
6. 18-Hydroxylase and 18-dehydrogenase
7. 17,20-Desmolase
8. Steroid sulphotransferase
9. 17β-Hydroxysteroid dehydrogenase
10. Aromatase
11. Steroid sulphatase
12. 5α-Reductase
13. 16α-Hydroxylase.

The Control of Steroid Biosynthesis

The main regulators of steroid hormone biosynthesis are the pituitary trophic hormones ACTH, LH and FSH. ACTH stimulates the adrenal cortex to produce glucocorticoids, adrenal androgens and aldosterone. The control of ACTH release is complex: a negative feedback loop exists while control from higher centres is effected through modulation of the production and release of corticotrophin releasing factor (CRF). Many different factors can influence steroid production in this way including stress and circadian rhythms. This regulatory mechanism is disturbed in disorders of the hypothalamic–pituitary–adrenal axis and thus investigation of the changes is important in reaching a diagnosis. Control of adrenal steroid biosynthesis is also probably influenced by adrenal structure and the vascular arrangement of the adrenal gland (Hornsby, 1985).

In addition to ACTH, aldosterone secretion is controlled by plasma sodium and potassium concentrations and the renin–angiotensin system. ACTH has only a minor role in normals but is important in salt-losing congenital adrenal hyperplasia. Aldosterone and the renin–angiotensin system are inter-related by a feedback loop: a fall in aldosterone giving rise to sodium loss and hence release of renin from the kidney. This in turn produces increased levels of angiotensin II which directly stimulates the zona glomerulosa of the adrenal cortex to synthesise aldosterone. Control of the gonadal synthesis of steroids by FSH and LH is discussed in Chapter 32 (p. 841).

CATABOLISM AND EXCRETION OF STEROIDS

Prior to excretion, steroids undergo complex degradative steps which can involve reduction, oxidation, hydroxylation, side chain cleavage and conjugation to form glucuronides or sulphates. It is not surprising therefore, in view of the large number of steroid hormones and precursors and the different possible degradative pathways, that a very large number of individual steroid metabolites can be found in urine. As an example, the neutral steroid metabolites of cortisol following an intravenous injection of ^{14}C-cortisol are given in Table 31.2.

TABLE 31.2

Main Neutral Steroid Metabolites of Cortisol in Urine (after Fukushima *et al.*, 1960)

Metabolite	Conjugate	Mean Excretion (%)
Cortisol	Free	1·7
Cortisone	Free	1·7
Tetrahydrocortisol	Glucuronide	17·8
(3α,11β,17α,21-tetrahydroxy-5β-pregnan-20-one)		
Allotetrahydrocortisol	Glucuronide	9·5
(3α,11β,17α,21-tetrahydroxy-5α-pregnan-20-one)		
Tetrahydrocortisone	Glucuronide	24·1
(3α,17α,21-trihydroxy-5β-pregnane-11,20-dione)		
20α-Cortol	Glucuronide	1·9
(5β-pregnane-3α,11β,17α,20α,21-pentol)		
20β-Cortol	Glucuronide	4·5
(5β-pregnane-3α,11β,17α,20β,21-pentol)		
20α-Cortolone	Glucuronide	11·4
(3α,17α,20α,21-tetrahydroxy-5β-pregnan-11-one)		
20β-Cortolone	Glucuronide	8·2
(3α,17α,20β,21-tetrahydroxy-5β-pregnan-11-one)		
11-Oxoaetiocholanolone	Glucuronide*	3·1
(3α-hydroxy-5β-androstane-11,17-dione)		
11β-Hydroxyaetiocholanolone	Glucuronide*	3·9
(3α,11β-dihydroxy-5β-androstan-17-one)		
11β-Hydroxyandrosterone	Glucuronide*	1·0
(3α,11β-dihydroxy-5α-androstan-17-one)		
Other neutral steroids		11·4

* May also be excreted as sulphates, undetected by the techniques used.

Steroids are catabolised mainly in the liver but additional metabolism can occur in other tissues, e.g. skin and kidney and even the adrenal gland itself. The main route of excretion is in the urine but a percentage of steroid metabolites, particularly oestrogens and androgens, are excreted in the bile and undergo enterohepatic circulation. Excretion of steroid metabolites can be severely reduced in both liver and kidney disease and in the latter case faecal excretion is increased.

The modification of the steroid nucleus and conjugation to sulphate or glucuronic acid makes the hydrophobic steroid molecule more hydrophilic thus facilitating excretion in the urine. Early diagnostic work on patients with steroid disorders was essentially based on this urinary excretion of steroid metabolites. The large number of metabolites and the complexity of the separation techniques for individual identification gave rise to chemical methods which measured groups of steroids with a particular chemical structure or property. For reasons discussed below the analysis of steroid metabolites in this way has been largely abandoned but urine steroid analysis by GLC, with or without mass spectrometry, remains a useful method in the investigation of patients with inherited disorders of steroid biosynthesis or steroid-producing tumours.

The renal excretion of unmetabolised, unconjugated steroids is a potentially useful investigative technique. Evidence from studies of cortisol excretion has shown that non-protein bound cortisol in the blood is filtered at the glomerulus and a fraction reabsorbed in the renal tubule (Beisel *et al.*, 1964a,b). If the total quantity of cortisol in blood is increased there is an increase in the unbound fraction and thus increases in both filtration and reabsorption of cortisol by the kidney. The reabsorption of cortisol appears to be by passive diffusion and there is no evidence of a tubular maximum, thus in the absence of abnormalities of cortisol-binding globulin, the excretion of free cortisol in the urine is directly related to the plasma concentration.

For further details, see Peterson (1971).

MEASUREMENT OF STEROIDS IN BODY FLUIDS

Two main approaches have been used in the biochemical investigation of disorders of steroid metabolism; the analysis of steroids in plasma (or serum) and urine. More recently, the advantages of steroid estimation in saliva have been realised.

A variable proportion of the individual steroids in plasma is bound to serum proteins—cortisol-binding globulin, sex hormone-binding globulin and albumin—and the bound steroid molecules are probably biologically inactive. However, the techniques routinely used to measure plasma steroids include both the protein-bound and free fractions. With the exception of cortisol, which circulates at relatively high concentrations, most steroid hormones circulate in the nanomolar range and require assays which are both sensitive and specific. These criteria are usually met by immunoassay techniques.

One problem with the assay of steroids in plasma is that without multiple sampling the information obtained relates only to the time of sampling. Steroid hormones are frequently released in a pulsatile fashion which in turn may be superimposed on other physiological variations, e.g. circadian rhythms and the menstrual cycle. Interpretation of plasma steroid assays in the absence of externally administered dynamic stimuli or suppression needs to take account of the circumstances of taking the sample.

The analysis of urinary steroids can be performed relatively simply by group analysis (17-oxosteroids, 17-oxogenic steroids and 17-hydroxycorticosteroids) or by more complicated techniques involving separation by extraction and/or chromatography to identify individual steroid molecules. Urinary steroids are usually measured on a 24-hour collection with all the attendant problems. The advantage is, however, that the result represents an average excretion over 24 h. thus avoiding the problem of circadian variation of steroid concentrations.

The observation by Shannon *et al.* (1959) that cortisol could be measured in saliva and subsequent observations that it reflected the non-protein bound fraction in blood led to the proposal that measurement of salivary steroid concentrations could be clinically advantageous, especially in children. Advantages include the ability to do frequent measurements, as an out-patient if necessary, and to have results which directly relate to the physiologically active fraction of the steroid. This overcomes many of the disadvantages of plasma and urine assays.

Plasma Steroid Analysis

The analysis of plasma steroids is now almost universally performed by radioimmunoassay. Methodological details of radioimmunoassays of individual steroids will not be given here; readers are referred to Chapter 6 (p. 110) for a discussion of the principles of radioimmunoassay. Other techniques which may be used for some steroids include fluorimetry, GLC and HPLC as well as more recently developed non-isotopic immunoassays.

Radioimmunoassay

The major problems in steroid radioimmunoassay lie in the production of specific antisera, choice of isotope and labelled derivative. Steroids are not by themselves antigenic and in order to raise antisera they must be coupled to a larger antigenic carrier molecule, usually bovine serum albumin. Linkage first involves the synthesis of a derivative of the steroid so that it possesses a functional group which can react with the carrier protein. Examples include cortisol-3-(*O*-carboxymethyl) oxime and cortisol 21-hemisuccinate. The specificity of the antiserum produced depends to a large extent on the orientation of the steroid molecule to the protein and the accessibility of distinguishing groups. Careful selection of the linkage carbon or group, through which the steroid is coupled, is therefore very important. Examples of cross-reactions of several anti-cortisol antisera are shown in Table 31.3. It can be seen that linkage through C-21 using a hemisuccinate derivative produces antisera with low specificity with reference to differences at C-17, C-20 and C-21. Similar considerations should be taken into account when raising antisera to other steroids, e.g. 17α-hydroxyprogesterone, progesterone, testosterone, etc.

TABLE 31.3

Cross Reactivity of Anticortisol Antisera

| Steroid | Linking Carbon | | | |
	21	21	3	3
Cortisol	100	100	100	100
11-Deoxycortisol	9	100	7·1	3·8
Corticosterone	8	—	4·0	12·5
Cortisone	12	40	0·7	6·6
17α-Hydroxyprogesterone	2·5	56	0·01	0·06
Progesterone	1	28	0·01	0·001
Testosterone	0·3	13	0·01	0·001
Reference	A	B	C	D

References: A—Abraham *et al.* (1972), B—Ruder *et al.* (1972), C—Fahmy *et al.* (1975), D Dash *et al.* (1975).

Competitive protein-binding assays using cortisol-binding globulin as the ligand-binding protein have been used but poor cross-reactivity between circulating steroid molecules has led to their abandonment in favour of radioimmunoassay. Assays using monoclonal anticortisol antibodies have not been described but monoclonal antibodies to other steroids have been produced.

The original radioimmunoassays for steroids used tritium as the isotopic label. This had the advantage that the steroid and its labelled analogue were effectively immunologically identical. On the other hand, specific activities were low reducing the sensitivity and increasing counting times considerably so that the assays usually required extraction, purification and concentration steps. Furthermore, these assays required liquid scintillation counting which is expensive and not compatible with the radioimmunoassay of polypeptide hormones.

An alternative to tritium is iodine-125. This isotope reacts directly with steroids with a phenolic A ring, e.g. oestrogens, but in order to label the great majority of steroids some form of derivative is needed. It is possible to label the carrier protein of the immunogen but usually the steroid is coupled to histamine or tyramine which can be iodinated before or after coupling. In this case, the steroid and label are different and the affinity of the antibody for the label may be much higher than for the steroid. This is so particularly if the chemical bridges between steroid and protein, and steroid and histamine or tyramine are similar in structure. Most ^{125}I-steroid radioimmunoassays have adequate sensitivity and specificity and are the assays of choice for the determination of plasma cortisol as well as other steroids.

Steroid radioimmunoassays can be performed directly on a plasma sample or after some form of extraction or chromatographic prepurification. A substantial and variable proportion of the steroid hormone is bound to plasma proteins and in order to measure the total steroid concentration it is first necessary to displace the bound steroid. This can be achieved by raising the temperature, lowering the pH or by the addition of a chemical reagent which will compete for the binding sites. Extraction using organic solvents of different polarity has the advantage of allowing some purification while denaturing the binding proteins and of some concentration of steroid. Extraction with organic solvents can, however, cause difficulties with immunoassays causing high blanks and it is essential to check regularly for this type of error. Direct assays, which are much easier to perform, are replacing extraction assays as highly specific antisera have become available.

A large number of commercial kits is available for the radioimmunoassay of plasma steroids. Before use these should be carefully evaluated using a recommended protocol for kit evaluation (Percy-Robb et al., 1980; Fraser and Wilde, 1986). Special attention should be given to the specificity of the antiserum used, as diagnostic errors have been reported using commercial kits when high concentrations of abnormal steroids have been present in plasma.

Fluorimetric Assays

This method (Mattingly, 1962) is still in common use despite the greater accuracy of radioimmunoassay methods. Steroids which possess the 11-hydroxyl group fluoresce in the presence of concentrated sulphuric acid, the two main steroids being cortisol and corticosterone.

Reagents.
1. Methylene dichloride. Do not inhale vapour. Extract solvent successively with one tenth volume of concentrated sulphuric acid until the extracts are

no longer coloured. Wash with distilled water (200 ml/l) until washings are neutral. Distil after drying over sodium sulphate (b.p. 39–40 °C). Store in the dark. Alternatively the FDPC grade solvent (BDH Chemicals) is satisfactory without purification.
2. Concentrated sulphuric acid, analytical reagent grade.
3. Ethanol, analytical reagent grade.
4. Fluorescence reagent. Add 7 volumes concentrated sulphuric acid *slowly* to 3 volumes of ethanol while cooling under running water or with ice. If a yellow or brown colour develops, discard the ethanol and try a new batch. This reagent is stable up to 1 month stored in a stoppered glass container.
5. Stock standard. Dissolve 10·86 mg cortisol in 10 ml ethanol. Dilute 1 ml of this to 100 ml with ethanol. These solutions are stable for up to 1 year at 4 °C.
6. Working standard. Dilute 1 ml stock standard with 10 ml water to give a concentration of 3·0 μmol/l.

Apparatus. All glassware must be thoroughly cleaned initially with chromic acid followed by sodium metabisulphite. Always use a non-fluorescent detergent for subsequent washing. Ideally glassware should only be used for this purpose.

Technique. *Collection of blood*. Collect 10 ml blood into a heparinised tube; separate plasma as soon as possible. Store plasma at 4 °C for up to 1 week. Longer storage at − 20 °C should be in separate small volumes, each of which can be wholly used in the subsequent analysis. Unsatisfactory results are obtained if, after thawing, an aliquot is removed from a larger volume because of the precipitation of protein. Haemolysed plasma is unsuitable for analysis.

Pipette 2 ml plasma into a 20 ml stoppered tube and add 15 ml methylene dichloride. (Smaller volumes in proportion can be used for paediatric samples.) Shake for 2 min, centrifuge to separate phases and remove the plasma layer. Treat 2 ml water (blank) and 1 ml working standard plus 1 ml water in the same way. Keep batch sizes small as accurate timing is important to minimise non-specific interference. At zero time add 10 ml extract to 5 ml fluorescence reagent in a glass-stoppered tube, shake vigorously for 20 s and carefully remove the supernatant. Transfer acid extracts to separate cuvettes for reading. Repeat for blank, standard and samples at 1 min intervals. The fluorescence at 530 nm is read at exactly 12 min in a fluorimeter with excitation wavelength 470 nm.

Calculation. Plasma cortisol (nmol/l) =

$$\frac{(\text{Reading of test}) - (\text{Reading of blank})}{(\text{Reading of standard}) - (\text{Reading of blank})} \times \frac{3 \cdot 0 \times 1000}{2}$$

Notes.
1. On average only approximately 60% of the fluorescence measured in this way is due to cortisol. Results reported using the method are therefore, not surprisingly, higher than the more specific RIA methods. Results are best referred to as plasma 11-hydroxycorticoids. Despite this limitation, the fluorimetric technique gives adequate clinical results when investigating changes in individual patients, e.g. circadian rhythms or dynamic tests.
2. *Interferences*. Several drugs interfere: spironolactone, fucidic acid, mepacrine and vinblastine. Bilirubin also interferes, but can be removed by washing the plasma extract with 2·0 ml of 100 mmol/l sodium hydroxide before removing 10 ml for fluorimetry. Other interferences reported include benzyl alcohol in heparin anticoagulant, high plasma cholesterol and heavy smoking.

Reference ranges. Plasma 11-hydroxycorticosteroids (0900 h) by the above technique range from 220–750 nmol/l, mean 470 nmol/l.

High Performance Liquid Chromatography

Methods for measurement of steroids by HPLC have been reported for over 10 years (Heftman and Hunter, 1979). Routine assay of steroids in the clinical laboratory by this technique has, however, not been widely adopted. Considerable advantages can be obtained using HPLC including the simultaneous measurement of several steroids as well as of synthetic steroids. Ultraviolet, fluorescence and electrochemical detectors have all been used as well as techniques involving pre- and post-column derivatisation. Clinically useful methods can be performed simply using isocratic chromatography with ultraviolet detection, while HPLC can also be used to purify steroids prior to assay by RIA (Eibs and Schöneshöfer, 1984). The method described below is based on the method of Loche *et al.* (1984).

Reagents.
1. Methanol, HPLC grade.
2. Diethyl ether, anhydrous.
3. Water, chromatographically pure.
4. Standard steroids.

Equipment.
1. HPLC pump and injection valve.
2. Ultraviolet detector. If of fixed wavelength use 254 nm filter.
3. C18 Bondapak (Waters Chromatography Division) column, 10 μm particles (10 cm × 5 mm internal diameter).

Technique. Extract 0·5 ml serum or plasma with 2 ml diethyl ether in conical tubes. Snap-freeze aqueous phase and decant ether extract. Evaporate the ether to dryness and reconstitute with 300 μl of water–methanol (45/55, v/v). Inject 100 μl onto the column. Separation is achieved using water–methanol (45/55, v/v) at a flow rate of 1 ml/min. The retention times of various steroids using this system are given in Table 31.4. Quantitation of individual steroids is performed using either external or internal standards.

TABLE 31.4

Retention Times of Various Steroid Standards on HPLC
(Loche *et al.*, 1984)

Steroid	Retention Time (min)
6β-Hydroxycortisol	< 3·00
Aldosterone	3·90
Cortisol	5·72
21-Deoxycortisol	8·45
Dexamethasone	9·66
Cortisone	11·29
Corticosterone	11·58
11-Deoxycortisol	12·50
17α-Hydroxyprogesterone	29·01

Urine Steroid Analysis

Although methods for measuring urinary steroids as their glucuronide or sulphate conjugates have been described, it is usual to hydrolyse the conjugates before analysis by chemical or chromatographic means.

Hydrolysis of Conjugates

The choice of hydrolytic procedure is critical as steroids differ widely in their stability to these procedures. For example, 17-oxosteroids without a Δ^5-bond are relatively stable to hydrolysis with hot acid while other steroids are partially or completely destroyed. After hot acid hydrolysis, 60 % of dehydroepiandrosterone (DHA) sulphate is converted to derivatives other than DHA while 17-hydroxy-corticosteroids are almost completely destroyed. Hot acid can also modify steroids by chlorination or dehydration. Despite these disadvantages, hot acid hydrolysis is fast and complete.

Various techniques of mild acid hydrolysis of steroid sulphates have been described. The most common procedure is that of Burnstein and Lieberman (1958). Urine is brought to molar concentration with sulphuric acid and extracted three times with ethyl acetate. The combined extracts contain all the steroid sulphates together with sufficient sulphuric acid to hydrolyse them on standing at 37 °C overnight.

Minimal degradation of urinary steroids is obtained by using enzymic hydrolysis. A suitable technique is as follows. To 30 ml urine add 3 ml 5 mol/l acetate buffer, pH 4·6 (5 mol/l acetic acid: 5 mol/l sodium acetate, 2:3) followed by 1 ml *Helix pomatia* digestive juice (100 000 units sulphatase, 10 000 units β-glucuronidase). After incubation at 40 °C for 24 h a further incubation of 24 h is performed following the addition of 2 ml Ketodase (10 000 units β-glucuronidase). The disadvantages of enzymic hydrolysis include the long incubation times and the difficulty of ensuring that hydrolysis is complete.

The most frequently used method for the hydrolysis of corticosteroid glucuronide metabolites involves prior oxidation with metaperiodate which simultaneously removes the side chain at C-17 and replaces the glucuronide with a formyl group. Mild alkaline hydrolysis will then remove the formyl group without affecting the steroid molecule.

Group Reactions for Steroids

For many years group reactions for urinary steroids were the major analytical method for the study of adrenal pathology. These have now almost ceased to be performed for reasons described below and will only be briefly discussed here to clarify problems of nomenclature when reading the older literature. Readers wishing further details should refer to the 5th edition of this book.

C_{19} **Steroids, Oxosteroids.** The major constituents of the C_{19} urinary steroids are the metabolites of the adrenal and gonadal androgens and are measured by the Zimmermann reaction. After hydrolysis and drying, the steroid residue is reacted with *m*-dinitrobenzene in alkaline solution to give a purple colour. A small proportion of C_{19} derivatives of cortisol is also measured.

17-Oxosteroid   *m*-Dinitrobenzene   Coloured product

C_{21} **Steroids**. These steroids can be measured in different ways. Steroids with a dihydroxyacetone side chain (cortisol, cortisone, 11-deoxycortisol and their tetrahydro-derivatives) react with phenylhydrazine in sulphuric acid to give a yellow colour (Porter–Silber reaction). The steroids measured in this way are referred to as *17-hydroxycorticosteroids*. An alternative method is that of Norymberski which measures *17-oxogenic steroids*. After reduction of the 17-hydroxy-20-one-21-(hydroxy or deoxy) side chain with borohydride, which also converts the native 17-oxosteroids to 17-hydroxysteroids, the side chain is cleaved by metaperiodate. The resulting 17-oxosteroids can then be measured by the Zimmermann reaction. Steroids measured by this method include those with 17, 20,21-trihydroxy and 17,20-dihydroxy-21-deoxy side chains including cortol, cortolones and pregnanetriol.

The reasons for the demise of the urinary group steroid determinations, reviewed by Rudd (1983), are analytical and clinical.

Analytical.

1. Marked differences in molar absorption coefficients of products produced by different 17-oxosteroids in the Zimmermann reaction. Alteration in pattern of excretion may mask major changes in molar excretion and *vice versa*. Some Zimmermann chromogens are unstable and light-sensitive.

2. Solvents are hazardous, unpleasant and, in some cases, a serious fire risk. Other reagents are toxic.

3. Poor analytical precision means that CVs of approximately 25% are typically achieved. Inaccuracy of 24 h urine collections will add to this.

4. Specificity is often poor due to interfering chromogens, e.g. in neonates or in the presence of glucose. Correction for these problems may further reduce precision.

5. Poor sensitivity means that determination of 17-oxogenic and 17-oxo-steroids in neonatal urine is unreliable.

Clinical.

1. *Androgens.* Testosterone, the principal male androgen, has a C-17 hydroxyl group but only approximately 25–30% is converted to 17-oxosteroid which means that 70% of urinary oxosteroid is of adrenal origin in normal males. In females, almost all urinary oxosteroid is of adrenal origin. Thus urinary 17-oxosteroid excretion gives only a rough guide to adrenal androgen excretion and is totally inadequate for estimation of testicular function. In clinical situations where plasma testosterone is raised, e.g. polycystic ovary, increases in plasma testosterone concentration are not reflected by increased urinary 17-oxosteroid excretion. Lack of specificity and sensitivity means that the measurement of urinary 17-oxosteroid cannot be used to discriminate between normal and low steroid secretion rates.

2. *Glucocorticoids.* For a long time the measurement of 17-hydroxycorticoids or 17-oxogenic steroids in association with dynamic tests was the main analytical tool for the investigation of Cushing's syndrome. Crapo (1979), reviewing the literature on the performance of 17-hydroxysteroid measurements, found a false-positive incidence of 25% in obese patients and a false-negative rate of 11% in patients with Cushing's syndrome. Similarly, 17-oxogenic steroid determinations gave a false-negative result in 24% of patients with Cushing's disease. On the other hand, urine free cortisol determination and single dose dexamethasone tests gave 5 and 13% false-positive and 5·6 and 1·9% false-negative results in obese controls and patients with Cushing's syndrome respectively. Urinary estimation of glucocorticoid metabolites is unsuitable for screening for adrenal hypofunction and in short term tests with ACTH or Synacthen.

There is therefore almost no place for the group estimation of urinary steroid metabolites. These tests have been replaced by more specific urine (e.g. free cortisol, pregnanetriol) or plasma assays (e.g. cortisol, 17-hydroxyprogesterone, DHA and testosterone).

Urinary 11-Hydroxycorticosteroids

This fluorimetric method (Mattingly *et al.*, 1964) has a surprising degree of specificity.

Reagents.
1. As for plasma assay (p. 814).
2. Sodium hydroxide, 1 mol/l.

Technique. Collect a 24 h specimen of urine and keep it cool. If analysis is delayed, freeze an aliquot. Clear urine by centrifugation. Extract a 2 ml sample with 15 ml dichloromethane in a glass-stoppered tube; remove the upper aqueous layer by suction and shake well for 20 s with 2 ml sodium hydroxide. Stand (about 10 min) for layers to separate and remove the aqueous layer. Add 10 ml extract to 5 ml fluorescence reagent, shake vigorously for 20 s and remove the upper layer. Transfer acid layer to a cuvette and read the fluorescence at 530 nm in a fluorimeter with excitation at 470 nm. A standard should be treated in a similar manner.

Calculation. Urinary cortisol (nmol/24 h) =

$$\frac{\text{Reading of unknown}}{\text{Reading of standard}} \times 3{\cdot}0 \times \frac{\text{24 h urine volume (ml)}}{2}$$

Reference Ranges.
215–1030 nmol/24 h.
Mean—male, 630 nmol/24 h.
Mean—female, 490 nmol/24 h.

Urine Free Cortisol

The measurement of urine free cortisol is performed either directly, or after prior purification using solvent extraction or chromatography. In the first case, heavy reliance is placed on the specificity of the antibody or ligand-binding protein used. Murphy *et al.* (1981) compared seven different binding proteins (four antibodies; human, dog and horse cortisol-binding globulins) and showed that without purification by LH–20 chromatography all methods grossly overestimated the amount of free cortisol. Most of the interference is probably due to cortisol metabolites, e.g. cortisol sulphate and 20-dihydrocortisone which cross-react with most anticortisol antibodies and may co-elute with cortisol on LH–20 chromatography. Despite these problems the measurement of urine free cortisol is an extremely useful investigation for adrenocortical overactivity providing that each laboratory validates its own assay and derives a local reference range. Simple extraction with methylene chloride will reduce interferences substantially. Using dog cortisol-binding globulin in their assay Murphy *et al.* (1981) reported the normal ranges for urine cortisol given in Table 31.5.

Pregnanetriol

Pregnanetriol conjugates are extracted from urine and then hydrolysed. The free pregnanetriol is purified by chromatography on alumina and measured

TABLE 31.5

Urine Free Cortisol Excretion: Effect of LH–20 Chromatography (After Murphy *et al.*, 1981)

Group	Urine Free Cortisol (nmol/24 h)	
	Unchromatographed	Chromatographed
Men	94·9 ± 32·3	56·6 ± 26·5
Non-pregnant women	109 ± 21·2	38·6 ± 15·5
Late pregnancy	215 ± 101	105 ± 67·6
Children (2–12 y)	36·1 ± 8·8	21·5 ± 9·4

colorimetrically after reaction with sulphuric acid (Köber reaction). The method is essentially that of Bell and Varley (1960).

Reagents.

1. Benzene (spectrometric grade), saturated with distilled water.
2. Concentrated sulphuric acid.
3. Ammonium acetate buffer, pH 5·0. Dissolve 7·7 g ammonium acetate in 900 ml water, adjust pH with glacial acetic acid and make up to 1 litre.
4. Ketodase. Ox liver glucuronidase, 5000 Fishman units/ml (Warner Lambert Laboratories).
5. Alumina. Nominal activity grade 1 (Woelim Pharma GmbH, DD3340 Eschwege, West Germany). Store tightly capped. For details of preparation see below.
6. Ammonium sulphate.
7. Silver sand. Acid washed, 40–100 mesh.
8. Sodium hydroxide–saline solution. Dissolve 250 g sodium chloride in 1 litre of 1 mol/1 sodium hydroxide.
9. Extraction solvent. Ether–ethanol 3/1 v/v.
10. Elution solvents:
    A. Ethanol : water-saturated benzene, 8/992 v/v.
    B. Ethanol : water-saturated benzene, 30/970 v/v.
    C. Ethanol : water-saturated benzene, 100/900 v/v.
11. Stock standard. Dissolve 20·2 mg pregnanetriol in 100 ml ethanol to give a concentration of 600 μmol/l. Store in a stoppered glass container at $-20\,°C$.

Technique. *Sample.* Collect a 24 h urine specimen, store at 4 °C until analysis. Alternatively, use 10 ml of a random urine to establish the diagnosis of congenital adrenal hyperplasia in infants over 7 days of age. If random specimens are analysed from infants less than 7 days of age then there is a strong possibility of incorrect diagnosis.

Preparation of alumina. The activated alumina must be partially deactivated with water before use. Prepare 12 × 1 cm glass chromatographic columns with a porosity 1 sintered glass disc at the lower end and reservoir at the upper end. Occlude the lower end of the column and pour in 20 ml water-saturated benzene followed by 3 g alumina. After settling, tap to remove air and cover top with 0·5 g sand to protect the alumina. Allow the benzene to drain until the sand is just covered. Pipette 100 μl stock standard into two 50 ml glass tubes. Set one aside and into the other add 25 ml water-saturated benzene and run through a column, stopping the flow just before the liquid surface reaches the column top. Run 25 ml, 12 ml and 10 ml of elution solvents A, B and C respectively through the column collecting each fraction separately (fractions 1, 2 and 3). Follow with 20 ml of elution solvent C and collect 4 × 5 ml fractions (fractions 4, 5, 6 and 7). Measure the pregnanetriol content of the individual fractions (see below) and calculate each as a percentage of the total unchromatographed standard.

At least 95 % should be recovered in fraction 3 if the alumina is to be usable. If the pregnanetriol elutes in later fractions or remains uneluted then deactivation is necessary. Deactivation is achieved by adding 1 ml water to 100 g alumina in a closed container and shaking for 3 h after which the alumina is retested and the process repeated until the correct elution profile is achieved. If pregnanetriol elutes mainly in fractions 1 and 2, this indicates excessive deactivation. Store the deactivated material in a tightly-stoppered container.

Analysis of samples. Take 100th of the urine volume or 5 ml whichever is the greater and make up to 10 ml if less than 20 ml, or 20 ml if between 10 and 20 ml, using distilled water. If a random urine is used take 10 ml. Place the urine in a separating funnel and dissolve 0·5 g ammonium sulphate per ml urine; shake well. Extract 3 times with half the sample volume of extraction solvent, allowing separation of the phases and collecting the organic phase. Pool the extracts and evaporate in a boiling water bath under reduced pressure.

Dissolve the residue in 10 ml ammonium acetate buffer and hydrolyse the conjugates with 5000 units glucuronidase for 4 h at 37 °C. After cooling, extract 3 times with 10 ml water-saturated benzene, pool and save organic phases. Wash the pooled organic phase with 10 ml sodium hydroxide-saline solution, followed immediately by three washes with 10 ml distilled water. Prepare columns as described above and run the washed benzene extract through the column, stopping the flow when benzene just reaches the sand; discard the eluate. Wash column with 20 ml elution solvent B, stopping the flow when the solvent reaches the sand and again discarding the eluate. Elute the pregnanetriol with 15 ml elution solvent C and save the complete eluate. Evaporate to dryness under reduced pressure in a boiling water bath and dry in a desiccator for 1 h.

Add 3 ml concentrated sulphuric acid to the residue, mix well and incubate at 25 °C for 1 h. Measure absorbance at 400, 435 and 470 nm against a concentrated sulphuric acid blank. Discard the alumina from the column; it can only be used once. Take 100 μl standard (0·06 μmol) in 30 ml water-saturated benzene through the whole chromatographic procedure.

Calculation. An Allen correction is applied:

$$\text{Corrected absorbance} = 2A_{435} - (A_{400} + A_{470})$$

Urinary pregnanetriol (μmol/24 h) =

$$\frac{\text{Corrected absorbance of unknown}}{\text{Corrected absorbance of standard}} \times 0{\cdot}06 \times \frac{24 \text{ h urine volume}}{\text{sample volume}}$$

When a 10 ml random specimen has been used then the calculation is:

Urinary pregnanetriol (μmol/l) =

$$\frac{\text{Corrected absorbance of sample}}{\text{Corrected absorbance of unknown}} \times 6$$

If corrected absorbance of the sample is greater than that of the standard, repeat using a reduced sample volume.

Reference Ranges.

Age (years)	Range (μmol/24 h)
0–1	less than 0·3
2–5	0·3–0·6
5–7	0·6–1·2
7–puberty	less than 3·0
Adult	less than 6·0

Random urine (age 7–60 days), less than 0·3 μmol/l.

Notes.

1. Observe full safety regulations when using concentrated sulphuric acid and benzene. If desired, toluene may be used in place of benzene throughout.
2. The ethanol should be aldehyde-free.

GLC of Urinary Steroids

Although the use of group urinary steroid analysis has declined, the measurement of individual steroids in urine remains an important tool in the investigation of patients with inherited disorders of steroid biosynthesis and may also prove useful in studying patients with adrenal tumours. Measurement of atypical steroid metabolites in the latter case is helpful both diagnostically and in monitoring therapy or the reappearance of tumour. These methods require a high degree of technical skill and are best carried out in a laboratory processing sufficient samples to maintain the required skills and obtain a wide clinical experience. As such methods are beyond the scope of this volume, interested readers are referred to Shackleton and Honour (1976) and Shackleton *et al.* (1981).

Salivary Steroids

The pioneering work of Shannon *et al.* (1959) using chemical analysis, and their later studies using isotope dilution and competitive protein binding for the measurement of steroid hormones in saliva was ignored by clinical chemists and endocrinologists until the late 1970s when several groups became interested in saliva as a body fluid suitable for analysis. The key to the expansion of interest was the development of highly sensitive radioimmunoassays for steroids which could measure the concentrations of steroid hormones in saliva.

The advantages of salivary steroid measurement are as follows:

1. *Measures 'free' steroid fraction.* As steroid hormones are bound in varying degrees to specific binding globulins, the biological activity of the hormone is primarily due to the unbound or 'free' fraction. Plasma steroid assays measure both fractions and changes in plasma steroid concentration may be brought about not only by alterations in secretion and metabolism of the steroid but also by physiological or pathological variation in its binding globulin, e.g. in pregnancy, oral contraceptive or other oestrogen therapy, androgen therapy and liver disease. A measure of the free steroid fraction overcomes the problem of variable protein binding but methods for plasma are technically difficult and time-consuming. Only the free steroid hormone in plasma is able to enter the

saliva and therefore the salivary steroid concentration can be used as a direct estimation of plasma free steroid (Walker *et al.*, 1984; Table 31.6).

TABLE 31.6

Comparison of Plasma Free Steroid Fraction with Saliva: Plasma Ratio For Steroid Hormones (After James and Few, 1985)

Steroid	Mean Free Steroid (%)	Saliva: Plasma × 100%
Testosterone	2	1
Oestradiol	2	1
Progesterone	2·5	1
Cortisol	4	5
Androstenedione	8	12
Oestriol	10	10
Aldosterone	33	25

2. *Non-invasive technique.* Many endocrine studies require repetitive samples over hours or days. Salivary collection avoids the problems of repeated venepuncture or venous cannulae. It is therefore of particular advantage in paediatrics and allows physiological as well as pathological studies to be pursued ethically.

3. *Avoids hospitalisation.* Salivary steroids are to a large extent stable at room temperature for several days. Patients can collect salivary specimens at home and mail them to the laboratory. This saves both the patient and the physician time as results of tests can be made available for the patient's attendance at hospital. It is of particular use in monitoring ovulation using progesterone and in monitoring treatment of patients with congenital adrenal hyperplasia using 17α-hydroxyprogesterone.

4. *Avoids stress.* Tests of adrenocortical function are influenced by many factors of which stress is an important one. The absence of invasive techniques and other factors such as hospitalisation reduces stress to a large extent.

5. *Decreases blood loss.* Investigation of patients with adrenal disorders, especially Cushing's syndrome, may require a large number of investigations. The total quantity of blood withdrawn can be substantial and should be avoided in children.

6. *Technical advantages.* The protein content of saliva is mainly enzymes and glycoprotein which have no steroid binding properties. Direct steroid assays can therefore be performed more easily without the need for heat treatment, blocking agents, etc. Standards can be made up in buffer and the need to obtain steroid-free plasma is removed.

The main disadvantages of saliva steroid assays include the need for more sensitive assays as steroid levels in saliva vary between 1–25 % of plasma values. Another potential problem is the metabolism of steroids by enzymes in the salivary glands. Cortisol can be converted to cortisone by 11β-dehydrogenase which is present in large quantities in salivary gland cells. However, this has not proved to be a practical problem in the clinical situation. Salivary assays are less suitable when blood is required for analysis of other hormones not measureable in saliva or some other biochemical parameter.

Neutral steroids enter saliva by diffusing through cells. Although early data suggested that the concentration of these steroids was dependent on flow rate, more recent results show that within the range of flow rates achieved, either unstimulated or stimulated, there is no measurable effect of flow rate (Vining *et al.*, 1983). On the other hand, steroid conjugates such as DHA sulphate do not enter saliva by diffusion but by ultrafiltration through tight junctions between salivary acinar cells and their salivary concentration varies inversely with flow rate.

Saliva is an easy fluid to collect. Most subjects, especially children, can produce sufficient saliva on demand but occasionally stimulation using citric acid crystals or chewing on an inert object is required to induce a satisfactory flow. A number of simple precautions are needed when collecting saliva. Ideally, tooth brushing should be avoided and the mouth rinsed well with water 5 minutes before collection. Contamination with gingival blood may give rise to falsely elevated salivary steroid concentrations and hence the method is not suitable if the patient has gum or other mouth diseases. One further pitfall in collection is exogenous steroid in the form of therapy which can be present in the mouth in high concentration sufficient to cross-react in the assay. Samples of saliva should therefore be taken before the patient takes any steroid therapy. On receipt in the laboratory, saliva should be centrifuged to remove debris. The viscosity of saliva can be reduced considerably by freezing and thawing and this facilitates pipetting.

Salivary assays have been described for cortisol, progesterone, 17α-hydroxyprogesterone, aldosterone, testosterone, dehydroepiandrosterone sulphate, oestriol, oestradiol and some synthetic steroids. Walker *et al.* (1984) have reviewed physiological studies of salivary cortisol in infants and children which show a high degree of correlation between plasma and saliva results. Peters *et al.* (1982) used salivary cortisol estimation in the investigation of abnormalities of the hypothalamic–pituitary–adrenal axis and demonstrated that saliva can substitute for blood in both adrenal stimulation and suppression tests.

Immunoassay of Adrenocorticotrophic Hormone

ACTH is synthesised in the pituitary as part of a larger molecule, pro-opiomelanocortin. This molecule is cleaved into a group of related peptides: N-terminal pro-opiomelanocortin, ACTH, β- and γ-lipotropins, α-, β- and γ-MSH, β-endorphin and CLIP (corticotrophin-like intermediate lobe peptide, 18–39 ACTH). Many of these peptides appear in plasma in pathological conditions, e.g. Cushing's syndrome and in several cases, cross-reactions with ACTH immunoassays can occur.

ACTH immunoassays remain difficult; many commercial kits are poorly validated with inadequate detection limits, problems with cross-reactivity and lack of parallelism with standards. They require extraction procedures using talc, silicic acid or glass which removes interfering substances and also allows the concentration of ACTH before assay (Ratcliffe and Edwards, 1971). These assays can distinguish low normal levels. Occasionally, more useful clinical information can be obtained by chromatography of the plasma to elucidate the molecular weight of the circulating ACTH. High molecular weight ACTH has been found both in ectopic ACTH secretion, in patients with pituitary-dependent Cushing's disease and even in severely ill patients with no primary disturbance of the hypothalamic–pituitary–adrenal axis (Howlett and Rees, 1985).

Samples for ACTH estimation should be collected into cooled plastic tubes with lithium heparin anticoagulant, centrifuged within 5 min and stored in plastic tubes after snap-freezing at $-20\,°C$ until assayed. All contact with glass should be avoided. It has been suggested that ACTH is more stable than previous studies have indicated and that endogenous ACTH may be stable for up to 2 h at room temperature. If this proves to be the case, the assay of ACTH will be considerably facilitated.

A reliable measurement of ACTH is extremely useful in the differential diagnosis of Cushing's syndrome. Laboratories proposing to measure ACTH should make every attempt to validate their assay both technically and clinically. A poor assay will give dangerously misleading information.

Reference Range. This is method dependent but with a specific assay the reference range for basal plasma ACTH at 0900 h is 4·4–17·6 pmol/l.

DISORDERS OF THE HYPOTHALAMIC–PITUITARY–ADRENAL AXIS

Disorders of the adrenal gland are manifest by the clinical signs and symptoms of excess or deficient production of glucocorticoids, mineralocorticoids or adrenal androgens. The disorders may be present singly or in combination, e.g. in steroid 21-hydroxylase deficiency there is glucocorticoid deficiency together with androgen excess and a variable deficiency of mineralocorticoid. The minor physiological actions of a steroid may become important when it is present in excess, e.g. the mineralocorticoid effect of cortisol in Cushing's syndrome. These facts should be kept in mind especially as the investigational methods for disorders of the hypothalamic–pituitary–adrenal axis are divided for convenience into those which affect the three groups of steroids.

Glucocorticoid Excess

Excessive production of cortisol results in the clinical picture of Cushing's syndrome. The patients are usually obese and manifest decreased carbohydrate tolerance with hyperglycaemia and glycosuria. Protein catabolism is increased leading to thinning of the skin and osteoporosis. Some patients with ectopic ACTH secretion may present with a different picture of severe weight loss and metabolic alkalosis. This probably represents in part the primary pathology (malignancy) in these patients as other patients with ectopic ACTH production present with classical Cushing's syndrome.

The causes of Cushing's syndrome are summarised in Table 31.7. Primary adrenal disease and excess ACTH due to hypothalamic and pituitary disease account for about 80 % of cases of Cushing's syndrome. The remainder arise from ectopic production of ACTH from benign and malignant tumours in many organs. Accurate diagnosis is therefore essential and laboratory investigations alone are not sufficient. In particular, considerable reliance is placed on radiology including ultrasonic scans and computerised tomography (Howlett and Rees, 1985).

The laboratory investigation of Cushing's syndrome falls into two distinct phases: the demonstration of excessive cortisol production and the differential diagnosis of the aetiology.

Biochemical Diagnosis of Cushing's Syndrome

This is based (Crapo, 1979) on the use of simple tests: absence of diurnal variation of cortisol, increased excretion of urinary free cortisol or absence of the

TABLE 31.7
Aetiology of Cushing's Syndrome

---

1. *Hypothalamic–Pituitary*
   (a) Basophil adenoma
   (b) Corticotroph hyperplasia
   (c) Functional defect (normal histology)
2. *Adrenal*
   (a) Tumours
       (i) benign
       (ii) malignant
   (b) Nodular adrenal hyperplasia
   (c) Micronodular adrenal hyperplasia
3. *Ectopic ACTH*
   (a) Benign tumour, e.g. carcinoid adenoma
   (b) Malignant tumour, e.g. oat-cell carcinoma of lung
4. *Ectopic CRF—corticotrophin-releasing factor*
5. *Iatrogenic*
   (a) ACTH therapy
   (b) Glucocorticoid therapy
6. *Alcohol-induced*

---

suppression of cortisol secretion by low doses of dexamethasone. In all of these tests, false-positive and false-negative results occur and it may be necessary to use more than one test or to repeat the tests at intervals if clinically indicated. The diurnal rhythm of cortisol is particularly prone to interference from stress due to venepuncture, hospital admission, illness and psychiatric disorders especially depression. Out-patient salivary cortisol measurement overcomes some of these problems.

Two forms of dexamethasone suppression test are used. The simpler is to give 1 mg dexamethasone at midnight and measure the plasma cortisol concentration at 0900 h the next day. More reliable results follow the administration of 8 doses of 0·5 mg dexamethasone every 6 h. In the latter test, either urine free cortisol excretion during the second 24 h period or the plasma cortisol 6–8 h after completion of the course may be measured. Both tests can be done on out-patients; in the latter case suitable timings must be worked out (Kennedy *et al.*, 1984). Some patients with pituitary Cushing's disease will, however, suppress even with these low doses of dexamethasone. False results also occur if the patient fails to take the drug or if they have altered dexamethasone metabolism, e.g. increased hepatic clearance due to enzyme induction.

Differential Diagnosis of Cushing's Syndrome

Overproduction of cortisol due to either excess ACTH or autonomous secretion cause abnormalities of the feed-back control loop. Investigation of these perturbations will in most cases lead to the correct diagnosis.

Basal ACTH Secretion. The finding of very low or undetectable plasma ACTH with a sensitive and reliable assay indicates that the patient has primary adrenal pathology (tumour or nodular hyperplasia). On the other hand, a high plasma ACTH concentration indicates a hypothalamic–pituitary cause or ectopic ACTH production. Although patients with the latter condition usually have the higher plasma ACTH concentrations, there is substantial overlap between the two groups. However, very high plasma ACTH concentrations are indicative of an ectopic source of ACTH. Abnormal molecular forms of ACTH and circulating ACTH precursors have been found in both groups of patients but predominantly in ectopic ACTH production. On the other hand, pituitary tumours associated with unusual molecular forms of ACTH are usually large and invasive and relatively easily diagnosed.

Insulin Tolerance Test. This test is useful in distinguishing patients with severe depression with absent diurnal rhythm and lack of suppression by dexamethasone from patients with Cushing's syndrome.

Insulin (0·1–0·2 units/kg) is given intravenously after an overnight fast. Blood samples are taken for cortisol and glucose measurement before the insulin is given and at 15, 30, 60, 90 and 120 min thereafter. The test is invalid if the blood glucose fails to fall to 2·2 mmol/l or less. In normal subjects the rise in plasma cortisol concentration should be at least 250 nmol/l and a minimum value of 500 nmol/l should be reached. A normal rise is found in depressed patients but the majority of patients with Cushing's syndrome fail to show a rise. If growth hormone response is measured during this test, it too is frequently found to be suppressed in Cushing's syndrome.

Metyrapone Test. Administration of the drug metyrapone (metopirone; 2-methyl-1, 2-bis-(3′-pyridyl)-propan-1-one) inhibits cortisol biosynthesis at the 11β-hydroxylase step, i.e. the conversion of 11-deoxycortisol to cortisol. The reduction in plasma cortisol concentration activates the feed-back loop giving rise to release of ACTH and increased stimulation of the adrenal cortex. Either plasma ACTH or 11-deoxycortisol can be measured in this test but where assays for these substances are not readily available, urinary 17-oxogenic steroids can also be measured. Metyrapone, 750 mg, is given 4-hourly for 24 h. Blood is taken at 0, 1, 2, 3 and 24 h. If urine is being collected then 24 h collections should be made on the day preceding the test, the test day and the following day. Patients sometimes suffer from nausea, dizziness and vomiting which can be reduced by giving the drug with milk. In pituitary-dependent Cushing's disease there is an exaggerated response (greater than 200%) of basal ACTH, 11-deoxycortisol or urinary 17-oxogenic steroids compared to normals. Patients with primary adrenal pathology show no response. Some patients with ectopic ACTH syndrome also show an exaggerated response to metyrapone thus limiting the value of the test (Howlett and Rees, 1985).

Dexamethasone Suppression Test. In pituitary-dependent Cushing's disease negative-feedback control is not totally suppressed. Rather a relative resistance of the ACTH-secreting cell to cortisol is present. This is exploited by the use of the two-stage dexamethasone suppression test. The first stage is to give 0·5 mg dexamethasone 6 hourly for 48 h followed secondly by 2 mg dexamethasone 6 hourly for an additional 48 h. Plasma ACTH and cortisol are measured at the start of the test and at 0800 to 0900 h each day. Suppression at low doses effectively rules out Cushing's syndrome; while failure to suppress on the higher dose indicates that ectopic ACTH syndrome or primary adrenal pathology is the likely diagnosis. Unfortunately, as with all tests used in the diagnosis of Cushing's syndrome, the picture is not clear-cut and a number of patients with pituitary-dependent Cushing's disease do not suppress and may even show a rise in plasma cortisol in the high dose dexamethasone test. Patients with ectopic ACTH syndrome and adrenal tumours may also show a paradoxical rise in cortisol production. This is probably due to the tumours having their own intrinsic biological rhythm for the production of ACTH and cortisol and the changes seen depend on when in the cycle the test is carried out. Thus patients with ectopic ACTH syndrome may also show suppression with high dose dexamethasone.

CRF Test. The place of the administration of corticotrophin-releasing factor (CRF) in the differential diagnosis of Cushing's syndrome is not clear. Responses of plasma ACTH and cortisol concentration appear to be highly variable (Orth, 1984).

Selective Venous Catheterisation. The measurement of plasma ACTH concentrations at selected venous sites can occasionally prove useful if other means of localising the site of origin of the ACTH have failed. It is important to take peripheral venous samples for ACTH simultaneously to compensate for the pulsatile release of ACTH.

A flow diagram of the investigation of ACTH-dependent Cushing's syndrome is shown in Fig. 31.3 (Howlett and Rees, 1985).

Glucocorticoid Deficiency

The signs and symptoms of glucocorticoid deficiency are variable and depend on the nature, severity and duration of the cause. Adrenocortical disease should be suspected in any patient with unexplained weight loss, malaise, vomiting, hypoglycaemia, severe circulatory collapse, hypotension, dehydration, vitiligo or pigmentation. In addition, the relationship of adrenal failure to other endocrine disease should be remembered. Acute adrenal failure is an emergency that must be treated before there is time to undertake comprehensive laboratory endocrine tests.

Glucocorticoid deficiency can either be due to disease of the adrenal gland or be secondary to a failure of ACTH secretion as a consequence either of a hypothalamic–pituitary disorder or suppression of the pituitary by the long-term administration of exogenous steroids. The last group should cause no diagnostic difficulty but there is sometimes a need to assess the activity of the hypothalamic–pituitary–adrenal axis after the withdrawal of steroid therapy.

Primary adrenal failure is relatively easily diagnosed by measurement of plasma ACTH concentration and by the Synacthen test. Due to lack of feedback inhibition by cortisol, the plasma ACTH concentration will be elevated. Synacthen (tetracosactrin: 1–24 ACTH) stimulates the adrenal to produce cortisol. It is given by intramuscular injection in either a short-acting or long-acting (Synacthen Depot) form. The former is a solution containing 250 μg/ml, the latter is a suspension of the hexa-acetate adsorbed on to zinc phosphate and contains 1 mg Synacthen per ml. Absence of a cortisol response to short-acting Synacthen indicates adrenal failure but not the aetiology. In secondary adrenal failure the administration of Synacthen Depot over several days will stimulate the adrenal gland to produce cortisol. The insulin tolerance test can be used to test pituitary ACTH reserve but this test must be performed with great care as patients with glucocorticoid deficiency are hypersensitive to insulin-induced hypoglycaemia.

Short Synacthen Test. Inject 250 μg Synacthen intramuscularly after taking a blood sample for basal cortisol concentration. Further blood samples are taken 30 and 60 min later. The normal cortisol response is a rise of at least 220 nmol/l to a minimum plasma concentration of 550 nmol/l. Alternatively, Synacthen may be given intravenously with a single sample taken 30 min later. The paediatric dose of Synacthen is 5 μg/kg body weight.

Long Synacthen Test. The test may be carried out over 3 or 5 days. Synacthen Depot (1 mg) is given intramuscularly each morning and blood samples are taken

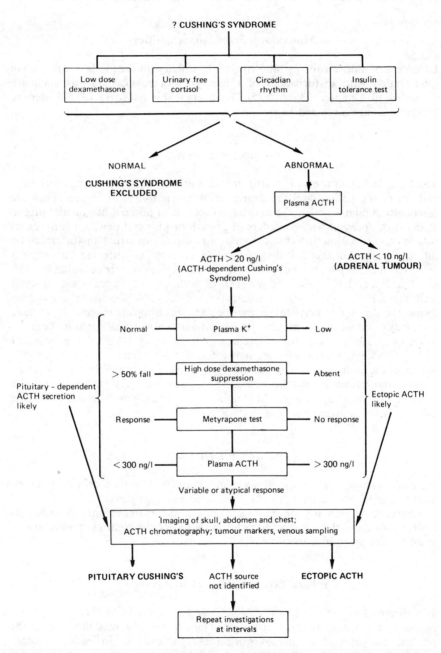

Fig. 31.3. Flow Diagram of a Strategy for the Diagnosis of Cushing's Syndrome. (Modified from Howlett and Rees, 1985 with permission.)

24 h later for cortisol determination. Patients with secondary adrenal failure will show a steady rise in plasma cortisol concentration throughout the test.

Mineralocorticoid Abnormalities

Disorders of aldosterone metabolism, both primary and secondary, are closely inter-related with disturbances of electrolyte homeostasis and as such are discussed in Chapter 23 (p. 575). The very rare disorders of aldosterone biosynthesis are discussed below.

Androgen Excess

The signs and symptoms of androgen excess are variable depending on the age and sex of the patient and the degree of oversecretion of androgen. They are essentially similar whether the androgen excess is of adrenal or gonadal origin. Patients can present with disorders of growth or pubertal development, sexual precocity, virilisation in females, acne, hirsutism, menstrual disturbances or infertility. The differential diagnosis may require measurement of plasma testosterone, dehydroepiandrosterone, dehydroepiandrosterone sulphate, androstenedione, LH, FSH and ACTH as well as the appropriate imaging techniques. Patients with high concentrations of dehydroepiandrosterone and/or its metabolites, e.g. 16α-hydroxydehydroepiandrosterone are more likely to have large malignant adrenal tumours whereas patients with adrenal adenomas excrete lower quantities of adrenal androgens and on capillary GLC of urine steroids 11β-hydroxyandrosterone is frequently found. Biochemical diagnosis of the source of the androgen and the nature of the tumour is limited by some overlap between the various groups. Stimulation and suppression tests are not of proven value in the identification of the origin of the androgenic steroid in female patients with hirsutism.

Androgen Deficiency

Adrenal androgen deficiency is only manifest in children with delayed puberty. This is usually associated with congenital adrenal hypoplasia.

Reference ranges for plasma testosterone, androstenedione, dehydroepiandrosterone and dehydroepiandrosterone sulphate throughout childhood and in adults are given in Table 31.8.

Inborn Errors of Steroid Biosynthesis

Inborn errors of metabolism (Finkelstein and Shaefer, 1979; New *et al.*, 1983; Addison, 1987) have been identified for eight of the enzymes involved in the adrenal biosynthesis of steroid hormones (Table 31.9). In addition, other inherited defects of peripheral steroid metabolism (5α-reductase and steroid sulphatase deficiencies) have been identified. The overall incidence of many of these disorders is very low but steroid 21-hydroxylase deficiency is one of the more common inborn errors of metabolism with reported incidences in Caucasian populations varying between 1:5000 and 1:15000 live births. High

TABLE 31.8

Age-related Reference Ranges for Some Important Androgens

Age	Androstenedione (nmol/l)		Dehydroepiandro- sterone (nmol/l)		Dehydroepiandro- sterone Sulphate (μmol/l)	Testosterone (nmol/l)	
	M	F	M	F	M + F	M	F
3–7 d	0·6–1·5	0·6–2·0	—	—	—	0·7–18	0·4–1·0
7 d–1 m	0·1–3·4	0·2–2·4	1·5–20	3·0–20	0·6–9·0	3·0–12	0·1–1·0
1 m–1 a	0·1–2·4	0·1–0·8	0·3–10	0·6–6·0	0·1–1·0	0·1–10	0·1–0·6
1–4 a	0·1–0·9	0·1–0·6	0·4–3·0	0·7–1·6	0·1–1·8	0·1–0·5	0·1–0·6
4–10 a	0·1–1·1	0·4–1·6	0·4–10	0·4–10	0·1–3·7	0·1–0·9	0·1–0·7
P1	0·2–3·3	0·3–2·5	0·9–11	0·4–7·0	0·4–4·8	0·2–0·6	0·1–0·6
P2	0·3–4·0	0·5–4·1	1·8–20	2·0–60	1·0–7·0	0·3–2·5	0·2–1·5
P3	0·6–5·4	1·0–5·6	4·5–22	4·4–65	2·0–7·5	1·0–30	0·6–1·9
P4	1·0–5·0	2·5–7·0	6·5–25	6·0–60	2·5–9·0	3·0–30	0·7–2·2
P5	1·6–4·8	2·7–9·4	8·0–25	7·5–58	3·0–12	10–30	0·8–2·8
Adult	2·0–8·0	2·8–10	7·0–35	2·5–35	1·5–15	13–38	0·7–2·4

These ranges have been derived from several sources in the literature, they should be used for guidance only in view of the problem of between-laboratory standardisation. P1–P5 Pubertal staging according to Tanner (1962). m = month, a = year.

incidences are found in Alaskan Eskimos (1:1500) and in particular in Yupik Eskimos (1:500).

The clinical presentation of this group of diseases is brought about by a combination of deficient production of one or more steroid hormones, increased production of other normal steroid hormones due to excess ACTH secretion as a consequence of removal of feed-back inhibition and, lastly, the metabolic effects of steroids not normally present in blood. Classically presenting in the neonatal period, increased understanding and improved methodology have revealed that some of the disorders are very variable and may also present in infancy, late childhood and early adulthood. Presentation is with one or more of the following signs and symptoms: electrolyte disturbances, ambiguous genitalia, postnatal virilisation, hypertension, premature or delayed puberty, abnormal menstruation, infertility and hirsutism.

Androgens play a major role in pre-natal sexual development. Increased or reduced androgen production at the crucial stages of sexual differentiation give rise to varying degrees of genital abnormality when the genetic sex and fetal androgen concentration are working in opposite directions (Saenger, 1984). Thus in steroid 21-hydroxylase deficiency, the increased androgen secretion will lead to masculinisation of the female, while a male infant is often thought to possess normal genitalia although hyperpigmentation of the scrotum and a large penis are not infrequently present.

Diagnosis. Investigation of a suspected steroid biosynthetic disorder is particularly urgent in the neonatal period when infants are at risk if the condition is associated with salt depletion or if there are problems of gender assignment. The symptoms of salt depletion (dehydration, vomiting, etc.) are non-specific but the patients will have hyponatraemia and hyperkalaemia. The earliest and most suitable test is the measurement of plasma 17α-hydroxyprogesterone, a test which can be performed as soon as 24 h after birth. This will detect the most common

TABLE 31.9

ACTH, Renin, Steroid Hormones and their Metabolites in Plasma and Urine in the Individual Disorders of Steroid Biosynthesis

Deficient Enzyme	Increased in Urine	Decreased in Urine	Increased in Plasma	Decreased in Plasma
20,22-Desmolase		Oxosteroids (Absent) Oxogenic Steroids (Absent) Pregnanetriol	ACTH Renin	Cortisol Aldosterone Testosterone
3β-Hydroxysteroid dehydrogenase	Oxosteroids Pregnanetriol		ACTH Renin 17α-Hydroxypregnenolone Pregnenolone DHA	Δ⁴Steroids Aldosterone
17α-Hydroxylase	Pregnanediol Pregnanetriol	Oxosteroids(±)	ACTH(±) Progesterone 11-Deoxycorticosterone Corticosterone Pregnenolone	Renin 17-Hydroxyprogesterone Cortisol Testosterone Aldosterone
21-Hydroxylase	Oxosteroids Pregnanetriol Pregnanetriolone 17-Hydroxypregnanolone		ACTH Renin 17α-Hydroxyprogesterone 21-Deoxycortisol DHA Androstenedione Testosterone	

Enzyme				
11β-Hydroxylase	Oxosteroids Tetrahydro-11-deoxycortisol Tetrahydro-11-deoxycorticosterone			ACTH Renin 11-Deoxycortisol 11-Deoxycorticosterone Androstenedione Testosterone
Corticosterone methyl oxidase Type I	11-Dehydrocorticosterone	Tetrahydroaldosterone Tetrahydro-11-dehydro-18-hydroxycorticosterone		Renin Corticosterone
Corticosterone methyl oxidase Type II	11-Dehydrocorticosterone Tetrahydrocorticosterone Tetrahydro-11-dehydro-18-hydroxycorticosterone	Tetrahydroaldosterone	Aldosterone	Renin
17β-Hydroxysteroid dehydrogenase	Oxosteroid(±)		Androstenedione	Testosterone(±) (increased androstenedione: testosterone ratio) DHT(±)

inborn error of steroid biosynthesis, 21-hydroxylase deficiency, in which the concentration of 17α-hydroxyprogesterone exceeds 50 nmol/l. Alternative measurements in urine, pregnanetriol and the 11-oxygenation index (the ratio of 11-deoxy-17-oxosteroids to 11-hydroxy-17-oxosteroids), are often unreliable until the patient is 7–10 days old. Furthermore the collection of 24 h urines in neonates is difficult and is made even more so when the genitalia are abnormal. Plasma 17α-hydroxyprogesterone is sometimes raised in sick premature infants to concentrations similar to many cases of 21-hydroxylase deficiency. These infants are frequently hyponatraemic and repeated investigation may have to be undertaken. Reference ranges for plasma 17α-hydroxyprogesterone are given in Table 31.10.

TABLE 31.10
Plasma 17α-Hydroxyprogesterone Reference Ranges

Age	17α-Hydroxyprogesterone (nmol/l)	
1 d	5·0–30	
2–7 d	0·5–30	
7 d–1 m	0·6–10	
1 m–4 m	< 6·0	
4 m–10 a	< 3·0	
	M	F
10–15 a	0·5–2·5	1·0–5·0
Adult	< 6·0	

d = day, m = month, a = year.

The second most common steroid biosynthetic defect, 11-hydroxylase deficiency, usually presents later in childhood and can be diagnosed by measuring plasma 11-deoxycortisol concentration. Investigation of the other disorders including inborn errors of aldosterone biosynthesis require sophisticated steroid measurements using capillary GLC and should be performed, or the results confirmed, by an experienced laboratory. A summary of the major biochemical abnormalities in the different inborn errors of steroid biosynthesis is given in Table 31.9 (p. 832).

Monitoring of Therapy. Patients with steroid biosynthetic defects which result in deficient production of glucocorticoid and mineralocorticoid are treated by replacement therapy. There are considerable problems in both over- and under-treatment especially in childhood. Clinical management of therapy is probably the more important but the clinician can be helped by biochemical monitoring.

The objective of giving glucocorticoid replacement is 2 fold: replacement of the physiological function of cortisol and the abolition of excess androgen production by feed-back inhibition of ACTH secretion. Urinary 24 h pregnanetriol excretion will give an overall picture of the efficacy of therapy in suppressing adrenal activity but if the result is abnormally high then this will not indicate at what time of day the patient has 'escaped' from control. Alternative methods have involved measurement of plasma androgens and 17α-hydroxyprogesterone on a single occasion but this has the same disadvantage. A profile of adrenal activity throughout the day can be obtained by the use of salivary or blood-spot 17αhydroxyprogesterone determinations and this allows optimal adjustment of therapy.

Mineralocorticoid replacement can be assessed by measurement of plasma renin activity. In patients who are difficult to control, optimisation of mineralocorticoid replacement often leads to a reduction in cortisol requirement and improvement in overall control.

REFERENCES

Abraham G. E., Buster J. E., Teller R. C. (1972). *Anal. Lett*; **5**: 757.

Addison G. M. (1987). In *The Inherited Metabolic Diseases*. (Holton J. B., ed) p. 326. Edinburgh: Churchill Livingstone.

Beisel W. R., *et al.* (1964a). *J. Clin. Endocr. Metab*; **24**: 887.

Beisel W. R., DiRaimondo V. C., Forsham P. H. (1964b). *Ann. Int. Med*; **60**: 641.

Bell M., Varley H. (1960). *Clin. Chim. Acta*; **5**: 396.

Burnstein S., Lieberman S. (1958). *J. Am. Chem. Soc*; **80**: 5235.

Crapo L. (1979). *Metabolism*; **28**: 955.

Dash R. J., England B. E., Midgely A. R., Niswender G. D. (1975). *Steroids*; **26**: 647.

Eibs G., Schöneshöfer M. (1984). *J. Chromat*; **310**: 386.

Fahmy D., Read G. F., Hillier G. (1975). *Steroids*; **26**: 267.

Finkelstein M., Shaefer J. M. (1979). *Physiol. Rev*; **59**: 353.

Fraser C. G., Wilde C. E. (1986). *Commun. Lab. Med*; **2**: 1.

Fukushima D. K., *et al.* (1960). *J. Biol. Chem*; **235**: 2246.

Gower D. B. (1979). *Steroid Hormones*. London: Croom Helm.

Heftman E., Hunter I. R. (1979). *J. Chromat*; **165**: 283.

Hornsby P. J. (1985). In *The Adrenal Cortex*. (Anderson D. C., Winter J. S., eds) p. 1. London: Butterworths.

Howlett T. A., Rees L. H. (1985). *Ann. Clin. Biochem*; **22**: 550.

International Union of Pure and Applied Chemistry, IUPAC (1969). *Biochem. J*; **113**: 5.

James V. H. T., Few J. D. (1985). *Clinics in Endocrinology and Metabolism*; **14**: 867.

Kennedy L., *et al.* (1984). *Brit. Med. J*; **289**: 1188.

Loche S., *et al.* (1984). *J. Chromat*; **317**: 377.

Makin H. L. (1984). *Biochemistry of Steroid Hormones*, 2nd ed. Oxford: Blackwell Scientific Publications.

Mattingly D. (1962). *J. Clin. Pathol*; **15**: 374.

Mattingly D., Dennis P. M., Pearson J., Cope C. L. (1964). *Lancet*; **2**: 1046.

Murphy B. E. P., Okouneff L. M., Klein G. P., Ngo S. C. (1981). *J. Clin. Endocr. Metab*; **53**: 91.

New M. I., Dupont B., Grumbach K., Levine L. S. (1983). In *The Metabolic Basis of Inherited Disease*, 5th ed. (Stanbury, J. B., *et al.*, eds) p. 973. New York: McGraw Hill.

Orth D. N. (1984). *New Engl. J. Med*; **310**: 649.

Percy-Robb I. W. *et al.* (1980). *Ann. Clin. Biochem*; **17**: 217.

Peters J. R., Walker R. F., Riad-Fahmy D., Hall R. (1982). *Clin. Endocrinol*; **17**: 583.

Peterson R. E. (1971). In *The Human Adrenal Cortex*. (Christy N. P., ed) p. 87. New York: Harper and Row.

Ratcliffe J. R., Edwards C. R. W. (1971). In *Radioimmunoassay Methods*. (Kirkham K. E., Hunter W. M., eds) p. 502. Edinburgh: Churchill Livingstone.

Riad-Fahmy D., Read G., Hughes I. A. (1979). In *Hormones in Blood*, 3rd ed. (Gray C. H., James V. H. T., eds) Vol. 3, p. 179. New York, London: Academic Press.

Rudd B. (1983). *Ann. Clin. Biochem*; **20**: 65.

Ruder H. J., Guy R. L., Lipsett M. B. (1972). *J. Clin. Endocr. Metab*; **35**: 219.

Saenger P. (1984). *J. Pediat*; **104**: 1.

Shackleton C. H. L., Honour J. W. (1976). *Clin. Chim. Acta*; **69**: 267.

Shackleton C. H. L., Taylor W. F., Honour J. W. (1981). *An Atlas of Chromatographic Profiles of Neutral Adrenal Steroids in Health and Diseases*; Delft: Packard-Becker BV.

Shannon I. L., Prigmore J. R., Brooks R. A., Feller R. P. (1959). *J. Clin. Endocr;* **19**: 1477.

Tanner J. M. (1962). *Growth at Adolescence,* 2nd ed. Oxford: Blackwell Scientific Publications.

Vining R. F., McGinley R. A., Symons R. G. (1983). *Clin. Chem;* **29**: 1752.

Walker R. F., Joyce B. G., Dyas J., Raid-Fahmy D. (1984). In *Immunoassays of Steroids in Saliva.* (Read G. F., Riad-Fahmy D., Walker R. F., Griffiths K., eds). p. 308. Cardiff: Alpha-Omega.

32

OESTROGENS, PROGESTOGENS AND ANDROGENS—GONADAL FUNCTION TESTS

Androgens, oestrogens and progesterone are secreted in varying degrees by both the gonads and the adrenal cortex. Following secretion they may undergo peripheral conversion in, e.g. liver, skin, muscle or adipose tissue. The production rate (PR) of a particular hormone (amount of hormone entering the circulation per unit time) has two components: glandular secretion of the hormone and peripheral conversion of a pre-hormone to the hormone. The PR is related to the plasma concentration (C) and metabolic plasma clearance rate (MCR) such that PR = MCR × C. The concept of clearance is discussed in Chapter 29 (p. 767).

OESTROGENS

The three major oestrogens are oestrone (E1), oestradiol-17β (E2) and oestriol-16α,17β (E3). Fig. 32.1 illustrates their biosynthesis from androstenedione and

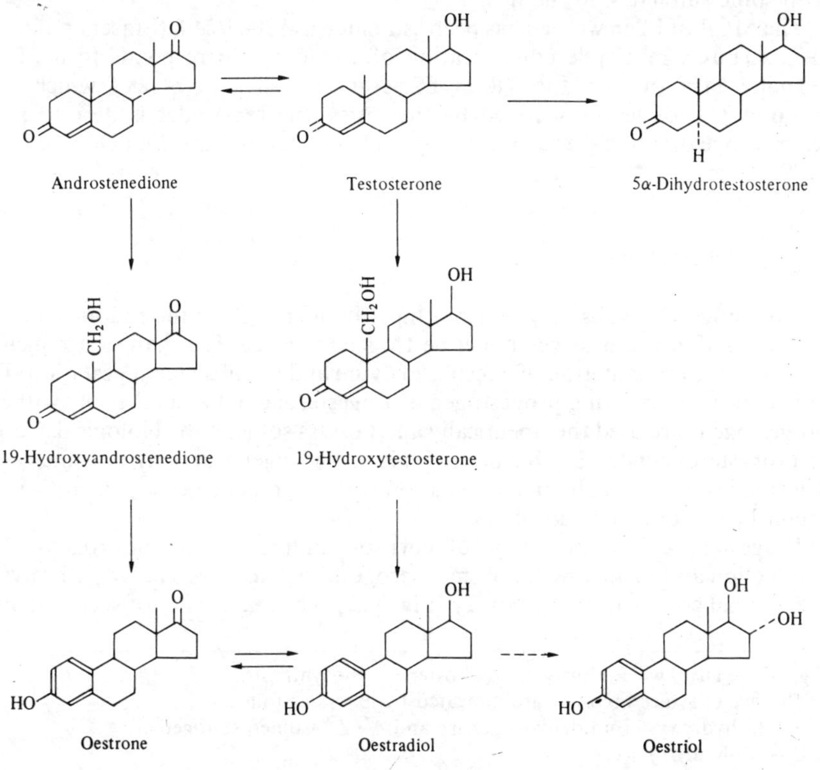

Fig. 32.1. Biosynthesis of Oestrogens and Dihydrotestosterone.

testosterone through the 19-hydroxy intermediates. The major site of oestrogen production is the ovary but the adrenal cortex and the Sertoli cells of the testis also produce small quantities of oestrogens. In the ovary the formation of E3 from E1 or E2 is only a minor pathway but in pregnancy an additional route for oestriol synthesis becomes available (Chapter 33, p. 858) when this steroid becomes the major oestrogen produced. The sites of production in the ovary in the non-pregnant state are the Graafian follicle and, following its rupture, the corpus luteum. Of the three major oestrogens, E2 is biologically the most potent and accounts for most of the oestrogenic activity in the non-pregnant woman of reproductive age. The adrenal cortex is not an important source of E2 in women during their reproductive phase as indicated by the unchanged plasma E2 concentrations following dexamethasone suppression of the hypothalamic–pituitary–adrenal axis (Abraham, 1974; Abraham and Chakmakjian, 1973). In the post-menopausal woman, the most important oestrogen is E1 produced by the peripheral conversion, mainly in adipose tissue, of androstenedione secreted from the adrenal cortex (Grodin *et al.*, 1973). The plasma oestrogens are mainly protein-bound, probably less than 5 % being in the free form. Normal plasma contains all three oestrogens and E1 is also present as its sulphate. Oestriol sulphate is present during pregnancy. Circulating E2 is specifically bound to sex hormone binding-globulin (SHBG) and only loosely bound to albumin (Dunn *et al.*, 1981), whereas E1 and oestrone sulphate are almost exclusively bound to albumin. Some E2 is converted into E1 and E3 during metabolism and all are excreted as conjugates, mainly glucosiduronates with some sulphates, in the urine.

The MCR of E2 in women has been estimated as 1200 l/24 h (Fraser and Baird, 1974). Thus a mid-cycle concentration of 1·1 nmol/l corresponds to a PR of 1·3 μmol/24 h. In men, the PR of E2 is about 160 nmol/24 h of which only 44 nmol/24 h or less is secreted by the testes; the remainder is derived from testosterone or adrenal androgens by peripheral metabolism (MacDonald *et al.*, 1979).

PROGESTOGENS

A progestogen is a substance which brings about changes in the endometrium of the uterus after this has been under oestrogen influence. The changes are such as to favour the implantation of a fertilised ovum and its subsequent gestation. The only naturally-occurring progestogen is progesterone but a number of synthetic progestogens are used therapeutically and possess some of the biological actions of progesterone with variable oestrogenic or androgenic activity in some cases. These substances, usually in combination with a synthetic oestrogen, are widely prescribed as oral contraceptives.

Progesterone is a precursor of cortisol, androgens and oestrogens. The production and further metabolism of progesterone follows similar pathways in the adrenal cortex, testis and ovary (Fig. 32.2). The major sites of secretion into

Fig. 32.2. The Two Pathways of Testosterone Biosynthesis.
The five enzymes involved are indicated by letters as follows:
A→3β-hydroxysteroid dehydrogenase and Δ^5–Δ^4 isomerase together,
B—17α-hydroxylase,
C—C17-20 lyase,
D—17β-hydroxysteroid dehydrogenase.

Pregnenolone → A → Progesterone

Pregnenolone → B → 17α-Hydroxypregnenolone

17α-Hydroxypregnenolone → A → 17α-Hydroxyprogesterone

Progesterone → B → 17α-Hydroxyprogesterone

17α-Hydroxypregnenolone → C → Dehydroepiandrosterone

17α-Hydroxyprogesterone → C → Androstenedione

Dehydroepiandrosterone → A → Androstenedione

Dehydroepiandrosterone → D → Δ⁵-Androstenediol

Androstenedione → D → Testosterone

Δ⁵-Androstenediol → A → Testosterone

the circulation are the corpus luteum of the ovary and, in pregnancy, the placenta. A small amount is secreted by the adrenal cortex in both sexes and by the testes in men. Progesterone occurs in the plasma mainly bound to protein (98 % of total concentration, the proportion remaining constant throughout the menstrual cycle). A major fraction is bound to cortisol-binding protein (CPB) and a minor fraction bound to low affinity sites on albumin and other plasma proteins (Westphal *et al.*, 1977).

ANDROGENS

The major androgens are testosterone, dihydrotestosterone (DHT), androstene-dione, dehydroepiandrosterone (DHA) and dehydroepiandrosterone sulphate (DHAS). The pathways of androgen synthesis are illustrated in Fig. 32.2.

Androgens in Women

In women, quantitatively the most important androgens are androstenedione and DHAS. Androstenedione is secreted in approximately equal amounts by the adrenal cortex and ovaries (Abraham, 1974) with a PR of 11·5 μmol/24 h and MCR of 2100 l/24 h (Bardin and Lipsett, 1967). The mean plasma concentration of androstenedione changes during the menstrual cycle like E2, rising from 4·20 nmol/l in the early follicular phase to an ovulatory peak of 6·90 nmol/l, subsiding to a mid-luteal plateau of 5·03 nmol/l and falling premenstrually (DeVane *et al.*, 1975; Kim *et al.*, 1974). There is also a diurnal variation of about 50 % which is synchronous with cortisol (Givens, 1978).

Both DHA and DHAS are weak androgens the roles of which are undefined except in pregnancy when they serve as precursors for E3. The PR of DHAS is estimated to be 20 μmol/24 h (MacDonald *et al.*, 1965) and DHA 2·5 μmol/24 h. Over 90 % of DHAS (Abraham and Chakmakjian, 1973) and over 80 % of DHA (Abraham, 1974) production is accounted for by adrenal secretion, the remainder by ovarian secretion. The plasma concentrations are again partly under ACTH control and parallel cortisol but do not change greatly during the menstrual cycle. The mean concentrations are: DHA 14 nmol/l, DHAS 5·5 μmol/l (Abraham, 1974; DeVane *et al.*, 1975). The possibility of a further pituitary hormone influencing adrenal androgen production has not been resolved. Low plasma concentrations are found prepubertally which increase at puberty. They decline markedly in the 4th and 5th decades.

The MCR and PR of testosterone are approximately 600 l/24 h and 0·8 μmol/24 h respectively (Bardin and Lipsett, 1967). About 35 % of the PR is accounted for by secretion from the adrenal cortex and the ovaries, and about 65 % by peripheral conversion, mainly in androgen-sensitive tissues such as skin, by the reduction of androstenedione at C17 (Fig. 32.1, p. 837) (Kirschner and Bardin, 1972). In the normal menstruating woman, the mean plasma concentration of testosterone in the early follicular phase is 1·1 nmol/l (DeVane *et al.*, 1975) with only a small diurnal variation (Givens, 1978). It increases slightly at mid-cycle (Kim *et al.*, 1974) and is doubled on oral contraceptive regimens due to an increase in SHBG (Easterling *et al.*, 1974). The fraction of testosterone not bound to plasma proteins is 1·4 % (Dunn *et al.*, 1981). The PR of DHT is approximately 190 nmol/24 h of which the majority originates from the peripheral metabolism of androstenedione (Ito and Horton, 1971).

Androgens in Men

In men, quantitatively the most important androgen is testosterone. The PR is 24 μmol/24 h, 95% being secreted by the testes (Horton and Tait, 1966). About 50% of testosterone is excreted as 17-oxosteroids in the urine and 50% metabolised to more polar compounds and excreted as conjugates. Testosterone is the major precursor for the synthesis of the potent androgen DHT in target organs by the key enzyme 5α-reductase (Fig. 32.1, p. 837). The PR of DHT is 1·0 μmol/24 h, the majority being contributed by peripheral conversion and only a small amount by testicular secretion (Horton and Tait, 1966; Ito and Horton, 1970; Ito and Horton, 1971). Approximately 44% of circulating testosterone is bound to SHBG, 50% is bound to albumin and 2·2% circulates in the unbound form (Dunn *et al.*, 1981).

In men the PR of androstenedione is 7·0–10·5 μmol/24 h (Horton and Tait, 1966) and the plasma concentration 4·03 ± 1·22 nmol/l (Thorneycroft *et al.*, 1973). The PR of DHAS is 18·8 μmol/24 h (MacDonald *et al.*, 1965); the plasma concentration ranges from 1·9 to 3·5μmol/l (Vermeulen, 1979).

OTHER HORMONES CONCERNED WITH GONADAL FUNCTION

Both *follicle stimulating hormone* (FSH) and *luteinising hormone* (LH) are glycoproteins containing α and β sub-units. The α sub-units are identical, containing a single polypeptide chain of 89 amino acids with two carbohydrate side chains. The β sub-units of FSH and LH both contain polypeptide chains of 115 amino acids but with little homology. The carbohydrate side chains also differ. Microheterogeneity in the carbohydrate side chains is observed in both hormones and is probably due to differing extraction techniques. LH and human chorionic gonadotrophin (HCG) share considerable homology throughout the β sub-units. The secretion of FSH and LH, like other anterior pituitary hormones, is under the control of the hypothalamus and is subject to negative and positive feed-back at both the hypothalamic and pituitary levels by the secretory products of the gonads. A single decapeptide, *gonadotrophin releasing hormone* (GnRH, also known as LH/FSH–RH), is secreted by neurones in the hypothalamus and acts as the releasing hormone for both FSH and LH when it reaches the anterior pituitary by passing along the hypothalamic–hypophyseal portal system. The release of FSH and LH occurs within a few minutes of the arrival of GnRH, the relative proportion of LH and FSH probably being influenced by the local steroid hormone milieu in both the hypothalamus and anterior pituitary. In both sexes the secretion of LH and FSH is pulsatile.

Before puberty the production of the gonadotrophins is low but an early sign of the onset of puberty is a fluctuating but sub-threshold secretion of FSH and LH. Once more marked and sustained secretion occurs, there is gonadal growth in both sexes. The gonadotrophins initiate development of secondary sexual characteristics and, in normal girls, the onset of menstruation.

In women the dwindling ovarian function at the menopause is associated with an increased release of FSH and LH as negative feed-back becomes less effective. The situation in men is less abrupt but older men have higher outputs of gonadotrophins on average. Biologically active gonadotrophins are excreted in the urine of the post-menopausal woman and may be partially purified and used therapeutically under the name of human menopausal gonadotrophins (HMG).

Prolactin consists of a single polypeptide chain of 198 amino acids with a molecular weight of 21 000. It is secreted by the dopamine receptor-containing lactotroph cells of the anterior pituitary. Secretion is under the tonic inhibitory control of dopamine synthesised in hypothalamic neurones and secreted into the hypothalamic–hypophyseal portal system. It is pulsatile in nature with no fixed periodicity, is maximal during early sleep and is minimal at 1000 h. Prolactin secretion is stimulated by the suckling reflex, physical trauma and TRH, and is augmented by oestrogens. The role of psychological stress is not entirely clear (Koninckx, 1978; Brooks et al., 1986). Dopamine receptor-blocking drugs (e.g. phenothiazines) and dopamine-depleting drugs (e.g. α-methyldopa) cause an increased prolactin secretion. Dopamine agonists, such as bromocriptine, are used therapeutically to suppress secretion.

Prolactin receptors are present on the cell surface of many tissues, including the ovary, testis and mammary gland. The only well-defined physiological roles for prolactin are the initiation and possibly the maintenance of lactation.

SEX HORMONE BINDING GLOBULIN

Sex hormone-binding globulin is a β globulin (molecular weight, 100 000), composed of two dissimilar sub-units both containing substantial amounts of carbohydrate. In plasma, various dimeric complexes are probably present. SHBG contains one high affinity binding site for DHT, testosterone or E2 per molecule, the affinity for the last being about one order of magnitude less than for testosterone. The affinity for DHT is about twice that for testosterone. Androstenedione and DHAS are not bound to SHBG. In normal men and women 97·8 % and 98·6 % respectively of the circulating testosterone is protein-bound—the majority to SHBG and albumin (Dunn et al., 1981). Thus alterations in the plasma concentration of SHBG markedly affect the MCR of testosterone. The protein is synthesised in the liver and has structural similarities with the androgen-binding protein (ABP) synthesised in the testis. For more detailed discussions of SHBG see Anderson (1974), Siiteri et al. (1982) and Siiteri and Simberg (1986).

HORMONAL CHANGES DURING THE NORMAL MENSTRUAL CYCLE

Cyclical changes occur in E2, progesterone, FSH, LH and hypothalamic activity during the menstrual cycle. The changes are well documented but the details of control are still not fully understood (Fig. 32.3).

The average length of the cycle is 28 days, the first day being the day of onset of the menstrual flow. Ovulation occurs on average on the 14th day. The period up to ovulation is the *proliferative phase* and the remainder of the cycle is the *luteal phase*. During the proliferative phase a Graafian follicle enlarges and eventually ruptures and in the same phase the endometrium undergoes changes. Initially the superficial layer is shed during the menstrual flow but then proliferation occurs and the endometrium thickens. Following ovulation, the luteal phase is characterised by the formation of the corpus luteum and the further thickening and glandular development of the endometrium to prepare it for the implantation of an ovum which has been fertilised and undergone early development during its passage down the Fallopian tube.

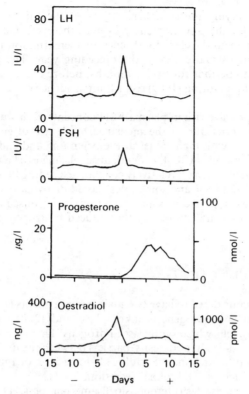

Fig. 32.3. Hormonal Changes During the Normal Menstrual Cycle.
Median concentrations in plasma (after Kletzky *et al.*, 1975). Day 0 is the day of the LH peak.

At the start of the cycle the circulating plasma concentrations of E2 and progesterone are low and the anterior pituitary releases increasing quantities of FSH and LH. These, but especially FSH, stimulate the development of several follicles but usually only one is selected for eventual rupture. The developing follicle produces an increasing output of E2 with some depression of FSH and LH output. Towards the end of the follicular phase the rapidly growing follicle produces an exponential rise in E2 production. This triggers, by positive feedback, an abrupt release of GnRH from the hypothalamus and an abrupt pituitary release of LH and FSH. A final growth spurt of the follicle results in its rupture and ovulation about 30 h later. The pre-ovulatory peak of plasma E2 is followed by a fall. LH activity assists in the formation and early maintenance of the corpus luteum in the luteal phase. Progesterone, which has been present in low concentration in the plasma during the follicular phase, now appears in increasing quantities over the next 4 or 5 days reaching a peak shortly after the middle of the luteal phase. A second peak of plasma E2 occurs around this time. This is probably secreted by the corpus luteum but some may come from follicles which were stimulated but did not rupture. This increasing output of E2 and progesterone suppresses FSH and LH release and the corpus luteum, which relies on LH for its support, starts to decay. As it does so there is a rapid fall in the plasma concentration of E2 and progesterone. This is associated with spasm of the arterioles supplying the superficial layers of the thickened endometrium leading to their sloughing with haemorrhage as the cycle ends.

The term, menopausal, refers to absence of menstruation for three months following some menstrual cycles in the preceding year. The post-menopausal woman has had no periods for twelve months. Before these stages, many cycles may be anovular and Doring (1969) records an incidence of 12 % in women aged 41 to 45.

There is a progressive rise in plasma FSH concentration with increasing age. LH and FSH patterns during the menstrual cycle are often atypical in pre-menopausal women with high values at the beginning and end of the cycle and absent peaks at mid-cycle. After the menopause, plasma FSH and LH concentrations are increased and remain relatively constant exceeding those seen in most of the normal menstrual cycle and sometimes exceeding ovulatory peak concentrations. The increased gonadotrophin secretion is a consequence of ovarian follicular failure as demonstrated by the reduced oestrogen and progesterone output.

TESTICULAR FUNCTION

The testis can be considered to have two main compartments (1) the seminiferous tubules in which spermatogenesis takes place and (2) the interstitial tissue containing Leydig cells which synthesise androgens. There is an anatomically ill-defined barrier (so called 'blood–testis' barrier) between the interstitial tissue and the seminiferous tubular lumen. Sertoli cells form part of this barrier and are responsible for much of the luminal secretion.

Leydig cells synthesise testosterone, small amounts of DHT and androstenedione, the majority of which enter the circulation. Some testosterone and androstenedione is taken up by Sertoli cells. These cells contain androgen receptors, and though not capable of *de novo* steroid synthesis, synthesise DHT and E2 from the androgen precursors.

FSH binds to high affinity specific receptors on the Sertoli cell membranes and, in the presence of testosterone, stimulates ABP synthesis via the cyclic AMP intracellular signalling system. ABP has similar physical characteristics to SHBG and appears to function as a transport protein for testosterone within the testis. Both FSH and testosterone are required for spermatogenesis. LH acting by a similar mechanism stimulates androgen synthesis in Leydig cells. Cell surface receptors for FSH are also present on Leydig cells. FSH probably increases the number of LH receptors on the Leydig cell membrane and consequently modulates the LH stimulation of androgen synthesis in these cells. Testicular function is thus complex and integrated.

The secretion of FSH and LH from the pituitary is pulsatile. The plasma concentration of testosterone fluctuates throughout the day in an ill-defined manner, though the highest plasma concentration is observed in the early morning. Pituitary LH secretion is subject to negative feed-back inhibition by testosterone, probably at both the hypothalamic and pituitary levels. FSH secretion is inhibited in a similar fashion at the pituitary level by inhibin, a poorly characterised protein, probably secreted by Sertoli cells.

There is no abrupt cessation of testicular function comparable with the decline in ovarian function in women. Testosterone secretion, production of viable spermatozoa and sexual potency may continue into old age. There is, however, some reduction in testosterone secretion in older males and the FSH and LH values are rather higher.

PRINCIPLES INVOLVED IN GONADAL FUNCTION TESTS

The mainstay of investigation is the measurement of individual plasma hormone concentrations by immunoassay techniques. Unfortunately such measurements give little information concerning hormone production or clearance rates. The practical details of particular immunoassays are beyond the scope of this book. The pituitary and gonadal hormones may show diurnal variation, monthly variation and age-related changes in plasma concentrations, and be secreted episodically. As a consequence the interpretation of individual values may be difficult.

Group steroid assays and assays of specific hormones or their metabolites in 24 h urine collections were discussed in the 5th edition of this book. They are no longer commonly performed, and with the advent of satisfactory methods for the measurement of individual hormones in plasma probably should be abandoned (Rudd, 1983).

A proper assessment of the hypothalamic–anterior pituitary–gonadal axis may involve the stimulation of the different organs involved and the determination of their secretions or the consequences of such secretions. The more commonly used dynamic tests are the GnRH test, clomiphene stimulation test and oestradiol benzoate stimulation test. The ovaries may also be directly stimulated in the treatment of infertility where there is potential for normal ovarian function.

For further information concerning the clinical aspects of particular endocrine problems textbooks such as Hall *et al.* (1980) or Wilson and Foster (1985) should be consulted. For paediatric problems, Brook (1981) and Clayton and Round (1984) are useful.

ANALYTICAL METHODS FOR BASAL SECRETION STUDIES

Determination of Oestradiol in Plasma

Since their initial introduction (Jaing and Ryan, 1969; Abraham *et al.*, 1970; Mikhail *et al.*, 1970), RIA methods have been improved by developing more specific antisera. The oestrogens themselves are not immunogens but become so when covalently linked to a protein, usually bovine serum albumin (BSA). The position on the steroid nucleus at which the linkage is made is important. If a characteristic group is employed to create the linkage it is only poorly recognised by the antiserum and hence discrimination between steroids differing in respect of the characteristic group may be poor. Thus E2 possesses two characteristic hydroxyl groups at C-3 and C-17β. If either of these is converted to the hemisuccinate and then linked to BSA, some specificity is lost. Thus E2-17β-succinyl-BSA produces antibodies which cross react with E1 (71 %), E2-17α (42 %) and E3 (12 %) making a chromatographic separation step essential (Schiller and Brammall, 1974).

More specific antisera have used steroid antigens linked at C-6 or C-11 thus leaving the determinants in rings A and D intact. Kuss and Goebel (1972) prepared the 6-carboxymethoximes of E1, E2 and E3 and used these to form an amide link to the lysine amino groups in BSA. Antisera to E2-6-

carboxymethoxime-BSA are highly specific and only cross react significantly with C-6 substituted-E2 (Doerr *et al.*, 1973; Exley and Moore, 1973; Loriaux *et al.*, 1973). Although such steroids occur in urine they are probably not present in significant amounts in plasma. Linkage to BSA using a succinyl group linked at C-11 has been used for 11α-hydroxy-E2 (Onikki and Adlercreutz, 1973) and for 11β-hydroxy-E2 (England *et al.*, 1974). The antiserum to the 11β variant seems to have the higher specificity. The most specific antisera can be used on simple organic solvent extracts of plasma without further purification. Commercial assays for E2 without an extraction step are available but have not been fully evaluated. While many workers have used tritiated E2 for the assay, it is possible to use radio-iodine labelled products of higher specific activity and which are easier to count (Chapter 9, p. 217). Thus England *et al.* (1974) conjugated the hemisuccinate of 11β-hydroxy-E2 with tyrosine methyl ester and then radio-iodinated the tyrosine group. Lindberg and Edqvist (1974) found that iodination of ring A of the oestrogen could lead to loss of immunoreactivity and preferred to conjugate E2-6-carboxymethyloxime with ^{125}I-tyramine.

INTERPRETATION

A wide variation in E2 levels is seen in apparently normal females (DeVane *et al.*, 1975; Kim *et al.*, 1974; Landgren *et al.*, 1980; Shaaban and Klopper, 1973). Each group reports a relatively wide range at any stage of the menstrual cycle and there is some disagreement between authors. In part, this may be due to the use of different antisera but many ranges are based on relatively few cycles. Also Kletzky *et al.* (1975) have shown that the E2 figures at any stage of the cycle are not distributed in a Gaussian fashion but are better represented as a 'log normal' distribution (Chapter 10, p. 240). They give the 95 % ranges and median values for each day in 22 women: early follicular, 41–470 (median 137) pmol/l; late follicular, 74–1000 (median 270) pmol/l. Landgren *et al.* (1980) give the 91 % ranges for various stages of the menstrual cycle in 68 women: early follicular, 150–370 pmol/l; pre-ovulatory peak, 690–2120 pmol/l; luteal maximum, 480–1180 pmol/l.

In general, the lowest values occur at the very end and beginning of the cycle with a progressive increase after day 6 to the ovulatory peak. The wide variation of peak concentration is partly due to its relatively short duration and the true peak may be missed if samples are only collected every 24 h. Thorneycroft *et al.* (1974) measured the plasma concentrations of E2 and other hormones at 4 hourly intervals in 4 normal women around the period of ovulation. In all cases the E2 peak preceded that of LH.

The clinical value of plasma E2 measurements in women is severely limited, mainly due to the wide variations seen throughout the menstrual cycle. Their use is largely confined to pre-pubertal problems, post-menopausal bleeding and the monitoring of infertility therapy. The plasma FSH concentration is not elevated with adequate oestrogenisation. A practical assessment of 'oestrogen status' is the progesterone challenge test (Hull *et al.*, 1979). Following a 5 day course of oral medroxyprogesterone acetate (a synthetic progestogen), withdrawal bleeding normally occurs. Absent or scanty bleeding indicates oestrogen deficiency.

Few values for other oestrogens are available in the normal cycle. E1 shows similar changes to E2 but they are less marked. In the early follicular phase, the mean values are: 193 pmol/l (DeVane *et al.*, 1975) and 108 pmol/l (Kim *et al.*, 1974). The last-named authors also quote mean values for the mid-cycle and mid-luteal phase peaks of 300 pmol/l.

Following the menopause, the mean plasma E2 concentration is 53·5 pmol/l (Judd *et al.*, 1974), which is less than that seen in the normal early follicular phase.

The mean plasma E1 concentration is 112 pmol/l (Judd *et al.*, 1974) and subject to diurnal variation.

The median plasma E2 concentration in normal men has been given as 63 pmol/l (Doerr, 1973) and a 95 % range of 35–101 pmol/l. Doerr (1976) reported a median plasma E1 concentration in normal men of 103 pmol/l and a 95 % range of 54–197 pmol/l. The values increase with increasing age.

Determination of Progesterone in Plasma

RIA methods for progesterone have been developed and as with E2, the specificity of the antiserum depends on the nature of the steroid linkage to BSA. Antisera raised to progesterone linked to BSA through position 20 (Midgley and Niswender, 1970) or position 3 (Furuyama and Nugent, 1971) show cross-reaction with related steroids and a chromatographic separation is required. The same need is apparent using 11-deoxycortisol linked to BSA through position 21 as there is well-marked cross reaction with deoxycorticosterone and 17α-hydroxyprogesterone (Abraham *et al.*, 1971). Greater specificity is shown by antisera raised to progesterone linked to BSA by the 11α-hemisuccinate group (Midgley and Niswender, 1970; Furr, 1973). Appreciable cross-reaction occurs with epimers of 11-hydroxyprogesterone but these are very poorly extracted into light petroleum. Some cross-reaction occurs with 5α-dihydroprogesterone (10%) and 5β-dihydroprogesterone (5·1 %). While these substances are extracted into light petroleum, they do not appear to be present in plasma (Furr, 1973). Interference from other steroids in the extract is likely to be less than 1%.

Non-extraction methods using anilino-naphthalene sulphonic acid (ANS) or danazol (a synthetic steroid) to strip progesterone from binding proteins, predominantly CBG, are now generally available. The majority use antisera to 11α-hemisuccinate conjugates. Both [^{3}H]progesterone or ^{125}I-labelled progesterone 11α-glucuronyl tyramine can be used as tracer, the latter becoming more popular. The bridge used for the iodinated tracer and that used for antiserum production should be dissimilar (Corrie *et al.*, 1981). Fluoroimmunoassays and enzyme-linked immunoassays are now available. Progesterone can also be measured in saliva (Walker *et al.*, 1979; Petsos *et al.*, 1986) which may have advantages when monitoring patients throughout the menstrual cycle. A review of progesterone assays and their performance is given by Wood *et al.* (1985).

INTERPRETATION
The plasma progesterone concentration has been determined throughout the menstrual cycle by numerous workers including Abraham *et al.* (1972), Shaaban and Klopper (1973) and Kletzky *et al.* (1975), the last authors demonstrating a 'log normal' distribution. During the follicular phase the values are usually less than 3 nmol/l, which is below the detection limit of many assays. Ovulation is followed by a mid-luteal phase peak (day 21 or 7 days post-ovulation) of 30–80 nmol/l in fertile cycles. In the investigation of infertility, values greater than 30 nmol/l can be used to indicate that ovulation has occurred (Hull *et al.*, 1982b), though values greater than 80 nmol/l may be associated with infertile cycles. If the menstrual cycle is irregular it may be advisable to measure plasma progesterone concentrations on days 19, 20 and 21. Abraham *et al.* (1974) suggested that the sum of any three results on different days should be greater than 48 nmol/l even if one of them was as low as 9·5 nmol/l. Increasingly, ultrasonography is being used

to measure the growth of Graafian follicles in the assessment of ovulation (Kerin *et al.*, 1981).

Following the menopause, the plasma progesterone concentration is reduced to 0·57 ± 0·20 (SD) nmol/l (Abraham *et al.*, 1971).

In men, the concentration of progesterone in plasma is low. Abraham *et al.* (1971) give a range of 0·75 ± 0·20 (SD) nmol/l. Similar values are quoted by Swain (1972).

Determination of Testosterone in Plasma

RIA methods have used antisera prepared against BSA linked to testosterone 3-oxime (Furuyama *et al.*, 1970) or testosterone 17-hemisuccinate (Thorneycroft *et al.*, 1973) thereby blocking one of the characteristic groups in testosterone. Most antisera cross react appreciably with DHT, androstenedione, Δ^4- and Δ^5-androstenediols. Solvent extracts have therefore often been purified further by solvent partition (Furuyama *et al.*, 1970) or by chromatography (Dufau *et al.*, 1972; Thorneycroft *et al.*, 1973; Pirke and Doerr, 1975).

To date most assays have incorporated a solvent extraction step using diethyl ether. Although direct assays have been reported (Pratt *et al.*, 1975) these have not found general acceptance. The displacement agents used have been, E2, ANS, pH and heat treatment. Direct assays are available commercially but the displacement conditions are often unknown and their performance has not been fully evaluated (Wheeler *et al.*, 1986).

Testosterone assays and their performance have been reviewed by Ismail *et al.* (1986).

INTERPRETATION

The plasma testosterone concentration in men remains relatively constant over the age range 18 to 50 years, but declines somewhat later. Pirke and Doerr (1975) found a median concentration of 20·3 nmol/l at age 22 to 61 and 14·7 nmol/l at age 69 to 93 years. The corresponding ranges were 10·9 to 33·4 nmol/l and 6·8 to 23·0 nmol/l. Vermeulen (1979) quotes a range of 9·7 to 41 nmol/l. There is, however, a marked fluctuation in plasma testosterone concentrations, with several broad peaks during the 24 h period. The lowest concentrations occur at 0100 h and 1500 h with the highest concentration at 0500 h, up to twice that at the nadir (Pirke and Doerr, 1975). There are also slow cyclical variations with mean periodicity of 3 weeks and an amplitude of 9 to 28 % (mean 17) around the individual average value (Doering *et al.*, 1975).

Much lower values are seen in pre-pubertal boys. Lee *et al.* (1974) found that the testosterone increase followed the increase in LH and the start of gonadal growth and was followed by growth of the penis and pubic hair. The mean values for successive years from ages 10 to 17 inclusive were 1·4, 3·0, 7·5, 11·7, 13·2, 17·3, 18·7 and 31·2 nmol/l.

The plasma concentration of DHT in normal men is about 10 % that of testosterone and responds in parallel to testosterone during the day and following stimulation or suppression tests (Pirke and Doerr, 1975). Much lower concentrations (0·5–1·0 nmol/l) occur in normal menstruating women and the adrenal cortex contributes approximately half (Abraham, 1974).

Vermeulen (1979) gives the following plasma androgen concentrations (mean ± 1SD nmol/l) for women during the menstrual cycle: testosterone; follicular, 1·2 ± 0·17; midcycle ± 2 day, 1·5 ± 0·24; luteal 1·3 ± 0·21: DHT; follicular, 0·79 ± 0·14; midcycle, 0·89 ± 0·14; luteal, 0·83 ± 0·14: androstenedione;

follicular, $5\cdot0 \pm 2\cdot3$; midcycle, $7\cdot7 \pm 1\cdot6$; luteal, $4\cdot2 \pm 0\cdot84$: DHA; follicular, $19\cdot1 \pm 3\cdot1$; midcycle, $19\cdot1 \pm 2\cdot6$; luteal; $18\cdot0 \pm 2\cdot3$: DHAS (μmol/l); follicular, $3\cdot1 \pm 1\cdot2$; midcycle, $3\cdot1 \pm 1\cdot0$; luteal, $2\cdot8 \pm 1\cdot4$. Following the menopause, the mean plasma concentrations of testosterone and androstenedione are $0\cdot69$ and $2\cdot6$ nmol/l respectively (Thorneycroft *et al.*, 1973).

The measurement of plasma androgen concentrations is of limited value in the investigation of the polycystic ovary syndrome and idiopathic hirsutism in women. Although the androgen production rates in hirsute women are increased, usually due to ovarian secretion (Kirschner *et al.*, 1976), the plasma androgen concentrations show a large overlap with respect to normal women (André and James, 1974). The concentration of free testosterone is generally increased (Kirschner *et al.*, 1976), in part due to a decreased plasma SHBG concentration. Improved separation of the two groups has been claimed by measuring testosterone and SHBG concurrently (Carter *et al.*, 1983). A recent onset accompanied by a plasma testosterone concentration greater than 7 nmol/l is suggestive of an androgen secreting tumour of the adrenal cortex or ovary.

The polycystic ovary syndrome is a mixed group of related conditions. In its full form there is hirsutism, amenorrhoea, infertility and ovarian abnormalities in the form of follicular cysts and a thickened capsule preventing ovulation. The condition may be discovered during investigations for infertility and is often diagnosed by laparoscopy or ultrasonography. DeVane *et al.* (1975) and Duignan (1976) in detailed studies found increased mean plasma concentrations of LH, E1, testosterone, androstenedione and DHAS but no significant increase in FSH, E2, or DHA. This suggests the possibility of both ovarian and adrenal involvement with peripheral formation of E1 from androstenedione. These findings, and an increased ovarian venous testosterone concentration, are similar to idiopathic hirsutism. Congenital adrenal hyperplasia is discussed in Chapter 31 (p. 830).

Determination of Gonadotrophins

For many years bioassays were used to measure FSH and LH, usually in urine. Such assays were laborious and often did not discriminate clearly between the two types of activity. With the development of RIA and other more recent immunological techniques using monoclonal antibodies, considerable improvements in specificity and sensitivity have been achieved (e.g. Hunter *et al.*, 1984). In most immunoassays for LH there is considerable cross-reaction with HCG. The commonly used standards for FSH are the 1st and 2nd International Reference Preparations (IRP) 69/104 and (IRP) 78/459 respectively, with assigned potencies for FSH of 10 and LH 25 IU/ampoule. These preparations are two batches of the same human pituitary bulk preparation. They were originally developed for bioassays but are now used for RIA determinations of FSH. The purity is low and they contain TSH, and α and β sub-units. The usual LH standard for RIA is IRP-68/40 derived from a human pituitary preparation. The purity is 95 % with only small FSH and TSH contamination. The assigned potency for LH is 77 IU/ampoule. The 2nd IRP-HMG, derived from the urine of post-menopausal women, was originally developed for urinary gonadotrophin assays and subsequently used for RIA determinations in plasma. It is no longer available. Reference materials for α and β sub-units are available from the National Institute for Biological Standards and Control. For further details concerning standards see Bangham (1983). Gonadotrophin assays and their performance have been comprehensively reviewed by Butt (1979; 1983).

INTERPRETATION

Agreement between immunological methods for the steroid hormones is fairly good but is less satisfactory for peptide hormones including LH and FSH. Variations in the relative activity of different antisera to different parts of the hormone molecule and the use of different standards contribute to the difficulties. Hence 'normal ranges' vary from one laboratory to another. The various studies on LH agree that there is a mid-cycle peak of plasma LH. When results for different cycles and different women are combined by superimposition of the peaks, the mean values show a clearly defined peak of relatively short duration of about 48 h on average (Thorneycroft *et al.*, 1974). The results for an individual cycle can be less clear cut and fluctuating concentrations around the period of ovulation may give the appearance of a broader peak or of several peaks. Fluctuation of plasma LH concentration is also seen during the 24 h period in males suggesting that episodic release of the hormone may be common (Boyer *et al.*, 1972). These peaks, including the ovulatory peak, can be of only a few hours duration in any one individual. These factors sometimes may make it difficult to be sure when or whether ovulation has occurred on the basis of plasma LH measurements alone. In the case of FSH there is general agreement that there is an ovulatory peak of plasma concentration which is relatively transient and usually less marked than that of LH.

According to Kletzky *et al.* (1975) the distribution of LH and FSH values is log normal at all stages of the cycle. They quote for LH the following 95 % ranges (and median) in IU/l related to 2nd IRP-HMG: follicular, 10·0–31·5 (18·0); ovulatory peak (day 0), 30·0–86 (50·0); days − 1 and + 1, 15·0–36·0 (23·0); luteal, 9·8–29·0 (17·0). For FSH, the values in the same units are: follicular, 6·0–17·0 (10·0); ovulatory peak (day 0), 17·0–40·0 (26·0); days − 1 and + 1, 6·2–22·5 (12·0); luteal, 4·3–15·0 (8·0). Landgren *et al.* (1980), using IRP 69/104 as standard, give the 91 % ranges for plasma LH in IU/l at various stages of the menstrual cycle in 68 women as; early follicular, 1·0–3·5; pre-ovulatory peak, 13–36; mean luteal phase, 1·1–4·3. The corresponding values for FSH (IU/l) using the same standard are; 0·9–4·0; 2·5–16; 1·5–3·3. At the menopause the plasma FSH and LH concentrations increase on average 8-fold and 2-fold respectively (Wide *et al.*, 1973).

Gonadotrophin values in men are similar to those in women during the early follicular phase. After the age of 40–50 years there is a progressive increase in gonadotrophin values but only the FSH concentration attains statistical significance (Wide *et al.*, 1973).

The differentiation between hypergonadotrophic (primary gonadal failure) and hypogonadotrophic hypogonadism (secondary gonadal failure) is often possible by measuring plasma FSH and/or LH. Reduced secretion as a consequence of anterior pituitary or hypothalamic disease may be difficult to differentiate from low normal values with some present methods. In these circumstances the GnRH test is often helpful. Abnormally high values are seen with a normal hypothalamus and pituitary released from negative feed-back suppression by primary gonadal failure.

—

Determination of Prolactin

Prior to the introduction of the 1st prolactin IRP 75/504 standard (650 mIU/ampoule) a variety of standards was used. However, this material is no longer generally available and a new reference preparation is awaited. Prolactin assays and their performance have been comprehensively reviewed by Franks (1979; 1983).

INTERPRETATION
Franks *et al.* (1975) using prolactin standard VLS No 1, reported a mean plasma prolactin concentration during the follicular phase of normal menstruating women as 7·0 μg/l with a range of 3·0–15 μg/l (approximately 60–300 mIU/l). There was no significant difference in the values obtained from this group and a group of post-menopausal women. There is a small mid-cycle peak thought to be due to increased E2 production. The plasma prolactin concentration increases during pregnancy to reach a maximum in the third trimester. Cowden *et al.* (1979a) using IRP 75/504 standard reported a mean value of 168 mU/l and upper 95th centile of 340 mU/l in healthy adults, with no sex difference. In contrast Guyda and Friesen (1973) reported the mean value for adult men to be 66% of that for women. The values in childhood are similar to adult male values with no sex difference (Cowden *et al.*, 1979a; Guyda and Friesen, 1973), though there is an increase at puberty in girls (Thorner *et al.*, 1977). The mean value for infants under 3 months of age is 4 133 mU/l (Cowden *et al.*, 1979a).

Hyperprolactinaemia (values greater than the appropriate reference range) should always be documented on at least two occasions because of the episodic secretion of prolactin and the uncertain effects of venepuncture and 'stress'. Values up to 700 mU/l should be treated with caution and a thorough history of drug therapy, including the contraceptive pill and dopamine receptor-blocking drugs, obtained. Hypothyroidism should always be considered.

The main causes of hyperprolactinaemia are macro- or micro-adenoma of the anterior pituitary gland and 'functional' hyperprolactinaemia (idiopathic hyperprolactinaemia). The differentiation between the latter two conditions may be difficult. Dynamic tests involving TRH, metoclopramide and other drugs have been advocated (Cowden *et al.*, 1979a; Cowden *et al.*, 1979b) but these have not found universal acceptance in clinical practice (Jacobs, 1981; Shalet *et al.*, 1981). Basal plasma prolactin concentrations greater than 700 mU/l are unlikely to be due to 'stress' and values greater than 1000 mU/l are likely to be associated with a pituitary tumour. Hyperprolactinaemia is a common cause of female infertility (Jacobs, 1975). Prolactinomas occurring in males may result in impotence and/or oligospermia. Chronic renal failure is often accompanied by hyperprolactinaemia.

Determination of Sex Hormone-binding Globulin

Assay methods for plasma SHBG include binding capacity assays using DHT as ligand followed by precipitation (Anderson *et al.*, 1976; Rosner, 1972) and various immunological techniques, including RIA (Cheng *et al.*, 1983; Khan *et al.*, 1982) and radial immunodiffusion (Earnshaw *et al.*, 1982). Such assays are not generally available. At present there is no SHBG reference preparation.

INTERPRETATION
There is a large variation in the results obtained by different workers (Khan *et al.*, 1982). Rosner (1972) using a binding capacity assay reports the mean DHT (nmol) bound per litre of plasma; men, 32; women, 63; pregnant women, 427. Cheng *et al.* (1983) report the plasma SHBG concentration (mean ± SD nmol/l)

in a small number of subjects; men, 18 ± 9; women, 54 ± 13, women in late pregnancy, 374 ± 55. There is no discernible variation throughout the menstrual cycle. Prepubertally the values are similar to those in adult women. In both sexes the values decline with the onset of puberty but rise in late female puberty. There is a small increase in men with increasing age. Increased values are seen in patients with hyperthyroidism, cirrhosis of the liver, in male hypogonadal hypogonadism and male patients treated with oestrogens. Decreased concentrations occur in hirsute women, patients with the nephrotic syndrome and patients treated with androgens. The main use of this investigation is discussed above.

INVESTIGATIONS USING DYNAMIC TESTS

GnRH Test

Besser *et al.* (1972) found that after an intravenous dose of 100 μg of synthetic GnRH, plasma LH rose significantly reaching peak levels in 20 to 30 min. Plasma FSH responses were slower and smaller, often not moving outside the normal basal range. The mean responses were similar for males and for females in the early follicular phase of the cycle but there were marked individual variations. Similar results are reported by others and occur also with higher doses (Crosignani *et al.*, 1974). The responses are relatively constant for the individual and bigger LH increases are associated with a definite FSH response (Shahmanesh *et al.*, 1975). The release of gonadotrophins might be expected to be followed by an increase in gonadal hormone output. In the male, the plasma testosterone response is variable and may not be helpful, but in the female, plasma E2 increases to a maximum about 6 h after stimulation and the response has been used as a test by Katz and Carr (1974). The gonadotrophin increase is greatest in females near the time of ovulation, diminishes during the luteal phase and is least in the follicular phase (Shaw *et al.*, 1974). Also the greater increases are accompanied by an increased LH/FSH ratio (Yen *et al.*, 1972). In the male at least, the response varies at different times of the day being maximal at 0600 h and 1800 h and minimal at 1200 h (Schwarzstein *et al.*, 1975).

The protocol for the test varies between authors but a typical one is as follows (Edwards and Besser, 1974); A 100 μg dose of GnRH is administered intravenously as a bolus between 0800 h and 1000 h. Blood samples are taken before and 20 and 60 min afterwards for LH and FSH assay. In adult males the LH concentration rises 7- to 8-fold and FSH 2-fold above the basal levels. The peak concentrations usually occur at 20 min. If the 60 min value is greater than the 20 min value, the response is said to be delayed. The response in women is qualitatively similar but varies in magnitude with the stage of the menstrual cycle and is dependent on circulating steroid concentrations particularly E2 (Shaw *et al.*, 1974). The LH response is 3- to 4-fold greater in the luteal phase than in the follicular phase with the greatest response in the pre-ovulatory phase. The FSH responses are similar but less marked.

Unfortunately the test does not distinguish between primary hypothalamic and primary pituitary failure (Mortimer *et al.*, 1973; Jacobs, 1975) unlike the situation with TRH. It appears that an adequate store of gonadotrophins in the anterior pituitary, released during the test, requires the tonic effect of the releasing hormone and is also affected by the steroid milieu. Repeated stimulation with releasing hormone eventually results in a normal response if the pituitary is intact. There is little to be gained in performing a GnRH test if the basal values are high.

However, the test can be used to exclude primary pituitary disease (Marshall *et al.*, 1972).

Clomiphene Stimulation Test

Clomiphene citrate initiates the hypothalamic release of GnRH by modifying the feedback control of circulating oestrogens or testosterone. It acts as an oestrogen antagonist at E2 receptor sites in the hypothalamus. The usual dose for dynamic studies is 50 mg taken orally and twice daily for 5 to 7 days. Plasma samples are collected at intervals which vary with different workers. After collecting basal

clomiphene

samples, the frequency of plasma sampling is not greater than once daily at various times between the 3rd and 19th day. The response of LH is more marked than that of FSH and so is the more useful determination. Alternatively, plasma E2 or progesterone concentrations can be determined. An adequate response to GnRH, but a failure to respond to clomiphene is suggestive of a hypothalamic lesion. Clomiphene citrate is used in the assessment and treatment of infertility (Hull *et al.*, 1982a). An indication of whether ovulation has occurred can be obtained by measuring plasma progesterone concentration in the luteal phase.

Oestrogen Provocation Test

For ovulation to occur the hypothalamus must respond to the rapidly rising plasma E2 concentration in the late follicular phase by provoking the release of GnRH, resulting in the pre-ovulatory surge of LH (positive feed-back). The oestrogen provocation test is used to test the integrity of this mechanism (Shaw *et al.*, 1975). After collecting a basal blood sample, oestradiol benzoate (1 mg) is given by intramuscular injection and further samples are collected at 8, 24, 32, 48, 56 and 72 h. The plasma E2 concentration is maximal at 8 h and in normal female subjects the plasma LH concentration is maximal at 48–72 h. A small increment in FSH occurs at the same time.

HCG Stimulation Test

HCG may be used in females in the therapeutic induction of ovulation. In males it has been employed to demonstrate the presence of testicular tissue, when this is in doubt, to assess the Leydig cell reserve in the testis and to assess its possible therapeutic use in hypogonadotrophic states. The dose used varies considerably, 1000 to 5000 IU daily for 1–4 days. Marshall (1975) uses a dose of 2000 IU i.m. on days 0 and 3 and collects plasma for testosterone measurement on days 0, 3 and 5. The normal response is a rise to 150–300 % of the basal level on either day 3 or day 5. The peak value is usually greater than 35 nmol/l. DHT shows smaller increases (Pirke and Doerr, 1975).

REFERENCES

Abraham G. E. (1974). *J. Clin. Endocr. Metab*; **39**: 340.

Abraham G. E., Chakmakjian Z. H. (1973). *J. Clin. Endocr. Metab*; **37**: 581.

Abraham G. E., Maroulis G. B., Marshall J. R. (1974). *Obstet. Gynec*; **44**: 522.

Abraham G. E., Odell W. D., Edwards K., Purdy J. M. (1970) *Acta Endocrinol*; Suppl; **147**: 332.

Abraham G. E., Odell W. D., Swerdloff R. S., Hopper K. (1972). *J. Clin. Endocr. Metab*; **34**: 312.

Abraham G. E., Swerdloff R., Tulchinsky D., Odell W. D. (1971). *J. Clin. Endocr. Metab*; **32**: 619.

Anderson D. C. (1974). *Clin. Endocrinol*; **3**: 69.

Anderson D. C., et al. (1976). *Clin. Endocrinol*; **5**: 657.

André C. M., James V. H. T. (1974). *Steroids*; **24**: 295.

Bangham D. R. (1983). In *Immunoassays for Clinical Chemistry*, 2nd ed. (Hunter W. M., Corrie J. E. T., eds) p. 27. Edinburgh: Churchill Livingstone.

Bardin C. W., Lipsett M. B. (1967). *J. Clin. Invest*; **46**: 891.

Besser G. M., et al. (1972). *Brit. Med. J*; **3**: 267.

Boyer R. M., et al. (1972). *J. Clin. Endocr. Metab*; **35**: 73.

Brook C. G. D., ed. (1981). *Clinical Paediatric Endocrinology*. Oxford: Blackwell Scientific Publications.

Brooks J. E., et al. (1986). *Clin. Endocrinol*; **24**: 653.

Butt W. R. (1979). In *Hormones in Blood*, 3rd ed., Vol. 1. (Gray C. H., James V. H. T., eds) p. 411. New York, London: Academic Press.

Butt W. R. (1983). In *Hormones in Blood*, 3rd ed., Vol. 4. (Gray C. H., James V. H. T., eds) p. 148. New York, London: Academic Press.

Carter R. D., et al. (1983). *Ann. Clin. Biochem*; **20**: 262.

Cheng C. Y., et al. (1983). *J. Clin. Endocr. Metab*; **56**: 68.

Clayton B. E., Round J. M., eds. (1984). *Chemical Pathology and the Sick Child*. Oxford: Blackwell Scientific Publications.

Corrie J. E. T., Hunter W. M., Macphersen J. S. (1981). *Clin. Chem*; **27**: 594.

Cowden E. A., Ratcliffe W. A., Beastall G. H., Ratcliffe J. G. (1979a). *Ann. Clin. Biochem*; **16**: 113.

Cowden E. A., et al. (1979b). *Lancet*; **1**: 1155.

Crosignani P. G., et al. (1974). *Amer. J. Obstet. Gynecol*; **120**: 376.

DeVane G. W., Czekala N. M., Judd H. L., Yen S. S. C. (1975). *Amer. J. Obstet. Gynecol*; **121**: 496.

Doering C. H., Kraemer H. C., Brodie H. K. H., Hambing D. A. (1975). *J. Clin. Endocrin. Metab*; **40**: 492.

Doerr P. (1973). *Acta Endocrinol*; **72**: 330.

Doerr P. (1976). *Acta Endocrinol*; **81**: 655.

Doerr P., Goebel R., Kuss E. (1973). *Acta Endocrinol*; **73**: 314.

Doring G. H. (1969). *J. Reprod. Fertil*; Suppl; **6**: 77.

Dufau M. L., Catt K. J., Isuruhara T., Ryan D. (1972). *Clin. Chim. Acta*; **37**: 109.

Duignan N. M. (1976). *Brit. J. Obstet. Gynaecol*; **83**: 593.

Dunn J. F., Nisula B. C., Rodbard D. (1981). *J. Clin. Endocr. Metab*; **53**: 58.

Earnshaw R. J., Bowen M., Levell M. J. (1982). *Clin. Chim. Acta*; **123**: 175.

Easterling W. E. Jr., Talbert L. M., Potter H. D. (1974). *Amer. J. Obstet. Gynecol*; **120**: 385.

Edwards C. R. W., Besser G. M. (1974). *Clinics Endocrin. Metab*; **3**: 475.

England B. G., Niswender G. D., Midgley A. R. Jr. (1974). *J. Clin. Endocr. Metab*; **38**: 42.

Exley D., Moore B. (1973). *J. Steroid Biochem*; **4**: 257.

Franks S. (1979). In *Hormones in Blood*, 3rd ed., Vol. 1. (Gray C. H., James V. H. T., eds) p. 279. New York, London: Academic Press.

Franks S. (1983). In *Hormones in Blood*, 3rd ed., Vol. 4. (Gray C. H., James V. H. T., eds) p. 109. New York, London: Academic Press.

Franks S., et al.(1975). *Clin. Endocrinol*; **4**: 597.

Fraser I. S., Baird D. T. (1974). *J. Clin. Endocr. Metab*; **39**: 564.

Furr B. J. A. (1973). *Acta Endocrinol*; **72**: 89.

Furuyama S., Mayes D. M., Nugent C. A. (1970). *Steroids*; **16**: 415.

Furuyama S., Nugent C. A. (1971). *Steroids*; **17**: 663.

Givens J. R. (1978). *Clin. Obstet. Gynaecol*; **21**: 115.

Grodin J. M., Siiteri P. K., MacDonald P. C. (1973). *J. Clin. Endocr. Metab*; **36**: 207.

Guyda H. J., Friesen H. G. (1973). *Pediat. Res*; **7**: 534.

Hall R., Anderson J., Smart G. A., Besser G. M. (1980). *Fundamentals of Clinical Endocrinology*, 3rd ed. London: Pitman Medical.

Horton R., Tait J. F. (1966). *J. Clin. Invest*; **45**: 301.

Hull M. G. R., Knuth V. A., Murray M. A. F., Jacobs H. S. (1979). *Brit. J. Obstet. Gynaecol*; **86**: 799.

Hull M. G. R., Savage P. E., Bromham D. R. (1982a). *Brit. Med. J*; **284**: 1681.

Hull M. G. R., *et al*. (1982b). *Fertil. Steril*; **37**: 355.

Hunter W. M., *et al*. (1984). *Ann. Clin. Biochem*; **21**: 275.

Ismail A. A. A., *et al*. (1986). *Ann. Clin. Biochem*; **23**:135.

Ito T., Horton R. (1970). *J. Clin. Endocr. Metab*; **31**: 362.

Ito T., Horton R. (1971). *J. Clin. Invest*; **50**: 1621.

Jacobs H. S. (1975). *Postgrad. Med. J*; **51**: 209.

Jacobs H. S. (1981). *Progress in Obstetrics and Gynaecology*. (Studd J., ed); **1**: 263.

Jaing N. S., Ryan R. J. (1969). *Proc. Mayo Clinic*; **44**: 461.

Judd H. L., Judd G. E., Lucas W. E., Yen S. S. C. (1974). *J. Clin. Endocr. Metab*; **39**: 1020.

Katz M., Carr P. J. (1974). *J. Obstet. Gynaecol. Brit. Cwlth*; **81**: 791.

Khan M. S., Ewen E., Rosner W. (1982). *J. Clin. Endocrinol*; **54**: 705.

Kerin J. F., *et al*. (1981). *Brit. J. Obstet. Gynaecol*; **88**: 81.

Kim M. H., Hosseinian A. H., Dupon C. (1974). *J. Clin. Endocr. Metab*; **39**: 706.

Kirschner M. A., Bardin C. W. (1972). *Metabolism*; **21**: 667.

Kirschner M. A., Zucker I. R., Jespersen D. (1976). *New Engl. J. Med*; **294**: 637.

Kletzky O. A., Nakamura R. M., Thorneycroft I. H., Mishell D. R. Jr. (1975). *Amer. J. Obstet. Gynecol*; **121**: 688.

Koninckx P. (1978). *Lancet*; **1**: 273.

Kuss E., Goebel R. (1972). *Steroids*; **19**: 509.

Landgren B.-M., Unden A.-L., Diczfalusy E. (1980). *Acta Endocrinol*; **94**: 89.

Lee P. A., Jaffe R. B., Midgley A. R. Jr. (1974). *J. Clin. Endocr. Metab*; **39**: 664.

Lindberg P., Edqvist L. E. (1974). *Clin. Chim. Acta*; **53**: 169.

Loriaux D. L., Guy R., Lipsett M. B. (1973). *J. Clin. Endocr. Metab*; **36**: 788.

MacDonald P. C., *et al*. (1965). *J. Clin. Endocr. Metab*; **25**: 1557.

MacDonald P. C., *et al*. (1979). *J. Clin. Endocr. Metab*; **49**: 905.

Marshall J. C. (1975). *Clinics Endocrin. Metab*; **4**: 545.

Marshall J. C., *et al*. (1972). *Brit. Med. J*; **4**: 643.

Midgley A. R. Jr., Niswender G. D. (1970). *Acta Endocrinol*; Suppl; **147**: 320.

Mikhail G., Wu C-H., Ferin M., van der Wiele R. L. (1970). *Steroids*; **15**: 333.

Mortimer C. H., *et al*. (1973). *Brit. Med. J*; **4**: 73.

Onikki S., Adlercreutz H. (1973). *J. Steroid Biochem*; **4**: 633.

Petsos P., Ratcliffe W. A., Heath D. F., Anderson D. C. (1986). *Clin. Endocrinol*; **24**: 31.

Pirke K. M., Doerr P. (1975). *Acta Endocrinol*; **79**: 357.

Pratt J. J., Wiegman T., Lappoln R. E., Woldring M. G. (1975). *Clin. Chim. Acta*; **59**: 337.

Rosner W. A. (1972). *J. Clin. Endocr. Metab*; **34**: 983.

Rudd B. T. (1983). *Ann. Clin. Biochem*; **20**: 65.

Schiller H. S., Brammall M. A. (1974). *Steroids*; **24**: 665.

Schwarzstein L., *et al*. (1975). *J. Clin. Endocr. Metab*; **40**: 313.

Shaaban M. M., Klopper A. (1973). *J. Obstet. Gynaecol. Brit. Cwlth*; **80**: 776.

Shahmanesh M., Ellwood M., Nelson E., Hartog M. (1975). *Postgrad. Med. J*; **51**: 59.

Shalet S. M., Chapman A. J., Whitehead E., Beardwell C. G. (1981). *Postgrad. Med. J*; **57**: 485.

Shaw R. W., Butt W. R., London D. R., Marshall J. C. (1974). *J. Obstet. Gynaecol. Brit. Cwlth*; **81**: 632.

Shaw R. W., Butt W. R., London D. R., Marshall J. C. (1975). *Clin. Endocrinol*; **4**: 267.

Siiteri P. K., *et al.* (1982). *Recent Prog. Horm. Res*; **38**: 459.
Siiteri P. K., Simberg N. H. (1986). *Clinics Endocrin. Metab*; **15**: 247.
Swain M. C. (1972). *Clin. Chim. Acta*; **39**: 455.
Thorner M. O., *et al.* (1977). *Clin. Endocrinol*; **7**: 463.
Thorneycroft I. H., Ribiero W. O., Stone S. C., Tillson S. A. (1973). *Steroids*; **21**: 111.
Thorneycroft I. H., *et al.* (1974). *J. Clin. Endocr. Metab*; **39**: 754.
Vermeulen A. (1979). In *Hormones in Blood*, 3rd ed., Vol. 3. (Gray C. H., James V. H. T., eds) p. 355. New York, London: Academic Press.
Walker R. F., Read G. F., Riad-Fahmey D. (1979). *Clin. Chem*; **25**: 2030.
Westphal U., Stroupe S. D., Cheng S.-L. (1977). *Ann. N.Y. Acad. Sci*; **286**: 10.
Wheeler M. J., Shaikh M., Jennings R. D. (1986). *Ann. Clin. Biochem*; **23**: 303.
Wide L., Nillius S. J., Gemzell C., Roos P. (1973). *Acta Endocrinol*; Suppl; **173**: 1.
Wilson J. D., Foster D. W., eds (1985). *William's Textbook of Endocrinology*, 7th ed. Philadelphia: W. B. Saunders.
Wood P., *et al.* (1985). *Ann. Clin. Biochem*; **22**: 1.
Yen S. S. C., Vanden Berg G., Rebar R., Ehara Y. (1972). *J. Clin. Endocr. Metab*; **35**: 931.

33

TESTS IN PREGNANCY

Biochemical tests which may assist the clinician during a patient's pregnancy may be grouped into two types. The first group, generally known as function tests, are aimed at establishing the integrity of the feto-placental unit in order to assess the progress of the pregnancy. The second group comprises specific diagnostic tests, looking for fetal problems such as congenital abnormalities, lack of lung maturity or damage due to Rhesus incompatibility. These may require special treatment before or after birth or specific action immediately, e.g. termination of pregnancy.

Feto-placental function tests are based on the pattern of output of hormones and proteins by the fetus and placenta during pregnancy. The information provided by many different biochemical products of pregnancy has been evaluated (Wilde and Oakey, 1975). The confirmation of pregnancy itself relies on the detection in urine of chorionic gonadotrophin (HCG). Once pregnancy is established, production of the peptide, human placental lactogen (HPL), and of specific placental proteins provides an opportunity for monitoring. Although progesterone is produced in large quantities by the placenta its measurement has proved of little value in pregnancy assessment. The assay of its urinary metabolite, 5β-pregnanediol, has fallen into disuse. The determination of oestrogens provides the only means of assessing the function of the feto-placental unit as a whole since the major pregnancy oestrogens require the activity of both the fetus and the placenta for their production.

Interpretation of function tests is made difficult by the variety of clinical conditions affecting them. Tests may be used to provide reassurance that no intervention is required, and this can be predicted with reasonable confidence when results are within the range found in uncomplicated pregnancies. On the other hand, when used to indicate that the fetus is compromised, the prediction of abnormality is much less reliable because there are many causes of fetal demise, and the effect of different clinical conditions (intra-uterine death, eclampsia, Rhesus isoimmunisation, diabetes, etc.) on feto-placental metabolism is varied. Most fetal deaths are attributable to causes other than feto-placental insufficiency (Vinall et al., 1980a,b) and function tests could not be expected to predict them.

These uncertainties have given rise to some scepticism about the usefulness of biochemical monitoring in pregnancy (Zlatnick et al., 1979; Shaxted, 1980; Rosenberg et al., 1982). This view has coincided with improvements in physical monitoring techniques and there has therefore been a decline in biochemical monitoring. Complete withdrawal of the laboratory service may not necessarily worsen stillbirth and mortality rates (Chamberlain, 1984). Such conclusions, however, do not go unchallenged and assays are still performed in significant numbers and are considered worthwhile if used appropriately, e.g. when intrauterine death from continuing placental insufficiency is likely to occur but the fetus is sufficiently mature to stand a reasonable chance of survival if delivered (Vinall et al., 1980a).

Tests of feto-placental function are performed either on serum or urine. The choice depends upon such factors as production rates, clearance rates, pool sizes, circadian variation and the variety and choice of metabolites (Klopper, 1976). The half-life of the analyte being measured should be sufficiently short to permit changes in its production rate to be recognised quickly so that action can be taken. Placental proteins appear in only trace quantities in urine and therefore serum assays are required. For oestrogens, serum and urine assays are used. Serum methods have become common because of the ease of collection and the rapid provision of results, but only one point in time within a complex metabolic process is being sampled. Urine estimations provide a longer-term view of the process but this must be balanced against the inconvenience and inaccuracies of urine collections and the delays before results are available.

The second group of tests in pregnancy is aimed at the detection of specific problems of the fetus itself. The tests are predominantly carried out on amniotic fluid. Bilirubin levels give an indication of Rhesus sensitisation. Phospholipid measurements provide information about the maturity of the fetal lungs and the risk of perinatal respiratory distress syndrome. Alphafetoprotein (AFP) assays and examination of acetylcholinesterase isoenzymes are used in the detection of neural tube and ventral wall defects, normally following unusually high maternal serum AFP levels. Other fetal abnormalities may be found by examining cells from amniotic fluid but this is not normally the province of the clinical biochemistry laboratory. However, the antenatal detection of Down's syndrome, which has hitherto been based on chromosome studies, may be assisted by the finding of low AFP levels in maternal serum (Cuckle and Wald, 1984).

OESTROGENS

Oestrogen assays are widely used in monitoring the progress of pregnancy. Oestrone (E1), oestradiol (E2) and oestriol (E3) are all produced by the feto-placental unit but E3 has received most attention. The metabolism of the oestrogens in pregnancy is reviewed in detail by Levitz and Young (1977) and Goebelsmann (1979). In outline, the androgen DHA-sulphate, largely produced by the growing fetal adrenal glands, is subjected to placental sulphatase and aromatase activities to produce mainly E1 and E2. The E3 arises from that fraction of precursor androgen which first undergoes 16α-hydroxylation in the fetal liver before further modification. In plasma, more than 90% of E3 is in the form of conjugates, particularly 16-glucosiduronate (20%), 3-sulphate,16-glucosiduronate (40%), 3-sulphate (15%) and 3-glucosiduronate (15%). This conjugation occurs principally in the maternal liver but also in the intestine where glucuronyl transferase is active. The enterohepatic circulation of oestrogens accounts for a substantial proportion of plasma and urine conjugates. Evidence of E3-16-glucosiduronate formation by the kidney is also to be found (Buchan and Klopper, 1979; Rock *et al.*, 1981). The renal clearance of these conjugates differs markedly so that the proportions in plasma and urine are quite different (Young *et al.*, 1976; Alexander *et al.*, 1979). No unconjugated oestrogens appear in urine and the glucosiduronates (mainly 16-) account for about 85% of the urinary E3, the sulphates accounting for 15%. This complexity of oestrogen metabolism gives rise to a wide choice of possible fractions and metabolites to assay. No good evidence exists to show that one analyte gives better clinical information than another, and assays have been chosen largely for their speed and convenience.

Determination of Maternal Urinary Oestrogens

Fractionation of urinary conjugates of the three major oestrogens is time-consuming and gives little additional information. Therefore 'total oestrogens', reflecting the predominant E3-glucosiduronates, are usually measured. The end-point of the reaction is the pink colour obtained when the phenolic group of the oestrogen molecule reacts with Köber reagent (a mixture of a phenol, often quinol, and sulphuric acid). This colour can be extracted into chloroform containing 4-nitrophenol or trichloracetic acid to form highly fluorescent products (Ittrich, 1958) increasing the sensitivity and specificity of the method. Direct fluorimetric measurement of the material, without extraction, is also possible (see below). The oestrogen conjugates are first hydrolysed (by acid in automated methods) and the urine is diluted prior to quantitation. Several manual and automated methods are described in the 5th edition of this book. Only automated methods are now used routinely and they are usually based on those of Hainsworth and Hall (1971) and Lever *et al.* (1973). There follows the description of an automated method for a Technicon AutoAnalyzer II system recommended by a working party of the DHSS Advisory Committee on the Assessment of Laboratory Standards (1981).

The method described assumes that the urine specimen is a complete 24 h collection. The inaccuracies of such collections and the time taken for their completion has led to the determination of 'oestrogen/creatinine ratios' on early morning urine specimens. The creatinine may be assayed separately or incorporated into the oestrogen manifold (Rao, 1977; Phillips *et al.*, 1978; Phillips, 1979).

Automated Method for Pregnancy Oestrogens (based on Lever *et al.*, 1973)

The urine is diluted, mixed with Köber reagent containing quinol and ferrous sulphate in sulphuric acid and heated to 130 °C. The resultant mixture is diluted with a solution of trichloracetic acid and chloral, cooled and passed directly through the flow cell of the fluorimeter.

Reagents. All chemicals should be of analytical reagent grade if available.
1. Alkaline diluent, 50 mmol/l sodium hydroxide. Dilute 10 ml of a 40 g/l solution to 2 l with distilled water.
2. Köber reagent. Solution A. Add 28 g quinol to 450 ml concentrated sulphuric acid and dissolve by swirling occasionally for 30 min at room temperature. Solution B. Add, *with cooling and careful mixing*, 560 ml concentrated sulphuric acid to 165 ml distilled water containing 7 g ferrous sulphate in solution. Add solution A to solution B *with cooling and careful mixing*.
3. Fluorescence reagent. Dissolve 100 g trichloracetic acid and 200 g chloral hydrate in 1 litre distilled water. Sticky oily globules may form on standing. To keep the system free from particulate matter, use a 001 sintered glass filter in the reagent line. Prepare fresh reagent weekly and filter through Whatman No. 2 paper before storing.
4. Oestriol stock standard, 2·5 mmol/l. Dissolve 144 mg oestriol (Sigma E1253) in 200 ml ethanol.
5. Working standards. If analyses are to be carried out on 24 h urine specimens, then standards in the range 25 to 100 μmol/l are required. For early morning urines, these values should be doubled. Dilute the stock standard with 100 mmol/l sodium hydroxide and prepare fresh working standards weekly.

Apparatus. The manifold is shown in Fig. 33.1. A Technicon Sampler II with an electronic timer or a cam checked for accuracy and a Pump III with air bar are appropriate. The sampling rate is 40/h with a sample wash ratio of 2:1. The heating bath must be capable of maintaining a temperature of 132 °C within 1 °C; a Skalar oil bath is suitable. The fluorimeter is a Locarte LFM4 with thallium lamp (emission 535 nm), flow cell, no excitation filter and 560 nm emission interference filter. Many recorders are suitable but a few are incompatible giving irregular spiky peaks.

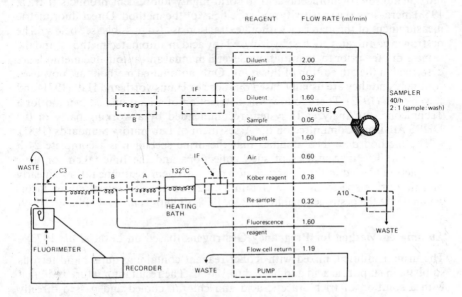

Fig. 33.1. Flow Diagram for AutoAnalyzer II Method for Urinary Oestrogen Determination.
All pump tubes are Tygon except for the Köber reagent and flow cell return which are Acidflex. A10 = T connector, 116-B034-01; C3 = debubbler, 116-0202-03; IF = injection fitting, 116-0489-01. The heating bath coil is 6·9 ml volume and 2·0 mm i.d.; the other coils are: A, 20 turn, 1·6 mm i.d., 196-0002-01; B, 20 turn, 2·0 mm i.d., 157-B095-01; C, 20 turn, 2·0 mm i.d., 157-0248-01.

Technique. Place reagent leads into reagents, switch on all modules except the sampler, and pump reagents through the system until a steady baseline is seen on the recorder. Set the baseline to approximately 5% of the full scale deflection. Switch on the sampler, sample three cups of the highest working standard and set the peak heights to approximately 90% full scale deflection. Sample the standards, controls and urine specimens. Read the unknowns from the standard curve and correct the results for the 24 h urine volume. It may be more convenient to predilute urines to 2 litres if the volume is less than this to simplify calculations for the majority of specimens.

At the end of the run, first switch off the heating bath and then pump all lines free of reagent before turning off the other modules. With time, charred organic matter may accumulate in the heating bath coil. This coil should therefore be washed weekly at room temperature with a dilute solution of RBS 25 (Chemical Concentrates RBS Limited) prepared by diluting 20 ml concentrated RBS 25 to 1 litre with water.

Notes.
1. Some substances in urine produce spurious results. The most important is glucose where the recovery of oestrogens falls with increasing glucose concentration. The apparent oestrogen output is reduced by 40 % at a glucose concentration of 110 mmol/l (20 g/l) according to Campbell and Gardner (1971). Every urine should be tested for the presence of glucose before being analysed.
2. Glucose is best removed by reduction to sorbitol using sodium borohydride (Little *et al.*, 1975). Incubate 5 ml urine for 1 h at 37 °C with 0·5 ml sodium borohydride, 500 g/l in 100 mmol/l sodium hydroxide, and one drop of octan-2-ol to prevent frothing. Add 0·5 ml glacial acetic acid to remove excess borohydride. When calculating the oestrogen output, make allowance for the additional dilution of urine resulting from this procedure.
3. Other interfering substances are much less common. Mandelamine (methanamine mandelate) liberates formaldehyde during acid hydrolysis. Aldehydes react with oestriol giving derivatives which do not react with the Köber reagent. Aspirin, excreted as the glucosiduronate, interferes in high dosage if hydrolysis is accomplished enzymatically using glucuronidase (Adlercreutz, 1975).

INTERPRETATION

The interpretation of pregnancy oestrogen results is complex. It is possible to produce 95 % probability ranges of oestrogen excretion in normal pregnancy (Hull *et al.*, 1975; McFadyen *et al.*, 1980) at each week of gestation. However, great inter-individual variation makes valid interpretation of results from one person difficult. Also this range may be inappropriate when comparing results from patients with specific problems such as diabetes, Rhesus isoimmunisation, hypertension or intra-uterine growth retardation. Correct interpretation demands an awareness of the precise clinical question being asked. The aim may be to seek reassurance that the pregnancy can safely be left to continue, it may be to predict 'high risk' in the future, or it may be to decide when to deliver a baby already known to be at risk.

Single assays on individual subjects are usually valueless. A trend must be established by repeated estimations, continuously falling values indicating that the fetus may be in impending danger. If the assay is to predict, rather than reflect impending demise, then frequent sampling and rapid availability of results are required. In the case of diabetic mothers, the fetus may rapidly become compromised and frequent sampling intervals are particularly important.

Fig. 33.2 shows action limits applicable to oestrogen excretion (Heys *et al.*, 1968). Only the lower values are of interest. Results within the 'borderline' zone suggest that more active monitoring is required. Those below this zone imply that the baby may need to be delivered. There are, however, many exceptions to this oversimplification where oestrogen excretion remains low throughout monitoring with no associated fetal detriment. This emphasises the importance of looking for trends rather than acting on the basis of cut-off values. But when a falling trend is noticed within the 'normal' range, intervention may not be required unless values drop into the 'borderline' zone.

A number of clinical situations which directly cause low oestrogen excretion must be recognised. If the fetus has already died the excretion will of course be low. Since the fetal adrenal gland is required for the production of precursor androgens, fetal adrenal hypoplasia, whether due to fetal anencephaly or to other congenital defects, is associated with low values (Dean *et al.*, 1977). A similar effect

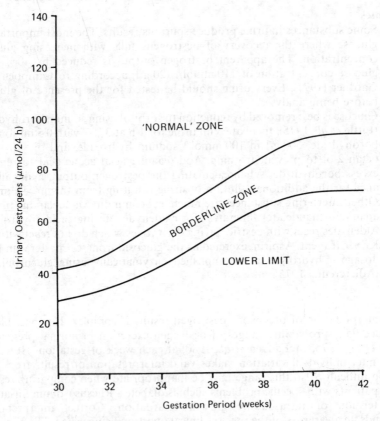

Fig. 33.2. Action Limits for Urinary Oestrogen Excretion (after Heys *et al.*, 1968).

can be seen if the mother is taking corticosteroids as these cross the placenta and suppress the output of ACTH from the fetal pituitary. Doses below the equivalent of 75 mg of cortisol per day are unlikely to be the cause of low oestrogen excretion. The congenital absence of placental sulphatase also leads to low oestrogen excretion since DHA sulphate cannot be utilised (Oakey, 1978; Harkness *et al.*, 1983). Penicillin and its analogues interfere with the production and excretion of oestrogens. This is thought to act in the gut by interfering with the substantial enterohepatic circulation of oestrogens (Buchan and Klopper, 1979). High oestrogen excretion is found in multiple pregnancies.

Determination of Maternal Serum Oestrogens

The need for rapidly available results without the delays and inaccuracies inherent in urine collections has led to the widespread use of serum assays. Radioimmunoassays are available as commercial kits for 'total' oestriol and for 'unconjugated' oestriol. The former assays involve acid or enzyme hydrolysis of conjugates followed by the determination of the total unconjugated oestriol. The latter assays rely on antisera that do not recognise oestriol conjugates. Almost half of the oestriol produced by the feto-placental unit finds its way into the maternal bile (Adlercreutz, 1974) and is likely to re-enter the plasma from the gut as a conjugate. There is no clear evidence to suggest that one method is clinically superior to the other.

INTERPRETATION

Maternal serum oestriol results can be interpreted in much the same way as described for urinary oestrogens with the added complication that only a single point in time is being examined and fluctuations may occur during the day. These changes have been estimated to be between 5 and 30 per cent (Masson and Wilson, 1972; Townsley *et al.*, 1973; Goebel and Kuss, 1974; Klopper, 1975; Katagiri *et al.*, 1976). Kit manufacturers usually supply ranges by which to interpret results but these are often 95 % confidence intervals for uncomplicated pregnancies rather than criteria for action.

HUMAN PLACENTAL LACTOGEN IN MATERNAL SERUM

Human placental lactogen (HPL) is produced only in the syncytial layer of the placental trophoblastic tissue and its measurement is therefore a test of placental rather than feto-placental function. For a review of its biosynthesis and regulation see Chatterjee and Munro (1977). It is a single chain polypeptide of 191 amino acids with a monomeric mol. wt. of 21 600. Between 0·3 and 1 g are secreted daily in the third trimester, largely into the maternal circulation where a mean concentration of about 6 mg/l is maintained. Clearance from plasma is rapid and shows two components, one with a half-life of 10–15 min and the other with a half-life of 30–60 min (Beck *et al.*, 1974). No diurnal rhythm has been demonstrated so that blood samples may be taken at any time. Estimates of random day-to-day variations are between 4 % and 12 % (Houghton *et al.*, 1982). The advantages of HPL over oestrogen assays are the less complex metabolism, the independence from effects of corticosteroid or ampicillin treatment and the lack of confusion by fetal adrenal hypoplasia and placental sulphatase deficiency. Its disadvantages relate to its assessment of the mass of functional placental tissue rather than to the integrity of the fetus itself. Thus, if placental mass is small, as it tends to be with a 'small for dates' fetus, or large, as with diabetic pregnancies, the HPL may be low or high regardless of the condition of the fetus.

Compared with many polypeptide hormones, the concentrations of HPL in plasma are very high. Thus many robust and simple radioimmunoassay techniques are available for its determination.

INTERPRETATION

HPL can be determined in plasma or serum early in pregnancy. There is a progressive increase to a plateau at 36 to 40 weeks. Typical average values are 0·1 mg/l at 9 weeks, 1 mg/l at 15 weeks, 3 mg/l at 26 weeks, 5 mg/l at 32 weeks and 6 mg/l at the plateau. The concentrations in unaffected pregnancies at each period of gestation are distributed in log-normal fashion and this should be allowed for when calculating lower limits.

The usefulness of HPL determinations has been discussed by Letchworth and Chard (1972), Wilde and Oakey (1975), Gartside and Tindall (1975) and Spellacy *et al.* (1976). When used in the first and second trimester (particularly up to 20 weeks) it is helpful in distinguishing patients with threatened abortion who require hospital care from those whose pregnancies are not in immediate danger. After 20 weeks, the prediction is much less reliable, particularly in Rhesus-sensitised and diabetic pregnancies. In pregnancies complicated by toxaemia the HPL levels are often low, but this is not always associated with fetal distress. Many patients with mild toxaemia have lower HPL concentrations than patients with severe pre-eclamptic toxaemia. Falling HPL levels predict some cases of fetal death but some deaths are accompanied by continuing normal levels. Letchworth and Chard (1972) found that 70% of women with three or more subnormal HPL results (less than 4 mg/l) during the last 6 weeks of pregnancy had fetal distress or neonatal asphyxia if pregnancy was prolonged.

OTHER PROTEINS AND ENZYMES

Human chorionic gonadotrophin (HCG) is produced by the placenta and is excreted in the urine from early in pregnancy; it is used for its detection. Peak production occurs between the 7th and 10th weeks of gestation. HCG estimations have not proved useful in managing pregnancy.

Several other polypeptides have been isolated from the placenta and identified in detectable amounts in maternal serum. They are known as 'pregnancy-associated plasma proteins' (PAPP) A, B and C. The latter is also known as Schwangerschaftsprotein-1 (SP-1) or 'pregnancy specific beta-1 glycoprotein'. These proteins are secreted by the placental syncytiotrophoblast. Their function is unknown although a possible involvement in the generation of pre-eclampsia has been described (Hughes *et al.*, 1980). Their half-life tends to be rather long (1 to 4 days) and they have as yet no advantages over HPL assays.

There is undoubtedly a relationship between high levels of AFP in maternal serum and the birth of underweight babies (Brock *et al.*, 1977, 1980; Wald *et al.*, 1980) but the predictive value of such assays is not sufficiently good for early detection of the condition. Chard *et al.* (1986) found that the test misses five of every six cases of low birthweight.

The placental enzymes, heat-stable alkaline phosphatase and cystine amino-peptidase (oxytocinase), have occasionally been used to monitor placental activity but they are rarely used now.

BILIRUBIN IN HAEMOLYTIC DISEASE

Neonatal or intrauterine deaths are risks in pregnancies of Rhesus-sensitised women although the advent of anti-D immunoglobulin prophylactic treatment of Rh negative mothers (to prevent sensitisation) has dramatically reduced the incidence of fetal death. Only 3 in every 1000 stillbirths and perinatal deaths are now due to this cause (Urbaniak, 1985). Many amniotic fluids from such pregnancies have a yellow-green colouration due to the presence of bilirubin or other intermediate products of haem metabolism. Bilirubin in amniotic fluid decreases in normal pregnancy becoming undetectable by about the 36th week (Mandelbaum *et al.*, 1967). When there is fetal damage caused by Rhesus isoimmunisation, the bilirubin concentration is raised, the level being proportional to the damage. The measurement of bilirubin in amniotic fluid by direct spectrophotometry or by colorimetry after diazotisation can be used to assess the need for intra-uterine transfusions or early delivery of the baby.

Direct Spectrophotometry (Whitfield *et al.*, 1970)

Liley (1961) showed that there is a good correlation between peak absorption at 450 nm and the severity of haemolytic disease. Background absorption is accounted for by reading at 365, 450 and 550 nm.

Technique. Centrifuge the amniotic fluid (collected in tubes covered with black paper to exclude light) for 20–30 min. Filter through Whatman No. 42 paper. Transfer to a spectrophotometer cuvette of 1 cm path and scan against a water blank from 350–700 nm. An instrument enabling a 5-fold scale expansion facilitates calculations. Draw a straight line between absorbance readings at 365 and 550 nm and record the difference (A_{450}) between this line and the peak absorbance at 450 nm. With this technique the errors due to instrumental factors can be large (Burnett, 1972). A spectrophotometer capable of reading to 0·001 absorbance units is required, and its ability to give a straight baseline with a blank should be established. Manual graphing procedures should be avoided if errors are to be minimised.

INTERPRETATION

The A_{450} values can be used directly to predict haemolytic disease with the aid of the action line prepared by Whitfield *et al.* (1970) from which the need to deliver early or to perform fetal blood transfusion can be considered according to the A_{450} and the stage of gestation (Fig. 33.3).

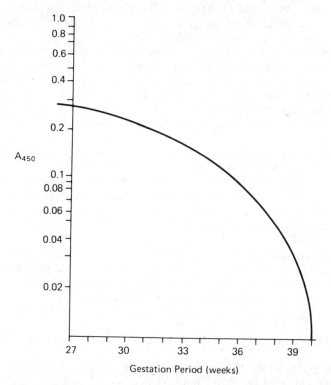

Fig. 33.3. Action Line for Haemolytic Disease (after Whitfield *et al.*, 1970). Results above the line require action.

Care must be taken in accurately assessing the A_{450} value due to bilirubin because of considerable absorption by non-bilirubin substances which obscure the bilirubin peak and in some cases even give negative A_{450} results. The interference may be caused by haemoglobin and its derivatives (methaemoglobin, methaemalbumin and oxyhaemoglobin), pigments, meconium staining or turbidity of the fluid. Corrections for some of these have been described (see the 5th edition of this book).

Blood product contamination can be reduced by extracting the fluid into chloroform containing aniline, 10 g/l, and reading the absorbance at 453 nm against a solvent blank. The usual colorimetric methods for bilirubin in serum lack the sensitivity required, but Watson *et al.* (1965) modified the Lathe and Ruthven method by avoiding dilution of the sample. Kapitulnik *et al.* (1970) used a modification of the method of Malloy and Evelyn using a 1 in 3 instead of a 1 in 10 dilution. For details of these methods see the 5th edition of this book.

PHOSPHOLIPIDS IN AMNIOTIC FLUID

The development of respiratory distress syndrome (RDS or hyaline membrane disease) is a common problem in immature neonates. This has to be borne in mind when early induction of labour is being contemplated and a balance has to be struck between the respiratory hazards and the risk of allowing the pregnancy to continue. Adequate expansion of the alveoli of the normal lung at birth depends in part on the presence of surfactant. As the lung matures this material accumulates and passes into the amniotic fluid.

The increasingly widespread use of ultrasound and other physical monitoring techniques has improved estimations of gestational age and maturity, and improvements in neonatal care have increased the survival rate of immature babies. Therefore the need for biochemical assessment of lung maturity is declining (James *et al.*, 1983; Turnbull, 1983). Nevertheless, the measurement of the phospholipids constituting lung surfactant can be used as an index of fetal lung maturity.

Dipalmitoyl lecithin is an important component of surfactant and appears in the amniotic fluid in increasing amounts from about 35 weeks gestation. The absolute concentration of lecithin, the ratio of lecithin to sphingomyelin, assumed to be produced at a constant rate by extra-pulmonary sources (L/S ratio) and the proportion of phosphatidyl glycerol are most commonly used. Other chemical and physical methods are discussed by Freer and Statland (1981) and Harvey and Parkinson (1980).

Methods for amniotic fluid lipid analysis involve extraction into methanol-chloroform followed by chromatographic separation on silica gel. The separated phospholipids can be quantitated chemically by measuring their phosphorus content or by direct area or densitometric measurement.

Determination of Amniotic Fluid L/S Ratio (Gotelli *et al.*, 1978)

The lipids extracted by chloroform–methanol are partially purified by cold acetone extraction before chromatography.

Reagents.
1. Methanol, chloroform, glacial acetic acid and acetone, all of analytical reagent grade.

2. Mobile phase: chloroform–methanol–glacial acetic acid–water, 75/25/7/4 v/v.
3. Staining reagent. Dissolve 10 g dodecamolybdophosphoric acid in 500 ml distilled water.
4. Sodium chloride solution, 20 g/l.
5. Acid stannous chloride solution. Dissolve 20 g stannous chloride in 55 ml concentrated hydrochloric acid and make up to 500 ml with distilled water, filtering if necessary.
6. Standards. These are available with different L/S ratios from Sigma.

Technique. Centrifuge the amniotic fluid specimen at 900 *g* for 5 min. Pipette duplicate 1 ml quantities of samples and standards into separate glass-stoppered tubes and add 1 ml methanol and 2 ml chloroform to each. After thorough mixing, cool in a freezer or on ice before centrifuging. Carefully recover the bottom, chloroform layer and evaporate to dryness at 65 °C under a stream of nitrogen. Cool, and carefully wash the precipitate twice by adding 200 μl ice-cold acetone, discarding the washings after each addition. Dry the residue and transfer with 10 μl chloroform to a small spot on a 10 × 10 cm silica gel thin-layer chromatography plate, alongside standards. Develop the chromatogram until the solvent nears the top of the plate. Remove the plate and after drying, stain for 3 min, followed by a saline wash for 15 min. Develop the colour for 5 min in the stannous chloride reagent, then wash the plate with saline and dry thoroughly. Measure the ratio of lecithin to sphingomyelin by scanning densitometry of the coloured spots.

INTERPRETATION

The selection of a critical L/S ratio to differentiate between maturity and immaturity is difficult as the risk of RDS increases continuously as the ratio decreases. Although a ratio of 2·0 is traditionally used as the critical value or action limit, there are considerable problems in using figures taken uncritically from the literature since apparently small differences in technique can give quite different results. There is debate about the need for acetone fractionation and methods which omit this step often give different results from those which include it. Lecithin and sphingomyelin do not respond to all staining procedures equally and so different visualisation methods may affect the results. Most studies show that amniotic fluid can be stored for short periods at − 20 °C without affecting the results but this may not be true for other storage conditions. Differences are certainly attributable to changes in centrifugation speeds and times.

The production of consistent results therefore depends on meticulous attention to detail and action limits selected by the laboratory should be validated by comparison with the occurrence of RDS in the cases analysed. The combination of data from many sources gives an approximate guide to the potential of the technique. In such a study (Harvey and Parkinson, 1980) when the ratio exceeded 2·0, the chance of RDS occurring was about 1 in 50, whereas between ratios of 1·5 and 2·0 it was 1 in 3, and below a ratio of 1·5, it was 3 in 4. In the editor's laboratory, using the method described above, the L/S ratio action limit above which there is an RDS probability of 1 in 50 is 2·4.

In pregnancies complicated by maternal diabetes or Rhesus haemolytic disease (Whitfield and Sproule, 1974) false prediction of maturity is not uncommon. The interpretation is also complicated if the amniotic fluid is stained with blood or meconium; the phospholipid composition of serum is quite different from that of amniotic fluid. Changes in amniotic fluid volume may affect the results in diabetic pregnancies in which lecithin may be produced without incorporation into mature lung surfactant. In such pregnancies it is often desirable to perform further tests, especially the measurement of phosphatidyl glycerol (PG) in amniotic fluid. Fortunately PG can be determined by the same chromatographic procedure as is used for the L/S ratio (Gotelli *et al.*, 1978). In this case the density of the PG spot is expressed as a percentage of the total phospholipids. Blood contamination has no effect on PG, the presence of which almost always indicates lung maturity.

There is good evidence to suggest that lung maturation is influenced by fetal adrenocortical activity (Harvey and Parkinson, 1980) and that it can be stimulated by exogenous administration of corticosteroids 24 h before delivery. A similar role has been postulated for thyroxine.

Simpler Methods for Assessing Lung Maturity. Because of the lengthy nature of the techniques for L/S ratio measurement, attempts have been made to find quicker ways of predicting lung maturity. Sbarra *et al.* (1978) showed that the amniotic fluid absorbance at 650 nm was correlated with its L/S ratio. If cells and debris are removed first and allowance is made for the effect of other large molecules such as protein, then the remaining turbidity is attributable to surfactant, the particulate size of which scatters light.

After centrifuging the amniotic fluid, the absorbance of the undiluted supernatant is determined at 650 nm against a water blank. The protein absorbance is then determined in the same way after mixing 0·1 ml of centrifuged liquor with 3·5 ml sulphosalicylic acid, 30 g/l, and leaving for 10 min. The difference reflects surfactant concentration and can be used to predict the L/S ratio if a sufficient number of amniotic fluids is examined by both techniques to provide an estimate of the level of confidence which can be attached to the simpler measurement. In practice, those fluids in which unequivocally high L/S ratios are predicted can be rapidly selected leaving those where doubt as to the L/S ratio exists to be examined by the longer procedure of chromatography.

The method is unsatisfactory if the fluid is not fresh or is stained with blood or meconium.

TESTS FOR NEURAL TUBE DEFECTS

Neural tube defects (NTDs) occur in 2–4 births per 1000 in the UK. They represent a failure, during embryonic development, in the closure of part of the neural tube, giving rise to anencephaly, encephalocoele or spina bifida, depending on the location and type of lesion (Davidson and Young, 1981). Some lesions are 'closed', being covered by a layer of skin, but in those that are 'open' (which tend to be associated with more severe consequences), components of extracellular fluid and of neural tissue may leak into amniotic fluid. Two of these components have proved useful in the detection of these defects. The first, AFP, is an α_1-globulin originating from the fetal liver and yolk sac. Its concentration in fetal plasma reaches a maximum between 12 and 16 weeks of gestation and then declines steadily to term. The second, acetylcholinesterase (AChE), arises from exposed neural tissue. Its activity is independent of gestational age.

The inherent risk and the inconvenience of amniocentesis rule out the possibility of analysing amniotic fluid in pregnancies other than those in which the probability of a defect is significantly increased. This is the case if a previous child had a NTD, one of the parents or a sibling is affected or the mother has been found to have high blood AFP levels. The measurement of maternal serum AFP is thus a screening test for NTD.

The temporal pattern of AFP concentration in maternal blood differs from that in amniotic fluid or fetal blood. While the levels in the latter are falling from 16 weeks of gestation, the maternal blood levels continue to rise until the third trimester. The (UK) Collaborative Study (1977) on maternal serum AFP assays concluded that blood samples should be taken for screening after 16 completed weeks of gestation and preferably before the end of the 18th week. Samples taken later than 22 weeks leave little time for termination of pregnancy if subsequent tests show there to be an abnormality. Perhaps of more importance is the lack of a substantial quantity of data after 20 weeks with which to compare results.

Screening programmes for NTDs have been reported from a number of centres (Wald *et al.*, 1979; Brock, 1982; Ferguson-Smith, 1983; Roberts *et al.*, 1983). There is need for rapid and effective communication between laboratory, obstetrician and ultrasonographer, and the laboratory should have a large database of results related to pregnancy outcome to assist in the interpretation of unusual results. Screening is therefore best carried out by laboratories specially equipped and staffed to provide a service on a regional or sub-regional basis. Blood samples taken at 16–18 weeks gestation act as the initial screen. Since the diagnostic capabilities of amniotic fluid AFP assays decrease with gestational age, these blood results must be available quickly. Before amniocentesis is considered, such causes of raised serum AFP as twins and incorrect gestational dating must be ruled out usually by ultrasound scanning and by repeating the assay. Improvements in ultrasound scanning have increased the rate of detection of NTDs at this stage without requiring amniocentesis (Campbell and Pearce, 1983), but ultrasound is unlikely to replace maternal serum AFP assays which can pinpoint the population at risk. After appropriate screening, the diagnosis depends on the measurement of AFP and analysis of AChE in amniotic fluid.

The impact of screening programmes on the birth rate of NTD babies is hard to judge. Certainly the incidence of such births has declined over the last decade or more (Owens *et al.*, 1981; Carstairs and Cole, 1984; Lorber and Ward, 1985). A poor quality diet in early pregnancy appears to be related to the occurrence of NTDs. Supplementing the diet at this time with vitamins (Pregnavite Forte F) seems to reduce the incidence (Smithells *et al.*, 1983). Although the importance of these findings is still not clear and although an active ingredient has not been identified, the use of such supplements may have had some impact. Nevertheless, it is most probable that screening has made a significant contribution to the decline in the incidence of NTDs.

Determination of Maternal Serum AFP

Serum AFP is measured by radioimmunoassay. The relatively high concentrations have enabled simple and robust methods to be developed. Many commercial kits are available but these can be expensive if large populations are to be screened. Assays can be developed by laboratories as inexpensive antisera and iodinated AFP are available from within the National Health Service. Standards can be prepared by adding graded quantities of fetal cord serum to a pool of male serum and calibrating in repeated assays against the International Reference Preparation 72/227. The assay needs to measure concentrations in the range 20–200 k U/l (1 kU is approximately equivalent to 1 μg). Methods have been described by Vince *et al.* (1975), Leek *et al.* (1975) and Brock *et al.* (1974).

INTERPRETATION

The AFP concentration above which action is required is determined by reference to the number of misclassifications expected at any given concentration and the seriousness of the consequences of misclassification. An action limit that is too low results in a high amniocentesis rate and most fluids will be from unaffected pregnancies. One that is too high results in open NTDs being missed. Action limits are different for each week of gestation if AFP concentration is used. It is preferable to quote limits as multiples of the median concentration in unaffected pregnancies (MOMs) at each week of gestation.

Table 33.1, from data in the UK Collaborative Study (1977), shows the detection rates for open spina bifida and anencephaly at different MOMs. The proportion of unaffected pregnancies above these limits is also shown as are the odds of there being an open NTD present when the incidence is 2 in 1000 births. Screening laboratories tend to use cut-off points within the range 2·0 to 2·5 MOMs (Ferguson-Smith, 1983). Those laboratories using a low cut-off may have a policy of requiring a second blood sample if the first is high. This eliminates some of the non-NTD causes of raised levels and reduces the amniocentesis rate. Testing a further specimen, correcting estimates of gestational age and avoiding amniocentesis in twin pregnancies and threatened abortions reduce the proportion requiring amniocentesis to 1–2 % or less (Ferguson-Smith *et al.*, 1978). Those laboratories using a high cut-off value may not require a second blood sample before amniocentesis but may miss more cases of NTD.

TABLE 33.1

Percentage of Singleton Pregnancies with Maternal Serum AFP Levels at 16 to 18 Weeks of Gestation Equal to or Greater than the Specified Multiples of the Normal Median and the Odds of an Abnormality

	Multiple of the Normal Median				
	2·0	2·5	3·0	3·5	4·0
Anencephaly	90	86	84	82	76
Open Spina Bifida	91	79	70	64	45
No NTD	7·2	3·3	1·4	0·6	0·3
Odds at incidence 2 in 1000	1:41	1:21	1:10	1:4	1:3

Elevated maternal serum AFP levels are found in many circumstances in the absence of a NTD. The most common is an error in gestational dating. In all cases where the maternal serum AFP is raised, the gestational dating should be reviewed, preferably with the aid of ultrasound scanning (Roberts *et al.*, 1979; Wald *et al.*, 1982). Such scanning should also detect multiple pregnancies in which the mean AFP concentration is higher than in singleton pregnancies. Feto-maternal haemorrhage, whether spontaneous or induced by amniocentesis, also gives elevated levels (Hay *et al.*, 1979; Dallaire *et al.*, 1980) as does intra-uterine death. Rarer causes which do represent fetal abnormality are ventral wall defects (exomphalos and gastroschisis), renal defects (agenesis, nephrotic syndrome, Potter's syndrome), duodenal and oesophageal atresias, imperforate anus and some chromosome abnormalities including Turner's syndrome. See Brock (1981) for details.

Amniotic Fluid AFP

The concentration of AFP in amniotic fluid is approximately 100 times greater than in maternal serum. Thus, by diluting amniotic fluid specimens, AFP can be determined by radioimmunoassay alongside maternal serum specimens provided that linearity checks are satisfactory and that an appropriate diluent that does not bias the results can be found.

Other techniques used are radial immunodiffusion and Laurell 'rocket' electrophoresis. The basis of these methods is described on pages 93 and 104. An outline of a rocket method is given below.

Electrophoretic Determination of Amniotic Fluid AFP

Reagents.
1. Tank buffer, 100 mmol/l, pH 8·6. Dissolve 12·51 g diethylbarbituric acid, 70·08 g sodium barbitone, 1·54 g calcium lactate and 5 ml thymol solution (50 g/l in isopropyl alcohol) in 4 l distilled water.
2. Gel buffer, 25 mmol/l, pH 8·6. Dissolve 4·43 g diethylbarbituric acid, 28·03 g sodium barbitone, 4·1 g calcium lactate and 4·0 g sodium azide in 4 l distilled water.
3. Wash solution. Mix 2 l industrial methylated spirit, 400 ml glacial acetic acid and 1·6 l water.
4. Staining solution, 5 g/l Coomassie Brilliant Blue in wash solution.
5. Sample diluent. Dissolve 90 g sodium chloride and 1 g sodium azide in 1 litre water.
6. Standards. Fetal cord serum or an amniotic fluid with a high AFP can be used as standards. Dilute in sample diluent to provide a range of standards up to 40 MU/l. They must be accurately calibrated against the International Reference Preparation 72/227 using the same gel system.

Technique. *Preparation of Gels.* Make up a 20 g/l aqueous agarose solution (Agarose—pure 0201–00, Koch–Light), boiling gently until the agarose has dissolved. Mix with an equal volume of gel buffer and add 400 μl of AFP antiserum (Mercia DAKO A008) per 100 ml of gel solution, maintaining the temperature at 55 °C. The volume of antiserum required may differ with each lot number. Pour 25 ml of the mixture on to each glass plate (17·5 cm × 9 cm) on a levelling table, allow to cool and store at 4 °C until required.

Analysis of Samples. Pipette 3 μl sample into each 2 mm diameter hole punched in the gel (22 holes per plate). Place the plate on the tank platen and hang strips of Whatman No. 1 paper from each side into the tank buffer to act as wicks. Run the plates at 15–16 mA constant current overnight. Keep the tank platen at 5 °C with circulated cooled water. Remove and dry the plates. Place in the staining solution for 1–2 min, then rinse with water and destain using the wash solution. After drying the plate a standard curve is drawn relating the height of the 'rocket' to the standard concentration. Unknowns are read from the graph.

INTERPRETATION

The Second UK Collaborative Study on AFP in Relation to Neural Tube Defects (1979) provides data for the interpretation of amniotic fluid AFP levels. Action limits are again based on MOMs. The report recommends different cut-off values according to the stage of gestation. The values for 16–18 weeks and for 19–21 weeks are 3·0 and 3·5 MOMs respectively. At these limits 99 % of open NTDs are detected and less than 1 % of unaffected pregnancies are included. The prevalence of open NTDs amongst mothers who had amniocentesis at these weeks in the Collaborative Study was 2·7%. In these circumstances the predictive value of a positive test is 80%. Improving on this prediction depends upon choosing only high risk pregnancies for amniocentesis by careful elimination of other causes of raised serum AFP concentrations.

Raised levels of amniotic fluid AFP arise from the same non-NTD causes as raised serum AFP. In addition, contamination of amniotic fluid with fetal blood, which has a high AFP concentration, gives rise to falsely elevated values. However, the contamination itself may be indicative of fetal problems especially if it is old, haemolysed blood from an earlier fetal bleed. If blood cells are present in the amniotic fluid a count should be performed to determine the number and the proportion of fetal cells present. Wald and Cuckle (1980) have suggested a correction that may be applied to account for fetal blood contamination, but it is based on average values of fetal blood AFP concentrations and is not recommended. Occasionally the sample is maternal urine rather than amniotic fluid. Its high urea concentration and low AFP result should help to avoid confusion.

Cholinesterase Isoenzymes

Analysis of cholinesterase isoenzymes in amniotic fluid is of value in conjunction with AFP assays to increase the degree of diagnostic certainty (Collaborative Acetylcholinesterase Study, 1981). Polyacrylamide gel electrophoresis (PAGE) is used to separate and identify the isoenzymes (Smith *et al.*, 1979; Seller and Cole, 1980). The following method employs vertical slab gels and LKB apparatus.

Electrophoretic Identification of the Isoenzymes

Reagents.
1. Electrode buffer, pH 8·9. Prepare a stock solution of 9·5 g Tris and 28·8 g glycine per litre distilled water. Dilute 1 part with 9 parts distilled water for use.
2. Resolving gel buffer, pH 8·3. Dissolve 36·3 g of Tris, 0·23 ml N, N, N', N'-tetramethylethylenediamine (TEMED) in water, add 10 ml concentrated hydrochloric acid and make to 100 ml with distilled water.
3. Stacking gel buffer, pH 6·7. Dissolve 5·98 g Tris, 0·5 ml TEMED in water, add 48 ml hydrochloric acid, 1 mol/l and make to 100 ml with distilled water.
4. Sample buffer. Mix 25 ml reagent (3), 10 ml glycerol and 10 mg bromophenol blue and dilute to 100 ml with distilled water.
5. Cholinesterase incubation buffer, pH 6·9. Dissolve 24·4 g maleic acid and 12·5 g sodium hydroxide in about 900 ml distilled water, adjust to pH 6·9 with sodium hydroxide, 100 g/l, and make up to 1 litre.
6. Resolving gel monomer solution. Dissolve 30 g acrylamide (electrophoresis grade) and 0·81 g N, N'-methylene-bisacrylamide (BIS) in distilled water and make up to 100 ml. Store in the dark.
7. Resolving gel initiator. Prepare freshly by dissolving 0·14 g ammonium persulphate in 100 ml distilled water.
8. Stacking gel monomer solution. Mix 6·4 g acrylamide, 0·24 g BIS and 12·5 ml reagent (3) with distilled water and dilute to 100 ml. Store in the dark.

9. Stacking gel initiator solution. Mix 51 mg ammonium persulphate, 2 mg riboflavin, 0·5 ml TEMED and 12·5 ml reagent (3) with distilled water and make up to 100 ml. Store at 4 °C in the dark where it is stable for about 2 weeks.
10. Cholinesterase preincubation solution. Dissolve, with warming, 135 g sodium sulphate in a mixture of 300 ml reagent (5) and 600 ml distilled water. Adjust to pH 6·9 with 10 mol/l sodium hydroxide.
11. Cholinesterase incubation solution. Mix 80 ml reagent (5), 8 ml cupric sulphate solution (30 g $CuSO_4$, $5H_2O$ per litre), 0·8 ml magnesium chloride solution (97 g/l) and 152 ml distilled water. Dissolve in this, 360 mg glycine and 36 g sodium sulphate, warming if necessary. Adjust to pH 6·9 with 10 mol/l sodium hydroxide. Prepare freshly for each gel and immediately before use add 280 mg of the enzyme substrate, acetylthiocholine iodide.

Technique. *Preparation of resolving gel slab.* For each gel mix 4 ml reagent (2), 8·5 ml reagent (6) and 3·5 ml distilled water and degas. Degas 16 ml reagent (7) separately. Mix the degassed solutions and pour into the gel former. Carefully overlay the surface with methanol containing bromophenol blue and leave to polymerise.

Preparation of stacking gel. Degas reagents (8) and (9) separately. Pour off any liquid overlying the resolving gel. Insert a 20 place sample comb between the glass plates. Gently mix 9 ml reagent (8) and 3 ml reagent (9) per gel and pipette on to the top of the resolving gel. Polymerisation is initiated by riboflavin in the presence of light. Using an x-ray viewer as a source of light, polymerisation is complete in about 30 min. The sample comb is then carefully removed. The sample wells are washed with diluted stacking gel buffer (1 part reagent (3) plus 7 parts water) before use.

Electrophoresis. Dilute the amniotic fluid samples 1:1 with reagent (4) and pipette 100 μl into each well. Blanks (reagent (4)), a positive control (fluid from a mother carrying an NTD fetus) and a negative control (fluid from an unaffected pregnancy) should be included on each gel. Assemble the apparatus and add the electrode buffer to the upper buffer reservoir. Electrophoresis is performed at 500 V with a current of 20 mA until the bromophenol blue dye front has travelled about 7·5 cm (approx. 5 h) maintaining the gel at 10 °C throughout. Dismantle the apparatus and wash the gel four times in 200 ml of the pre-incubation solution. Place the gel in 120 ml of the cholinesterase incubation solution and leave overnight in the dark. Discard the solution and wash with water. The banding pattern can now be observed and compared with those of the positive and negative controls.

INTERPRETATION

The band nearer the origin shows the activity of non-specific esterases and the faster, so-called 'NTD band', shows AChE. Confirmation of the identity of this band is obtained by demonstrating inhibition when a specific AChE inhibitor (Sigma A9013) is included in the cholinesterase incubation solution. This can be achieved by duplicating specimens on the gel and cutting the gel into two, incubating part with the inhibitor (0·5 ml of a 3 mg/l solution in 120 ml incubation solution) and part without.

The Collaborative Acetylcholinesterase Study (1981) found that only 4 of 813 NTDs which were detected by raised AFP levels were missed by PAGE of AChE. Three-quarters of the 63 cases of ventral wall defects which were highlighted by AFP showed an AChE band and none of the 11 cases of congenital nephrosis showed a band. About half of the other abnormalities detected by AFP (Turner's and Potter's syndromes or miscarriage) showed a band. Of particular importance, however, was the observation that of 125 unaffected pregnancies incorrectly identified by raised AFP only 8 showed a positive AChE band. This shows the value of AChE as a secondary test to reduce the number of false-positives identified by AFP. Its value as a primary test is yet to be proven, as it also misclassifies some pregnancies.

Early hopes that bloodstaining of the amniotic fluid has little effect on this assay have proved disappointing. Gross bloodstaining gives a streaky pattern that is difficult to interpret. Barlow *et al.* (1982) studied the effects of adding graded quantities of fetal blood to amniotic fluids and concluded that erythrocyte concentrations less than about 60×10^6 cells/ml are unlikely to give false-positive results. Such conclusions may depend substantially on the sensitivity of the PAGE method used, and it is recommended that great care is taken in interpreting positive gels if there is any sign of blood contamination, either maternal or fetal.

Promising results have emerged recently suggesting that ventral wall defects may be distinguishable from NTDs by the relative intensities of the two cholinesterase bands (Goldfine *et al.*, 1983; Wald *et al.*, 1984). The ratio of AChE to pseudocholinesterase bands measured by densitometry was less than 0·15 when the fetus had a ventral wall defect and was greater than this with NTDs, but the number of cases studied is still small and further work is required to confirm these results.

REFERENCES

Adlercreutz H. (1974). *New Engl. J. Med*; **290**: 1081.

Adlercreutz H. (1975). *Lancet*; **1**: 1386.

Alexander S., *et al.* (1979). *J. Clin. Endocr. Metab*; **49**: 588.

Barlow R. D., Cuckle H. S., Wald N. J., Rodeck C. H. (1982). *Brit. J. Obstet. Gynaecol*; **89**: 821.

Beck J. S., Melvin J. M. O., Hems G. (1974). *J. Reprod. Fertil*; **38**: 451.

Brock D. J. H. (1981). In *Amniotic Fluid and its Clinical Significance*. (Sandler M., ed) p. 169. New York, Basel: Marcel Dekker.

Brock D. J. H. (1982). *Brit. Med. J*; **285**: 365.

Brock D. J. H., Barron L., Raab G. (1980). *Brit. J. Obstet. Gynaecol*; **87**: 582.

Brock D. J. H., Bolton A. E., Scrimgeour J. B. (1974). *Lancet*; **1**: 767.

Brock D. J. H., *et al.* (1977). *Lancet*; **2**: 267.

Buchan P. C., Klopper A. (1979). *Brit. J. Obstet. Gynaecol*; **86**: 713.

Burnett R. W. (1972). *Clin. Chem*; **18**: 150.

Campbell D. G., Gardner G. (1971). *Clin. Chim. Acta*; **32**: 153.

Campbell S., Pearce J. M. (1983). *Brit. Med. Bull*; **39**: 322.

Carstairs V., Cole S. (1984). *Brit. Med. J*; **289**: 1182.

Chamberlain G. (1984). *Lancet*; **1**: 1171.

Chard T., *et al.* (1986). *Brit. J. Obstet. Gynaecol*; **93**: 36.

Chatterjee M., Munro H. M. (1977). *Vitamins and Hormones*; **35**: 149.

Collaborative Acetylcholinesterase Study. (1981). *Lancet*; **2**: 321.

Collaborative Study on Alpha-feto Protein in Relation to Neural Tube Defects, 1. (1977). *Lancet*; **1**: 1323.

Collaborative Study on Alpha-feto Protein in Relation to Neural Tube Defects, 2. (1979). *Lancet*; **2**: 651.

Cuckle H., Wald N. J. (1984). *Lancet*; **1**: 926.

Dallaire L., Belanger L., Smith C. J. P., Kelleher P. C. (1980). *Brit. J. Obstet. Gynaecol*; **87**: 856.

Davidson P. M., Young D. G. (1981). *Brit. J. Hosp. Med*; **19**: 222.
Dean L., Abell D. A., Beischer N. A. (1977). *Brit. Med. J*; **274**: 257.
Ferguson-Smith M. A. (1983). *Brit. Med. Bull*; **39**: 365.
Ferguson-Smith M. A., *et al.* (1978). *Lancet*; **1**: 1330.
Freer D. E., Statland B. E. (1981). *Clin. Chem*; **27**: 1629.
Gartside M. W., Tindall V. R. (1975). *Brit. J. Obstet. Gynaecol*; **82**: 303.
Goebel R., Kuss E. (1974). *J. Clin. Endocr. Metab*; **39**: 969.
Goebelsmann U. (1979). *Clinics in Obstet. Gynaecol*; **6**: 223.
Goldfine C., Miller W. A., Haddow J. E. (1983). *Brit. J. Obstet. Gynaecol*; **90**: 238.
Gotelli G. R., *et al.* (1978). *Clin. Chem*; **24**: 1144.
Hainsworth I. R., Hall P. E. (1971). *Clin. Chim. Acta*; **35**: 201.
Harkness R. A., Taylor N. F., Crawfurd M. A., Rose F. A. (1983). *Brit. Med. J*; **287**: 2.
Harvey D., Parkinson C. E. (1980). In *Laboratory Investigation of Fetal Disease.* (Barron
    A. J., ed) p. 267. Bristol: J. Wright and Sons.
Hay D. L., *et al.* (1979). *Brit. J. Obstet. Gynaecol*; **86**: 516.
Heys R. F., Scott J. S., Oakey R. E., Stitch S. R. (1968). *Lancet*; **1**: 328.
Houghton D. J., *et al.* (1982). *Brit. J. Obstet. Gynaecol*; **89**: 831.
Hughes G., Bischof P., Wilson G., Klopper A. (1980). *Brit. Med. J*; **280**: 671.
Hull M. G. R., Braunsberg H., Irving D. (1975). *Clin. Chim. Acta*; **58**: 71.
Ittrich G. (1958). *Z. Physiol. Chem*; **312**: 1.
James D. K., Tindall V. R., Richardson T. (1983). *Brit. J. Obstet. Gynaecol*; **90**: 995.
Kapitulnik J., Kaufmann N. A., Blondheim S. H. (1970). *Clin. Chem*; **16**: 756.
Katagiri H., Distler W., Freeman R. K., Goebelsmann U. (1976). *Amer. J. Obstet. Gynecol*;
    124: 272.
Klopper A. (1975). *Postgrad. Med. J*; **51**: 227.
Klopper A. (1976). In *Hormone Assays and their Clinical Application.* (Lorraine J. A., Bell
    E. T., eds) p. 73. Edinburgh: Churchill Livingstone.
Leek A. E., Ruoss C. F., Kitau M. J., Chard T. (1975). *Brit. J. Obstet. Gynaecol*; **82**: 669.
Letchworth A. T., Chard T. (1972). *Lancet*; **1**: 704.
Lever M., Powell J. C., Peace S. M. (1973). *Biochem. Med*; **8**: 188.
Levitz M., Young B. K. (1977). *Vitamins and Hormones*; **35**: 109.
Liley A. W. (1961). *Amer. J. Obstet. Gynecol*; **82**: 1359.
Little A. J., Aulton K.; Payne R. B. (1975). *Clin. Chim. Acta*; **65**: 167.
Lorber J., Ward A. M. (1985). *Arch. Dis. Childh*; **60**: 1086.
Mandelbaum R., La Croix G. C., Robinson A. R. (1967). *Obstet. Gynecol*; **29**: 471.
Masson G. M., Wilson G. R. (1972). *J. Endocrinol*; **54**: 245.
McFadyen I. R., Worth H. G. J., Wright D. J. (1980). *Brit. J. Obstet. Gynaecol*; **87**: 490.
Oakey R. E. (1978). *Clin. Endocrinol*; **17**: 403.
Owens J. R., Harris F., McAllister E., West L. (1981). *Lancet*; **2**: 1032.
Phillips S. (1979). *Med. Lab. Sciences*; **36**: 293.
Phillips S. D., Salway J. G., Payne R. B., Macdonald H. N. (1978). *Clin. Chim. Acta*; **89**: 71.
Rao L. G. S. (1977). *Brit. Med. J*; **275**; 874.
Roberts C. J., *et al.* (1979). *Brit. Med. J*; **278**: 981.
Roberts C. J., *et al.* (1983). *Lancet*; **1**: 1315.
Rock R. C., Chan D. W., Perlstein M. T. (1981). *Clinics in Lab. Med*; **1**: 157.
Rosenberg K., Grant J. M., Hepburn M. (1982). *Brit. J. Obstet. Gynaecol*; **89**: 12.
Sbarra A. J., Selvaraj R. J., Cetrulo C. L. (1978). *Amer. J. Obstet. Gynecol*; **130**: 788.
Seller M. J., Cole K. J. (1980). *Brit. J. Obstet. Gynaecol*; **87**: 1103.
Shaxted E. J. (1980). *Brit. Med. J*; **280**: 684.
Smith A. D., *et al.* (1979). *Lancet*; **1**: 685.
Smithells R. W., *et al.* (1983). *Lancet*; **1**: 1027.
Spellacy W. N., Buhi W. C., Birk S. A. (1976). *Obstet. Gynecol*; **47**: 446.
Townsley J. D., *et al.* (1973). *J. Clin. Endocr. Metab*; **36**: 289.
Turnbull A. C. (1983). *Brit. J. Obstet. Gynaecol*; **90**: 993.
Urbaniak S. J. (1985). *Brit. Med. J*; **291**: 4.
Vinall P. S., Oakey R. E., Scott J. S. (1980a). *Eur. J. Obstet. Gynecol Reprod. Biol*; **11**: 17.
Vinall P. S., Oakey R. E., Scott J. S. (1980b). *Eur. J. Obstet. Gynecol Reprod. Biol*; **11**: 25.

Vince D. J., McManus T. J., Ferguson-Smith M. A., Ratcliffe J. G. (1975). *Brit. J. Obstet. Gynaecol*; **82**: 718.

Wald N. J., Cuckle H. (1980). *Brit. J. Hosp. Med*; **18**: 473.

Wald N. J., Cuckle H., Boreham J., Turnbull A. C. (1980). *Brit. J. Obstet. Gynaecol*; **87**: 860.

Wald N. J., Cuckle H., Boreham J., Turnbull A. C. (1982). *Brit. J. Obstet. Gynaecol*; **89**: 1050.

Wald N. J., *et al.* (1979). *Brit. J. Obstet. Gynaecol*; **86**: 91.

Wald N. J., *et al.* (1984). *Brit. J. Obstet. Gynaecol*; **91**: 882.

Watson D., Mackay E. V., Trevella W. (1965). *Clin. Chim. Acta*; **12**: 500.

Whitfield C. R., Lappin T. R. J., Carson M. (1970). *J. Obstet. Gynaecol Brit. Cwlth*; **77**: 791.

Whitfield C. R., Sproule W. B. (1974). *Brit. J. Hosp. Med*; **12**: 678.

Wilde C. E., Oakey R. E. (1975). *Ann. Clin. Biochem*; **12**: 83.

Young B. K., Jirku H., Kadner S., Levitz M. (1976). *Amer. J. Obstet. Gynecol*; **126**: 38.

Zlatnick F. J., Varner M. W., Hauser K. S. (1979). *Obstet. Gynecol*; **54**: 205.

34

ADRENALINE, NORADRENALINE AND RELATED COMPOUNDS

The secretion of adrenaline by the adrenal medulla has been known since the end of the last century. Its formula shows that it has the two phenolic groups of catechol and is an amine, hence the term catecholamine. Other catecholamines related to adrenaline are noradrenaline and 3-hydroxytyramine (dopamine), both intermediates in the formation of adrenaline from tyrosine (see Fig. 34.1). Tyrosine is first hydroxylated at position 3 to give 3,4-dihydroxyphenylalanine (dopa) which is decarboxylated to form dopamine. Hydroxylation on the side chain produces noradrenaline, into the amino group of which a methyl group is finally introduced to give adrenaline. Both adrenaline and noradrenaline are physiologically active pressor amines. Catecholamines are found in the urine partly free and partly conjugated as glucuronides and sulphates.

The adrenal medulla is not the only tissue capable of producing catecholamines. The endings of adrenergic nerve fibres of the autonomic nervous system secrete noradrenaline and localised collections of neurones within the brain secrete noradrenaline or dopamine. Adrenaline secretion appears to be entirely from the adrenal medulla.

Several tumours share a common ancestry being derived embryologically from the neural crest. Of these the phaeochromocytoma has long been known to produce catecholamines. Its site of occurrence is most commonly in the adrenal medulla but it may arise anywhere along the sympathetic chain, a property which sometimes makes location very difficult. Actively secreting carotid body and glomus jugulare tumours in the neck have been described. All these tumours are usually histologically benign but can cause severe, sometimes fatal, disturbances. They are associated with hypertension, often paroxysmal in type, and other manifestations of sympathetic overactivity such as severe headache and sweating. Their diagnosis is important since surgical removal usually relieves the hypertension and avoids the serious consequences of sudden excessive release of catecholamines. Tumours arising in adults from sympathetic ganglia, called ganglioneuromas, also secrete catecholamines in some cases and are benign. A highly malignant tumour in children is the neuroblastoma which usually secretes very large amounts of catecholamine metabolites. These are present in urine although the excretion of the biologically active free amines is not greatly increased. Dopamine excretion may be much increased in certain cases of neuroblastoma and malignant phaeochromocytoma. See Gjessing (1968) for a discussion of the origin of the various neural crest tumours.

THE DETERMINATION OF CATECHOLAMINES

Since the previous volume of this text, there have been significant advances in the measurement of catecholamines and their metabolites. Biological methods of measurement are no longer used and the standard chemical methods for free catecholamines have been supplanted by radioenzymatic assays and high

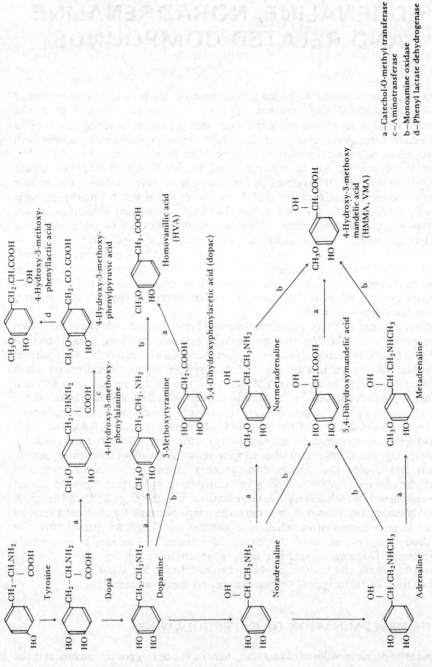

Fig. 34.1. Catecholamine Formation and Degradation.

a–Catechol-O-methyl transferase
c–Aminotransferase
b–Monoamine oxidase
d–Phenyl lactate dehydrogenase

performance liquid chromatography (HPLC) with fluorescent or electrochemical detection. Radioenzymatic assays are both expensive and time-consuming and will not be discussed further.

HPLC methods of measuring catecholamines and their metabolites in urine are now being adopted by many hospital laboratories, though many still use conventional chemical methods. These older methods highlight the reactivity of the catecholamines and explain their instability in biological fluids and during sample preparation. For this reason we give a brief summary of the chemical principles involved, and provide detailed descriptions of a limited number of methods. Interested readers are referred to the 5th edition of this book.

Chemical methods have been reviewed by Persky (1955) and Varley and Gowenlock (1963). Some determine only adrenaline and noradrenaline, others include dopamine. Oxidation converts adrenaline into adrenochrome and in alkaline solution this changes into adrenolutine (Fig. 34.2), the trihydroxyindole reaction. Adrenolutine has a yellowish-green fluorescence which however disappears rapidly in presence of oxygen. Noradrenaline is converted into similar compounds, noradrenochrome and noradrenolutine.

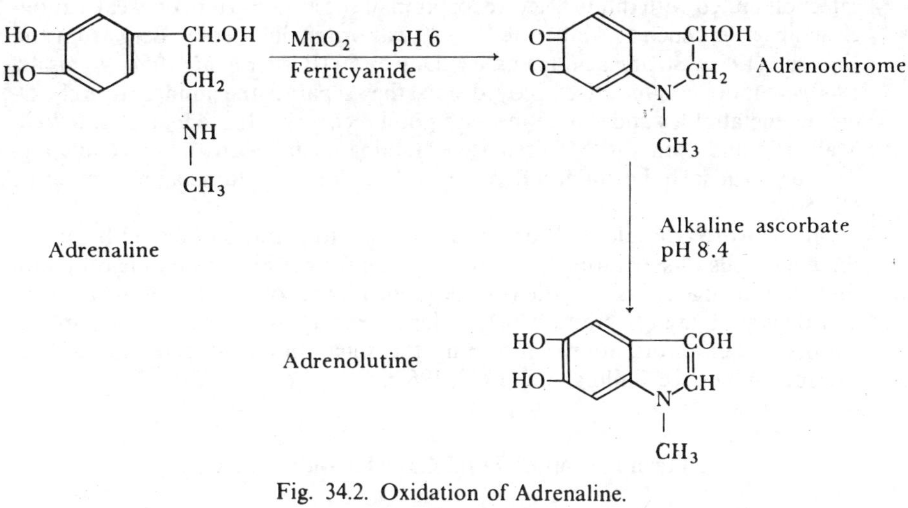

Fig. 34.2. Oxidation of Adrenaline.

Several different oxidising agents have been employed, including manganese dioxide (Lund, 1949), and ferricyanide (Von Euler and Floding, 1955; Sobel and Henry, 1957). With iodine (Von Euler and Hamberg, 1949) used for colorimetric determination of catecholamines in tissues, coloured 2-iodo derivatives of the adrenochromes are obtained. Crout (1961) used the trihydroxyindole reaction for the fluorimetric determination of catecholamines as did Griffiths *et al.* (1970) for determining plasma adrenaline and noradrenaline. All the agents oxidise both adrenaline and noradrenaline at a pH above 5 but only adrenaline is oxidised below pH 4, a property used for their differential estimation. The pink-coloured quinones produced by this oxidation can be transformed to highly fluorescent derivatives by the addition of alkali and the exclusion of oxygen. Alternatively, adrenaline and noradrenaline may be measured separately using differential spectrofluorimetry, reading at different activating and emission wavelengths (Vendsalu, 1960).

An alternative to the trihydroxyindole reaction is the condensation of the two *o*-quinone groups of adrenochrome with ethylenediamine in alkaline solution (Weil-Malherbe and Bone, 1952) in which adrenaline readily undergoes auto-oxidation. Dopamine, catechol and some of its derivatives, which may be present in urine, also give a strongly fluorescent product in this reaction.

SEPARATION OF CATECHOLAMINES FROM BIOLOGICAL FLUIDS

Regardless of assay technique, it is necessary to separate catecholamines from contaminating substances. It is fortunate that catecholamines have two reactive sites, the catechol and amine groups. Either or both have been used to extract catecholamines from biological fluids.

On stirring a solution containing catecholamines with alumina at pH 8·4, the catechol group is adsorbed (Lund, 1949; Weil-Malherbe and Bone, 1952). The alumina must be activated and the catecholamine protected from auto-oxidation by EDTA. The alumina is then separated by decantation, washed, and the catechols eluted with dilute acid. Adsorption of the amine group on weak cation-exchange resins such as Amberlite IRC 50 was originally used by Bergstrom and Hanssen (1951). Strong acid resins, e.g. Dowex 50 (Bertler *et al.*, 1958; Vendsalu, 1960) are more commonly employed since they separate the amines from the *O*-methyl metabolites and dopamine with good recovery (Haggendal, 1963). Weil-Malherbe and Bone (1957) first used alumina to take up the catechols and Zeocarb to adsorb the amines; Renzini *et al.* (1970) used alumina and Amberlite CG 50.

The trihydroxyindole reaction can be applied to extracts obtained by any of these methods of separation. The ethylenediamine method is suitable only with the ion-exchange resins as little is to be gained by adsorbing the total catechols and then applying a method which is dependent upon the catechol group.

For further information concerning the separation and determination of catecholamines see Callingham (1963, 1967).

Determination of Total Catecholamines in Urine

In this modification of the method of Bell, Horrocks and Varley, given in the 2nd edition of this book, catecholamines are adsorbed from untreated urine on to a column of Amberlite IRC 50, eluted and condensed in alkaline solution with ethylenediamine and the resulting fluorescence is read.

Reagents.
1. Sulphuric acid, 500 mmol/l.
2. Sodium hydroxide, 1 mol/l.
3. Amberlite IRC 50 (A.R., Aldrich Chemical Company), acid form.
4. Phosphate buffer, pH 6·5, 500 mmol/l. Mix 318 ml of a solution of $Na_2HPO_4,2H_2O$ (89·07 g/l) and 682 ml of KH_2PO_4 solution (69·085 g/l).
5. Ethylenediamine dihydrochloride, 2 mol/l. Dissolve 26·6 g in water and make up to 100 ml. Ethylenediamine dihydrochloride can be prepared from freshly distilled ethylenediamine. Dissolve 50 ml in 200 ml ethanol and mix with 1500 ml ethanolic hydrochloric acid containing 150 ml concentrated acid. Filter the crystals with suction, wash with ethanol and dry in an

incubator (Weil-Malherbe and Bone, 1954). Ethylenediamine dihydrochloride as bought can be recrystallised from ethanol (700 ml/l with water).

6. Ammonia, sp. gr. 0·88.
7. Solid sodium chloride.
8. Isobutanol.
9. Hydrochloric acid, 6 mol/l.
10. Sodium hydroxide, 10 mol/l.
11. Orthophosphoric acid, sp. gr. 1·75.
12. Stock standard solutions. (a) Adrenaline, 600 μmol/l. Dissolve 11·0 mg adrenaline in 10 ml of 1 mol/l hydrochloric acid and make to 100 ml with water. (b) Mixed standard. Dissolve 11·0 mg adrenaline, 19·1 mg noradrenaline bitartrate and 11·4 mg dopamine hydrochloride in separate 100 ml volumes of 10 mmol/l hydrochloric acid and mix in the ratio of 1:2·2:8·5 adrenaline, noradrenaline and dopamine. These are the mean proportions found in the urine of normal persons. The mixed standard contains 600 μmol/l.
13. Standard solutions for use. Dilute the stock standards 1 to 100 with water. The solutions then contain 6 μmol/l.

Technique. Collect a 24 h specimen of urine into a bottle containing 50 ml of 500 mmol/l sulphuric acid and measure the volume. Take 1/100th of this, making to about 15 ml for smaller volumes, and adjust to pH 6·5 with 1 mol/l sodium hydroxide.

Prepare a 5 × 1 cm column of the resin and wash in turn using a flow rate of about 5 ml/min with (1) 50 ml reagent (1); (2) 50 ml water; (3) 50 ml reagent (2); (4) 50 ml water; (5) 50 ml reagent (4); (6) 50 ml water.

Alternatively the resin can be prepared in bulk as follows. Wash with water, stand, and decant. Stir with 5 volumes of reagent (9) for 30 min, remove excess acid and wash several times with water, decanting each time. Add 3 volumes of water followed by 2 volumes reagent (10) added over 15 min while stirring mechanically. Wash again several times with distilled water. Then suspend the resin in an equal volume of water and add reagent (11) until the pH remains at 6·5 while stirring continuously for 30 min. For use place the required amount of the resin into the column, drain, and wash with 25 ml water.

Run the urine, adjusted to pH 6·5, through the column at a rate of 2 to 3 ml/min. Follow with 50 ml water. Then elute the adsorbed catecholamines with reagent (1). Discard the first 5 ml and collect the next 20 ml.

Fluorimetry. Measure 5 ml (≡ 1/400th of the total urine volume) of the eluate into a glass-stoppered tube and 0·5 ml of the diluted adrenaline standard plus 4·5 ml water into a similar tube (or 1·5 ml of mixed standard plus 3·5 ml water). To each, add 0·5 ml reagent (5) and 1 ml reagent (6). Place in a water bath at 50 °C for 20 min, cool, add solid sodium chloride (2 to 3 g) and 6 ml isobutanol, stopper, shake thoroughly for 3 min and then centrifuge to separate the layers. Remove the isobutanol layer for fluorimetry. For the blanks take a further 5 ml eluate (test blank), 0·5 ml standard plus 4·5 ml water (standard blank) and 5 ml water (reagent blank) and to each add 1 ml reagent (6). Heat in the water bath at 50 °C for 20 min, cool, and add 0·5 ml reagent (5) and proceed as described for the test and standard. Read against the reagent blank in the fluorimeter activating at 436 nm and reading fluorescence at about 530 nm.

Blanks are only required if an abnormally high result is obtained. Then it is particularly important to carry through a test blank since urines occasionally contain substances which fluoresce on addition of ammonia. The catecholamines are destroyed when heated with ammonia before adding the ethylenediamine thus allowing the fluorescence from other substances to be measured.

Calculation. Urinary total catecholamines (μmol/24 h) as adrenaline

$$= \frac{\text{Reading of unknown}}{\text{Reading of standard}} \times 0.5 \times \frac{6}{1000} \times 400, \text{ i.e.} \times 1.2$$

$$\text{or} = \frac{\text{Reading of unknown}}{\text{Reading of standard}} \times 3.6 \text{ (for mixed standard)}$$

Subtract any urine blank from the total test reading.

Notes.

1. In the above technique only the free catecholamines are determined (see also Macmillan, 1957) and this is preferable. Most earlier workers used a period of heating at pH 1 to 2 to hydrolyse conjugated catecholamines. To do this adjust the urine to pH 1·5 with more 500 mmol/l sulphuric acid, transfer to a small bottle, stopper firmly, heat in a boiling water bath for 20 min, cool, and adjust to pH 6·5 with 1 mol/l sodium hydroxide. Proceed as described above. The result then gives free and conjugated amines.

2. Adrenaline gives a 3-fold greater fluorescence than noradrenaline and dopamine. The ratio varies with the instrument used.

INTERPRETATION

In 422 hypertensive patients without phaeochromocytoma Bell (1960) found the daily urinary excretion of total unconjugated catecholamines was 0 to 1·3 μmol, with a mean of 0·46 μmol. The distribution was skew at the upper end, 5 % having values over 0·87 μmol and 1·5 % over 1·12 μmol. In 11 patients with phaeo-chromocytoma the two lowest results were 1·09 and 1·75 μmol, the remainder varying from 3·3 to 22 μmol.

Since the fluorescence given by adrenaline is approximately three times that of the other catecholamines, results expressed in terms of the mixed standard are numerically about three times greater than those given above. So almost all patients with hypertension not due to phaeochromocytoma will have values below 3·3 μmol/24 h.

In phaechromocytoma if the hypertension is paroxysmal considerable varia-tions in catecholamine excretion occur and amounts near to and possibly within the normal range can be obtained when the blood pressure is at its lowest. The excretion in one patient varied between 3·3 and 13·6 μmol/24 h while a patient who excreted 1·1 μmol/24h between attacks put out 11 μmol/24 h during a severe hypertensive phase. On the other hand, a patient whose hypertension did not vary much excreted between 5·2 and 6·0 μmol/24 h.

Over 70 % of the urinary catecholamines are unconjugated and the figure is similar in normal, hypertensive and phaeochromocytoma patients (Bell, 1960). Occasionally, large amounts of conjugated dopamine are found while the unconjugated catecholamine excretion remains normal. Crout and Sjoerdsma (1959) showed that ingestion of bananas produced increased excretion of conjugated noradrenaline and dopamine (also of 5-hydroxyindole acetic acid) which could reach several μmol. Because of this occasional finding it is considered preferable to determine only the free catecholamines.

Increased catecholamine excretion occurs after exercise and as a response to pain or stress including anaesthesia. Various drugs alter catecholamine metabo-lism and hence their excretion. Increases occur when patients are given phenothiazines, monoamine oxidase inhibitors, theophylline \or aminophylline; decreases occur after reserpine.

Direct interference during the fluorimetric procedure is reported. Tetracyclines, erythromycin and ampicillin are interfering antibiotics, and chloral and formaldehyde may sometimes cause problems. More important, however, are various drugs used in the treatment of hypertension which may cause false positives when hypertensive patients are investigated. The drugs involved are guanethidine and, especially, methyldopa. It is desirable that all drugs be withdrawn before the urine is collected. In particular, interference from methyldopa may persist for several days.

Measurement of Urinary Free Catecholamines Using HPLC with Electrochemical Detection.

Many HPLC methods are described for the measurement of urinary free catecholamines. The following procedure is used to measure noradrenaline, adrenaline and dopamine in urine and plasma at Hope Hospital, Salford. Catecholamines are adsorbed from the urine with activated alumina, eluted with acid, separated by reverse-phase ion-pair chromatography and measured by electrochemical detection.

Measurement is based on the ability of catecholamines to be reversibly oxidised to their corresponding *o*-quinones. Three electrodes, set at different potentials and arranged in series, cause sequential oxidation and reduction which screens out interfering compounds. Less selective detection systems will require more extensive sample preparation.

Reagents.
1. Extraction buffer, 1 mol/l Tris buffer pH 8·6, with 20 g/l EDTA.
2. Hydrochloric acid, 20 mmol/l.
3. Acetic acid, 100 mmol/l.
4. Mobile phase: 100 mmol/l citrate/phosphate buffer, pH 3·2, containing 4 mmol/l 1-heptanesulphonic acid (the ion-pair reagent), 0·2 mmol/l EDTA, 11 % methanol, 4 % acetonitrile. Filter through a 0·2 μm membrane under vacuum to degas before use.
5. Stock standard solutions (1 mmol/l) of noradrenaline, adrenaline, dopamine and 3,4-dihydroxybenzylamine (DHBA, the internal standard) are prepared in 20 mmol/l hydrochloric acid. These individual solutions may be stored at 4 °C for up to 6 months.
6. Intermediate standards (20 μmol/l). Dilute separately, 2 ml of each stock standard to 100 ml with reagent (2). These solutions are stable for up to 3 months at 4 °C.
7. Prepare working standards from the intermediate standards immediately before use and do not store. For the internal standard (100 nmol/l) dilute 0·5 ml to 100 ml with reagent (3). For the mixed catecholamine standards, dilute 1 ml noradrenaline, 0·4 ml adrenaline and 5 ml dopamine solutions to 50 ml with reagent (3). This 'top standard' contains 0·4, 0·16 and 2·0 μmol/l of noradrenaline, adrenaline and dopamine respectively. Prepare three more standards by doubling dilutions of the top standard with reagent (3). The zero standard (blank) is reagent (3) alone.
8. Ascorbic acid solution, prepare freshly by dissolving 50 mg in 100 ml water.
9. Activated alumina is prepared as described by Anton and Sayre (1962).

Apparatus.
1. Spherisorb ODS-2 5 μm analytical column 250 × 4·6 mm.

2. Kratos dual piston high pressure pump with pulse damper.
3. ESA Coulochem electrochemical detector Model 5100 A with conditioning cell Model 5021 (conditioning cell set at $+0.35$ V) and analytical cell Model 5011 (detector 1 set at $+0.05$ V, detector 2 set at -0.35 V).
4. Pye Unicam CDP 4 computing integrator.

Technique. Keep all tubes, reagents and samples at 4 °C in a cold tray. To 4 ml polystyrene tubes add (1) 1.5 ml distilled water; (2) 0.1 ml ascorbic acid solution; (3) 0.2 ml working internal standard; (4) 25 μl sample or standard; (5) 50 mg alumina; (6) 0.5 ml extraction buffer.

Cover the rack of tubes with 'clingfilm' and vortex the tubes for 10 min, avoiding any contact of the tube contents with the clingfilm to reduce the risk of introducing interfering organic substances. Centrifuge at 2500 rpm at 4°C for 30 s and aspirate the supernatant using a glass pipette to minimise contamination. Wash the alumina with 2 ml distilled water. Vortex for 20 s, centrifuge at 2500 rpm for 30 s at 4°C and aspirate the supernatant. After repeating this water wash, add 250 μl reagent (3) to the alumina. Vortex for 120 s. Centrifuge at 2500 rpm at 4°C for 10 min. Carefully remove this acid eluate and inject onto the HPLC column.

Calculation. The ratio of peak heights of the catecholamines to the peak heights of the internal standard (DHBA) is linear over a wide range (10 − 2000 nmol/l). Using five standards, the concentration of catecholamines in the unknowns is calculated by linear interpolation.

INTERPRETATION

In a series of 150 non-phaeochromocytoma hypertensive patients, all had total free catecholamine excretion (noradrenaline + adrenaline) less than 2.0 μmol/24 h. Most excreted less than 0.6 μmol/24 h, with only one non-phaeochromocytoma patient producing more than 1.3 μmol/24 h (1.8 μmol/24 h). Seven of eight known phaeochromocytoma patients had excretion rates between 2.0 and 6.0 μmol/24 h. One phaeochromocytoma patient produced 1.8 μmol in 24 h. There was minimal drug interference in the assay despite the broad range of medication received by these patients. Drugs affecting catecholamine metabolism should still be withdrawn (p. 882).

Determination of Adrenaline and Noradrenaline in Tissue Extracts

Occasionally the measurement of the catecholamine content of tissue extracts may help confirm the diagnosis of phaeochromocytoma. In the 5th edition, an iodine oxidation method was described. If the more sensitive and specific HPLC electrochemical detection methods are available, the above procedure can be simplified.

A small piece of fresh unfixed tissue (100–1000 mg) is accurately weighed into a known volume of 1 mol/l hydrochloric acid in a 20 ml glass specimen container. The catecholamines are extracted by shaking intermittently and storing for 24 h in the dark. Alternatively, the acidified specimen may be sent by post to another centre for analysis.

After centrifugation the catecholamines are extracted from a buffered aliquot of the acid and their concentration is measured using HPLC with electrochemical detection. Assuming complete extraction of catecholamines from the tissue, catecholamine content (mg/g) can be calculated as:

$$\frac{\text{Total volume of extract (ml)}}{\text{Weight of tissue (g)}} \times \text{Catecholamine concentration (mg/ml)}$$

INTERPRETATION

Normal adrenal tissue contains up to 1·0 mg catecholamines/g of which 90% is adrenaline. Phaeochromocytomas contain greatly increased amounts of catecholamines with noradrenaline predominating. Thus of 31 tumours investigated, 25 contained more noradrenaline than adrenaline with a range of 1·1 to 22·5 mg/g tissue. Adrenaline was barely detectable in 18 tumours but was the predominant material in 6 with a range from 1·1 to 11·0 mg/g tissue. In only 1 of these 31 tumours was noradrenaline not detected. In contrast, ganglioneuromas and neuroblastomas (see later) possess no storage capacity and values of the order of 100 to 200 μg/g tissue are usually found.

DETERMINATION OF CATECHOLAMINE METABOLITES

Methods are also available for determining certain metabolites of adrenaline and noradrenaline. The pathways by which these are formed are shown in Fig. 34.1 (p. 878). Noradrenaline and adrenaline are converted by catechol-*O*-methyl transferase into normetadrenaline and metadrenaline (also termed normetanephrine and metanephrine), then by the action of monoamine oxidase into 4-hydroxy-3-methoxy-mandelic acid (HMMA), often incorrectly termed vanillylmandelic or vanilmandelic acid (VMA). Alternatively, though quantitatively less so, oxidation to 3,4-dihydroxy-mandelic acid may occur first followed by conversion to HMMA.

Dopamine is metabolised along similar lines through 3-methoxytyramine to homovanillic acid (4-hydroxy-3-methoxy-phenylacetic acid). In certain patients with malignant phaeochromocytoma or neuroblastoma, atypical or deranged metabolism can occur whereby large amounts of dopa enter the circulation. Dopa can be decarboxylated in the kidney so that large amounts of dopamine are excreted in the urine, or it can be methylated and then undergo transamination to the corresponding keto acid, 4-hydroxy-3-methoxy-phenylpyruvic acid, which is unstable and is converted to the corresponding hydroxy acid, 4-hydroxy-3-methoxy-phenyllactic acid. This may be detected in small amounts in the urine of many neuroblastoma patients.

Determination of Metadrenaline and Normetadrenaline in Urine
(Pisano, 1960; Crout et al., 1961)

Pisano (1960) developed a relatively simple method for determining normetadrenaline and metadrenaline in urine. These compounds are adsorbed on to Amberlite CG 50, eluted with ammonia and converted to vanillin by oxidation with periodate, the vanillin formed being read at 350 and 360 nm.

Vanillin

Reagents.
1. Hydrochloric acid, 6 mol/l.
2. Sodium hydroxide, 2·5 mol/l.
3. Sodium hydroxide, 10 mol/l.
4. Amberlite CG 50, 100 to 200 mesh, Rohm and Hass (Aldrich Chemical Company Limited). This is a chromatographic grade of the IRC 50 resin

used for total catecholamine determination. Obtain the acid form and purify as follows. Suspend in about 3 volumes of water, stir for 10 min, then allow to stand for 30 min and discard the supernatant. Repeat the process several times until the supernatant is clear after standing 10 to 15 min. Add 3 volumes of water followed by 2 volumes of reagent (3) over a period of 15 min while stirring mechanically. Continue stirring for a further 2 h. Remove excess hydroxide by decanting and wash the resin well with several changes of water. To clear further, add 5 volumes of reagent (1), stir for about 30 min, remove excess acid and wash several times with distilled water with decanting. Reconvert to the alkaline form by repeating the stirring with reagent (3) for 30 min. Wash several times with distilled water. Then suspend the resin in an equal volume of water and add glacial acetic acid stirring continuously until the pH remains at 6·0 to 6·5 for 30 min. When the acetic acid is added the pH drops sharply but on stirring rises slowly until equilibrium is reached. This last stage is critical so sufficient time must elapse to ensure the pH remains at the correct level. Once prepared the resin keeps well.

After use the resin can be regenerated by first converting to the acid form, then to the sodium form.

5. Ammonia, 4 mol/l. Mix 100 ml ammonia (sp. gr. 0·88) with 360 ml water.
6. Sodium periodate solution, 20 g/l. Dissolve 100 mg $NaIO_4$ in 5 ml water as required.
7. Sodium metabisulphite, 100 g/l water. Kept stoppered, this is stable at 3 °C for at least 1 month.
8. Standard solution of normetadrenaline, 1 mmol/l. Dissolve 22·0 mg normetadrenaline hydrochloride (Normetanephrine, Sigma) in 100 ml hydrochloric acid, 10 mmol/l. This contains the equivalent of 183 mg/l of free base.

Technique. Collect a 24 h specimen in acid as for total catecholamines, filtering if necessary. Transfer one 200th of this into a capped test tube, add 1/10th its volume of hydrochloric acid and place in a boiling water bath for 20 min. Cool, adjust to pH 6·0 to 6·5 with reagent (2) and dilute to approximately 20 ml with water.

Prepare a column of resin about 5 × 1 cm and wash with 15 ml water to remove the buffer solution. Apply the hydrolysed urine at a flow rate not exceeding 1 ml/min. Then wash the column with 15 to 20 ml water and elute with ammonia until 10 ml of eluate is obtained. Take two 4 ml aliquots. To one (the test), add 100 μl periodate, mix and allow oxidation to proceed for 1 min. Then add 100 μl metabisulphite to remove excess periodate. To the other (the blank), add 100 μl metabisulphite, then 100 μl periodate. For the standard add 100 μl normetadrenaline standard (that is, 0·1 μmol) to 10 ml ammonia and treat as the test solution. Read each test against its own blank and the standard against an ammonia blank at 350 and 360 nm. Pisano uses the reading at 360 nm for the calculation (see note below).

Calculation. Urinary normetadrenaline + metadrenaline (μmol/24 h) (expressed as normetadrenaline)

$$= \frac{\text{Reading of unknown}}{\text{Reading of standard}} \times 0·1 \times 200$$

$$= \frac{\text{Reading of unknown}}{\text{Reading of standard}} \times 20$$

Notes
1. The reading at 360 nm should be approximately 75% of that at 350 nm. Interfering substances, e.g. *p*-octopamine, which oxidises to 4-hydroxy-benzaldehyde with a peak at 330 nm, if present, can reduce the reading at 360 nm to about 50% that at 350 nm. Such readings should be regarded with suspicion.
2. *Drug interference*. Altered excretion of metadrenalines occurs following administration of drugs which alter catecholamine metabolism. *Monoamine oxidase inhibitors* reduce HMMA formation and increase metadrenaline excretion. Increased output also occurs with the phenothiazine, *prochlorperazine*, which reduces the uptake of noradrenaline by tissues. *Levodopa* reduces the excretion.
Other drugs interfere with the method itself. *Phenothiazines* and the tricyclic antidepressant, *imipramine*, have caused trouble. It is desirable to withdraw these drugs before the investigation, if possible. A different, potentially serious source of interference (Johnson *et al.*, 1972) is methyl glucamine (*meglumine*) which occurs in radiographic contrast media in combination with iodinated substances. Meglumine salts are replaced by sodium salts of these iodinated compounds in other contrast media which do not interfere. Meglumine is adsorbed onto the resin, is eluted with the metadrenaline fraction and then competes for periodate preventing vanillin formation and so giving falsely low results. If this interference is suspected, read also at 330 and 300 nm. If the reading at 330 nm exceeds that at 350 nm and is similar at 300 nm meglumine interference is likely and the result is unreliable. Further specimens are best obtained after a lapse of at least 3 days but internal standards can be employed if necessary. *Labetalol* (Trandate) gives spuriously high results (Hamilton *et al.*, 1978) as a result of periodate oxidation to 4-hydroxy-3-carbamidobenzaldehyde.

INTERPRETATION
The daily excretion in normal persons is less than 5·5 μmol. In patients with phaeochromocytoma, Pisano (1960) reported a daily excretion of 16·5 to 620 μmol, Bell (1960) of 15 to 165 μmol.

Simplification of the Pisano Method for Metadrenaline and Normetadrenaline (Yates and Weinkove, 1986)

The following modification of the Pisano (1960) method simplifies the analytical technique, standardises the procedure and improves precision and accuracy. All samples and standards pass through the extraction procedure and a single container is used for hydrolysis and resin extraction of metadrenalines. The increased throughput allows the use of duplicate samples from patients and a full standard curve with control specimens in each analytical run.
Reagents. These are unchanged apart from some concentrations but wherever possible all chemicals are of 'analytical' grade. Altered reagents are as follows:
1. Hydrochloric acid, 2 mol/l.
2. Sodium hydroxide, 1 mol/l.
8. Normetadrenaline stock standard, 1 mmol/l. Dissolve 22 mg normetadrenaline hydrochloride (Sigma) in 100 ml hydrochloric acid, 100 mmol/l, and store at 4 °C.
9. Normetadrenaline intermediate standard, 0·1 mmol/l. Prepare freshly by diluting 1·0 ml stock standard to 10 ml with deionised water.
10. Control samples. Prepare by adding known amounts of normetadrenaline to freshly-voided acidified urine. When available, urine from patients known

to have phaeochromocytoma may be used. In all cases acidify the urine and store in separate small amounts at $-20\,°C$. The metadrenalines are stable for at least 6 months under these conditions.

Technique. Collect a 24 h urine sample as before. Analyse all patients' urines in duplicate. Transfer 10 ml quantities of urine from patients, controls and from a normal volunteer to glass screw-capped 'universal' containers (25 ml). Prepare a five point calibration curve (0–20 μmol/l) by adding 0, 0·5, 1·0, 1·5 and 2·0 ml intermediate standard to five 10 ml portions of the normal acidified urine and bring the final volume in each container to 12 ml with deionised water. Corrections are made later for the endogenous metadrenaline and normetadrenaline in the normal urine.

Add 1·0 ml reagent (1) to each container and mix. The *control* and *unknown* samples only are then hydrolysed by heating in a boiling water bath for 20 min. After cooling, adjust the pH of all samples, including the standards, to pH 6·0–6·5 using reagent (2). Add 5 ml resin slurry to every container, cap securely and place on a rotary mixer for 20 min. Allow the resin to settle for 5 min, then aspirate and discard the supernatant. Wash the resin by mixing with 10 ml deionised water for 5 min. After allowing the resin to settle, aspirate and discard the supernatant once more. Elute the metadrenalines from the resin by adding 8·0 ml reagent (5) to each container and placing on the rotary mixer for 20 min. After allowing the resin to settle, carefully transfer two 3·0 ml portions of the extract to two 10 ml disposable test tubes, labelled 'test' and 'blank'.

Add 0·1 ml fresh reagent (6) to the 'test' solution with rapid mixing, followed exactly 1 min later by 0·1 ml reagent (7) and another thorough mix. Treat the 'blank' tubes with the same reagents but in the *reverse* order. Read each unknown, standard and control against its own blank in a recording spectrophotometer over the 330 to 360 nm range.

Calculation. Plot a standard curve using the absorbance readings at 360 nm. A line parallel to this but passing through the origin is then drawn as the calibration line. This corrects for the amount of unconjugated metadrenaline and normetadrenaline present in the non-hydrolysed standards. Use the calibration line to determine the concentration (μmol/l) of unknowns and controls. Convert the results to output in μmol/24 h by multiplying the concentration by the 24 h urine volume in litres.

Interfering drugs and their metabolites are distinguished from vanillin by the criteria described earlier for the Pisano method.

INTERPRETATION

Using this method, the upper limit of the reference range is 10 μmol/24 h. Most phaeochromocytoma patients have excretion rates greater than 15 μmol/24 h. This modification does not, however, reduce the effect of interference by such drugs as labetalol, atenolol, sotalol, or those containing phenolphthalein. False positive results may be excluded by careful examination of the absorption curve. When interference is significant, it is preferable to measure the urinary output of unconjugated catecholamines.

This modification of the Pisano method has proved to be economical, rugged and reliable during a two year period of operation.

Determination of Urinary 4-Hydroxy-3-Methoxy-Mandelic Acid

Sandler and Ruthven (1959, 1961) extracted HMMA from urine by adsorbing it on to Dowex IX 2 ion-exchange resin in the acetate form, followed by elution, whereas Pisano *et al.* (1962) used direct solvent extraction. In either case, periodate was used to oxidise the HMMA to vanillin which was, assayed spectrophotometrically. Two-dimensional chromatography has been used for semi-quantitative work (Gitlow *et al.*, 1960; Robinson *et al.*, 1959).

Method of Pisano *et al.*, 1962 (See also Sandler and Ruthven, 1963)

HMMA is extracted from acidified urine into ethyl acetate, then back-extracted with alkali and oxidised to vanillin with periodate. After purification by further extraction, the vanillin is quantitated. An internal standard is used as HMMA recovery varies from one urine to another.

Reagents.
1. Hydrochloric acid, 6 mol/l.
2. Sodium chloride.
3. Ethyl acetate.
4. Potassium carbonate, 1 mol/l.
5. Sodium periodate, $NaIO_4$, 20 g/l. Dissolve 1 g in 50 ml water. Prepare freshly each week.
6. Sodium metabisulphite solution, 100 g/l in water. Keep refrigerated and prepare freshly each week.
7. Acetic acid, 5 mol/l. Dilute 30 ml glacial acetic acid to 100 ml with water.
8. Phosphate buffer, 1 mol/l, pH 7·5. Add approximately 45 ml 1 mol/l potassium hydroxide (56 g/l) to 50 ml 1 mol/l potassium dihydrogen phosphate (136 g KH_2PO_4/l) until the pH is 7·5.
9. Cresol red indicator, 400 mg/l in water.
10. Toluene.
11. HMMA standard, 3 mmol/l (594 mg/l) in water.

Technique. Collect a 24 h specimen of urine into a bottle containing 10 ml hydrochloric acid. Keep this cool. The volume of urine taken depends on the volume of specimen and the result expected. For a suspected normal value use 5 ml urine and transfer this amount to three 50 ml glass stoppered tubes. These are 'test', 'test plus standard', and urine 'blank' tubes. To the 'test plus standard' tube add 50 μl (that is, 0·15 μmol) of standard solution and to each tube 500 μl hydrochloric acid, sufficient solid sodium chloride (about 3 g) to saturate the solution and 25 ml ethyl acetate. Stopper and shake mechanically for 5 min to extract the phenolic acids. Centrifuge and transfer 20 ml of the ethyl acetate layer to a second glass stoppered tube and extract the phenolic acids into 1·5 ml potassium carbonate by shaking for 3 min. Centrifuge again and carefully transfer 1 ml of the carbonate layer to a third tube. To the 'test' and 'test plus standard' tubes, add 100 μl periodate solution and place all three tubes in a water bath at 50 °C for 30 min to convert the HMMA into vanillin. Cool, and add to all tubes 100 μl metabisulphite solution; then add 100 μl periodate to the 'blank' tube. Neutralise with 300 μl acetic acid and 600 μl phosphate buffer. Check the pH; it should be below 8·8, i.e. yellow to a drop of cresol red. Shake for 3 min with 25 ml toluene to extract the vanillin. Centrifuge and transfer 20 ml of the toluene layer to a further 50 ml glass stoppered tube and extract the vanillin into 4 ml potassium carbonate. Centrifuge and read against a carbonate blank at 360 nm.

Calculation. Urinary 4-hydroxy-3-methoxy-mandelic acid (μmol/l) =

$$\frac{\text{Reading of 'test'} - \text{Reading of 'blank'}}{\text{Reading of 'test + standard'} - \text{Reading of 'test'}} \times \frac{0\cdot15 \times 1000}{\text{Volume of urine used (ml)}}$$

For a normal urine using 5 ml this becomes

$$\frac{\text{Reading of 'test'} - \text{Reading of 'blank'}}{\text{Reading of 'test} + \text{standard'} - \text{Reading of 'test'}} \times 30$$

INTERPRETATION

Pisano *et al.* (1962) gave the reference range for daily excretion as 9·0 to 35·5 μmol. Much increased values, up to 2650 μmol, were found in patients with phaeochromocytoma.

The recovery of added HMMA varies from about 50 to 90% depending on other urinary constituents. Drugs such as clofibrate excreted as glucuronides compete for the periodate so that incomplete oxidation occurs. The blank is usually of little significance, but random urine samples from children with a neuroblastoma occasionally contain large amounts of vanillin-like material. Green and Walker (1970) showed that dietary vanillin contributes little to the blank and that a vanillin-free diet is not necessary. Restriction of bananas and chocolate is desirable. Certain drugs, e.g. nalidixic acid (Negram), increase values by direct interference which can be corrected for by the blank procedure (Elder, 1968).

Drugs which alter catecholamine metabolism may alter the excretion of HMMA. Decreases are seen after the administration of monoamine oxidase inhibitors, guanethidine, levodopa and imipramine. Variable effects occur after reserpine and phenothiazines.

Summary.

Phaeochromocytoma. Now that determinations of catecholamines, normetadrenalines and HMMA can be carried out comparatively simply, we can compare the results in patients with phaeochromocytoma. Although HMMA is present in largest amounts, a better indication of relative value is to express each daily excretion in relation to the upper reference limit. Thus Crout *et al.* (1961) found in 15 of 23 patients that free catecholamines show the greatest relative increase above normal, and HMMA the least. We have found that during hypertensive phases the free amines are most increased, though all three determinations show diagnostic increases, while during quiescent periods the determination of the metadrenalines is the most sensitive.

Kelleher *et al.* (1964) also found determination of metadrenalines easier and more helpful than that of HMMA. On the other hand Sandler (1964), while accepting that the metadrenalines undergo the largest proportional increase, thought their estimation (Pisano, 1960) to be more tedious than that of HMMA. A simplified metadrenaline assay (Yates and Weinkove, 1986) may help although it does not overcome greater relative interference by substances absorbing at wavelengths of 330 to 340 nm (Georges and Whitby, 1964).

Although gross increases in catecholamine excretion, usually associated with phaeochromocytoma, can be detected by the methods described, 14 of 49 urine specimens from the Manchester Royal Infirmary series of patients with raised metadrenaline output had a catecholamine (adrenaline plus noradrenaline) excretion of less than 1·2 μmol/24 h. Sheps *et al.* (1966) also reported normal urinary catecholamines in 7 of 28 cases. The older chemical methods are subject to interference by methyldopa used in the treatment of hypertension which further reduces its value in the routine screening for phaeochromocytoma. Drug interference was rarely encountered at Hope Hospital (Salford, UK) with the urinary free catecholamine assays using HPLC with electrochemical detection.

Determination of metadrenaline excretion on 89 urines from 23 of the Manchester Royal Infirmary patients with proven phaeochromocytoma gave a mean figure of 38 μmol/24 h, 5·4 times the upper limit of 7·0 μmol/24 h for non-phaeochromocytoma hypertensive patients. Only 3 results were less than 14 μmol/24 h, twice the non-phaeochromocytoma upper limit. The mean excretion of HMMA in 78 urines from 19 of these patients was 81·5 μmol/24 h, 2·04 times the upper limit of the non-phaeochromocytoma range of 40 μmol/24 h. Fifty-one results (65 %) were less than 80 μmol/24 h and 11 (14 %) less than 50 μmol/24 h, a value exceeded on several occasions by non-phaeochromocytoma patients on first admission to hospital.

This confirms that metadrenaline excretion is relatively more increased in phaeochromocytoma. In our opinion it is less subject to interference than the HMMA estimation and is the preferred screening test for phaeochromocytoma. This was also the view of Sheps *et al.* (1966) after reviewing the results from 18 patients with phaeochromocytoma. The statement by Crout *et al.* (1961) that an excretion of less than 5·5 μmol/24 h of metadrenalines in a patient with sustained hypertension can be taken to exclude phaeochromocytoma, and values of over 13·7 μmol/24 h to be diagnostic for this, would appear to be valid. For intermediate values they recommend determination of the free amines. If the hypertension is paroxysmal but metadrenaline excretion is normal, it is unlikely that surgical intervention is justified. We would advise repeating the metadrenaline assay on urine samples collected during or following the hypertensive episode and measuring free catecholamines in these specimens.

Sensitive plasma catecholamine assays by radioenzymatic or HPLC methods may be useful in the patient with paroxysmal hypertension and normal urine findings. Blood samples could be collected during the hypertensive episode, although phaeochromocytoma patients do not have to be hypertensive to have raised plasma catecholamines. Because of catecholamine instability the plasma must be separated and frozen within the hour and stored at $-20\,°C$. Plasma catecholamines could then be measured at centres with a special interest.

Plasma catecholamines can also be measured when it is impossible to collect adequate urine specimens, as in oliguric patients and small babies. The measurement of plasma catecholamines in blood obtained by catheterisation of the vena cava at various levels has been used in the localisation of catecholamine-secreting tumours. A new radionuclide, radiolabelled MIBG (metaiodobenzyl-guanidine), which is taken up by catecholamine-producing tissue, has reduced the need for multiple venous sampling for localising phaeochromocytomas (Sisson *et al.*, 1981).

To date there is no single reliable assay in urine or plasma which can be used to exclude a phaeochromocytoma. This is not helped by the fact that clinicians are notoriously poor at suspecting the diagnosis. A 50-year survey of post mortem material in the US showed that the majority of phaeochromocytomas were missed, or discovered accidentally at surgery for unrelated conditions (Beard *et al.*, 1983). Since 90 % of these tumours are histologically benign and surgically curable, this places an extra burden on the laboratory to ensure the reliability of their assay methods. A recent examination of the results of an external quality assurance scheme in the UK (Weinkove *et al.*, 1986) showed poor laboratory performance. The authors confirmed previous findings (reported in the 5th edition of this book) that the metanephrine assay was more reliable than the more popular HMMA assays, although both showed poor reproducibility. They also demonstrated that laboratories doing the test more frequently fared better than the less active. Hopefully, new cheaper and more specific analytical methods for catecholamines and their metabolites may allow many more patients to be screened for this rare but curable condition.

There is still considerable discussion about the seleotion of suitable biochemical methods for the diagnosis of phaeochromocytoma (see review by Duncan and Smythe, 1985).

Neuroblastoma. Neuroblastoma is the most common malignant soft tissue tumour of childhood and presents most commonly as an abdominal mass. Although many tumours synthesise and secrete large amounts of the metabolites of noradrenaline and dopamine, they less frequently show manifestations of catecholamine excess. The excretion of these substances has been studied (see Voorhess and Gardner, 1960, who give several earlier references). Several workers report a marked increase in the excretion of HMMA, but in a smaller proportion of cases dopamine appears to be excreted in the largest amount. Bell (1968) from a study of 34 cases recognised variable excretion patterns as regards catecholamines, metadrenalines and HMMA. Some showed an increase in all three, while others showed a predominant increase in one of the analytes. In no case in which a neuroblastoma was shown to be present were tests for both HMMA or total catecholamines normal.

For reviews of various aspects of catecholamines see Varley and Gowenlock (1963), Bohun (1966) and Landsberg (1977).

REFERENCES

Anton A. H., Sayre D. F. (1962). *J. Pharmac. Exp. Ther*; **138**: 360.

Beard C. M. *et al.* (1983). *Mayo Clinic Proc*; **58**: 802.

Bell M. (1960). *Thesis for the Degree of M.Sc.*, Manchester University.

Bell M. (1968). In *Recent Results in Cancer Research*, Vol. 13, Tumours in Children. (Marsden H. B. and Steward J. K., eds) p. 138. Berlin: Springer-Verlag.

Bergstrom S. and Hansson G. (1951). *Acta Physiol. Scand*; **22**: 87.

Bertler J., Carlson A., Rosengren E. (1958). *Acta Physiol. Scand*; **44**: 273.

Bohun C. (ed) (1966). *Recent Results in Cancer Research*, Vol. 2, Neuroblastomas—Biochemical Studies. Berlin: Springer-Verlag.

Callingham B. A. (1963). In *The Clinical Chemistry of Monoamines*. (Varley H., Gowenlock A. H., eds) Amsterdam: Elsevier.

Callingham B. A. (1967). In *Hormones in Blood*, 2nd ed. (Gray C. H., Bacharach A. L., eds) p. 519. New York, London: Academic Press.

Crout J. R. (1961). *Standard Methods in Clinical Chemistry*, Vol. 3. (Seligson D., ed) p. 62. New York, London: Academic Press.

Crout, J. R., Pisano J. J., Sjoerdsma A. (1961). *Amer. Heart J*; **61**: 375.

Crout J. R., Sjoerdsma A. (1959). *New Engl. J. Med*; **261**: 23.

Duncan M. W., Smythe G. A. (1985). *Clin. Biochem. Revs*; **6**: 62.

Elder G. H. (1968). *Clin. Chim. Acta*; **19**: 507.

Georges R. J., Whitby L. G. (1964). *J. Clin. Pathol*; **17**: 64.

Gitlow S. E. *et al.* (1960). *J. Clin. Invest*; **39**: 221.

Gjessing L. R. (1968). In *Advances in Clinical Chemistry*, Vol. 11. (Bodansky O., Latner A. L., eds) p. 82. New York, London: Academic Press.

Green M., Walker G. (1970). *Clin. Chim. Acta*; **29**: 189.

Griffiths J. C., Laing F. Y. T., McDonald T. J. (1970). *Clin. Chim. Acta*; **30**: 395.

Haggendal J. (1963). *Acta Physiol Scand*; **44**: 273.

Hamilton C. A., Jones D. H., Dargie H. J., Reid J. L. (1978). *Brit. Med. J*; **2**: 800.

Johnson L. R., Reese M., Nelson D. H. (1972). *Clin. Chem*; **18**: 209.

Kelleher J. H., Walter G., Robinson R., Smith P. (1964). *J. Clin. Pathol*; **17**: 399.

Landsberg L. ed. (1977). *Clinics in Endocrinology and Metabolism*; **6**: 525.

Lund A. (1949). *Acta Pharmacol*; **5**: 75, 121, 231.

Macmillan M. (1957). *Lancet*; **1**: 715.

Persky H. (1955) In *Methods of Biochemical Analysis*, Vol. 2. (Glick D., ed) p. 57. New York: Interscience.

Pisano J. J. (1960). *Clin. Chim. Acta*; **5**: 406.

Pisano J. J., Crout J. R., Abraham D. (1962). *Clin. Chim. Acta*; **7**: 285.

Renzini V., Brunori C. A., Valori C. (1970). *Clin. Chim. Acta*; **30**: 587.

Robinson R., Ratcliffe J., Smith P. (1959). *J. Clin. Pathol*; **12**: 541.

Sandler M. (1964). *J. Med. Lab. Technol*; **21**: 306.

Sandler M., Ruthven C. R. J. (1959). *Lancet*; **2**: 113, 1034.

Sandler M., Ruthven C. R. J. (1961). *Biochem J*; **80**: 78.

Sandler M., Ruthven C. R. J. (1963). Broadsheet, No. 44 (NS), Association of Clinical Pathologists, London.

Sheps S. G., Tyce G. M., Flock E. V., Maher F. T. (1966). *Circulation*; **34**: 473.

Sisson J. C. *et al.* (1981). *New Engl. J. Med*; **305**: 12.

Sobel C., Henry R. J. (1957). *Amer. J. Clin. Pathol*; **27**: 240.

Varley H., Gowenlock A. H. eds. (1963). *The Clinical Chemistry of Monoamines*. Amsterdam: Elsevier.

Vendsalu A. (1960). *Acta Physiol. Scand*; **49**: Suppl. 173.

Von Euler U. S., Floding I. (1955). *Acta Physiol. Scand*; **33, suppl.** **118**: 45.

Von Euler U. S., Hamberg U. (1949). *Science*; **110**: 561.

Voorhess M. L., Gardner L. I. (1960). *Lancet*; **2**: 651.

Weil-Malherbe H., Bone A. D. (1952). *Biochem. J*; **51**: 311.

Weil-Malherbe H., Bone A. D. (1954). *Biochem. J*; **58**: 132.

Weil-Malherbe H., Bone A. D. (1957). *J. Clin. Pathol*; **10**: 138.

Weinkove C., Lomax K., Swift A. (1986). *Commun. Lab. Med*; **2**: 86.

Yates P., Weinkove C. (1986). *Ann. Clin. Biochem*; **23**: 487.

35

VITAMINS

The following laboratory methods for measuring vitamin deficiencies have used (1) the determination of the vitamin in blood or urine, either under ordinary conditions or after test doses, (2) the determination in serum or urine of metabolic products derived from the vitamin, (3) the determination in serum or urine of a substance the concentration of which is influenced by the amount of the vitamin in the body. For further information see Barker and Bender (1980 and 1982), various chapters in *Advances in Clinical Chemistry*, e.g. Davis and Icke (1983) and Truswell (1985).

Vitamins are organic compounds required for reproduction, health and growth and these essential dietary components are only needed in very small quantities. The diseases due to deficient diets have been studied in man from the 17th century. In the Western World with its mixed diet, serious deficiencies are rarely observed except in people with food fads, in patients with malabsorption or massive loss of blood or in patients receiving haemodialysis, parenteral nutrition or certain drugs, e.g. oral contraceptives. However, excessive use of some vitamins may be found. In poorer communities, severe deficiencies can occur.

The original division into fat-soluble, i.e. A, D, E and K, and water-soluble, i.e. B-complex and C, is still useful. Thus the former, being insoluble in water, are carried in the plasma attached to protein and so are not excreted in the urine. They are also stored in substantial amounts in some tissues, particularly the liver, so that a deficiency arises less quickly than with the water-soluble vitamins which are not often stored to any appreciable extent (vitamin B_{12} is a notable exception) so that any excess uptake is usually rapidly excreted in the urine. Whereas a deficiency of fat-soluble vitamins can arise in conditions in which there is impaired absorption of fat alone, more general malabsorption can affect the absorption of both fat-soluble and water-soluble vitamins.

When the existence of vitamins was first recognised, their chemical structures were unknown and they were distinguished alphabetically, sometimes differently in different countries. However, the use of the names of vitamins, based on their chemical nature or occasionally on their physiological behaviour, is preferable.

Initially, under the guidance of the League of Nations, the biological activity of the vitamins was based on international units (IU). These are less used now as we know, e.g. that 1 IU of β-carotene (provitamin A) corresponds to $0.60\ \mu g$ or 1.1 nmol of the pure substance. However, as vitamins are prescribed therapeutically in mass units, rather than in molar ones, the former will be used in this text.

Table 35.1 describes the nomenclature of the vitamins required by man, and their general roles. It is unusual to develop a single vitamin deficiency; several deficiencies are likely to occur together. The table, however, gives details of the features of individual deficiencies. Recommended dietary intakes are published by the National Research Council, Committee on Dietary Allowances (1980). Table 35.1 also gives an indication of the principal analytical methods available and of the availability of loading tests for assistance in making clinical diagnoses.

RETINOL (VITAMIN A) AND CAROTENES

Retinol is present in the rods of the retina as the aldehyde *retinal*, and is combined with protein to form *rhodopsin* (visual purple) which is required for vision in dim light. Vitamin A occurs in two natural forms: vitamin A_1 (retinol) and vitamin A_2 (3-dehydroretinol) which has an additional double bond in the β-ionene ring and is biologically less active.

R = CH₂OH for retinols, CHO for retinals, CO₂H for retinoie acids:

β-Carotene (provitamin A)

Retinol is derived from fish, dairy products and such animal tissues as liver. It is often added to margarine during manufacture. The provitamins, carotenes, can be converted into retinol in the wall of the small intestine and in the liver by a NADH-dependent enzymic reaction. Carotenes are derived from plant sources which include vegetables (carrots, lettuce, turnip, etc.) and fruits (peaches, oranges, etc.) Retinol is stored in the liver and to a lesser extent in the kidneys whereas carotenes accumulate in adipose tissue.

The carotenoids include α, β, γ carotenes and cryptoxanthine, which contains only one β-ionene ring. Theoretically, β-carotene with its double β-ionene ring might be expected to produce two molecules of retinol but in practice only one is formed, although the yield is higher than for the other carotenoids. The stability of the vitamin and provitamins depends on the presence of antioxidants.

Determination of Retinol and Carotenes in Serum

In the previous edition, the method used was based on the Carr–Price reaction using antimony trichloride in chloroform (Kimble, 1938–39; Kaser and Stekol, 1943), but this has the disadvantage of forming insoluble antimony oxychloride in the presence of moisture. A more convenient reaction uses trifluoroacetic acid (TFA) instead of antimony trichloride to produce a blue colour as before (Neeld and Pearson, 1963; Dugan *et al.*, 1964). A correction for the colour contribution by carotenes is still required.

Determination of Serum Retinol and Carotenes Using TFA (Bradley and Hornbeck, 1973)

Proteins are precipitated with alcohol and the retinol and carotenes extracted into light petroleum. After reading the intensity of the yellow colour due to carotenes, the light petroleum is evaporated and the residue dissolved in chloroform before

TABLE 35.1

Vitamins Required by Man

Common Name	Chemical Name	General Roles	Clinical Deficiency in Man	Principal Methods*	Loading Test?
Fat-soluble					
A_1 A_2	Retinol 3-Dehydroretinol Carotenes	Vision, growth and reproduction (Provitamins)	Xerophthalmia, keratomalacia, nyctalopia	C H	Yes
D_2 D_3	Ergocalciferol Cholecalciferol Other sterols	Calcification of bones and teeth (Provitamins)	Rickets (young), osteomalacia (adult)	R H	
E	Tocopherols (α, β, γ & δ)	Anti-oxidant for cell membranes and lipids (unsaturated)	Lipid peroxidation (RBC fragility), haemolytic anaemia (newborn)	C H O	
K_1 K_2 K_3	Phylloquinone Menaquinones Menadione	Blood clotting system (Provitamin)	Increased clotting time, haemorrhagic disease of the new born	C O	Yes

Water-soluble

B_1	Thiamine, aneurine	Thiamine pyrophosphate is cocarboxylase in carbohydrate metabolism	Beri beri, Wernicke–Korsakoff encephalopathy	F E O	Yes
B_2	Riboflavin	Electron carrier as FAD, FMN in redox reactions	Angular stomatitis, dermatitis, photophobia	F E	Yes
B_6	Pyridoxine, pyridoxal and pyridoxamine	Pyridoxal phosphate is a co-factor for deaminases and decarboxylases	Dermatitis, epileptiform convulsions, hypochromic anaemia	C F O	Yes
Niacin	Nicotinic acid, nicotinamide	Electron carrier as NAD^+, $NADP^+$ in redox reactions	Pellagra—dermatitis, dementia and diarrhoea	F	
Folic acid	Pteroylglutamic acid	Co-factor in metabolism of purines & pyrimidines	Megaloblastic anaemia	CB O	
B_{12} group	Cobalamins (various)	Co-factor in nucleic acid synthesis, amino & branched chain oxo-acid metabolism	Megaloblastic anaemia, CNS degenerations, psychiatric disorders	CB O	Yes
Biotin	Biotin	Carboxylation co-factor		R CB O	
Pantothenic acid		Coenzyme A component	Burning feet syndrome	R O	
C	Ascorbic acid	Connective tissue formation.	Scurvy	C H O	Yes

* C = colorimetric, F = fluorimetric, R = radio-immunoassay, H = high performance liquid chromatography, CB = competitive protein binding. E = enzymatic, O = other, e.g. prothrombin time, dark adaptation.

carrying out the colour reaction. Allowance is made for the carotene contribution to the reaction.

Reagents.

1. Ethanol, 950 ml/l, analytical reagent grade.
2. Light petroleum, analytical reagent grade, b.p. 40 to 60 °C.
3. Chloroform, anhydrous, analytical reagent grade.
4. TFA reagent. Mix 1 volume TFA, analytical reagent grade, with 2 volumes chloroform just before use. The reagent is stable for 4 h at 25 °C.
5. Retinol stock standard, 160 mg/l. Transfer 18·35 mg retinyl acetate (all-*trans*, Eastman Organic Chemicals) to a 100 ml volumetric flask and dilute to volume with chloroform.
6. Retinol working standards. Dilute 10·0 ml stock standard to 100 ml with chloroform. Then dilute 2·5, 5·0, 7·5 and 10·0 ml amounts of this solution to 100 ml with chloroform to obtain working standards with concentrations, 0·4, 0·8, 1·20 and 1·60 mg/l. These standards are stable for one week at 4 to 8 °C in the dark.
7. β-Carotene stock standard, 200 mg/l. Dissolve 20·0 mg synthetic crystalline β-carotene (Sigma Chemical Company) in about 4 ml chloroform and dilute to 100 ml with light petroleum.
8. β-Carotene working standards. Dilute 10·0 ml stock standard to 100 ml with light petroleum. Then dilute 2·5, 5·0, 10·0, 15·0 and 20·0 ml amounts of this solution to 100 ml with light petroleum to obtain working standards with concentrations of 0·5, 1·0, 2·0, 3·0 and 4·0 mg/l. Working standards are stable for only a few hours at 25 °C and should be made freshly for each analysis.

Technique.   Prepare all standards and carry out all analytical operations in low actinic glassware or in subdued light. Perform analyses in duplicate.

Specimen collection. The patient should be fasted and the blood sample collected should be free from haemolysis and protected from light. Freshly separated serum can be stored at $-20\,°C$ for at least two weeks in the dark.

Analysis. Pipette 1.0 ml serum into a 15 ml glass-stoppered centrifuge tube, add 2·0 ml ethanol, stopper and mix well with a vortex mixer. Add 3·0 ml light petroleum and place the stoppered tubes in a mechanical shaker for 10 min to extract the retinol and carotenes into the petroleum phase. Centrifuge the tubes for 10 min at 2500 g. Carefully transfer 2·0 ml of the upper, light petroleum phase or 2·0 ml of each carotene working standard into a dry cuvette, 10 mm optical path length, and read the absorbance (A_{450}) at 450 nm against a light petroleum blank. Do this without delay to prevent solvent evaporation and destruction of carotenoids by light.

Evaporate the contents of the cuvettes to dryness in a 50 °C water bath with the aid of a fine stream of nitrogen. Remove the cuvettes, drying each carefully to avoid marking them, and add 100 μl chloroform to each, mixing briefly with a vortex mixer. Also prepare cuvettes containing 100 μl of each retinol working standard. Add 1·0 ml TFA reagent to a blank cuvette containing 100 μl chloroform, mix and use it to zero the spectrophotometer at 620 nm. Add forcefully, to facilitate immediate mixing, 1·0 ml TFA reagent to each of the other cuvettes in turn, recording the absorbance (A_{620}) at exactly 2 s after adding the reagent. As TFA is a strong acid with an irritant vapour take care to avoid spilling or splashing it. The best results are obtained if the TFA reagent is added from an automatic pipette linked to a recording spectrophotometer. This allows the absorbance to be read at the peak or inflection point after the initial surging peak caused by the introduction of the TFA reagent.

Calculations.

$$\text{Serum carotene (mg/l)} = \frac{A_{450} \text{ of unknown}}{A_{450} \text{ of standard}} \times \text{concentration of standard} \times 3$$

$$\text{Serum retinol (mg/l)} = \frac{A'_{620} \text{ of unknown}}{A'_{620} \text{ of standard}} \times \text{concentration of standard} \times \frac{3}{2}$$

where $A'_{620} = A_{620} - F \cdot A_{450}$ and F is determined as follows:

The magnitude of F varies between laboratories and is best determined individually. To do this treat 2·0 ml of each of the carotene working standards in the same way as the 2·0 ml of the light petroleum extract in the full method and measure A_{620} for each. Determine F as A_{620}/A_{450} for each working standard and calculate the mean value.

Other Analytical Methods

HPLC methods using reverse-phase columns and an ultraviolet detector (Bieri *et al.*, 1979) are more rapid and can identify and quantitate retinol and the individual carotenes. Such methods may be the reference techniques in the future.

INTERPRETATION

The reference range for serum or plasma retinol in the fasting subject is 0·30 to 0·65 mg/l (Yudkin, 1941; Haig and Patek, 1942; Sinclair, 1947; Krebs, 1950). Values above 0·3 mg/l appear to indicate that there are appreciable reserves in the liver and they correlate well with retinol intake. Values over 1·40 mg/l have been found in patients with retinol toxicity.

The reference range for carotenes is between 0·5 and 2·0 mg/l though somewhat higher limits were suggested by Campbell and Tonks (1949), and Krebs and Hume (1949) gave a lower limit of 0·2 mg/l. The concentration is greatly influenced by the dietary intake of carotenes and large quantities can produce blood levels over 5 mg/l. Such *carotenaemia* causes a yellow skin pigmentation which may be mistaken for jaundice. High concentrations are found in hypothyroid states where conversion to retinol is decreased and in patients with hyperlipidaemia associated with diabetes, or with chronic renal disease. Low values occur often in patients with the malabsorption syndrome (Wenger *et al.*, 1957).

Daily Requirements. Adult man appears to need 500 to 600 μg retinol or twice this amount of carotene daily. During pregnancy and lactation, women need a further 200 μg retinol daily. Increased needs also occur at growth spurts in childhood. Even on a reasonable dietary intake of the usual nutrients, it has been suggested that these contain only about 300 μg retinol and dietary supplements may thus be considered. Increased needs occur in stress and exercise (Rodriguez and Irvin, 1980).

Retinol Deficiency. Several disorders are described. Interference with rhodopsin production leads to poor dark-adaptation or night blindness, nyctalopia, and later to retinal degeneration. Retinol is needed to maintain normal epithelial integrity. In deficiency, there is an increased incidence of dental and respiratory infections. Corneal changes, keratomalacia, and impaired lacrimal gland secretion leading to dryness of the conjunctivae, xerophthalmia, also interfere with vision. Retinol deficiency affects growth of bones in the skull with the risk of cranial nerve compression. Optic nerve compression may cause blindness and auditory nerve compression may result in deafness in the more extreme cases. A specific anaemia responding only to retinol replacement has been described.

Retinol Toxicity. Although this was originally described in Eskimos eating large quantities of polar bear livers, toxicity may arise from excessive intake of pharmaceutical preparations of retinol. Acute toxicity occurs when levels exceed 1·4 mg/l but chronic toxicity characterised by bone and joint pain, weight loss and a variety of non-specific symptoms may be very difficult to diagnose.

Retinol Absorption Tests. These have been used in the past for the study of malabsorption states but are not now regarded as satisfactory (see Chapter 27).

International Unit. Pharmaceutical preparations are sometimes still labelled in IU. One IU of retinol has the activity of 0·344 μg of retinol acetate, 0·30 μg of retinol or 0·60 μg of β-carotene.

Retinol Binding Protein. This is usually measured in serum or plasma by RIA and is present in a concentration of 40 to 50 mg/l. It has been used to assess the nutritional status with regard to retinol. Decreased concentrations of the binding protein are found in liver diseases where protein synthesis is impaired, in renal diseases with proteinuria, in malnutrition and malabsorption and in some thyroid disorders.

CHOLECALCIFEROL (VITAMIN D$_3$)

Cholecalciferol is the naturally occurring member in man of a group of substances which are potentially able to cure rickets. It is also known as vitamin D$_3$ and although some is present in the diet, an important contribution comes from the conversion by ultraviolet irradiation of the provitamin, 7-dehydrocholesterol, present in the skin. Ring B cleavage produces pre-cholecalciferol and this is then rearranged to form natural cholecalciferol. Another provitamin of lesser importance is ergosterol, found in ergot, yeast and other fungi. This sterol, on exposure to ultraviolet light, undergoes similar changes to form pre-ergocalciferol and then ergocalciferol (vitamin D$_2$). At least another 10 compounds exist which are converted by ultraviolet irradiation into products with antirachitic activity.

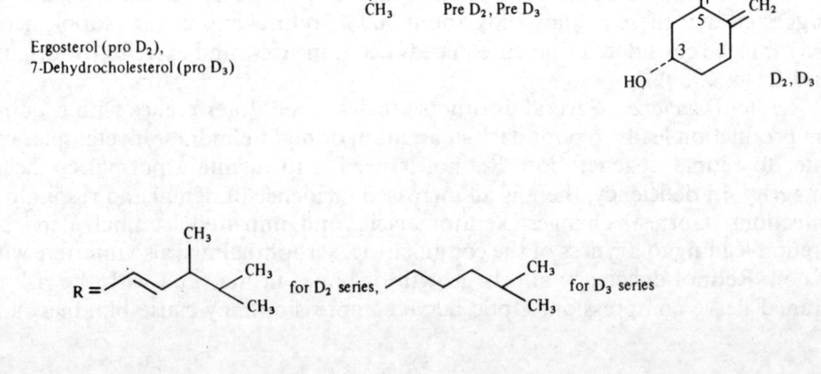

Ergosterol (pro D$_2$),
7-Dehydrocholesterol (pro D$_3$)

Pre D$_2$, Pre D$_3$

D$_2$, D$_3$

R = for D$_2$ series, for D$_3$ series

Cholecalciferol is present in only a few foods: egg yolk, fortified margarine and oily (sea) fish provide the main sources. High concentrations are found in fish liver oils. The dietary intake is tenuous and with the reduced action of ultraviolet light in the winter in Northern countries, potential deficiency is a real problem. Also in order to be efficiently absorbed with dietary fat in the form of chylomicrons, vitamin D requires the presence of bile salts, pancreatic lipase and a normal intestinal mucosa. Disorders affecting any of these also compromise an adequate supply of the vitamin.

The vitamin is not itself biologically active, but 1,25-dihydroxycholecalciferol (DHCC) into which it is converted is a potent hormone in calcium metabolism (Chapter 24). Cholecalciferol is first hydroxylated at C-25 in the liver and then circulates to the kidney where hydroxylation at C-1 takes place.

Methods for the Determination of Cholecalciferol and its Derivatives

As the concentrations of these substances in the plasma are very low, no chemical methods are available. Determinations by biological methods have now given way to HPLC and radioimmunoassay methods, the details of which are beyond the scope of this book. They are usually performed in a few centres only. A non-haemolysed sample of blood should be taken, sufficient to yield 5 ml of serum. This should be separated as soon as possible and stored at $-20\,°C$ until assayed.

INTERPRETATION

The reference ranges for 25-hydroxycholecalciferol and DHCC are 5 to 30 $\mu g/l$ and 20 to 50 ng/l for North West England (Dr E. B. Mawer, personal communication).

Daily Requirements. Only 2·5 μg of cholecalciferol is needed daily to prevent obvious rickets but for optimal growth 10 to 20 μg is required. Adults over the age of 25 probably require only 5 μg daily with double this intake during pregnancy or lactation.

Clinical Significance. Disorders of calcium metabolism which arise from deficiency or excess of the vitamin are discussed in more detail in Chapter 24. Deficiency leads to rickets in children and to osteomalacia in adults. Resistance to vitamin D therapy occurs if the conversion to DHCC is impaired by congenital or acquired conditions. In children with autosomal recessive vitamin D-resistant rickets, adequate responses may only occur with doses of 30 to 50 mg daily (Scriver, 1979). Inappropriately high intake of the vitamin leads to hypercalcaemia.

International Unit. Pharmaceutical preparations may be labelled in IU. One IU is the activity of 25 ng of cholecalciferol.

THE TOCOPHEROLS (VITAMIN E)

Vitamin E activity is shown by four naturally occurring tocopherols, α, β, γ and δ, with the general formula below, of which α-tocopherol is the most potent.

	α	β	γ	δ
R_1	Me	Me	H	H
R_2	Me	H	Me	H
R_3	Me	Me	Me	Me

The Tocopherols

Also, four tocotrienols occur with three double bonds in the side chain at C-3′,7′ and 11′. All are synthesised in plants, e.g. sunflower seeds, African violet and are especially abundant in vegetable oils (Janiszowska and Pennock, 1976). The viscous oils are soluble in fat solvents, stable to acid and heat without oxygen, but labile to alkaline solutions and to ultraviolet light.

Tocopherols are absorbed in the small intestine, enter the blood via the lymphatic system associated with chylomicrons and very low density lipoproteins and are mainly stored in adipose tissue. Small amounts of their metabolites are excreted in the urine.

Vitamin E appears to be a protector (antioxidant) for unsaturated, fatty acyl moieties of lipid within membranes where free radical damage can occur, e.g. hydrogen peroxide production by flavoprotein oxidase. This is reflected in the fragility of the red cell membrane.

Determination of Serum Tocopherol (Baker and Frank, 1968).

Serum tocopherols can be measured by their reduction of ferric to ferrous ions which then form a red complex with α,α'-dipyridyl. Tocopherols and carotenes are first extracted into xylene and the absorbance is read at 460 nm to measure the carotenes. A correction for the carotenes is made after adding ferric chloride and reading at 520 nm.

Reagents.
1. Absolute alcohol, aldehyde-free.
2. Xylene.
3. α,α'-Dipyridyl, 1·20 g/l in n-propanol.
4. Ferric chloride solution, 1·20 g $FeCl_3$, $6H_2O$/l in ethanol. Keep in a brown bottle.
5. Standard solution of DL-α-tocopherol, 10 mg/l in ethanol.

Technique. Into three stoppered centrifuge tubes measure 1·5 ml serum, standard or water (blank) respectively. To the test and blank add 1·5 ml ethanol and to the standard 1·5 ml water. Add 1·5 ml xylene to each tube, stopper, mix well and centrifuge. Transfer 1·0 ml of each xylene layer into a clean stoppered tube, carefully excluding any protein or ethanol. Add 1·0 ml dipyridyl reagent to each tube, stopper and mix. Pipette 1·5 ml of the mixture into colorimeter cuvettes and read the absorbance (A_{460}) of the test and standard against the blank at 460 nm. Then, in turn, beginning with the blank add 0·33 ml ferric chloride solution, mix, set the wavelength to 520 nm and 1·5 min after mixing read the absorbance (A_{520}) of the test and standard against the blank.

Calculation.

$$\text{Serum tocopherols (mg/l)} = \frac{A' \text{ of unknown}}{A' \text{ of standard}} \times 10$$

where $A' = A_{520} - 0.29 \times A_{460}$

Other Analytical Methods

The above method can be modified by adding nitrous acid which forms a yellow colour with all the tocopherols and tocotrienols except for the α-forms. The difference between the total measured by ferric chloride reduction and that measured by the nitroso reaction gives a measure of the amount of α-tocopherol plus α-tocotrienol.

The different tocopherols and tocotrienols can be separated and identified by gas chromatography and HPLC (Bieri *et al.*, 1979). The vitamin E status can be indirectly assessed by measuring the haemolysis of erythrocytes previously treated with hydrogen peroxide, dialuric acid or isotonic saline-phosphate buffer (Sauberlich *et al.*, 1974).

INTERPRETATION

The mean serum tocopherol concentration in healthy adults is 11 mg/l with a range from 6 to 19 mg/l. Lower figures, 2 to 4 mg/l, are found in infants but rise to adult levels later in childhood. The maternal plasma tocopherol is increased during pregnancy but the neonate has a much lower concentration and premature infants in particular are born with quite inadequate reserves.

Daily Requirements. The α-form is the most active biologically. There are probably adequate amounts of the vitamin in a mixed diet of 2000 to 3000 kcal. This contains the equivalent of 7 to 13 mg of α-tocopherol. Infants should receive 3 mg daily, older children 8 mg/day and after the age of 10 years the recommended daily intake is 10 mg with a 3 mg supplement during pregnancy.

Deficiency States. Those arising in premature or low-birth-weight babies are characterised by irritability, oedema and a haemolytic anaemia which responds specifically to treatment with α-tocopherol. Later in life, malabsorption states may be associated with serum tocopherol levels as low as 1 mg/l and in those with severe malabsorption this may result in increased red cell fragility, increased urinary excretion of creatinine due to muscle loss and in ceroid pigment deposition in the small intestinal musculature. In abetalipoproteinaemia, the chronic deficiency of tocopherol has been suggested as a factor in the later development of degenerative disorders of the central nervous system.

Other States. Increased plasma levels of 15 to 38 mg/l have been reported in association with hypercholesterolaemia but there is no evidence of toxic effects. Indeed doses of up to 300 mg daily have been used therapeutically, without detriment, in the treatment of such conditions as intermittent claudication, habitual abortion, sterility, muscular dystrophies and degenerative disorders of the central nervous system. In some cases the intention is to protect the individual against chemical oxidants. Any evidence for the value of such therapy is inconclusive (Lancet, 1974).

International Unit. One IU is the activity of 1·0 mg synthetic DL-α-tocopherol acetate.

VITAMIN K

Several vitamins K exist but all are derived from the synthetic product, 2-methyl-1,4-naphthaquinone, menadione, sometimes known as vitamin K_3. Other forms involve addition of a hydrocarbon chain at C-3.

C-3 substituents

2-Methyl-1,4-naphthoquinone

The only form in plants, of which green vegetables are the main dietary source, is 3-phytylmenadione, phytomenadione, phylloquinone or vitamin K_1. Bacteria are able to synthesise a range of products, the menaquinones or vitamins K_2, in which the side chain is composed of 4 to 13 isoprenyl units. Menadione itself is activated by conversion in the body to compounds of the K_2 class when administered therapeutically in reduced form as sodium menadiol diphosphate (Synkavit).

The absorption of vitamins K is similar to that of fats and other fat-soluble substances. It is stored in the liver where half of it is of type K_2 and is thought to originate in the colon where it is synthesised by bacteria. As a consequence, the daily dietary requirement of vitamin K is uncertain.

Vitamin K is a co-factor for the hepatic synthesis of various enzymes or precursors in the blood coagulation cascade process. These are prothrombin (factor II), proconvertin (factor VII), thromboplastin component (factor IX) and Stuart–Prower factor (factor X). The vitamin is not incorporated into the molecule but appears to be responsible for post-translational modification of glutamyl residues resulting in increased biological activity.

Analytical Methods. These usually involve measurement of the 'prothrombin time', the time taken for fresh citrated plasma to clot after addition of calcium and thromboplastin. This is increased if there is a deficiency of one or more of the four factors just described. Various methods are available and are usually carried out in haematology laboratories. For details see Dacie and Lewis (1978).

Vitamin K Deficiency. Once the level of prothrombin and related factors has fallen below 5% of the normal, there is a danger of serious overt bleeding. Deficiency is rarely due to poor dietary intake but the bacterial contribution is compromised in long-term antibiotic therapy and during the neonatal period. Fat malabsorption for any reason increases the risk of vitamin K deficiency, particularly if protracted. Even adequate absorption may be ineffective if hepatic synthesis of the coagulation proteins is impaired by liver disease or immaturity (p. 742).

Coumarins and other substances are used therapeutically as vitamin K antagonists in anticoagulation treatment. Occasionally, dietary coumarins may also produce haemorrhagic disease for the same reason.

Vitamin K Excess. Excess of natural vitamin K is uncommon and without obvious effect but excessive administration of menadione can cause a haemolytic anaemia with Heinz bodies in the red cells.

THIAMINE (VITAMIN B_1)

Thiamine, the first of the 'B group' of water-soluble vitamins to be recognised, is a pyrimidyl-substituted thiazole alcohol. It acts as a coenzyme in the form of its pyrophosphate ester, thiamine pyrophosphate (TPP), the coenzyme of three important enzymes. Pyruvate dehydrogenase complex (carboxylase) catalyses the decarboxylation of pyruvate with the eventual formation of acetyl co-enzyme A as the last step of the glycolytic pathway. Transketolase and transaldolase occur in carbohydrate metabolism via the pentose monophosphate shunt. They respectively transfer glycol aldehyde (a 2C fragment) and dihydroxyacetone (a 3C fragment) as described later (p. 908).

Thiamine pyrophosphate

Thiamine occurs in cereals and in animal foods such as liver, heart and kidney. Up to 5 mg of thiamine is actively transported daily into the jejunal mucosal cells in which it is converted into TPP. Only about 30 mg of thiamine is stored in body tissues, particularly in skeletal muscle.

Analytical Methods

The direct chemical determination of thiamine in plasma is difficult because of the low concentration and more indirect measurements of thiamine nutritional status have usually been employed. These include the measurement of thiamine or its metabolites in the urine, the investigation of the cocarboxylase activity by measuring pyruvate in blood, and the measurement of red cell transketolase activity with and without added TPP.

Determination of Thiamine in Urine by the Thiochrome Reaction (Johnson *et al.*, 1945)

Thiamine is oxidised by alkaline ferricyanide to the tricyclic derivative, thiochrome, which is extracted into butanol and measured fluorimetrically.

Thiochrome

Reagents.
1. Activated Decalso or Permutit. There is considerable variation between different samples. A product is required which will adsorb thiamine well and settle out rapidly. When about 200 mg are shaken with water in a 10 ml measuring cylinder all the particles should settle rapidly to the bottom in not more than 2 min. To obtain a suitable product, suspend material which will pass a 100-mesh sieve in acetic acid (10 ml/l water) in large cylinders. Within 2 min the heavier particles will have separated from the lighter ones and will have sunk to the bottom. Separate the particles by decanting. Boil the heavy granules three times with the dilute acetic acid with settling and decanting between fresh additions of acetic acid. Wash the product with distilled water and dry at 110 °C. If addition of potassium ferricyanide results in the formation of a blue colour, wash the product in a warm, fairly strong, solution of hydrochloric acid. Carry out test runs with synthetic thiamine. The activity of a satisfactory product remains constant for months if it is kept dry.
2. Potassium chloride solution, approximately 250 g/l.
3. Sodium hydroxide solution, 150 g/l.
4. Potassium ferricyanide solution, 2·5 g/l, prepared fresh daily.
5. Isobutanol or *n*-butanol. This should give almost no blank. Test each new batch before use.
6. Acetic acid, approximately 10 ml/l in water.
7. Stock standard thiamine chloride solution, 40 mg/l. Dissolve 4·48 mg thiamine chloride hydrochloride in 100 ml water.
8. Working standard, 400 μg/l. Dilute 1 ml stock standard to 100 ml with water and add 400 mg oxalic acid.

Technique. Collect urine in glass vessels and store in amber bottles, adding 100 mg oxalic acid for every 25 ml urine. Measure 2 ml urine (0·5 ml if the result is likely to be high), 2 ml working standard and 2 ml water (as blank) into glass-stoppered test tubes and to each add about 200 mg of the activated Decalso or Permutit and mix with ten rapid shakes. The adsorption is optimal at pH 3 to 6, which is assured by use of the oxalic acid. Now add about 8 ml acetic acid and mix by inversion ten times. Stand for a short time and remove the supernatant fluid. Repeat this washing process which is important since, if ineffective, the final fluorescence has a silvery-blue admixture to the true thiochrome mauve, thus giving unsatisfactory readings. If this happens, carry out further washes; the thiamine is firmly adsorbed so that repeated washings only remove interfering substances.

Add 0·5 ml potassium chloride solution and shake gently, taking care to avoid splashing the solid too far up the side of the tube. Elution is complete within 30 s. Add 0·1 ml potassium ferricyanide and 0·25 ml sodium hydroxide, shaking gently after each addition. Add 2 ml isobutanol, stopper and shake vigorously for about a minute (25 shakes up and down). Stand or centrifuge for a short time to allow separation of the two phases. Transfer the supernatant fluid to a cuvette and read in the fluorimeter at 435 nm using excitation at 365 nm and zeroing with the blank extract.

Calculation.

$$\text{Urinary thiamine chloride } (\mu g/l) = \frac{\text{Reading of unknown}}{\text{Reading of standard}} \times \frac{800}{V}$$

where V = volume of urine (ml) taken for analysis.

INTERPRETATION

Thiamine excretion is greatly affected by variations in the dietary intake and absorption but also by the analytical method used. Suggested daily excretion rates for the above method are 50 to 500 μg although Melnick (1942) regarded less than 90 μg as evidence of deficient intake. Concentrations of less than 50 $\mu g/l$ may be considered as abnormal and those below 20 $\mu g/l$ indicate extreme abnormality. More reliable results are claimed if the excretion after a loading dose of thiamine is measured. Melnick and Field (1942) gave intravenously 0·35 mg thiamine per m^2 of body surface area and collected urine for the next 4 h. At least 50 μg should be excreted in that time. Najjar and Holt (1940) gave adults a somewhat higher dose of 1 mg intravenously and suggested a minimum excretion of 110 μg in the following 4 h while Mason and Williams (1942) gave 1 mg orally and found that over 100 μg was excreted in the next 24 h.

Other metabolites of thiamine in urine have also been measured (Neal, 1970).

Determination of Blood Pyruvate

This simple but less sensitive investigation has either been used as a single test or as part of a pyruvate tolerance test. Thiamine deficiency reduces TPP activity and thereby retards the catabolism pyruvate so that its concentration in the blood tends to increase. Pyruvate is now measured enzymically using lactate dehydrogenase.

Enzymic Determination (Gloster and Harris, 1962; Boehringer leaflet)

The conversion of pyruvate to lactate by lactate dehydrogenase

$$CH_3.CO.COO^- + NADH + H^+ \rightarrow CH_3.CHOH.COO^- + NAD^+$$

proceeds almost to completion at pH 6·9 and its course can be followed by the change in absorbance at 340 nm due to NADH. The method given is a modification of that published by Boehringer.

Reagents.

1. Trichloracetic acid, 100 g/l in hydrochloric acid, 500 mmol/l.
2. Phosphate buffer, 1·1 mol/l. Dissolve 19·14 g dipotassium hydrogen phosphate in 100 ml glass-distilled water.
3. Reduced nicotinamide adenine dinucleotide. Dissolve 5 mg in 1 ml glass-distilled water. This is best made freshly but can be kept for a few days at 4 °C.
4. Lactate dehydrogenase, 0·75 mg enzyme protein in 1 ml ammonium sulphate solution. This and the previous reagent can be obtained from the Boehringer Corporation (London) Limited.
5. Pyruvate standard, 250 μmol/l. Dissolve 2·35 mg lithium pyruvate in 100 ml water.

Technique. Take about 5 ml blood into a syringe. Avoid venous stasis and, especially, activity of forearm muscles (Braybrooke *et al.*, 1975). At once inject the blood into 5 ml trichloracetic acid contained in a weighed centrifuge tube. Shake the tube well and reweigh to obtain the weight of blood added. From this the volume can be obtained by dividing by 1·060, the specific gravity. Alternatively it may be thought that the volume of blood can be measured with sufficient accuracy in the syringe. Centrifuge at 2000 r.p.m. for 10 min. Add 0·7 ml phosphate buffer to 2 ml supernatant fluid and to 2 ml water (as blank) and transfer 2 ml to 10 mm quartz cuvettes. Add a further 1 ml phosphate buffer and then 50 μl NADH.

Mix well by stirring. After 2 min read the absorbance at 340 nm against the blank. Repeat the reading 1 min later to ensure a steady state. This reading should be between 0·500 and 0·800, then add 50 μl lactate dehydrogenase and mix well with a glass rod. Read the absorbance after 2 min and at minute intervals for a further 3 min until no further change occurs. For normal bloods taken from resting persons a difference in absorbance (ΔA) between 0·050 and 0·100 is usually obtained. Check at intervals by putting the pyruvate standard through the procedure.

Calculation. If v ml of blood is taken then $2v/(5+v)$ ml of blood is present in 2 ml of the supernatant fluid; 0·7 ml of phosphate is added to this and 2 ml taken; the final volume is 3·1 ml. At 340 nm in a 10 nm cuvette a ΔA of 0·100 is equivalent to 16·1 nmol pyruvate per ml of reaction mixture. Hence:

$$\text{Blood pyruvate (μmol/l)} = \frac{5+v}{2v} \times \frac{2 \cdot 7}{2 \cdot 0} \times \frac{\Delta A}{0 \cdot 100} \times 3 \cdot 1 \times 16 \cdot 1$$

$$= 337 \times \frac{(5+v)}{v} \times \Delta A$$

Note. Sets of reagents for this enzymic determination can be obtained from Boehringer. In this case the blood is taken into an equal volume of perchloric acid (5 ml of the 70% acid diluted to 100 ml with redistilled water) instead of trichloracetic acid.

INTERPRETATION

The reference range for blood pyruvate by this method is 34 to 80 μmol/l. In marked thiamine deficiency, values up to 220 to 300 μmol/l are found. Increases in pyruvate have also been reported in diabetes mellitus, congestive heart failure, diarrhoea and other digestive disturbances, severe liver damage and in some acute infections.

Bueding *et al.* (1941) suggested using the increase in blood pyruvate which results from taking glucose. In normal persons, this reaches a maximum in an hour and returns to normal limits within 3 h. In thiamine deficiency a greater increase occurs and a longer time is required for the return to normal. This test is said to show abnormal results before the fasting blood pyruvate is increased. Blood for determination of pyruvate is taken fasting, and 30 min, 1 h and 2 h after giving 50 g glucose orally as in the glucose tolerance test. The rise in pyruvate should not produce a blood level of more than about 100 μmol/l; a greater rise is evidence in favour of thiamine deficiency.

Technique Using Red Cell Transketolase Activity (Brin, 1967)

Transketolase catalyses the reversible transfer of a 2-carbon moiety from a donor carbohydrate possessing an oxo group to an acceptor carbohydrate possessing an aldehyde group. The enzyme requires the presence of Mg^{2+} and TPP. Various methods have been described. Brin's sequence of changes can be summarised as follows:

ribose phosphate + xylulose phosphate $\xrightarrow{\text{transketolase}}$
(C_5) $\qquad\qquad\qquad (C_5)$

sedoheptulose phosphate + glyceraldehyde phosphate $\xrightarrow{\text{transaldolase}}$
(C_7) $\qquad\qquad\qquad\qquad (C_3)$

erythrose phosphate + fructose phosphate
(C_4) $\qquad\qquad\quad (C_6)$

Then erythrose phosphate + ribose phosphate $\xrightarrow{\text{transketolase}}$
(C_4) $\qquad\qquad\qquad (C_5)$

fructose phosphate + glyceraldehyde phosphate
(C_6) $\qquad\qquad\qquad (C_3)$

And 2 glyceraldehyde phosphate $\xrightarrow{\text{transaldolase}}$ fructose phosphate
(C_3) $\qquad\qquad\qquad\qquad\qquad\qquad\qquad (C_6)$

Overall there are 6 $C_5 \to 5$ C_6 since in order to get two molecules of glyceraldehyde phosphate the first five lines have to be doubled.

Plasma and white cells are removed from heparinised blood by centrifugation and washing with saline. The packed cells require weighing before haemolysis, achieved by adding an equal volume of water and freezing and thawing the sample once. The haemolysate is incubated with ribose-5-phosphate with and without the addition of TPP. When there is a deficiency of the latter, the rates of pentose disappearance and hexose formation are diminished. Either pentose can be determined using the orcinol reaction or, alternatively, hexose is measured by the anthrone reaction. The coefficient of variation between duplicates is 5 to 10 %. Alternatively, an enzyme-linked NADH method is available (Bayoumi and Rosalki, 1976).

The ranges of the TPP enhancing effect (%) are: normal, 0 to 15; marginally deficient, 15 to 25; severely deficient, usually with clinical abnormalities, greater than 25. No sex differences in response have been found.

Thiamine and Disease.

Daily Requirements. The need for thiamine is correlated with the amount of carbohydrate metabolised. It increases in muscular activity, pregnancy, lactation, prolonged fevers and in hyperthyroidism. The adult allowance has been suggested as 0·5 mg thiamine per 1000 kcal intake. Other suggested daily requirements are 0·4 mg for infants, increasing to 2·0 mg in adults. Some of the vitamin is destroyed during cooking at high temperatures, by alkalies and by sulphite (preservative).

Thiamine Deficiency. Severe deficiency causes the disease known as beri-beri but milder forms of deficiency are more common. Beri-beri was endemic in the Far East when the diet was mainly polished rice as thiamine is located in the rice husk. In the exudative form of beri-beri, impaired myocardial contractility leads to ventricular dilatation and congestive cardiac failure, sometimes with accompanying pericardial effusion. A less severe, 'dry' form is more usual in Western countries and occurs most often in alcoholics. The clinical features are peripheral neuropathy, extreme muscular weakness, anxiety and mental confusion.

RIBOFLAVIN (VITAMIN B$_2$)

Riboflavin, 7,8-dimethyl-10-(1'-D-ribityl) isoalloxazine, contains a ribitol group attached to a flavin (isoalloxazine). It is more heat-resistant than thiamine and in solution gives an intense yellow-green fluorescence and undergoes photodegeneration. These properties led to its discovery as the second member of the 'B group' of vitamins.

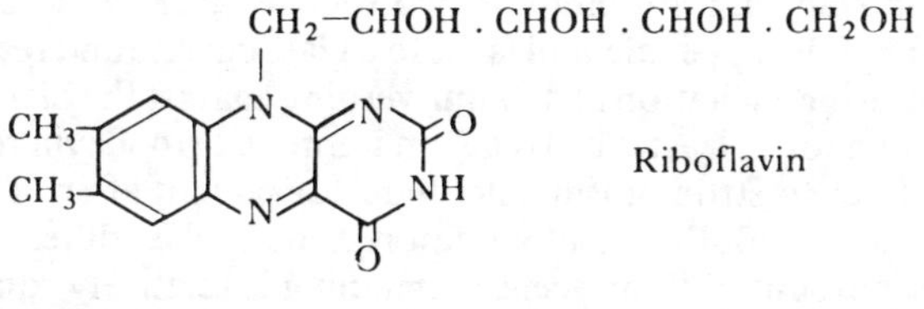

$$CH_2{-}CHOH . CHOH . CHOH . CH_2OH$$

Riboflavin

Riboflavin is involved as a coenzyme, either as its monophosphate, flavin mononucleotide (FMN) or linked with adenosine phosphate in flavin adenine dinucleotide (FAD). FMN is present in cytochrome-c-reductase and L-amino acid oxidase while FAD occurs in D-amino acid oxidase, xanthine oxidase and succinate dehydrogenase.

These two coenzymes are absorbed in the jejunum with the aid of bile salts. The body absorbs up to 25 mg of riboflavin daily but riboflavin stores are minimal. The flavoproteins are metabolised intracellularly and thyroid hormones are involved in the regulating mechanism.

Analytical Methods

Two schools of thought exist as to whether riboflavin itself should be measured, or whether the biochemical activities of the coenzymes should be studied. The nutritional status has therefore been assessed either by measuring riboflavin in urine, if necessary after a loading dose of the vitamin, or by measuring the activity of the FAD-dependent glutathione reductase in freshly lysed erythrocytes (Sauberlich *et al.*, 1972; Bayoumi and Rosalki, 1976).

Determination of Riboflavin in Urine (Slater and Morell, 1946)

After oxidising interfering substances with permanganate, riboflavin is extracted into an acetic acid–pyridine–butanol mixture and measured fluorimetrically.

Reagents.
1. Dry, powdered oxalic acid.
2. A mixture of equal volumes of pyridine and glacial acetic acid.
3. Potassium permanganate solution, 40 g/l.
4. Hydrogen peroxide solution, '10 volumes %'.
5. Isobutanol or *n*-butanol. Check each batch to ensure that there is no significant fluorescence in ultraviolet light.
6. Anhydrous sodium sulphate.
7. Stock standard riboflavin solution, 40 mg/l.
8. Working standard, 1·0 mg/l. Dilute 2·5 ml stock standard to 100 ml with water and add 400 mg oxalic acid.

Technique. Collect a 24 h urine specimen as described for thiamine. Carry out all operations in diffuse light. Measure 0·5 ml urine, working standard and water (blank) into separate 10 ml glass-stoppered test tubes and add 0·5 ml reagent (2) to each followed by one drop of the permanganate solution. Shake for 1 min, add two drops of hydrogen peroxide to remove excess permanganate and again shake gently. If the purple colour is not destroyed within 10 s, add a further drop of peroxide and warm to 21 °C. Add 1·5 ml butanol, stopper and shake vigorously up and down 25 times over 1 min. Stand to allow the layers to separate, add a small amount of sodium sulphate, rotate between the hands until the alcohol layer clears and stand for a minute or two for the layers to separate fully.

Transfer 1 ml of the upper alcohol layer to a glass cuvette and read at 535 nm in the fluorimeter using excitation at 450 nm, zeroing against the blank. The alcohol extracts are stable for at least 2 h. To get an improved riboflavin reading, expose the alcohol extract to strong ultraviolet light for 60 min after taking the initial reading and then read the residual fluorescence. The difference is due to riboflavin. The amount of fluorescence remaining is relatively constant at about half the initial reading in most urines collected without a loading dose of riboflavin.

Calculation.

$$\text{Urinary riboflavin (mg/l)} = \frac{\text{Reading of unknown}}{\text{Reading of standard}}$$

INTERPRETATION

The daily excretion is greatly influenced by the riboflavin content of the diet. On a satisfactory intake, the output is 0·5 to 0·8 mg/day. Tests based on the administration of a fixed dose of riboflavin are more satisfactory than those taken under basal conditions. If 16 μg riboflavin/kg body weight is given intravenously, at least 25 % of the dose should be excreted within 4 h (Najjar and Holt, 1941; Axelrod *et al.*, 1941).

Interference by other fluorescent materials in urine may sometimes cause confusion. More elaborate chromatographic separative techniques have been used in an effort to improve specificity (Haworth *et al.*, 1971).

Determination of Erythrocyte Glutathione Reductase Activity (Sauberlich *et al.*, 1972)

Glutathione reductase activity in an erythrocyte haemolysate is measured, with and without addition of FAD, by spectrophotometric determination of the rate of NADPH consumption.

$$\text{Apoenzyme} + \text{FAD} \rightarrow \text{Holoenzyme}$$

$$\text{G.S.S.G} + \text{NADPH} + \text{H}^+ \xrightarrow{\text{holoenzyme}} 2\,\text{GSH} + \text{NADP}^+$$

Reagents.
1. Sodium chloride solution, 150 mmol/l.
2. Potassium phosphate buffer, 100 mmol/l, pH 7·4.
3. NADPH solution, 2 mmol/l. Dissolve 16·6 mg of the tetrasodium salt of NADPH in 10 ml of 10 g/l sodium bicarbonate solution. Prepare fresh daily.
4. Oxidised glutathione solution, 7·5 mmol/l. Prepare daily by dissolving 46 mg glutathione in 9·9 ml double-distilled water and 100 μl sodium hydroxide solution, 1 mol/l.
5. FAD solution, 300 μmol/l. Dissolve 2·4 mg of the monosodium salt of FAD in 10 ml double-distilled water. Prepare fresh daily.
6. EDTA solution, 80 mmol/l. Dissolve 1·5 g dipotassium EDTA in 50 ml double-distilled water.

Technique. *Sample preparation.* Collect venous blood from a fasting subject, using EDTA or heparin as anticoagulant and chill on ice. Mix 200 μl blood with 1·0 ml cold saline, centrifuge and remove the supernatant. Repeat this twice more. Immediately prior to the assay, add 1·5 ml distilled water, mix and centrifuge to obtain a dilute haemolysate. Store in ice until ready for the assay.

Enzyme activity measurement. This is performed in two optical cuvettes, 1 and 2. Add 100 μl FAD solution to cuvette 1 and 100 μl distilled water to cuvette 2. To cuvette 1 add 2·0 ml phosphate buffer, 50 μl EDTA solution, 100 μl haemolysate and 100 μl glutathione solution. Mix and equilibrate the cuvette at 37 °C for 8 min and then add 100 μl NADPH solution. Measure the decrease in absorbance (ΔA_1) at 340 nm against a water blank over a 10 min period. Carry out the same steps for cuvette 2 to obtain ΔA_2.

Calculation. Results are expressed as an 'activity coefficient' (AC), the proportionate increase in enzyme activity resulting from FAD addition *in vitro*. Thus

$$AC = \Delta A_1 / \Delta A_2$$

INTERPRETATION
The AC figures suggested are: less than 1·2, acceptable vitamin level; 1·2 to 1·4, mild deficiency; greater than 1·4, significantly deficient. The test cannot be performed on erythrocytes deficient in glucose-6-phosphatase.

Riboflavin and Disease

Daily Requirements. These are based on age, activity, pregnancy and lactation. The minimal quantities required are 1·0 to 1·6 mg and on a reasonable diet, the quantities available are usually about twice this. Based on energy consumption, man needs about 0·6 mg per 1000 kcal daily. Foods rich in riboflavin are meat, fish and offal, with lesser amounts in butter, cheese and eggs. Fruit and vegetables supply little, other than green beans and peas.

Riboflavin Deficiency. Two possible causes of riboflavin deficiency exist. There is the possibility of inadequate formation of FAD in the intestinal mucosal cells if these are diseased, or there is inadequate dietary intake of the vitamin or inadequate absorption as part of a malabsorptive state. Although some bacterial synthesis of riboflavin occurs in the colon, it is not certain whether this is available to any significant degree. Riboflavin deficiency rarely occurs as an isolated disorder and its features are not clearly defined. Combined deficiency occurs in closed populations with inadequate nutritional care.

The features of deficiency appear in tissues of ectodermal origin. The eyes may show lacrimation, corneal vascularisation, keratitis or cataract formation; the oral mucosa shows inflammation, angular stomatitis or glossitis; the skin shows features such as pruritus and dermatitis. Other features claimed to be attributable to riboflavin deficiency are a normocytic, normochromic anaemia and a reduced conversion of tryptophan to nicotinic acid.

PYRIDOXINE (VITAMIN B_6)

Three members of the B_6 group occur naturally and are chemically related. They are pyridoxine itself, pyridoxamine and pyridoxal; all are pyridine derivatives.

$$\text{HO} \begin{array}{c} R \\ \\ \\ H_3C \end{array} \quad CH_2-O- \left\{ \begin{array}{l} \text{H, vitamin} \\ PO_3H_2, \text{ phosphate} \end{array} \right. \qquad \begin{array}{l} R = CH_2OH \text{ for pyridoxine} \\ CH_2NH_2 \text{ for pyridoxamine} \\ CHO \text{ for pyridoxal} \end{array}$$

Any dietary vitamins present as their 5-phosphate esters are hydrolysed by intestinal alkaline phosphatase before the free vitamins are absorbed. They are converted to pyridoxal-5-phosphate (PLP) which is a coenzyme for several enzymes involved in protein, fat and carbohydrate metabolism. Important ones are the transaminases (p. 499) and decarboxylases. PLP is also the coenzyme for kynureninase (EC 3.7.1.3), which catalyses the conversion of kynurenine and 3-hydroxykynurenine to anthranilic acid and 3-hydroxyanthranilic acid respectively during tryptophan catabolism. The blocks resulting from pyridoxine deficiency are shown in Fig. 35.1. Xanthurenic and kynurenic acids are normally excreted in small amounts only, but increases are found in pyridoxine deficiency. They are partly converted to 8-hydroxyquinaldic and quinaldic acids respectively. PLP is also required in the formation of δ-aminolaevulinic acid from glycine and succinyl coenzyme A at the start of haem synthesis (p. 642).

The vitamin is widely distributed in most vegetables and animal tissues but particularly good sources are cereals, liver and potatoes. There are significant losses during exposure to ultraviolet light or cooking of foods. The main catabolite of these vitamins is 4-pyridoxic acid, derived by oxidation of the CHO group in pyridoxal to COOH. It is excreted in the urine.

Analytical Methods

PLP has been measured in plasma using radioactive tyrosine and its apo-decarboxylase (Reynaulds, 1983). The suggested reference range is 5 to 23 μg/l.

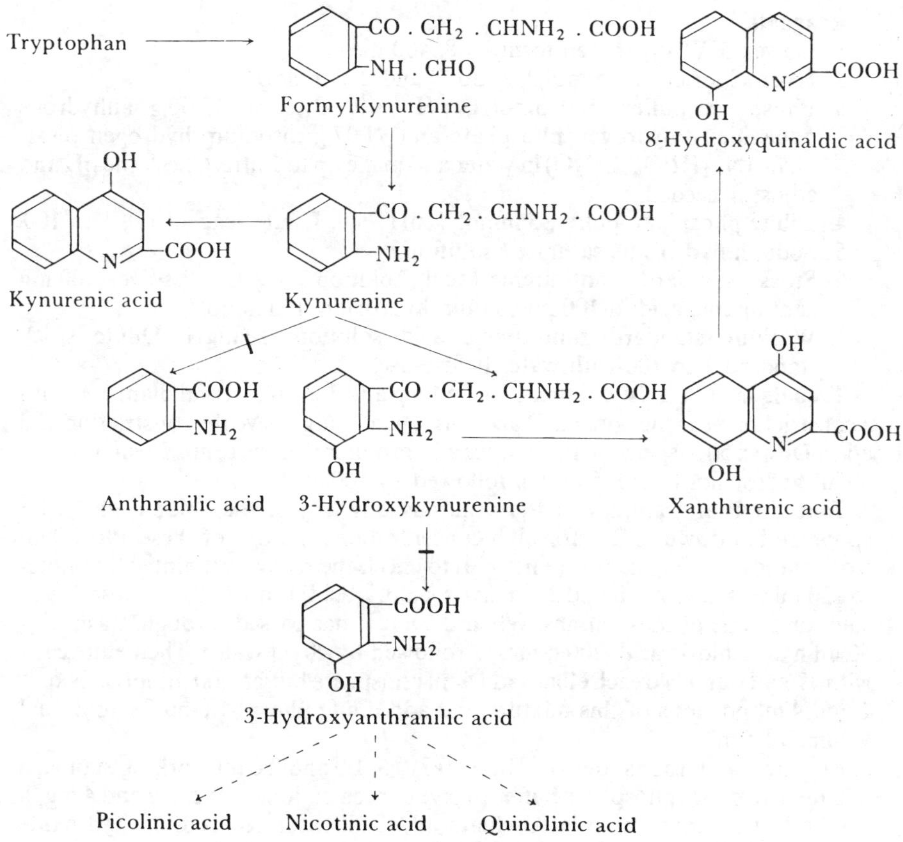

Fig. 35.1. The Catabolism of Tryptophan via the Kynurenine Pathway.
The blocks in pyridoxine deficiency are indicated by bars on the arrows.

Direct measurement of the urinary excretion of 4-pyridoxic acid is possible using HPLC. In deficiency states the concentration is below 0·8 mg/l.

Indirect methods require simpler equipment. A consequence of pyridoxine deficiency is the accumulation of 3-hydroxykynurenine, kynurenine, xanthurenic acid and 8-hydroxyquinaldic acid, kynurenic acid and quinaldic acid. The measurement of xanthurenic acid in the urine, often after giving a dose of tryptophan, is used most often. Chromatographic and colorimetric methods have been devised but fluorimetry is preferable.

Other indirect methods measure the activity of erythrocyte aspartate or alanine aminotransferase before and after the addition of PLP *in vitro*, thus reflecting the biological activity intracellularly (Bayoumi and Rosalki, 1976). A methionine loading test has also been used but requires the availability of an amino acid analyser (Hegsted *et al.*, 1976).

Fluorimetric Determination of Xanthurenic Acid (Satoh and Price, 1958)

After absorption on to a column of Dowex 50 in H⁺ form, xanthurenic and kynurenic acids are eluted with water to leave interfering substances on the column. The xanthurenic acid is measured fluorimetrically in alkaline solution in which the fluorescence of kynurenic acid is slight.

Reagents.
1. Dowex 50W (hydrogen form) × 8, 400 mesh.
2. Hydrochloric acid, 5 mol/l, 1 mol/l and 200 mmol/l.
3. Phosphate buffer, 500 mmol/l, pH 7·40. Dissolve 13·00 g anhydrous potassium dihydrogen phosphate and 71·97 g disodium hydrogen phosphate (Na_2HPO_4, $2H_2O$) in water and make up to 1 litre. Check the pH and adjust if needed.
4. Dilute phosphate buffer, 5 mmol/l, pH 7·40. Dilute reagent (3), 1 to 100.
5. Sodium hydroxide, saturated solution.
6. Stock standard xanthurenic acid solution, 1 g/l. Dissolve 100 mg xanthurenic acid in 100 ml sodium hydroxide, 100 mmol/l.
7. Working standard xanthurenic acid solution, 10 mg/l. Dilute stock standard 1 to 100 with water before use.

Technique. Use glass columns, 15 cm long and 1·2 cm external diameter, with a constriction near the bottom. Place a glass wool plug above the constriction and add a Dowex 50 suspension to produce a 3 cm column of the resin. Wash this with 50 ml hydrochloric acid, 5 mol/l, followed by 100 ml water.

Take duplicate samples of the urine, usually 5% of the volume of a 24 h specimen but down to 2% for high concentrations. To one of these add 1·0 ml stock standard (1 mg xanthurenic acid) to check the recovery. Dilute all samples to 120 ml with water and add 30 ml hydrochloric acid, 1 mol/l. Mix and add each solution to one of the columns. When the liquid has passed through, wash with 50 ml hydrochloric acid, 200 mmol/l, followed by 20 ml water. Then elute each with 396 ml water. To each eluate add 4 ml phosphate buffer, 500 mmol/l. Take 1, 2 and 4 ml portions of this mixture and add dilute phosphate buffer to a final volume of 5 ml.

Prepare standards as follows. Dilute 0·1, 0·5, 1·0 and 2·0 ml working standard to 5 ml with dilute phosphate buffer to give concentrations of 0·2, 1, 2 and 4 mg/l. To 5 ml of standard or diluted eluate add 5 ml saturated sodium hydroxide solution, mix, stand for at least 1 h, centrifuge and read in the fluorimeter against a blank of half-saturated sodium hydroxide solution, with excitation at 370 nm and emission at 525 nm.

Calculation. If v ml of eluate is diluted to 5 ml then

Eluate concentration (mg/l) =

$$\frac{\text{Reading of unknown}}{\text{Reading of standard}} \times \text{concentration of standard} \times \frac{5}{v}$$

If x per cent of the 24 h volume is taken,

Urinary xanthurenic acid (mg/24 h) = Concentration in eluate $\times \dfrac{40}{x}$

Notes.
1. A recovery of added xanthurenic acid of 95 ± 5% should be obtained.
2. Although kynurenic acid fluoresces in acid solution, its fluorescence in alkali is slight and interference is unlikely unless its excretion is very high.

Tryptophan Loading Test. After collecting a basal 24 h urine, Price *et al.* (1965) give 2 g L-tryptophan in orange juice or, in the case of young children 0·1 g/kg body weight up to a maximum of 2 g, and collect urine passed during the next 24 h into a bottle containing 25 ml hydrochloric acid, 1 mol/l. Alternatively, since the greatest increase of xanthenuric acid occurs in the first 12 h after taking the tryptophan, collect two 6 h specimens before and two after doing so.

INTERPRETATION

Normal persons excrete 1 to 3 mg xanthurenic acid daily and 2 to 11 mg in the 24 h after the tryptophan dose. In pyridoxine deficiency the response to tryptophan is greater; up to 60 mg may be excreted in 24 h.

Pyridoxine and Disease

Daily Requirements. These have been suggested as 0·5 to 1·2 mg varying proportionately with the dietary protein intake.

Pyridoxine Deficiency. Dietary deficiency rarely occurs in isolation and is usually combined with deficiencies of other vitamins of the B complex. Some drugs specifically interfere with pyridoxine metabolism. Isoniazid can form hydrazones with pyridoxal and PLP while D-cycloserine and penicillamine inactivate PLP by forming thiazolidine derivatives. A naturally-occurring antagonist, 4-deoxypyridoxine, has occasionally been found in the diet.

In addition to the increased excretion of tryptophan metabolites discussed above, disordered homocystine metabolism (p. 392) may be revealed as cystathioninuria and homocystinuria. After a marked deficiency of the vitamin has existed for 3 or 4 weeks, convulsions are common in children as a consequence of diminished formation of γ-aminobutyric acid from glutamic acid, a process which requires PLP. Other changes which have been ascribed to pyridoxine deficiency include dermatitis, glossitis, cheilosis, lymphopenia and a chronic anaemia which may be sideroblastic.

The various conditions usually respond to a daily dose of pyridoxine of 5 to 50 mg.

PANTOTHENIC ACID

This B vitamin is synthesised by most plants and micro-organisms from L-valine and β-alanine (from L-aspartate) as its structure indicates.

$$HOCH_2 . C(CH_3)_2 . CH(OH) . CO . NH . CH_2 . CH_2 . COOH$$

The biological activity depends on its combination with ATP and cysteine to form coenzyme A, a process requiring folate and biotin. Coenzyme A plays important roles in carbohydrate, fat and amino acid metabolism.

Pantothenic acid is widely distributed in animal products, vegetables and cereals, partly as coenzyme A. Pantothenic acid is heat-labile and up to 50 % can be lost during food preparation.

Analytical Methods

Pantothenic acid is excreted as such in the urine, the output being proportional to the dietary intake (Sauberlich *et al.*, 1974). Chemical analytical methods are relatively complex and involve radioimmunoassay, gas chromatography or HPLC. Coenzyme A in plasma may be measured enzymatically.

Daily Requirements. An intake of 4 to 7 mg is usually adequate to balance losses but more is needed during pregnancy, lactation or when there are high energy requirements.

Pantothenate Deficiency. Selective deficiency of the vitamin has only been achieved when volunteers were given the antagonist, methylpantothenic acid, or semi-synthetic diets. The subjects became irrascible and developed postural hypotension, tachycardia, constipation and peripheral neuropathy.

BIOTIN

Biotin, previously referred to as vitamin H, is bio-tetrahydro-2-oxothienol-(3,4-d)-imidazoline-4-valeric acid.

$$
\begin{array}{ccc}
& CO & \\
NH & & NH \\
| & & | \\
HC & \rule{1cm}{0.4pt} & CH \\
| & & | \\
H_2C & & CH.(CH_2)_4.COOH \\
& S & \\
\end{array}
$$

The –COOH group reacts readily with the ε-amino group of lysine to form biocytin and similarly with lysyl residues in proteins. It is also firmly bound by avidin, an egg-white protein. After linkage to lysyl groups in certain apoenzymes, it is a co-factor in several reactions involving carboxylases and transcarboxylases, (McCormick and Olson, 1984). In the presence of ATP and bicarbonate, the carboxylases introduce a –COOH group into the substrate. Thus pyruvate is converted to oxaloacetate while other substrates are acetyl-, propionyl- and β-methylcrotonyl-coenzyme A. Transfer of a –COOH group converts methylmalonyl-coenzyme A and pyruvate into propionyl-coenzyme A and oxaloacetate when catalysed by a specific transcarboxylase. These are all key reactions in carbohydrate and fat metabolism.

The best dietary sources are offal, milk and eggs, with lesser amounts in meat, cereals and fruit. Biotin is easily oxidised in food preparation to an inactive sulphoxide. Some hydrolysis of bound biotin occurs in the gut and biocytin and biotin are absorbed in the jejunum after which the erythrocytes hydrolyse biocytin to biotin. Colonic micro-organisms can synthesise biotin and this seems to be available to the body as the daily urinary biotin excretion exceeds the dietary intake of biotin 3- to 6-fold.

Analytical Methods

Lactobacillus pantarium has been used for the microbiological determination of biotin in urine and in proteolytic digests of whole blood. Radioimmunoassay methods have also been devised but no simple techniques exist.

Daily Requirements. These are uncertain but 100 to 200 μg is suggested for adults and 35 μg for young children. Based on energy use, the figure is 50 μg per 1000 kcal.

Biotin Deficiency. Isolated biotin deficiency is only likely if large quantities of raw egg white are eaten (Sauberlich *et al.*, 1974). Low levels in association with other deficiencies may occur in the elderly, in alcoholism, pregnancy and if energy expenditure is high. The features are nausea, anorexia, vomiting, depression and skin changes. These may be a dry scaly dermatitis in adults but a seborrhoeic dermatitis has been noted in infants.

NICOTINIC ACID, NIACIN

Nicotinic acid in the form of its amide, nicotinamide, is a component of two important co-enzymes, nicotinamide adenine dinucleotide (NAD^+) and nicotinamide adenine dinucleotide phosphate ($NADP^+$). These are found in almost all cells and are the hydrogen acceptors for numerous oxido-reductases.

| Nicotinic Acid | Nicotinamide | 1-Methylnicotinamide |

Nicotinic acid and nicotinamide present in food are readily absorbed from the jejunum and appear in the blood and cerebrospinal fluid. Little is stored as such but most cells convert them to NAD^+ and $NADP^+$. The degradation of these coenzymes by microsomal deaminase releases nicotinic acid which is excreted in the urine mainly as 1-methylnicotinamide with some 1-methyl-3-carboxamide-6-pyridone.

Analytical Methods

Simple methods have been used to determine the urinary excretion of 1-methylnicotinamide as this substance seems to give the best index of nicotinic acid nutritional status. It reacts with ketones in alkaline solution to form fluorescent derivatives. These are more stable in acid solution (Pelletier and Campbell, 1962; György and Pearson, 1967). Alternatively the native fluorescence of 1-methylnicotinamide can be measured simultaneously with the determination of thiamine in urine. Urinary metabolites can be separated by HPLC if required.

Determination of 1-Methylnicotinamide in Urine (Johnson *et al.*, 1945; see also Hochberg *et al.*, 1945: Huff and Perlzweig, 1947).

1-Methylnicotinamide is adsorbed at pH 4·5 on to a column of synthetic zeolite, eluted with potassium chloride, made alkaline and extracted into butanol and measured fluorimetrically.

Reagents. 1 to 5. These are the same as reagents 1, 2, 3, 5 and 6 described on (p. 905) for thiamine determination.

   6. Stock standard 1-methylnicotinamide chloride solution, 100 mg/l in water.

   7. Working standard, 5 mg/l. Dilute 5 ml stock standard to 100 ml with water and add 400 mg oxalic acid.

Technique. Collect urine as for thiamine and proceed as described for thiamine up to the first removal of the supernatant fluid. Wash once more only, using 8 ml acetic acid, and remove the supernatant. Add 500 μl potassium chloride solution and shake gently. Then add 2·0 ml butanol and 250 μl sodium hydroxide solution. Stopper at once and shake up and down 25 times over 1 min. Centrifuge and transfer 1 ml of the upper, butanol layer to a fluorimeter cuvette.

Take fluorimetric readings with excitation wavelength at 360 nm and emission set at 460 nm, not earlier than 5 min after adding the alkali. After adjusting the sensitivity, zero the instrument with the blank extract.

Calculation.

$$\text{Urinary 1-methylnicotinamide (mg/l)} = \frac{\text{Reading of unknown}}{\text{Reading of standard}} \times \frac{10}{V}$$

where V = volume of urine (ml) taken for analysis.

INTERPRETATION

The average daily excretion of 1-methylnicotinamide, when nicotinic acid intake is satisfactory, is 7 mg with a range of 3 to 17 mg.

Daily Requirements. These are uncertain as colonic bacteria also contribute to the daily uptake in addition to the dietary intake of the vitamin and of tryptophan. Balance studies suggest a daily dietary intake of 15 to 20 mg for adults and 4 mg for young children, with gradual increase to adult levels by the age of 15. The requirements are increased in exercise. The vitamin is found in meat and offal especially and to a lesser extent in fruit, vegetables and cereals.

Nicotinic Acid Deficiency. The classical deficiency state is pellagra, originally described in people subsisting on maize. The disease is characterised by pigmented dermatitis in areas of skin exposed to sunlight, diarrhoea with widespread inflammation of epithelial surfaces, and by dementia.

This may appear as a secondary manifestation in carcinoid syndrome and in Hartnup disease (p. 394). Both diminish the amount of tryptophan available for conversion to nicotinic acid in the body. As maize protein is also deficient in tryptophan this amino acid appears to be an important source of nicotinic acid in metabolism (Fig. 35.1, p. 913). The diminished production of nicotinic acid by colonic bacteria may contribute to deficiency symptoms if antibiotic therapy is prolonged.

FOLIC ACID

The molecule of folic acid shows three features, a pteridine group linked by *p*-aminobenzoic acid to glutamic acid, and is referred to as pteroylglutamic acid (PGA). *p*-Aminobenzoic acid is an essential growth factor for many micro-organisms which synthesise PGA.

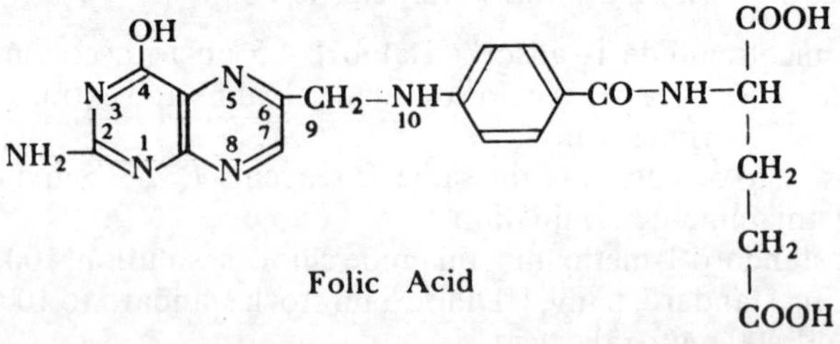

Folic Acid

The metabolic role of folate is of considerable importance and largely involves 5,6,7,8-tetrahydrofolate (THF), a molecule which can accept or donate various 1-carbon fragments such as methyl ($-CH_3$), methylene ($=CH_2$), methenyl ($=CH-$), formyl ($-CHO$) and formimino ($-CH:NH$). This activity involves the N atoms at positions 5 and 10. The various molecules permit cyclical regeneration of THF (Fig. 35.2). The main source of the 1-carbon fragments is serine.

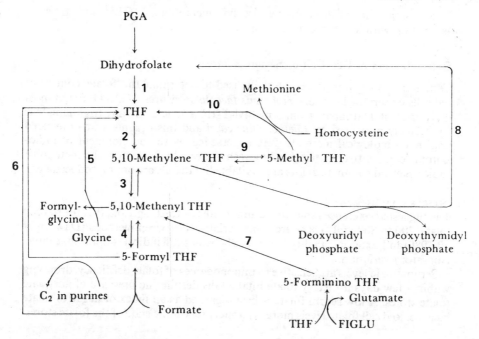

Fig. 35.2. Folate Metabolism.
The enzymes are: **1.** folate reductase, **2.** serine hydroxymethyl transferase, **3.** 5,10-methylene THF dehydrogenase, **4.** 5,10-methenyl THF cyclohydrolase, **5.** glycinamide-diribonucleotide transformylase, **6.** 5-formyl THF synthetase, **7.** 5-formimino THF reductase, **8.** thymidylate synthetase, **9.** 5,10-methylene THF reductase, **10.** 5-methyl THF methyltransferase.

Four points are of special interest: (1) 5,10-methylene-THF is involved in the synthesis of thymine residues in deoxyribonucleic acid (DNA), (2) 5-methyl-THF is only effectively recycled in the presence of the appropriate methyl-transferase, an enzyme requiring vitamin B_{12} as its prosthetic group, (3) the formimino group only enters the scheme through formiminoglutamic acid (FIGLU), a degradation product of histidine and this requires a supply of THF, (4) dihydrofolate is reduced by folate reductase which is antagonised by aminopterin and amethopterin, which are therefore effective cytotoxic drugs.

PGA and its derivatives—triglutamate, polyglutamates and THF occur in green leaf vegetables. The polyglutamates require hydrolysis by conjugases before absorption which occurs in the jejunum. About 20 % of the daily uptake of folate, 300 to 500 μg, is derived from dietary sources and the rest is synthesised by intestinal bacteria. Some folate is stored in the red cells, the concentration in which is about 20 times that in the plasma. The total body stores, mainly in the form of 5-methyl-THF, amount to 15 mg, enough for 75 to 150 days.

Analytical Methods

The methods used have fallen into the two groups: direct and indirect. The direct determination of folate in red cells or serum is possible and is now often performed in haematology laboratories. The main indirect method has been the determination in the urine of the histidine metabolite, FIGLU, sometimes in association with a loading dose of histidine.

Determination of Red Cell or Serum Folate

Certain micro-organisms were initially used to determine the 'folate' content of red cells or serum. Thus, *Streptococcus faecalis* measures PGA, THF and most derivatives of THF apart from 5-methyl-THF. The last and any triglutamate is additionally measured by *Lactobacillus casei* and this organism was preferred until microbiological methods were superseded by the development of radio-isotopic competitive protein binding techniques which are now the method of choice. Several commercial kits are available but details are not reproduced here.

INTERPRETATION

The suggested reference range for serum folate is 4 to 20 μg/l and that for red cell folate, 200 to 800 μg/l. There are some variations between methods (Dawson *et al.*, 1980) and External Quality Assurance Schemes still indicate appreciable inter-laboratory variation.

Serum folate levels are sensitive to minor degrees of folate deficiency, dropping within a few days if dietary folate intake falls despite the presence of adequate folate stores. A low serum folate is best regarded as an index of negative folate balance. Red cell folate levels more accurately reflect the state of the folate stores.

Determination of FIGLU and Histidine Loading Tests

These investigations have become obsolescent with the development of satisfactory isotopic methods for the direct determination of folate. The catabolism of histidine to FIGLU is shown in Fig. 35.3. As the further utilisation of FIGLU involves THF (Fig. 35.2, p. 919) it accumulates in folate deficiency and is excreted in increased amounts in the urine. This is more obvious if the pathway is stressed by administration of histidine orally.

Methods for the determination of FIGLU have included cellulose acetate electrophoresis and enzymatic techniques. Details appear in the 5th edition of this book but are not included again because of the diminishing importance of the investigation. The histidine loading tests studied the increase in FIGLU excretion, either during 8 h after giving 15 g histidine, or during 24 h after giving 5 g morning, midday and evening.

In the 24 h test, the daily excretion of FIGLU increases from 0·6 to 30 mg in the normal nutritional state to 185 to 2050 mg in folate deficiency (Luhby *et al.*, 1959). A considerably increased excretion is seen in some patients with malignant disease (Noeypatimanond *et al.*, 1966) but increases of lesser degree are found in pernicious anaemia. In megaloblastic anaemia, treatment with folate or vitamin B_{12}, as appropriate, reduces FIGLU excretion to normal.

Folate and Disease

Daily Requirements. The adult requires 300 to 500 μg in total of which 100 to 200 μg is needed in the diet. Increased needs are present in pregnancy and in stress.

Folate Deficiency. Folate deficiency of subclinical degree is common. Body stores are inadequate to protect against long-term inadequacy of supply but are a buffer against transient deficiencies. Poor intake of foods rich in folate, especially

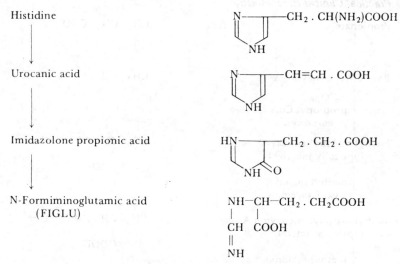

Fig. 35.3. Histidine Catabolism.

green-leaf vegetables, is important particularly if there are increased needs for folate. This is the case in pregnancy, haemolytic anaemia, liver disorders and malignancy. Malabsorption of water-soluble materials from the intestine, especially if this affects the jejunum, is important and may produce rapid deficiency in coeliac disease, sprue or loss of small intestine by surgical excision. Broad spectrum antibiotic therapy, if prolonged, greatly diminishes the bacterial synthesis of folate in the colon and contributes to deficiency. Other drugs such as phenytoin and barbiturates interfere with enzymes of the folate cycle and may cause deficiency symptoms.

The main clinical effect of deficiency is a megaloblastic anaemia as a consequence of impaired formation of DNA during erythrocyte maturation. As vitamin B_{12} deficiency causes a similar type of anaemia, further discussion is deferred until this vitamin has been considered.

THE COBALAMINS (VITAMIN B_{12})

Cobalamins have a complex structure not reproduced here. Trivalent cobalt in the form of Co^+ is present at the centre of a porphyrin ring which is linked to a ribonucleotide whose organic base is dimethylbenzimidazole. The usual form isolated has CN^- linked to the Co^+ and is referred to as cyanocobalamin; if OH^- replaces CN^-, hydroxycobalamin results. As with other B vitamins, further conversion is needed before coenzyme activity is apparent. If CN^- is replaced by a 5-deoxyadenosyl group, the product, deoxyadenosylcobalamin, has coenzyme activity as does methylcobalamin.

Important coenzyme functions of the cobalamins include:

1. Coenzyme for 5-methyl-THF methyltransferase (Fig. 35.2) which allows 5-methyl-THF, the storage form of folate, to enter the folate cycle;
2. Coenzyme in the methylation of soluble ribonucleic acid (RNA);
3. Coenzyme in the conversion of methylmalonylcoenzyme A to succinylcoenzyme A (and hence succinate) by methylmalonyl CoA mutase (Fig. 35.4).

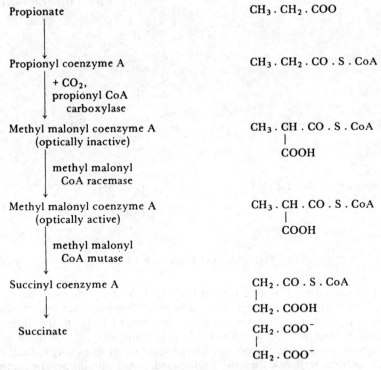

Fig. 35.4. The Conversion of Propionate to Succinate.

Function (1) involves vitamin B_{12} in folate metabolism particularly in the formation of DNA and so both these vitamins, when deficient, lead to a similar megaloblastic anaemia. Function (3) was formerly used in the chemical, indirect assessment of vitamin B_{12} deficiency. Its involvement with fatty acid metabolism may account for the neurological effects of vitamin B_{12} deficiency.

Vitamin B_{12} is present in the diet in many animal tissues, especially in liver, but also in milk and eggs. Its intestinal absorption with calcium ions requires combination with intrinsic factor, a glycoprotein secreted at the cardiac end of the stomach, and takes place in the terminal ileum. In the mucosal cells it is mainly converted to deoxyadenosylcobalamin. This is transported to the liver in combination with the α-globulin, transcobalamin I, where it is stored, unlike other B vitamins. The liver contains 3 to 6 mg, a supply sufficient for about 5 years. As required, a β-globulin, transcobalamin II, transports the vitamin to the bone marrow.

Analytical Methods

The vitamin has been measured directly in the serum or red cells and indirectly by measuring the urinary excretion of methylmalonic acid, often after a valine load.

Direct Methods. Microbiological assays using *Lactobacillus leichmanii* or *Euglena gracilis* were originally used but have been superseded by radio-isotopic competitive protein binding methods. Alternatively, the intestinal absorption of vitamin B_{12} can be studied by isotope methods (Dacie and Lewis, 1978). Doses of

0·5 to 2 mg of vitamin B_{12} labelled with ^{57}Co or ^{58}Co are given orally with and without intrinsic factor. One mg of non-radioactive vitamin is also given parenterally to reduce undue storage of absorbed isotope. Unabsorbed vitamin may be measured in the stools, or absorption studied by hepatic uptake or urinary excretion of the isotope. The latter, the Schilling test, shows excretion of over 33 % of the isotopic dose in the next 24 h in normal persons.

Competitive Protein Binding Assays. These require release of the vitamin from binding proteins in the serum initially, in some cases by treatment with hot acid. Various commercial kits are available for such assays (Dawson *et al.*, 1980; Waters *et al.*, 1981) which are more often carried out in haematology laboratories. The results of External Quality Assurance Schemes suggest the need for careful control of details of the technique.

Indirect Method. The conversion of propionate to succinate (Fig. 35.4) depends on the coenzyme activity of vitamin B_{12}. If necessary, the pathway can be stressed by the administration of valine which is metabolised to propionate. With the development of satisfactory direct methods for the measurement of vitamin B_{12}, this indirect method is now used infrequently and has therefore not been included here. Details are available in the 5th edition of this book if needed.

INTERPRETATION

The reference range for vitamin B_{12} in serum is 200 to 1000 ng/l. It is desirable that each laboratory establishes its own reference range by comparison of the vitamin level with other haematological findings (Dawson *et al.*, 1980).

Dietary deficiency of vitamin B_{12} is unusual but is described in vegans. More important is intrinsic factor deficiency. This is typically seen in the gastric atrophy found in classical pernicious anaemia but congenital deficiency occurs rarely while total gastrectomy results in acquired deficiency. Direct interference with absorption is seen in terminal ileal abnormalities, e.g. Crohn's disease. The Schilling test carried out with and without intrinsic factor allows discrimination between intrinsic factor deficiency and impairment of absorptive site. Utilisation of dietary vitamin B_{12} by bacteria colonising the small intestine reduces the amount available for absorption. This occurs in some cases of steatorrhoea, particularly those associated with the 'blind-loop' syndrome or tropical sprue. Infestation with the fish tapeworm also causes similar losses. Whatever the cause of the deficiency, the liver stores protect the body from the consequences of deficiency for several years.

Increased serum vitamin B_{12} values have been noted in liver cell necrosis, presumably due to release from the damaged hepatic stores.

Daily Requirements. These have been suggested as 3 to 30 µg, with a possible increase during growth and pregnancy.

Consequences of Deficiency. Deficiency of vitamin B_{12} or of folate results in disordered haemopoiesis. Unlike folate deficiency, however, vitamin B_{12} deficiency leads to disordered function of nervous tissue, recognised clinically as subacute combined degeneration of the spinal cord.

Deficiency of folate itself, or deficiency of vitamin B_{12} which impairs the folate cycle, retards DNA synthesis. Cell cytoplasmic functions which depend on RNA are unaffected. The outcome is delayed maturation of cell nuclei and increased cell size. In the red cell precursors in the marrow, cytoplasmic formation of haemoglobin continues but the normal nuclear changes during red cell maturation are delayed. The resulting megaloblast replaces the normal cell, the normoblast. Altered maturation also affects leucocyte and platelet precursors. In consequence the number of red cells, polymorphs and platelets in the peripheral blood is reduced. The red cells are larger than usual, are often distorted and are more readily haemolysed. Both folate and vitamin B_{12} deficiency thus lead to increases in serum bilirubin, urinary urobilinogen and serum lactate dehydrogenase. In many cases serum iron is increased.

The lowest serum B_{12} values are seen in pernicious anaemia, falling as the severity of the anaemia increases. Figures of 10 to 110 ng/l are recorded. Subnormal results occur in other causes of vitamin B_{12} deficiency and about half the cases of folate deficiency have reduced B_{12} levels which rise to normal on folate therapy. True vitamin B_{12} deficiency requires replacement of the vitamin, often by parenteral injection. This is important for the well-being of the central nervous system. Folate is ineffective in this role.

ASCORBIC ACID (VITAMIN C)

L-Ascorbic acid, a water-soluble vitamin, is a modified hexose with strong acidic and reducing properties. In solution, ascorbate is readily oxidised by air to dehydro-L-ascorbate, especially in the presence of metallic ions such as Cu^{2+}. Both forms are biologically active and are interconvertible in the body. The rate of oxidation of ascorbate *in vitro* increases with increasing pH but above pH 5, dehydroascorbate also undergoes further oxidation, ring opening and loss of biological activity. The product is dioxo-L-gulonate which is subsequently cleaved to L-threonate and oxalate. Animals other than man, primates and the guinea pig can synthesise ascorbate from glucose; the exceptions lack L-gulonolactone oxidase.

| L-Ascorbic acid | Dehydro-L-ascorbic acid | Dioxo-L-gulonic acid | L-Threonic acid |

The mode of action of ascorbate is unclear. It is necessary for the development of cartilage, bone and dentine. The vitamin is a cofactor for protocollagen hydroxylase which is involved in the hydroxylation of proline during connective tissue maturation. L-Ascorbate is also involved in relation to Fe(II)-enzyme systems in the metabolism of tyrosine and dihydroxyphenylalanine and in microsomal drug metabolism.

The best dietary sources of the vitamin are citrus fruits, berries, tomatoes, raw cabbage and other green vegatables. Losses during processing and cooking can be considerable. In man, ascorbate and dehydroascorbate are readily absorbed from the stomach and ileum into the circulation. Ascorbate diffuses passively into many cells but platelets, adrenal and retinal cells possess active transport mechanisms. Dehydroascorbate diffuses freely into cells and is stabilised as ascorbate. The vitamin is excreted in the urine as ascorbate, dehydroascorbate and catabolites such as oxalate.

Analytical Methods

The more common methods rely either on the reducing properties of ascorbate or the ketonic properties of dehydroascorbate.

Redox titration of ascorbate with 2,6-dichlorophenolindophenol in acid solution involves reduction of this dye to a colourless leucobase while ascorbate is oxidised to dehydroascorbate. The latter, if present initially, can only be measured if it is first reduced to ascorbate in acid solution by hydrogen sulphide. Other reducing substances may be present, particularly in urine, which also react, thus impairing the specificity of the method.

2,6-dichlorophenolindophenol
(oxidised form)

colourless leucobase
(reduced form)

Dehydroascorbate forms a hydrazone with 2,4-dinitrophenylhydrazine. The product is red in acid solution and is measured colorimetrically. In this case, the ascorbate must first be oxidised to dehydroascorbate by shaking with activated charcoal or copper sulphate solution. Other ketones may interfere by forming hydrazones.

In blood and urine the vitamin is mainly present as ascorbate in fresh samples. Immediate redox titration or preservation of the ascorbate in strongly acid solution until titration is possible is thus important with the first type of method.

Determination of Urinary Ascorbate by Titration with 2,6-Dichlorophenolindophenol (Harris and Ray, 1935).

Reagents.
1. Glacial acetic acid.
2. Solution of 2,6-dichlorophenolindophenol. Weigh out accurately 40 mg of the dye and dissolve in 100 ml distilled water. One ml of this solution is equivalent to 0·2 mg ascorbate. Since the keeping qualities of the solution are poor, prepare freshly at frequent intervals. It should not be kept in use for more than a week. BDH Chemicals supply tablets of the dye which when dissolved in 5 ml water provide the same solution.

   Solutions of dye can be checked against an ascorbic acid solution of known concentration. Dissolve 40 mg pure dry ascorbic acid in 100 ml acetic acid (100 ml glacial acid diluted to 1 litre with water). Dilute 5 ml of this to 100 ml with the acetic acid. Titrate 0·5 ml of the dye with this solution. Five ml should be required to decolourise it.

Technique. Pipette 0·5 ml dye solution into a test tube (15 × 2·5 cm) and add 1 ml glacial acetic acid. Run in the urine slowly, with constant shaking, until the red colour has been discharged. Note the urine volume required.

Calculation. As 0·5 ml of dye reacts with 0·1 mg ascorbic acid

$$\text{Urinary ascorbate (mg/l)} = \frac{100}{\text{ml urine required}}$$

Alternative Technique. Mix a portion of the urine with one-ninth its volume of glacial acetic acid and determine the volume required to decolourise 0·5 ml dye. This ensures a uniform concentration of acetic acid. Then,

$$\text{Urinary ascorbate (mg/l)} = \frac{111}{\text{ml urine required}}$$

Notes.
1. The urine must be titrated fresh, that is within a few minutes of being passed, unless acetic acid is added immediately in the proportion of 1 part to 9 parts of urine. Such acidified urine will keep for several hours. The determination is most often done on urine specimens collected as part of saturation tests (see below) which can be titrated at once. A rather large amount of acetic acid is required to protect 24 h specimens, the determination of ascorbic acid in which is not very convenient.
2. Other reducing substances, particularly sulphydryl compounds, which may be present react more slowly than ascorbic acid at pH 3 so that the method is sufficiently accurate for most clinical purposes. In saturation tests, because of the greater quantity of ascorbate often present, the effect of these interfering substances is much less important.

INTERPRETATION

The daily output of ascorbate, usually about 20 to 30 mg, is about half the daily intake. The minimum intake that protects against scurvy is about 60 mg. In deficiency states, urinary ascorbate is almost absent. The small amounts measured are probably due to other reducing substances. The 24 h excretion is not a good index of the deficiency state and a saturation test is preferable.

Ascorbic Acid Saturation Tests

These tests assume that if the previous intake of the vitamin has been insufficient, the tissues will take up quite large amounts when ascorbic acid is given so that little or none will be excreted in the urine. Persons whose intake has been adequate will excrete appreciable amounts of this added vitamin. Various dosages have been used, the ascorbic acid has been given orally and intravenously, and different times for urine collection have been used. The test described is almost identical to that of Harris and Abbasy (1937).

Technique. An oral dose of 11 mg ascorbic acid/kg body weight is used, giving an average dose for adults of about 700 mg. This may be given in water, either fasting or 2 to 3 h after a meal. Only one specimen of urine is collected covering the period 4 to 6 h after the dose when excretion is maximal. Thus, the test can be carried out as follows:

1000 h Give the ascorbic acid dissolved in about 150 ml water.

1400 h Empty the bladder completely and discard the urine.

1600 h Empty the bladder completely and estimate the ascorbate content almost immediately as described above.

Repeat the test daily until a normal response is obtained.

INTERPRETATION

In a normal nutritional state for ascorbate, an output of about 50 mg should be obtained on the first or second day. In mild deficiency states, 6 to 10 days may elapse before this output is achieved. In severe deficiency, 14 to 21 days may be needed. In deficiency states, the apparent excretion of up to 2 mg ascorbate is attributable to other reducing substances and stays constant until the deficiency has almost been corrected when the ascorbate content of the urine specimen rises rapidly towards 40 to 50 mg, the amount found in a normal state. Urines rich in ascorbate should be diluted 5- to 10-fold with water before titration, otherwise errors may arise.

The test has been criticised but is convenient and satisfactory in practice. Any ascorbate deficiency is being treated during the test and the effects may be apparent clinically.

Determination of Plasma Ascorbate by 2,6-Dichlorophenolindophenol Titration

Reagents.
1. Trichloracetic acid solution, 100 g/l, *or* freshly prepared metaphosphoric acid solution, 50 g/l.
2. Solution of 2,6-dichlorophenolindophenol. Prepare as for the urine method and then dilute this, 5 ml to 25 ml, when 1 ml = 40 μg ascorbate.

Technique. Separate plasma immediately after collecting the blood. Thoroughly mix 4 ml plasma and 4 ml reagent (1) and centrifuge. Pipette 200 μl of the dye solution into a test tube and titrate with the supernatant until the reddish colour is discharged.

Calculation. As 200 μl dye is equivalent to 8 μg ascorbate,

$$\text{Plasma ascorbate (mg/l)} = 16/\text{ml titration}$$

Notes.
1. While metaphosphoric acid has advantages over trichloracetic acid, even the solid form is unstable once the reagent bottle has been opened. The stability of trichloracetic acid is satisfactory.
2. Blood can be collected into heparin, EDTA or oxalate. The plasma is best separated and titrated at once but if necessary, the protein-free supernatant can be stored for a few hours at $-20\,^{\circ}$C. Alternatively 4 to 5 ml of blood can be collected into a test tube containing one drop each of potassium cyanide solution (50 g/l) and potassium oxalate solution (200 g/l).

INTERPRETATION

Plasma ascorbate levels are of limited value in assessing the severity of deficiency of this vitamin. On an adequate diet, plasma ascorbate levels are between 4 and 20 mg/l, and frequently 8 to 14 mg/l. Values below 2 mg/l suggest marked deficiency. Ascorbate disappears more rapidly from the plasma than from the cells when a diet is low in vitamin C and the leucocytes appear to be the last to be depleted. The determination of leucocyte ascorbate has been used as a better index of severe deficiency.

Determination of Leucocyte Ascorbate (Denson and Bowers, 1961; Gibson *et al.*, 1966)

Blood is diluted with a saline/EDTA/dextran mixture in which the red cells form rouleaux and settle out rapidly on standing. The leucocytes and platelets remain suspended and are recovered by centrifugation. After extraction into trichloracetic acid, ascorbate is measured by the 2,4-dinitrophenylhydrazone method.

Reagents.

1. Diluent. Mix 200 ml sodium chloride solution, 8·5 g/l, 50 ml dextran, 60 g/l, and 2 ml sodium edetate, 100 g/l. Measure 12·5 ml portions into screw-cap containers and autoclave for 15 min at a pressure of 5 psi (35 kPa).
2. Trichloracetic acid solution, 50 g/l.
3. Colour reagent. Mix the following solutions in the proportions 20/1/1; 2,4-dinitrophenylhydrazine, 22 g/l in sulphuric acid, 10 mol/l; thiourea, 50 g/l water; copper sulphate, 6 g $CuSO_4,5H_2O/l$ water.
4. Sulphuric acid. Add 650 ml concentrated acid to 350 ml water.
5. Standard ascorbic acid solution, 10 mg/l in reagent (2).

Technique. Collect 6 to 10 ml venous blood and add at once to a container of diluent. Mix and allow the red cells to settle for 30 min before removing the supernatant. Mix this well and then centrifuge 10 ml for 15 min at 3000 r.p.m. Discard the supernatant, allowing the tube to drain for 30 s before adding 1·3 ml trichloracetic acid to the leucocyte-platelet deposit. Mix thoroughly, centrifuge and transfer 1·0 ml supernatant to a small test tube. In other tubes place 1·0 ml trichloracetic acid (blank), 0·5 ml trichloracetic acid plus 0·5 ml standard, and 1·0 ml standard. To each tube add 0·3 ml colour reagent and incubate at 37 °C for 4 h. Cool in iced water, add 2 ml sulphuric acid slowly, mix and read the absorbance at 520 nm, against the blank.

Carry out a leucocyte count on the remainder of the original leucocyte suspension using a 1 in 50 dilution in a Coulter counter. Subtract the background blank.

It is preferable to carry out the chemical and cytological measurements in duplicate.

Calculation.

$$\text{Supernatant ascorbate content (mg/l)} =$$

$$\frac{\text{Reading of unknown}}{\text{Reading of standard}} \times 5 \text{ or } 10$$

The factor depends on the standard used. If required, the linearity can be checked by using other volumes of the standard and making each up to 1·0 ml with trichloracetic acid.

Buffy layer (leucocyte + platelet) ascorbate ($\mu g/10^8$ leucocytes)

$$= \frac{\text{Supernatant ascorbate (mg/l)} \times 1·3}{\text{Leucocyte count}/\mu l \text{ supernatant}}$$

INTERPRETATION

The ascorbate concentration in leucocytes and platelets is similar in normal blood. If the number of either of these is abnormal, the above method gives a misleading estimate of the leucocyte ascorbate concentration. This can be estimated from the buffy layer result by dividing by 2·0 if the platelet and leucocyte counts are normal (Gibson *et al.*, 1966). In thrombocytopenia with normal leucocyte numbers, the factor is reduced to 1·3 and this figure may be used in relative thrombocytopenia, when the leucocyte count increases disproportionately to that of the platelets. In thrombocythaemic states, absolute or relative, the factor becomes 3·0.

The reference range for the buffy layer is 21 to 57 $\mu g/10^8$ leucocytes and for the leucocytes alone it is 11 to 21 $\mu g/10^8$ leucocytes.

Ascorbate and Disease

Daily Requirements. Ideally these are 100 to 200 mg in adults but 70 mg is sometimes taken as the minimum. Young children require about half the adult intake initially with an increase to adult levels by the onset of puberty.

Ascorbate Deficiency. The classical deficiency disease is scurvy, described originally in subjects whose diet lacked fresh fruit and vegetables. The deficiency leads to weakening of collagen in the walls of small blood vessels with the development of wide-spread haemorrhages in response to minimal trauma. Interference with collagen maturation is also apparent in the delayed healing of wounds and in the development of osteoporosis. In addition, an ascorbate-dependent anaemia is described.

Although florid scurvy is unusual in the UK, sub-clinical deficiency is not uncommon particularly among the very young and the elderly whose diet may be deficient in ascorbate-rich foodstuffs. This is more likely to happen in the winter. The body stores of the vitamin are small and in the absence of intake are likely to be depleted in 4 weeks. Ascorbate deficiency is said to be more common in patients with peptic ulcer, diabetes and epilepsy but this may well be a reflection of their dietary habits or drug therapy.

Massive doses of the vitamin have been given in an attempt to prevent or ameliorate the common cold. Opinions vary as to the efficacy but very large doses are partly excreted unchanged in the urine and partly metabolised to oxalate with the possible consequence of formation of calcium oxalate stones in the renal tract.

REFERENCES

Axelrod A. E., Spies T. D., Elvehjem C. A., Axelrod V. (1941). *J. Clin. Invest*; **20**: 229.

Baker H., Frank O. (1968). *Clinical Vitaminology*, p. 172. New York: Wiley.

Barker B. M., Bender D. A., eds (1980). *Vitamins in Medicine*, 4th ed., Vol. 1, London: William Heinemann Medical Books.

Barker B. M., Bender D. A., eds. (1982). *Vitamins in Medicine*, 4th ed., Vol. 2, London: William Heinemann Medical Books.

Bayoumi R. A., Rosalki S. B. (1976). *Clin. Chem*; **22**: 327.

Bieri J. G., Tolliver T. J., Catignani G. L. (1979). *Amer. J. Clin. Nutr*; **32**: 2143.

Bradley D. W., Hornbeck C. L. (1973). *Biochem. Med*; **7**: 78.

Braybrooke J., Lloyd B., Nattrass M., Alberti K. G. G. M. (1975). *Ann. Clin. Biochem*; **12**: 252.

Brin M. (1967). In *Newer Methods of Nutritional Biochemistry*, Vol. 3, (Albanese A., ed) p. 407. New York, London: Academic Press.

Bueding E., Stein M. H., Wortis H. (1941). *J. Biol. Chem*; **137**: 793.

Campbell D. A., Tonks E. L. (1949). *Brit. Med. J*; **2**: 1499.

Committee on Dietary Allowances. (1980). *Dietary Allowances*, 9th ed., National Academy of Sciences, Washington, D.C.

Dacie J. V., Lewis S. M. (1978). *Practical Haematology*, 6th ed. Edinburgh: Churchill Livingstone.

Davis R. E., Icke G. C. (1983). *Advances in Clinical Chemistry*; **23**: 93.

Dawson D. W., *et al.* (1980). *J. Clin. Pathol*; **33**: 234.

Denson K. W., Bowers E. F. (1961). *Clin. Sci*; **21**: 157.

Dugan R. E., Frigerio N. A., Siebert J. M. (1964). *Anal. Chem*; **36**: 114.

Gibson S. L. M., Moore F. M. L., Goldberg A. (1966). *Brit. Med. J*; **1**: 1152.

Gloster J. A., Harris P. (1962). *Clin. Chim. Acta*; **7**: 206.

György P., Pearson W. N., eds. (1967). *The Vitamins*, Vol. VI and VII. New York, London: Academic Press.

Haig C., Patek A. J. (1942). *J. Clin. Invest*; **21**: 377.

Harris L. J., Abbasy M. A. (1937). *Lancet*; **2**: 1429.

Harris L. J., Ray S. N. (1935). *Lancet*; **1**: 71, 462.

Haworth C., Oliver R. W. A., Swaile R. A. (1971). *Analyst*; **96**: 432.

Hegsted D. M., *et al.*, eds. (1976). *Nutrition Reviews' Present Knowledge in Nutrition*, 4th ed., The Nutrition Foundation Inc., Washington, D.C.

Hochberg M., Melnick D., Oser B. L. (1945). *J. Biol. Chem*; **158**: 265.

Huff J. W., Perlzweig W. A. (1947). *J. Biol. Chem*; **167**: 157.

Janiszowska W., Pennock J. F. (1976). *Vitamins and Hormones*; **34**: 77.

Johnson R. E., Sargent F., Robinson P. F., Consolazio F. C. (1945). *Ind. Eng. Chem. Anal. Ed*; **17**: 384.

Kaser M., Stekol J. A. (1943). *J. Lab. Clin. Med*; **28**: 904.

Kimble M. S. (1938–9). *J. Lab. Clin. Med*; **24**: 1055.

Krebs H. A. (1950). *Ann. Rev. Biochem*; **19**: 420.

Krebs H. A., Hume E. M. (1949). *MRC Special Report Series*, No. 264, Medical Research Council, London.

Lancet leading article. (1974). *Lancet*; **2**: 26.

Luhby A. L., Cooperman J. M., Teller D. N. (1959). *Proc. Soc. Exp. Biol. Med*; **101**: 350.

McCormick D. B., Olson A. E. (1984). In *Nutrition Reviews' Present Knowledge in Nutrition*, 5th ed. (Ohlson R. E., McCormick D. B., Olson A. E., eds) p. 217. The Nutrition Foundation Inc., Washington, DC.

Mason H. L., Williams R. D. (1942). *J. Clin. Invest*; **21**: 247.

Melnick D. (1942). *J. Nutr*; **24**: 139.

Melnick D., Field H., Jr. (1942). *J. Nutr*; **24**: 131.

Najjar V. A., Holt L. E., Jr. (1940). *Bull. Johns Hopk. Hosp*; **67**: 107.

Najjar V. A., Holt L. E., Jr. (1941). *Science*; **93**: 20.

Neal R. A. (1970). In *Proceedings, Workshop on Problems of Assessment and Alleviation of Malnutrition in the U.S.* (Hansen R. G., Munro H. N., eds) p. 129. National Institutes of Health, Bethesda.

Neeld J. B., Pearson W. N. (1963). *J. Nutr*; **79**: 454.

Noeypatimanond S., Watson-Williams E. J., Isräels M. C. G. (1966). *Lancet*; **1**: 454.

Pelletier O., Campbell J. A. (1962). *Anal. Biochem*; **3**: 60.

Price J. M., Brown R. R., Yess N. (1965). In *Advances in Metabolic Disorders*, Vol. 2. (Levine R., Luft R., eds) p. 159. New York, London: Academic Press.

Reynaulds R. D. (1983). *Fed. Proc*; **42**: 665.

Rodriguez M. S., Irvin M. I. (1980). In *Nutritional Requirements in Man*. (Irvin M. I., ed) p. 75. The Nutrition Foundation Inc., Washington, D.C.

Satoh K., Price J. M. (1958). *J. Biol. Chem*; **230**: 781.

Sauberlich H. E., *et al.* (1972). *Amer. J. Clin. Nutr*; **25**: 756.

Sauberlich H. E., Skala J. H., Dowdy R. P. (1974). In *Laboratory Tests for the Assessment of Nutritional Status*, pp. 74, 88, 91. Florida: CRC Press Inc.

Scriver C. R. (1979). *Nutrition and the Medical Doctor*; **5**: 2.

Sinclair H. M. (1947). In *Recent Advances in Clinical Pathology*, 1st ed. (Dyke S. C., ed) p. 180. London: Churchill Livingstone.

Slater E. C., Morell D. B. (1946). *Biochem. J*; **40**: 644, 652.

Truswell A. S. (1985). *Brit. Med. J*; **291**: 1033, 1103.

Waters H. M., *et al.* (1981). *J. Clin. Pathol*; **34**: 972.

Wenger J., Kirsner J. B., Palmer W. L. (1957). *Amer. J. Med*; **22**: 373.

Yudkin S. (1941). *Biochem J*; **35**: 551.

36

DRUGS AND POISONS

INTRODUCTION

This chapter is divided into three parts, each dealing with a particular aspect of toxicology. The structure of each part is broadly similar, that is a short introduction describing relevant pharmacology, followed by a concise description and comparison of associated methodology and the final major portion dealing more fully with the determination and interpretation of individual compounds or classes of compound. A brief outline of each part follows. Units for drug concentration are not universally agreed. *Mass* units are used here.

1. Therapeutic Drug Monitoring

There are differences in the rate of metabolism of many drugs between individuals and for long-term treatment of chronic disorders it is important to maintain the plasma concentration of a drug between certain limits for optimal activity. Individual adjustment of dose to match the rate of metabolism is needed to avoid low concentrations which would result in inadequate control, or abnormally high ones with the possibility of toxic effects.

This part covers the pharmacology, determination and interpretation of plasma concentration data for those drugs for which there is a sound pharmacological reason for controlling therapy by measurement of plasma concentrations.

2. Acute Poisoning and Emergency Methods

Drugs may be taken in large doses in acute poisoning. Most of these cases are of self-poisoning, not done with suicidal intent but in an effort to attract attention to problems which loom large in the mind of the patient. A minority are true suicidal attempts and a similar number may be accidental or homicidal poisonings. Death may occur in self-poisoning and in all cases is more likely the larger the dose of the poison. In many cases there will be no specific therapy but proper management, in an intensive care unit for the more serious cases, is assisted by recognition of the poison. This can involve examination of blood, urine and gastric aspirate. It is often sufficient to perform qualitative analyses, but in a few cases actual determination of drug concentration is necessary. The publication *Hospital Treatment of Acute Poisoning* (DHSS, HM (68) 92, 1968) required hospital laboratories to be capable of determining salicylate, barbiturates and iron in blood or gastric aspirate, ethanol and carboxyhaemoglobin in blood. Screening tests for phenothiazines in urine were also required.

In addition to these, there are a few other instances where knowledge of the plasma concentration will materially affect therapy and, ultimately, the outcome. A brief discussion is also included of those drugs in which a knowledge of the plasma concentration does not usually affect the treatment.

3. Drugs of Abuse

Drug abuse is now a serious problem in this country and urine testing for drugs of abuse is an essential part of the treatment of drug abusers. The techniques described may also be of use to those who wish to identify the drugs involved in cases of acute poisoning. Identification of some inhaled solvents or ingested purgatives is included in this section.

Sources of Information

The subject of toxicology can not be dealt with adequately in a single chapter in a book of this nature; hence further information on methodology and interpretation must be sought in the vast literature on the subject. Especially useful are the books or reviews by Richens and Marks (1981), Bochner *et al.* (1978), Vale and Meredith (1981), Baselt (1982), Dreisbach (1980), Moffat (1986), and Stead and Moffat (1983).

The local units of the Regional Drug Information Service are staffed by experienced, highly qualified pharmacists who have ready access to a large amount of relevant information on all aspects of toxicology and therapeutic drug monitoring. The clinical chemist involved in providing a toxicology service will find it well worth while establishing a good working relationship with the staff of these units. A list of the Regional Drug Information Units with telephone numbers is given in Table 36.1.

The structures, synonyms and applications of approximately 10 000 compounds are listed in the Merck Index (1976) and details of a large number of drugs including composition, uses, doses, metabolism, etc., are given in Martindale (1982). An up-to-date list of ethical drugs is published monthly as the Monthly Index of Medical Specialities (MIMS) by Haymarket Publishing Limited, London. Fuller details of all current drugs are contained in the British National Formulary published jointly, each year, by the British Medical Association and the Pharmaceutical Society.

The above texts are the essential minimum for the hospital biochemistry laboratory wishing to assist the medical staff with the toxicological problems with which they are frequently faced.

PART 1. THERAPEUTIC DRUG MONITORING

Pharmacology

Administration and Absorption. Drugs may be administered by a variety of routes. Those drugs for which assays of plasma concentration will be required are most often administered intravenously (i.v.) or orally. Intravenous administration usually results in immediate, effective and predictable plasma concentrations, but its use is generally restricted to hospitalised patients. Oral administration, while generally convenient for the patient and not requiring medical supervision, usually results in very variable plasma concentrations. These depend mainly on (1) the physico-chemical properties of the drug, e.g. its stability at gastric and intestinal pHs; (2) the product formulation, e.g. how rapidly and completely the tablet disintegrates; (3) timing of the dose in relation to ingestion of food; and (4) the integrity of intestinal absorption mechanisms.

TABLE 36.1
Regional Drug Information Service.

Local Unit	Telephone Number
Aberdeen	0224–681818 Extension 2316
Belfast	*0232–240503 Extension 2032
Birmingham	*021–554 3801
Bristol	0272–20256 Direct line·
Cardiff	0222–759541 Direct line
	*0222–569200 Direct line
Dublin	*0001–745588 Direct line
Dundee	0382–60111 Extension 2351
Edinburgh	*031–229 2477 Extension 2234
	*031–228 2441 (SPIB Viewdata)
Glasgow	041–552 3535 Extension 4407/4486
Guildford	0483–504312 Direct line
Inverness	0463–234157 Extension 288
Ipswich	0473–712233 Extension 4322/4323
Leeds	*0532–430715 Direct line
Leicester	0533–555779 Direct line
Liverpool	051–236 4620 Extension 2126/7/8
London (Guy's Hospital)	*01–407 7600 Extension 2568
	*01–635 9191
London (London Hospital)	01–247 5454 Extension 147/62
London (Northwick Park)	01–423 4535 Direct line
Manchester	061–276 6270 Direct line
	061–276 6110 Direct line
Newcastle	0632–321525 Direct line
	*0632–325131
Reading	0734–875111 Extension 302
Southampton	0703–780323 Direct line
Sutton Coldfield	021–378 2211 Extension 3565

* Poisons Information Centres

Distribution. While absorption into the blood stream is taking place, the drug is also distributed into various 'compartments' depending on its lipid solubility, pKa, the pH of body fluids, the extent of protein binding and regional blood flow. Water-soluble drugs are generally confined to the extracellular space whereas lipid solubility enables drugs to pass into intracellular spaces. Many drugs also become bound in varying degrees to plasma and tissue proteins. Yet others are selectively concentrated in specific tissues. Pharmacologists use the concept of 'apparent volume of distribution' to indicate that proportion of the total body load of drug which is present in the blood. An apparent volume of distribution, Vd, of less than 0.3 l/kg body weight suggests that most of the drug is present in the plasma (e.g. salicylate $Vd = 0.2$ l/kg of body weight) whereas a large apparent volume of distribution (> 3 l/kg body weight) suggests that most of the drug is bound to tissues (e.g. digoxin $Vd = 10$ l/kg).

The mass of drug which is absorbed and the relative rates of its absorption and distribution determine the maximum plasma concentration and the time after ingestion at which this maximum is achieved.

Elimination. Drugs may be removed from the body by a number of processes and routes. The most common process is simple hepatic modification, e.g.

acetylation or hydroxylation followed by conjugation with, e.g., glucuronic acid to form a less toxic, more water-soluble compound which can be excreted in the urine. Drugs which are already strongly polar are frequently excreted unchanged and others which cannot readily be rendered water-soluble are excreted predominantly in the bile.

These three phases, i.e. absorption, distribution and elimination, are common to all drugs and are reflected in the changes in plasma drug concentration following oral ingestion as shown in Fig. 36.1. This curve does not represent any particular drug. Those with rapid absorption and distribution phases and slow elimination are typified by digoxin(p. 965), while others have distribution and elimination phases which are indistinguishable.

Half-time. The elimination of a drug from plasma may be classified according to its half-time ($t_{\frac{1}{2}}$), which is analogous to the half-life of radioactive decay, and is the time required for the plasma concentration of a drug to fall to half its value. The dosage interval is generally a multiple or sub-multiple of the plasma half-time of the drug to be prescribed, and is usually chosen to minimise the difference between peaks and troughs in plasma concentration. This is important if the drug exhibits a narrow 'therapeutic window', i.e. the concentration range between the minimum effective concentration and the toxic threshold.

Account must be taken of these pre-dose troughs and post-dose peaks when sampling blood for concentration measurement. For most drugs the ideal time to sample blood is immediately pre-dose. This is especially true for drugs such as digoxin which have a very high but transient post-absorption peak well into the toxic range. For those drugs in which peak and trough concentrations do not differ by more than 20%, timing of blood sample is perhaps less critical.

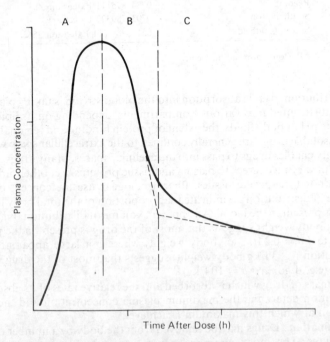

Fig. 36.1. The Change of Drug Concentration with Time.
The three phases are: A, absorption; B, distribution; C, elimination.

When drug treatment is started or when the dosage is changed, it will be seen from Fig. 36.2 that at least 5 half-times must elapse before the dosage change has exerted its full effect and a new 'steady state' is established. In the case of phenytoin, which has a mean $t_{\frac{1}{2}}$ of 20 h, this will be 5×20 h, i.e. 4–5 days. From the foregoing, it would be misleading therefore to adjust a patient's therapy on a measure of the plasma concentration made too soon after a previous dosage change whether this was an increase (Fig. 36.2(A)) or a decrease (Fig. 36.2(B)).

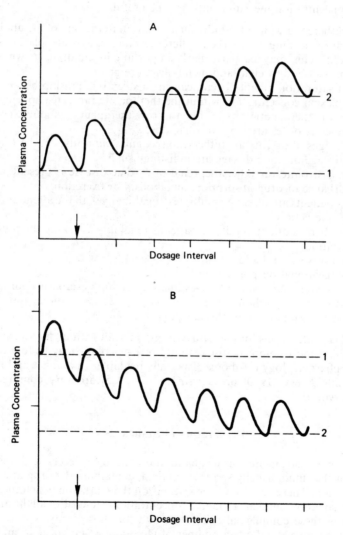

Fig. 36.2. Changes in Drug Concentration after Adjustment of Dose.
The time intervals on the horizontal axis are "half-times"; 1 = previous steady state concentration; 2 = new steady state concentration.
A. Dose increased at arrow. B. Dose decreased at arrow.

Rationale of Therapeutic Drug Monitoring

Therapeutic drug monitoring imposes a considerable drain on laboratory resources and must be held tightly in check if the indiscriminate use of expensive resources is to be avoided. It is essential, therefore, to have a clear laboratory policy as to which drugs will be monitored by plasma assay, under what circumstances and how frequently. To aid the laboratory in these decisions, Richens and Warrington (1979) outlined the relevant pharmacology of a number of commonly used drugs and suggested the following list of criteria against which the request for an assay should assessed.

Drug concentration measurements may be useful:

1. when there is a wide inter-individual variation in the rate of metabolism of the drug, leading to marked differences in steady-state plasma concen-trations. This may be particularly important in children, in whom dif-ferences in body weight and metabolism are great.
2. when saturation kinetics occur, causing a steep relationship between dose and plasma concentration within the therapeutic range (e.g. phenytoin).
3. when the therapeutic ratio is low (narrow therapeutic window), i.e. when therapeutic doses are close to toxic doses.
4. when signs of toxicity are difficult to recognise clinically, or where signs of overdosage or underdosage are indistinguishable.
5 when gastrointestinal, hepatic, renal or cardiac disease is present, causing disturbance of drug absorption, metabolism or excretion.
6. when patients are receiving multiple drug therapy with the attendant risk of drug interaction.
7. when there is doubt about the patient's reliability in taking the prescribed medication.

To this list we would add:

8. for educational purposes.
9. for research purposes; e.g. re-evaluation of long-established drugs pre-viously used without the benefits of concentration monitoring. Antidepressants fall into this category.

Special considerations for individual drugs are dealt with under the particular drug name. A more complete discussion of pharmacology may be found in any standard pharmacology text book. Especially readable is Laurence and Bennett (1980) while Avery (1980) or Gilman *et al.* (1985) are very comprehensive reference works.

Preparation of Standards

Calibration of instruments for the quantitation of drugs in body fluids requires a sample of that fluid, usually serum or plasma, containing the drug at a known concentration. There are a few preparations on the market in which the analyst can be reasonably confident about the concentrations stated. For all the drugs not included in these commercial calibrators and for those analysts who wish to prepare their own standards a number of factors must be borne in mind.

1. Parent drugs and metabolites are not yet all available in catalogues. Where we have been able to locate these, they are included in the method descriptions. For drugs and metabolites not so listed it is necessary to write to the manufacturer. The process of obtaining a supply is rather lengthy and

usually involves signing a form to affirm that the compound supplied will not be used in treatment. Our practice is to request a small amount (0·5–1·0 g) for standardisation purposes. In many instances this is provided *gratis*.

2. It is essential to remember that therapeutic ranges usually apply to the base material of a drug and not its salt. The reader will have seen both 'valproate' and 'valproic acid' referred to in the literature. When preparing standards using salts, therefore, allowance must be made for the difference in molecular weights.

3. Usually only small amounts of the drug and its metabolite will be available in solid form from which to prepare standards; hence it is important to conserve the material. Our practice is to prepare 100 ml of a stock solution in an appropriate solvent, e.g. methanol and to store this at 4 °C. As soon as the stock solution is prepared, a small, accurately measured volume of this is evaporated to dryness and redissolved in a solvent, e.g. 0·1 mol/l hydrochloric acid for which Moffat (1986) quotes an absorption coefficient for the drug in question. The figure obtained should be close to Moffat's quoted value and, if recorded, can be used to check the concentration of the stock solution on subsequent occasions, after warming to room temperature.

The nominal concentration of the stock solution is usually 100–200 mg/l. This concentration avoids the necessity to weigh amounts less than 10 mg, provides concentrations high enough for checking absorption coefficients and aids the conservation of small supplies of material.

4. Preparation of the serum standard is achieved by evaporating to dryness in one flask the appropriate quantities of all the compounds to be included in the standard. The dried material is then dissolved in drug-free serum. This is subdivided into suitable volumes and stored at −20 °C.

Quality Assurance

There are now several commercial control sera available which cover a wide range of drugs and concentrations. These should be employed in all assays, as with other analytical methods in clinical chemistry, in order to monitor changes in calibration and precision between batches. There are also several quality assurance schemes for the most common drug assays, and it is clearly in the interest of a laboratory providing a therapeutic drug monitoring service to participate in these schemes. In addition to monitoring the performance of an assay they assist in the choice of method in terms of bias and precision. For some drugs no commercial material and no QC scheme exists. Drug-free serum which has been 'spiked' with the drug (and, if appropriate, the metabolite) of interest can be subdivided and frozen to serve as a control material if nothing else is available.

The low specificity of some assay techniques and the close similarity of structure and pharmacology of many drugs makes the provision of a reliable, routine assay service very difficult at times. Unrelated drugs having the same retention times after chromatographic methods have been applied, provide a major source of error for which the analyst must be constantly on the alert. Interferences of this nature, when discovered, must be reported in the relevant press to alert all users of the same method to the problem. The availability of two methods based on different analytical principles for the same drug, such as high performance liquid chromatography (HPLC) and an immunoassay method, can be very useful in resolving these difficulties. The development of ultraviolet detectors for HPLC which can perform an absorbance scan over a range of wavelengths is potentially useful in avoiding misidentification of a sample peak.

ANTIASTHMATICS

Theophylline

Theophylline (1,3-dimethylxanthine) is used to relieve asthma and to decrease the chance of apnoea in premature infants. It acts by relaxing bronchial smooth muscle and will therefore lessen the likelihood of bronchospasm.

The drug is usually administered orally, after which it is rapidly absorbed, however it may also be given by intravenous infusion should occasion demand. Theophylline is rapidly distributed to tissues, has an apparent Vd ranging from 0·3 to 0·7 l/kg body weight and is 40–65 % protein-bound. It is metabolised to other methylxanthines, especially caffeine, which also have bronchodilator properties. A number of metabolic conversions are involved, some of which are saturable and these cause a greater-than-predicted increase in plasma theophylline concentration following a dosage increment. Elimination, therefore, does not follow strict zero-order kinetics, it is decreased with diminished hepatic or renal function and also by the concurrent administration of other drugs. Theophylline elimination is enhanced by cigarette smoking. In the neonate caffeine can also be metabolised to theophylline. .

Side-effects of theophylline therapy include nausea, headaches and insomnia, usually observed at the start of therapy and avoided by slowly increasing the dose. The concentration-related effects include vomiting, diarrhoea, tremor and cardiovascular effects and death as the concentration rises (Jacobs *et al.*, 1976).

The relevant pharmacological parameters are given in Table 36.2 and theophylline metabolism is shown in Fig. 36.3.

TABLE 36.2
Pharmacological Data for Antiasthmatics.

	Therapeutic Range (mg/l)	Toxic Threshold (mg/l)	Half-time (h)	Vd (h)
Theophylline				
Adults	5–20	25	3–11	0·3–0·7
Neonates			approx. 30	
Caffeine				
Adults	10–20	25	2·3–4·5	0·4
Neonates			approx. 100	
'Total xanthines' in neonates, i.e. theophylline + caffeine		25		

Methodology

A number of immunoassays are available for the determination of theophylline such as the EMIT assay by Syva and the Fluorescence Polarisation Assay produced by Ames for the Fluorostat and by Abbott for the TDx system. The

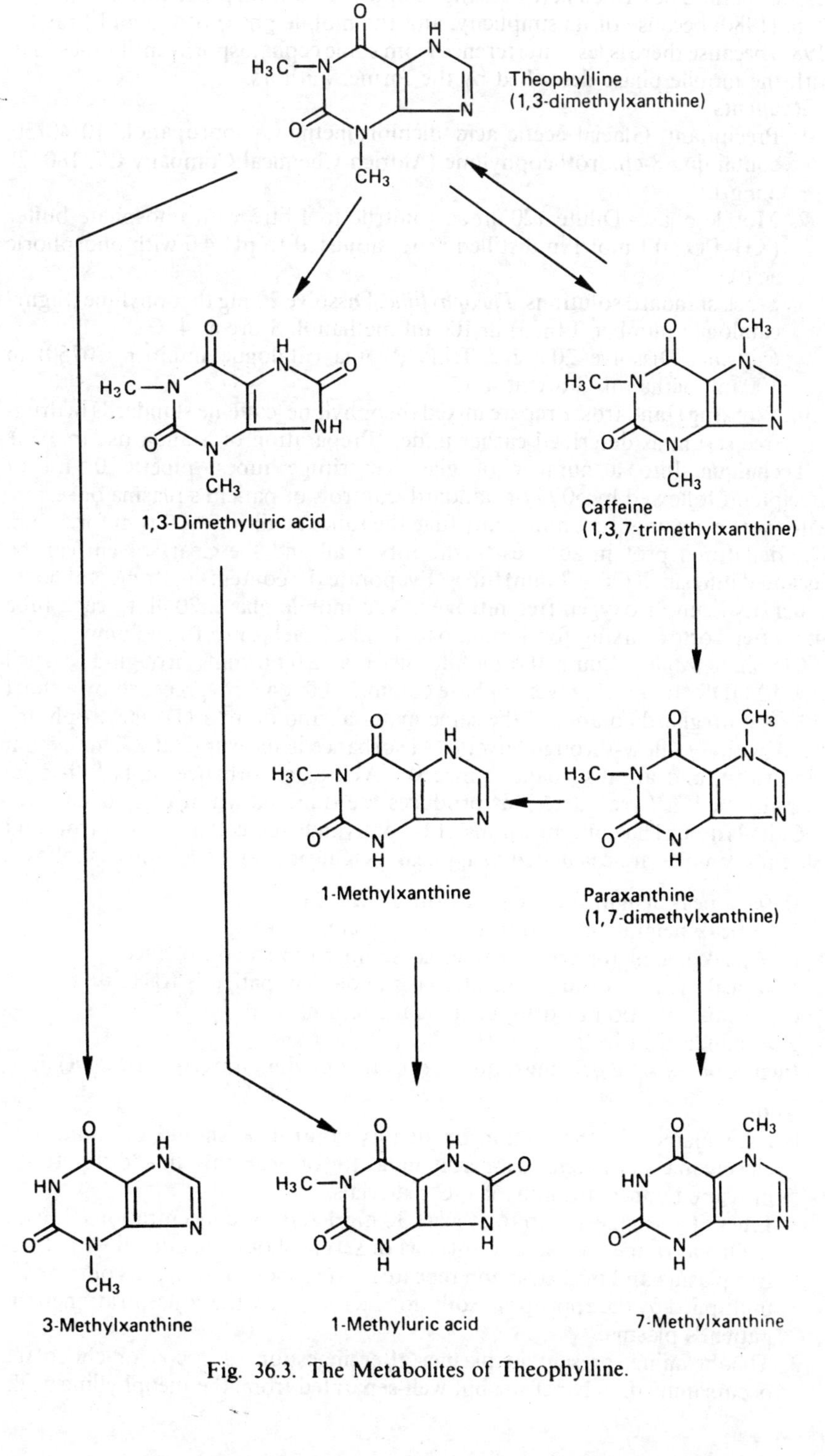

Fig. 36.3. The Metabolites of Theophylline.

HPLC method described here uses the sample preparation procedure of Weidner *et al.* (1980) because of its simplicity, and the mobile phase of Ou and Frawley (1982) because there is less interference from some cephalosporin antibiotics than with the mobile phase described by the former authors.

Reagents

1. Precipitant. Glacial acetic acid–dichloromethane–isopropanol, 10/40/50, containing 8-chlorotheophylline (Aldrich Chemical Company C7, 180–7), 2 mg/l.
2. Mobile phase. Dilute 120 ml acetonitrile to 1 litre with phosphate buffer (KH_2PO_4 0·1 mol/l in distilled water adjusted to pH 4·0 with phosphoric acid).
3. Stock standard solutions. *Theophylline.* Dissolve 20 mg theophylline (Sigma catalogue number T1633) in 100 ml methanol. Store at 4 °C.
   Caffeine. Dissolve 20 mg caffeine (Sigma catalogue number C0750) in 100 ml methanol. Store at 4 °C.
4. Working standards. Prepare mixed theophylline/caffeine standards in drug-free serum as described earlier under 'Preparation of Standards', (p. 936).

Technique. Into a number of glass centrifuge tubes, pipette 0·5 ml of precipitant followed by 50 μl of standard, controls or patient's plasma or serum. After vortex mixing for 1 min, centrifuge the tubes at about 2000 rpm for 5 min. The denatured protein adheres to the tube wall and the clear solvent can be decanted into small (70 × 7 mm) tubes. Evaporate the contents to dryness at 60 °C under a stream of oxygen-free nitrogen. Add mobile phase, 20 μl, to each tube and, after vortex mixing for 1 min, load 10 μl of each onto the column.

Chromatography. Pump the mobile phase at 2·0 ml/min through a Partisil type 10 ODS (10 μ C18) reverse-phase column, 200 × 4 mm, preceded by a short (40 × 4 mm) guard column of the same material, and on to a UV spectrophotometer with 8 μl flow-through cuvette. Absorbance is measured at 272 nm, 8 nm bandwidth, and an absorbance range 0·1 AUFS (absorbance units full-scale) output to a 1 mV recorder. This produces the trace shown in Fig. 36.4.

Calculation. The concentrations of theophylline and caffeine in controls and patient's samples are calculated using peak height or peak area ratios as follows:

If Ds = peak height (or area) of drug in standard trace;
Dt = peak height (or area) of drug in patient's trace;
Is = peak height (or area) of internal standard in standard trace;
It = peak height (or area) of internal standard in patient's trace;
Cd = concentration of drug in standard serum;
R = standard ratio for drug D;
then $R = (Is \times Cd)/Ds$ mg/l and serum theophylline (mg/l) = $(Dt \times R)/It$.

Notes.

1. As explained in the section on quality control, R should be monitored closely in every batch, as an early indicator of problems, in addition to the measured concentrations of QC materials.
2. Linearity is achieved up to at least 30 mg/l and for concentrations outside the linear range, the patient's plasma or serum should be diluted with drug-free plasma and the extraction repeated. The concentration thus obtained is multiplied by the appropriate dilution factor to give the concentration in the patient's plasma.
3. Theobromine, present in plasma after ingestion of cocoa or chocolate, occurs immediately before, but well-separated from, the theophylline peak.

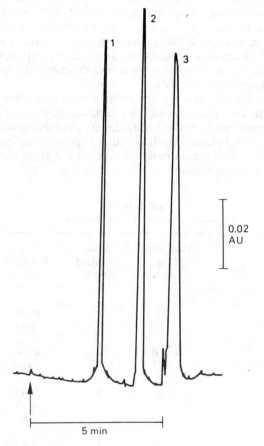

Fig. 36.4. The Separation of Theophylline by HPLC.
1 = Theophylline; 2 = 8-chlorotheophylline (internal standard); 3 = caffeine. The arrow indicates the time of injection.

4. As with all HPLC methods, the life of the analytical column is improved if a short 'pre-column' is used. Considerable economies are possible if the mobile phase is recycled. Reducing the flow-rate of the mobile phase to about 0·2 ml/min after use allows the system to remain in 'stand-by' mode for emergency assays especially out of hours. It is then simply a matter of resetting the flow to 2 ml/min, turning on the photometer and recorder and the system is ready to receive the extracted samples for analysis.

ANTICONVULSANTS

The more common anticonvulsant drugs used in various forms of epilepsy are hydantoins, succinimides, oxazolidones and barbiturates. These and other anticonvulsants have structural similarities as shown in Fig. 36.5 (A–D). Phenytoin, primidone, carbamazepine and phenobarbitone are the most commonly used drugs for the treatment of *grand mal* attacks and are often used in combination. The succinimides and oxazolidones are mainly used to control *petit mal* attacks. Some of the other drugs may act by modifying the metabolism of the major anticonvulsants. The benzodiazepines are mainly used i.v. to achieve early control in status epilepticus although modern views favour the use of i.v. phenytoin. With the exception of phenytoin, all the above anticonvulsants have linear dose–concentration response curves, i.e. doubling the dose causes a doubling of the plasma concentration.

With all anticonvulsants, there is often a wide variation in plasma concentration with time in any individual patient. This variation may have several sources, e.g. variation in compliance from day to day, dietary changes, variation in sample time in relation to dose, between-batch variation in pharmaceutical preparation and analytical error. The clinician must take account of these variations when interpreting plasma concentrations.

TABLE 36.3
Pharmacological Data for Anticonvulsants.

	Therapeutic Range (mg/l)	Toxic Threshold (mg/l)	Half-time (h)	Mean Vd (l/kg)
Carbamazepine				
Adults	5–12	15	10–30	1·4
Children			8–19	
Ethosuximide				
Adults	40–100	150	40–60	0·7
Children			30	
Phenobarbitone				
Adults	15–30	40	50–150	0·9
Children			40–70	
Neonate < 5 days			200	
Phenytoin				
Adults	7–20	25	7–60†	0·6
Neonate < 2 days			80	
Primidone	5–10*	25	3–20	0·6
Valproate	50–100	200	6–20	0·2

† = crude estimate due to concentration–dependent kinetics.
* = interpretation requires knowledge of phenobarbitone concentration.

Carbamazepine

Pharmacology

Carbamazepine is used prophylactically in both adults and children with generalised tonic-clonic (*grand mal*) and partial seizures. It is thought to restrict the speed of epileptic discharge by reducing post-tetanic potentiation (Julien and Hollister, 1975). It has also been shown to have a wide spectrum of other actions including sedative, anticholinergic and antidiuretic effects some of which may explain its side-effects. The most common of these are dose-related and include ataxia, diplopia, drowsiness and blurred vision (Livingston *et al.*, 1974). Less commonly, skin reactions, haematological changes and some hepatic effects have been described.

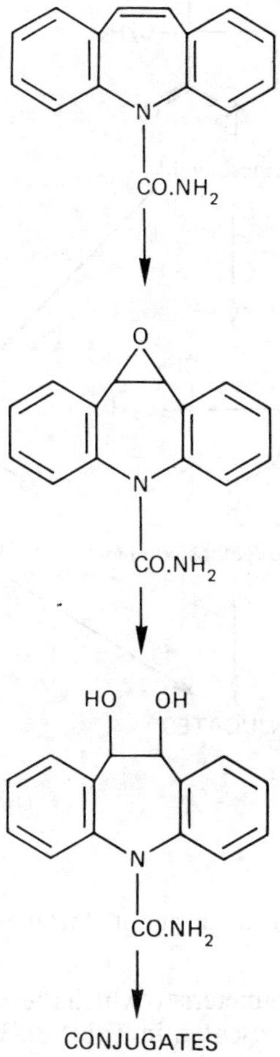

Carbamazepine

Carbamazepine
10, 11-epoxide

10, 11-Dihydroxy-
carbamazepine

CONJUGATES

Fig. 36.5A. Carbamazepine and its Metabolites.

Absorption of carbamazepine is slow and variable following an oral dose; the peak is reached within 2 to 24 h. It is highly lipophilic and distributes rapidly with an apparent Vd ranging between 0·96 and 2·0 l/kg body weight. Carbamazepine is metabolised to its 10,11-epoxide which is reported to have anticonvulsant properties in rats although this is not yet established in humans (Frigerio and Morselli, 1975) and which constitutes about 30–50% of the total plasma carbamazepine concentration in chronically treated patients. The usefulness of measuring plasma concentrations of the epoxide, although strongly advocated by some groups, is not yet thoroughly established. The major metabolite in urine is the trans-10,11-dihydroxide which constitutes about 20% of the daily excretion (Fig. 36.5A, above).

Carbamazepine induces its own elimination and hence dosage is gradually increased at the commencement of therapy. Phenytoin and phenobarbitone also induce carbamazepine metabolism and there is a higher elimination rate in children and in women during pregnancy. Elimination, which is almost entirely (99%) hepatic, is diminished in liver disease.

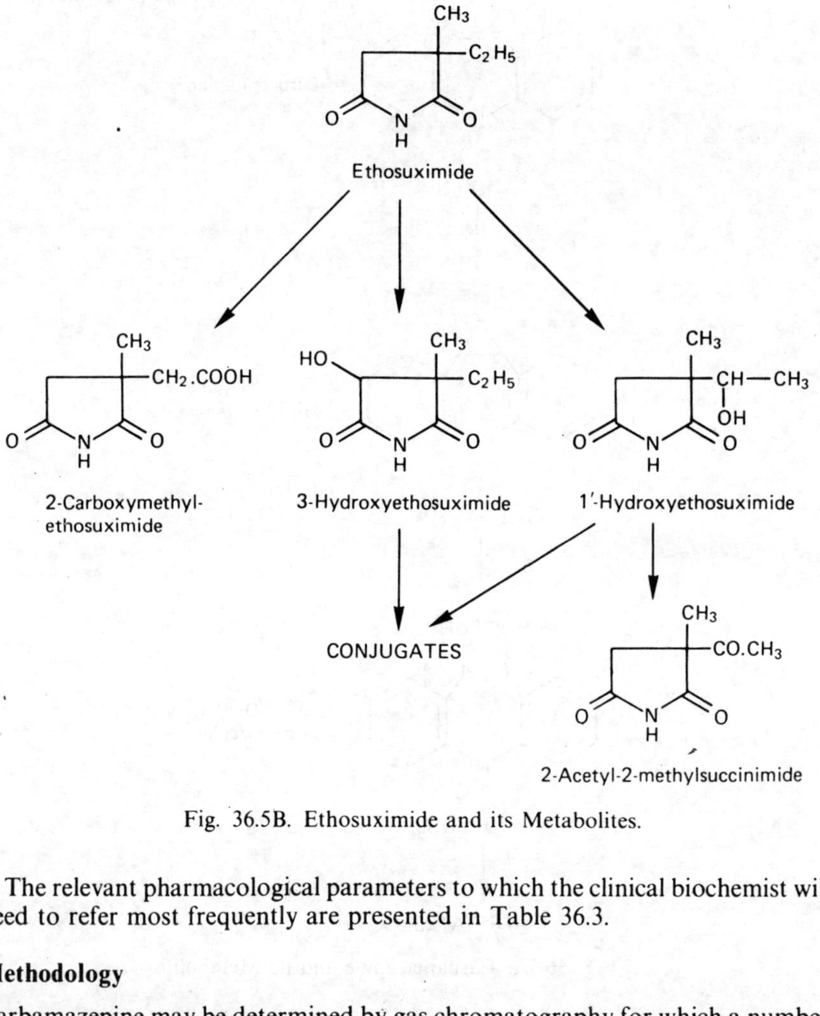

Fig. 36.5B. Ethosuximide and its Metabolites.

The relevant pharmacological parameters to which the clinical biochemist will need to refer most frequently are presented in Table 36.3.

Methodology

Carbamazepine may be determined by gas chromatography for which a number of methods exist (Morselli and Frigerio, 1975). The most popular current methods however are the homogeneous immunoassays, e.g. EMIT (enzyme multiplied immunoassay) outlined on p. 125 and described fully by Schottelius (1978) and also HPLC which is described here. The major advantage of chromatographic methods is that they allow simultaneous multiple drug determinations on a single sample. Hence, the method described here includes the determinations of some other anticonvulsants and so will be referred to in later sections.

Determination of Anticonvulsants by HPLC

Anticonvulsant drugs are extracted from buffered plasma into chloroform containing an internal standard. After evaporating the chloroform, the drugs are redissolved in mobile phase, separated on a reverse-phase column and detected by their UV absorption. The method is linear to about twice the upper limit of the therapeutic range for each drug.

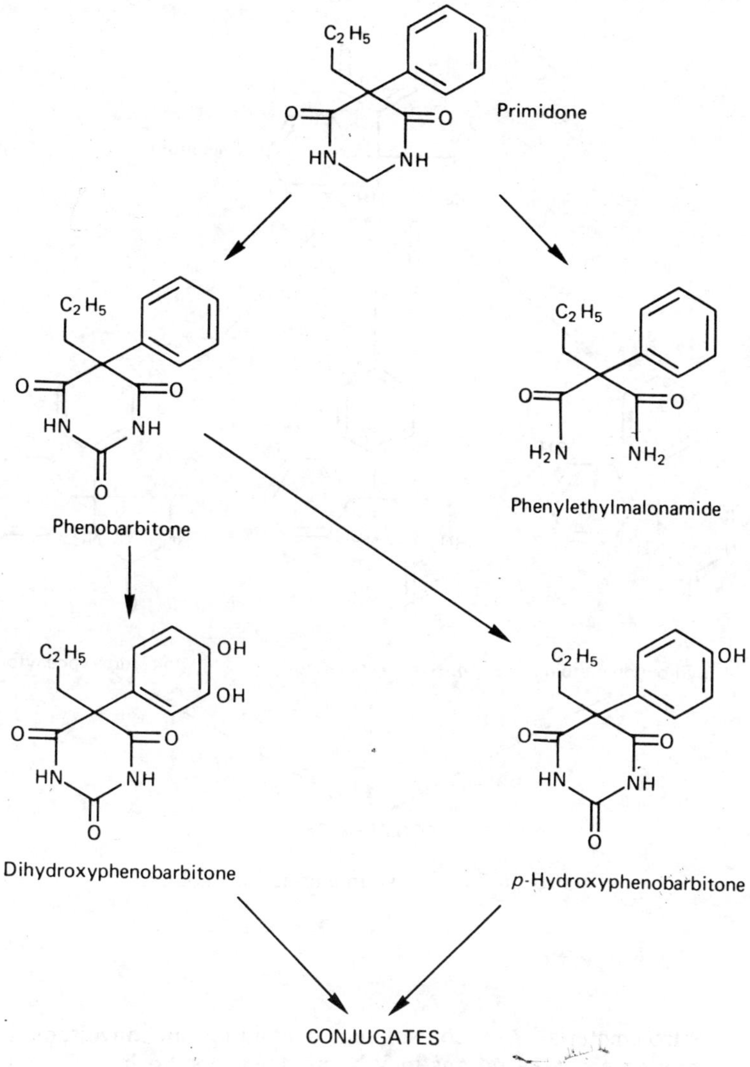

Fig. 36.5C. Primidone, Phenobarbitone and Their Metabolites.

Reagents.
1. Phosphate buffer, 100 mmol/l KH_2PO_4, pH 8·0.
2. Stock internal standard solution, 20 mg methyl diphenylhydantoin in 100 ml chloroform; stable indefinitely at 4 °C.
3. Extractant. Dilute 20 ml stock internal standard to 1 litre with chloroform.
4. Serum standard, serum containing each of the drugs to be assayed at a concentration of 20 mg/l. This can be prepared by weighing pure drug substance and dissolving in drug-free serum, or a commercial preparation such as Seronorm Pharmaca AED (Nyegaard and Company, Oslo) can be used. After preparation or reconstitution, portions of about 110 μl can be stored at − 20 °C and thawed when required for use.

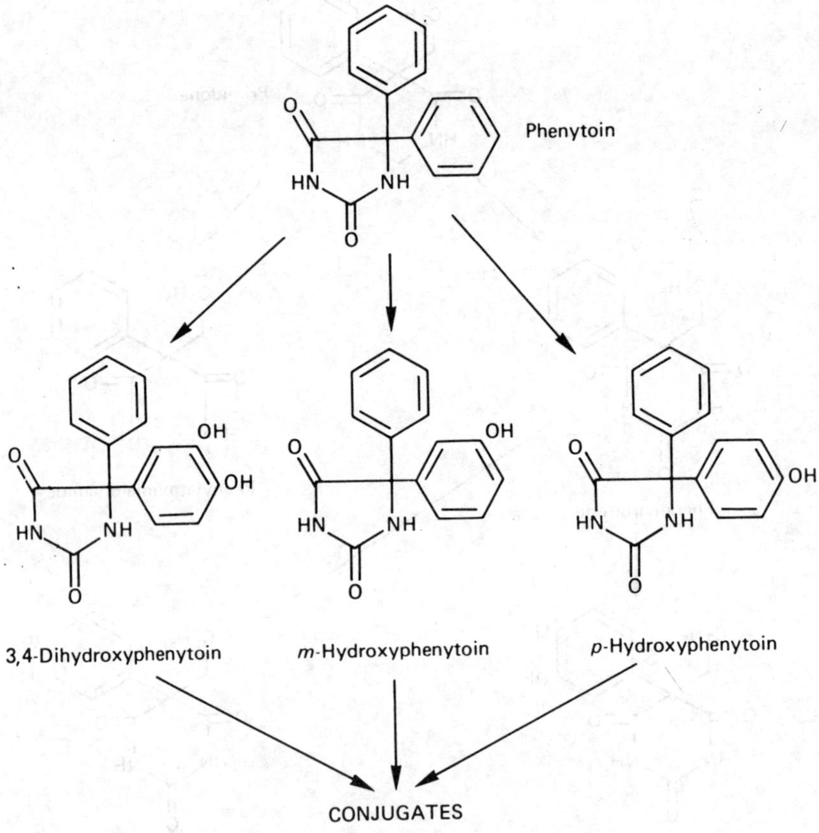

Fig. 36.5D. Phenytoin and its Metabolites.

5. Control material. Any control sera containing anticonvulsant drugs at appropriate concentrations may be used, e.g. Lyphochek TDM Control (Biorad, Watford, Herts).
6. Mobile phase, acetonitrile (chromatography grade) 300 ml, tetrahydrofuran (chromatography grade) 70 ml, glacial acetic acid 0·5 ml, diluted with distilled water to 1 litre. This solution should then be lightly 'degassed' by applying a vacuum from a venturi pump until it 'boils' and then maintaining this for a further 30 s. The base line produced by this mobile phase should be free from 'noise'. Distilled water, unlike deionised water, is virtually gas-free and particle-free if it is fresh and therefore will not usually need filtering. If collected in a reservoir, it is important to check that algae are not present since such particles cause base-line 'noise'.

The position of the carbamazepine peak can be altered in relation to the other peaks by adjusting the amount of tetrahydrofuran used in the mobile phase. A decrease in the tetrahydrofuran concentration delays the elution of this drug.

Technique. To 100 μl buffer in 10 ml glass centrifuge tubes, add 100 μl of patient's serum, standard serum or control serum. After mixing for a few seconds add 1 ml extractant, vortex-mix for 1 min and then centrifuge for 5 min at 2000 rpm. Transfer the lower extractant layers carefully by Pasteur pipette to small (70 × 7 mm) glass tubes and evaporate the extractant under oxygen-free nitrogen at a temperature not exceeding 65 °C. To each tube add 100 μl mobile phase and, after vortex-mixing for 30 s, load 10 μl onto the column.

The HPLC conditions are as follows: Mobile phase is pumped at 1·5 ml/min through a Partisil 5 ODS (5 μ, C18 silica) column, 125 × 4 mm preceded by a guard column (20 × 4 mm) of the same material, and then through a UV detector set at 205 nm, 8 nm bandwidth, range 0·1 AUFS, the signal from which is sent to a 1 mV chart recorder or integrator. A typical trace is shown in Fig. 36.6. The calculation of results for each drug from peak height or area ratios is as described under theophylline in the previous section.

Considerable economies can be achieved by recycling the mobile phase as 1 litre of mobile phase will produce satisfactory base-line, peak shape and separation for 2–4 weeks depending on the number of samples analysed. When not in use, the flow rate is decreased to about 0·2 ml/min.

Ethosuximide

Pharmacology

Ethosuximide is an antiepileptic drug which is effective against *petit mal* (absence) seizures and totally inactive in *grand mal*. Unlike phenytoin, it prevents the spread of low frequency repetitive neuronal discharges in the cerebral cortex (Englander *et al.*, 1979).

The drug is well absorbed following oral administration resulting in peak plasma concentrations within 2 to 4 h. A syrup is available for children unable to take the gelatin capsules. The mean Vd is 0·62 and 0·69 l/kg body weight respectively in adults and children. Less than 1 % of the circulating drug is protein-bound and therefore salivary concentrations closely resemble plasma concentrations (Horning *et al.*, 1977).

Ethosuximide is extensively metabolised in the liver (Fig. 36.5B, p. 944) by a variety of demethylation and hydroxylation reactions, although the pathway is not yet fully established (Glazko, 1975), and about 30 % of the drug is excreted unchanged. None of the recognised metabolites have antiepileptic activity and there is no induction of hepatic enzymes by ethosuximide. If ethosuximide is added to the therapeutic regimen of a patient with steady-state concentrations of phenytoin, these will rise. It is unclear whether this is due to competition for a common elimination process or inhibition of the enzymes involved.

The most common side-effects of ethosuximide are gastric upset, nausea, vomiting and anorexia. These occur early in therapy in about 20 % of patients and are minimised by taking the drug with food. Some patients also report headache, fatigue, lethargy and dizziness early in therapy and these symptoms usually disappear with time. Rarely, skin rashes and fever are reported while bone marrow depression and the presence of antinuclear antibodies have been observed in some patients.

Ethosuximide has a linear dose–plasma concentration curve which increases in steepness throughout childhood and hence the dosage required to maintain the desired plasma concentration is not strictly related to body weight. The major reason for frequent monitoring, once satisfactory control and its associated plasma concentration is achieved, however, is that of patient compliance. Most

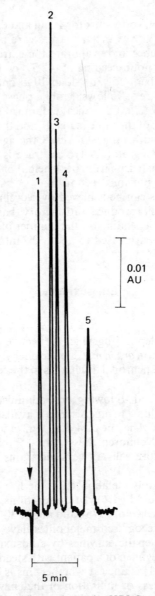

Fig. 36.6. The Separation of Anticonvulsants by HPLC.
  1 = Primidone; 2 = phenobarbitone; 3 = carbamazepine; 4 = phenytoin; 5 = MPPH
(internal standard). The arrow indicates the time of injection.

patients on ethosuximide are children; their weight gain is not continuous; the
ethosuximide is required prophylactically to prevent the occurrence of absence
seizures which are not easy to recognise and the daily dose of up to 1·5 or even
1·75 g (6 or 7 capsules) may be unacceptably large. Some of these factors may
contribute to the prescribed dose being inadequate and some to the patient's
reluctance to comply. Table 36.3 (p. 942) presents the relevant pharmacological
parameters.

Methodology

A variety of GLC methods exists for the determination of ethosuximide. A relatively simple one is the method by Harvey and Sherwin (1978) using a column of OV17. An EMIT method is also available from Syva UK Limited.

The GLC method described later (p. 953) for valproate also separates ethosuximide in about 6 min after loading the extracted sample onto the column. Results are calculated as previously described (p. 940).

Phenobarbitone

Pharmacology

Phenobarbitone has been in continuous use for over 80 years as an anticonvulsant effective in all types of epilepsy except *petit mal*. It is thought to act by decreasing the excitability of the entire nerve cell by increasing the threshold for electrical stimulation. Not surprising, perhaps, is the general sedation which it causes as one of its major side-effects, although young children often show irritability and hyperactivity when on phenobarbitone therapy. Less common side-effects are dermatitis, nausea and vomiting but these are minimised by gradually increasing the dose until control with therapeutic plasma concentrations is achieved.

Absorption of phenobarbitone is moderately rapid and complete but is variable and gives peak plasma concentrations in 2 to 18 h post-dose. It is distributed throughout most tissues and is approximately 50% protein-bound with an apparent Vd of 0·7 to 1·0 l/kg body weight. Approximately 70% of a dose is metabolised in the liver to *p*-hydroxyphenobarbitone (Fig. 36.5C, p. 945) which has no anticonvulsant properties. Urine of patients on chronic phenobarbitone therapy contains sulphate and glucuronide conjugates of both phenobarbitone and its metabolites. The elimination of the drug is faster in children than adults. Phenobarbitone is a well-recognised hepatic enzyme inducer and therefore enhances the elimination of phenytoin as well as itself. Elimination is decreased in hepatic and in renal disease. To aid interpretation of analytical results, the relevant pharmacological data are presented in Table 36.3 (p. 942).

Methodology

Methods for determination of phenobarbitone, in order of popularity in the UK, are immunoassay (e.g. the EMIT assay system, Syva UK Limited), HPLC, described fully in this chapter under carbamazepine and GLC which is fully detailed in the 5th edition of this book (volume 2, page 301) to which the reader is referred.

Primidone

Pharmacology

Primidone is rapidly absorbed following an oral dose and peak plasma concentrations are achieved in 1 to 3 h. Only a small proportion, approximately 20%, is protein-bound and the apparent Vd is 0·6 l/kg body weight. Primidone is metabolised by the liver to phenobarbitone and phenylethylmalonamide (Fig. 36.5C, p. 945) both of which have antiepileptic properties. Two-thirds of a dose of primidone is conjugated and excreted unchanged and one-third is metabolised as above.

It has never been satisfactorily shown whether primidone possesses anti-epileptic properties apart from those of its metabolites, hence the commonly held view that only phenobarbitone needs to be measured in patients on primidone or mixed primidone plus phenobarbitone therapy.

The plasma primidone-phenobarbitone ratio in patients treated solely with primidone is usually between 0·1 and 0·25. A lower ratio than this will be found in patients treated with phenobarbitone in addition to primidone, and a higher ratio in a patient whose compliance is suspect and who has 'topped up' with primidone a few hours before attending for blood sampling.

Overall, even if primidone is quantitated in plasma, it is necessary also to measure phenobarbitone since this is the figure on which the clinician adjusts the patient's therapy. See Table 36.3 (p. 942).

Methodology

The methods available are generally identical to those for other anticonvulsants and the HPLC method described under carbamazepine will easily quantify primidone.

Phenytoin

Pharmacology

Phenytoin, 5,5-diphenylhydantoin, is the most widely used drug for the treatment of most forms of epilepsy except *petit mal* for which it is ineffective. It is gaining popularity as the primary drug in the treatment of status epilepticus (Wilder *et al.*, 1977), or the prophylactic prevention of the seizures which frequently accompany pre-eclamptic toxaemia of pregnancy (Robertson, 1982).

The mode of action of phenytoin, like all anticonvulsants, is unknown but it has been shown to impair the release of pre-synaptic transmitter (Epslin, 1957) and elevate threshold potentials by interfering with calcium ion transport (Woodbury, 1977) in the cerebral cortex of rats.

Apart from the concentration-related effects of toxicity, the side-effects of phenytoin include such diverse reactions as hypocalcaemia and osteomalacia, megaloblastic anaemia, peripheral neuropathy, various skin rashes, hepatitis and malformations of infants born to women on phenytoin therapy. All these effects are of much lower frequency than the most common ones reported with other anticonvulsants.

Phenytoin is almost completely absorbed giving peak plasma concentrations within 3 to 9 h after an oral dose. It may be administered i.v. at not more than 50 mg/min for the safe and rapid treatment of status epilepticus due to its rapid penetration of brain tissue. More than 90% of plasma phenytoin is protein-bound and it has an apparent Vd of 0·5 to 1·2 l/kg body weight.

Phenytoin is extensively metabolised by the liver to hydroxyphenytoins (Fig. 36.5D, p. 946) which are the predominant forms found in the urine. Unlike all other anticonvulsants, the dose–plasma concentration curve is non-linear because the hydroxylating enzyme can be saturated and hence the metabolism follows Michaelis–Menten and not first-order kinetics.

A graph of dose versus plasma concentration for a series of patients (Fig. 36.7) shows that once saturation of the metabolising enzyme is achieved, a small

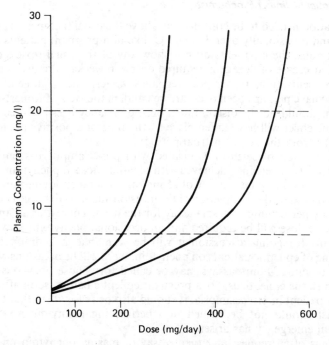

Fig. 36.7. Changes in Plasma Phenytoin Concentration with Dose.
The therapeutic range lies between the horizontal broken lines. The different curves indicate individual variations in response.

increment in dose causes a large increment in plasma concentration but enzyme saturation occurs at different plasma concentrations between patients. Phenytoin is therefore the example *par excellence* of plasma concentration monitoring being essential for patient management.

The saturation kinetics of phenytoin mean that the elimination, and hence the $t_{1/2}$, are concentration-dependent. Quoted values for $t_{1/2}$ range from 10 to 90 h but most frequently 20–40 h.

Mawer *et al.* (1974) demonstrated that 40% of patients on phenytoin had sub-therapeutic plasma concentrations and that by careful adjustment of dose, based on the judicious use of plasma concentration measurements, the seizure frequency in these patients could be significantly reduced. To assist the 'fine tuning' of dosage a 25 mg tablet of phenytoin is now available. Status epilepticus is more conveniently handled by phenytoin alone than by the use of diazepam or phenobarbitone (Ferguson, 1982). This is probably because the use of a single drug, i.v., gives predictable plasma concentrations and, from these, a convenient transfer to predictable oral dosing is possible once the seizures are under control and the patient is conscious.

Robertson (1982) investigated the decrease in plasma phenytoin concentration which occurs at constant dosage, as pregnancy proceeds. He concluded that this was due to increases in Vd, the free phenytoin fraction and hepatic metabolism. Despite the progressive increases in dose necessary to maintain a steady plasma concentration throughout pregnancy, the patient's fit-frequency usually increased and only when the plasma concentration was actually increased progressively did the patient remain seizure-free. In many patients the plasma concentration needed to be considerably above the usual therapeutic range, over 20 mg/l and occasionally over 30 mg/l. Unlike non-pregnant patients with high concentrations, these patients do not show any of the usual toxic signs. Once delivered, decrease of dosage is required over 4–6 weeks to return the patient's plasma concentrations to her pre-pregnancy values. The teratogenic effects of phenytoin have perhaps been over-stressed and, in the view of Robertson (1982), phenytoin should not be discontinued once pregnancy is established since any teratogenic effect will have taken place by the time of a positive pregnancy test (6–8 weeks from the last menstrual period).

The prevention of seizures associated with pre-eclamptic toxaemia of pregnancy is most conveniently achieved with a loading dose of phenytoin (18 mg/kg body weight) i.v. in saline at a rate of 25 mg/min. Therapeutic concentrations are usually achieved by the completion of the infusion and it is advisable to check that this is so by performing a plasma assay for the drug. Thereafter an appropriate maintenance dose will be required and an occasional phenytoin assay required.

From the foregoing discussion it will be seen that in addition to regular monitoring of epileptic patients on phenytoin, there will be occasions when more frequent or out-of-hours assays may be called for. Those occasions are (1) a patient in status epilepticus, (2) a pregnant epileptic patient soon after delivery and (3) a patient in pre-eclampsia. It should also be self-evident that the clinical biochemist should not be rushed into performing phenytoin assays simply because an emergency has arisen.

Clinicians often request an urgent assay of plasma phenytoin on a patient having frequent fits in the belief that these can be caused by toxic concentrations of phenytoin. There is no convincing evidence for this view. Such a patient, who was previously seizure-free on phenytoin, more often has an inadequate plasma phenytoin concentration and the clinician may need to act accordingly. Careful discussion of the clinical data with the clinician, bearing in mind the relevant pharmacology and especially the long $t_{1/2}$ of phenytoin, will avoid unnecessarily frequent assays being performed at unsocial hours, and inappropriate clinical action due to misinterpretation of data. The relevant pharmacology is summarised in Table 36.3 (p. 942).

Methodology

The GC determination of phenytoin is given in detail in the 5th edition of this book (Vol. 2, p. 301). The most popular current methods are EMIT and HPLC for which full details are given under carbamazepine.

Valproate

Pharmacology

Sodium valproate (sodium 2-propylpentanoate), the newest anticonvulsant, is claimed to be effective against *grand mal* as well as *petit mal* types of epilepsy. It is thought to act by increasing the brain concentration of gamma-aminoisobutyric acid (GABA) which is a natural inhibitory neurotransmitter in the CNS (Pinder *et al.*, 1977). GABA is then thought to prevent the spread of convulsive activity. However, the anticonvulsant effect of valproate has also been demonstrated without a concomitant increase in GABA.

The most common side-effects are mainly related to the commencement of therapy and are nausea, vomiting, diarrhoea and sedation. Less commonly the patient complains of hair loss and loss of appetite, while laboratory investigation may reveal elevated liver enzyme activities, decreased fibrinogen concentration and inhibited platelet aggregation. Rarely, thrombocytopenia and pancreatitis may be observed but clinically the most serious effect is hepatotoxicity. Occasionally, this has led to hepatic coma and death (Suchy *et al.*, 1979).

There is marked variation of valproate pharmacokinetics between patients. The drug is rapidly absorbed giving peak plasma concentrations 1 to 3 h after an oral dose. It is distributed rapidly into highly perfused organs and extracellular water and is highly protein-bound. Valproate is metabolised in the liver to produce 8 to 10 metabolites, mostly inactive, the main one of which, 2-*n*-propyl-3-oxo-pentanoic acid, also exhibits antiepileptic activity. All these metabolites, after glucuronidation, appear in the urine together with about 5 % of the dose as unchanged drug.

The dose–plasma concentration curve is non-linear, but unlike phenytoin, produces a less-than-predicted increment in plasma concentration for each increment in the dose. In common with all anticonvulsant drugs, the elimination of valproate is diminished in hepatic and renal disease. The elimination of valproate is enhanced, and therefore previously stable plasma concentrations are decreased, by addition of phenobarbitone, phenytoin or carbamazepine to a patient's therapy.

Due to its short $t_{1/2}$, pre-dose trough and post-dose peak plasma concentrations of valproate are more widely divergent than with other antiepileptic drugs and therefore the timing of blood samples is more critical. Some authorities advocate the determination of both peak and trough concentrations at steady state in order to assess the dosage but it is generally agreed that the pre-dose trough concentration is an adequate guide and obviously a single sample is easier to obtain and less traumatic for young patients. The relevant pharmacological parameters are given in Table 36.3 (p. 942).

Methodology

Valproate has little useful UV absorption and therefore HPLC methods using UV detection tend to be rather insensitive. The principal methods are therefore EMIT and GLC of which there are numerous examples. The methods of Chard, (1976) and Williams (1985) are both suitable and the latter, modified to allow the simultaneous determination of ethosuximide, is fully described here.

Reagents.
1. Extractant. Mix together 40 ml each of chloroform, ethyl acetate and methanol. Add 15 mg α,α-dimethyl-β-methylsuccinimide (Aldrich Chemical Company, 16, 350–3) as an internal standard.
2. Sulphamic acid solution, 2 mol/l in water.
3. Serum standards containing sodium valproate and ethosuximide at 50, 100 and 200 mg/l (p. 936) are used. Sodium valproate may be obtained from Reckitt and Colman, Dansome Lane, Hull HU8 7DS and ethosuximide from Parke–Davis and Company, Mitchell House, Southampton Road, Eastleigh, Hants. SO5 5RY.

Technique. Into the requisite number of labelled Eppendorf paediatric tubes pipette 100 μl of standards, controls and patients' sera followed by 20 μl sulphamic acid solution to all tubes. Mix gently and then add 200 μl extractant to all tubes. Vortex mix for 10 s and immediately centrifuge. Inject 2 μl of the lower phase from each tube onto the GC column.

Gas chromatography. Silanise a 2 m × 2 mm glass column and pack with 10 % SP1000 on Supelcoport 80–100 mesh (Supelco number 1–1761). The glass wool at the column ends must be phosphoric acid-washed and dried before use. The carrier is nitrogen at 50 ml/min and the operating temperature is initially 185 °C for 2 min and then programmed to rise at 20 °C/min to 250 °C for a final time of 3 min, but should be adjusted to give the best resolution for each column. The injection port temperature is 150 °C. A flame ionisation detector is used at a temperature at 250 °C and the trace obtained is shown in Fig. 36.8.

Since the method linearity changes with the age of the column, a range of standards is required, as described above. After analysis, the peak height ratio

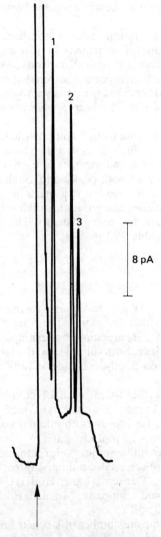

Fig. 36.8. The Determination of Valproate and Ethosuximide by Gas Chromatography. 1 = Valproate; 2 = internal standard; 3 = ethosuximide. The arrow indicates the time of injection.

(valproate peak height)/(internal standard peak height) for each standard is plotted against standard concentration. The peak height ratios for controls and patients' samples are then calculated and the graph used to read off the concentrations in mg/l.

Note. Sulpelcoport is supplied by Supelchem, R. B. Radley and Company Limited, London Road, Sawbridgeworth, Herts, CM21 9JH.

ANTIDEPRESSANTS

Pharmacology

This group of drugs is widely prescribed as 'tricyclic antidepressants' in the more severe forms of depression. The several members may be subdivided into different groups but share the common chemical feature of having two benzene rings joined by a seven-membered ring (Table 36.4). The latter is a cycloheptene in the dibenzocycloheptenes, but contains one or two nitrogen atoms in the dibenzazepines and dibenzdiazepines respectively. Others contain an oxygen or sulphur atom in the seven-membered ring. A basic side-chain is attached to the central ring in all cases and these drugs are found amongst the basic group in the usual extraction procedures.

The group as a whole is rapidly absorbed and the drugs enter the tissues leaving only a small quantity in the circulation. They are readily metabolised in the liver and the conjugated metabolites are rapidly cleared by the kidney. An important step in metabolism is demethylation. Thus imipramine is converted to desipramine and amitriptyline to nortriptyline. The urine contains mainly metabolites (Fig. 36.9).

The rate of metabolism shows wide individual variation so that the plasma concentration may vary widely from one patient to another on a constant dose. Thus Braithwaite and Widdop (1971) found a 15-fold range for amitriptyline and a 12-fold range for nortriptyline under such conditions. In view of this, methods

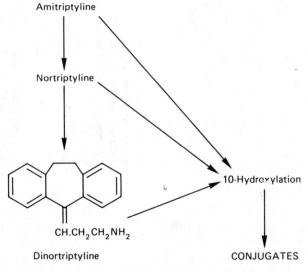

Fig. 36.9. The Metabolism of Amitriptyline.

TABLE 36.4

Tricyclic Antidepressants

Dibenzazepines

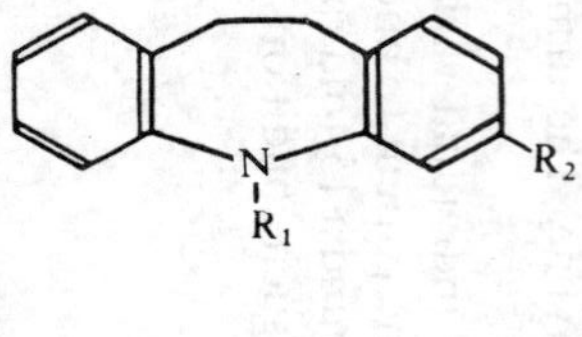

	R_1	R_2
Clomipramine (Anafranil)	$-CH_2.CH_2.CH_2N(CH_3)_2$	Cl
Desipramine (Pertofran)	$-CH_2.CH_2.CH_2NHCH_3$	H
Imipramine (Berkomine, Dimipressin, Ethipram, Norpramine, Praminal, Tofranil)	$-CH_2.CH_2.CH_2N(CH_3)_2$	H
Opipramol (Insidon)	$-CH_2.CH_2.CH_2.N$⟨N.CH_2.CH_2.CH_2OH⟩ 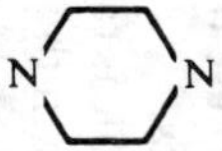	H
Trimipramine (Surmontil)	$-CH_2.CH(CH_3).CH_2N(CH_3)_2$ (also extra double bond in 7-membered ring)	H

Dibenzocycloheptenes

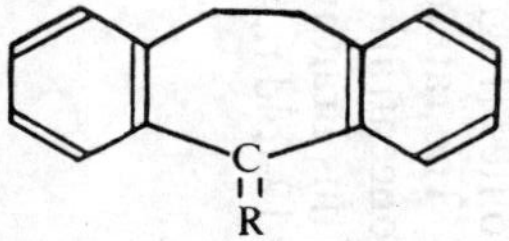

R

$=CH.CH_2.CH_2N(CH_3)_2$

$=CH.CH_2.CH_2NHCH_3$

$<^{CH_2.CH_2.CH_2NHCH_3}_{H}$

Amitriptyline (Laroxyl, Lentizol, Saroten, Tryptizol)
Nortriptyline (Allegron, Aventyl, Motival)
Protriptyline (Concordin)

Compare the *antihistamine*,
cyproheptadine (Periactin)

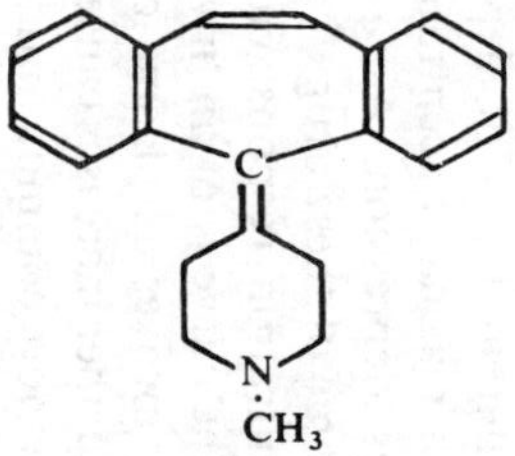

Dibenzdiazepine
Dibenzepin (Noveril)

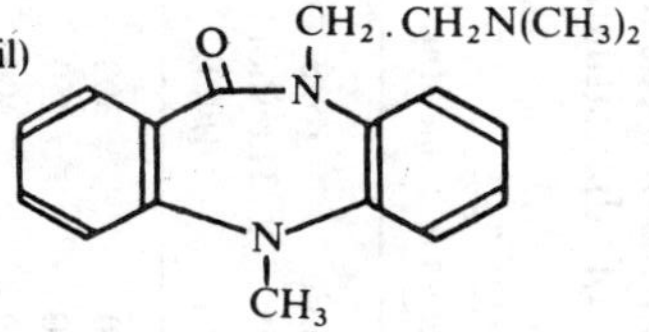

$CH_2.CH_2N(CH_3)_2$

CH_3

Dibenzthiepin and Dibenzoxepin

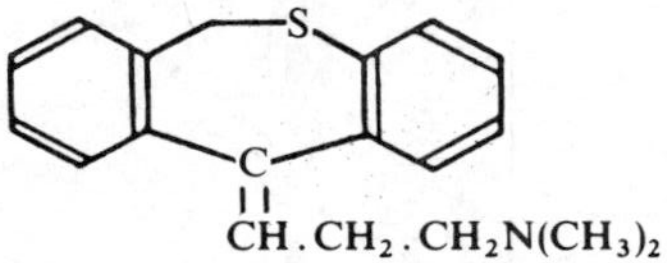

$CH.CH_2.CH_2N(CH_3)_2$

Dothiepin (Prothiaden)

$CH.CH_2.CH_2N(CH_3)_2$

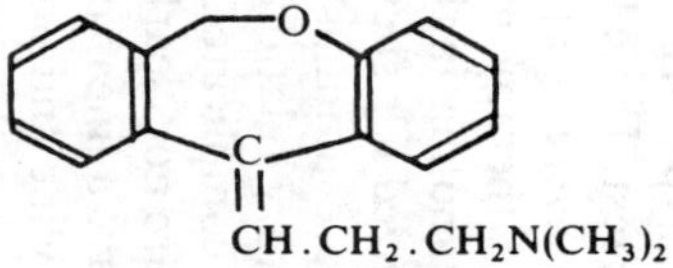

Doxepin (Sinequan)

have been developed for monitoring plasma concentrations to achieve better therapeutic control. It is claimed (Kragh-Sørensen *et al.*, 1973) that for nortriptyline the optimal concentration in plasma is 175 μg/l with less satisfactory effects at higher or lower figures. The prescription of these substances to depressed patients is associated with the risk of deliberate self-poisoning. The ingestion of more than 1 g is likely to have serious effects. The clinical features are especially centred on the nervous and cardiovascular systems. There may be hallucinations, hyper-reflexia, convulsions and varying degrees of unconsciousness but rarely profound coma. Depression of respiration, dilation of pupils, dryness of the mouth and urinary retention are seen. The cardiovascular effects include tachycardia, hypotension and a tendency to develop severe arrhythmias leading to cardiac arrest. These features become apparent within an hour or two after ingestion and severe symptoms rarely persist for longer than 18 to 24 h. Intensive supportive therapy may be needed during this time and the rapid detection of the metabolites in the urine may aid in the detection of the cause of poisoning and the need for such care.

Antidepressants are administered for different types of depressive illness although a satisfactory relationship between plasma concentration and effect exists only for uncomplicated endogenous depression. As a consequence, therapeutic ranges are not clearly defined. Some of these drugs, e.g. imipramine and desipramine, have a linear plasma concentration–response curve while with others, e.g. amitriptyline and nortriptyline, the curve is of an 'inverted U' type. This means that the antidepressant effect improves as plasma concentrations increase but beyond a certain concentration further increases cause a lessening of the effect. Pharmacological parameters of the more common antidepressants are summarised in Table 36.5.

Authorities are divided on the usefulness of measuring plasma concentrations of antidepressants but clarification of the situation may come with the

TABLE 36.5
Pharmacological Parameters of Some Antidepressants.

Antidepressant	Therapeutic Range* (μg/l)	Toxic Threshold (μg/l)	Half-time (h)	Vd (l/kg)
Amitriptyline	50–150	300	8–51	20–45
Nortriptyline	50–150	250	15–90	20–57
Clomipramine	100–500	400	20–84	
Desmethylclomipramine	200–1000			
Dothiepin	20–60	1000	11–40	20–92
Desmethyldothiepin	10–50		22–60	
Doxepin	50–150	100	8–25	9–33
Desmethyldoxepin	30–100		33–80	
Imipramine	10–110	300	8–20	20–40
Desipramine	20–330	400	12–54	25–59
Mianserin	15–70	500	6–39	approx. 13
Desmethylmianserin	5–25			
Protriptyline**	70–250	500	3–8 (days)	15–31

* Therapeutic ranges for antidepressants are not yet thoroughly established, consequently there is wide variation in the ranges quoted by different sources.
** Protriptyline does not have a desmethyl-metabolite.

accumulation of data with good clinical audit of patients on therapy. The major situations requiring plasma monitoring of antidepressant plus active metabolite are whenever they are used in patients who (1) are elderly, because of wider variability in plasma concentrations and an increased vulnerability to adverse effects; (2) have cardiac disease, because of an association between depression and increased risk of circulatory disorders and because toxic concentrations affecting cardiac conduction can arise even from very low doses in poor hydroxylators; (3) develop marked side-effects on modest dosages; (4) do not respond after an appropriate length of time on a standard dosage regimen. Measurement of plasma concentrations can also assist in achieving therapeutic plasma concentrations in the shortest possible time.

All antidepressants have moderate to long half-times and hence show little post-dose peak and trough fluctuations. While as a general rule, pre-dose samples give the most reproducible results, sample timing in relation to time of dose is probably unimportant. The possibility of unstable metabolites necessitates that samples should be separated as soon as possible after venesection and the serum stored frozen until analysed.

Methodology

Many methods have been published for the assay of antidepressants indicating that the determination of these drugs is not without problems. Most methods have been concerned with the determination of one drug and its major metabolite in plasma. This is generally unsatisfactory since most clinical biochemists will be required to determine a number of these drugs and their metabolites. Solvent extraction at an alkaline pH is common to most of the published methods of which the earliest ones were relatively non-specific spectrophotometric or spectrofluorimetric assays while the later and better ones employ GLC or HPLC.

Many GLC methods require derivatisation of the compounds to produce adequate separation and to diminish on-column losses; some require multiple extraction steps to eliminate non-specific interference and use an electron-capture detector to provide adequate sensitivity for routine therapeutic monitoring.

In the last 10 years many HPLC methods have appeared including either ion-pair partition, adsorption or reverse-phase liquid chromatography mostly using UV detection. The sensitivity of these methods is similar to that of GLC and the methods are generally simpler since derivatisation is usually avoided.

Recently, immunoassays using either isotopic or non-isotopic labels have become available but two separate assays are required if the metabolite concentration is to be determined in addition to the parent drug. The current immunoassays mostly determine parent plus metabolite as a single concentration. The method described below is the normal-phase HPLC method of Blakesley *et al.* (1986).

Collection of Samples. Brunswick and Mendells (1977) demonstrated that 'Vacutainers', if used to collect blood for tricyclic antidepressants, caused falsely low concentrations to be obtained due to the presence of a plasticiser eluting from the rubber stopper. Two other studies (Wood *et al.*, 1979; Danon and Chen, 1979) suggested that heparin or lipoproteins also cause a decrease in plasma concentration of tricyclic antidepressants and therefore serum or whole blood should be used. Our experience suggests that the difference in concentration between serum and heparinised plasma is probably not significant, but serum yields a cleaner solvent extract.

Determination of Tricyclic Antidepressants by HPLC

Reagents.
1. Extraction solvent. Add 15 ml amyl alcohol, analytical reagent grade to 985 ml heptane, HPLC grade (Fisons).
2. Internal standard, butriptyline 2 mg/l in 5 mmol/l sulphuric acid.
3. Sodium carbonate solution, 1 mol/l.
4. Sulphuric acid, 200 mmol/l.
5. Sodium hydroxide solution, 2 mol/l.
6. Methyl t-butyl ether, HPLC grade (Fisons).
7. Methanol, HPLC grade (Fisons).
8. Standards. Stock solutions of the antidepressants are prepared in 5 mmol/l sulphuric acid. Working standards are prepared in drug-free serum to cover the range 0 to 300 μg/l. See the section on preparation of standards (p. 936).

Technique. Into 25 ml glass-stoppered tubes pipette 2 ml of each of the standards, controls and patients' sera. Add 200 μl internal standard solution, 2 ml sodium carbonate and 10 ml extraction solvent. Stopper and mix by rotation for 5 min and then centrifuge at 3000 rpm for 5 min. Pipette 1·2 ml sulphuric acid into the same number of clean conical centrifuge tubes and transfer to these the solvent layer from the extracting tubes. Stopper these tubes and mix by rotation for 5 min and then centrifuge for 1 min at 500 rpm. Discard the solvent layer and add 1 ml sodium hydroxide and 200 μl methyl t-butyl ether. Vortex mix for 10 s and then centrifuge for 1 min at 500 rpm. Using a 2 ml syringe and a blunt needle, remove the aqueous layer and load 50 μl of the organic layer onto the column.

Chromatography. An HPLC column $100 \times 4·5$ mm and packed with 5 μm diameter silica particles is required and is installed into a conventional HPLC system of pump, injection valve (with 50 μl loop) and UV detector. The column must not have been previously used with aqueous mobile phases and should be pre-conditioned by pumping 500 ml methanol (HPLC grade) containing 500 μl perchloric acid. The working mobile phase consists of 500 ml methanol (HPLC grade) containing 40 μl perchloric acid and is pumped at 2 ml/min for analysis. Extreme care should be taken when changing from a reverse-phase method to the normal-phase method for tricyclic antidepressants to prevent water entering the column. The column may be left filled with working mobile phase when removed from the instrument and does not need the pre-conditioning step to be repeated.

The method is linear to 300 μg/l for all the antidepressants listed in Table 36.6, which presents retention times relative to butriptyline. The authors list optimal wavelengths (204–213 nm) for each drug and metabolite. However, a single wavelength of 207 nm is satisfactory. The photometer output is connected to a 1 mV recorder and produces the trace shown in Fig. 36.10 at 0·08 AUFS.

Lithium

Pharmacology

Simple preparations of lithium are rapidly absorbed and produce peak plasma concentrations at about 1 h post-dose after which there is rapid distribution into tissues ($t_{1/2}$ about 70 min) followed by a slow elimination phase with a half-time of 8 to 20 h. Controlled-release preparations delay the time at which the peak concentration is reached and reduce the pre- and post-dose concentration differences.

TABLE 36.6

Relative Retention Times for Antidepressants with Respect to Butriptyline.

n-Desmethylclomipramine	0·66
Procyclidine	0·67
Nortriptyline	0·69
Maprotyline	0·75
Desipramine	0·75
Butriptyline	1·00
Trimipramine	1·11
Protriptyline	1·15
Clomipramine	1·20
Amitriptyline	1·29
Imipramine	1·44
Mianserin	1·48
Doxepin	1·53

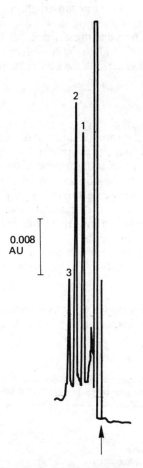

Fig. 36.10. The Separation of Antidepressants by HPLC.

1 = Desmethyldothiepin; 2 = butriptyline (internal standard); 3 = dothiepin. The arrow indicates the time of injection.

The major effect of lithium is against manic-depressive illness but there is also a significant risk of nephrotoxicity (Amdisen, 1975) and a slightly lower risk of hypothyroidism (Amdisen, 1978; Amdisen and Schou, 1978), both at relatively low plasma lithium concentrations. Since lithium is eliminated by the kidney without metabolic modification, slight renal impairment leads to accumulation of the drug and further toxic effects. This cycle of events, once established, can become rapidly fatal due, most commonly, to the combined effects of impaired renal function, dehydration and a hypothyroid state.

The wide inter-individual differences in dosage requirements, the narrow margin of safety and the rapidity with which a potentially toxic situation can escalate to a fatality are the prime reasons for measuring serum concentrations of lithium. The clinical aspects of lithium therapy are complex and the reader is referred to the excellent review by Amdisen (1981), or the major text on lithium therapy by Johnson (1980).

Collection of Blood. Timing of blood sample in relation to time of dose is critical because of the rapid decrease in plasma concentration during the distribution phase. Amdisen (1973) proposed sampling blood in the morning 12 ± 0.5 h after the last lithium evening dose in an attempt to standardise the procedure. The long elimination half-time dictates that measurement of the 12 h serum lithium concentration should not be considered earlier than one week after any dosage adjustment unless serious toxicity is suspected.

Methodology

Flame photometry is the method of choice for lithium determination and most modern instruments provide automatic dilution of sample and direct read-out of lithium results. The use of lithium as the internal standard for the determination of sodium and potassium means that some instruments require prolonged washing before a satisfactory base-line reading can be obtained. The potassium used as internal standard in lithium estimations may also be difficult to remove when the instrument is returned to its normal role for sodium and potassium assays. For these reasons, many laboratories will prefer to have an instrument used solely for lithium determination.

A fuller discussion of instrumentation and details of a method using flame emission are given in the 5th edition of this book and in Chapter 7.

INTERPRETATION

The important concentration ranges for serum lithium are given in Table 36.7, but apply only to samples collected at 12 ± 0.5 h after an evening dose. Samples

TABLE 36.7
Important Concentration Ranges (mmol/l) for Serum Lithium.
(Samples taken 12 ± 0.5 h post-dose)

*Therapeutic range	0·3–1·3
Warning range	1·3–1·5
Slight to moderate poisoning	1·5–2·5
Substantial risk of severe intoxication	2·5–3·5
Life-threatening intoxication	above 3·5

* There is a welcome tendency for medical practitioners to aim for lower concentrations and narrower ranges than in the past.

collected at other times will be difficult to interpret because of the wide variation in kinetics between different lithium preparations and between patients.

\Since impairment of glomerular filtration by lithium may precede a toxic episode, it has been suggested by Johnson (1980) and by our own observations that measurement of serum creatinine in addition to lithium may detect early changes in GFR. There is, however, evidence to suggest that the primary renal effect is on the tubule and not the glomerulus. Hansen and Amdisen (1978) divide lithium intoxication into three types; (1) intoxication which develops in spite of unchanged dosage and which is caused by impaired renal elimination of lithium; (2) intoxication caused by prescription of a dosage inappropriately high for the patient; (3) acute ingestion of a dose in excess of the daily requirement. The signs and symptoms of lithium poisoning, which include nausea, vomiting, confusion, seizures and coma, may be delayed for 2 to 3 days during which time permanent mental, neurological or renal damage may have occurred (Amdisen *et al.*, 1974). A routine 12 h post-dose serum lithium result which is above the toxic limit of 1·5 mmol/l should alert the clinician to take appropriate action. A patient who presents with signs of toxicity may need dialysis as assessed by the criteria below and hence an emergency assay of lithium may be required.

Criteria for dialysis treatment in lithium intoxication are described by Amdisen (1981) and may be rationalised in the following manner. The patient should be admitted for observation and either a 12 h post-dose blood sample submitted for analysis or an estimate of the 12 h post-dose concentration made from the lithium concentration of a blood sample drawn urgently at a known time. Dialysis should be considered when the 12 h post-dose lithium concentration (or its estimate) is greater than 1·5 mmol/l and one or more of these additional criteria are met:

1. another lithium estimation 3 h after the first shows a decrease of less than 10%;
2. if the 12 h post-dose concentration (or its estimate) is in the range 2·5 to 3·5 mmol/l;
3. urgent dialysis is required if the 12 h post-dose concentration (or its estimate) is greater than 3·5 mmol/l;
4. dialysis should be repeated if the serum lithium exceeds 1·0 mmol/l during the rebound phase after dialysis is discontinued.

A fuller discussion is provided by Richens and Marks (1981) and by Johnson (1980).

CARDIOACTIVE DRUGS

The number of drugs available for the treatment of cardiac arrhythmias is large and it is strongly argued that for a few of these, therapy should be controlled with the aid of plasma concentration measurements. Adjustments in therapy are especially difficult for several reasons: (1) there is no general agreement on what constitutes an acceptable end-effect; (2) although some monitoring can be done by electrocardiography, the first indication of toxicity may be cardiac arrest; (3) it is frequently difficult to know whether a change in cardiac function is due to the drug employed, a non-specific effect or the result of other disease processes; (4) as cardiac function changes during therapy, either improving or worsening, so the metabolism (hepatic and renal handling) may change; (5) patient's poor compliance.

Many physicians feel that it has not been rigorously established that the monitoring of plasma concentrations of amiodarone, disopyramide, lignocaine, or quinidine is useful except as an indicator of poor compliance. Therefore, procainamide, its metabolite N-acetyl procainamide, digoxin and propranolol are probably the only drugs in this group where measurement of plasma concentration to control therapy is rather more thoroughly established as useful.

The structures and metabolism of common cardioactive drugs are presented in Fig. 36.11A–C and relevant pharmacological parameters in Table 36.8.

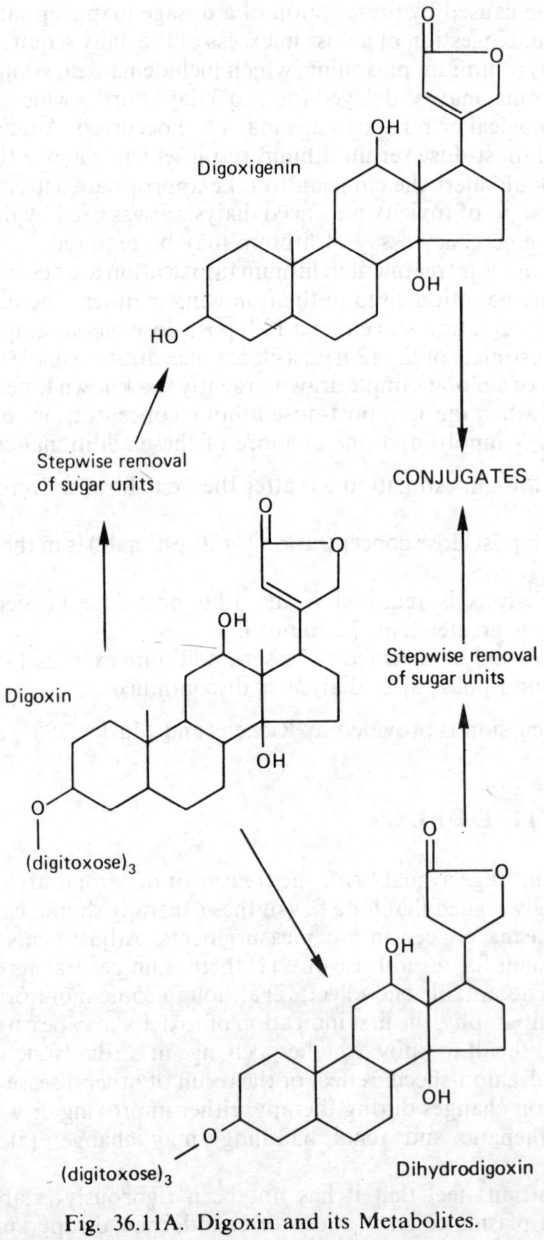

Digoxigenin

Stepwise removal
of sugar units

CONJUGATES

Digoxin

Stepwise removal
of sugar units

(digitoxose)$_3$

(digitoxose)$_3$

Dihydrodigoxin

Fig. 36.11A. Digoxin and its Metabolites.

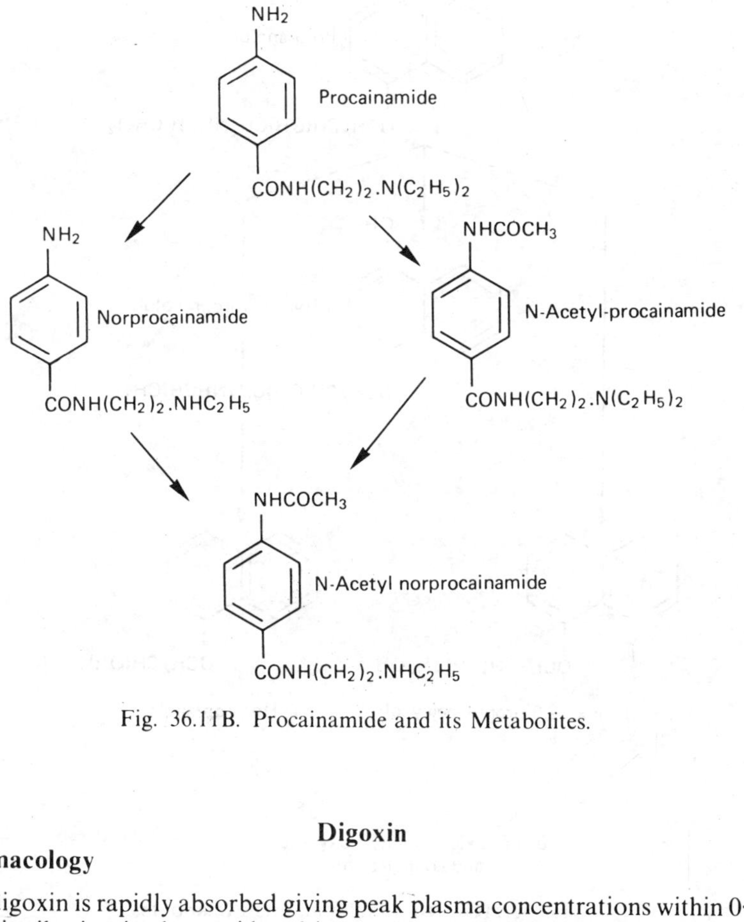
NH2
Procainamide
CONH(CH2)2.N(C2H5)2
NH2
Norprocainamide
CONH(CH2)2.NHC2H5
NHCOCH3
N-Acetyl-procainamide
CONH(CH2)2.N(C2H5)2
NHCOCH3
N-Acetyl norprocainamide
CONH(CH2)2.NHC2H5

Fig. 36.11B. Procainamide and its Metabolites.

Digoxin

Pharmacology

Oral digoxin is rapidly absorbed giving peak plasma concentrations within 0·5 to 2 h. Distribution is also rapid and is usually complete by about 6 h post-dose. Most of the body burden of digoxin is extravascular with less than 1 % remaining in the circulation. By about 6 h after an oral dose the plasma concentration has returned almost to the pre-dose value as shown in Fig. 36.12. During this elimination phase the plasma concentration falls slowly with a half-time ranging from 33 to 51 h. It is essential to sample blood for assay either immediately pre-dose or during the elimination phase, i.e. more than 6 h post-dose, in order to avoid the early post-dose peak in plasma concentration. Elimination is mainly by glomerular filtration and tubular secretion; a small proportion is eliminated by non-renal routes.

Jelliffe (1971) and others have shown that a plasma potassium concentration below 3·5 mmol/l increases the sensitivity of the response to digoxin. It is possible that a low plasma magnesium may have the same effect. It is essential, therefore, to measure plasma potassium and creatinine whenever plasma digoxin is assayed so that changes in these may serve as an early warning of possible digoxin toxicity if appropriate measures are not taken.

Digoxin has a narrow margin of safety. The therapeutic range, 0·8 to 2·0 μg/l, is the range of plasma concentration within which the benefits of digoxin are associated with the lowest incidence of toxicity. However, in a study (Aronson *et al.*, 1978) of two groups totalling 71 patients who showed no toxicity, 21 (29·6 %)

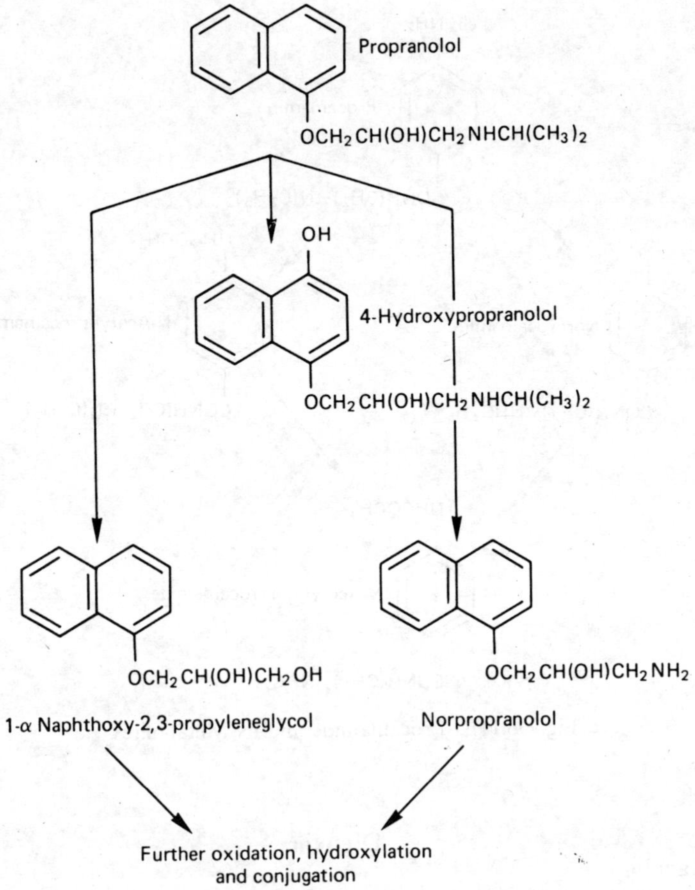

Propranolol

$OCH_2CH(OH)CH_2NHCH(CH_3)_2$

OH

4-Hydroxypropranolol

$OCH_2CH(OH)CH_2NHCH(CH_3)_2$

$OCH_2CH(OH)CH_2OH$

1-α Naphthoxy-2,3-propyleneglycol

$OCH_2CH(OH)CH_2NH_2$

Norpropranolol

Further oxidation, hydroxylation
and conjugation

Fig. 36.11C. Propranolol and its Metabolites.

TABLE 36.8

Pharmacological Data for Cardioactive Drugs.

	Therapeutic Range (µg/l)	Toxic Threshold (µg/l)	Half-time (h)	Vd (l/kg)
Digoxin	0·8–2·0	> 3·0*	33–51	5–10
Infants < 7 days old				
Premature			approx. 90	
Term			approx. 52	
Procainamide	4·0–10·0	16·0	2–5	3·3–4·8
Propranolol				
(β blocker)	30–260	2000	2–4	3–5
(anti-hypertensive)	50–1000			

* Toxicity may commence with concentrations within the therapeutic range (see text) but is most probable with concentrations greater than 3·0 µg/l.

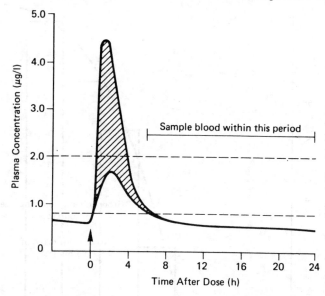

Fig. 36.12. Changes in Plasma Digoxin Concentration Following an Oral Dose.
The therapeutic range lies between the two horizontal broken lines. The arrow indicates the time of the dose.

had plasma digoxin concentrations greater than 2.0 $\mu g/1$ and 8 (11·3%) had plasma concentrations greater than 3.0 $\mu g/l$. Conversely, in a group of 12 patients showing toxicity, 8 (75%) had plasma digoxin concentrations less than 3.0 $\mu g/l$ and 7 (58%) had plasma concentrations less than 2.0 $\mu g/l$ (Fig. 36.13). These results suggest that the emergency assay of plasma digoxin concentration in suspected toxicity is likely to be of very little value and that the physician should act on his clinical assessment of the patient and a knowledge of the plasma potassium and creatinine. This view is supported by the work of Morgan (1984).

Methodology

Many methods for measurement of plasma digoxin have been published. Most have never been used routinely except in a few laboratories. The advent of reagent kits for the radioimmunoassay of digoxin using ^{125}I-label has encouraged most clinical biochemistry laboratories to provide the assay routinely and there are now several kits on the market. There are also some non-isotopic immunoassay kits available typified by the EMIT assay for digoxin manufactured by Syva UK.

Recently, Soldin (1986) drew attention to the cross-reactivity between some available anti-digoxin antibodies and eleven naturally-occurring lipids and three steroid hormones. He also pointed out that digoxin metabolites only lose their ability to cross-react with the antibodies used in assays with the opening of the lactone ring attached to C-17 of the sterane nucleus. A naturally-occurring digoxin 'endoxin' has also been postulated by Gruber *et al.* (1980).

The presence of naturally-occurring digoxin-like material has been demonstrated in the plasma of patients with renal disease (Craver and Valdes, 1983) and in neonates (Valdes *et al.*, 1983) so in these situations some methods will produce misleadingly high results (Graves *et al.*, 1983). It is clearly important to

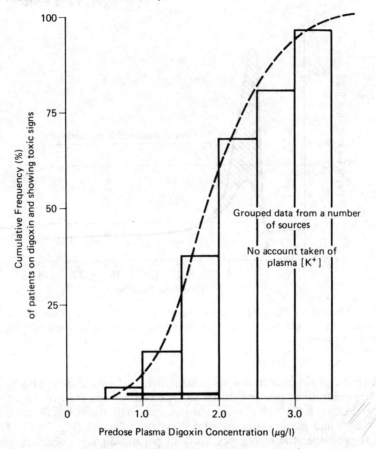

Fig. 36.13. The Frequency of Digoxin Toxicity in Relation to the Plasma Concentration.

choose a method which estimates as little as possible of the endogenous digoxin-like material. Of the six methods studied by Graves and colleagues, the radioimmunoassay method manufactured by Becton–Dickinson and the 'Immophase' method made by Corning Medical showed less than $0.05\,\mu g/l$ interference. In the other four methods (Beckmann 'RIAphase', Clinical Assays 'Gamma Coat', New England Nuclear 'Rainen Digoxin RIA' and Syva 'EMIT-CAD') the interference was unacceptably high.

The Becton–Dickinson antibody-coated tube assay for digoxin is described here and consists of packs of antibody-coated tubes, a bottle of buffered, labelled antigen (3-O-succinyl digoxigenin tyrosine-^{125}I) and a range of calibrators. The antibody has a very high association constant directed primarily towards the antigenic determinants on the C and D rings of the steroid part of the digoxin molecule. Performance of the assay involves pipetting, in duplicate, $50\,\mu l$ amounts of each calibrator, control serum and patient's plasma into appropriately marked tubes, adding 1 ml of labelled antigen, vortex-mixing and incubating at $37\,^\circ C$ for at least 15 min (1 h is the recommended time). The labelled antigen competes with the digoxin present in calibrators, controls or patient's samples for the binding sites on the immobilised antibody during the incubation period. After incubation, the tube contents are poured away and the tubes rinsed twice with 1 ml of water by vortexing and decanting. The label bound to the tubes is determined by counting in a gamma-counter for 3 min and the results are determined by plotting digoxin concentration against either percentage label binding or logit. Alternatively, a gamma-counter can be used which will calculate and print out the results directly in units of concentration.

Procainamide

Pharmacology

Procainamide is a local anaesthetic which is also useful in the management of ventricular arrhythmias. It is absorbed rapidly giving peak plasma concentrations at about 30 min following i.m. injections and at about 1 h following an oral dose. The drug is also distributed and eliminated rapidly, having a plasma half-time in the range 2·5 to 4·5 h. Although most (50 to 60%) of a dose of procainamide is excreted unchanged in the urine, 10 to 15% appears as the active metabolite N-acetyl procainamide (NAPA) in slow acetylators and 20 to 25% in fast acetylators. The remainder is excreted as p-aminobenzoic acid and its conjugate. N-Acetylprocainamide has the same potency as procainamide, reaches peak plasma concentrations at 45–90 min after an oral dose of the parent drug and has a plasma half-time of about 6 h.

The reasons for measuring plasma concentrations of procainamide are (1) the very variable relationship between oral dose and concentration or effect; (2) the narrow therapeutic window of 4 to 10 mg/l; (3) frequent (every 3 to 4 h) dosing is necessary, because of the short $t_{1/2}$, and omission of a dose may have serious consequences; (4) modification of pharmacokinetics due to changes in gastrointestinal, hepatic or renal functions.

The relevant pharmacological parameters are given in Table 36.8 (p. 966), and the structure and metabolism shown in Fig. 36.11B (p. 965).

Methodology

Clearly, N-acetyl procainamide concentrations should be considered together with those of procainamide in any clinical situation and hence the assay method employed should quantify both. A variety of methods exists for the quantitation of procainamide and its metabolite and the most common of these are (1) GLC after derivatisation; (2) EMIT—there are separate reagent kits for parent drug and metabolite; (3) HPLC—the reverse-phase method of Rocco *et al.* (1977) is ᵗescribed here.

Reagents.
1. Sodium hydroxide solution, 1 mol/l.
2. Stock internal standard solution. Dissolve 100 mg N-propionyl procainamide (Sigma catalogue number P6523) in methylene chloride, analytical reagent grade, and make to 100 ml.
3. Extractant. Dilute 2 ml stock internal standard solution to 1 litre with methylene chloride, analytical reagent grade.
4. Standards. Serum standards are required at the concentrations 5, 10, 20 and 30 mg/l for both procainamide (Sigma catalogue number P9391) and N-acetyl procainamide (Sigma catalogue number A5513).

Technique. Into the appropriate number of labelled glass centrifuge tubes ᵖipette 100 μl of standard, control or patients' serum. To each add 100 μl sodium hydroxide solution and 500 μl extractant. The tubes are vortex-mixed for 1 min and then centrifuged for 5 min. Transfer the lower organic layers by Pasteur pipette to clean tubes (70 × 7 mm) and evaporate the solvent under oxygen-free nitrogen. Redissolve the residue in 100 μl mobile phase and load 10 μl onto the column.

Chromatography. Mobile phase. To 400 ml methanol (HPLC grade) add 10 ml of glacial acetic acid, analytical reagent grade, and dilute to 1 litre with fresh distilled water. Adjust the pH to 5·5 with sodium hydroxide solution, 10 mol/l. Mobile phase is pumped at 2·0 ml/min through a HPLC column, 300 × 4 mm, packed with 10 μm C18 reverse-phase material. A guard column (40 × 4 mm) packed with the same material and preceding the analytical column protects the latter and extends its life. The column effluent is passed to a UV spectrophotometer, wavelength 280 nm, 8 nm bandwidth and the signal from this output is displayed on a 1 mV recorder. At 0·1 AUFS a trace as shown in Fig. 36.14 is obtained.

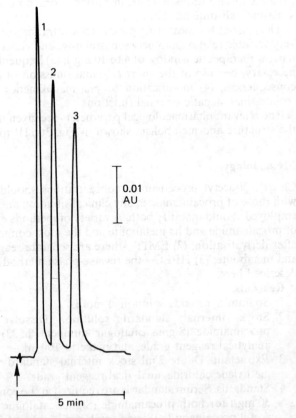

Fig. 36.14. The Separation of Procainamide by HPLC.
1 = Procainamide; 2 = *N*-acetylprocainamide; 3 = *N*-propionylprocainamide (internal standard). The arrow indicates the time of injection.

Propranolol

' **Pharmacology**

Propranolol is a beta-adrenergic blocking agent with a number of functions in heart disease including use as an anti-arrhythmic. It is rapidly absorbed following an oral dose and gives peak plasma concentrations within 60 to 90 min. It is also rapidly distributed and eliminated, after extensive metabolism, with a plasma half-time of approximately 3 h. Some of its metabolites are pharmacologically active, the major one being 4-hydroxypropranolol. The metabolism of propranolol is shown in Fig. 36.11C (p. 966).

There is a large individual variation in the dose–response curve and in the dose–plasma concentration time curve for this drug. Hence, it is useful to measure plasma concentrations in those patients who fail to respond to conventional doses. In addition, apart from demonstrating poor compliance, plasma concentration measurements are useful in assisting dosage adjustment in patients with progressive renal disease.

The relevant pharmacological data are presented in Table 36.8 (p. 966).

Methodology

The usual preparations of propranolol are racemic mixtures in which the *l*-isomer is 60 to 100 times more potent as a beta-blocker than the *d*-isomer. Hepatic metabolism does not handle the two isomers identically and hence the relative concentrations of parent and metabolites varies in a complex manner. It is usual to measure propranolol only, although some authorities advocate measuring the 4-hydroxy metabolite too.

An EMIT method for propranolol is available as is a variety of GLC and fluorescence methods. The reverse-phase HPLC method of Hackett and Dusci (1979) is described here.

Reagents.
1. Phosphate buffer, KH_2PO_4, 45 mmol/l, adjusted to pH 3·0 with phosphoric acid.
2. Sodium hydroxide, 5 mol/l.
3. Solvent mixture. Dilute 15 ml isoamyl alcohol, analytical reagent grade, to 1 litre with *n*-heptane, analytical reagent grade.
4. Stock internal standard solution. Dissolve 2 mg promazine (Sigma catalogue number P6656) in solvent mixture and make up to 100 ml.
5. Extractant. Dilute 10 ml stock internal standard solution to 1 litre with solvent mixture.
6. Standards. Serum standards covering the range 200, 400 and 600 μg/l for propranolol (Sigma catalogue number P0884) are required. See the section on preparation of serum standards (p. 936).
7. Mobile phase. Dilute 350 ml acetonitrile (HPLC grade) to 1 litre with the phosphate buffer.

Technique. *Glassware.* Stoppered centrifuge tubes (150 × 20 mm), conical glass centrifuge tubes and their stoppers must be silanised before use by immersion in dichlorodimethylsilane in toluene, 100 g/l, for 10 min. This procedure should be performed in a fume chamber. The tubes are emptied, rinsed in toluene followed by methanol and then heated in an oven at 110 °C for 30 min. Probably, any silanising procedure in current use for gas chromatograph columns will suffice.

Into the appropriate number of silanised tubes pipette 2 ml of standard, control and patients' serum or plasma. To each add 100 μl sodium hydroxide and 12 ml extractant. Stopper the tubes, shake mechanically for 5 min and then centrifuge at 2000 rpm for 5 min. Transfer 10 ml of the solvent layer to a conical tube and evaporate under oxygen-free nitrogen. To each tube add 50 μl mobile phase and vortex-mix for 1 min. After standing at room temperature for 10 min, vortex-mix a second time. Following this, 10 μl from each tube is loaded onto the column.

Chromatography. Mobile phase is pumped through a column 300 × 4 mm filled with 10 μm C18 reverse-phase material and on to a UV spectrophotometer set at 230 nm wavelength, 8 nm bandwidth, 0·05 AUFS. The output is fed to a 1 mV recorder. A guard column (40 × 4 mm) inserted before the analytical column will extend the life of the latter. A specimen trace is shown in Fig. 36.15. The mobile phase can be recycled for economy.

Acetylator Status

Pharmacology

Several drugs containing an aromatic amino group are metabolised by *N*-acetylation. Genetic polymorphism for this type of metabolism has been

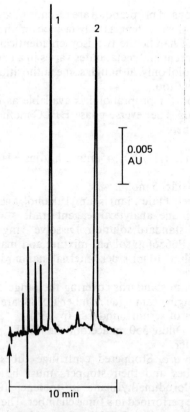

Fig. 36.15. The Separation of Propranolol by HPLC.
1 = Propranolol; 2 = promazine (internal standard). The arrow indicates the time of injection.

demonstrated for such drugs as dapsone, hydrallazine, phenelzine, procainamide, sulphadimidine, the amino-metabolite of nitrazepam, and isoniazid. The *N*-acetyltransferase enzyme is present in the liver and gastrointestinal mucosa and subjects may be classified as 'slow' or 'fast' acetylators depending on the rate at which they metabolise sulphadimidine or isoniazid (Evans *et al.*, 1960). The metabolism of isoniazid is shown in Fig. 36.16.

Unlike the mixed-function oxidase enzyme system, *N*-acetyltransferase appears not to be induced by the drugs being metabolised. Hence it has been suggested that the slow acetylators will accumulate the drug concerned and develop adverse reactions, while the fast acetylators will respond poorly to a standard regimen, but not all authorities agree on this.

The isoniazid acetylator phenotype pattern varies with ethnic group, ranging from 100% fast acetylators in Canadian Eskimos to 18% in Egyptians. The figure for the UK white population is 40% (Lunde *et al.*, 1977). Slow acetylators are of autosomal homozygous recessive genotype but the fast acetylators are of two genotypes: heterozygous or homozygous dominant, the latter having significantly lower serum isoniazid concentrations on a standard dose than the former (Gilman *et al.*, 1985).

Opinions differ on the usefulness of assessing acetylator phenotype. If there is a good correlation between the plasma concentration of a drug and its clinical effect, and if a specific assay for the drug is available, then occasional direct monitoring should enable the clinician to adjust therapy satisfactorily.

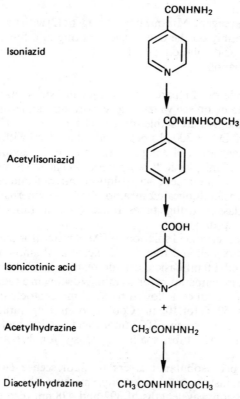

Fig. 36.16. The Metabolism of Isoniazid.

Conversely, establishing the acetylator status of the patient before therapy starts may enable the clinician to prescribe appropriately without recourse to frequent plasma assays.

Isoniazid is the drug most commonly used to determine acetylator status. Its application, fluorimetric assay (Miceli *et al.*, 1975) and interpretation of the results are described here.

Determination of Acetylator Status

Following venepuncture (5 ml without anticoagulant), give the patient 10 mg isoniazid per kg body weight as a single oral dose and collect further blood samples 2, 4 and 6 h later. Each specimen must reach the laboratory within 4 h of venesection. On receipt, the serum is separated and deproteinised at once.

Reagents.
1. Dissolve in deionised water, 5·2 g sodium acetate (CH_3COONa, $3H_2O$), 154 mg sodium metabisulphite, 480 mg sodium hydroxide and dilute to 100 ml.
2. Dissolve in deionised water, 20·4 g sodium acetate (CH_3COONa, $3H_2O$), 616 mg sodium metabisulphite, 1·76 g sodium hydroxide and dilute to 100 ml.
3. Salicylaldehyde solution. Working in a fume cupboard, dissolve 225 μl salicylaldehyde in 10 ml absolute ethanol and dilute to 100 ml with deionised water.
4. Basic aldehyde reagent. Mix one part of reagent (2) with two parts of reagent (3). Prepare freshly on the day of use, working in a fume cupboard.
5. Trichloracetic acid solution, 50 g/l.
6. 2-Mercaptoethanol.
7. Isobutanol.
8. Isoniazid standards. Prepare 100 ml aqueous stock standard, 100 mg/l. Dilute this with deionised water to give working standards of 1, 2, 4, 6 and 8 mg/l. All standards are stable for 2 weeks at 4 °C.
9. Control serum. Dilute 300 μl stock standard to 10 ml with drug-free serum to give a concentration of 3 mg/l. Prepare immediately before use.

Technique. Into 10 ml plastic tubes pipette 500 μl fresh serum (control or patient's), add 4·5 ml trichloracetic acid solution, mix well and centrifuge at high speed for 5 min. Transfer duplicate 2 ml amounts of the supernatants into each of two 10 ml conical glass centrifuge tubes. If necessary the tubes may be stored in the deep-freeze for up to 3 weeks.

Add 4·5 ml trichloracetic acid solution to 500 μl water (for the blank) or 500 μl of each standard, mix well and transfer duplicate 2 ml amounts to 10 ml glass centrifuge tubes. Add 1·0 ml basic aldehyde reagent to all tubes, mix well and allow to react at room temperature for 10 min. Working in a fume cupboard, add 2·0 ml reagent (1) to all tubes, followed by 80 μl mercaptoethanol and mix well before incubating at 50 °C for 10 min. Cool to room temperature and adjust the pH to 5·45–5·75 if necessary, using 100 mmol/l acid or alkali and a pH meter. Add 3·0 ml isobutanol to each tube, shake vigorously for 30 s and centrifuge at 2000 rpm for 5 min.

Transfer the upper, isobutanol layers to fluorescence cuvettes and after adjustment of the instrument's sensitivity, measure the fluorescence using excitation and emission wavelengths of 392 and 478 nm respectively.

Calculation. Plot the fluorimeter readings of the blank and standards against concentration to obtain a standard curve from which the control and test results can be read.

Plot the logarithm of the concentration (y axis) against the time of sampling after the oral dose (x axis) and extrapolate the line linearly to zero time. Note the intercept concentration and determine the time at which half this concentration is achieved (Fig. 36.17). This is the plasma isoniazid half-time.

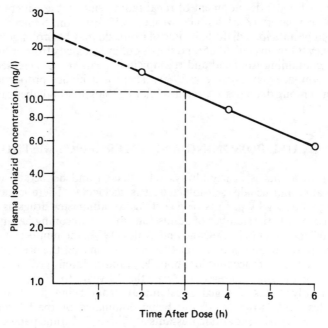

Fig. 36.17. Determination of the Half-time of Isoniazid.

Extrapolation to zero time gives an intercept concentration of 23·0 mg/l. The time corresponding to 23/2 or 11·5 mg/l is 3·0 h.

Notes.
1. Isoniazid condenses with salicylaldehyde under the reaction conditions to produce a fluorescent product which can be extracted into isobutanol.
2. Salicylaldehyde produces an irritant vapour and containment in a fume cupboard is desirable.
3. Serum deproteinisation no later than 4 h after venesection is essential for the satisfactory performance of this investigation.

INTERPRETATION

Fast acetylators have a mean plasma isoniazid half-time of about 60 (range 45 to 80) min following a single oral dose (Avery, 1980) and can be distinguished from slow acetylators whose mean $t_{1/2}$ is 180 (range 140–200) min (Bartells and Spring, 1975; Avery, 1980).

Evans (1960) reported that fast acetylators have isoniazid concentrations of less than 2·5 mg/l, 6 h after an oral dose of 10 mg/kg body weight. Plasma concentrations above 2·5 mg/l indicate slow acetylation. He also reported that fast acetylators excrete only 3% of unchanged drug in their urine, whereas slow acetylators may excrete as much as 30%.

Reidenberg *et al.* (1973) concluded that renal impairment does not affect isoniazid elimination half-time. Slow acetylators may, however, accumulate toxic concentrations of drugs which are metabolised by acetylation if their renal function is impaired. The half-time of isoniazid in anuric patients is about 17 h (Avery, 1980). Some workers have suggested that acetylator phenotype could be a determinant for the development of renal failure since these patients are often also slow acetylators (Karlsson and Molin, 1975; Fine and Sumner, 1975).

As might be anticipated, the half-time of isoniazid may be prolonged in hepatic insufficiency (Gilman *et al.*, 1985) and the risk of liver toxicity from antitubercular regimens containing isoniazid and rifampicin appears to be increased in those who are slow acetylators (Avery, 1980). There is a higher proportion of fast acetylators among diabetics, especially children, than in non-diabetic individuals (Avery, 1980).

PART 2. ACUTE POISONING AND EMERGENCY METHODS

Poisoning in adults is nearly always self-inflicted and deliberate, whereas in children, although usually self-inflicted, it is accidental. There is, however, an increasing tendency by parents or guardians to administer drugs as a form of child abuse. While the number of admissions due to poisoning has increased to over 100 000 per annum in England and Wales (1978), the number of deaths has remained approximately constant at 4000 per annum over the previous 12 years. Children under 5 years account for about 20% and children aged 5 to 14 years for about 6% of the total admissions. Over the 10 years to 1978, the pattern of poisons involved has changed substantially from being dominated by the barbiturates (15% down to 5%) to being dominated by the benzodiazepines (15% up to 30%), tricyclic antidepressants (4% up to 12%) and paracetamol (2% up to 12%). Most deaths due to poisoning occurred outside hospital so that fewer than 1000 (0·6%) cases died after admission. This proportion might have been higher without medical intervention although this assertion is probably impossible to substantiate. Of all deaths, carbon monoxide, barbiturates and analgesics each account for 20 to 25%, while antidepressants and tranquillisers each account for 5 to 10%. About 60% of all poisonings involved more than one compound and ethanol featured prominently in the majority.

Organisational Considerations

The hospital clinical biochemistry laboratory intending to help the physician with suspected poisoning cases needs to establish the following:

1. *Personnel.* A senior clinical biochemist should be responsible for the service to be provided, including liaison with clinicians and help with interpretation of results and should also be available out of hours for handling queries.
2. *Ward Instructions.* The laboratory should declare, in printed form, which assays are available and when, and the specimens required for analysis.
3. *Reference Support.* The district general hospital laboratory should establish a good working relationship with a larger laboratory which has additional facilities for poison detection and quantitation. This referral laboratory

should be reasonably close, e.g. within an hour's travel, so that specimens can be quickly transported there for analysis, especially out of hours. In addition, the district laboratory should establish contact with the nearest Poisons Information Service and its own Regional Drug Information Unit (Table 36.1, p. 933) which will be staffed by a Principal Pharmacist and have ready access to information in journals, text books, manufacturers' data and computer files.

4. *Analyses.* The laboratory should establish appropriate methods for the analyses detailed later.

The Clinical Request

In all instances the medical staff should be encouraged to request analysis for the drug or poison which their clinical examination of the patient and their experience lead them to suspect is involved. Requests to the biochemistry laboratory for 'Drug screen;? overdose' are unrealistic, unhelpful and should be discouraged. The requesting physician in all circumstances, but especially if he is unsure of the appropriate analyses to be undertaken, should discuss the circumstances of the case and his clinical findings with the clinical biochemist responsible for providing the toxicology service. This procedure will usually enable the most appropriate assays to be commenced without delay and, in many instances, allow the appropriate therapy to be instituted immediately. The clinical biochemist will also be able to consult other nearby toxicology services for analytical assistance, if required, at an early stage.

A useful guide when discussing acute poisoning problems with medical staff is the table of clinical signs related to single drug poisoning in the paper by Lockett (1978).

Material for Analysis

Most investigations are carried out on blood, urine, vomit or gastric aspirate, removed before gastric lavage commences. Occasionally tablets, capsules, etc. recovered from the stomach or found in the patient's possession may be submitted. These can often be identified from their size, colour and markings using the 'Tablident' drug identification system marketed by Edwin Burgess Publications Limited (Longwick Road, Princes Risborough, Aylesbury, Bucks., HP17 9RR) and usually in the possession of Regional Poisons Information Units and occasionally of hospital pharmacies.

Urine has the advantage that it is often available in large quantities. Many drugs are not excreted as such but the urine may contain several metabolites, some of which can be detected by simple qualitative tests. Extraction procedures and more elaborate methods of detection and quantitation are possible but variable metabolism between individuals may make interpretation difficult. One advantage is that drugs can usually be detected in the urine, often as metabolites, for some time after they have become undetectable in the blood.

Blood can usually be obtained and is best anticoagulated so that the maximum volume can be extracted if necessary. Some drugs are rapidly removed from the circulation by the tissues, making identification or quantitation more difficult. The blood concentration is only important in the treatment of a few types of poisoning. The simpler qualitative tests are not usually applicable and more elaborate qualitative or quantitative methods are required. Metabolites are often present in the circulation but these usually present few problems.

Gastric aspirate, if removed within an hour or two of ingestion of the poisoning agent, often contains this in relatively high concentration and in a chemically unchanged form. Sometimes tablet residues or characteristic odours can aid identification. Separation from other components of gastric contents usually requires extraction procedures.

Pharmacology

To be effective, an ingested poison has to be absorbed from the gastrointestinal tract. This is a time-dependent process which can often be speeded up by alcohol, slowed by either concomitant ingestion of other drugs or by clinical use of adsorbants and delayed if sustained-release preparations are ingested.

Distribution to the tissues is also time-dependent and can sometimes be delayed by appropriate therapy to chelate the ingested poison or enhance its elimination.

Metabolism is often a saturable process and may also produce toxic metabolites as, e.g. in paracetamol or methanol poisoning. Metabolism and elimination are also very dependent on hepatic and renal function. Some poisons will inhibit these directly by toxic action or indirectly by, e.g. decreasing cardiac output and hence hepatic or renal perfusion. It is important, therefore, when interpreting plasma concentrations to be aware of the limitations of a single data point. A blood specimen collected too soon after ingestion may yield a misleadingly low concentration or even negative results.

Most instances of poisoning involve more than one agent and the finding of one drug in high concentration does not preclude the presence of another, possibly more toxic, compound requiring much more urgent attention. It is in this regard that discussions between a senior clinical biochemist and the clinician can be especially useful.

It is also necessary for the laboratory to know what therapy has already been instituted prior to the request. Drugs administered to the patient before specimens are collected will almost certainly be present in them and may interfere positively or negatively in the analysis for the causative agent. A sound practice is to encourage the clinician to collect urine and blood samples on all admissions, whether or not poisoning is suspected at that stage, so that pre-therapy specimens are available for later use if needed. Timing of subsequent specimens depends on the suspected or demonstrated poison and is discussed under the individual poisons.

The assays described here should all be available at one laboratory in each region. The simpler, more commonly requested assays should be available in every district general hospital dealing with acute poisoning. In both instances, the only assays described are those the results of which will materially aid diagnosis and affect the treatment of the poisoned patient.

ALCOHOLS

Ethanol

This is one of the most common agents affecting cerebral function and is readily available. Although death from acute ethanol poisoning itself is uncommon, alcohol is often taken with other drugs and potentiates their effects sometimes with fatal results.

Measurement of its concentration is rarely required urgently except to monitor the treatment of methanol or ethylene glycol poisoning. GC is the best analytical method (p. 982) since these two other alcohols can be determined simultaneously. An enzymic method (Sigma kit) is available for ethanol alone or a dichromate method may be used (see 5th edition). The 'osmolar gap' method below is non-specific but useful if ethanol is the only alcohol present.

Screening Test for 'Alcohol' (Coakley *et al.*, 1983).

Macarulla and Mendia (1961) demonstrated a large 'osmolar gap' or difference between measured and calculated plasma osmolalities in subjects with high plasma ethanol concentrations. Thirteen or more formulae have been proposed over the years for calculating ethanol concentration from the osmolar gap but none has proved entirely satisfactory. Thus Redetzki *et al.* (1972) suggested that discrepancies were due to the presence of lactic acid and other osmotically active compounds in the plasma of patients intoxicated with ethanol. However, Bhagat *et al.* (1985) demonstrated that discrepancies also exist between the measured and calculated concentrations of ethanol in solutions of sodium chloride, suggesting that ethanol alters the degree of dissociation of sodium chloride in solution, in addition to depressing the freezing point. The errors involved are small and unlikely to be misleading if the test is used as a screen for 'alcohol'. It must be remembered that high values will also be obtained following ingestion of methanol, isopropanol and ethylene glycol and, to a lesser extent, in lactic or ketoacidoses. Similarly, high values will be obtained due to the underestimation of sodium in plasma with gross lipaemia or the presence of a paraprotein unless an ion-selective electrode is used.

The algorithm of Bhagat *et al.* (1985) using concentrations in mmol/l is:

$$\text{Calculated osmolality} = 1 \cdot 89[\text{Na}^+] + 1 \cdot 38[\text{K}^+] + 1 \cdot 03[\text{Urea}] + 1 \cdot 08[\text{Glucose}] + 7 \cdot 45 \text{ mmol/kg}$$

$$\text{Osmolar gap} = (\text{Measured osmolality}) - (\text{Calculated osmolality})$$

$$\text{'Alcohol' concentration (mg/l)} = (\text{Osmolar gap}) \times 34 \cdot 2 - 183$$

Concentrations calculated to be less than 200 mg/l should be reported as not detected.

Ethylene Glycol

Ethylene glycol (ethane-1,2-diol) is a colourless, odourless, water-soluble liquid with wide commercial application but used most commonly, alone or in various combinations with methanol, as a car radiator anti-freeze.

After ingestion, ethylene glycol is metabolised to acetaldehyde, glycolate, oxalate and lactate as shown in Fig. 36.18. These products inhibit a number of processes including oxidative phosphorylation, cellular respiration and glucose metabolism. Acidosis results from the production of glycolate, oxalate and lactate. Hypocalcaemia and renal damage may also result from oxalate formation.

The amount of ethylene glycol ingested and the delay before treatment is instituted determine the degree of poisoning and the outcome. Patients who have ingested ethylene glycol appear to be inebriated but without smelling of alcohol; they may also be comatose and have a large anion gap. In the first 12 h after ingestion there may be nausea, vomiting and haematemesis and a variety of

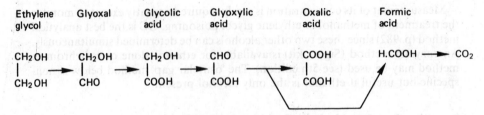

Fig. 36.18. The Metabolism of Ethylene Glycol.

neurological signs and symptoms, nystagmus, convulsions, depressed reflexes and coma. In the untreated patient the following 12 h shows involvement of the cardiorespiratory system including tachycardia, hypertension, pulmonary oedema and congestive cardiac failure. Involvement of the renal system follows with acute tubular necrosis and death may occur at any time.

Adequate treatment depends on early diagnosis and hence demonstration and quantitation of ethylene glycol in the blood is essential. Following gastric lavage to prevent further absorption, appropriate measures for the ensuing respiratory distress and shock are instituted together with bicarbonate infusion to correct the metabolic acidosis. Starting as early as possible, ethanol should be infused as a competitive inhibitor of glycol metabolism in amounts sufficient to produce blood ethanol concentrations between 1000 and 2000 mg/l. Once the concentration of blood ethanol is known following an initial dose, a new loading dose (L) is calculated as follows:

Let W = the patient's body weight (kg);
D = the measured ethanol concentration (mg/l);
V = the volume of distribution of ethanol = 0·6 l/kg;
then for a target blood ethanol concentration of 1500 mg/l,
$L = (W \times V \times (1500 - D))/1000$ g ethanol; or $L/0·8$ ml of ethanol.

The blood ethanol and glycol concentrations should be measured after 3 to 4 h to ensure that the ethanol concentration is adequate and that the glycol concentration is falling. The half-time for the ethylene glycol should be calculated. A half-time as short as 3 h suggests that the ethanol concentration is insufficient to inhibit ethylene glycol metabolism. The necessity for repeat assays will depend on circumstances but every 6 h is probably sufficient in most instances.

Occasionally, haemodialysis or haemoperfusion are used in an attempt to remove the glycol more rapidly. However, glycol and oxalate are not readily removed by either of these procedures whereas the protecting ethanol is. Hence if dialysis or haemoperfusion are used, the ethanol infusion rate will need to be increased to balance this loss. The oxalate may persist in the body long after the glycol has been removed and therefore acid–base status and plasma calcium should continue to be monitored for some time.

Methodology

Several colorimetric and gas chromatographic methods have been described. The one below uses the same analytical column as the ethanol/methanol method but with a different internal standard and a higher column temperature. It allows a simple, rapid changeover between the determinations of ethanol and ethylene glycol.

Determination of Ethylene Glycol (Mowatt, 1986).

Reagents.
1. Internal standard. Heptan-2-one, 100 mg/l in water. Store at 4 °C.
2. Sodium tungstate solution, 100 g/l.
3. Sulphuric acid, 330 mmol/l.
4. Ethylene glycol standard. Weigh accurately 100 mg ethylene glycol, dissolve in water and make to 100 ml. Prepare freshly immediately before use.

Technique. Into appropriately labelled glass centrifuge tubes pipette 200 μl each of patient's serum or plasma, standard solution and water. Add to each tube 200 μl internal standard, 200 μl sodium tungstate and 200 μl sulphuric acid solutions. Vortex-mix thoroughly and centrifuge for 5 min at 2000 rpm. Inject 1 μl of each supernatant onto the gas chromatograph column.

Gas Chromatography. A silanised glass column 2 m × 4 mm is packed with Poropak-Q, 80–100 mesh. The carrier is nitrogen at 50 ml/min and the operating temperature 220 °C, injection port temperature, 250 °C and the detector temperature, 350 °C. A flame ionisation detector is used and the output from the electrometer is connected to a 1 mV recorder. A standard trace is shown in Fig. 36.19. The method is linear to 2000 mg/l. If the glycol concentration is higher than the standard, dilute the serum with water and re-analyse.

INTERPRETATION
Clinical intervention is necessary when the plasma ethylene glycol concentration exceeds 300 mg/l as such figures have been associated with fatalities. It is essential that satisfactory hydration and renal function are maintained and that the blood ethanol concentration remains between 1000 and 2000 mg/l until the ethylene glycol concentration falls below 50 mg/l. Measurements of ethanol and ethylene glycol concentrations should be made 6 hourly until the glycol is undetectable.

Methanol

Methanol poisoning is seen in those who ingest methanol-containing 'antifreeze' solutions or, sometimes, 'methylated spirits'. Ingestion may be deliberate but is sometimes accidental as the imbiber believes erroneously that the alcohol ingested is ethanol. Methanol is occasionally ingested accidentally by children.

Depending on the time since ingestion, patients present with a variety of symptoms: headache, dizziness, abdominal pain, blurred vision, nausea, vomiting, or impaired consciousness leading to coma. Methanol is readily metabolised to formaldehyde and formate, both of which may be implicated in the gastric and neurological symptoms. Investigation usually reveals a marked metabolic acidosis with a large anion gap, hyperglycaemia and, occasionally, a raised amylase level as a consequence of pancreatic damage.

Treatment involves gastric lavage, if ingestion is recent, correction of the metabolic acidosis by bicarbonate, and the infusion of ethanol as a competitive inhibitor of methanol oxidation. The principles are similar to those discussed for ethylene glycol poisoning. The laboratory is therefore required to measure the blood methanol and ethanol concentrations in order to monitor progress and to assist in the adjustment of ethanol infusion rates.

Occasionally, the severity of the poisoning requires haemodialysis especially if the blood methanol concentration exceeds 500 mg/l or if the metabolic acidosis

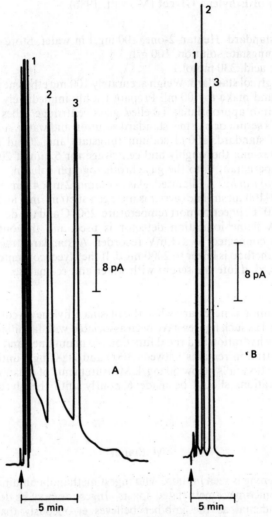

Fig. 36.19. The Gas Chromatographic Separation of Alcohols.
A. 1 = Ethanol; 2 = ethylene glycol; 3 = heptan-2-one (internal standard).
B. 1 = Methanol; 2 = ethanol; 3 = n-propanol (internal standard).
The arrows indicate the times of injection.

or neurological abnormalities prove refractory. Blood methanol concentrations below 50 mg/l may be discounted.

Methodology

The GC method for blood ethanol and methanol differs only slightly from that for ethylene glycol. To 200 μl blood add 3 ml internal standard (n-propanol, 1 : 5000) and 300 μl each of reagents (2) and (3). The standard contains ethanol and methanol, each in a concentration of 1000 mg/l. The column temperature is 165 °C and that of the detector is 250 °C. Other details are unchanged from p. 981.

A standard trace is shown in Fig. 36.19 above.

ANALGESICS

These pain-relieving drugs are, in many cases, readily available to the general public. They are in common use and form an important group of drugs associated with fatal poisoning. Those most frequently encountered are the various forms of salicylate and paracetamol.

Aspirin and Other Salicylates

The salicylate most often employed therapeutically is acetyl salicylate (aspirin); a few preparations contain salicylamide. Both are rapidly hydrolysed to salicylic acid so the parent is rarely found in plasma beyond 3 h after ingestion. Aspirin is a component in a number of mixed preparations involving purines, alkaloids and other drugs. A common preparation used in the elderly is benorylate, a compound of aspirin and paracetamol which yields these two components after absorption from the gastrointestinal tract.

In adults, moderately severe poisoning occurs following intake of 50, or more, 300 mg aspirin tablets. Unlike poisoning with many other agents, the patient is normally mentally alert but is usually restless and may complain of tinnitus and abdominal pain. Hyperventilation lasting several hours as a result of drug stimulation of the respiratory centre is usually obvious. The body temperature is increased and sweating occurs. Many patients vomit. The combination of losses of salt and water may result in dehydration with a reduction in urinary volume and rate of salicylate elimination (Brown, 1971). The movement of potassium into cells and the increased urinary loss accounts for the hypokalaemia which is sometimes seen. The blood pH is usually normal or slightly increased as the respiratory alkalosis is compensated by a metabolic acidosis due to increased metabolism and the nature of the drug. The P_{CO_2} falls to below 25 mmHg (3·3 kPa) with a base deficit in over half the cases of moderately severe poisoning.

More severe poisoning in adults leads to shock, intravascular haemolysis, reduced prothrombin concentrations and the possibility of acute renal failure. The metabolic acidosis may be exacerbated by poor tissue perfusion and the blood pH may fall as low as 7·10. This is often associated with drowsiness, a bad prognostic sign. In such severe poisoning there is a danger of pulmonary oedema or sudden respiratory or cardiac arrest. The toxic effects, unlike the clinical signs, are related to the circulating salicylate concentration, the determination of which plays an important part in the early clinical assessment and subsequent monitoring.

The clinical picture in children is somewhat different in that the metabolic acidosis is usually marked and persistent and of a greater degree than the initial respiratory alkalosis. The blood pH falls and the child may be drowsy or even unconscious. Hypokalaemia may be less marked but hypoglycaemia may sometimes occur. Again it is necessary to know the plasma salicylate concentration to assess therapy. The principles of treatment are the removal of residual drug from the stomach, the correction of water and electrolyte deficiencies, correction of low blood pH if present and the rapid elimination of salicylate by the kidney. If renal function is satisfactory, forced alkaline diuresis should be used in the more severe cases of salicylate poisoning. Dialysis is frequently employed in less severe forms and in young children.

Determination of Serum Salicylate (Trinder, 1954)

This method, still the most popular in the UK, depends on the purple colour produced by the reaction of ferric ions with the phenol group in salicylic acid.

Reagents.
1. Colour reagent. Dissolve 40 g mercuric chloride in 850 ml water, warming if necessary. When cold, add 120 ml hydrochloric acid, 1 mol/l, and 40 g ferric nitrate, $Fe(NO_3)_3,9H_2O$. When this has dissolved make up to 1 litre with water. The reagent is stable indefinitely at room temperature.
2. Standard solution, 200 mg/l as salicylic acid. The standard solution prepared from sodium salicylate and available from BDH Chemicals (cat. no. 230683S) is convenient and reliable.

Technique. Into plastic tubes pipette 1·0 ml serum, 1·0 ml water (for the blank) or 1·0 ml standard. Add 5·0 ml colour reagent, stopper and shake *vigorously*. Centrifuge at 2000 rpm for at least 2 min before transferring each supernatant fluid to a cuvette using a Pasteur pipette. Read against the blank at 540 nm.

Calculation.

$$\text{Serum salicylate (mg/l)} = \frac{\text{Reading of unknown}}{\text{Reading of standard}} \times 200$$

Notes.
1. The expected absorbance for the standard is $0\cdot34 \pm 0\cdot01$.
2. If the absorbance of the unknown exceeds 0·8, reanalyse using 0·5 ml serum, 0·5 ml water and 5·0 ml reagent.
3. If 1 ml serum is not available, either use 0·5 ml with 2·5 ml colour reagent, or follow the procedure in note (2) if a high result is expected. Do not alter the ratio of sample volume to colour reagent.
4. Measure the absorbance of the supernatant from the patient's serum only if it shows some purple colour. Results are unreliable below 10 mg/l and are best reported as 'salicylate not detected'.

INTERPRETATION
The therapeutic range of salicylate for analgesic purposes is approximately 50 to 150 mg/l and as an anti-inflammatory agent is approximately 100 to 350 mg/l. Toxic signs may be observed at almost any concentration in chronic usage and especially over 200 mg/l. Deliberate poisoning usually results in concentrations in excess of the upper therapeutic limit, occasionally over 1000 mg/l in severely poisoned patients, and alkaline diuresis should be considered for concentrations greater than 500 mg/l in adults or over 300 mg/l in children.

When the blood sample is collected more than 12 h after ingestion, the serum salicylate concentration may be relatively low and a better indication of the toxic effects is given by the serum potassium concentration and the blood acid–base data.

Paracetamol

Paracetamol, *p*-acetylaminophenol, is the pharmacologically active metabolite of phenacetin and acetanilide. It has been introduced as a safer drug than phenacetin which has a cumulative toxic effect on the kidney. Paracetamol, which avoids some of the undesirable gastric irritant effects of aspirin, is readily available to the public and is increasingly involved in attempted self-poisoning. Like aspirin, paracetamol and phenacetin are available in proprietary preparations in combination with other drugs. A combination very common in self-poisoning cases is co-proxamol, Distalgesic (paracetamol and dextropropoxyphene).

Paracetamol is excreted in the urine partly in conjugated form as the phenolic sulphate or glucosiduronate. Both the free and the conjugated forms may undergo hydrolysis of the acetylamino group liberating the amine. Excretion is rapid and paracetamol in therapeutic doses is quickly cleared, with a mean half-time of 2·5 h, making accumulation very unlikely. However, after ingestion of a large amount of paracetamol, the metabolising system becomes overloaded possibly due to exhaustion of the supply of thiol residues or saturation of the metabolising enzymes and a toxic intermediate metabolite accumulates resulting in hepatic necrosis after a few days (Fig. 36.20).

Many patients recover satisfactorily but the degree of liver damage is related to the dose taken and the time which elapses between ingestion and any necessary treatment. The overall mortality is about 1% and it is generally held that

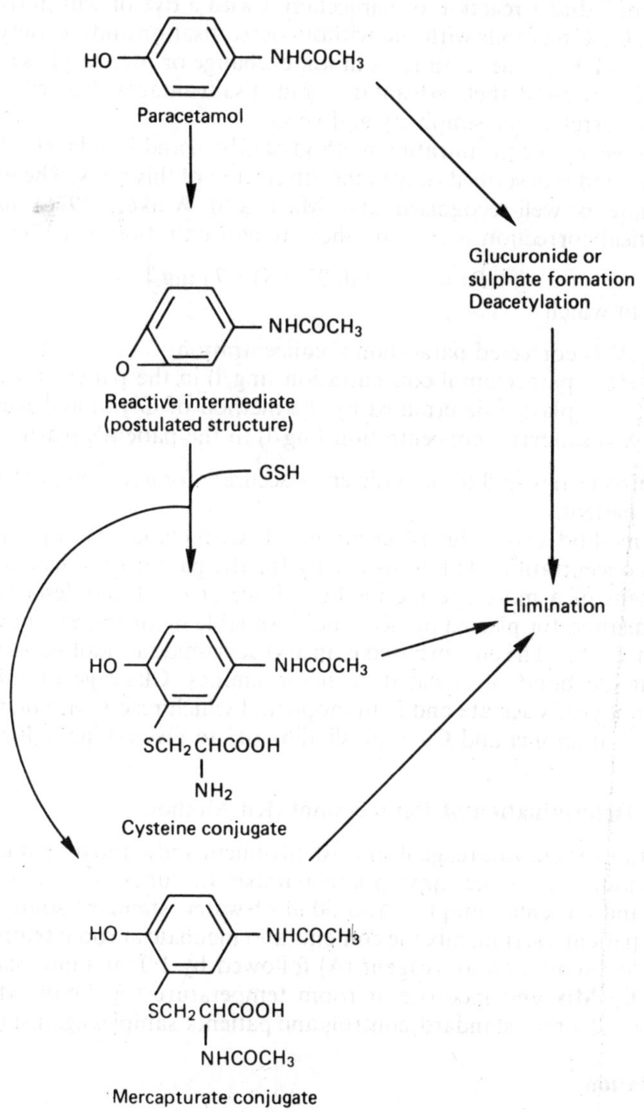

HO —⟨ ⟩— NHCOCH₃

Paracetamol

Glucuronide or
sulphate formation
Deacetylation

NHCOCH₃

O

Reactive intermediate
(postulated structure)

GSH

Elimination

HO —⟨ ⟩— NHCOCH₃

SCH₂CHCOOH
|
NH₂

Cysteine conjugate

HO —⟨ ⟩— NHCOCH₃

SCH₂CHCOOH
|
NHCOCH₃

Mercapturate conjugate

Fig. 36.20. The Metabolism of Paracetamol.
GSH = glutathione.

treatment with N-acetylcysteamine as a source of thiol groups protects against liver damage. N-Acetylcysteamine is less toxic than cysteamine, previously used, but still carries a finite risk. As many cases are relatively mild it is desirable to be able to detect paracetamol ingestion and measure the plasma concentration achieved as an emergency investigation.

Methodology

Wiener (1978) reviewed methods then available for the determination of plasma paracetamol. These were as follows: spectrophotometric (Routh *et al.*, 1968; Dordoni *et al.*, 1973); a variety of colorimetric methods based on conversion to p-aminophenol; direct reaction of paracetamol with a dye or with nitrous acid; a number of GLC methods with and without derivatisation and a variety of HPLC methods involving either cation- or anion-exchange or reverse-phase chromatography. He reviewed their advantages and disadvantages, linearity, precision, recoveries, correlations, simplicity and speed.

For emergency use the nitration method of Glynn and Kendal (1975) has been widely used and is described fully in the 5th edition of this book. The interference by salicylate is well-recognised and Mace and Walker (1976) suggested a mathematical correction based on salicylate concentration which is

$$Pc = Pd - [(0.07 \times S) + 7] \text{ mg/l}$$

in which

Pc = corrected paracetamol concentration;
Pd = paracetamol concentration (mg/l) in the patient's
    plasma determined by the method of Glynn and Kendal;
S = salicylate concentration (mg/l) in the patient's plasma.

This correction is said to be sufficiently accurate for assessment of the acutely poisoned patient.

As the method also includes certain non-toxic metabolites of paracetamol in the final concentration, its low specificity for the parent drug has hastened the development of a more specific method. Price *et al.* (1983) described a rapid enzymic method for plasma paracetamol (available in kit form from Cambridge Life Sciences Plc). The enzyme used is an aryl acylamide amidohydrolase, specific for the amide bond of acylated aromatic amines. Cleavage of this bond in paracetamol yields acetate and p-aminophenol which reacts with o-cresol in the presence of ammonia and Cu^{2+} at alkaline pH to give a blue indophenol dye.

Enzymic Determination of Paracetamol (Kit Method)

Reconstitute the enzyme reagent with 10 ml diluent and stand for 5 min. Dispense 500 μl amounts into the appropriate number of tubes for blank, standard, controls and patients' samples. Add 50 μl of water, standard solution, control serum or patient's serum, mix the contents and incubate at room temperature for 5 min. Add 1.0 ml o-cresol reagent (A) followed by 1.0 ml ammoniacal copper reagent (B). Mix and incubate at room temperature for 4 min. Measure the absorbance, A, of the standard, controls and patients' samples against the blank at 615 nm.

Calculation.

$$\text{Serum paracetamol (mg/l)} = \frac{A(\text{Test})}{A(\text{Standard})} \times \text{Standard concentration}$$

Note. It is claimed that there is no interference from common metabolites of paracetamol, or from 32 varied drugs at a concentration of 1 mmol/l, or from salicylate at a concentration of 5 mmol/l.

INTERPRETATION

There is much individual variation in the susceptibility of patients to the hepatotoxic action of paracetamol (Wright and Prescott, 1973). Previous induction of the hepatic microsomal enzyme systems by alcohol or by drugs such as barbiturates renders the patient more susceptible. Since paracetamol alone produces neither coma nor specific early signs and symptoms, the severity of poisoning cannot be determined on clinical grounds. Also, clinical evidence of liver damage does not become apparent for many hours and abnormal liver function tests, even aminotransferase activities, may not be demonstrable until 24 h or more after ingestion while maximal abnormalities may be delayed for several days (Stewart and Simpson, 1973).

The early assessment of the likely severity of paracetamol poisoning and the need for early therapeutic intervention thus depends on measurement of the paracetamol concentration in the plasma. It is important not to determine this too soon after ingestion since absorption may be incomplete and a misleadingly low concentration will result. The physician must be certain that 4 or more hours

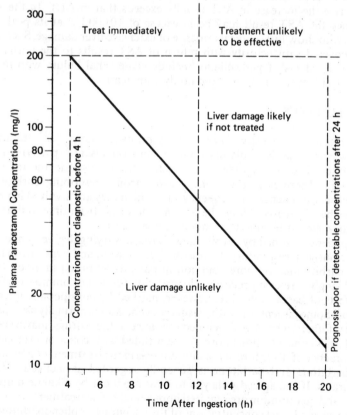

Fig. 36.21. 'Action Lines' for Treatment in Paracetamol Overdosage (see text).

have elapsed since ingestion. In case of doubt a repeat assay 2 to 4 h after the first one will indicate the magnitude and direction of change.

Prescott *et al.* (1976) and Stewart *et al.* (1979) have both produced plasma concentration-time curves with added 'action lines' (Fig. 36.21) which indicate the likelihood of liver damage developing in relation to a particular plasma paracetamol concentration up to 12 and 24 h after ingestion. An early suggestion (Prescott *et al.*, 1971) that estimation of paracetamol half-time could indicate the degree of liver damage has not been widely accepted since prolonged half-times can also be due to saturation of the metabolising enzymes. There are suggestions, however, that patients with paracetamol concentrations close to, but below, the action line and who also have prolonged paracetamol half-times (i.e. greater than 4 h) will benefit from *N*-acetylcysteamine therapy.

The patient in whom the time of ingestion is not known with certainty presents a particular diagnostic problem if the plasma paracetamol concentration is raised. A second plasma paracetamol assay 4 h after the first enables the half-time to be calculated and a value greater than 4 h suggests enzyme system saturation or liver damage, as outlined above, and indicates that a considerable period of time may have elapsed since ingestion and therefore the patient is probably at risk.

The degree of liver damage can be followed satisfactorily using enzyme determinations. Suitable enzymes are aspartate aminotransferase (AST), alanine aminotransferase (ALT) and gamma-glutamyltranspeptidase (GGT). The determination of prothrombin time is also important in the more severe cases. In the acute phase the increase in AST usually exceeds that in ALT. In the author's experience the AST result may be in excess of 10 000 U/l at its peak even in patients who show little clinical evidence of extensive liver damage. Such patients have recovered satisfactorily with return of AST results to the normal range. Other toxic effects of paracetamol include acute renal failure with its typical biochemical features and, less commonly, pancreatitis.

BARBITURATES

Barbiturates are widely used as hypnotics, some as tranquillisers. Phenobarbitone has been discussed under 'Anticonvulsants' (p. 949) in Part 1 of this chapter. The very short-acting barbiturates are used in the induction of anaesthesia. There has been a move away from prescribing barbiturates as tranquillisers and hence the frequency with which they are involved in poisoning incidents has decreased. None-the-less they do occur from time to time and the laboratory should be able to recognise these drugs.

The patient poisoned by barbiturates shows, in varying degrees, impaired level of consciousness, respiratory depression, hypotension and hypothermia. Deaths due to barbiturate are more common in patients admitted in grade IV coma. Table 36.9 gives relevant pharmacological data for some common barbiturates. The effects of barbiturates are, however, marked by considerable inter-subject variation. Some patients die with plasma concentrations normally associated with recovery. Others, who have developed tolerance to these drugs, may be conscious with plasma concentrations normally associated with coma or even death.

The practice of using forced alkaline diuresis in the treatment of poisoning with phenobarbitone and barbitone is generally regarded as ineffective for other barbiturates. If the agreed policy is to treat a patient by alkaline diuresis then identity and quantitation are required immediately. The treatment will usually be initiated when plasma concentrations of the barbitone or phenobarbitone exceed 100 mg/l.

TABLE 36.9

Pharmacological Data for Barbiturates.

Barbiturate	Therapeutic Range* (mg/l)	Half-time (h)	Vd (l/kg)
Amylobarbitone	2–12	8–40	approx. 1
Barbitone**	5–30	approx. 48	0·4–0·6
Butobarbitone	2–15	approx. 40	approx. 0·8
Cyclobarbitone	2–10	8–17	approx. 0·5
Heptabarbitone**	1–4	6–11	approx. 1
Hexobarbitone**	1–5	3–7	approx. 1
Methylphenobarbitone	5–15	50–60	2–3
Pentobarbitone	2–10	15–48	0·7–1·0
Phenobarbitone	15–30	15–150	0·5–1·2
Quinalbarbitone	2–10	19–34	0·6–1·9

* Included in this table to indicate potency. Varying degrees of toxicity develop with concentrations up to about 5 times the upper therapeutic limit. Beyond this, fatalities become much more likely. If dependence has developed, much higher concentrations may be encountered without fatalities.

** Now withdrawn but may still be available from illegal sources.

Many serious barbiturate poisonings are handled successfully by intensive supportive therapy and hence the only requirement of the biochemistry department is to demonstrate the presence of a barbiturate (an immunoassay will achieve this very quickly) and provide other common biochemical assays as the need arises. The identity and quantitation of the barbiturate can usually be left until later.

Whichever policy is adopted for handling these patients, the laboratory has a role in assessment of the adequacy of respiration and tissue perfusion by performing blood gas analysis and in monitoring electrolyte and fluid balance during diuretic therapy.

Methodology

A variety of methods for the determination of barbiturates is given in the 5th edition of this book. A satisfactory method for the identification and quantitation of barbiturates by HPLC is given below. The identity of the barbiturate should be separately confirmed by another technique, e.g. TLC, since HPLC methods are generally non-specific.

Reagents.

1. Phosphate buffer, 500 mmol/l KH_2PO_4 solution, adjusted to pH 7·5.
2. Phosphate buffer, 10 mmol/l KH_2PO_4 solution, adjusted to pH 8·0.
3. Diethyl ether.
4. Mobile phase: 60/40, reagent (2)/acetonitrile.
5. Stock standard solutions. Dissolve 25 mg of each of the barbiturates listed in Table 36.9 (above) in methanol or chloroform as appropriate and make to 100 ml. Store at 4 °C.
6. Mixed serum standard. Pipette 2 ml of each stock solution into a single test tube and evaporate off the solvents. Dissolve the residues in 10 ml of drug-

free serum, divide into 250 μl amounts and store frozen. The concentration of each drug is 50 mg/l.

Technique. Into 4 appropriately labelled glass-stoppered tubes pipette 200 μl drug-free serum (blank), serum standard, control serum, or patient's serum. Add 200 μl pH 7·5 buffer and 2 ml diethyl ether, stopper and vortex-mix for 1 min. Remove stoppers and centrifuge at 2000 rpm for 2 min. Transfer the ether (upper) layers to clean dry conical tubes and evaporate under nitrogen at 60 °C. Wash down the tube sides with 200–300 μl ether and re-evaporate. Dissolve the residues in 200 μl of mobile phase and load 10 μl onto the column.

Chromatography. Pump the mobile phase at 1 ml/min through a column (250 × 4 mm) packed with 10 μm C18 reverse-phase material and preceded by a guard column (40 × 4 mm) packed with the same material. The column effluent is monitored by a spectrophotometric detector, wavelength 200 nm, 8 nm band width, range 0·1 AUFS connected to a 1 mV recorder. A mixed standard trace is shown in Fig. 36.22.

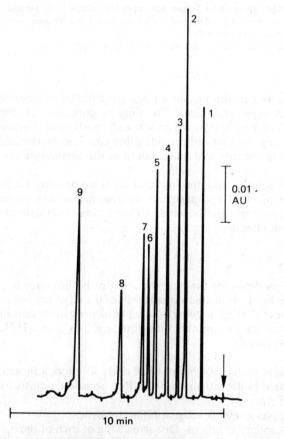

Fig. 36.22. The Separation of Barbiturates by HPLC.
1 = Barbitone;   2 = phenobarbitone;   3 = butobarbitone;   4 = cyclobarbitone;
5 = heptabarbitone;   6 = amylobarbitone;   7 = pentabarbitone;   8 = quinalbarbitone;
9 = methaqualone.

The method is linear to approximately 50 mg/l for each drug. Serum with concentrations higher than this should be diluted with drug-free serum and re-extracted. The detection limit is approximately 2 mg/l.

CARBON MONOXIDE

Non-smokers exhibit a background carboxyhaemoglobin saturation of less than 2%, and in smokers this figure is reportedly as high as 6%. Carbon monoxide has 200 times the affinity for haemoglobin than does oxygen. So air containing carbon monoxide in a concentration of 0·1% will convert half the haemoglobin into carboxyhaemoglobin if breathed for an hour. At twice this atmospheric concentration, death may supervene within a few hours. Carbon monoxide is implicated in fatal poisoning either accidentally or with deliberate intent. Domestic gas supplies in the UK are now entirely natural gas and therefore virtually free from carbon monoxide. Carbon monoxide is formed, however, when carbonaceous matter is burnt in oxygen-poor conditions, e.g. car exhaust fumes liberated in a closed garage or leakage from the flue of a solid-fuel stove or gas fire.

In the absence of anaemia, toxic effects such as headache and lassitude appear at about 20% saturation with carbon monoxide. More severe symptoms with muscular weakness, giddiness, fainting attacks and dyspnoea develop as the saturation increases towards 50%. Loss of consciousness occurs at 50 to 80% with a fatal outcome if exposure continues, the length of time required shortening at the higher concentrations. Removal from the carbon monoxide atmosphere allows fairly rapid breakdown of carboxyhaemoglobin with reformation of oxyhaemoglobin. The important irreversible effects on cerebral function depend on the degree and duration of impaired oxygenation of the brain. The half-time of carbon monoxide is 4 to 5 h at atmospheric oxygen tension. Administration of pure oxygen decreases the half-time to approximately 80 min and hyperbaric oxygen at 3 atmospheres decreases the half-time to 24 min.

A method for the determination of carboxyhaemoglobin is given on p. 665. Samples of blood for analysis should be taken without delay after removal from the toxic atmosphere and should be anticoagulated with sodium fluoride in a sealed tube filled to the brim to prevent loss of carbon monoxide.

DIGOXIN

Approximately 25% of patients on digoxin therapy and exhibiting, in varying degrees of severity, toxic signs and symptoms have plasma digoxin concentrations within the therapeutic range of 0·8 to 2·0 μg/l. Conversely, about 25% of patients with plasma digoxin concentrations between 2·0 and 3·0 μg/l show no evidence of toxicity. Consequently, the diagnosis of digoxin toxicity is primarily a clinical problem to which an emergency assay of plasma digoxin contributes very little. (See the section on digoxin in Part 1 of this chapter for a fuller discussion.)

The large apparent *Vd* for digoxin indicates that at least 90% of the body burden of digoxin is tissue-bound which means that all forms of dialysis and haemoperfusion contribute very little to its elimination. The only exception to this is the patient who is anuric or has very little residual renal function.

Wellcome Medical Division have recently introduced a preparation of a digoxin-binding antibody, Digibind, which can be administered to patients suffering from digoxin toxicity. The preparation is given i.v., renders plasma digoxin concentrations undetectable within 1 or 2 min and causes marked improvements in cardiac rhythm within 15–30 min if the dysrhythmia was due to digoxin. The material is very expensive.

The most appropriate assays which the biochemistry laboratory can perform are plasma potassium and acid–base determinations, since it is essential to maintain normokalaemia and high urine outputs and normal homeostasis until the emergency has passed.

IRON

Acute iron poisoning is an occasional though decreasingly common problem encountered in children. It arose because parents did not recognise iron preparations as dangerous but is becoming less of a problem due to increased awareness and the introduction of child-proof tablet containers. Deliberate excess ingestion of iron preparations is occasionally encountered in adults.

Within 12 h of ingesting large amounts of iron preparations, epigastric pain, nausea and vomiting are observed. Haematemesis often occurs which, if severe, leads to circulatory failure. In severe poisoning there may be confusion, convulsions, pulmonary oedema, metabolic acidosis and cyanosis. Renal or hepatic failure may develop with consequent fatal outcome.

Treatment with desferrioxamine after gastric lavage should be prompt and success depends very largely on maintenance of urine output to allow adequate excretion of the iron chelate (see Vale and Meredith (1981) p. 176).

Method for Serum Iron Determination

Any routine method for serum or plasma iron is appropriate although some involving automatic analysers for the analysis of large routine batches may be difficult to operate out-of-hours or impossible to start up quickly enough to provide an emergency assay. There are several kit methods on the market but the assay may be required so infrequently that many time-expired kits would be discarded unused.

The following method is recommended for emergency use since it is technically simple, although care is required in its execution, and the reagents are stable for long periods at room temperature.

Reagents.
1. Trichloracetic acid, 300 g/l.
2. Thioglycollic acid. Dilute 80 ml of the acid to 100 ml with deionised water.
3. Sodium acetate solution. Dissolve 58 g $CH_3COONa,3H_2O$ in deionised water and make to 100 ml.
4. Bathophenanthroline reagent. Dissolve 15 mg bathophenanthroline in isopropanol and make to 100 ml with the same solvent.
5. Hydrochloric acid, concentrated.
6. Standard in serum. It is most convenient to use a commercial lyophilised material for this since absolute accuracy is not required; Ortho 'Normal' is suitable. It should be reconstituted according to the manufacturer's instructions and the quoted concentration used in the calculation given below.

Technique. Into four 10 ml plastic tubes appropriately labelled, pipette 2 ml each of water, serum standard, control serum and patient's serum. To all tubes add 3 ml of deionised water, followed by 1 drop of hydrochloric acid and 1 drop of thioglycollic acid solution; cap and mix. Add 1 ml trichloracetic acid solution *and stir well using a glass rod*. Centrifuge at 2000 rpm for at least 5 min. Transfer 3 ml clear supernatant from each tube to labelled clean tubes and add 0·4 ml sodium acetate solution. Cap, mix well and then add 2 ml bathophenanthroline reagent. Cap and mix thoroughly and then read the absorbances (A) of all tube contents against the blank at 510 nm.

$$\text{Serum iron } (\mu\text{mol/l}) = (A\,(\text{test})/A\,(\text{standard})) \times \text{Standard concentration}$$

INTERPRETATION

The toxic threshold for plasma iron in children is 90 μmol/l and in adults 145 μmol/l. Concentrations higher than these indicate moderate to severe poisoning requiring treatment with parenteral desferrioxamine (Matthew and Lawson, 1979). Plasma iron concentration should be assayed at 12 and 24 h after the initiation of treatment in order to monitor progress. Depending on these concentrations, further treatment and additional assays may be necessary. A close watch should be kept on the effects of any fluid and electrolyte loss, changes in acid–base status and on renal and hepatic function depending on the severity of the poisoning.

PARAQUAT

This quaternary ammonium base, used as a herbicide, continues to be implicated in accidental and deliberate poisoning. It is related to another weedkiller, diquat. They are much more toxic in man than the original animal work suggested. Paraquat is available in liquid and solid formulations sometimes in conjunction with other herbicides. The liquid preparations, usually only available to commercial growers, are more concentrated and hence more dangerous. A dose of 3 g is likely to be lethal and is contained in only 15 ml of the most potent preparations. Accidental poisoning has occurred as a result of storing liquids containing paraquat in unlabelled or mislabelled domestic bottles.

After a single oral dose, acute ulcerative damage occurs in those parts of the skin and mucous membranes in contact with the poison. More serious effects on the liver, kidney and heart occur 2 or 3 days later. Later still, signs of pulmonary dysfunction appear with dyspnoea and pulmonary oedema leading to a progressive fatal pulmonary fibrosis.

Ingestion of paraquat is still associated with a high mortality and the outcome is still more dependent on the amount ingested than on treatment. Paraquat is absorbed rapidly from the gut giving peak plasma concentrations within 1 h. Thereafter the concentration falls precipitately due to very rapid distribution into tissues and equally rapid clearance from the blood by renal elimination. Paraquat is retained in the tissues for much longer and its slow redistribution is responsible for the prolonged low plasma concentrations.

The mechanism of the toxic action of paraquat has not yet been thoroughly resolved, but since paraquat can be readily reduced by electrons from the electron transport chain, it is believed to form an unstable free radical. This free radical in turn interacts with oxygen to produce the very toxic superoxide. Superoxide dismutase, which exists to cope with the small amounts of endogenous superoxide, is overwhelmed by the large amount of superoxide produced by the ingested paraquat and the excess superoxide produces the lipid free radicals which are finally responsible for the tissue damage. This damage commences immediately paraquat is ingested and presumably continues while paraquat remains in the tissues.

If less than 4 h have elapsed since ingestion, then gastric lavage is appropriate therapy. A 30% suspension of Fuller's earth (250 ml) and a 5% suspension of magnesium sulphate are usually left in the stomach after lavage and this dose is repeated every 4 h until faecal samples are negative with the dithionite test. Whole gut irrigation, forced diuresis, peritoneal dialysis and haemodialysis have not been conclusively shown to be effective in all cases of paraquat poisoning. Similarly, recent suggestions for the use of low tension oxygen therapy, administration of superoxide dismutase and D-propranolol, steroids and immunosuppressant drugs have been shown not to effect the outcome significantly. If the patient presents more than 8 h after ingestion, Vale and Meredith (1981) suggest that haemoperfusion be considered.

Most seriously poisoned patients die from multiorgan failure and relatively few from pulmonary fibrosis alone. Since there is no specific therapy for paraquat poisoning, the assay is an approximate but useful prognostic indicator (Proudfoot *et al.*, 1979) during the first 24 h after ingestion (Table 36.10). More recently, Hart *et al.* (1984), using data from 219 cases of paraquat poisoning, have produced a contour map showing probability of survival based on plasma concentration and time since ingestion. In addition to intensive supportive therapy it is useful to monitor pulmonary, renal and hepatic functions for a number of days until the clinician is satisfied that the patient is out of danger.

TABLE 36.10
Toxicity of Paraquat.

Time after ingestion (h)	Maximum plasma concentration compatible with survival (mg/l)
8	0·65
12	0·50
16	0·40
20	0·35
24	0·30

Qualitative Test for Paraquat in Urine or Faeces

A blue colour is produced by reduction with alkaline dithionite.

Reagents.
1. Sodium hydroxide solution, 1 mol/l.
2. Sodium dithionite reagent. Dissolve 100 mg of the solid in 10 ml sodium hydroxide immediately before use.

Technique. Add 1 ml dithionite reagent to 1 ml urine or a centrifuged faecal suspension. A strong blue colour indicates the presence of paraquat, diquat or both. The natural colour of the urine produces a greenish colour with lower concentrations. Then the sensitivity may be improved by shaking with alumina and decanting before testing with dithionite.

Note. Berry and Grove (1971) increased the urine volume to 5 ml and detected 1 mg/l in clear urine and 1·5 mg/l in cloudy specimens.

Determination of Paraquat in Serum or Plasma

A chromatographic method is described in the 5th edition of this book, but the most satisfactory method in terms of sensitivity and precision is probably radioimmunoassay which is available in a few centres. The method given here is by Jarvie and Stewart (1979) in which the paraquat is extracted from serum and reduced by alkaline dithionite to give a blue colour. Peak identification and absorbance measurement is made easier with the use of a scanning spectrophotometer with second derivative facility.

Reagents.

1. Extraction solvent. Add 50 ml water-saturated isobutyl methyl ketone to 50 ml water-saturated isobutanol. In this, dissolve 0·5 g sodium dodecyl sulphate.
2. Sodium chloride solution, 2·5 mol/l.
3. Sodium hydroxide solution, 300 mmol/l.
4. Sodium dithionite reagent. Dissolve 0·3 g $Na_2S_2O_4$ in 10 ml reagent (3). Prepare freshly immediately before use.
5. Stock standard, 200 mg/l. Dissolve 27·6 mg paraquat dichloride (1,1'-dimethyl-4,4'-bipyridylium chloride, Aldrich cat. no. 85, 617–7) in water and make to 100 ml. This solution is equivalent to 200 mg of paraquat ion per litre. It is unstable and should not be stored after preparation of the serum standards. *NB: This compound is harmful by skin absorption and inhalation.*
6. Intermediate standard, 2 mg/l. Take 0·5 ml stock standard solution and make to 50 ml with drug-free serum.
7. Working standards. Make 0·5, 1·0, 2·5 and 5·0 ml amounts of intermediate standard up to 10 ml with drug-free serum to give concentrations of 0·1, 0·2, 0·5, 1·0 and 2·0 mg/l. Divide into 2·5 ml amounts and store frozen.

Technique. To 2 ml drug-free serum (blank), each working standard and patient's serum in 15 ml glass-stoppered tubes, add 2 ml deionised water. Mix and add 10 ml extraction solvent. Stopper the tubes and mix gently by inversion for 5 min taking care to avoid formation of emulsions; a haematology mixer is ideal for this. Centrifuge at 3000 rpm for 5 min. Carefully transfer 8 ml of each solvent phase to clean 10 ml glass-stoppered tubes. Add 0·8 ml reagent (2) to each tube, shake vigorously for 5 min and centrifuge for 2 min at 3000 rpm. Carefully aspirate the solvent phase and transfer 0·7 ml of the aqueous phase to small (e.g. 70 × 7 mm) glass tubes and process each tube individually as follows: Add 100 μl reagent (4) to the first tube, mix briefly, transfer to a spectrophotometer cuvette and immediately scan the absorbance profile between 460 and 380 nm. Generate the second derivative of the absorbance scan and either produce a hard copy for measurement with a millimetre ruler or cause the spectrophotometer to display the second derivative difference between the peak and trough corresponding to the absorbance inflection at 397 nm, (see Fig. 36.23). Add 100 μl reagent (4) to the second tube and repeat the process of scanning etc. Process all the tubes in this way. When differences are obtained for all the standards, plot these against concentration and read the patient's serum paraquat concentration from the graph.

THEOPHYLLINE

The pharmacology of theophylline is described in Part 1 of this chapter. With mild theophylline toxicity, clinical features may include nausea, abdominal pain.

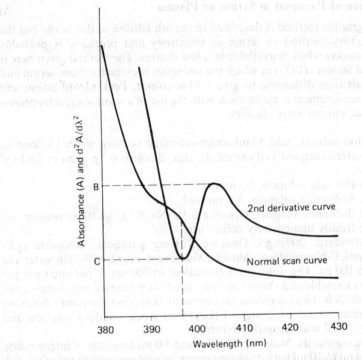

Fig. 36.23. Spectrophotometric Curves in the Determination of Paraquat.
The trough and peak of the second derivative curve correspond to the inflection at 397 nm. The difference between B and C is plotted against concentration. For technical reasons the derivative curve is displaced slightly to the right.

vomiting, agitation, tremor, hyperventilation and tachycardia. In severe cases, cardiac arrhythmias, hypotension, convulsions, impaired consciousness and cardiorespiratory arrest may occur. One reported case (Burgan *et al.*, 1982) resembled acute pancreatitis.

The most recent views on the treatment of theophylline poisoning suggest gastric aspiration and lavage should be performed if less than 10 h have elapsed since ingestion. Children should, instead, be given ipecacuanha. Activated charcoal should then be given if there is no vomiting. In all cases a blood sample should be taken on admission and assayed for theophylline. If the concentration is greater than 20 mg/l a repeat assay after 4 h will indicate whether theophylline continues to be absorbed. This is important since the peak plasma concentration may be delayed 10 or more hours with slow-release preparations of the drug.

Peritoneal and haemodialysis are ineffective in removing theophylline, but Park *et al.* (1983) use charcoal haemoperfusion for all patients with a plasma theophylline concentration of 60 mg/l or more, 4 h after ingestion. They consider haemoperfusion if any three of the following risk factors are present:

1. patient over 60 years of age;
2. liver disease or cardiac failure present;
3. plasma theophylline concentration greater than 50 mg/l;
4. theophylline plasma half-time greater than 24 h.

This last criterion requires two plasma theophylline concentrations (A and B) to be determined at a known time interval (T) of at least 4 h and with the second concentration (B) lower than the first (A). The half-time can be calculated using the formula:

$$t_{1/2} = (T \times \log 2)/(\log A/B)$$

The risk of cardiac arrest requires continuous electrocardiographic monitoring, and the biochemistry laboratory will also be required to assist in guarding against hypokalaemia, acidosis and dehydration. Theophylline should be assayed about every 6 h during haemoperfusion.

Methodology

The HPLC method for theophylline described earlier (p. 940) is suitable for emergency use and can provide an answer in about 1 h. One of the immunoassays may be more convenient, however, if the necessary equipment is to hand, as the answer can be available in a short space of time. The cost per test is considerably higher than HPLC.

PART 3. DRUGS OF ABUSE

Drug Dependence

All substances ingested for their psychotropic effect carry some potential for dependence. The degree of dependence is governed by the substance involved, the frequency and duration of its use and the psychological make-up of the subject.

Drugs of abuse may be classified according to many criteria. The Misuse of Drugs Act (1971) divides drugs into three classes: Class A includes drugs such as heroin, cocaine and lysergides and offences against the Act involving these drugs carry the most serious penalties. Class B drugs include cannabis and amphetamines and offences involving these attract less severe punishment. Class C includes, among others, Mandrax.

A more satisfactory classification based on the principal effect produced by the drug is used here.

1. **Stimulants**. These produce an increase in physical and mental activity. Users feel alert and confident and tiredness is either banished or is less marked. The reasons given for using stimulants are usually a desire to 'keep going' at all-night parties, to counteract the soporific effect of other drugs, or because they promote a sense of superiority and confidence. In addition to habituation, users run the risk of showing aggressive, sometimes violent, antisocial behaviour, of feeling anxious, frightened and isolated and of imposing a continuous strain on the heart. Included in this group are cocaine, sympathomimetic (anorectic) amines, e.g. amphetamines, and the antidepressants.

2. **Depressants**. They exert a slowing effect on the activity of the body and brain. The user does not feel depressed but enjoys intense feelings of relaxation and well-being with a lessening of pain sensation and anxiety. Not all have the same intensity of effect but all carry the risk of habituation, achievement of toxic concentrations, very deep coma and death. All, with the exception of alcohol, are available on prescription for a range of medical conditions.

This group of compounds has two main divisions: The hypnotic/sedative group includes ethanol, barbiturates, benzodiazepines, phenothiazines, antihistamines and several other tranquillisers. The narcotic/analgesic group includes alkaloids and synthetic drugs, e.g. heroin, morphine, codeine, methadone, pethidine and dextropropoxyphene.

3. **Hallucinogens**. Also called psychotomimetics, they cause a wide range of psychological effects—pleasant to very frightening hallucinations giving rise to severe, though usually temporary, mental disturbances. This group includes, in increasing order of potency, the cannabinoids, the amphetamine-like compound mescaline and the lysergides. Major risks associated with the use of the hallucinogens, especially LSD, are the unpredictability of effects, the frequency of severe mental disturbances (i.e. 'bad trips') and the severe distortions of perception which lead to foolish actions (e.g. the imagined ability to fly) often with fatal results.

4. **Solvents**. These 'deliriants' are often used for their psychotropic effect mainly by young adolescent boys. The effects of inhaling solvents, usually immediate and short-lived, are light-headedness, relaxation, well-being, blurred vision, confused thinking, loss of memory and, occasionally, hallucinations. Since solvents are usually 'huffed', i.e. inhaled from a plastic bag, the most common causes of death are from unconsciousness and consequent suffocation or from physical injury during loss of control. Cardiac arrest is also associated with solvent abuse, particularly with aerosol propellants which are mainly fluorocarbons. There is evidence, too, that chronic solvent abuse can cause damage to liver, kidney, bone marrow and brain.

Rationale of Drug Abuse Screening

It is now recognised that symptoms of psychiatric illness can be mimicked by the use of certain drugs and many psychiatrists will request a urine screen in certain cases to assess drug use. Drug users who are referred, by their general practitioner or by the courts, to drug-dependence clinics are accepted for treatment usually on the basis of a verbal contract between themselves and the psychiatrist. This contract, of which urine testing is an important part, is based on a clear understanding, by both sides, of what is involved in the treatment and on mutual trust. The usual programme is as follows.

On acceptance, tests on two separate urine specimens must show the presence of the drug(s), and/or metabolites, which the patient claims to be abusing. After commencement of treatment, the urine testing is intended to confirm that the patient does not break the contract either by resuming the use of the abused drug(s), by using a different drug or by not taking the drug of treatment if one has been prescribed. Some psychiatrists advocate daily testing of the patient's urine during therapy but two or three times per week is probably sufficient since the usual doses and the fact of long half-times ensures that most drugs will be detectable in urine up to 3 days, and possibly longer, after use (see Table 36.11).

Specimens for Analysis

Obtaining suitable specimens is fraught with difficulty. Many patients occasionally try to deceive the clinician, for a variety of reasons, about their history of drug abuse, the drug used, the dose, or the frequency of dosing (Connell and Mitcheson, 1984). For example, in order to obtain methadone to pass to others, a patient who is not an opiate user will substitute a urine from one who is when

TABLE 36.11

Persistence of Drugs and/or Metabolites in Urine after Discontinuing Intake; TLC Methods with a Sensitivity of Approximately 1 mg/l.

Drug/metabolite	Plasma $t_{1/2}$ (h)	Persistence in urine (Days)
Amphetamines	12–34 (Urine pH dependent) (Refer to Table 36.9)	Up to 3
Barbiturates		
'short-acting'	< 40	Up to 2
'long-acting'	> 40	Up to 14
Benzodiazepines	(Refer to Table 36.13)	
'short-persistence, high-potency'		Up to 14
'long-persistence, low-potency'		Up to 28
Cannabinoids*	14–38	Up to 21
Cocaine/benzoylecgonine		Up to 3
Methadone	15–55	Up to 3
Morphine	1–7	Up to 3

* Immunoassays probably more sensitive.

asked to produce a specimen for testing. This can often be discovered by alert nursing staff who are suspicious of the temperature of the 'freshly voided' urine.

Some patients are asked to stop the use of drugs and are not prescribed a replacement, such as methadone, during their treatment. Often they will continue to abuse drugs and will substitute a sample from a non-user, or a sample of some other liquid (e.g. Lucozade!) or merely dilute their own urine with warm water from the washbasin tap. Any suspicious fluids can be investigated appropriately, e.g. by measuring glucose, urea or osmolality. Urines suspected of being a single specimen divided among a group of patients (a common occurrence) can be shown to be so by measurement of sodium, potassium, urea and creatinine.

In some circumstances a volume diuresis contrived to coincide with urine collection at the clinic can also cause false negative tests. Clearly, ingested drugs will produce metabolites and so any urine specimen containing only the parent drug when metabolites are also expected has probably been 'spiked' to convince the clinician that the illicit drug has been used or that methadone is being taken. All suspicious and low osmolality urines should be reported as such to the requesting psychiatrist.

Urine Screening Tests for Drugs of Abuse

Factors to be taken into account when selecting techniques for screening urine for drugs of abuse are (1) the number of samples to be processed annually, (2) the range of drugs to be covered, (3) the turn-around time required, (4) equipment available, (5) staff available, (6) available budget, and (7) other relevant local considerations. Methods currently favoured follow.

Immunoassays

These are usually 'kit' methods based on the availability of an antibody directed towards a particular drug or group of drugs and linked to an indicator reaction, such as an enzyme assay, which can be followed in a simple spectrophotometer. The 'EMIT-ST' marketed by Syva UK Ltd is a portable system of reagents for detecting commonly abused drugs and incorporates sampling and diluting devices and an end-point photometer all housed in an attaché case. A test is reported as positive if the concentration of the drug in the sample equals or exceeds the limit of detection. Against the convenience, simplicity and portability of the system must be set its cost, currently about 10 times that of TLC, the limited shelf-life of reagents, the high initial capital outlay (currently similar to that of an HPLC system), the ready interference by the presence of blood, protein, bilirubin, and some cross-reactivity with dissimilar drugs present in high concentration. For fuller details the manufacturer's publications should be consulted.

Thin-Layer Chromatography

These methods are technically straightforward and several extraction, development and location procedures are described in the 5th edition of this book. The most difficult aspect, however, is interpretation due mainly to the presence of metabolites. An essential aid to interpretation, therefore, is a collection of urines from patients who have ingested known, single drugs. Extracts from these urines can then be subjected to the selected procedure and a file of R_f and locating reactions can be built up. Moffat (1986) gives a great deal of data on parent compounds but almost nothing on metabolites. The TLC procedures in Moffat (1986) or in edition 5 will identify most abused drugs except benzodiazepines and cannabinoids. These are dealt with in a later section.

A comprehensive system for the identification of abused drugs by TLC is the 'TOXILAB' system marketed by Mercia Diagnostics, Mercia House, Broadford Park, Shalford, Guildford, Surrey GU4 8EW. This system comprises a number of 'kits' of reagents and materials for separating and identifying barbiturates, basic drugs, benzodiazepines and cannabinoids. The methods involved are all broadly similar, consisting of extraction tubes containing buffer salts and an extraction solvent mixture, thin-layer plates of glass-fibre matting with the standard mixtures pre-loaded in position, and a system for evaporating the solvent extracts to concentrate the extracted drug onto small glass-fibre discs which are then pressed into place on the TLC plate.

After development and location, the R_fs and colours of each spot are compared with photographs of chromatograms of known drugs and metabolites and this allows identification of the unknown drugs to be made. The cost per sample is similar to other TLC systems although the initial outlay is high. The system, however, works extremely well even in relatively inexperienced hands. The presence, in a specimen of urine or blood, of any of the drugs listed in the system's compendium can usually be confirmed within an hour of receiving the specimen.

Multisolvent Thin-layer Chromatography

A different approach to comprehensive identification of drugs by TLC is described by Stead et al. (1982). They investigated the resolving power of four different solvent systems for basic drugs and four for acidic and neutral drugs, in identifying commonly prescribed or abused drugs or drugs involved in accidental or deliberate poisonings. In this system a series of reference compounds is chromatographed in order to calculate relative R_fs. For basic drugs, the combined use of three solvent systems enables identification of an unknown with a high degree of certainty. A series of locating agents is used to confirm the findings by R_f. The major problem, as with all chromatography systems, lies in obtaining reproducible retention data.

The system works reasonably well, in our experience, if care is exercised in making and checking the developing solvents in order to obtain reproducible R_fs. We store all the R_f data in a computer file. The R_fs obtained using the three solvent systems are entered into a BASIC program which then scans the file and produces a list of likely matches. The staining reactions and clinical circumstances relating to the specimen under investigation help in identifying the unknown. In general, however, metabolites are not easily identified.

Gas Chromatography

Many laboratories with a large workload choose GC for drug abuse work, and the 5th edition contains methods for amphetamines, barbiturates and basic drugs. The use of GC is satisfactory for identification of a wide range of parent drugs but interpretation is again complicated by metabolites. A collection of 'positive urines' as recommended for TLC greatly aids this process.

Flannagan (1983) overcame this problem by the use of two GC columns packed with different materials, OV1 and Poly A103. A simple alkaline extract into chloroform was injected onto each column to yield two chromatograms. Most drugs are unlikely to have the same R_t on both columns so that a co-eluting pair on one column is usually readily resolved on the other. Flannagan constructed a table of R_t values for drugs and metabolites using this system which greatly assists the identification of unknown drugs detected in urine.

Method Selection

Many workers feel that a more satisfactory approach, especially for basic drugs, is to use several methods each dedicated to one particular group of drugs. With TLC, although the capital outlay is small, this approach is likely to be time-consuming whereas with GC or HPLC, although the throughput may be rapid, the capital outlay will be large since one dedicated instrument is likely to be required for each group of compounds.

The literature detailing individual methods is vast and the reader is referred to Fishbein (1982) Volume 4, and publications such as the *Journal of Chromatography*, the *Journal of Chromatographic Science* and the *Journal of Analytical Toxicology* if this approach is desired.

Four groups of drugs are not readily resolved by the above general screening methods. These are benzodiazepines, cannabinoids, solvents and purgatives. The last although not causing dependence are none-the-less abused. Each of these is discussed in detail here.

BENZODIAZEPINES

The benzodiazepine group of drugs is widely prescribed. Some are mild tranquillisers, particularly chlordiazepoxide, diazepam, lorazepam, medazepam and oxazepam. Some are employed as hypnotics. Clonazepam is still occasionally prescribed as an anticonvulsant and diazepam is sometimes used in the initial treatment of status epilepticus. The current benzodiazepines are shown in Table 36.12. These drugs are widely distributed to patients, are often taken in deliberate self-poisoning attempts and are readily available to drug abusers in a variety of forms and from a wide variety of sources on the illegal market.

TABLE 36.12
Structural Relationships of Currently Available Benzodiazepines
(proprietary name given in parentheses)

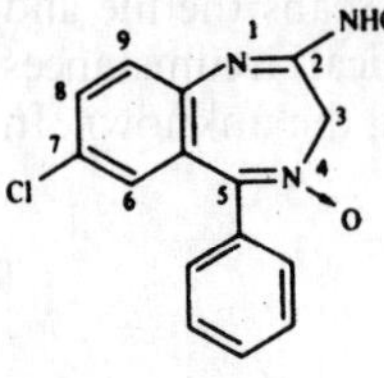

chlordiazepoxide (Librium)

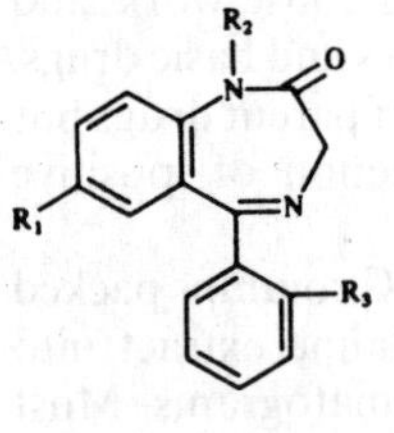

R_1	R_2	R_3	
NO_2	H	Cl	clonazepam (Rivotril)
Cl	CH_3	H	diazepam (Valium)
NO_2	CH_3	F	flunitrazepam (Rohypnol)
Cl	$(CH_2)_2N(C_2H_5)_2$	F	flurazepam (Dalmane)
NO_2	H	H	nitrazepam (Mogadon)
Cl	$CH_2\!\!-\!\!\triangleleft$	H	prazepam (Centrax)

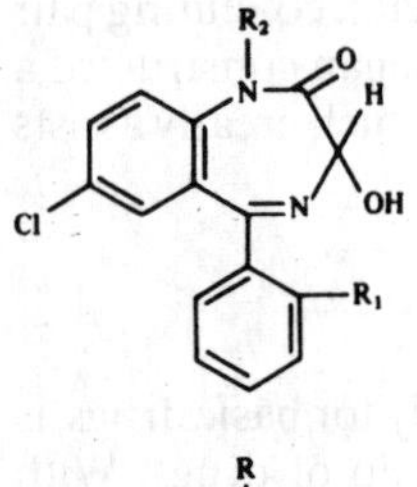

R_1	R_2	
Cl	H	lorazepam (Ativan)
Cl	CH_3	lormetazepam (Loramet)
H	H	oxazepam (Serenid)
H	CH_3	temazepam (Euhypnos)

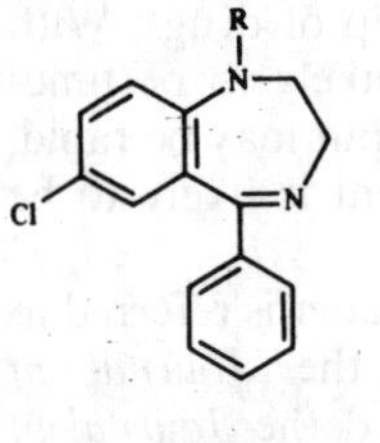

R	
CH_3	medazepam (Nobrium)

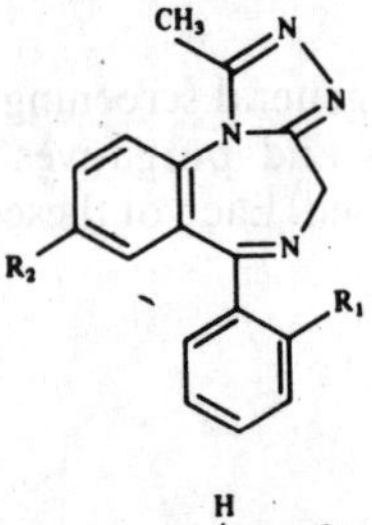

R_1	R_2	
H	Cl	alprazolam (Xanax)
Cl	Cl	triazolam (Halcion)

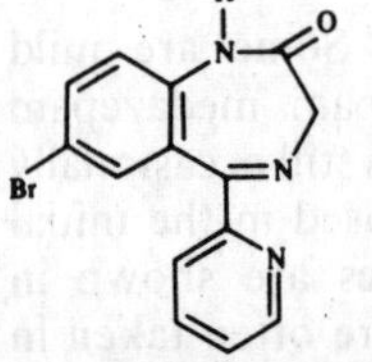

bromazepam (Lexotan)

bromazepam
(Lexotan)

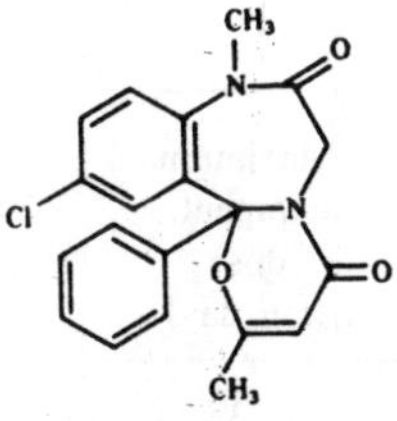

ketazolam
(Anxon)

ketazolam (Anxon)

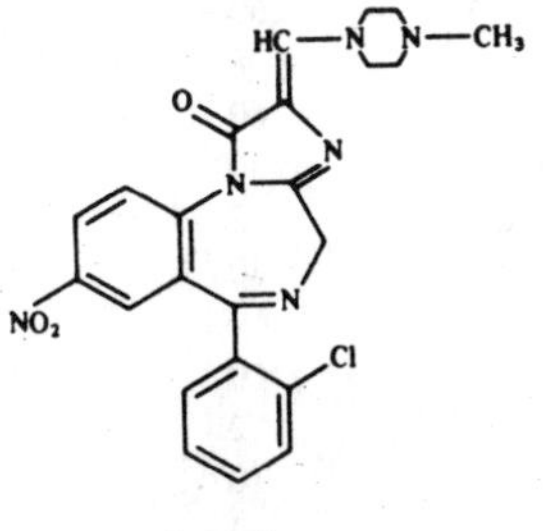

loprazolam
(Dormonoct)

loprazolam (Dormonoct)

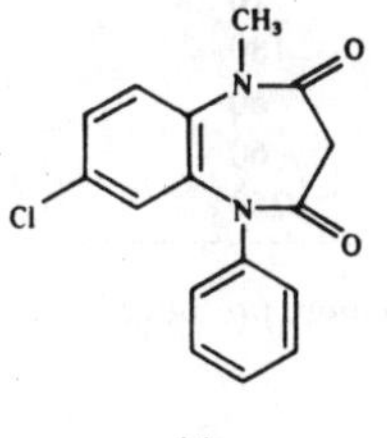

clobazam
(Frisium)

clobazam (Frisium)

The major effect of benzodiazepines is of relaxation tending to drowsiness. In excess, varying degrees of unconsciousness result and when ingested with alcohol, barbiturates or antidepressants there is a summation of effects leading in some instances to marked respiratory depression, profound coma and death.

Table 36.13 reveals that they fall broadly into two groups depending on the elimination half-time. There is probably no preference among drug abusers for one type over another. Most illegal users take whatever is available. The drugs with the longest half-times will probably be detectable in the urine for a longer period after use, but this depends to some extent on the dose involved. Most of these drugs also produce pharmacologically-active metabolites.

Detection Methods

Simple procedures for screening urine for benzodiazepines are described in the 5th edition of this book. The nitration method described there is satisfactory for plasma as well as urine. If, however, it is desired to identify the benzodiazepines it is necessary to resort to GC or HPLC. The former technique requires a sensitive detector, usually an electron-capture detector, while the latter technique may

TABLE 36.13

Relevant Pharmacological Data for Benzodiazepines

Benzodiazepine	Half-time (h)	Vd (l/kg)	Maximum therapeutic dose (mg/day)
Alprazolam	6–12	approx. 1	3
Bromazepam	8–19	approx. 0·9	9
Chlordiazepoxide*	5–30	0·3–0·6	100
Clobazam	10–58	approx. 1	60
Clonazepam	18–45	2–4	8
Clorazepate*	approx. 2		60
Diazepam*	20–100	0·5–2·5	30
Flunitrazepam	10–70	approx. 4	2
Flurazepam	2–3		30
(desalkylflurazepam)	2–5 days		
Ketazolam*	1·5		60
Loprazolam	4–11		2
Lorazepam	9–24	1–2	10
Lormetazepam	approx. 10	approx. 5	2
Medazepam*	1–2		40
Nitrazepam	18–38	2–4	10
Oxazepam	4–25	0·5–2	180
Prazepam*	40–100	0·5–2·5	60
Temazepam	3–38	approx. 1	60
Triazolam	1·5–3	1–2	250

*Major metabolite, usually diazepam or desmethyl diazepam, with much more prolonged half-time.

require the facility of solvent programming. The reverse-phase method of Lensmeyer *et al.* (1982) separates all common benzodiazepines and their pharmacologically active metabolites by use of a ternary solvent gradient system.

For most drug abuse or acute poisoning situations it is adequate to demonstrate the presence of metabolites in the patient's urine. The following simple method is based on the acid hydrolysis of these drugs to their corresponding 2-aminobenzophenones. After chromatographic separation they are diazotised and coupled to form an azo-dye. The method is only suitable for those benzodiazepines in which the substituent on the N–1 atom adjacent to the benzene ring is hydrogen (Table 36.12, p. 1002). They form primary amines which can be diazotised.

Reagents.

1. Hydrochloric acid, concentrated.
2. Light petroleum, b.p. 40–60 °C.
3. Methanol.
4. Sulphuric acid, 9 mol/l.
5. Sodium nitrite solution, 10 g/l. Prepare freshly.
6. Ammonium sulphamate solution, 50 g/l.
7. N-(1-Naphthyl)ethylenediamine hydrochloride solution, 5 g/l.
8. A positive control. This can be a urine from a patient known to be taking a benzodiazepine or normal urine to which is added oxazepam and nitra-

zepam (1 ml of a solution of 10 mg of each of these in 100 ml HCl, 1 mol/l, added to 9 ml urine).

9. Developing solvent: chloroform–acetone: 4/1 by volume.

Technique. Into two glass-stoppered boiling tubes (150 × 30 mm) pipette 10 ml test urine and a known positive. To both add 3 ml concentrated hydrochloric acid. Place the tubes in a boiling water bath for 15 min, remove and cool. To both tubes add 10 ml light petroleum, stopper and shake mechanically for 5 min. Centrifuge the tubes for 5 min at 2000 rpm and transfer the solvent layers as completely as possible to conical tubes. Evaporate to dryness under oxygen-free nitrogen at not more than 60 °C. Dissolve the residues in 100 μl methanol and transfer to discrete spots at one end of a thin-layer chromatography plate (silica gel G 250 × 100 mm). Develop until the solvent almost reaches the top of the plate; remove and dry.

Spray the plate with sulphuric acid and dry using warm air. Then successively spray with the sodium nitrite, ammonium sulphamate and naphthyl-ethylenediamine solutions drying with warm air between each application. Aminobenzophenones produce a violet/purple colour at a concentration of about 1 μg/ml, i.e. 'therapeutic' concentrations, but the test is not specific. GC or HPLC methods are required to identify individual benzodiazepines as outlined earlier.

CANNABINOIDS

The common source of cannabinoids is marihuana which is usually smoked but may be ingested. The principal cannabinoid is Δ^9-tetrahydrocannabinol of which a few milligrams are required to produce the desired effects. The smoke from about 0·5 g of the resin needs to be inhaled to achieve this dose. The major effects of the drug are euphoria, hallucination, distortions of perception and sedation. Deaths sometimes result directly from the toxic effects of the drug but the most common fatalities are due to accidents resulting from the hallucinations or the altered view of reality which the individual obtains.

Plasma concentrations are usually in the range up to 100 μg/l after an adequate dose. Those concentrations are achieved within 10–15 min by inhalation. The effects last a considerable period of time; tetrahydrocannabinol has an elimination half-time of 14 to 38 h and is present predominantly in the tissues, Vd = 4–14 l/kg. Metabolism of tetrahydrocannabinol is extensive producing two active metabolites, 11-hydroxy- and 8β-hydroxytetrahydrocannabinols, both in low concentration, and two or three further metabolites without any psycho-tropic activity. The metabolism is shown diagrammatically in Fig. 36.24.

A variety of TLC systems exists for the demonstration of cannabinoids in urine. Quantitation requires GC or HPLC and several methods have been described. The urine specimens from drug dependence clinics, however, can be adequately handled by a simple, reliable TLC method such as the system described here.

Detection of a Tetrahydrocannabinol Metabolite (Tetlow and McMurray, 1984)

After alkaline hydrolysis of the glucuronide of 11-nor-Δ^9-tetrahydrocannabinol-9-carboxylic acid (Δ^9-THC-COOH), the latter is coupled with a stable diazonium salt (Fast Blue BB) to form an azo-dye with indicator properties. The authors claim excellent correlation with the EMIT cannabinoid screen.

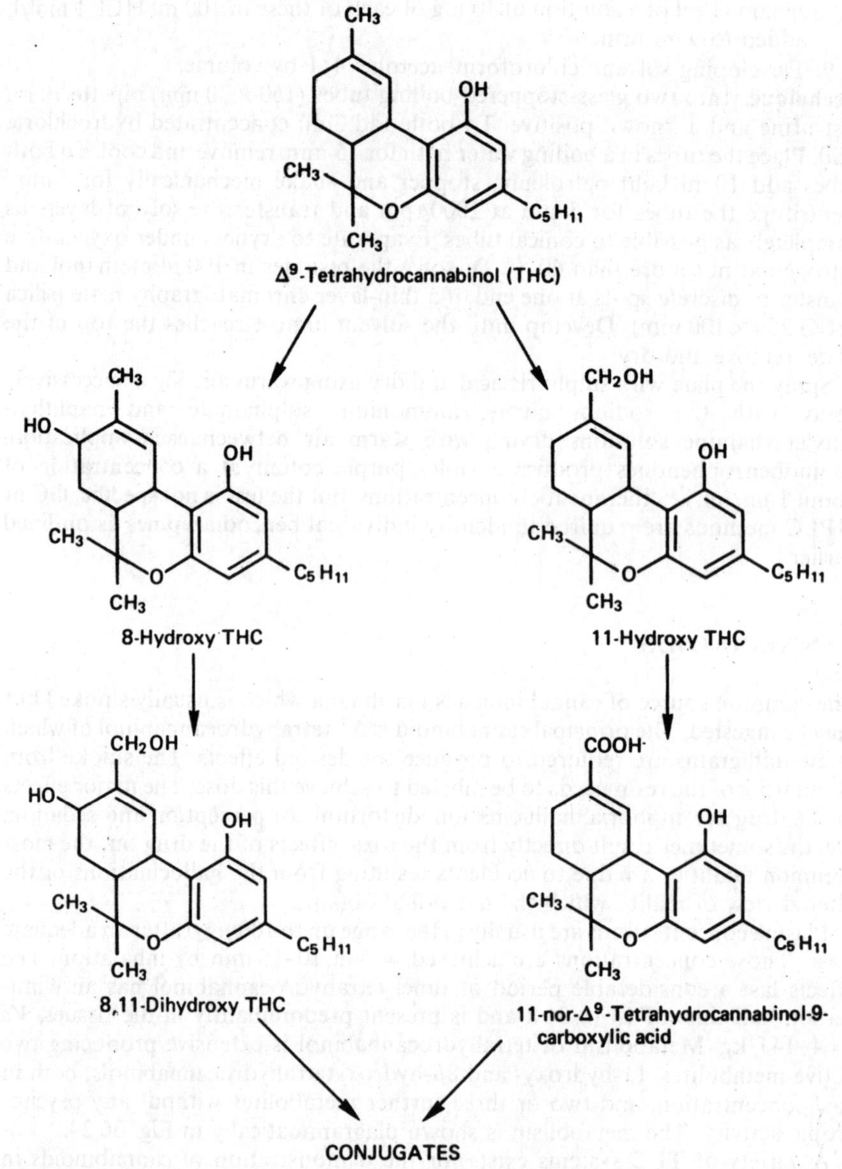

Fig. 36.24. The Metabolism of Δ⁹-Tetrahydrocannabinol.
The C_5H_{11} group is *n*-pentyl. Both α and β-forms of 8-hydroxy-THC occur but only the β-form is active.

Reagents.
1. Potassium hydroxide solution, 11·8 mol/l.
2. Maleic acid solution, 2 mol/l.
3. Ethyl acetate–hexane, 1/9 by volume.
4. Methanol.

5. Developing solvent: heptane–acetone–glacial acetic acid: 70/30/0·8 by volume.
6. Fast Blue BB salt solution, containing 250 mg in 250 ml dichloromethane. This solution is stable for up to 2 weeks in a dark bottle.
7. Diethylamine.
8. Hydrochloric acid, 1 mol/l.
9. A suitable positive control. This can be obtained from the TOXILAB THC system or, alternatively, known positive urines can be subdivided and stored frozen.

Technique. To 10 ml urine add 0·85 ml potassium hydroxide and leave for 15 min at room temperature to hydrolyse the glucuronide. Adjust the pH of the mixture to 2·0 to 2·5 by adding maleic acid and extract the Δ^9-THC-COOH into 10 ml ethyl acetate/hexane. Evaporate the extract to dryness at 40 °C under vacuum and dissolve the residue in 15 μl methanol. This is then applied to the TLC plate (Schleicher and Schuell, type F 1500, ref. no. 394632) near one end and after drying, the plate is developed using reagent (5).

After drying, dip the plate in the Fast Blue BB solution, dry for 60 s and then expose to an atmosphere of diethylamine for 15 s. Place the plate under a stream of cold air for 3 to 5 min until the diethylamine smell disappears. At this stage, the Δ^9-THC-COOH appears as a red spot with R_f 0·3, which allows initial identification of positive urines. When the plate is dipped in the hydrochloric acid, the spot turns purple with some loss of intensity but as the plate dries, the intensity increases while the background colour fades.

PURGATIVES

Purgative abuse is most common among middle-aged women who often present with a variety of symptoms including weight loss, diarrhoea and muscle weakness. Hypokalaemia is almost always present and the low concentration of urinary potassium indicates an extra-renal loss. Since the dietary intake of potassium is rarely inadequate, purgative abuse should be rigorously excluded before embarking on the the use of expensive and time-consuming tests to diagnose much less common disorders such as Bartter's syndrome.

Purgatives are classified by their mode of action into four groups (Table 36.14). Commercial preparations often contain a mixture of members of one or more groups. Potassium loss is caused primarily by the members of group 4 only. Occasionally, in the investigation of weight loss, loose stools are obtained in which the fat content is normal and the patient is normokalaemic. The possibility of purgative abuse in these instances should not be overlooked since any of the purgatives of groups 1 to 3 may be involved. At present it is not easy to demonstrate the use of any of the members of groups 1 and 2, although oil droplets may be seen on the surface of a centrifuged sample of faeces indicating the presence of group 1 purgatives.

It is insufficient merely to test for phenolphthalein since it is present in fewer than one third of the preparations in which saline cathartics or contact cathartics are the active ingredients and in only one quarter of 64 preparations on the market. It is therefore equally important to examine the urine and faeces for anthraquinones and related contact cathartics and it is occasionally necessary to examine faeces for increased magnesium concentrations. The structures of some of the stimulant cathartics are presented in Fig. 36.25.

TABLE 36.14

Classification of Purgatives

Group	Active components
1. Emollients	Dioctyl sodium sulphosuccinate
	Dioctyl calcium sulphosuccinate
	Mineral oils, e.g. liquid paraffin
	Glycerine
2. Bulk formers	Methyl cellulose
	Sodium carboxymethyl cellulose
	Ispaghula or sterculia preparations
	Tragacanth
	Bran
	Lactulose
3. Saline cathartics	Magnesium sulphate
	'Milk of Magnesia'
	Magnesium citrate
	Sodium phosphates
	Sodium sulphate
	Sodium potassium tartrate
4. Contact (or stimulant) cathartics	Castor oil
	Phenolphthalein
	Senna
	Cascara
	Bisacodyl
	Danthfon
	Aloes, aloin
	Colocynth
	Rhubarb

Stimulant Cathartics

The following method of de Wolff *et al.* (1981) involves the pretreatment of urine with β-glucuronidase at pH 5·0 to hydrolyse conjugates. Urine and faeces are applied to 'Extube' extraction columns to separate the purgatives from interfering materials. The purgatives are eluted using a chloroform/isopropanol mixture and applied to TLC plates which, after developement, are visualised by UV light and also by spraying with alkali.

Reagents and Materials.

1. Silica gel coated plates, 10×20 cm, with fluorescent indicator and concentrating zone (Merck cat. no. 13728).
2. 'Extube' extraction columns (types Tox-Elute, TE3020 and Clin-Elute, CE1003 from Analytichem International).
3. β-Glucuronidase from bovine liver, activity approximately 10^6 units/g (Sigma, cat. no. G 2051). Dissolve 50 mg in 10 ml water to give an activity of 5000 units/ml. Prepare freshly for use. Store the solid desiccated at $-20\,°C$.
4. Methanol–water mixture: 88/30.
5. Chloroform, AR.
6. Ethanol, absolute alcohol.
7. Sodium hydroxide solution 6 mol/l.
8. Hydrochloric acid, 6 mol/l.

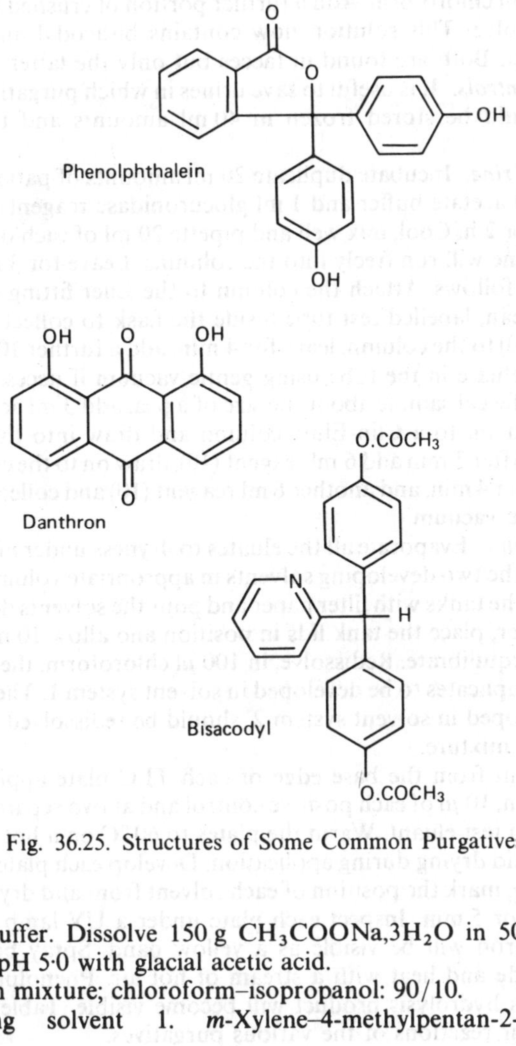

Phenolphthalein

Danthron

Bisacodyl

Fig. 36.25. Structures of Some Common Purgatives.

9. Acetate buffer. Dissolve 150 g $CH_3COONa,3H_2O$ in 500 ml water and adjust to pH 5·0 with glacial acetic acid.

10. Extraction mixture; chloroform–isopropanol: 90/10.

11. Developing solvent 1. *m*-Xylene–4-methylpentan-2-one–methanol: 30/30/3.

12. Developing solvent 2. *n*-Hexane -toluene–acetic acid: 30/10/10.

13. Buchner flask, 500 ml, with a wide neck fitted with a rubber stopper through which is fitted a long, wide bore needle with a Luer fitting. It should be possible to stand a test tube in the flask to collect the 10–15 ml of eluant through the needle.

14. *Drug reference solutions.* Weigh out sufficient of each crushed tablet to contain 2 mg of its active ingredient and dissolve in its appropriate solvent as follows.

(a) Dorbanex (contains danthron). Dissolve in 10 ml chloroform.

(b) Senokot (contains senna). Dissolve in methanol–water: 7/3.

(c) Veracolate (contains phenolphthalein). Dissolve in 1 ml ethanol, then make to 10 ml with chloroform.

(d) Dulcolax (contains bisacodyl). Dissolve in 2 ml ethanol, add 20 μl sodium hydroxide solution and heat at 70 °C for 30 min. After cooling, adjust to pH 7·0 using the hydrochloric acid (requires about 20 μl) and add 8 ml chloroform. Add a further portion of crushed tablet and shake to dissolve. This solution now contains bisacodyl and its hydrolysis product. Both are found in faeces but only the latter in urine.

15. *Positive controls.* It is useful to save urines in which purgatives are detected. These should be stored frozen in 40 ml amounts and thawed prior to analysis.

Technique. *Urine.* Incubate duplicate 20 ml amounts of patient's and control urines with 2 ml acetate buffer and 1 ml glucuronidase reagent in covered glass tubes at 56 °C for 2 h. Cool, mix well and pipette 20 ml of each onto a Tox-Elute column. The urine will run freely into the columns. Leave for 3 min. Elute from each column as follows. Attach the column to the Luer fitting on the Buchner flask, place a clean, labelled test tube inside the flask to collect the eluate. Add 10 ml reagent (10) to the column, leave for 4 min, add a further 10 ml reagent (10) and collect the eluate in the tube using gentle vacuum if necessary.

Faeces. To a faecal sample about the size of a pea, add 3 ml acetate buffer and vortex-mix. Pour on to a Clin-Elute column and draw into the column using gentle vacuum. After 3 min add 6 ml reagent (10), draw on to the column as before and, after a further 4 min, and another 6 ml reagent (10) and collect the eluate, still using only gentle vacuum.

Chromatography. Evaporate all the eluates to dryness under nitrogen at 37 °C. Prepare each of the two developing solvents in appropriate volumes for the tanks to be used. Line the tanks with filter paper and pour the solvents down the sides to saturate the paper, place the tank lids in position and allow 10 min for the tank atmospheres to equilibrate. Redissolve, in 100 μl chloroform, the residues of one of each pair of duplicates to be developed in solvent system 1. The second of each pair, to be developed in solvent system 2, should be redissolved in 100 μl of the methanol–water mixture.

To a line 5 mm from the base edge of each TLC plate apply 10 μl of each reference solution, 10 μl of each positive control and at two separate positions 2·5 and 10 μl of each test eluant. Warm the plates to 60 °C on a hot plate and use a stream of air to aid drying during application. Develop each plate to within 20 to 30 mm of the top, mark the position of each solvent front and dry the plates in an oven at 120 °C for 5 min. Inspect each plate under a UV lamp having 366 nm emission. Danthron will be visible as a yellow band. Spray both plates with sodium hydroxide and heat with a stream of hot air. Phenolphthalein, senna, bisacodyl and its hydrolysis product will become visible. Table 36.15 gives R_f values and colour reactions of the various purgatives.

INTERPRETATION

Anthraquinone-related purgatives can be detected after minimal dose for up to 32 h in urine. In faeces, all can be detected for up to two days after ingestion except for bisacodyl which cannot be detected beyond about 18 h. Simple alkalinisation of urine only demonstrates unconjugated phenolphthalein (Heitzer *et al.*, 1968) yet it is present, like the other contact cathartics, mainly in a conjugated form. Hydrolysis is therefore a pre-requisite of a thorough investigation of this group of purgatives.

Saline Cathartics

Magnesium salts are those most commonly employed in saline cathartics but they are not absorbed to any great extent and hence, after ingestion, increased

TABLE 36.15
Thin-layer Chromatographic Behaviour of Purgatives

Purgatives	System 1 R_f relative to phenolphthalein	System 2 R_f relative to senna	Fluorescence at 366 nm	Colour	Colour after NaOH spray
Bisacodyl	0·98				Purple
Bisacodyl hydrolysis product	0·71				Purple
Danthron	1·38	1·38	+ +	System 1: orange System 2: yellow	Red/Purple
Phenolphthalein	1·00	0·08			Violet
Senna		1·00	+ +	Yellow	Pink/Red

concentrations of magnesium can be readily demonstrated in faeces (Wilcock, 1983).

Homogenise 4 g portions of faeces with water to a total volume of 50 ml for 30 min, then centrifuge at 4000 rpm for 5 min. The clear supernatants, after dilution by 1 in 200 in lanthanum chloride solution, are subjected to analysis by atomic absorption flame photometry for magnesium (see p. 605).

Subjects who have ingested minimum doses of magnesium salts within the previous 36 h have faecal magnesium concentrations within the range 96 to 615 (mean 371) μmol/g dried faeces, significantly higher than a control group of subjects taking either no medication or ingesting minimum doses of other groups of purgatives. The faecal magnesium concentrations for the control group are 42 to 130 (mean 89·6) μmol/g dried faeces.

If a thorough search for the presence of stimulant cathartics proves negative, and there is still strong clinical suspicion of purgative abuse, then the estimation of faecal magnesium may indicate that 'Magnesia' is involved.

SOLVENTS

Solvent abuse is not a new phenomenon. The sniffing of ether and chloroform was popular and fashionable among middle and upper class adults in the 19th century. Today it is most popular among young teenage boys in the UK and among very young children in some Third World countries. In some areas of affluent countries it has reached epidemic proportions. Although recently solvent abuse has been increasing in the UK, increased public awareness of the problem and a policy of making solvent-based products unavailable to minors, should contribute significantly to a decrease in the incidence of cases.

Solvents are available in such products as adhesives, dry-cleaning and stain-removing agents, deodorants, pain-relieving and fire-extinguishing aerosols, typewriter correcting fluids, duplicator fluids, cigarette lighter refills of various types, shoe dyes, hair lacquers, nail polish removers and many other products. The solvents employed in these products include acetone, toluene, trichloro-ethylene, trichloroethane, ethanol, methanol, tetrachloromethane, tetrachloro-ethylene, methylene chloride, amyl acetate, and butane. Manufacturers are not legally obliged to state the formulation of products on the packaging and are free to change the formulation at any time without giving prior notice or warning. Hence, there will obviously be other solvents involved in the future and even today some products contain more than one solvent.

Gas chromatography provides the most comprehensive method for separating and identifying solvents, and that described by Oliver and Watson (1977) is presented in detail here. The small, inexpensive infrared vapour analysers recently introduced may prove useful within the context of solvent abuse.

Detection of Solvents by Gas Chromatography

A glass column $2 \text{ m} \times 3 \text{ mm}$ i.d. is packed with 10% Carbowax 400 on Chromosorb W, 80–100 mesh. Nitrogen is used as the carrier at a flow rate of 60 ml/min. The column temperature is 70 °C isothermal and the injection port temperature is 150 °C. A flame-ionisation detector (250 °C) is used and the output connected through the amplifier to a 1 mV recorder.

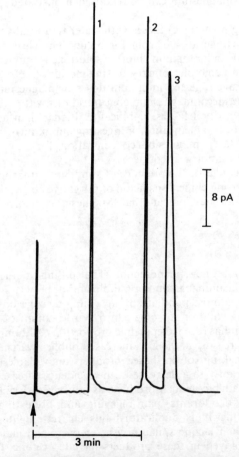

Fig. 36.26. Separation of Solvents by Gas Chromatography.
1 = Acetone; 2 = ethanol; 3 = toluene. The arrow indicates the time of injection.

Retention times can be determined by injection of 1 μl of aqueous solutions or suspensions of each solvent at an approximate concentration of 1000 mg/l. An example of the trace obtained is shown in Fig. 36.26.

Heparinised blood samples are required in capped glass tubes filled to the brim to prevent solvent loss. Using a 5 ml disposable syringe and needle, 5 ml of blood under test is transferred to a 25 ml conical flask which is fitted with a screw cap having a rubber septum. The sealed flask is placed in a 60 °C water bath for 45 min to liberate the solvent.

Using a gas syringe fitted with a valve, 1 ml of the vapour from the flask is injected onto the GC column. Table 36.16 gives approximate retention times relative to ethanol for some commonly encountered solvents. The identity of solvents in commercial products can be determined in some instances by pipetting 1 ml of the product into an open vial placed inside a sealed polythene bag. After allowing a few minutes for evaporation to occur, 1 ml of the vapour in the bag is injected onto the column. This technique can be used to establish a relationship between an unidentified peak obtained on a patient's sample and a sample of the solvent thought to have been inhaled.

TABLE 36.16

Approximate Retention Times and Toxic and Fatal Concentrations of some Solvents in Man.

Solvent	R_t (ethanol = 1·00)	Toxic (mg/l)	Fatal (mg/l)
Acetone	0·48	200	550
Tetrachloromethane	0·52		
Ethyl acetate	0·58		
Benzene	0·70		0·94
Formaldehyde	0·85		
Trichlorethylene	0·87		
Isopropanol	0·94	3400	
Ethanol	1·00	1500	3500
Chloroform	1·04	70	390
Perchloroethylene	1·04		
Toluene	1·18		10 000
1,2-Dichloroethane	1·35		
Butan-2-ol	1·58		
1,4-Dioxan	1·67		
n-Amyl alcohol	3·68		

A trace of acetone is sometimes seen depending on the time of day with respect to meals. Concentration data are sparse and unreliable. Concentrations greater than 1 mg/ml indicate recent inhalation but the very short half-times indicate that blood samples should probably be collected within about one hour after inhalation in order to detect the solvent.

Ramsey and Flannagan (1982a) described a GLC method for solvents, including aerosol propellants, on 0·3% Carbowax 20 M on Carbopack C, 80–100 mesh, using flame ionisation and electron-capture detectors. They produced retention data using this system for almost 200 compounds in this class. The same authors (1982b) described a method using HPLC to detect and quantify the metabolites of various solvents in urine. They reported on the urine concentrations of hippurate (metabolite of toluene and cresols) and of o- and p-toluric acids (metabolites of the xylenes). Hippurate/creatinine ratios greater than 1 strongly support a diagnosis of toluene abuse.

In a study of 290 cases of solvent abuse, Francis et al. (1982) found no association between blood concentrations of solvents and the clinical signs and symptoms shown in those patients.

ACKNOWLEDGEMENTS

The author wishes to acknowledge the considerable assistance in the provision of information that he has received from: Dr J. Strang, North Western Regional Consultant for Drug Dependence; Dr M. Ashton, Institute for the Study of Drug Dependence; Dr D. Leitch, John Rylands University Library, Manchester; Dr F. Leach and Mrs E. Saddler, Northwest Region Drug Information Unit. The following persons kindly provided details of their methods: Miss C. Mowatt, Tameside General Hospital; Mr A. V. Tetlow, Hope Hospital, Salford; Mrs L. H. Wilcock, Manchester Royal Infirmary; Mr A. Williams, Park Hospital, Manchester.

REFERENCES

Amdisen A. (1973). Brit. Med. J; 2: 240.
Amdisen A. (1975). Dan. Med. Bull; 22: 277.
Amdisen A. (1978). J. Anal. Toxicol; 2: 193.
Amdisen A. (1981). In Therapeutic Drug Monitoring. (Richens A., Marks V., eds) Chapter 11A. Edinburgh: Churchill Livingstone.
Amdisen A., Gottfries C. G., Jacobson L., Winblad B. (1974). Acta Psych. Scand; Suppl. 255: 25.
Amdisen A., Schou M. (1978). In Side Effects of Drugs Annual, Vol. 2. (Dukes M. N. G., ed) p. 17. Amsterdam: Excerpta Medica.
Aronson J. K., Grahame-Smith D. G., Wigley F. M. (1978). Quart. J. Med; 47: 111.
Avery G. S. ed. (1980). Drug Treatment. Principles and Practice of Clinical Pharmacology and Therapeutics, 2nd ed. Edinburgh: Churchill Livingstone.
Bartells H., Spring P. (1975). Chemotherapy; 21: 1.
Baselt R. C. (1982). Disposition of Toxic Drugs and Chemicals in Man, 2nd ed. California: Biomedical Publications.
Berry D. J., Grove J. (1971). Clin. Chim. Acta; 34: 5.
Bhagat C. I., Beilby J. P., Garcia-Webb P., Dusci L. J. (1985). Clin. Chem; 31: 647.
Blakesley J. D., Howse C. Q., Spencer-Peat J., Wood D. C. F. (1986). Ann. Clin. Biochem; 23: 552.
Bochner F., Carruthers G., Kampmann J., Steiner J., eds. (1978). Handbook of Clinical Pharmacology. Boston: Little, Brown and Co.
Braithwaite R. A., Widdop B. (1971). Clin. Chim. Acta; 35: 461.
Brown S. S. (1971). Ann. Clin. Biochem; 8: 98.
Brunswick D. J., Mendells, J. (1977). Communications in Psychopharmacology; 1: 131.
Burgan T. H. S., Gupta I., Bate C. M. (1982). Brit. Med. J; 284: 939.
Chard C. R. (1976). In Clinical and Pharmacological Aspects of Sodium Valproate in the Treatment of Epilepsy. (Legg N. J., ed). Tunbridge Wells: MCS Consultants.
Coakley J. C., Tobgui S., Dennis P. M. (1983). Pathology; 15: 321.
Connell P. H., Mitcheson M. (1984). Brit. Med. J; 288: 767.
Craver J. L., Valdes R. (1983). Ann. Int. Med; 98: 483.
Danon A., Chen Z. (1979). Clin. Pharmacol. Ther; 25: 316.
de Wolff F. A., de Hass E. J. M., Verweij M. (1981). Clin. Chem; 27: 914.

DHSS (HM(68)92). (1968). *Hospital Treatment of Acute Poisoning*. London: HMSO.
Dordoni B., Willson R. A., Thompson R. P. A., Williams R. (1973). *Brit. Med. J*; **3**: 86.
Dreisbach R. H. (1980). *Handbook of Poisoning: Prevention, Diagnosis and Treatment.* California: Lange Medical Publications.
Englander R. N., Johnson R. N., Brickley J. J., Hanna G. R. (1979). *Neurology*; **29**: 96.
Epslin D. W. (1957). *J. Pharmacol. Exp. Therap*; **120**: 301.
Evans D. A. P., Manley K. A., McKusick V. A. (1960). *Brit. Med. J*; **2**: 485.
Ferguson I. T. (1982). In *Epilepsy Forum*-3. p. 17. Eastleigh, Hants: Parke-Davis Medical.
Fine A., Sumner D. J. (1975). *Brit. J. Clin. Pharmacol*; **2**: 475.
Fishbein L., ed. (1982). *Chromatography of Environmental Hazards*, Vols 1–4. New York: Elsevier.
Flannagan R. J. (1983). PhD Thesis. University of London.
Francis J., *et al.* (1982). *Human Toxicol*; **1**: 271.
Frigerio A., Morselli P. L. (1975). In *Advances in Neurology*, Vol. 2. (Penry J. K., Daly D. D., eds) p. 295. New York: Raven Press.
Gilman A. G., Goodman L. S., Rall T. W., Murad F., eds. (1985). *Goodman and Gilman's Pharmacological Basis of Therapeutics*, 7th ed. London: Collier Macmillan.
Glazko A. J. (1975). *Epilepsia*; **16**: 367.
Glynn J. P., Kendal S. E. (1975). *Lancet*; **1**: 1147.
Graves S. W., Brown B. A., Valdes R. (1983). *Ann. Int. Med*; **99**: 604.
Gruber K. A., Whitaker J. M., Buckalew V. M. Jr. (1980). *Nature*; **287**: 743.
Hackett L. P., Dusci L. J. (1979). *Clin. Toxicol*; **15**: 63.
Hansen H. E., Amdisen A. (1978). *Quart. J. Med*; **47**: 123.
Hart T. B., Nevitt A., Whitehead A. (1984). *Lancet*; **2**: 1222.
Harvey C. D., Sherwin A. L. (1978). In *Antiepileptic Drugs—Quantitative Analysis and Interpretation*. (Pippinger C. E., Penry J. K., Kutt H., eds) p. 87. New York: Raven Press.
Heitzer W. D., Warshaw A. L., Waldman T. A., Laster L. (1968). *Ann. Int. Med*; **68**: 840.
Horning M. G., *et al.* (1977). *Clin. Chem*; **23**: 157.
Jacobs M. H., Senior R. M., Kessler G. (1976). *J. Amer. Med. Assoc*; **235**: 1983.
Jarvie D. R., Stewart M. J. (1979). *Clin. Chim. Acta*; **94**: 241.
Jelliffe R. W. (1971). *Fed. Proc*; **30**: 284.
Johnson F. N., ed. (1980). *Handbook of Lithium Therapy*. Lancaster: MTP Press.
Julien R. M., Hollister R. P. (1975). In *Advances in Neurology*, Vol. 11. (Penry J. K., Dal D. D., eds) p. 263. New York: Raven Press.
Karlsson E., Molin L. (1975). *Acta Med. Scand*; **197**: 299.
Kragh-Sørensen P., Åsberg M., Eggert-Hansen C. (1973). *Lancet*; **1**: 113.
Laurence D. R., Bennett P. N. (1980). *Clinical Pharmacology*, 5th ed. London: Churchill Livingstone.
Lensmeyer G. L., Rajani C., Evenson M. A. (1982). *Clin. Chem*; **28**: 2274.
Livingston S., Pauli L. L., Berman W. (1974). *Diseases of the Nervous System*; **35**: 103.
Lockett S. (1978). *Brit. J. Hosp. Med*; **19**: 200.
Lunde P. K. M., Frislid K., Hansteen V. (1977). *Clinical Pharmacokinetics*; **2**: 182.
Macarulla F. M., Mendia B. (1961). *Rev. Med., E. G. Navarra*; **5**: 32.
Mace P. F. K., Walker G. (1976). Lancet; **2**: 1362.
Martindale (1982). *The Extra Pharmacopoeia*, 28th ed. (Reynolds J. E. F., ed). London: The Pharmaceutical Press.
Matthew H., Lawson A. A. H. (1979). *Treatment of Common Acute Poisonings*, 4th ed. p. 129. Edinburgh: Churchill Livingstone.
Mawer G. E., *et al.* (1974). *Brit. J. Clin. Pharmacol*; **1**: 163.
Merck Index, The (1976). *An Encyclopaedia of Chemicals and Drugs*, 9th ed. (Windholz M., ed). Rahway, New Jersey: Merck & Co.
Miceli J. N., Olson W. A., Weber W. W. (1975). *Biochem. Med*; **12**: 348.
Moffat A. C., ed. (1986). *Clarke's Isolation and Identification of Drugs*, 2nd ed. London: Pharmaceutical Press.
Morgan D. B. (1984). *Ann. Clin. Biochem*; **21**: 449.
Morselli P. L., Frigerio A. (1975). *Drug Metabolism Review*; **4**: 97.
Mowatt C. (1986). Personal communication.

Oliver J. S., Watson J. M. (1977). *Lancet*; **1**: 84.

Ou C. N., Frawley V. L. (1982). *Clin. Chem*; **28**: 2157.

Park G. D., *et al.* (1983). *Amer. J. Med*; **74**: 961.

Pinder R. M., Brogden R. N., Speight T. M., Avery G. L. (1977). *Drugs*; **13**: 81.

Prescott L. F., Wright N., Roscoe P., Brown S. S. (1971). *Lancet*; **1**: 519.

Prescott L. F., *et al.* (1976). *Lancet*; **2**: 109.

Price C. P., Hammond P. M., Scawen M. D. (1983). *Clin. Chem*; **29**: 358.

Proudfoot A. T., Stewart M. S., Levitt T., Widdop B. (1979). *Lancet*; **2**: 330.

Ramsey J. D., Flannagan R. J. (1982a). *J. Chromatog*; **240**: 423.

Ramsey J. D., Flannagan R. J. (1982b). *Human Toxicology*; **1**: 299.

Redetzki H. M., Koerner T. A., Hughes J. R., Smith A. G. (1972). *Clin. Toxicol*; **5**: 343.

Reidenburg M. M., Drayer D., DeMarco A. L., Bellow C. T. (1973). *Clin. Pharmacol. Therap*; **14**: 970.

Richens A., Marks V., eds. (1981). *Therapeutic Drug Monitoring*. Edinburgh: Churchill Livingstone.

Richens A., Warrington S. (1979). *Drugs*; **17**: 488.

Robertson I. G. (1982). In *Epilepsy Forum*-3. p. 9. Eastleigh, Hants: Parke-Davis Medical.

Rocco R. M., Abbott D. C., Giese R. W., Karger B. L. (1977). *Clin. Chem*; **23**: 705.

Routh I. J., Shore N. A., Arrendonde E. G., Paul W. D. (1968). *Clin. Chem*; **14**: 882.

Schottelius D. D. (1978). In *Antiepileptic Drugs—Quantitative Analysis and Interpretation.* (Pippinger C. E., Penry J. K., Kutt H., eds) p. 95. New York: Raven Press.

Soldin S. J. (1986). *Clin. Chem*; **32**: 5.

Stead A. H., *et al.* (1982). *Analyst*; **107**: 1106.

Stead A. H., Moffat A. C. (1983). *Human Toxicology*; **3**: 437–464.

Stewart M. J., Adriaenssens P. I., Jarvie D. R., Prescott L. F. (1979). *Ann. Clin. Biochem*; **16**: 89.

Stewart M. J., Simpson E. (1973). *Ann. Clin. Biochem*; **10**: 173.

Suchy F. J., *et al.* (1979). *N. Engl. J. Med*; **300**: 962.

Tetlow V. A., McMurray J. R. (1984). Personal communication.

Trinder P. (1954). *Biochem. J*; **57**: 301.

Valdes R., Graves S. W., Brown B. A., Landt M. (1983). *J. Pediatr*; **102**: 947.

Vale J. A., Meredith T. J., eds. (1981). *Poisoning. Diagnosis and Treatment.* London: Update Books.

Weidner N., *et al.* (1980). *Amer. J. Clin. Pathol*; **73**: 79.

Wiener K. (1978). *Ann. Clin. Biochem*; **15**: 187.

Wilcock L. H. (1981). Personal communication.

Wilder B. J., *et al.* (1977). *Ann. Neurol*; **1**: 511.

Williams A. (1985). Personal communication.

Wood M., Shand D. G., Wood A. J. J. (1979). *Clin. Pharmacol. Therap*; **25**: 103.

Woodbury D. M. (1977). In *Scientific Approaches to Clinical Neurology.* (Goldensohn E. S., Appel S. H., eds) p. 693. Philadelphia: Lea and Febiger.

Wright N., Prescott L. F. (1973). *Scot. Med. J*; **18**: 56.

FURTHER READING

Connell P. H. (1968). In *Symposium on the Scientific Basis of Drug Dependence.* The Biological Society, London.

Connell P. H. (1972). Drug Abuse and Social Issues—2nd International Symposium, *International Pharmacopsychiatry*; **7**: 199.

DHSS. (1984). *Guidelines of Good Clinical Practice in the Treatment of Drug Dependence.* Department of Health. London: HMSO.

DHSS. (1985). *Drug Misuse: Prevalence and Service Provision.* Department of Health. London: HMSO.

HMSO. (1965). *Drug Addiction—The Second Report of the Interdepartmental Committee,* SO Code 32–531. London: HMSO.

Home Office. (1985). *Tackling Drug Misuse: A Summary of the Government's Strategy,* London: HMSO.

Strang J. (1983). *Lancet*; **2**: 400.

APPENDICES

INDICATORS

The following well-tried indicators are available from several manufacturers either in solid form or as prepared solutions.

	pH range	Colour change
Phenol red (acid range)	0·0–2·0	pink to yellow
Cresol red (acid range)	0·2–1·8	red to yellow
m-Cresol purple (acid range)	0·6–2·4	red to yellow
Thymol blue (acid range)	1·2–2·8	red to yellow
Bromophenol blue*	2·8–4·6	yellow to blue
Methyl orange*	2·8–4·6	red to yellow
Methyl orange, screened	3·0–4·6	violet to green
Congo red*	3·0–5·0	blue to red
Bromocresol green*	3·8–5·4	yellow to blue
Methyl red*	4·2–6·3	red to yellow
Chlorophenol red*	4·8–6·8	yellow to red
Litmus*	5·0–8·0	red to blue
Bromocresol purple*	5·2–6·8	yellow to purple
Bromothymol blue*	6·0–7·6	yellow to blue
Neutral red	6·8–8·0	yellow to red
Phenol red	6·8–8·4	yellow to red
Cresol red	7·2–8·8	yellow to red
m-Cresol purple	7·6–9·2	yellow to purple
Thymol blue	8·0–9·6	yellow to blue
Phenolphthalein*	8·3–10·0	colourless to purple-red
Thymolphthalein	9·3–10·5	colourless to blue
Alizarin yellow GG	10·0–12·0	colourless to yellow
Tropaeolin O	11·1–12·7	yellow to orange

The following mixed indicators are supplied by BDH Chemicals Limited.

'4460'	4·4–6·0	red to green
'4·5'	3·5–6·0	orange-red to blue
'6676'	6·6–7·6	orange to violet
'7785'	7·7–8·5	green to purple
'9011'	9·0–11·0	yellow to violet-grey
'1113'	11·0–13·0	yellow to red-purple

Several wider range mixed indicators are useful for approximate determination of pH. They are available from BDH Chemicals Limited.

BDH '4080'	4·0–8·0	red-yellow-bluish green
BDH '678'	5·0–10·0	orange-green-grey-violet
BDH '1014'	10·0–14·0	green-pink-orange
BDH 'Full Range'	1·0–14·0	red to violet (spectral colours)
BDH 'Universal Indicator'	4·0–11·0	red to violet (spectral colours)

Some indicators, indicated by * in the list above, are also supplied in paper form. Other narrow-range papers (2 pH units) are available. Between them, they cover the whole range from pH 0 to 14.

BUFFER MIXTURES

The following mixtures are suitable for general purposes. In each case details are given for making 1 litre of solution. ΔpH/°C refers to the rate of change of pH with temperature. The ionic strength (I) is in mmol/l as is the osmolarity.

1. *KCl-HCl (Clark and Lubs) at 20 °C*

pK = 1·33 ΔpH/°C $\approx$ 0   I = 147 to 57 (pH 1 to 2·2)
Osmolarity = 294 to 114

Volume (ml) 200 mmol/l hydrochloric acid to be added to 250 ml of 200 mmol/l potassium chloride followed by dilution to 1 litre with water.

pH	ml	pH	ml	pH	ml
1·0	485	1·6	131·5	2·2	35·5
1·2	322·5	1·8	84		
1·4	207·5	2·0	53		

2. *Glycine-HCl (Sørensen) at 18 °C*

pK = 2·35 ΔpH/°C $\approx$ 0   I = 100 to 189 (pH 1·2 to 3·6) Osmolarity = 200 to 289

Volume (ml) of glycine-sodium chloride mixture, 100 mmol/l of each, to be diluted to 1 litre with 100 mmol/l hydrochloric acid.

pH	ml	pH	ml	pH	ml
1·2	150	2·2	583	3·2	856
1·4	287	2·4	645	3·4	903
1·6	382	2·6	702	3·6	945
1·8	457	2·8	756		
2·0	523	3·0	808		

3. *Phthalate-HCl (Clark and Lubs) at 20 °C*

pK_1 = 2·95 ΔpH/°C = 0·001   I = 50 (constant)
Osmolarity = 147 to 103

Volume (ml) of 200 mmol/l hydrochloric acid to be added to 250 ml of 200 mmol/l potassium hydrogen phthalate followed by dilution to 1 litre with water.

pH	ml	pH	ml	pH	ml
2·2	233·5	2·8	132	3·4	49·8
2·4	198	3·0	101·5	3·6	30·0
2·6	165	3·2	74·0	3·8	13·2

4. *Acetate-acetic acid (Walpole) at 23 °C*

pK = 4·76 ΔpH/°C = −0·004   I = 7 to 90 (pH 3·6 to 5·6)
Osmolarity = 107 to 190

Volume (ml) of A: 200 mmol/l acetic acid and volume (ml) of B: 200 mmol/l sodium acetate to be diluted to 1 litre with water.

pH	A	B	pH	A	B	pH	A	B
3·6	463	37	4·4	305	195	5·2	105	395
3·8	440	60	4·6	255	245	5·4	88	412

pH	A	B	pH	A	B	pH	A	B
4·0	410	90	4·8	200	300	5·6	48	452
4·2	368	132	5·0	148	352			

5. *Phthalate-NaOH (Clark and Lubs) at 20 °C*

$pK_2 = 5·41$ $\Delta pH/°C = 0·001$ $I = 51$ to 144 (pH 4·0 to 6·2)
Osmolarity = 100 to 147

Volume (ml) of 200 mmol/l sodium hydroxide to be added to 250 ml of 200 mmol/l potassium hydrogen phthalate followed by dilution to 1 litre with water.

pH	ml	pH	ml	pH	ml
4·0	2·0	4·8	87·5	5·6	198·5
4.2	18·3	5·0	128·3	5·8	215·5
4.4	36·8	5·2	148·8	6·0	227·0
4·6	60·0	5·4	176·3	6·2	235·0

6. *Tris-maleate-NaOH (Gomori) at 23 °C*

pK's = 6·24, 8·08   I uncertain   Osmolarity = 107 to 187

Volume (ml) of 200 mmol/l sodium hydroxide to be added to 250 ml of tris [hydroxymethyl] aminomethane and maleic acid, 200 mmol/l of each, followed by dilution to 1 litre with water.

pH	ml	pH	ml	pH	ml
5·2	35	6·4	185	7·6	290
5·4	54	6·6	213	7·8	318
5·6	78	6·8	225	8·0	345
5·8	103	7·0	240	8·2	375
6·0	130	7·2	255	8·4	405
6·2	158	7·4	270	8·6	433

7. *Phosphate (Sørensen) at 18 °C*

$pK_2 = 7·20$ $\Delta pH/°C = -0·003$ $I = 77$ to 191 (pH 5·8 to 7·9)
Osmolarity = 139 to 195

Volume (ml) of 1/15 mol/l monopotassium phosphate to be diluted to 1 litre with 1/15 mol/l disodium phosphate.

pH	ml	pH	ml	pH	ml
5·80	920	6·85	475	7·40	192
5·90	901	6·90	446	7·45	175
6·00	878	6·95	418	7·50	159
6·10	847	7·00	389	7·55	143
6·20	814	7·05	361	7·60	130
6·30	776	7·10	334	7·65	118
6·40	733	7·15	308	7·70	106
6·50	682	7·20	280	7·75	95
6·60	625	7·25	256	7·80	85
6·70	565	7·30	232	7·90	68
6·80	504	7·35	211		

8. *Barbitone-HCl (Michaelis) at 23 °C*
pK = 7·98 $\Delta pH/°C = -0·008$ $I = 52$ to 99 (pH 6·8 to 9·6)
Osmolarity = 152 to 199

Volume (ml) of 100 mmol/l sodium barbitone to be diluted to 1 litre with 100 mmol/l hydrochloric acid.

pH	ml	pH	ml	pH	ml
6·8	522	7·8	662	8·8	908
7·0	536	8·0	716	9·0	936
7·2	554	8·2	769	9·2	952
7·4	581	8·4	823	9·4	974
7·6	615	8·6	871	9·6	985

9. Tris-HCl (Gomori) at 23 °C

pK = 8·08   ΔpH/°C = − 0·020   I = 44 to 5 (pH 7·2 to 9·0)
Osmolarity = 94 to 55

Volume (ml) of 200 mmol/l hydrochloric acid to be added to 250 ml of 200 mmol/l tris[hydroxymethyl] aminomethane and diluted to 1 litre with water.

pH	ml	pH	ml	pH	ml
7·2	221	8·0	134	8·8	41
7·4	207	8·2	110	9·0	25
7·6	192	8·4	83		
7·8	163	8·6	61		

10. Borate-KCl-NaOH (Clark and Lubs) at 20 °C

pK = 9·24   ΔpH/°C = − 0·006   I = 97 to 56 (pH 7·8 to 10)
Osmolarity = 153 to 194

Volume (ml) of 200 mmol/l sodium hydroxide to be added to 250 ml of boric acid–potassium chloride mixture, 200 mmol/l of each, and diluted to 1 litre with water.

pH	ml	pH	ml	pH	ml
7·8	13·3	8·6	60·0	9·4	160·0
8·0	20·0	8·8	82·0	9·6	184·3
8·2	29·5	9·0	107·0	9·8	204·0
8·4	42·8	9·2	133·5	10·0	219·5

11. Glycine-NaOH (Sørensen) at 18 °C

pK_2 = 9·78   ˙ΔpH/°C = − 0·025   I = 193 to 100 (pH 8·4 to 13·0)
Osmolarity = 293 to 208

Volume (ml) of glycine-sodium chloride mixture, 100 mmol/l of each, to be diluted to 1 litre with 100 mmol/l sodium hydroxide.

pH	ml	pH	ml	pH	ml
8·4	965	10·0	630	11·6	488
8·6	948	10·2	590	11·8	478
8·8	921	10·4	561	12·0	462
9·0	885	10·6	537	12·2	436
9·2	842	10·8	522	12·4	400
9·4	790	11·0	510	12·6	334
9·6	732	11·2	503	12·8	242
9·8	677	11·4	497	13·0	75

12. Na_2CO_3-$NaHCO_3$ (Delory and King) at 23 °C

pK_2 = 10·33   ΔpH/°C = − 0·008   I = 58 to 135 (pH 9·2 to 10·6)
Osmolarity = 104 to 143

Volume (ml) of A: 200 mmol/l sodium carbonate and B: 200 mmol/l sodium bicarbonate to be diluted to 1 litre with water.

pH	A	B	pH	A	B	pH	A	B
9·2	20	230	9·8	110	140	10·4	193	58
9·4	48	203	10·0	138	113	10·6	213	38
9·6	80	170	10·2	165	85			

13. *Wide range buffer, citrate-phosphate-borate-barbitone (Britton and Welford)* at 25 °C

pKs = 2·15, 3·13, 4·76, 7·20, 7·98, 9·24, 12·38. ΔpH/°C = 0 at pH 2·6 to − 0·020 at pH 12   I = uncertain   Osmolarity = 149 to 171.

Dissolve 6·004 g citric acid monohydrate, 3·888 g potassium dihydrogen phosphate, 1·767 g boric acid, and 5·263 g sodium barbitone (all 28·57 mmol/l) in water and make to 1 litre. Volume (ml) of 200 mmol/l sodium hydroxide to be added to 1 litre of the above solution.

pH	ml	pH	ml	pH	ml	pH	ml
2·6	20	5·0	271	7·4	558	9·8	793
2·8	43	5·2	295	7·6	586	10·0	808
3·0	64	5·4	318	7·8	617	10·2	820
3·2	83	5·6	342	8·0	637	10·4	829
3·4	101	5·8	365	8·2	656	10·6	839
3·6	118	6·0	389	8·4	675	10·8	849
3·8	137	6·2	412	8·6	693	11·0	860
4·0	155	6·4	435	8·8	710	11·2	877
4·2	176	6·6	460	9·0	727	11·4	897
4·4	199	6·8	483	9·2	740	11·6	920
4·6	224	7·0	506	9·4	759	11·8	950
4·8	248	7·2	529	9·6	776	12·0	996

14. *Zwitterionic biological buffers (Good) at 20 °C*

The buffers listed above have restrictions when used in the usual physiological pH range. Component ions may combine with reactants or products or may interfere with their determination. The following compounds which possess both acidic and basic groups ('zwitterions') cover the physiological range of pH, react very little with enzymes or substrates, do not enter cells and interfere to only a slight degree with spectrophotometric measurements. They are dissolved in water at the required concentration and the pH is adjusted by addition of acid or base.

Substance	pKa	pH range	pH/°C
2-(*N*-Morpholino) ethanesulphonic acid, MES	6·15	5·8–6·5	− 0·011
N-(2-Acetamido) iminodiacetic acid, ADA	6·62	6·2–7·2	− 0·011
Piperazine-*NN'*-bis (2-ethanesulphonic acid), PIPES	6·80	6·4–7·2	− 0·0085
N-(2-Acetamido)-2-aminoethanesulphonic acid, ACES	6·88	6·4–7·4	− 0·020
NN-(Bis-2-hydroxyethyl)-2-aminoethanesulphonic acid, BES	7·15	6·6–7·6	− 0·016
3-(*N*-Morpholino) propanesulphonic acid, MOPS	7·20	6·5–7·9	− 0·011
N-((Trishydroxymethyl)methyl)-2-aminoethanesulphonic acid, TES	7·50	7·0–8·0	− 0·020
N-2-Hydroxyethylpiperazine-*N'*-2-ethanesulphonic acid, HEPES	7·55	7·0–8·0	− 0·014
N-2-Hydroxyethylpiperazine-*N'*-3-propanesulphonic acid, EPPS	8·00	7·6–8·6	− 0·011
N-((Trishydroxymethyl)methyl)glycine, TRICINE	8·15	7·6–8·8	− 0·021
NN-(Bis-2-hydroxyethyl)glycine, BICINE	8·35	7·8–8·8	− 0·018
2-(Cyclohexylamino) ethanesulphonic acid, CHES	9·55	9·0–10·1	− 0·011
3-(Cyclohexylamino) propanesulphonic acid, CAPS	10·40	9·7–11·1	− 0·021

PROPERTIES OF COMMON LABORATORY REAGENTS

Reagent	Density[a] (kg/kg)	Sp. gr.	Concentration (mol/l)	Volume for[b] diluting (ml)
Acids				
Acetic, 'glacial'	> 0·99	1·048–1·051	17·4	115
Hydrochloric, 'concentrated'	0·36	1·18	11·7	172
Nitric, 'concentrated'	0·69–0·71	1·412–1·417	15·5–16·0	129–125
Orthophosphoric, '88%'	0·88	1·75	15·7	127
'10%'	0·095–0·105	1·015–1·057	1·02–1·13	—
Perchloric, '72%'	0·72	1·70	12·2	164
'60%'	0·60	1·54	9·2	218
Sulphuric, 'concentrated'	0·98	1·84	18·4	109
Bases				
Ammonia solution, 'concentrated'	0·35	0·880	18·1	111
'26%'	0·26	0·908	13·9	144
Other				
Hydrogen peroxide, '100 volumes'	0·28–0·29[c]	1·11	8·9	224
'20 volumes'	0·06[c]	1·02	1·8	—
'10 volumes'	0·03[c]	1·01	0·9	—

[a] = or 'per cent w/w ÷ 100'.
[b] = volume of reagent to be diluted to 1 litre with water to give a solution of concentration, 2 mol/l.
[c] = kg/l.

PROPERTIES OF COMMON SOLVENTS

Name	BP (°C)	Density (kg/l)
Diethyl ether	35	0·71
Dichloromethane	40	1·31
Carbon disulphide	46	1·27
Acetone	56	0·79
1,1-Dichloroethane	57	1·17
Chloroform	61	1·48
Methanol	65	0·79
n-Hexane	69	0·65
Ethyl acetate	77	0·90
Carbon tetrachloride	77	1·58
Ethanol	78	0·79
Benzene	80	0·88
Cyclohexane	81	0·78
Propan-2-ol (iso-propanol)	82	0·79
2-Methylpropan-2-ol (tert-butanol)	82	0.78
1,2-Dichloroethane	84	1·25
Trichloroethylene	87	1·48
Propan-1-ol (n-propanol)	97	0·80
Butan-2-ol (sec-butanol)	100	0·80
Water	100	1·00
Formic acid	101	1·21
1,4-Dioxane	101	1·03
2-Methylpropan-1-ol (iso-butanol)	108	0·80
Toluene	111	0·86
3-Methylbutan-2-ol	112	0·81
Pyridine	115	0·98
Pentan-3-ol	115	0·82
Butan-1-ol (n-butanol)	118	0·81
Acetic acid	118	1·05
Pentan-2-ol	119	0·81
2-Methoxyethanol (methyl cellosolve)	125	0·96
2-Methylbutan-1-ol	129	0·82
3-Methylbutan-1-ol	131	0·81
2-Ethoxyethanol (ethyl cellosolve)	136	0·93
Pentan-1-ol (n-amyl alcohol)	138	0·81
p-Xylene	138	0·86
m-Xylene	139	0·86
Acetic anhydride	140	1·09
2-Methylbutan-2-ol	142	0·81
o-Xylene	144	0·88
2-Methoxyethyl acetate (methyl cellosolve acetate)	145	1·00
Amyl acetate	149	0·88
Dimethylformamide	153	0·94
2-Ethoxyethyl acetate (cellosolve acetate)	156	0·97
Ethanolamine	170	1·01
Aniline	184	1·02
Dimethylsulphoxide	189	1·10
Ethylene glycol	197	1·11
Formamide	211	1·13
Nitrobenzene	211	1·21

ATOMIC WEIGHTS

Selected from the Table of Atomic Weights, 1967 (IUPAC) with revisions of 1971, which is based on the assigned mass of exactly 12 for ^{12}C. Some of the figures have been rounded off.

Element	Symbol	Atomic number	Atomic weight	Element	Symbol	Atomic number	Atomic weight
Aluminium	Al	13	26·98	Molybdenum	Mo	42	95·94
Antimony	Sb	51	121·75	Neon	Ne	10	20·18
Argon	Ar	18	39·95	Nickel	Ni	28	58·71
Arsenic	As	33	74·92	Nitrogen	N	7	14·01
Barium	Ba	56	137·34	Osmium	Os	76	190·2
Beryllium	Be	4	9·012	Oxygen	O	8	16·00
Bismuth	Bi	83	208·98	Palladium	Pd	46	106·4
Boron	B	5	10·81	Phosphorus	P	15	30·97
Bromine	Br	35	79·90	Platinum	Pt	78	195·09
Cadmium	Cd	48	112·40	Potassium	K	19	39·10
Caesium	Cs	55	132·91	Radium	Ra	88	226·03
Calcium	Ca	20	40·08	Radon	Rn	86	222
Carbon	C	6	12·01	Rubidium	Rb	37	85·47
Cerium	Ce	58	140·12	Scandium	Sc	21	44·96
Chlorine	Cl	17	35·45	Selenium	Se	34	78·96
Chromium	Cr	24	52·00	Silicon	Si	14	28·09
Cobalt	Co	27	58·93	Silver	Ag	47	107·87
Copper	Cu	29	63·55	Sodium	Na	11	22·99
Fluorine	F	9	19·00	Strontium	Sr	38	87·62
Gallium	Ga	31	69·72	Sulphur	S	16	32·06
Gold	Au	79	196·97	Tantalum	Ta	73	180·95
Helium	He	2	4·003	Technetium	Tc	43	98·91
Hydrogen	H	1	1·008	Tellurium	Te	52	127·60
Iodine	I	53	126·90	Thallium	Tl	81	204·37
Iridium	Ir	77	192·22	Thorium	Th	90	232·04
Iron	Fe	26	55·85	Tin	Sn	50	118·69
Krypton	Kr	36	83·80	Titanium	Ti	22	47·90
Lanthanum	La	57	138·92	Tungsten	W	74	183·85
Lead	Pb	82	207·2	Uranium	U	92	238·03
Lithium	Li	3	6·941	Vanadium	V	23	50·94
Magnesium	Mg	12	24·31	Xenon	Xe	54	131·30
Manganese	Mn	25	54·94	Zinc	Zn	30	65·38
Mercury	Hg	80	200·59	Zirconium	Zr	40	91·22

INDEX